# Principles of clinical medicine

# Principles of clinical medicine

Edited by

**P. John Rees** MA, MD, FRCP
Consultant Physician and Senior Lecturer in Medicine, United Medical
and Dental Schools, Guy's Hospital, London

and

**D. Gwyn Williams** MD, FRCP
Professor of Medicine, United Medical and Dental Schools, Guy's
Hospital, London

Edward Arnold
A member of the Hodder Headline Group
LONDON   BOSTON   MELBOURNE   AUCKLAND

First published in Great Britain 1995 by
Edward Arnold, a division of Hodder Headline PLC,
338 Euston Road, London NW1 3BH

Distributed in the Americas by
Little Brown and Company,
34 Beacon Street, Boston, MA 02108

Whilst the advice and information in this book is believed to be true and
accurate at the date of going to press, neither the authors nor the publisher
can accept any legal responsibility or liability for any errors or omissions
that may be made. In particular (but without limiting the generality of the
preceding disclaimer) every effort has been made to check drug dosages;
however it is still possible that errors have been missed. Furthermore,
dosage schedules are constantly being revised and new side effects
recognized. For these reasons the reader is strongly urged to consult the
drug companies' printed instructions before administering any of the drugs
recommended in this book.

*British Library Cataloguing in Publication Data*
A catalogue record for this book is available from the British Library

ISBN 0 340 563001 (Pb)

1 2 3 4 5 95 96 97 98 99

Photoset in 11/12 pt Garamond by Rowland Phototypesetting Limited
Bury St Edmunds, Suffolk
Printed and bound in Great Britain by The Bath Press Ltd, Avon

# Contents

# Preface

This new textbook of medicine has its origins in the short textbook of medicine with its lineage going back for many years. However, this is a new venture. Some authors remain from the previous book but all the chapters are new and there is a different pattern to this book. The importance of the basic science and techniques is acknowledged by some of the introductory chapters which will help students come to grips with aspects of genetics, immunology and molecular biology where advances have been so fast in the last few years.

Today's students also need to deal with broader aspects of medicine such as medical ethics, and they need to learn the skills of communication with their peers and patients, as well as newer areas such as clinical audit. These topics are briefly introduced early in the book.

The major part of the book still deals with the clinical problems in the major systems. Most chapters start with the basic aspects of symptoms, signs and investigations before covering the clinical disorders themselves. We have tried to link the basic science involved to the principles of clinical medicine and the practical aspects of the disorders and their management. We have purposely allowed such duplication between chapters to allow a complete account of certain topics to be rendered without having to cross refer to other chapters.

Tables and illustrations appear throughout the book. Rather than provide bare lists of causes or conditions we have tried to help the reader by highlighting the commoner causes or problems in the tables. These are shown by the addition of a second colour. The decision as to which items in the list are common is not done with accurate statistics. It is the clinical impression of the editors and the authors backed by appropriate information when this is available.

We hope that this new textbook of medicine will prove to be useful and enjoyable to students of medicine, nursing, dentistry and related professions. Practising clinical medicine is a privilege and a pleasure mixed sometimes with frustrations and pressures. The same attributes apply to the editing of medical textbooks, the privilege and pleasure of reading expert contributions, the frustrations and pressures of organization and deadlines. We are grateful to all the authors who are enthusiasts and experts in their subjects and in teaching, and we hope that some of their enthusiasm and expertise can be transmitted to our readers.

# Contributors

**Stephanie A. Amiel** BSc, MD, FRCP
Senior Lecturer, Unit for Metabolic Medicine, Diabetes, Endocrinology and Metabolism, United Medical and Dental Schools, London; Honarary Consultant, Guy's Hospital, London

**Rodney Grahame** MD, FRCP, FACP
Professor of Clinical Rheumatology, United Medical and Dental Schools, Guy's Hospital, London

**Anne S. Hamblin** PhD
Department of Pathology and Infectious Diseases, The Royal Veterinary College, London

**Terence J. Hamblin** DM, FRCP, FRCPath
Professor of Immunohaematology, University of Southampton Medical School

**Peter G. Harper** FRCP
Consultant Medical Oncologist, Guy's Hospital, London

**Roderick J. Hay** DM, FRCP, MRCPath
Mary Dunhill Professor of Cutaneous Medicine, St John's Institute of Dermatology, Guy's Hospital, London

**Brendan H. Hicks** BSc, MD, FRCP
Senior Lecturer in Medicine and Postgraduate Dean, United Medical and Dental Schools; Consultant Endocrinologist, Guy's Hospital, London

**R. John Jarrett**
Emeritus Professor of Clinical Epidemiology, United Medical and Dental Schools, Guy's Hospital, London

**Michael D. O'Brien** MD, FRCP
Physician for Nervous Diseases, Guy's Hospital, London

**Marcus E. Pembrey** BSc, FRCP
Mothercare Professor of Paediatric Genetics, Institute of Child Health, London

**Stephen H. Powis** BSc, MRCP
MRC Clinician Scientist Fellow and Honorary Senior Registrar, Renal Unit, Guy's Hospital, London

**P. John Rees** MA, MD, FRCP
Consultant Physician and Senior Lecturer in Medicine, United Medical and Dental Schools, Guy's Hospital, London

**Steven H. Sacks** BSc, PhD, FRCP
Director of Renal Research Laboratory, United Medical and Dental Schools, Guy's Hospital, London

**Hugh M. Saxton** FRCR, FRCP, DMRD
Emeritus Consultant Radiologist, Guy's Hospital, London

**Gordon E. G. Sladen** MA, DM, FRCP
Consultant Physician and Gastroenterologist, Lewisham Hospital, London

**Mark M. Smithies** MRCP
Consultant Physician, Intensive Care Unit, Guy's Hospital, London

**Ian D. Starke** MD, BSc, MSc, FRCP
Consultant Physician Lewisham Hospital, London; Senior Lecturer in Medicine of the Elderly, United Medical and Dental Schools, Guy's Hospital, London

**Adam D. Timmis** MD, FRCP
Consultant Cardiologist, The London Chest Hospital, London

**Glyn N. Volans** BSc, MD, FRCP
Director, National Poisons Unit and Consultant Physician, Guy's Hospital London

**James P. Watson** MD, FRCP, FRCPsych
Professor and Head, Department of Psychiatry, United Medical and Dental Schools, Guy's Hospital, London

**Mark L. Wilkinson** MD, BSc, FRCP
Consultant Physician, Gastroenterology Unit, Guy's Hospital London; Senior Lecturer, United Medical and Dental Schools, London

**D. Gwyn Williams** MD, FRCP
Professor of Medicine, United Medical and Dental Schools, Guy's Hospital, London

**Martin J. Wood** MA, FRCP
Consultant Physician, Department of Infection and Tropical Medicine, Birmingham Heartlands Hospital, Birmingham

# Medicine in today's world

1

It is now 30 years since the first edition of this book's predecessor, the *Short Textbook of Medicine*. The size and the content of the book have changed over that period to keep pace with the rapid developments in medicine and the changes in disease. New diseases such as acquired immune deficiency syndrome (AIDS) have appeared and others such as smallpox have been eradicated. Advances in areas such as genetics, molecular biology, pharmacotherapy and imaging have increased the options available for investigation and management.

In developed countries major causes of illness and death are degenerative diseases such as vascular disorders and malignant disease. Despite the established dangers around one-third of adults in developed countries continue to smoke and inappropriate use of alcohol is another preventable cause of acute and chronic illness. In many countries the tobacco industry provides employment in growing or manufacturing industries and the sales of tobacco bring in large revenues in the form of taxation. These factors may influence the energy and funds spent by governments in prevention of smoking and alcohol abuse. The health benefits from reduction in smoking bring economic benefits but are seen later than these short-term gains. These and other areas of prevention are important for the future health of these countries. Medical students and doctors should provide a lead in following a healthy lifestyle.

In less developed countries the priorities are different. Only one-quarter of the world's population lives in developed countries, yet these areas account for four-fifths of the world's income and there is little sign of any change. The dietary protein intake in many parts of Africa is less than that of the average domestic cat in the UK while across the world the ratio of doctors to patients varies 100-fold between countries. Yet the areas which are poorly supplied with medical care are those where poor nutrition and infectious diseases give the greatest potential for effective medical intervention.

In 1978 the World Health Organization conference at Alma Ata in Asia launched the drive for 'Health for All' by the year 2000. In fact the prospects look bleaker now than they did four or five years ago. Famine in the north-east areas of Africa continues and has extended. Although the human immunodeficiency virus (HIV) and acquired immune deficiency syndrome (AIDS) have produced great worries in Europe and North America where thousands have died, these numbers are small compared to the prospects in Africa, Asia and South America. In some countries in Africa the disease is likely to devastate the population particularly the young men and women who are most economically active. The treatments which provide some respite for sufferers in the west are out of reach of those in poorer countries.

In addition to traditional problems and HIV the increased ease of communication and travel across the world is speeding the introduction of diseases of urbanization and affluence to the less developed areas. The tobacco industry, seeing its traditional strongholds in slow decline, is seeking new opportunities in Asia and Africa and will target its advertizing in these areas. In the wake of such changes in diet and lifestyle our familiar western cardiovascular and respiratory disorders are beginning to appear.

The ease of international travel also allows diseases to move the other way and doctors in developed countries need to bear in mind infectious diseases from the tropics and elsewhere. Malaria is a common worry in those who take holidays or work in these areas.

In developed countries the costs of medical care continue to rise as more possibilities become available. Economic constraints are being applied and choices need to be made as the budget available for health care will not cover everything that doctors may wish to do and the public want to receive. In the past some new aspects of management and treatment have become part of regular practice without adequate evaluation but financial limits have increased the importance of a stricter evaluation of new developments and of current practices. Doctors need to have the skills to perform and interpret these assessments.

When investigations and treatments are established the audit of local practice is being used to test whether they are being delivered effectively. Hospitals in the UK are involved in the regular audit of clinical practice and delivery of care to ensure that they are providing the best care their facilities will allow. Audit often leads to adjustments in practice which can then be re-evaluated (page 14).

Many doctors and hospitals have always practised these techniques of critical evaluation. Commercial pressures will increase the demand for assessments in all branches of medicine: in primary care and public health as well as in acute hospitals. Resource decisions should depend upon evaluations of need in the community, the possibilities for prevention and intervention for these needs and the ability of the health system to deliver the appropriate care. Doctors need to play a prominent part in these decisions and will require management skills in order to be able to do this.

The medical world has an important part to play in speaking up on health matters to individual patients, local communities, nationally and internationally. The pace of change of the last 20 years and the scientific possibilities suggest that modern medical students can look forward to 30 or 40 years of working in which there will be changes in diseases and health care which are unimaginable now. The new student will need a critical and enquiring mind able to take in and assess the scientific advances which will appear. Together with this the basic skills of communication and rapport with patients need to be developed. These skills will always be necessary as patients provide the starting point for all medicine no matter how advanced, and most doctors spend most of their time with patients (page 10). In addition the new doctor will need extra skills in areas such as audit, management and information technology. This may seem a daunting task but will flow naturally from a basic grounding in scientific and clinical skills and a lively interest in medicine. This interest should be cultivated by approaching clinical problems from the skills seen everyday on the wards and in clinics. The patients act as the stepping stones to explore the social, scientific and clinical problems that they present.

The new knowledge and techniques available to medicine have heightened the importance of ethical aspects of medical practice. Ethics and medicine have long been related and in every field of practice ethical problems, old and new, will continue to be unavoidable for all individuals (page 6).

# **E**thics

2

Ethics may be defined as a person's or a group's rules of conduct based on morals. Medicine and ethics are inseparable. As our abilities to treat disease become more fundamental, more invasive, more complex and more successful, and as changing political pressures impact on medicine, the rate at which ethical questions in medicine arise seems to be rapidly increasing. This very brief chapter is not intended to answer these questions; its purpose is to highlight the fact that facing ethical matters is part of one's professional life if one cares for the sick in any capacity.

Consciously or unconsciously ethics are used in many different circumstances by all involved in patient care. While there may be broad agreement on what seem to be the most fundamental ethical questions (e.g. it is wrong to kill another human being), the individuals who contribute to that agreement represent a sum of single opinions which can vary widely (not everyone becomes a conscientious objector at a time of war). This room for individual variation will widen as the ethical questions to be answered become less clearly rooted in apparently simple issues of right versus wrong. Consequently one can be surrounded by conflicts of opinions on ethical matters, and it can be very difficult not to become confused. Our ethical views are a composite based on moral philosophy, religious beliefs, education and upbringing, and the cultural pressures, continually changing, of the society in which we live. Opinions can change quite quickly, for example, the acceptance of legal abortion in the UK during the last 25 years, and can differ markedly between nations simultaneously, for example, euthanasia is allowed under some circumstances in The Netherlands, but not in other European countries. These factors require a tolerance and respect for views held by others.

For anyone who looks after patients, either directly, for example, as a nurse or a doctor, or indirectly, for example, as a member of a committee deciding policies, ethical questions will be inescapable. The answers are sometimes obvious, but more usually they are not. They will be found by debate, pondering, and by not being afraid to change one's mind.

The different areas in which ethical questions arise are:

- **Individual:** in one-to-one relationships with a patient, or with a colleague.
- **Corporate:** as a member of a group which is making policies. The group may range from a unit, such as a group practice or a clinical department, to committees responsible to hospitals, health authorities, or directly to the government of the country.
- **As a member of society:** outside their professional activity, individuals make decisions which affect the ethics of health care, for example, when deciding how one will vote in political elections.

There are certain principles of ethics which are particularly helpful to define for those having to answer ethical questions in medicine:

- **Beneficence:** beneficial aims should be sought for individuals and society. Such a statement seems obvious, but all-out pursuit of beneficence in one field may have harmful effects in another, so a balance of good over harm is necessary.
- **Non-maleficence:** harm should not be imposed on individuals or groups. This statement appears even more obvious than the first, but nonetheless this principle arises frequently in medicine, such as when new techniques or drugs are being used. There is a learning curve during which mistakes will occur, and there are often unforeseen side effects. Most hospitals and medical schools have 'Research Ethics Committees' to give an opinion and advice on such matters, and when doing so they are applying the principle of non-maleficence.
- **Justice:** individuals must be considered and treated equally, and every person can expect his or her due.
- **Autonomy:** individuals are capable of making their own decisions from the evidence put before them; they may alter these decisions, and then act according to these decisions.

As stated above, this chapter does not set out to answer any ethical questions, but brief illustrations of some problems often faced in everyday practice follow.

## Choosing priorities in health care

Even the richest nations in the world are wrestling with the problem of ensuring the maximum benefit for their population within their finite budgets. Does one assess priorities on grounds of justice (every person can expect his or her due)? i.e. no treatment should be withheld from anyone (unless there are medical contraindications). Does one attempt to maximize beneficence by trying to do the most good for most people – what happens then to patients with rare diseases? However beneficence is employed, the principle of non-maleficence will be broken. Even trying to solve the problem by making health care available for everyone with no constraints will violate the principle of non-maleficence because to pay for that will use resources which would otherwise be spent on other important and worthwhile activities such as education and public transport. Not only are these of value in themselves, but they can also improve the health of individuals.

## Should a dying patient always be told their prognosis?

Not to do so would seem to withhold one of the most important and fundamental items of information a patient could receive, and to deny the patient's exercise of autonomy at a crucial stage in his/her life. Yet anyone who has cared for dying people will know of instances in which the knowledge of approaching death has ruined the remainder of that person's life, and that for some patients it may be better to withhold that information (following the principle of non-maleficence).

## Withholding treatment for a disease which would otherwise be fatal

Not to treat pneumonia in an elderly patient who has suffered a stroke causing irrecoverable dense hemiplegia and complete aphasia, but who is not unconscious, seems to be flying in the face of the principle of beneficence. One cannot say with certainty that the patient does not find his/her current quality of survival acceptable, nor can one discuss the implications of the decision with the patient, i.e. their autonomy is not being respected. But, aside from the issue of quality of life, should resources be directed to this patient and not, albeit indirectly, to other areas of health care such as neonatal intensive care units?

New techniques and new pressures will ensure that ethical questions will continually evolve, or old ones resurface. There is much debate within, and without, medicine on issues such as euthanasia, the use of human embryos for research, and the application of transgenic techniques. Despite the variation in individual and national opinions on these and other ethical questions, it is worth reminding ourselves that the application of ethics to medicine is not new. Hippocrates perceived 2000 years ago the need for a statement of personal rules to guide the physician – the Hippocratic Oath.

---

### THE HIPPOCRATIC OATH

I swear by Apollo the physician, and Aesculapius and Health, and All-heal, and all the gods and goddesses, that, according to my ability and judgement, I will keep this Oath and this stipulation – to reckon him who taught me this Art equally dear to me as my parents, to share my substance with him, and relieve his necessities if required; to look upon his offspring in the same footing as my own brothers, and to teach them this Art, if they shall wish to learn it, without fee or stipulation; and that by precept, lecture and every other mode of instruction, I will impart a knowledge of the Art to my own sons, and those of my teachers, and to disciples bound by a stipulation and oath according to the law of medicine, but to none other, I will follow that system of regimen which, according to my ability and judgment, I consider for the benefit of my patients, and abstain from whatever is deleterious and mischievous. I will give no deadly medicine to anyone if asked, nor suggest any such counsel; and in like manner I will not give to a woman a pessary to produce abortion. With purity and with holiness I will pass my life and practise my Art. I will not cut persons labouring under the stone, but will leave this to be done by men who are practitioners of this work. Into whatever houses I enter, I will go into them for the benefit of the sick, and will abstain from every voluntary act of mischief and corruption; and, further, from the seduction of females, or males, of freemen or slaves. Whatever, in connection with my professional practice, or not in connection with it, I see or hear, in the life of men, which ought not to be spoken of abroad, I will not divulge, as reckoning that all such should be kept secret. While I continue to keep this Oath unviolated, may it be granted to me to enjoy life and the practice of the Art, respected by all men, in all times. But should I trespass and violate this Oath, may the reverse be my lot.

# Communication

3

The commonest complaints from the public who come into contact with doctors concern problems of communication. Often these relate to lack of information or a feeling that the doctor is not interested or concerned. Many of them could have been avoided by improved communication initially and most others can be resolved by open discussion and explanation when they arise. Action should be taken to explore any problems as soon as they are suspected.

Many students are very nervous about their early contacts with patients. They worry that they are not going to know what questions to ask, how to keep the history going and how to react to problems which may arise. Some students express a feeling of embarrassment during one-to-one contact with patients. Communication skills are not unique to medical consultations, they are part of everyday family and social contact. Some people are naturally skilled at communicating with others and making them feel at ease and confident to talk about their problems. Some are more diffident and need to learn techniques which can improve their rapport with patients and enable them to acquire good clinical histories.

Many elements of communication skills can be taught and the various aspects can be developed during contact with patients. Most medical schools now have courses on communication skills. These may come very early or be associated with attachments in general practice or psychiatry. The earlier students can gain confidence in their abilities the better and the more they will gain from their contact with patients. Examiners at final and postgraduate examinations are instructed to look for evidence of communication skills.

One of the most important elements in communication with patients is the development of the patient's confidence:

- Confidence that the person to whom they are talking has the time and interest to want to know about their problems
- Confidence also in their professional qualities, to treat information seriously and confidentially and to have the knowledge and skills to help

Medical students are in the process of building up the knowledge and skills but they can show the appropriate interest and confidentiality from their first patient contact.

In counselling and in many ordinary doctor–patient contacts communication in itself is an important element of the treatment. There are some situations in which more advanced skills are needed. Examples are angry or distressed patients or relatives; patients who have a serious illness or who are dying; talking to parents of ill children; patients from different cultures and ethnic groups.

## Approaching patients

Patients are not obliged to help in the teaching of medical students by giving their histories or allowing students to perform minor procedures such as venesection. However, most are very happy to help. They should be aware of the status of the person dealing with them. This means that students and doctors should always introduce themselves to patients by name and state their position, medical student, registrar etc. and explain the reason for the interview.

Expectations of dress and manner change with time and area. In general many patients find it easier to deal with doctors and students who have the appearance they expect. This does not mean that pin stripe suits are essential wear. It does mean that clean, tidy clothes are necessary. Many patients may feel that medical competence is important while dress is irrelevant but some patients complain that they are unable to disclose personal details to someone wearing dirty jeans and trainers.

Whenever possible choose the setting for the medical interview to make the patient feel relaxed and able to communicate in private. Try to go into the interview knowing the patient's name and a few basic facts about them. Curtains around the bed in the middle of a ward may hide others from sight but they are not soundproof. Patients lying in bed in ill-fitting hospital pyjamas are rarely comfortable speaking to faces staring down on them from four feet above the bed. Try to get a more relaxed situation. In outpatients or surgery this will mean a quiet room with chairs four to six feet apart and easy eye contact with the patient without a grand desk in between. If the patient has to lie in bed then do not tower over them but get down to the same level in a position where you can talk easily together. If other people such as students and relatives need to be present make sure that everyone knows who is there and can take part in the conversation if necessary.

Doctors are often overstretched and have too little time to devote to each patient. Good interviewers develop the skill to make each patient feel that they are being given sufficient time. Students usually have fewer patients to see and can spend as much time as they need with patients. The skills to obtain the history in a restricted time will need to be developed for examinations and future sessions in outpatients and surgery.

There are plenty of ways to set up the interview badly. Common mistakes are:

1 Failure to introduce yourself
2 Being in too much of a hurry
3 Writing the whole time, no eye contact
4 Being distant from the patient by desk, space or mood
5 Being interrupted by the telephone etc.

## Questions

The opening of an interview should be encouraging and state what you want to know, usually all about the patient's medical problems. Make sure the patient knows what is expected of them otherwise you may miss some areas.

Open and closed questions are used in a conventional history. The account of the presenting problems should be explored with open questions which give the patient the chance to talk about their problems in their own words. This should be facilitated by the interviewer both verbally by encouraging phrases and signals and non-verbally by nodding and showing interest. During the interview you should listen to what the patient is telling you, this should generate ideas about the patient's problem which can be explored by subsequent lines of questioning. Early on students worry so much about their next question that they may fail to listen clearly and miss new avenues to explore.

Later in the interview you will want to sort out specific details with closed questions about precise timings or positions or types of pain etc.

Sensitive issues such as smoking, drinking alcohol, sexual habits, financial and emotional problems are usually best left until later in the interview when a rapport should have built up between patient and interviewer. If these are the main issues and the patient is uncomfortable then do not push them too fast, let the patient dictate the pace.

It is usually helpful to try to sum up the patient's story and relate it back to them and allow them to comment as necessary. This helps the patient to be sure that you have listened and they have got over the right message and helps you to know that you have received the history correctly and interpreted the patient's main worries.

## Other areas of communication

Communication is important in contact with other health professionals as well as patients and relatives. One element of this is efficient note keeping. The notes are an important record which are used subsequently in the patient's care and occasionally in legal disputes. Sometimes it is worth imagining what your notes would sound like read out in court. Flippant phrases and idiosyncratic abbreviations do not sound impressive, and rude personal comments should never be recorded.

Communication between general practitioners and hospital doctors is a regular occurrence and can also lead to misunderstandings. Communications to general practitioners should be prompt and legible. They should also be concise and to the point. Think what the general practitioner needs to know about a case, they are more likely to read and be helped by a clear description of events, results, conclusions and plans for future care than a rewrite of the full hospital clerking. The telephone and fax machines should be used to communicate urgent information.

When doctors ask for an opinion from a colleague, which is most often a general practitioner's referral to hospital, they should give the important parts of the history and express clearly the reason for the referral and specific questions which need to be answered. Drugs taken by the patient should be listed, the patient may know them as the 'little blue tablets' rather than as digoxin. Communication on request forms should be clear and contain all the appropriate history and the questions to be answered. It often helps to put yourself in the place of the recipient and see if you would find the information adequate.

Medical students can observe good and bad communication skills in practice by watching doctors and others at work. When you observe a history being taken think about the communication as well as the content, and see how they relate. You can pick up clues regarding the degree of comfort of interviewer and interviewee from their posture and movements. Look for non-verbal clues. See how the patient is encouraged to give their story. It will be more difficult to observe communication in difficult areas such as talking to dying patients or breaking bad news. Techniques can be learnt from suitable videos, role playing and communication courses. When advice is given see how well patients take in information and how written or visual information may help.

Remember that everyone can learn skills of communication and no-one can know enough, the learning goes on through regular patient contact.

# **A**udit

4

The original meaning of audit was an official examination of financial accounts, and this term has now been widely applied to a process of evaluation of procedures in medicine. Although audit in medicine is not new, it has become a much more important and prominent activity in the last 5–10 years. The proper recognition of the importance of audit arose from controlled trials of drugs, which began their now accepted and vital role in medicine only 40–50 years ago. The results of these controlled trials replaced clinical judgement and anecdote as the arbiters of treatment.

The meaning of medical audit has evolved to be quite distinct from controlled trials of drugs and similar applied clinical research. The Department of Health defines it as 'the systematic critical analysis of the quality of medical care, including the procedures used for diagnosis and treatment, the use of resources, and the resulting outcome and quality of life for the patient'. As well as improving the quality of care for patients, audit aims to ensure efficient use of resources, and to educate all involved in patient care. The distinctions between research and audit can be blurred. Table 4.1 lists some features which help to differentiate between the two processes.

**Table 4.1** Distinguishing between research and audit.

|  | Research | Audit |
| --- | --- | --- |
| Aim | To increase knowledge and/ or test a hypothesis | To define improvements in care and to effect them |
| Patient allocation | Random, to different groups | No random allocation |
| Placebo/new treatment | May be used | Not used |
| Patient selection | May be used | Not used |

The recent development of audit has resulted from various factors working together. These are the increased use of a scientific approach to solve medical problems, the requirement for ethical justification for performing invasive or dangerous procedures on patients, the growing and welcome desire by patients for more knowledge of the investigations and treatment given to them, and, particularly recently, the need to show that there is value for the money being spent on health care. Audit has extended to many facets of medicine beyond therapy, such as the efficacy of drugs or surgical procedures, the information given to patients and its retention by them, planning of appointment systems in general practitioners' surgeries and outpatient clinics, and the satisfaction of patients with less obvious, but nonetheless important, factors such as the attitudes of staff and hospital food. The process of audit therefore draws together nurses, doctors, dietitians, physiotherapists, pharmacists, administrators etc.

The process of audit can be briefly summarized as follows:

1 What should we be doing? – Decide what to audit
2 Are we doing it? – Do the audit
3 Where are we failing? – Analyse the audit
4 How can we get better? – Take steps to improve the situation
5 Did it work? – Repeat the audit, or selected parts

Audit is pointless unless its findings are acted upon to prevent needless wasteful or harmful practices, and therefore a necessary part of the practice of audit is to act upon the conclusions which it provides (a process known as 'closing the loop').

The importance attributed to audit is reflected in the fact that it has now become a necessary part of doctors' postgraduate training in the UK.

# Epidemiology

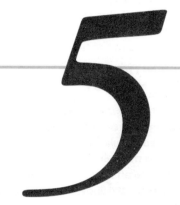

# INTRODUCTION

Epidemiology can be defined as 'the study of the distribution and determinants of health-related states and events in populations, and the application of this study to the control of health problems'. A definition given by the *Oxford English Dictionary* is 'that branch of medical science which treats of epidemics', which is true but inadequate, in that it describes only part, nowadays a small part, of the practice of epidemiology.

---

## DEFINITION AND PURPOSES OF EPIDEMIOLOGY

Epidemiology is the study of the distribution and determinants of health-related states or events in specified populations, and the application of this study to the control of health problems.

The practice of epidemiology – health surveillance and disease control in populations – is integral to public health practice. As a **research** method, epidemiology is used to test hypotheses about causes of disease, to measure health risks and to conduct experiments to investigate the efficacy of preventive, diagnostic or therapeutic regimens or procedures.

The purposes of epidemiology are to enlarge our understanding of factors that influence health-related states or events, so that the health of populations and individuals can be enhanced, protected or restored; to provide information and analyses to guide decisions affecting community health; and to respond to community concerns regarding health.

---

# HISTORY

The word epidemiology first appeared in the English language as part of the title of The London Epidemiological Society, founded in 1850. Amongst the members of this Society were two of the pioneers of the discipline – William Farr and John Snow – as well as two eminent physicians from Guy's Hospital, London – Richard Bright and Thomas Addison – whose fame, however, rests upon their clinical reputations. It was during the latter half of the nineteenth century that epidemiology gradually emerged as a distinct discipline with its own methods and philosophy, although with strong links with the sister disciplines of sociology, demography and biostatistics.

As in many other aspects of medicine, it is possible to trace the origins of epidemiology in the writings of Hippocrates. Thus, in *On Airs, Waters, and Places* stress is placed on the importance of considering the variety of environmental influences on diseases in humans. As we shall see, much of epidemiological research is concerned with environmental factors as well as constitutional and lifestyle factors and the interaction of these.

However, the philosophical basis for modern epidemiology, as for science in general, is to be found in the seventeenth century and in particular in the writings of Francis Bacon who developed the basis of inductive logic. The idea that mathematical relationships could be established for the physical universe suggested that a similar approach might be applied to the biological world. A notable attempt was made by John Graunt, a London haberdasher and a founding member of the Royal Society. He analysed the Bills of Mortality which were abstracts of christenings and burials based upon the parish registers which had commenced in 1538. From 1629 the annual bill was published regularly and included a breakdown of deaths by (apparent) cause. In 1662 Graunt published a monograph *Natural and Political Observations Mentioned in a Following Index and Made Upon the Bills of Mortality* in which he noted the effects of epidemics of plague, the excess of male births, seasonal variations in mortality, urban–rural differences in mortality and introduced the life table as in Table 5.1 which illustrates the high mortality rate in childhood and youth characteristic of the past which are still present in many countries. Three centuries later, the demographer David Glass commented that one of the outstanding qualities of Graunt's work was 'the search for regularities and configurations in mortality and fertility'.

**Table 5.1** The first life table. Adapted from John Graunt's monograph of 1662. The data are based on deaths recorded in London.

| Age | Deaths | Survivors |
| --- | --- | --- |
| 0 | – | 100 |
| 6 | 36 | 64 |
| 16 | 24 | 40 |
| 26 | 15 | 25 |
| 36 | 9 | 16 |
| 46 | 6 | 10 |
| 56 | 4 | 6 |
| 66 | 3 | 3 |
| 76 | 2 | 1 |
| 80 | 1 | 0 |

Following the development of mathematical (analytical) approaches to data came the notion of **control groups**. Thus in 1747 James Lind published probably the first **clinical trial**. He had formulated several hypotheses about scurvy and tested these by giving several treatments to different groups of sailors suffering from the disorder. Only those receiving oranges and lemons improved or recovered and Lind inferred that citric acid fruits could cure scurvy. By 1795 the Naval authorities had been convinced of this and required the inclusion of limes or lime juice in the sailors' diet; hence the soubriquet 'limeys' for British sailors, subsequently extended to any Briton.

Another early example of the analytical approach was the article by Pierre Charles-Alexandre Louis in 1835 which contributed to the demise of bleeding as a therapy. Louis analysed data from 77 patients with pneumonia and reported that a higher proportion of those bled in days 1–4 of the illness died compared with those bled during days 5–9. In fact the difference was not statistically significant and would probably not have been published in a respectable modern journal!

The other major development in the nineteenth century was the collection of routine statistics relating to population structure, mortality and morbidity. Systematic enumeration of the population (census taking) began in 1790 in the USA and in 1801 in France and Britain. In the UK subsequent censuses, of increasing complexity, have been held at ten-year intervals. The present system of registration of births and deaths dates from 1836, although failure to register did not become subject to penalty until 1855 in Scotland and 1875 in England and Wales.

In 1839 William Farr was appointed to the recently formed General Register Office and in his Annual Reports and other publications drew attention to many inequalities of health in terms of both mortality and morbidity. He also devised a system of classifying disease which was largely adopted by the International Statistical Congress in 1864. This was the forerunner of the International Classification of Disease (ICD) now compiled under the auspices of the World Health Organization (WHO).

The data gathered by Farr and others fuelled the activities of the Sanitary Movement, which culminated in the two major Public Health Bills of 1872 and 1875. These established a sanitary authority for every district and gave local authorities powers to deal with a number of environmental issues, including sewerage, the water supply and food quality.

# THE EPIDEMIOLOGICAL APPROACH

It is important to appreciate that the practice of epidemiology is not confined to professional epidemiologists. In the nineteenth century the most powerful exposition of the association between disease and dirt due to overcrowding, insanitary conditions and poverty, was provided by a civil servant – Edwin Chadwick. In this century excellent epidemiological studies within single general practices in the UK have been performed by William Pickles, John Fry and Julian Tudor Hart and by collaborating practices under the leadership of Clifford Kay. The Association of Rubella and Birth Defects was established as the result of studies by an ophthalmologist – N.M. Gregg. Denis Burkitt, a surgeon, discovered the lymphoma which now bears his name and subsequently described its epidemiological characteristics.

What these doctors had in common was the application of epidemiological methods and techniques to study the diseases or disorders in which they were specially interested.

These epidemiological methods fall into four broad categories and will be outlined using ischaemic heart disease (IHD), a major scourge of developed countries, as an example.

1 *Descriptive.* National mortality statistics can reveal differences in mortality rates both between and within countries, positive associations with age, higher rates in men than women at any given age and, in the UK, higher rates in certain ethnic groups, for example, in people of South Asian origin. These can be supplemented by population surveys and cohort studies which can identify risk factors for IHD such as raised levels of cholesterol and blood pressure, diabetes mellitus, family history of IHD and many others.

2 *Hypothesis testing.* 'Risk factor' simply means a statistically significant association with the disease and this does not necessarily mean that the factor is a 'determinant' of the disease. Epidemiological methods cannot definitely differentiate association from causation, but Bradford Hill has suggested a number of aspects of association which bear upon the interpretation. These include the strength of the association, consistency of association between studies, the temporal relationship of the association (i.e. which is the cart and which is the horse) and the biological plausibility of the factor being a determinant. Here one would also look for evidence from other disciplines, for example, experimental pathology. Examples for IHD would be its relationships with dietary fat consumption and smoking, which can lead to testable hypotheses for its aetiology and treatment.

## RISK FACTOR

An attribute or exposure that is associated with an increased probability of a specified outcome, such as the occurrence of a disease. **Not necessarily a causal factor**.

If there is good evidence that the association is causal, then the risk factor may properly be regarded as a **determinant**.

3 *Intervention.* If one believes that a raised serum cholesterol is a determinant of IHD then the hypothesis can be tested by an intervention study using appropriate diets and/or drugs which reduce the level of serum cholesterol.

4 *Development and refinement of methods.* In any of the categories 1–3 above it may be necessary to devise new, or refine old, methods of measurement, which may then require evaluation in a pilot study before embarking on a definitive study. Thus, there is a problem in estimating the prevalence of angina pectoris in a population because of systematic differences between observers, using conventional clinical history taking, in the responses obtained. To overcome interobserver variation, although not all other problems, standard questionnaires, for example, the Rose questionnaire, can be used, either administered by an observer or self-administered. Ideally, such questionnaires should be validated in the population which is to be studied.

# SCRUTINY OF ROUTINE DATA COLLECTIONS

## Mortality data

These data are derived from the certificate of the cause of death issued by a medical practitioner. The first part of the form records the condition directly leading to death, with antecedent conditions if appropriate. The second part is for other significant conditions contributing to death, but which were not related to the disease or condition actually causing death. Clearly, there is scope for different opinions about individual cases. In the UK the certificate is taken to the Registrar of Births and Deaths by an 'informant', who is required to provide additional information about the deceased: name, sex, marital status, maiden name of married women, date and place of birth, final occupation, usual address, and date and place of death. Official guidance is available to doctors and Registrars concerning the circumstances when cases should be referred to the Coroner. If the latter requires an autopsy, then the Coroner issues the death certificate on the basis of the autopsy report and any other relevant information.

The information is transcribed by the Registrar into a draft entry of death registration and a copy of this form is sent to the Office of Population Censuses and Surveys (OPCS) where the data are coded using a standard manual prepared by the WHO. The OPCS uses these coded data to produce a variety of national mortality statistics and the WHO uses the data from a number of contributing countries to produce international compilations of mortality statistics.

Since the time of John Graunt, mortality data have been much used as a source of epidemiological studies. However, there are several problems in evaluating the data. In countries with well-developed systems of data collection, all-causes mortality statistics are fairly reliable. Cause-specific mortality data are another matter. In the first place, the practitioner's opinion concerning the cause of death frequently involves a degree of speculation, particularly in the elderly where several organ systems may be diseased or disordered. Indeed several studies have demonstrated substantial differences between causes of death ascertained by clinicians and those ascertained by pathologists after an autopsy. Secondly, the coders at OPCS can only work with the data in the death certificate and if this is ambiguous they are required to exercise judgment in assigning an ICD code. Thirdly, most data published relate to the 'underlying' cause of death, i.e. the disease or injury that initiated the train of events leading to death.

Comparing mortality data over time may be affected by changes in certificating fashion and/or by improvements in medical knowledge which lead to more precise attribution. Furthermore, ICD codes are periodically revised and these may give rise to artefactual changes in cause-specific mortality data. In an international comparison of deaths ascribed to heart disease in 1985 it was noted that the proportion of heart diseases ascribed to 'other than ischaemic heart disease' differed widely, from 2% in Icelandic males to 59% in Japanese males. Part of this difference could be due to variation in the prevalence of other cardiac disorders, but equally variation in physicians' perception of cardiac disease may be responsible.

Finally, even if the national mortality data are regarded as valid, interpretation of trends may require additional information. Thus, in several countries IHD mortality rates have fallen substantially in the past 10–15 years. This does not necessarily imply that the incidence of IHD has fallen. It could be that improved treatment of those with evident IHD has produced a fall in mortality. In fact, evidence from the USA, where there have been several ongoing population studies, suggests that both the incidence of IHD and case-fatality rates have declined.

## USES OF MORTALITY STATISTICS

As outlined above, one may wish to look for trends over time or to compare rates between different countries. Within a country one might wish to look at associations with age, gender, ethnicity, socioeconomic status and geographical region. As age and gender are often important associations, in making comparisons between other groupings, some account must be taken of differences between the populations compared by their age and sex composition. This can be done by dividing into age- and sex-specific groups or by using a **Standardized Mortality Ratio** (SMR). By using relatively simple mathematics this provides a method of comparing the mortality in two or more populations allowing for any differences in age and sex composition (see the example in the box).

Standard Mortality Ratios for IHD in the UK indicate considerable regional variation with, for example, high rates in Scotland and northern England and low rates in the south, particularly south-west England. Only part of this variation can be explained by differences in social class or smoking habit, but environmental factors seem to be important. Thus data from the British Regional Heart Study on internal migration indicate that in migrants IHD rates are closer to those in the area of migration than to place of birth.

Mortality statistics are useful in raising important issues, for example, the substantial increase in asthma deaths observed in the 1960s, which may give rise to or support an hypothesis. In this context clinicians had already suggested the possible dangers of overuse of bronchodilator inhalations and the mortality data were compatible with such an hypothesis. However, routine data collections are not often satisfactory for testing hypotheses and this is usually better done by special studies.

# Other routine data collections

As well as mortality data, the OPCS collects and publishes data on births, marriages, abortions, migration and congenital abnormalities. Notifications of infectious diseases are also processed by OPCS and statistics appear in their weekly, quarterly and annual publications. Further information [including voluntary and anony-

## EXAMPLE

The crude death rates from lung carcinoma in Westshire and Eastshire are respectively 745 and 186 per million population. However, the population structure of the two counties is known to be different, so that some standardizing method is necessary in order to make a proper comparison. Rates could be standardized for both counties or the population of the whole country or, as in the example below, the population of Eastshire is taken as the 'standard' population. Its age-specific rates are calculated.

| Age group | Males | | | Females | | |
|---|---|---|---|---|---|---|
| | Number of deaths | Population | Rate | Number of deaths | Population | Rate |
| 0–39 | 45 | 1.5 million | 30 | 15 | 1.5 million | 10 |
| 40–59 | 720 | 600000 | 1200 | 105 | 700000 | 150 |
| 60+ | 1200 | 300000 | 4000 | 200 | 400000 | 500 |

These rates are then applied to the population of Westshire to derive the expected number of

deaths if the rates were the same in this population.

| Age group | Males | | | Females | | |
|---|---|---|---|---|---|---|
| | Rate | Population | Expected deaths | Rate | Population | Expected deaths |
| 0–39 | 30 | 1.4 million | 42 | 10 | 1.3 million | 13 |
| 40–59 | 1200 | 400000 | 480 | 150 | 400000 | 60 |
| 60+ | 4000 | 200000 | 800 | 500 | 300000 | 150 |
| Total | | | 1322 | | | 223 |
| | | | (1545) | | | |

The Standardized Mortality Ratio (SMR):

$$= \frac{\text{Observed number of deaths}}{\text{Expected number of deaths}} \times 100$$

$$= \frac{745}{1545} \times 100 = 48.2$$

Thus, taking into account age and sex distribution Westshire has slightly under half the mortality rate from carcinoma of the lung than Eastshire. (NB In practice narrower age bands would be used for the calculation.)

mous acquired immune deficiency syndrome (AIDS) notifications] on infectious diseases is published by the Public Health Laboratory Service in the regular Communicable Disease Reports. Much of this information is laboratory based. A special system exists for sexually transmitted diseases with data provided by the specialist clinics and collated by the British Cooperative Clinical Group. The routine collection of data in infectious disease is useful not only in monitoring trends but also in detecting outbreaks or epidemics and in assessing the effect of interventions such as immunization.

It was the routine reporting to the Centers of Disease Control in Atlanta, USA, and the recognition of a rise in incidence of pneumonia caused by *Pneumocystis carinii*, which led to the discovery of a disorder – AIDS – which has now become a major public health problem worldwide.

The survey division of OPCS performs specially commissioned *ad hoc* surveys as well as a number of regular surveys. The General Household Survey began in 1971 and a sample of approximately 15 000 households is studied annually, data being sought on a number of topics, which are changed from time to time. They include demographic variables, smoking and alcohol consumption and a section on health and use of the health services. The National Food Survey, also based on a sample of households, measures the amount and kind of food bought over one week, but excludes food bought and consumed outside the home. These data are supplemented by that obtained from the Family Expenditure Survey, which includes expenditure on food and alcohol.

The Health and Safety Executive collects and publishes data on industrial or workplace accidents – fatal and non-fatal – and on a number of diseases or poisonings related to occupational exposure.

## SURVEYS

Murphy's first law states that 'The information you have is not the information you want'. For epidemiologists routine data collections may be inadequate and information needs to be obtained by a survey – defined by the *Dictionary of Epidemiology* as 'an investigation in which information is systematically collected but in which the experimental method is not used'.

There are many ways of performing surveys and each has its own advantages and disadvantages. For example, if one wanted to know the distribution of heights and weights in a population, measurement by trained observers would be more accurate, but much more costly, than self-reporting. However, the latter may be adequate for certain purposes. By contrast, if one wanted to study the distribution of blood pressure levels in a population, this could only be done using measurements by trained observers.

Surveys may be predominantly descriptive, as in the OPCS surveys mentioned earlier. They may, however, be more focussed in the sense of looking for associations between a disease and variables thought or suspected to be related. Thus there are numerous studies relating the presence of IHD (measured as symptomatic disease and/or by electrocardiographic abnormalities) with a long list of variables or 'risk factors' such as family history, obesity, hypertension, smoking etc. Studies of this kind may provide data which bear upon the aetiology of disease.

Surveys may also be used in service planning. In order to plan services to meet needs rather than demand and to allocate resources accordingly, information, not usually available from routine data sources, is required about the frequency and severity of the various health problems in the particular community. Repeated surveys are required to monitor the effects of changes in the services provided.

## COHORT STUDIES

The word cohort is derived from the Latin *cohors* – the tenth part of a legion. When first introduced into epidemiology it referred to a birth cohort, i.e. a segment of the population defined by period of birth. The term has subsequently been used to describe any designated group, for example, an occupational group, or a group exposed to a common environmental insult and which is followed or traced over a period of time.

### Birth cohorts

A cross-sectional study might indicate an association of a disease with attained age. Such an association might be due to the effects of ageing and/or to an accumulation of environmental influences, but the possibility must be borne in mind that it might be due to the differing experience of age cohorts. Thus, in the 1970s postencephalitic Parkinsonism in the UK was a disease of elderly persons. This was due to the fact that the pandemic of encephalitis lethargica, the cause of this form of Parkinson's disease, reached its peak in the early 1920s and subsequently declined rapidly. Thus birth cohorts from 1930 onwards were not exposed to the causative agent. In a different context, if one plots the height of adults against attained age, there is a negative correlation. Most of this is due to the increase in height attained by successive generations over the past century.

---

### COHORT (OR GENERATION) EFFECT

Variation in health status that arises from the different causal factors to which each cohort in the population is exposed as the environment and society change. Each consecutive birth cohort is exposed to a unique environment that coincides with its life span.

Source: *A Dictionary of Epidemiology*. Oxford: Oxford University Press.

---

There are few long-term observational studies of birth cohorts. The classic study is the 'National Survey of Health and Development', now under the auspices of the Medical Research Council. This began as an investigation of the cost of childbirth and the working of medical and nursing services, to provide information for use in the design of the National Health Service. The subjects comprised over 16 000 births in England, Wales and Scotland during the week 3–9 March 1946.

Information for the study was collected by doctors and health visitors when the babies were eight weeks old. It showed not only the cost of having the baby, but that it was much more expensive, in terms of the proportion of income spent, for mothers in manual workers' families than for those who were better off. The study described the great range of risk to the life and health of mothers and babies, and found that risks were much greater for the poor than for others. It also revealed that only one in five mothers had received pain relief during childbirth, and this information was used to change the law to permit midwives to give pain relief without the need for a doctor to be present when she did so.

A follow-up study was designed to examine the health and progress of some of these babies. A third of the babies studied were selected for follow-up in the National Survey of Health and Development, since even this proportion amounted to a large population to study (5362 babies). Selection was carried out at random, but in such a way as to ensure a good representation of babies from all over the country and from all parts of society.

The study has provided a great deal of information about educational attainment, health and disease, and their interrelationship with social class and environmental factors. One observation – a negative association between birth weight and adult blood pressure levels – implies an effect of intrauterine environment upon blood pressure, an observation which has been extended by others to cardiovascular mortality, respiratory disease and, possibly, non-insulin-dependent diabetes mellitus. If the hypothesis concerning intrauterine environment is correct, then the possibility arises of influencing the incidence of chronic disease in adult life by addressing those factors which lead to low birth weight.

As mentioned earlier, the term cohort has been extended to describe any designated group of persons 'who are followed or traced over a period of time'. Such a group may be composed of people exposed to an environmental hazard, for example, radiation or asbestos. The population of Hiroshima was exposed to an atomic bomb in 1945 and the survivors have been studied to determine, amongst other things, the long-term effects of the radiation exposure. The degree of exposure can be crudely estimated by the individual's distance from the epicentre of the explosion. Table 5.2 shows the incidence of leukaemia in relation to the intensity of radiation (using the surrogate measure). Note the use of person-years of observation, a statistical device to take account of the fact that people lost to follow-up, for whatever reason, do not contribute the maximum of 11 years observation.

**Table 5.2** Incidence of leukaemia in residents of Hiroshima (1947–58) in relation to distance from the epicentre of the explosion.

| Distance from the epicentre (m) | Incidence rate per 1 million person-years at risk |
|---|---|
| 0–999 | 1366 |
| 1000–1499 | 308 |
| 1500–1999 | 42 |
| 2000–9999 | 28 |

Source: Brill AB et al. Ann Int Med 1962; **56**: 590.

A cohort may be defined by occupation, as in the study begun by Doll and Bradford Hill on British doctors in 1951. Here the cohort members were doctors on the Medical Register, living in the UK and who agreed to participate. The study was designed to examine, in particular, the relationship between smoking habit and subsequent disease experience. Table 5.3 shows one of the analyses in which male non-smokers are compared with heavy smokers, the latter defined as men smoking 25 or more cigarettes daily. Age-adjusted death rates are given for four major causes of death and the data converted into a relative risk (or rate ratio) and an attributable rate (the increment in the death rate associated with heavy smoking). The **relative risk** can be considered as the risk to the individual of heavy smoking and is greatest for chronic bronchitis/emphysema. The **attributable rate**, by contrast, is the increment in disease burden in the whole population which can be attributed to heavy smoking and is greatest for IHD. This is because the mortality rate due to IHD is substantial in non-smokers so that a modest relative risk gives rise to a high attributable risk.

## CASE–CONTROL (OR CASE REFERENT) STUDIES

These are commonly used as a preliminary test of hypotheses about the aetiology of a disease or, alternatively, as a means of generating such hypotheses.

The method is retrospective – looking back from effect to cause, thus departing from the experimental or cohort approach where effects or events are observed prospectively. Persons known to have the disease of interest (cases) are compared with those who are free of the disease (controls). Past histories and exposures to the suspected agent(s) are ascertained by direct questioning and/or by scrutiny of records. The simplest analysis compares the rates of exposure in cases and controls. More sophisticated statistics may be used to take account of associations between exposures (**confounding**).

---

**CONFOUNDING FROM THE LATIN *CONFUNDERE* – TO MIX TOGETHER**

When two or more variables are associated with an outcome, in particular when the variables are associated with one another, it may be difficult or impossible to isolate the 'effect' of any individual variable.

---

**Table 5.3** Relative and attributable risks of death from selected causes associated with heavy cigarette smoking by British male physicians 1951–61.

| Cause of death | Death rate | | Relative risk | Attributable risk |
|---|---|---|---|---|
| | **Non-smokers** | **Smokers** | | |
| Lung cancer | 0.07 | 2.27 | 32.4 | 2.20 |
| Other causes | 1.91 | 2.59 | 1.4 | 0.68 |
| Chronic bronchitis | 0.05 | 1.06 | 21.2 | 1.01 |
| Cardiovascular disease | 7.32 | 9.93 | 1.4 | 2.61 |

Source: Doll R, Hill AB. Br Med J 1964; **1**: 1399.

The method is relatively quick and cheap and is useful for the investigation of uncommon diseases. It also allows the evaluation of several aetiological factors acting synchronously or separately.

The major problem with the method is potential bias. A Canadian epidemiologist, David Sackett, identified 35 varieties! These fall into three main groups. First, selection bias. It is difficult to avoid differential selection of patients and controls. One way of attempting to minimize such bias is by having controls derived from more than one reference population. Second, information bias – in particular biased recall of exposures by patients in comparison with controls. Third, confounding factors. If recognized, these can to an extent be incorporated into the study design or be allowed for by statistical adjustments. If unknown then they are a potential source of bias.

An example of a successful case–control study is that of Vessey and Doll. In the mid-1960s, following the introduction of the combined oral contraceptives, case reports of fatal and non-fatal thromboembolism began to appear and these gave rise to considerable public alarm. However, the reports were difficult to evaluate as there was virtually no information on the incidence of such events, so the association with oral contraceptive use might have been no more than chance. The Medical Research Council's Statistical Research Unit used the case–control method to investigate the hypothesis of an association between oral contraceptive use and thromboembolism. Cases were women aged 16–40 years inclusive discharged from 19 general hospitals in the catchment area of the N.W. Metropolitan Regional Hospital Board with an appropriate diagnosis in the period 1964–66. There were several predetermined criteria for excluding certain categories. For each affected woman two control pateints were selected who had been diagnosed as suffering from an acute medical or surgical condition or had been admitted to hospital for an elective operation and who matched the affected patient with regard to hospital, date of admission, age and parity. Patients and controls were subsequently interviewed by the same investigator and inquiries made about the medical, obstetric, social, family and contraceptive history.

The data are presented in a standard way (as shown in the example opposite), i.e.

|  | *Diseased* | *Not diseased* |
|---|---|---|
| Suspected cause present | $a$ | $c$ |
| Suspected cause absent | $b$ | $d$ |
| Total | $a + b$ | $c + d$ |

The summary statistic obtained from this table is the odds ratio (O.R.) where:

$$O.R. = \frac{a \times d}{b \times c}$$

If there were no differences in exposure between cases and controls, then the O.R. equals 1. It is possible to calculate 95% confidence intervals for the O.R. and to adjust the O.R. for confounding variables. In this example an association was observed between oral contraceptive use and cigarette smoking. However, statistical adjustment for this made little difference to the O.R.

**EXAMPLE**

Oral contraception and thromboembolism

| | Cases | Controls |
|---|---|---|
| Users | 26 (*a*) | 10 (*c*) |
| Non-users | 32 (*b*) | 106 (*d*) |
| Total | 58 (*a* + *b*) | 116 (*c* + *d*) |

$$\text{O.R.} = \frac{a \times d}{b \times c} = \frac{26 \times 106}{32 \times 10} = 8.6$$

Source: Vessey M, Doll R. *Br Med J* 1968; **2**: 199.

This association has been confirmed by prospective studies and plausible biological mechanisms described. However, several case-control studies of a putative association between oral contraceptive use and breast cancer have yielded discrepant results. There are also salutary examples of case-control studies where the association went one way with one control group and the opposite way with a second!

## EXPERIMENTAL EPIDEMIOLOGY

There are two broad varieties of experimental epidemiology: (a) the clinical trial and (b) the community trial or experiment. In the clinical trial the efficacy of a drug or procedure or of prevention is tested in individual subjects. By contrast in a community trial a group of individuals is subjected to the trial drug or procedure and the collective results compared with those in an unexposed group or, less satisfactorily, with the same group's experience prior to the exposure. Examples of community trials include fluoridation of the water supply in an attempt to reduce the incidence/severity of dental caries and, more recently, the impregnation of 'mosquito nets' with insecticides in one or more villages in a malarial area in an attempt to reduce the incidence of nocturnal mosquito bites and thus of malaria.

The theory and practice of clinical trials is an area where the skills of statisticians, clinical pharmacologists and epidemiologists overlap in a complementary fashion.

# Molecular Biology

# *I*NTRODUCTION

The field of molecular biology has grown from the study of the chemistry of deoxyribonucleic acid (DNA) and includes an understanding of the way in which the coded instructions in the genetic material are translated into protein. Nowadays, the term is liberally applied to many aspects of cellular and physiological events which can be interpreted in molecular terms. In this chapter, we will keep to the original sense and discuss aspects of DNA and ribonucleic acid (RNA) technology which have found, or are likely to find, an application in medicine. We will explain the fundamental vocabulary of molecular biology and illustrate advances in diagnosis and therapy which have resulted from the new biology. We will then speculate about the potential of current research and its impact on the understanding of disease. The term molecular pathology has been used to describe the interpretation of disease at a molecular level. Molecular genetics is the definition, in molecular terms, of the inherited component of disease.

# *T*HE LANGUAGE OF MOLECULAR BIOLOGY

## *The human genome*

The human genome consists of approximately 3 × 10⁹ (3 billion) base pairs of DNA arranged on 23 pairs of chromosomes. The DNA sequence of individual genes is transcribed as messenger RNA (mRNA) and then translated into protein. However, the complete amino acid sequence of a protein is not usually encoded by a contiguous stretch of genomic DNA. Genes contain additional DNA sequences called **introns** which are spliced out of mRNA and are thus not represented in the final protein sequence (Fig. 6.1). The regions of the gene which do encode protein sequence are called **exons**. In the laboratory, molecular biologists often work with complementary DNA (cDNA). Complementary DNA differs from genomic DNA in that it is made directly from spliced mRNA by the enzyme reverse transcriptase, and thus does not contain introns.

## *Digesting DNA; restriction endonucleases*

Restriction endonucleases (or restriction enzymes) are used to reduce the vast amount of genomic DNA to fragments of a more manageable size. These enzymes, derived from micro-organisms, cleave double-stranded DNA at specific sites by recognizing unique oligonucleotide sequences (Table 6.1). For example, the enzyme EcoRI recognizes the sequence 5′-GAATTC-3′, cleaving between the

**Table 6.1** Some restriction endonucleases and the cleavage sequences which they recognize. The points at which cleavage of double-stranded DNA occurs are indicated by arrows. In some cases cleavage leaves an overhang of one strand of DNA, in other cases a blunt end is left. Restriction enzymes are named after the micro-organisms from which they were isolated; for example, BamHI was isolated from *Bacillus amyloliquefaciens H*.

| Restriction enzyme | Cleavage site |
|---|---|
| BamHI | G↓GATC C<br>C CTAG↑G |
| EcoRI | G↓AATT C<br>C TTAA↑G |
| HaeIII | GG↓CC<br>CC↑GG |
| HindIII | A↓AGCT T<br>T TCGA↑A |
| PstI | C TGCA↓G<br>G↑ACGT C |

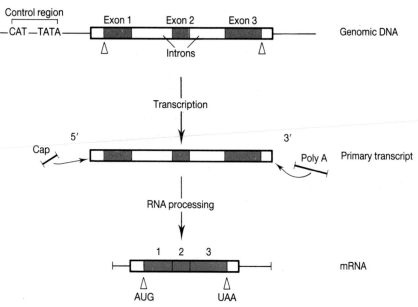

**Figure 6.1** Transcription of a typical gene. Coding sequences (exons) and intervening sequences (introns) are transcribed as a primary RNA transcript. A DNA cap and poly A tail are added and introns are spliced out to form a mature messenger RNA (mRNA) molecule. This has start (AUG) and stop (UAA) codons as shown. In the laboratory, molecular biologists use the enzyme reverse transcriptase to make complementary DNA (cDNA) from spliced mRNA. Complementary DNA does not contain introns. Note, however, that spliced mRNA (and cDNA) does contain sequence at both the 5′ and 3′ ends which is not eventually translated into protein.

nucleotides G and A. When a large amount of DNA, such as total human genomic DNA, is cut·by a specific enzyme, many different sized fragments are produced. Different restriction enzymes cut with different frequencies, depending upon how often an enzyme encounters its cleavage site. The less frequently it cuts, the greater the average size of fragments produced.

# DNA hybridization and Southern blot analysis

DNA fragments produced by restriction enzyme digestion can be separated according to size by electrophoresis in agarose (Fig. 6.2). Many techniques in molecular biology depend upon determining which of these fragments contains a specific DNA sequence, such as that encoding a particular gene. Southern blotting, a method developed to facilitate this, is named after its inventor E.M. Southern. Like many other techniques, it is based upon hybridization of nucleic acid. Double-stranded DNA can be separated, or denatured, into two complementary single strands by treatment with heat or alkali. Conversely, single-stranded DNA can form double-stranded DNA when it is allowed to re-anneal, or hybridize, under appropriate conditions.

In Southern blotting (Fig. 6.3), fragments of DNA are first separated by electrophoresis and transferred to a membrane with the ability to bind DNA. Membrane-bound DNA is denatured and hybridized with a specific fragment of radiolabelled DNA, often referred to as a 'probe'. Hybridization is extremely sensitive and will occur only between fragments of membrane-bound DNA whose sequence is complementary to the probe. Such fragments are then visualized by autoradiography (exposure of the membrane to X-ray film). If the conditions are made less stringent, the probe can also hybridize with membrane-bound DNA whose sequence is only partially complementary. Southern blotting can also be used to analyse genetic variation, or polymorphism, when this affects a restriction enzyme cleavage site. This results in varying DNA fragment sizes with **restriction fragment length polymorphism (RFLP)**. An example of this is seen in Fig. 6.3.

Larger

Smaller

**Figure 6.2** Fragments of DNA produced by restriction enzymes can be separated by electrophoresis through a porous gel made of agarose. Smaller fragments will move faster than larger fragments. Once visualized, sizes of fragments can be estimated by comparison with fragments of known size. In this illustration, two tracks are shown. Each contains the same DNA cut by a different restriction enzyme, resulting in two different patterns of fragments of varying size.

# Cloning DNA; plasmids and cosmids

In order to analyse and manipulate specific genes or stretches of DNA, methods have been devised to clone DNA. Fragments generated by restriction endonucleases are isolated and inserted into DNA from another biological source, referred to as the vector. The commonest vectors are bacter-

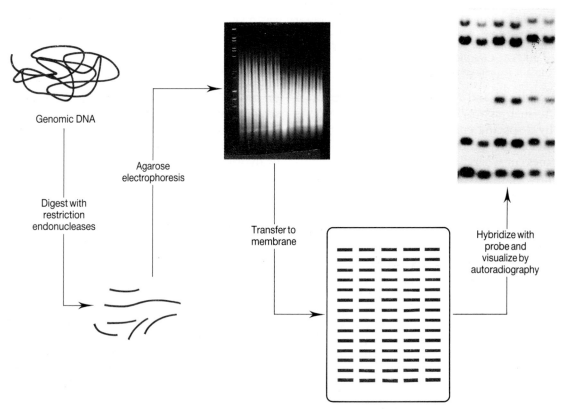

Genomic DNA

Digest with restriction endonucleases

Agarose electrophoresis

Transfer to membrane

Hybridize with probe and visualize by autoradiography

**Figure 6.3** Southern blotting. DNA is first cut with restriction enzymes and separated by electrophoresis through an agarose gel. The gel is placed on a piece of nitrocellulose membrane and buffer is allowed to flow from gel to membrane. This flow transfers the separated DNA fragments to the membrane, producing an exact mirror image of their position in the gel. The membrane is hybridized to a radiolabelled probe which binds to any complementary DNA sequences on the membrane. After washing to remove unhybridized probe, fragments containing such sequences can be visualized by autoradiography. Note that presence of the middle band is variable, the result of a restriction fragment length polymorphism (RFLP). This example is reproduced courtesy of Dr W. Foulkes.

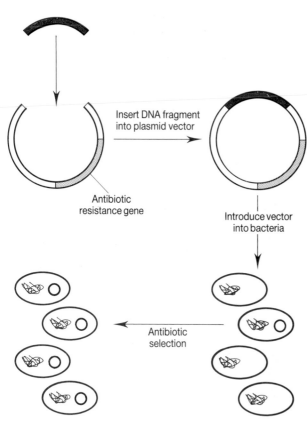

**Figure 6.4** Cloning DNA. The DNA fragment to be cloned is ligated into a plasmid vector containing an antibiotic-resistance gene (such as β-lactamase). The plasmid is introduced into bacteria which are then grown in a culture containing the antibiotic to which the plasmid confers resistance. Only those bacteria containing plasmids will survive and replicate. Bacteria can be cultured in bulk and large quantities of the cloned DNA fragment purified.

ial plasmids, which permit the insertion of small fragments of DNA, usually below 5 kb in size (Fig. 6.4). Cosmids are plasmids which have been manipulated to allow the insertion of much larger fragments of DNA. Vectors and their inserts can be grown in bacterial hosts, resulting in large quantities of the DNA fragment under analysis.

# Cosmid maps of the genome

Cloning techniques can be used to construct maps of chromosomal DNA. Instead of deliber-

ately cloning defined, single DNA fragments, random DNA libraries can be produced by inserting thousands of different uncharacterized fragments into multiple copies of the same vector. For example, if total human genomic DNA is digested by the enzyme Sa13a and cloned into a cosmid vector, the resulting library theoretically contains fragments covering the entire human genome. When plated out on agar, each individual bacterial colony contains cosmids with a single fragment insert. The DNA within these colonies can be transferred onto membranes for hybridization with specific probes.

If the probe is a known gene, colonies which hybridize should possess the gene. These cosmids can be isolated, their genomic DNA inserts digested with restriction enzymes and new probes prepared from each end. These probes can be used to detect yet further cosmids whose genomic inserts overlap the original cosmid. As more and more overlapping cosmids are isolated, an ever more extensive map can be constructed of the DNA surrounding the original gene. One of the eventual aims of the human genome project (see later) is to produce cosmid maps of each chromosome. Figure 6.5 shows a cosmid map of the class II region of the human major histocompatibility complex (MHC).

# Isolating genes from cDNA libraries

In order to isolate new genes, libraries are constructed which contain cDNA. For example, to isolate the human homologue of a mouse liver gene, mRNA is purified from human liver and used to make a human liver cDNA library (Fig. 6.6). As the human gene would probably be similar, but not identical, to the mouse gene the mouse gene could be used as a probe under non-stringent hybridization conditions. With luck, a colony could be identified containing a plasmid whose insert was the human version of the mouse gene.

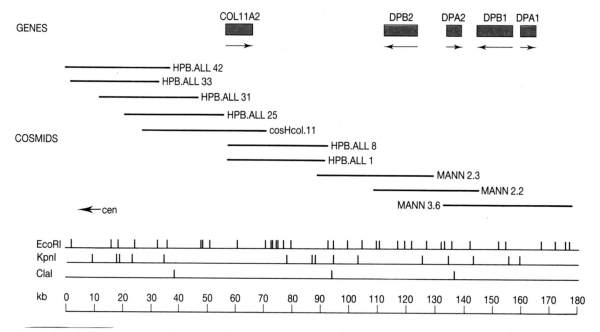

**Figure 6.5** Genomic DNA can be mapped by overlapping cosmids. This example illustrates cosmids covering a portion of the human major histocompatibility complex [the human leukocyte antigen (HLA) region]. The physical distance in kilobases is represented along the bottom. Above this are the location of restriction sites for the enzymes EcoRI, KpnI and ClaI. The position of individual genes (shown without their exon/intron structures) are shown at the top of the figure. Reproduced courtesy of Dr I. Hanson.

# Sequencing genes

Thousands of human genes have now been isolated in the form of cDNA clones. Determining the sequence of such clones is a simple matter. The most commonly used technique, the Nobel-prize winning dideoxynucleotide method developed by Sanger, is illustrated in Fig. 6.7. Once a new gene is discovered, its sequence can be compared with the ever increasing pool of known genes. Sequence homology may suggest that the

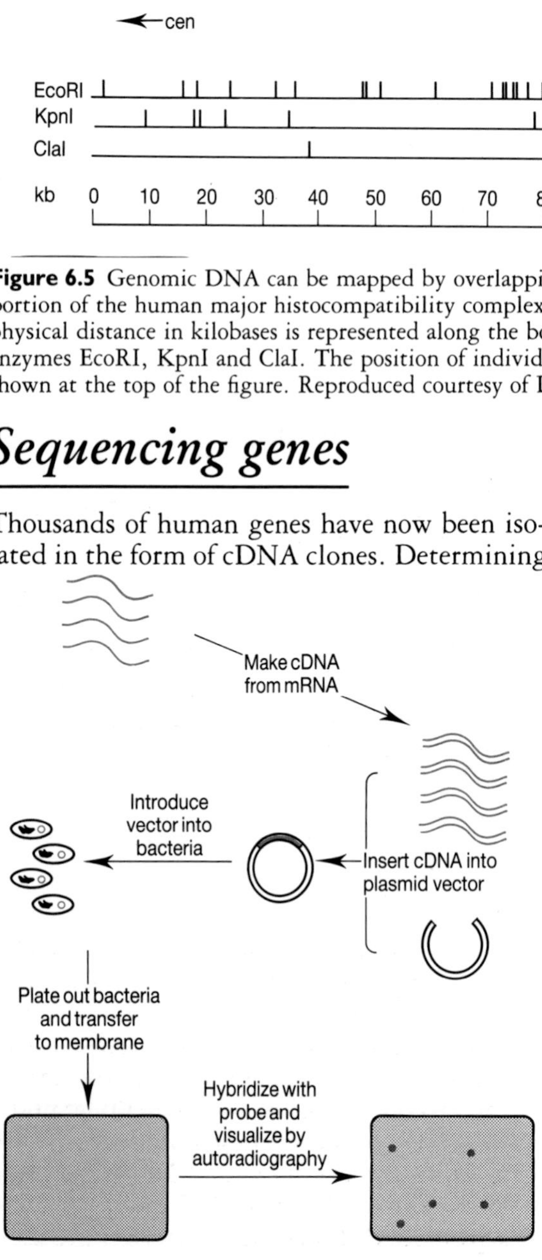

**Figure 6.6** Creation of a complementary DNA (cDNA) library. Complementary DNA is made from messenger RNA (mRNA) using reverse transcriptase and cloned into a plasmid vector. This is introduced into bacteria which are plated out on agar where they grow as single colonies. DNA from the colonies is transferred to nitrocellulose membranes and hybridized with an appropriate probe. Following autoradiography, the position of positive clones containing DNA which has hybridized with the probe can be determined by alignment with the original plates.

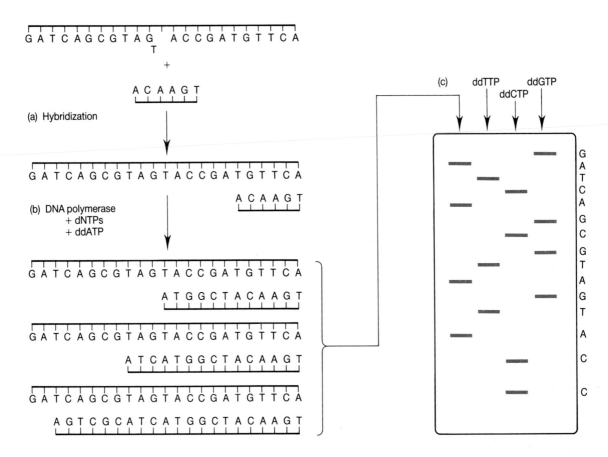

**Figure 6.7** Sequencing DNA. The Sanger sequencing protocol utilizes $2',3'$-dideoxynucleotides (ddNTPs) which, when incorporated into a growing DNA strand, block formation of phosphodiester bonds with other deoxynucleotides (dNTPs). (a) A short oligonucleotide primer is hybridized with the DNA to be sequenced. Note that the primer sequence is complementary to part of the DNA, for instance, to vector sequence immediately before the site at which an unknown complementary (cDNA) has been ligated and cloned. (b) DNA polymerase is used to make a complementary second DNA strand from the $3'$ end of the primer, adding one dNTP after another. (One of the dNTPs is radiolabelled to allow subsequent visualization.) When a ddNTP is added (ddATP in our illustration), the reaction stops. This results in a number of different length complementary strands, all ending with a ddATP complementary to a T on the template DNA strand. (c) The products of four polymerase reactions, each containing a different ddNTP, are separated by polyacrylamide gel electrophoresis and visualized by autoradiography. As shown, the DNA sequence can be read from the pattern of fragments.

new gene shares a similar function with a known gene. Similar techniques can also be used to sequence whole stretches of genomic DNA.

# The polymerase chain reaction

DNA amplification by polymerase chain reaction (PCR) has revolutionized molecular biology (Fig. 6.8). The value of the technique lies in its

ability to produce large quantities of DNA from minute amounts of starting material. In principle, the steps are as follows:

1 Oligonucleotide primers, about 20 nucleotides long, are synthesized in the laboratory such that one is complementary to one DNA strand at one end of the desired target sequence, whilst the other is complementary to the sequence of the other DNA strand at the other end of the target section of DNA.

2 Heating the patient's total DNA causes the two strands of the DNA double helix to separate and allows the primers to have access

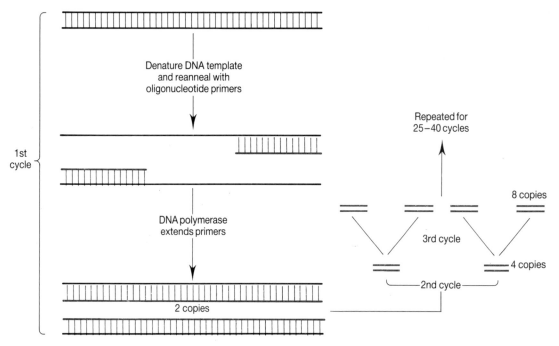

**Figure 6.8** The polymerase chain reaction (PCR). In each cycle, the double-stranded DNA template is separated by heating and cooling to allow the oligonucleotide primers to bind. DNA polymerase then extends the primers by adding free nucleotides (dNTPs). *Taq* DNA polymerase is usually used as it is stable at high temperatures. Theoretically, *n* cycles will result in $2^n$ copies of the target DNA, potentially an enormous amplification.

to the sequences at either end of the target DNA.

3 Cooling the DNA causes the primers to hybridize to the ends of the target DNA strands to form short double-stranded lengths of DNA that will be recognized by the DNA polymerase enzyme. Because of the short lengths involved, this primer pairing occurs ahead of full restoration of double-stranded DNA.

4 Warming the DNA in the presence of DNA polymerase and a supply of nucleotides causes this enzyme to start replicating the single-stranded DNA from the point where the primers have hybridized. In this way each target DNA sequence is doubled.

5 Repeating steps 2, 3 and 4 in the presence of thermal stable DNA polymerase and enough nucleotides and primer will lead to an exponential increase in copies of the target DNA sequence. Each newly synthesized strand will act as a template for primer hybridization in the next round of DNA replication.

Many modifications of the PCR technique have been developed for applications such as rapid DNA cloning, identification of mutations within genes, typing known polymorphisms within genes, and detection of DNA from infectious agents within blood or tissue.

# *Transferring genes*

One of the most exciting developments in molecular biology has been the introduction of techniques which transfer single genes into populations of cells or whole animals. These methods have primarily been used to study the functions of specific genes, but the same technology is being adapted for use in the treatment of human disease. **Transfection** is the introduction of a foreign gene into a cell line in culture. This is achieved by inserting a cDNA clone into an appropriate vector, which is then forced into the cell, either chemically or by an electric current. Genes can also be inserted into whole organisms, most commonly mice, to produce **transgenic** animals. In this technique, cDNA is microinjected into blastocysts, which are then reimplanted in the uterus. If the cDNA successfully integrates into the mouse genome, the resulting animal will be chimaeric; a proportion of its cells, including germ cells, will contain the foreign gene. Further cross-breeding will produce a mouse whose cells all contain the foreign gene. Similar technology has been used to produce 'knock-out' mice, animals in which specific genes have been deleted or rendered non-functional by disruption of their loci in embryonic cells.

# $D$IAGNOSIS USING MOLECULAR TECHNIQUES

Direct examination of DNA and sometimes RNA has the advantages of speed, accuracy and sensitivity which are crucial in diagnosis. Several different methods can be used, all with the object of identifying a particular stretch of genetic material. The following examples illustrate the scope and power of these techniques.

## Virology and microbiology

Many diagnostic laboratories are equipped to identify DNA or RNA sequences in foreign organisms. This is particularly useful for viruses and bacteria, for example, mycobacteria, cytomegalovirus (CMV), human immuno-deficiency virus (HIV-1), which are difficult to culture in the laboratory and whose identification has depended on examination of the host immune response. Use of PCR has gained rapid success because it can be used with great speed, specificity and sensitivity. DNA can be extracted from a small sample of blood or tissue and analysed using specific oligonucleotides. This has helped to recognize clinical infection with CMV which is notoriously difficult to isolate by culture methods. Detection of hepatitis C in the peripheral blood using PCR is virtual proof of infection, whereas the presence of antibody may be due to present or past infection. However, careful controls are needed with each PCR analysis in view of the extreme sensitivity of the method and the potential for error. Another technique which has entered the laboratory is *in situ* hybridization, employing short nucleotide probes to analyse tissues infected by virus. This allows direct tissue examination for the presence, for example, of CMV infection in transplant recipients.

## Tissue typing for transplantation

The immune response to donor tissue is focussed on the **human leukocyte antigen** (HLA) system of cell surface glycoproteins (page 84). These molecules are highly polymorphic, that is, different individuals have HLA molecules that differ in structure, and can be discriminated by antibodies and T-lymphocytes. Molecular analysis of the HLA genes on chromosome 6 (HLA-DR, -DQ, -DP, -B, -C and -A) has led to reclassification of the HLA system according to the number of genes coding for these molecules and the sequence variation in each of these genes. As a result, for example, individuals who were formerly typed as HLA-DR3 can be split into at least three groups according to differences in the fine structure of one of their two HLA-DR molecules. This level of refinement in HLA typing is likely to affect organ matching and is also helping to identify genes which influence susceptibility to autoimmune diseases (see later). DNA typing of HLA antigens is now legally required for proof of the relationship when a kidney transplant is performed between family members. Methods commonly employed are PCR and probing using non-isotopically labelled DNA fragments.

# Identity testing

The technique of genetic 'finger-printing' makes use of the presence of short DNA sequences which are repeated in tandem for a variable number of times on each of two chromosomes (variable number tandem repeats, VNTRs). The chromosome pair will give rise to two different sized fragments of DNA which can be cut out with a given restriction enzyme and identified by Southern blotting (Fig. 6.9). All individuals except identical twins can be distinguished by the fragment pattern so that paternity can be excluded if the putative father and child have no fragments in common. The accuracy of the technique is enhanced if more than one probe is used. The PCR can be used to amplify the segment of interest so that identity testing in forensic cases can be carried out on DNA from a small sample of semen, saliva, hair root or blood. The method has also been used to monitor the survival of donor cells after bone marrow transplantation. This method is an example of the way in which an anonymous segment of DNA can be used as a genetic marker.

# Carrier detection and prenatal diagnosis in genetic disease

The common genetic diseases, such as cystic fibrosis and muscular dystrophy, are caused by mutations in single genes (see below). The mapping of these diseases to particular loci makes it possible to screen for the diseases, and families can then practice zygote selection (see also Chapter 7, page 74). DNA from a sample of human chorionic villus may be examined at 9–13 weeks of pregnancy, or DNA may be taken from amniotic fluid cells at a slightly later stage. The advent of *in vitro* fertilization, and the ability to amplify a single copy of DNA from a single cell, have made it feasible to carry out preimplantation diagnosis of some X-linked disorders. Some diseases for which gene probes are available and permit genetic analysis are shown in Table 6.2.

(a)

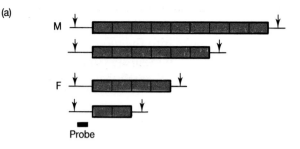
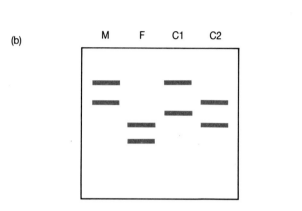

**Figure 6.9** The principle of paternity testing. (a) A short stretch of DNA, represented by the open rectangle, is repeated for a variable number of times in different people. The mother (M) has two alleles (one on each chromosome) which differ in length. The putative father (F) has two other alleles also differing in length. These are cut using a restriction enzyme with cutting sites as shown by the arrows. (b) Child 1 (C1) possesses neither of the alleles of the putative father and therefore paternity can be excluded. Paternity cannot be excluded in child 2 (C2) because the child has one allele which is the same as one from the putative father.

Diseases caused by point mutation, for example, the GAG to GTG substitution in the β-globin gene in sickle cell anaemia, can be detected by PCR amplification of the sequence containing the mutation. The PCR product can be probed using a short synthetic nucleotide specific for the altered sequence (allele specific oligonucleotide, ASO). Alternatively, the PCR product may be digested using a restriction enzyme (e.g. MstII) which has a cutting site in the normal sequence but not in the altered sequence and therefore generates a different number of fragments. Or, PCR primers can be designed so that they only bind to the altered sequence and therefore result in an amplification product only if the sequence is present. Large deletions, such as those in the β-thalassaemias

**Table 6.2** Some examples of diseases where molecular genetic diagnosis can be carried out.

| | Direct gene analysis | Linkage with gene probe |
|---|---|---|
| Sickle cell anaemia | X | |
| Thalassaemias | X | |
| Duchenne muscular dystrophy | X | |
| Cystic fibrosis | X | |
| Neurofibromatosis | X | |
| Lesch–Nyhan syndrome | X | |
| Polyposis of colon | X | |
| Huntingdon's disease | X | |
| Tay–Sachs disease | X | |
| Familial hypercholesterolaemia | X | |
| Haemophilia A | X | |
| Haemophilia B | X | |
| Adult polycystic kidney disease | | X |
| Atopic asthma | | X |

and Duchenne muscular dystrophy, may be recognized by the absence of fragments on RFLP analysis. Exact sizing of the missing fragment and hence better classification of the disease is made possible using gel electrophoresis modified for separation of large fragments of DNA (pulsed field gel electrophoresis).

### LINKAGE ANALYSIS

In diseases where the disease locus has not been fully identified and therefore cannot be directly examined, segregation analysis using DNA markers which are closely linked to the mutant gene may be used to predict whether a person is a carrier. DNA from affected family members must be available to show that the disease phenotype and the genetic marker are inherited together. This is only possible if the affected relative is heterozygous for the allele at the marker locus. An example is adult polycystic kidney disease (APCKD) where the mutant gene has been mapped to chromosome 16 and lies close to the α-globin gene cluster. A polymorphic segment of DNA in the α-globin gene cluster serves as an accurate reference point to detect the presence of the APCKD gene.

However, occasionally families with APCKD occur in which the disease phenotype is not linked to the α-globin gene, and therefore analysis with chromosome 16 markers may not be helpful. Another confounding feature is the rare occurrence of recombination, during meiosis, between the APCKD gene and the DNA marker. With a recombination fraction of 0.1, possession of the DNA marker will give a correct prediction of the inheritance of the mutant gene with 90% certainty. Markers on both sides of the APCKD locus improve the accuracy of diagnosis by reducing the effect of crossover between one of the DNA markers and the mutant gene.

## Molecular cytogenetics

Molecular probes can be used in conjunction with cytogenetic analysis to help detect gross chromosomal deletions and other abnormalities. Non-isotopic labels are attached to the DNA probes, so that they can be identified (on chromosomal spreads) by a further reaction. Commonly, the label is biotin, which can be visualized in a further step involving avidin that has been labelled with fluorochrome. Alternatively, the DNA probe may be labelled with digoxygenin, and the binding of the probe can be detected using antibody against digoxygenin, labelled with fluorochrome or peroxidase. This approach can detect trisomies, deletions (e.g. Duchenne muscular dystrophy), duplications and small translocations. In addition, X- and Y-specific probes may be used to demonstrate anomalies such as the presence of a Y sequence in XX males or absence of a Y sequence in XY females.

## Cancer

A number of probes have been developed from basic research which allow the detection of somatic mutations and other abnormalities in tumour cells. Point mutations in the *H-ras* oncogene can be recognized in human colon carcinoma. Other probes allow the detection of gene rearrangement in lymphoid cells, which help to establish the clonality and therefore malignant origin of the cells. Amplification of oncogenes can be detected in numerous tumours. These techniques are likely to play an increasing role in the classification and staging of tumours, and monitoring of therapy.

## THERAPEUTIC USES OF MOLECULAR BIOLOGY

Recombinant DNA technology – the ability to isolate and package genes so that they can be manipulated for different purposes – has given rise to a number of new treatments as well as more effective replacements for existing treatments.

## Molecular pharmacy

A large industry has grown up around the ability to clone peptides and proteins from the human genome and expand them in potentially unlimited quantities. These products are pure and are potentially free from the problem of viral contamination that has plagued the use of natural products such as growth hormone and factor VIII. The isolated clone, however, must first be manipulated to make a product which is biologically active and non-antigenic in humans. An example is recombinant human erythropoeitin (EPO) which has readily found use in the treatment of the anaemia of chronic renal failure. The product cannot be successfully made in bacterial cells since these lack the ability to glycosylate the peptide backbone of EPO which is in itself biologically inactive. The EPO gene has therefore been expressed in mammalian tissue culture cells (derived from the Chinese hamster ovary) since these can carry out the necessary post-translational modifications to the peptide molecule.

## Vaccines

The techniques of molecular biology have made it possible to manufacture new vaccines against previously unpreventable diseases and provide more effective replacements for existing vaccines. The antigenic portions of viral proteins must first be identified and isolated, using molecular cloning techniques. Production in viral and other constructs can then be scaled up and the protein or peptide elaborated in an antigenic form. A successful vaccine against hepatitis B was constructed in this way from the P25 component of the surface antigen of the virus. Great interest has focussed on the envelope protein (gp 120) of HIV-1 and a number of vaccines generated using different strategies are being assessed.

## Blocking peptides

The CD4 cluster differentiation antigen on the surface of lymphocytes acts as a receptor for HIV-1 which binds by its envelope glycoprotein, gp 120. Soluble forms of the CD4 protein have been developed by recombinant DNA technology. These block viral entry to T-lymphocytes, and are being assessed in clinical trials. It is hoped that smaller, blocking peptides will be devised as the precise structure of the domain of CD4 recognized by HIV becomes known. This approach also opens up new possibilities for immunosuppressive treatment based on the interference of the interaction between cell receptors and ligands which are important in the immune response.

## Synthetic antibodies

Mouse or rat monoclonal antibodies are used widely in laboratory diagnosis, but their therapeutic application is limited because rodent antibodies can provoke an immune response in humans and they may not work so well with human effector functions, such as complement. Attempts to produce human monoclonal antibodies by fusing human antibody cells with myeloma cell lines have only been partially successful. Hope has therefore been pinned on recombinant DNA technology to construct new monoclonal antibodies.

One approach has been to graft, by molecular cloning, the antigen binding site of existing rodent monoclonal antibodies onto the framework of human antibodies. The resulting 'humanized' antibody is still able to recognize the target antigen but acquires new effector functions which belong to the human portion of the antibody. An example is humanized anti-CD3 against the signal transduction component of the T-cell receptor, currently under evaluation as an immunosuppressive agent. Another, is a broadly reacting T-cell antibody (Campath I) used in the treatment of lymphomas. If the goal is achieved a new wave of therapeutic agents, more effective and less troublesome than their predecessors, will be produced.

A further step forward has made it possible to isolate the genes encoding the variable portions of the heavy and light chains of the antibody binding site, and to bring these together to create new antibody binding sites. These are expressed on the surface of bacteriophage particles. Antibody fragments with the desired specification can be selected and expanded for therapeutic and diagnostic use. With this technology, it is theoretically possible to sample the entire human antibody repertoire using a cDNA library derived from pools of B-cells, and in addition select novel combinations of heavy and light chains. This offers the exciting possibility of being able to retrieve antibodies against self components, such as tumour necrosis factor and immunoglobulins, which are normally deleted or suppressed during the development of the immune system, and put them to therapeutic use.

# Gene therapy

This refers to the packaging of a cloned gene and insertion into the genome of a recipient with a defective somatic gene. It would clearly be better to replace a defective function with a single treatment than with the missing protein. To achieve this, however, several problems need to be overcome. The new gene has to be delivered in such a way that it can be integrated into the host genome. It has to be expressed in the tissue in question. It must also come under the control of the regulatory machinery of the cell. These difficulties have been partly overcome using retroviral vectors. Viruses have the information for packaging foreign DNA into viral particles and for (randomly) inserting it into the host genome. Viral particles containing the cloned gene could, for example, be used to infect bone marrow cells in a patient with a potentially fatal defect, where no alternative therapy is available. One form of immunodeficiency due to adenosine deaminase deficiency has been successfully treated by inserting the missing gene into patients' lymphocytes and reinfusing them.

# Antisense technology

In this terminology, the coding strand of DNA is the sense strand. Transcription of this strand produces an RNA molecule with a complementary base sequence. (The only difference is that RNA has uracil instead of thymine.) If a synthetic oligonucleotide with the appropriate antisense sequence can be introduced into the cell, it will bind to the messenger RNA and, effectively, shut off the gene. One achievement of this technology has been the creation of a tomato with longer shelf-life. Another recent example is the use of an antisense oligonucleotide against the proto-oncogene, *c-myb*, to prevent proliferation and thickening in experimentally damaged vessel walls, providing a new route to cardiovascular therapy. A hope for the future is that antisense technology will have a role in controlling the proliferation of cancer cells and viruses.

# *T*HE MOLECULAR DISSECTION OF DISEASE

Diseases that are influenced by genetic factors can be divided into those with a simple inheritance, arising from mutation of a single gene (single gene disorders), and diseases, such as heart disease and diabetes, that are thought to arise from the influence of several genes interacting with the environment (polygenic disorders). A general aim of research using molecular biology has been (1) to identify the gene or genes involved in the pathogenesis of these diseases and (2) to understand the range of defects associated with abnormal gene function. A reverse approach, that is, to discover a new gene and then to search for a function of that gene and identify a disease when the gene is not properly expressed, may also illuminate disease mechanisms.

## *Single gene disorders*

The inherited disorders of haemoglobin illustrate the large variety of molecular defects that can cause a single disorder. In β-thalassaemia, over a hundred different mutations have been recognized. Many of the defects are due to point mutations, that is, substitution of single bases, some of which result in a single amino acid change in the β-globin chain. Other mutations result in an abnormally long or short (and functionally defective) β-globin, due to the disabling of a Stop codon or creation of a new one (UAG, UGA, UAA) in an inappropriate place. Other mutations cause abnormal processing of RNA due to the loss of a normal splice site or emergence of a new one (Fig. 6.10), leading to a reduction in β-globin synthesis. Others impair the addition of a poly-A tail to the finished transcript, reducing its stability and leading to a reduction in the amount of protein product. So called frameshift changes are caused when deletion or addition of one or two (but not three) bases throws the triplet codon sequence out of frame causing premature termination of the peptide at or beyond the point corresponding to

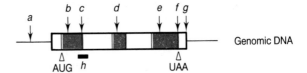

**Figure 6.10** Examples of point mutations in a hypothetical gene: *a* in the control region, causing reduced transcription; *b* in the coding region, causing an abnormal product; *c* at a splice site, leading to reduced synthesis; *d* in the coding region, creating a premature stop codon and early termination of protein synthesis; *e* deletion of one or two bases in the coding region resulting in a frameshift; *f* in a stop codon resulting in a long protein product; *g* in the poly A site causing a reduction in protein synthesis. A small deletion is represented at *h*.

the frameshift. Mutations in the regulatory region upstream of the gene (Fig. 6.10) can, as might be expected, lead to a reduced level of transcription. Larger deletions are more common in α-thalassaemia.

The drastic effect on function of a single base substitution is exemplified by sickle cell anaemia (page 611). Here, the change from GAG to GTG in the base sequence of the β-globin gene results in a protein with a single amino acid substitution (glutamic acid → valine). This causes an abnormal tendency for aggregation of the haemoglobin molecule in deoxygenated blood.

Progress was rapid with the haemoglobinopathies because the abnormal protein was already known and the gene could be analysed. Most mutations occur at common restriction enzyme sites and therefore RFLP analysis proved useful in the dissection of these diseases. Those defects with affected sites away from restriction enzyme sites were soon recognized by sequencing.

A different strategy was needed with diseases like cystic fibrosis and neurofibromatosis, because the identity of the abnormal gene was unknown before it was mapped. Linkage analysis using DNA markers for specific chromosomes was used to determine the genetic location of such diseases. The most useful genetic markers are those which are highly polymorphic, since if the disease trait and a particular allele at the marker locus coexist in the same family members, it is highly likely that the marker locus and disease gene are genetically linked. Once the gene has been located to its chromosome the next step is to obtain additional markers to saturate the chromosome region around the gene, so that the distance between flanking markers becomes increasingly smaller until the gene itself has been found. The process of narrowing the gap by examining progressively closer regions of flanking DNA is called chromosome walking.

The utility of this approach is exemplified by cystic fibrosis (page 295). In 1985 the gene was placed on chromosome 7 and four years later the gene was cloned. Since then its function in the transport of chloride ions across the luminal surface of some epithelial cells has been identified. A range of mutations that can affect gene function has been disclosed, making it possible to offer carrier detection and prenatal diagnosis. This approach of going backwards from abnormal function to the unmasking of the gene is called reverse, or positional, genetics.

# Polygenic disorders

More common diseases, such as diabetes, rheumatoid arthritis, atherosclerosis and hypertension, are said to be polygenic, that is, they involve more than one gene. Direct analysis of genes will help to tease out the single gene entities that predispose, and interact with the environment.

## AUTOIMMUNE DISEASES

It has been known for a long time that certain HLA class II antigens are increased in frequency in patients with particular diseases. But not all patients with these diseases have the HLA antigen in question and it was therefore difficult to interpret whether the antigen itself was important in predisposing to the disease or whether it was linked to another gene of greater significance. Identification of antigen specificities, such as DR3 which is associated with insulin-dependent diabetes, and DR4 which is assoc-

iated with rheumatoid arthritis, was by a relatively blunt methodology using antibodies or sometimes T-cells to type a patient's lymphocytes for HLA antigens. The ability to analyse gene structure directly has led to much more precise classification of the HLA antigens. Consequently, it has been possible to re-examine disease associations with particular HLA genes in a much more powerful way. This has led to the recognition, for example, that most patients with insulin-dependent diabetes have HLA-DQ molecules with similar structures at the cleft which binds antigenic peptide and presents it to T-lymphocytes. Other research has shown structural similarities in the HLA molecules possessed by patients with rheumatoid disease and in the HLA molecules of patients with pemphigus. These and other studies implicate the HLA genes themselves in the disease process.

At the same time progress has been rapid to clone and dissect the portions of T-lymphocytes (T-cell receptors) which combine with HLA-bound antigen peptide as a crucial step to antigen recognition. This has revealed that particular T-lymphocyte populations with certain structural motifs predominate in the abnormal immune response in certain autoimmune diseases such as multiple sclerosis and possibly rheumatoid arthritis. If this is true, then therapy could be directed against certain subsets of T-cells.

A third element which has profoundly influenced the comprehension of normal and altered immunity is the elucidation of the crystallographic structure of the HLA molecule. This information, together with the details of the primary sequences of different HLA molecules, in particular around the antigen binding cleft where the sequence varies between different individuals, will undoubtedly provide a cornerstone for the molecular analysis of disease, and construction of new treatments based on blocking or enhancing specific molecular interactions.

## INFECTIONS

Viral antigens are presented to the immune system as small peptides bound to HLA class I molecules. Molecular cloning and sequencing of viral proteins has helped to delineate the antigenic portions which bind to HLA and are seen by the immune system. HLA class I molecules are very polymorphic, and it would be expected that, since individuals with different HLA molecules respond differently to different antigens, certain HLA types would confer resistance to infection. This has only recently been confirmed, using molecular analysis, in Gambian children with malaria: those with B35 and DR13 are less likely to have life-threatening forms of malaria. The fine discriminating power of molecular techniques may allow other associations between HLA and particular infections to be uncovered, and therefore may yield better definition of risk factors and more successful disease prevention. Investigation of the genome of the organism itself has highlighted the enormous capacity of *Plasmodium falciparum* to undergo genetic recombination, and hence to generate resistant forms.

## DEGENERATIVE DISEASES

Familial combined hyperlipidaemia consists of raised blood cholesterol and fat levels, and probably accounts for about 10 per cent of premature coronary heart disease. Molecular analysis so far suggests that it is a heterogeneous condition, with different genes involved in different families. In some families the defect is related to the apolipoprotein, CIII, gene. The CIII protein is an inhibitor of lipoprotein lipase, which promotes uptake and clearance of fat from the blood. A defect of the lipoprotein gene itself has been implicated in at least one family. Thus, several markers may eventually identify individuals at risk on whom preventative efforts should be focussed.

## NEUROLOGICAL AND PSYCHIATRIC DISORDERS

Progress is being made with Alzheimer's disease for which specific mutations have already been shown in several families. Research into functional psychiatric disorders, using DNA markers, may lead to a better definition of the genetic component of some of the familial disorders, such as severe cyclical depression and schizophrenia. With the cloning of neuro-transmitters and their receptors, the nature of functional disturbances can be examined.

## CONGENITAL MALFORMATIONS

Study of the developmental biology of simple animals, such as the nematode worm and fruit fly, provides models for the understanding of human development and congenital malformations. One of the discoveries that helped to cement this view was the finding of homeobox genes, important for somatic development in animals from worms to humans. Elegant experiments on the ways in which mutations in these genes can cause abnormal development offer an understanding into the origin of human malformations.

## NEOPLASTIC DISEASES

Molecular analysis has shown that tumour development can involve the dysfunction of genes that control normal cell proliferation, differentiation and development. Wilm's tumour in childhood seems to involve the loss of controlled development of the nephron. Children with this disease have a deletion of a band on chromosome 11. The gene responsible (WT1) has been cloned and identified as a zinc finger protein, a regulatory gene whose product is dependent on zinc for its stability and has 'fingers' which bind to the DNA of another regulatory gene upstream of the target gene. Point mutations involving the amino acids on the zinc finger of the WT1 protein lead to tumour development. Thus, the disease involves underfunction of a normal regulatory gene, and therefore such genes are known as **tumour suppressor genes**.

Oncogenes, on the other hand, are overexpressed in many tumours. In chronic myeloid leukaemia the gene is expressed at the translocation point between chromosomes 9 and 11, on the so-called Philadelphia chromosome. In Burkitt's lymphoma, the abnormality of oncogene expression occurs at the translocation site of chromosome 8 into other chromosomes, at positions involved in the rearrangement immunoglobulin genes during B-cell maturation.

# Charting the human genome

The holy grail of medical genetics is to have a linear map of the human genome charting the positions of the genes and a catalogue of all the variations at each locus. Disease genes can then be mapped into place alongside known markers, using genetic and physical linkage studies. The **human genome project** (HUGO) is a coordinated effort to obtain such a map. One aspect of the work is to sequence new genes pulled out of cDNA libraries more or less at random. This way, the 5 per cent or so of the human genome which codes for useful proteins will eventually be sequenced. As each new sequence is obtained, it can be mapped into position on large chromosomal fragments of the human genome packaged into yeast chromosomes (yeast artificial chromosomes or YACs). Another aspect of the project is the pooling of data from different species, to take advantage of the close homology, for example, between humans and mice. Smaller genomes, such as that of the nematode, may also serve as a test bed for new methods of analysis in more complex organisms.

An example of what can be achieved is shown by a study of sequences in the mouse genome known as microsatellites. These consist of long arrays of dinucleotide repeats which show considerable allelic variation in the number of repeats, and serve as useful reference points for the mapping of genes. These sequences have already been used to identify two new genes that influence the onset of diabetes in the non-obese diabetic mouse.

# Molecular anthropology

Genes, and parts of genes, shared in different species provide a source of study to examine evolutionary pathways. Extensive analysis of the genes of the major histocompatibility complex has provided extraordinary insight into the origin of genetic diversity in the immune system of higher animals and will also provide a useful background for the study of immune diseases in animal models. It seems possible that organ donation for human transplantation will involve animals selected on the basis of homologies in the recipient and donor species.

## THE IMPACT OF MOLECULAR BIOLOGY ON SOCIETY

Since DNA cloning and DNA sequencing were invented in the mid-1970s, DNA technology has had a more immediate impact on medical practice than was first anticipated. New pharmaceuticals, vaccines and replacement treatments arising from molecular biology will be of enormous benefit to human beings. Sudden and imaginative changes can take place with the introduction of a new technique: witness the influence of PCR on routine diagnostic practice.

Old controversies about prenatal diagnosis and carrier detection have been brought back into the limelight. In the last ten years, the genes responsible for virtually all of the common, inherited diseases have been mapped. The implications of this for prenatal diagnosis and carrier detection overlap with the broader ethical and social issues raised by abortion and screening programmes.

New questions have been raised about how the information from research into the common polygenic diseases, such as diabetes and heart disease, will be used. Genetic risk could be computed for heart disease, cancer and psychiatric diseases, and those at special risk encouraged to modify their lifestyle favourably. What then: would the information be sought for use by insurance companies, education and employment agencies, and for what purposes? Some have expressed the fear that this would create a new genetic underclass.

The preparative steps for gene therapy have

been taken and the progress of the first patients treated with new genes, in the USA, is being carefully monitored. Few people would object to the idea of replacement of a defective somatic gene. The concept of altering the destiny of our offspring by carefully editing or inserting new genetic traits into germ cell DNA is a matter for future debate.

These are all good reasons for keeping society informed and involved with developments as they occur, and should not divert from one of the most fruitful periods of science and medicine.

# Medical Genetics

7

# *I*NTRODUCTION

Advances in molecular genetics are not just illuminating the rarer, simply inherited disorders, but are beginning to elucidate some of the common diseases, such as cancer, cardiovascular disease and diabetes. Inherited diseases are encountered in virtually all clinical disciplines and an understanding of gene activity at the cellular and molecular level is essential for the proper appreciation of the pathogenesis of many diseases. In short, genetics is an integral part of modern medicine.

# *T*HE NATURE OF THE HUMAN GENOME

Figure 7.1 shows the human genome as it has been viewed for the last few decades. Each chromosome is an enormous DNA double helix of complementary nucleotide sequences, where cytosine (C) pairs with guanine (G) and thymine (T) with adenine (A). The DNA molecule is bound into chromatin by coiling around a protein complex, called a nucleosome, about every 200 nucleotide base pairs (bp) and then packing further as a supercoil. There is now an international effort underway to map and sequence all the 50–100 000 genes that are incorporated in the 22 pairs of autosomes and X chromosomes that appear in Fig. 7.1, plus the Y chromosome. The most important Y-linked gene, SRY, which diverts early development along the male route by turning fetal gonads into testes, has already been cloned. However, apart from some genes concerned with spermatogenesis, there are presumably no other really important genes carried exclusively on the Y chromosome for the simple reason that half the human race manages very well without it! It follows that Y-linked genetic diseases do not feature large in medicine, and that most of the Y chromosome does not consist of expressed genes but some other form of DNA.

# *Most DNA is repetitive sequences*

Only a few per cent of the DNA comprising the whole human genome consists of genes encoding proteins. Much of the remainder is made up of repetitive DNA sequences, either dispersed throughout the genome like minisatellite DNA of 'DNA fingerprinting' fame or contained in huge blocks, such as the heterochromatin that flanks the centromere of each chromosome. Why the repeat sequences are there and what role they play in human disease is uncertain. What is certain is that this so-called 'junk DNA' cannot be dismissed as being of no medical importance. The dispersed, 300 bp long Alu sequence, which is repeated 500 000 to 1 million times throughout the human genome, can predipose to misalignment and unequal crossing over between chromosomes of the pair during egg or sperm formation causing gene deletions or

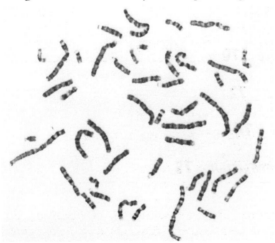

**Figure 7.1** A chromosome metaphase spread of a normal female stained with one of the Giemsa banding techniques.

duplications. Furthermore, the haphazard 'jumping' of an Alu sequence (via a transcribed RNA product) into the middle of the NF1 gene has been shown to be the causative mutation in a case of neurofibromatosis, and a disruptive insertion of a L1 repeat element into the factor VIII gene can cause haemophilia. Thus there is medical interest beyond just those nucleotide sequences that are transcribed and processed into messenger RNA molecules (mRNA) for translation into proteins, i.e. the coding sequences are illustrated in Fig. 7.2. Nevertheless, cloning these 'expressed' sequences is rightly a major goal of the human genome project and one that will have enormous impact on medicine. The ease with which one can proceed from the exon sequences (which can be cloned via mRNA) to characterizing the whole gene – introns, flanking untranscribed sequences and all – is largely dependent on the overall size of the gene. Figure 7.2 is a diagrammatic representation of the

smallest type of gene, such as β globin. As can be seen from Table 7.1, some genes and in particular their introns are enormously long sequences.

**Table 7.1** Variation in the size of genes.

| | Genomic size (kb) | cDNA (mRNA) | Number of introns |
|---|---|---|---|
| **Small** | | | |
| α-globin | 0.8 | 0.5 | 2 |
| β-globin | 1.5 | 0.6 | 2 |
| Insulin | 1.7 | 0.4 | 2 |
| Apolipoprotein E | 3.6 | 1.2 | 3 |
| **Medium** | | | |
| Collagen I pro-α-1 | 18.0 | 5.0 | 50 |
| Collagen I pro-α-2 | 38.0 | 5.0 | 50 |
| Collagen VII | | | |
| pro-α-1 | ~35 | 9.2 | 118 |
| Albumin | 25.0 | 2.1 | 14 |
| Adenosine | | | |
| deaminase | 32.0 | 1.5 | 11 |
| Factor IX | 34.0 | 2.8 | 7 |
| Low density | | | |
| lipoprotein | | | |
| receptor | 45.0 | 5.5 | 17 |
| **Large** | | | |
| Phenylalanine | | | |
| hydroxylase | 90.0 | 2.4 | 12 |
| **Giant** | | | |
| Factor VIII | 186.0 | 9.0 | 26 |
| Cystic fibrosis | | | |
| transmembrane | | | |
| regulator | ~250 | 6.5 | 26 |
| **Mammoth** | | | |
| Dystrophin | ~2400 | ~16 | 79 |

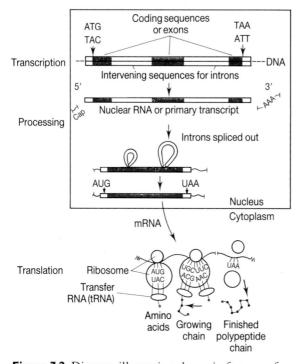

**Figure 7.2** Diagram illustrating the main features of transcription of a gene into a nuclear RNA molecule, the addition of a cap and a poly-A tail, the splicing out of the introns to produce the definitive messenger RNA (mRNA) molecule, and the translation of the mRNA into a polypeptide chain. The position of the translation initiation codon (AUG) and the termination codon (UAA) is indicated at both the DNA and RNA levels.

# An evolutionary perspective on gene sequences

Unique identifier sequences of human genes (expressed sequence tags) are now being generated at the rate of many thousands per year. What is instructive for an understanding of the human genome is how the thousands of short

**Table 7.2** Early results from random cDNA sequencing.

- Random primed cDNAs from human brain
- Automated partial sequencing, 400 ± 100 bp
- Searches on GenBank, Protein Information Resource and ProSite protein motif databases

| Database match | – | | | |
|---|---|---|---|---|
| | Human | | 197 | 32% |
| | (Mitochondrial genes | 67) | | |
| | (Repeated sequences | 59) | | |
| | (Ribosomal RNA | 28) | | |
| | (Other nuclear genes | 43) | | |
| | Non-human match | | 48 | 8% |
| | No database match | | 230 | 38% |
| | Polyadenylate insert | | 104 | 17% |
| | No insert | | 30 | 5% |
| | | | 609 | 100% |

Adapted from Adams et al. Science 1991; **252**:1651.

(approximately 400 bp) partial gene sequences that are generated are being sorted out in a meaningful way. That any sense at all can be made of these random DNA sequences is a consequence of the evolutionary process. As one might expect, human evolution is not so much a matter of design, but one of modification, reshuffling and rejigging pre-existing DNA sequences, the direction and speed of change being largely driven by natural selection. This process is enhanced by the separation of the coding sequences for the individual functional domains of large proteins by the intervening sequences of introns that divide up virtually all human genes (Fig. 7.2). It has also resulted in many entirely different genes sharing bits of DNA sequence as exons since useful protein domains are shuffled around during evolution and provide the evolutionary option of splicing together different exons to generate alternative proteins from a single gene.

A shared DNA sequence usually means shared function of the encoded protein domain. For example, all proteins that are translocated into the endoplasmic reticulum at the time of translation before being secreted need the same sort of signal peptide to guide this process; all proteins that extend through cell membranes need a hydrophobic domain that actually spans the

membrane, and so on. During evolution these shared DNA sequences of different genes tend to accumulate different neutral or adaptive changes, but still retain sufficient DNA sequence homology for computer searches to detect some similarity. This means that analysis of the nucleotide base sequence of a randomly cloned complementary DNA (cDNA) may well predict the gene's function and allow its tentative classification to a gene family.

Another evolutionary process that ran in parallel with exon shuffling was whole gene duplication. Once duplicated, the two genes could gradually develop slightly different, but still similar, functions. As further duplications occurred so a large gene family could emerge, such as the Ig superfamily embracing the immunoglobulin, human leukocyte antigen (HLA) and T-cell receptor genes amongst others. Gene families may remain clustered at one or two chromosomal locations, or become more dispersed. Some members of a gene family may accumulate disabling mutations, stop functioning and become a pseudogene; a troublesome relic of the past that predisposes to deletions and duplications by unequal crossing over. Thus on an evolutionary timescale, and indeed for some genes even over a few generations (as we shall see later), the human genome is far from fixed. Its structure reflects a dynamic process in which conservation of important sequences is set against a natural tendency for DNA replication and normal exchange between DNA molecules to go awry, with genetic disease as the consequence.

It is against this evolutionary perspective that the results of the first attempts at large scale random cDNA sequencing should be viewed (Table 7.2). In particular it should be noted that 8 per cent of the partial gene sequences were as yet unknown in human databases, but had homology with known eukaryotic genes. We share most of our genes with the mouse and the ability to use DNA sequence homology to move from humans to mouse (where precise models of genetic diseases can be discovered or engineered) and back again is becoming very important in the elucidation of molecular pathology and in developing new treatments.

# Types of genes, their regulation and role in development

There are three broad categories of genes:

1 Genes that have untranslated RNA as their product, for example, transfer RNA or ribosomal RNA, of which there are usually multiple copies in the genome.
2 Genes that encode protein transcription factors that bind DNA and have as their prime function the regulation of other genes, often in response to extracellular signals such as hormones.
3 Genes that encode proteins needed for tissue and cell structure, for example, collagen, myosin or myelin, and metabolism, for example, receptors or enzymes.

There are many metabolic and other functions that all cells require all the time, and the genes involved in these processes are known by the quaint term, housekeeping genes. Whilst their rate of transcription may be modulated, these genes are not permanently inactivated as part of differentiation. There are other genes that nearly all cells need on 'standby' to deal with acute stress, such as the genes for protein–tyrosine phosphatases induced by oxidative stress and heat shock, and then there are genes that are only expressed in a tissue-specific manner, such as those for haemoglobin. The determinant of which organs are significantly affected in a genetic disease is not solely a matter of which tissues express the mutant gene; there are many examples of widely expressed genes, where mutations seem to affect some tissues more than others.

remaining responsive to metabolic demands (including such complicated demands as wound healing, for example), gene expression inappropriate to the cell type must be avoided at all costs. This incredible balancing act is achieved by protein transcription factors interacting with each other and with specific DNA sequence motifs within (or beyond) the promoter region of the many genes involved. DNA sequences called enhancer elements that are central to cell type specific gene expression, may be located upstream, downstream or even within introns of the genes they regulate. Enhancers can be located several kilobases away from the gene concerned, posing the problem of how this DNA and the protein bound to it loops to make contact with the main transcription complex close to the gene. Also it poses particular problems for gene therapy involving the tissue-specific genes; the DNA inserted therapeutically has to have all the necessary regulatory elements for appropriate gene expression. Transcription factors characteristically have two distinct domains; a DNA-binding domain, and a transcription activation domain that contacts other transcription factors incorporated in the main transcription complex that forms around the TATAA sequence that is located about 20 bp upstream of the start site for transcription of most genes. Given DNA's fairly uniform structure, one might expect the amino acid sequence of the DNA-binding domain of different protein transcription factors to come from a rather limited range. In fact, many transcription factors employ one of four different DNA-binding domains; the helix-turn-helix homeodomain, zinc finger, leucine zipper and helix-loop-helix domains. These all have readily recognizable DNA sequences encoding them, which permit classification of gene sequences into the different transcription factor families.

# Transcription factors

The process of gradual cell and tissue differentiation during development demands a complicated system of molecular feedback mechanisms to regulate selective gene expression. Whilst

# DNA methylation

The long-term silencing of genes that underpins differentiation and the inactivation of one or other of the two X chromosomes in female cells (X-inactivation), is probably consolidated by shifts in DNA packing which limit the access of RNA polymerase, the enzyme responsible for gene transcription. To maintain differentiation such a mechanism must cope with successive cell divisions, since DNA replication is likely to disrupt protein–DNA binding. Here the methylation of DNA seems to play an important role in mammals (but not in lower animals). The selective methylation of DNA appears to be essential for mammalian development and the pattern of methylation can be preserved during DNA replication and cell division.

# Developmental genes

A group of developmental genes, usually encoding transcription factors, are of particular interest. So fundamental is the laying down of the body plan during early embryological development that the organization and sequence of key genes controlling morphogenesis are highly conserved between mouse and human, a fact that facilitated the genetic study of Waardenburg syndrome type 1, for example. This condition is characterized by deafness and pigmentary disturbances, typically a white forelock, and genetic linkage studies in affected families mapped the mutation to the q37 region of chromosome 2. A naturally occurring mutation in mouse, called Spotch because of its depigmented patches, was shown to be due to a mutation in the developmental gene, Pax3. The Pax family of developmental genes are so called because they all have a DNA motif termed 'paired'. Pax3 also has a homeodomain. Pax3 maps to that part of mouse chromosome 1 which is known to be homologous to human chromosome region 2q37. Thus the human PAX3 gene

(capitals are used for the human gene) became a prime 'candidate gene' for Waardenburg syndrome type 1. Mutations were duly found in some patients. Interestingly, one such mutation was an 18 bp deletion of a highly conserved (and therefore functionally important) 'paired' domain region of the gene and yet the clinical disorder was not particularly severe. Counter-intuitively it is emerging from studies in mice that to knock out completely one of these key developmental genes may not produce an embryonic lethal. They seem so important that back-up sets of genes have evolved reducing the impact of any one mutation. Many rarer congenital abnormalities may be due to mutations in such developmental genes. An example is provided by the Denys–Drash syndrome. This manifests as ambiguous genitalia (male pseudohermaphrodism), glomerulonephritis and a predisposition to Wilms's tumour and is caused by point mutations in the WT1 gene (commonly a mutation at nucleotide position 1180, resulting in an arginine to tryptophan change). The WT1 gene, encoding a 'zinc finger' DNA-binding protein and mapping to chromosome 11p13, was first defined as a tumour suppressor gene because its deletion predisposed to Wilms's tumour formation. This example emphasizes the links that can exist between genes involved in development and those mutant genes implicated in cancer. After all, in the final analysis, cancer is the loss of regulation of cell growth. The dominantly inherited pigmentary disturbance, piebaldism, is due to mutations in the *c-kit* proto-oncogene (mast/stem cell growth factor receptor), originally implicated in a leukaemia found in kittens. This last example also emphasizes how tissue specific the clinical effects can be despite widespread expression of a mutant gene, presumably because different tissues have different compensating or fallback systems.

## TOWARDS AN UNDERSTANDING OF GENETIC DISEASE

# Is a disease genetically determined?

Growth, development and the maintenance of health is a constant interaction between genes and environment, but it is the differences between people that matters in medicine. Given the same general environmental circumstances why was this child born deaf and the brother not, or why did this person develop diabetes mellitus when most people don't? Where the cause of the difference is primarily due to differences in genetic makeup, we say it is genetically determined. This phrase can be used to describe a condition due to a genetic change in a somatic cell which is then transmitted to progeny cells as proliferation proceeds, such as in a tumour. The term hereditary implies that all or some of the germ cells carry the mutation or relevant combination of genes. There is therefore the potential for these to be transmitted to offspring. In some disorders this potential may never be realized because the severity of the abnormality prevents long survival or reproduction. Thus the sporadic occurrence of a disorder does not tell us whether or not it is genetically determined.

There are three basic approaches to elucidating genetic factors in disease:

1 Twin studies, usually the comparison of concordance for the condition in monozygotic (identical, MZ) and dizygotic (DZ) twins. Whilst high or complete concordance in MZ, but much lower concordance in DZ twins, indicates hereditary determination, it says little about the number of genes involved.
2 Family studies and pedigree analysis are the cornerstone of medical genetics. The pattern of recurrence within families can indicate so-called 'monogenic' or Mendelian inheritance.
3 Direct analysis of chromosomes or genes.

A useful distinction when considering genetic factors in disease is the actual combination of particular genes inherited, **the genotype**, and the observable effect these genes produce in the individual, the corresponding **phenotype**. These terms are best limited to the discussion of one particular gene (or a few) and its effect.

# Loci and alleles

A meaningful classification of disease is essential for good clinical practice. As more and more genes are mapped and sequenced (or at least their exons and exon/intron junctions are sequenced), the closer we can get to a definitive classification of the simply inherited, or **Mendelian**, disorders. To date, nearly all the genetic variation in human populations seems to be confined to small changes in DNA sequences rather than in the actual position of a particular gene on the chromosome. This relatively constant chromosomal position is known as the gene locus, and since chromosomes and the genes they carry come in pairs, it is customary to regard the two gene sequences together as constituting the gene locus. Alternative genes that can occupy the same locus are called alleles. Obviously with only two DNA sites any one individual can only have two alleles at any one locus. However, in the whole population there may be numerous alleles, for example, over a 100 abnormal haemoglobins due to variants in the β-globin gene have been described.

Where the alleles at an autosomal locus are the same, the term **homozygous**, is used. Where one is the normal, common or 'wild type' allele and the other a variant or in the case of a disease a mutant, the individual is said to be **heterozygous**. Where an individual has two different mutant alleles, they are called **compound heterozygotes**. This terminology works well in clinical genetics where one is dealing with harmful mutations and simple Mendelian inheritance. Now that it is becoming possible to characterize the mutations in autosomal recessive disorders at the DNA sequence level, it turns out that many affected individuals are not homozygotes in the strictest sense, i.e. homoallelic, but compound heterozygotes. Nevertheless, because both alleles are clinically significant mutants, the person has no normally functioning allele and is clinically affected. In Britain, about 60 per cent of patients with cystic fibrosis are true homozygotes with a deletion of codon 508 of the cystic fibrosis transmembrane conductance regulatory (CFTR) gene on each chromosome 7, whilst the remainder are compound heterozygotes (e.g. delta 508 on one chromosome 7 and a point mutation at codon 551 on the other chromosome 7, or other combinations). In clinical genetics one needs to be able to describe the genotype in a meaningful way when it comes to DNA analysis, and so it is useful to use the term compound heterozygote for distinguishing these patients from healthy carriers or heterozygotes.

However, when dealing with highly polymorphic loci, with numerous normally functioning alleles (e.g. the HLA genes), the distinction between the terms heterozygotes and compound heterozygotes becomes meaningless and serves no purpose.

# Allelic heterogeneity

Different mutations of the same gene can sometimes produce different clinical outcomes; indeed, so different that, from the clinical point of view, there would be little to suspect that the two diseases were due to mutations at the same gene locus. Sickle cell disease, with its vasculo-occlusive painful crises, presents a very different clinical picture from the transfusion dependence of β-thalassaemia, yet both are due to mutations in the β-globin gene at 11p15. Sickle cell disease is unusual in that it always involves exactly the same mutation at codon 6 of the β-globin gene, usually on both the chromosomes of the pair, although sickle/thalassaemia compound heterozygotes may present a very similar clinical picture. However, β-thalassaemia is much more typical of genetic disease demonstrating considerable allelic heterogeneity, with over 100 different muta-

tions capable of producing a very similar clinical picture. Such allelic heterogeneity is the rule rather than the exception with most genetic diseases. The different classes of mutations and their effects on function are listed later, but it is easy to imagine that any mutation that effectively knocks out gene expression will produce the same result, whilst two mutations that modify the protein product in very different ways could result in quite distinct phenotypes which are regarded clinically as different diseases.

From the practical point of view, allelic heterogeneity limits mutation detection by DNA analysis as a simple diagnostic tool. It is now technically easy to detect a known DNA sequence change in a gene, but if the result is negative, one is left uncertain as to whether there is another mutation within that gene or one is looking at the wrong gene locus altogether. There are increasingly powerful methods for detecting DNA sequence mismatches between the known normal sequence and the patient's gene, but this can be laborious for genes with huge coding regions. It may be difficult to interpret any sequence differences that are discovered, because some amino acid changes in the gene product can be inconsequential polymorphisms and not the cause of the patient's disease. The term **polymorphism** is given to a DNA or amino acid sequence variation that occurs in 1 per cent or more of the population. It is purely an arbitrary definition based on frequency and does not imply either harmlessness or clinical significance. It is important to appreciate that interpreting DNA sequence changes, particularly those that just change an amino acid, often needs a substantial knowledge of the structure and function of the gene's protein product. There is a reverse side to this issue of the significance of DNA sequence polymorphisms. Just because a polymorphic change in a gene or protein occurs in healthy people does not mean that it cannot be a risk (or protective) factor with respect to a common disease of multifactorial causation, where genetic and environmental or lifestyle influences interact in a complicated manner. Thus the interpretation of the medical significance of DNA sequence polymorphisms also requires genetic epidemiology.

# Locus heterogeneity

This form of genetic heterogeneity refers to the apparent same clinical condition being due to mutations at entirely different gene loci. This causes difficulties when it comes to genetic counselling and predictive tests based on DNA analysis, whether by mutation detection or gene tracking. There are many diseases that are difficult, if not impossible, to distinguish clinically and yet are due to mutations at one of two or more gene loci. Table 7.3 lists a few important examples. These loci may be on one or more autosomes, and sometimes the X chromosome as well. Retinitis pigmentosa is an example of a disorder that can be inherited in either an X-linked or autosomal fashion.

**Table 7.3** Selected examples of locus heterogeneity.

| Disorder | Gene | Chromosomal location |
|---|---|---|
| Osteogenesis imperfecta type I | Collagen I A1 Collagen I A2 | 17q21.31–q22.05 7q21.3–q22.1 |
| Tuberose sclerosis | ? ? | 9q33–q34 16p13 |
| Epidermolysis bullosa simplex | Keratin 5 Keratin 14 | 12q11–13 17q12–21 |
| Retinitis pigmentosa | RP1 RP2 RP3 RP4 (RP5) RP6 RP7 RP8 RP9 | ? ? ? Rhodopsin ? Peripherin/ RDS protein ? ? | 8p11–q21 Xp11–3 Xp21.1 3q21–q24 Xp21.3–p21.2 6p21.1–ter 7q31–35 7p15.1–p13 |

# Classification of Mendelian disorders by locus

With the prospect of defining all single gene disorders at the DNA sequence level, there has to be a gradual convergence of the existing clinical classifications with the standardized listing of all monogenic disorders in McKusick's catalogue, *Mendelian Inheritance in Man*. This catalogue has been adopted as the main clinical listing for the **Human Genome Project** and is increasingly arranged on a gene locus basis, so it does seem logical for the primary classification of monogenic disorders also to be by gene locus. The role of the clinician will be to compare similar diseases, known to arise as a result of mutations at two different loci, to detect subtle differences in the clinical phenotype. These features will then serve as *clinical* guides to which gene locus is mutant in the patient and where DNA analysis should be focussed. It is likely that biochemical data or histological features will be an even better guide to which molecule is primarily involved in the pathogenesis of the disease and therefore which gene locus is mutant. For example, haemophilia A (factor VIII deficiency) had been distinguishable from haemophilia B (factor IX deficiency) by co-agulation studies long before the two X-linked loci were mapped to Xq27 and Xq28, respectively.

Whilst classification at the locus level will have to be incorporated into disease definitions, it will often be insufficient by itself for clinical purposes. As indicated above, two mutations in the same gene can sometimes give quite different diseases. One consequence of being able to define the mutation at the DNA level in individual patients, is that genotype/phenotype correlations can be studied. How useful these correlations will be in improving prognostic precision and management choice is unclear. Genetics has a habit of being more complicated than we first thought.

It should be noted that different mutations of the same gene locus can not only lead to different clinical manifestations but also different patterns of autosomal inheritance. One mutation may only produce disease in the homozygous state (**autosomal recessive inheritance**) whilst another does so in the heterozygous state (**autosomal dominant inheritance**). It follows that just because two diseases are inherited in a different Mendelian fashion one should not necessarily assume that different gene loci are involved.

# Multiloci mutations

So far we have only considered mutations affecting a single locus, but mutations may involve a few or many loci. Some of the past distinction between Mendelian disorders and structural (as opposed to numerical) chromosomal abnormalities was largely a reflection of the limitations of the methods employed for genetic analysis. With better cytogenetic resolution including fluorescent *in situ* hybridization, or FISH (discussed later), for defining microdeletions, duplications and other rearrangements, plus more extensive DNA sequences and better physical maps linking up neighbouring genes, the 'no man's land' of genome analysis from 50 kilobases (kb) to 5 megabases (mb) is beginning to yield its secrets. The mutation causing Charcot–Marie–Tooth disease (hereditary motor and sensory neuropathy, type 1) is a duplication of some 2 mb at 17p11.2, and there is a growing list of microdeletion syndromes

(Table 7.4). For the most part, disorders due to autosomal, multiloci mutations are transmitted (when the severity of their effect does permit child bearing) as autosomal dominant disorders. A syndrome due to a deletion of more than one neighbouring gene is called a contiguous gene disorder, with the combination of features being a reflection of the number of genes knocked out. Thus there are two main ways of disabling multiple genes to give a multifeature disorder: a contiguous gene deletion or a mutation in a developmental gene that is a transcription factor for several other genes further down the developmental pathway.

**Table 7.4** Selected microdeletion syndromes.

| Disorder | Chromosomal region |
|---|---|
| Angelman syndrome (page 63) | 15q11–13 |
| Di George syndrome (page 94) | 22q11.2 |
| Prader–Willi syndrome (page 63) | 15q11–13 |
| WAGR syndrome (page 69) | 11p13 |

# MUTATIONS AND THEIR EFFECTS

## Some DNA sequences are prone to mutation

The nature of some DNA sequences makes them liable to mutate. As indicated earlier, the cytosine of the dinucleotide CpG is often methylated, and 5-methyl-C naturally tends to deaminate to thymine. This results in a C to T substitution and is a potent cause of point mutations. Not only does it cause a substantial proportion of known mutations causing disease, but it accounts for the fact that the dinucleotide CpG is underrepresented in the genome.

The recent discoveries of the mutational events underlying the fragile X syndrome and myotonic dystrophy have illustrated just how unstable some stretches of trinucleotide repeats

(CGG and CTG, respectively) can be. The genetics of each disorder is described below (pages 61 and 59), but they share a progressive lengthening of the trinucleotide repeat sequence from one generation to the next and at some critical length this DNA becomes highly unstable in somatic cells expanding to enormous size (one can almost think of it as a DNA tumour). Whilst the number of repeats can get smaller, it does seem that there is some mechanism that makes increases more likely.

A third class of mutation-prone DNA sequence is on a larger scale and has already been mentioned. When homologous chromosomes (the paternally and maternally derived copy of a chromosome) pair up during the first division of meiosis, they must align precisely because recombination between chromatids of the pair will occur. If this crossing over takes place when the two chromosomes are misaligned, a chromatid with a deletion and one with a corresponding duplication will be generated. Misalignment seems to be more common when there are similar DNA sequences nearby. It may be a repeat sequence (e.g. Alu sequence) or a region where a duplication has been fixed during evolution (e.g. α-globin loci on chromosome 16,21-hydroxylase/C4 loci on 6).

# Mutations may be confined to a subset of cells

It is worth remembering that the patient we see represents the end result of an almost countless number of cell divisions, during which errors in DNA replication or chromosomal segregation can occur at any time. If a lethal mutation occurs in a cell in relatively differentiated tissue, it is of no significance. The cell dies and that's that. However, a mutation that perturbs the regulation of cell growth can predispose to cancer. When mutations at gene, or chromosomal, level occur early in development they can predispose to congenital disorders, with the end result being a reflection of:

1 How early the error occurred.
2 The extent to which the proliferative advantage of the normal cells over the mutant ones can offset the damage.
3 The degree to which the placental function is involved and therefore the chance of miscarriage.

**Somatic mosaicism** is the term used when an organism (derived from a single zygote) develops with two or more major cell lines of different genotypes. Somatic mosaicism may result in all or some of the germ cells carrying a mutation. When the mosaicism is confined to the gonads so that just some of the germ cells are affected, the term gonadal mosaicism is used.

# The effect of different types of mutation

The effects of different mutations fall into two broad categories: changes in protein structure and changes in the amount of normal protein.

## CHANGES IN THE STRUCTURE OF THE PROTEIN GENE PRODUCT

### Amino acid substitution or missense mutation

This is the simplest of mutations, usually caused by a single nucleotide base change that alters the codon. The impact this has on the function of the protein depends, of course, on how critical is the particular amino acid. The triple helix domain of all collagens has a glycine every third residue because this small amino acid packs neatly into the centre of the helix. Substitution of any larger amino acid tends to disrupt the helix and allow overhydroxylation etc. For this reason, many of the point mutations causing osteogenesis imperfecta are such glycine substitutions. The remarkable effect of the sickle mutation, a valine substitution for glutamic acid at the 6th residue of β-globin, stems from the fact that it enhances a pre-existing tendency of deoxyhaemoglobin molecules to aggregate.

### Loss or addition of one or a few codons

Provided the reading frame for translation of the RNA into polypeptide is preserved, a slightly modified protein can be produced. The most famous codon deletion is the 508 deletion in the CFTR gene; the commonest mutation in cystic fibrosis.

### Exon skipping

This can arise when there is a mutation that alters the recognition of the splice sites by the exon/intron splicing machinery. The messenger RNA (mRNA) and peptide contain an exon deletion, but there is no corresponding deletion in the genomic DNA.

### Unequal crossing over to produce a hybrid protein

This arises when homologous chromosomes misalign at meiosis.

## Truncated or novel peptides at the C terminus

A single base change towards the end of the translated region of a gene can sometimes create a Stop codon, which leads to a slightly truncated protein being produced. Alternatively, the base change may remove the normal Stop codon, converting it to a codon for an amino acid. This results in a novel, additional string of peptides until another Stop codon is reached. A deletion or addition of one or two bases (or any number of bases that is not a multiple of three) generates a shift in the reading frame. If this occurs close to the end of the gene, again a partially functional protein with a truncated or novel C terminus can be produced.

## Deletion within the gene

Provided the reading frame is maintained intact, small to large deletions within the gene can often result in a partially functional protein. The best known example is Becker muscular dystrophy, where some huge in-frame deletions of the dystrophin gene result in relatively minor effects on muscle function.

## CHANGES IN THE AMOUNT OR ABSENCE OF PROTEIN GENE PRODUCT

### Deletion

Obviously deletion of the whole of a gene results in no gene product. The phenotype in such a situation is a guide to what will happen with the many other types of mutation (considered below) that result in a 'knock out' of the gene. Interestingly, there are many situations in autosomal dominant disorders where the complete absence of a gene product from one allele is less troublesome than an altered protein. This phenomenon goes by several different names, such as protein suicide, included/excluded mutants or dominant negative effect, but in essence it is a case of a faulty gene product being more trouble than its worth when it comes to assembling multimeric proteins (Fig. 7.3). It is better to do without, or to use an unconventional but correctly formed protein as a partner. Osteogenesis imperfecta provides an illustration of why heterozygotes for a mutation causing an abnormal α-1 chain of type 1 collagen end up worse off than those heterozygous for an α-1 gene deletion. In the former situation, not half, but three-quarters of the collagen trimers 'include' one or two defective α-1 chains. It is better to build a thinner wall than lay half-baked bricks in three courses out of four.

## RNA that cannot be processed properly

The intron/exon boundaries have highly conserved DNA sequences, and mutations within one of these sequences can prevent the splicing out of an intron, which, of course, does not code for protein. Depending on the exact base change, there may be only abnormally spliced mRNA produced or a combination of abnormal and normal mRNA. In the latter case the end result will be a reduced amount of normal gene product. Another type of mutation which can produce a reduced amount of normal mRNA is a change in the polyadenylation site, so that the mRNA is somewhat unstable. The abnormal expansion of

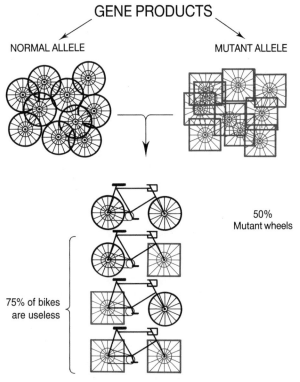

**Figure 7.3** A mechanism in dominant negative mutations. A bicycle with its two wheels can illustrate what can happen in a dimeric protein when one of two genes of the pair produces a mutant polypeptide chain – 75 per cent, not 50 per cent, of the protein molecules are defective.

the CTG repeat in the 3′ untranslated region of the myotonin protein kinase gene in myotonic dystrophy is thought to lead to reduced mRNA by defective RNA processing, at least in the classical young adult onset form.

### Premature Stop codons and frameshift mutations

When a Stop codon is generated by a base change in a codon relatively early in the gene sequence, then the severely truncated protein produced at translation is generally useless and unstable. In practice no recognizable gene product is produced. As indicated earlier, the deletion of one or two bases leads to a shift in the reading frame, generating a novel amino acid sequence from that point onwards. More often than not this frameshift results in a Stop codon within a short distance, so the protein in such mutations is usually severely truncated.

### Impaired or blocked transcription

Mutations in the special sequences upstream needed for the efficient assembly of various transcription factors and RNA polymerase usually result in a reduced level of gene product. The full mutation in fragile X, with marked expansion of the CGG repeat within the 5′ region of the FMR-1 gene, is associated with widespread DNA methylation, which appears to block transcription.

## MENDELIAN INHERITANCE

See Fig. 7.4.

# Autosomal dominant disorders

In medical genetics the term autosomal dominant refers to the situation where a monogenic disorder is manifest clinically in the heterozygous state. In Britain the overall incidence of autosomal dominant disorders is about 7 per 1000 live births; some of the more common conditions being adult polycystic kidney disease (mutation on chromosome 16), monogenic hypercholesterolaemia (chromosome 19), neurofibromatosis (chromosome 17), and Huntington's disease (chromosome 4). As each parent passes on only one chromosome of each pair to the child, any child of a person with an autosomal dominant disorder has a 1 in 2 chance of being affected. On average half will inherit the chromosome carrying the abnormal gene, and half the chromosome carrying the normal gene. Thus given enough offspring the condition can manifest in each generation and in both sexes, with only affected individuals able to pass it on.

Unfortunately in clinical practice the matter is complicated by variation in the expression of the gene and new mutation. Both points are illustrated by neurofibromatosis, which has an incidence of about 1 in 3000. The manifestations in someone carrying the gene vary from just a few characteristic pigmented patches on the skin, so-called *café au lait* spots, to gross disfigurement with a mass of cutaneous and subcutaneous tumours, and mental handicap. In neurofibromatosis, as in many autosomal dominant disorders, a mildly affected person has to be warned that any child inheriting the gene may not be so lucky as they have been. It can also be seen that a person with minimal manifestations may be regarded as normal, and give rise to the view that the condition has 'skipped a generation'. Taking variation in the expression of the gene one stage further, one can argue that in some situations there will be no manifestation of the gene carried by some family members; that is, the gene has less than 100 per cent penetrance. Reduced penetrance as a concept distinct from variable gene expression is not very helpful in practice. The important message is that one cannot give advice until a careful physical examination has been performed.

It is important, of course, to know the usual

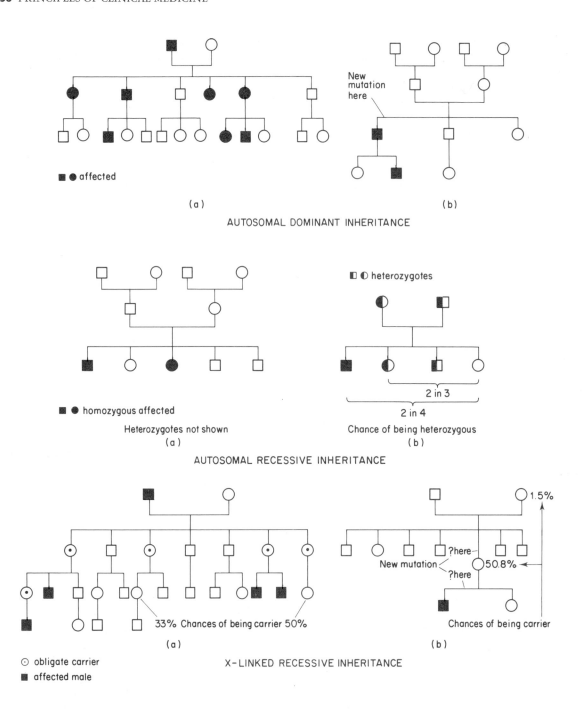

**Figure 7.4** Pedigrees illustrating Mendelian inheritance. **Autosomal dominant inheritance.** (a) On average 50 per cent of the offspring of an affected individual are affected; there is male-to-male transmission. (b) In severe disorders new mutations will be frequently encountered. **Autosomal recessive inheritance.** (a) Affected individuals are usually confined to one sibship, with a 1 in 4 recurrence risk if both parents are healthy. (b) The healthy sibs of an affected individual have a 2 in 3 chance of being a carrier. **X-linked recessive inheritance.** (a) No male-to-male transmission; daughters of an affected male and females in the direct line between two affected males are obligate carriers. For other females the chance of being a carrier is influenced by the number of normal sons. (b) In X-linked lethal disorders overall one-third of affected males and half of carrier females represent new mutations. The probability of this being the case is influenced by the number of normal males in the pedigree.

age of onset of the disease because quite a proportion of autosomal dominant disorders only manifest later in life, often after carriers of the gene have completed their families. Huntington's disease is a degenerative disorder of the brain, particularly of the basal ganglia, with an average age of onset of about 40 years. The discovery of the trinucleotide repeat expansion mutation on chromosome 4 allows presymptomatic detection of those carrying the mutation with all its attendant psychological and management problems.

All dominant disorders have to start at some time as new mutations in the ovum or sperm. The more severe the type of disease, the less likely the patient is to reproduce, and the greater proportion of affected individuals will be the result of a new mutation. In the mild dominant disorders, or those of late onset, the vast majority of patients have inherited it from an affected parent. New mutations and the variable gene expression can combine to create difficult clinical decisions. If a single child in the family has overt neurofibromatosis, the apparently healthy parents will want to know the risk to their further children. If it is decided the child is the result of a new mutation, then the risk of recurrence is very low. However, if an examination reveals convincing minimal signs of neurofibromatosis in one parent, then the couple face a 1 in 2 risk with each pregnancy. This demonstrates the importance of knowing what are the minimal signs of the disorder, and the difficulties that could arise in doubtful cases. Occasionally neither parent shows evidence of the disease but they have two affected children. If this occurs in a disorder expected to exhibit full penetrance, the explanation is likely to be gonadal mosaicism. This has been directly demonstrated by DNA analysis of the sperm in a man who, although healthy himself, had two children with severe osteogenesis imperfecta by different women. A proportion of his sperm showed a type 1 collagen $\alpha$-1 chain mutation.

It is estimated that about half the cases of neurofibromatosis are due to new mutations, and this represents an estimated mutation rate of about $10^{-4}$; that is, 1 in 10 000 germ cells mutate per generation, or 1 in 5000 babies have neurofibromatosis as a result of a new mutation. This is one of the highest mutation rates in humans; estimated mutation rates for dominant (and X-linked conditions) usually lie between $10^{-5}$ and $10^{-6}$.

# Myotonic dystrophy and anticipation

Myotonic dystrophy is a disease that has long fascinated clinicians. It is inherited as an autosomal dominant, but also shows the phenomenon of **anticipation**, in which there is increased severity/earlier age of onset with successive generations. The grandparent may just have cataracts and not be diagnosed until their offspring present with classical myotonia in early adult life (indeed it is sometimes difficult to decide which grandparent is the affected one!). The grandchild on the other hand is often congenitally affected, particularly if the transmitting parent is the mother. Recognized by physicians since 1911 and formally demonstrated by Julia Bell in 1947, who compared sib and parent/child age-of-onset correlations, anticipation has in recent years been largely dismissed as being due to ascertainment bias. Discovery of the expanding CTG repeat as the mutational basis of myotonic dystrophy also provided a molecular genetic explanation for the anticipation. There is a fair correlation between the age of onset and the length of the CTG repeat in the untranslated 3′ end of the DM gene, which even holds true on the rare occasion in which there is a reversal of the usual progression on transmission to give a *reduction* rather than an expansion in the repeat. It should be stressed, however, that unlike fragile X, expansion of the repeat can occur in both male and female transmissions although sperm do not carry the largest expansions explaining the fact that congenitally affected babies nearly always inherit the DM mutation from an affected mother, not father. The other striking feature of myotonic dystrophy is that DNA marker evidence indicates that all families share a particular ancestral chromosome 19 (or rather the DM gene region of it), raising the question of what it is that triggers expansion to very high levels (over 1000 repeats) after many generations of slight expansion (40–60 repeats) above the normal (5–30 repeats).

# Autosomal recessive disorders

In autosomal recessive inheritance the disorder is only manifest clinically when the patient has a double dose of the abnormal gene (i.e. in the homozygous or compound heterozygous state). The patient has no normal allele at the particular locus involved, having inherited one abnormal gene from each parent. Usually both parents are heterozygous. Rarely one or even both parents are themselves affected homozygotes. In the usual situation, where both parents are heterozygous, a child has a 1 in 4 chance of being an affected homozygote, there is a 2 in 4 chance of being a heterozygote like the parents, and a 1 in 4 chance of being normal.

In Britain the overall incidence of autosomal recessive disorders is about 2.5 per 1000 live births, and the commonest is cystic fibrosis. About 1 in 2500 are affected and about 1 in 25 people are heterozygotes, or carriers of the gene. The mutant CFTR gene (on chromosome 7) results in the loss of normal cyclic adenosine monophosphate (cAMP)-mediated apical chloride conductance of a wide variety of epithelial cells. This causes a generalized alteration in mucus, with blocked pancreatic ducts leading to digestive problems, and blockage in the bronchial tree causing recurrent chest infections. A great number of autosomal recessive disorders are caused by an absent or inactive enzyme, preventing a step in a critical metabolic pathway – the so-called 'inborn error of metabolism' first elucidated by Garrod in the early years of this century. The clinical features of many inborn errors of metabolism are the result both of the accumulation of substances before, and a deficiency of substances beyond, the enzyme block.

The heterozygous state can be detected by biochemical tests in many autosomal recessive disorders and this can play an important part in genetic counselling. This fact also raises the question of whether a condition is truly recessive, if the gene produces a detectable effect in the heterozygous state. In practice the heterozygote is generally healthy, and there is such a vast difference between the clinical manifestation in the heterozygous and the abnormal homozygous state that the use of additional categories such as intermediate or codominant disorders is unhelpful. Sickle cell anaemia and β-thalassaemia major (Cooley's anaemia) can be regarded as autosomal recessive disorders even though the heterozygote or sickle cell trait may have some *in vivo* sickling of the red cells with extreme anoxia, and people with β-thalassaemia trait may be slightly anaemic.

The incidence at birth of a recessive disorder in a population depends primarily on the incidence of the heterozygous state. Obviously early death will modify the frequency with which it is encountered in an older population, and a changing rate of cousin marriage can also have an effect. The extent to which new mutations maintain the frequency of heterozygotes for different recessive disorders is difficult to estimate, but natural selection has played the predominant role in sickle cell disease and the thalassaemias. The sickle cell trait affords some protection against malaria, and analysis of DNA around the sickle gene locus indicates that about 80 per cent of West Africans with the sickle cell trait inherited the gene from a common ancestor.

First cousins share one-eighth of their genes in common and therefore they have a slightly increased chance of having children with recessive disorders compared with unrelated parents in the same population. Direct comparison between populations is not valid because a high cousin marriage rate over many generations tends to reduce the frequency of harmful recessive genes by natural selection.

# X-linked recessive disorders

X-linked recessive inheritance produces a characteristic family pedigree, where males are affected and the gene is passed on by unaffected females. Using simple diagrams of the X and Y chromosome it is easy to satisfy oneself that an abnormal gene carried on one of the X chromosomes in a female will be passed on to half her daughters, who would be heterozygous like herself, and to half her sons who would manifest the disease because they have no compensating X. An affected male would produce only heterozygous daughters, but cannot pass the gene on to his sons, who only receive his Y chromosome. In a population where the X-linked red-cell enzyme defect glucose-6-phosphate dehydrogenase (G6PD) deficiency is common, an affected man may have an affected son, but only because his wife is also a heterozygote. In such a mating each girl has a 50 per cent chance of being an affected homozygote.

In some X-linked disorders a proportion of female heterozygotes are mildly affected, and this is the case with G6PD deficiency. Cytochemical staining of the red cells shows that about half are G6PD-deficient and half are normal. The explanation (the Lyon hypothesis) lies in the fact that only one of the X chromosome pair is active in any one cell. The random inactivation of one or other X chromosome occurs in each cell early in embryonic development, and thereafter the descendants of a particular cell have the same inactive X. By chance, some women heterozygous for G6PD deficiency have the normal X chromosome inactivated in 80–90 per cent of their cells, and can therefore develop haemolysis, like the affected hemizygous males, when exposed to certain drugs such as sulphonamides and antimalarials.

In Britain the incidence of X-linked disorders is about 1.4 per 1000 male live births. Two important examples are Duchenne muscular dystrophy (1 in 4000 males) and the fragile X syndrome (1 in 2000). Duchenne muscular dystrophy (DMD) is due to mutations in the dystrophin gene that result in no protein product in the muscle (when there is a reduced amount or truncated dystrophin present, the patient suffers the milder Becker muscular dystrophy). The dystrophin gene has the distinction of being the largest gene yet described in the human. It has 79 exons distributed over about 2400 kb within the p21 region of the X chromosome. About 60 per cent of boys with DMD have intragenic deletions, which are readily detected by DNA analysis. The presence of the normal X chromosome makes detection of deletions in female carriers more difficult, although new molecular genetic methods, such as FISH outlined later, look very promising. As a group, carriers have a higher plasma creatine kinase (CK) level. Creatine kinase measurement, pedigree analysis taking into account the presence of healthy males, and mutation detection and gene tracking by DNA analysis are used in various combinations to determine the carrier status of female relatives seeking help. The overlap in the distribution of CK values between DMD carriers and normal women is a reflection of the random X-inactivation process described above, with some carriers being 'favourably' inactivated. This is a general problem with biochemical carrier testing in X-linked disorders and serves to emphasize how important DNA analysis is in clinical genetics.

The term X-linked dominant has been used for the very few rare conditions where the heterozygous female is regularly affected. However, the hemizygous male is always more severely affected, and in some instances, such as incontinentia pigmenti affected males rarely survive gestation to be born, so only female patients are encountered in clinical practice.

## FRAGILE X SYNDROME

The fragile X syndrome, the commonest inherited form of mental retardation, gets its name from the unstainable gap or 'fragile site' seen at Xq27.3 in 5–50 per cent of cells, when lymphocytes are cultured in folic acid-deficient or other special medium (Fig. 7.5). It is still not clear how the mutational events cause the fragile site. However, discovery of the role of expansion of the polymorphic CGG repeat at the 5′ end of the FMR1 gene in causing the mental retardation has explained both the unusual inheritance of this condition and revolutionized genetic services for affected families. A striking feature of many pedigrees is that affected cousins have inherited the condition from the maternal grandfather who is fragile-site-negative and clinically normal. It is now known that these 'normal transmitting males' carry a premutation which corresponds to a small expansion of the CGG repeat from the normal range of 5–?50 to ?50–200 repeats. The daughters of normal transmitting males are also phenotypically normal because the premutation only progresses

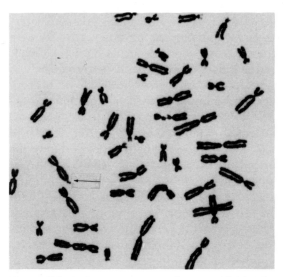

**Figure 7.5** A chromosome metaphase spread (simple unbanded stain) showing the appearance of the fragile site (arrowed) of Xq27.3 associated with the fragile X mental retardation syndrome.

with mental retardation is characterized by a massive expansion of the CGG repeat sequence. It seems that when a critical repeat size is reached the DNA becomes somatically unstable, so that different cells have different sized CGG repeat expansions and give a smear rather than a discrete band on DNA analysis. About 30–50 per cent of sisters of affected males are clinically affected (showing the full mutation on one X), although on average the intellectual deficit is less than in males.

DNA analysis now allows much more reliable prenatal diagnosis for those who want it and simple carrier testing for female relatives of affected individuals. To date, testing earlier generations in affected families has not revealed the progression from normal to premutation. Where a female relative has a premutation of more than 90 repeats, then progression to the full mutation on transmission of that X chromosome seems inevitable. Preliminary studies on the general population indicate that most X chromosomes have about 30 CGG repeats and about 1 in 750 have a premutation that is unstable on transmission.

to the full mutation when transmitted by a female, not a male. (This is in contrast to the situation in myotonic dystrophy.) As illustrated in Fig. 7.6, the full mutation which correlates

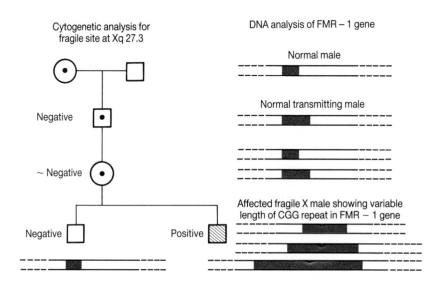

**Figure 7.6** A schematic representation of the progression from premutation to the full mutation in a fragile X pedigree. Full expansion of the CGG repeat (blocked in segment) results in intellectual impairment and the appearance of fragile sites on appropriate cytogenetic examination.

# Non-classical inheritance

We have already noted that myotonic dystrophy and the fragile X syndrome do not exactly follow the classical patterns of Mendelian inheritance, in that the mutation, and as a consequence the severity of the disease, progresses with successive generations. We cannot yet explain why only affected mothers, not fathers, produce a baby with congenital myotonic dystrophy, or why progression from premutation to full mutation in fragile X only occurs in females, but parent-of-origin effects are turning out to be an important component of the variation in gene expression seen in many diseases.

## Genomic imprinting

The term genomic imprinting refers to different expression of a normal gene, depending on the sex of the parent who transmits it. When this is observed, it implies that the gene carries a 'tag', or imprint, that was placed during spermatogenesis or oogenesis and can modulate gene expression in the developing embryo. The imprint may act to silence the allele from one parent, so that normal development is dependent solely on the function of the allele from the other parent. That this silencing is not a DNA mutation, is shown by the fact that the *same* gene transmitted in a later generation by someone of the opposite sex is no longer silenced; the imprint has been erased at some time between generations. As with many normal phenomena, imprinting is most clearly revealed when the system goes wrong. There are three informative situations: large pedigrees, microdeletions and uniparental disomy.

Dominant transmission of a mutation involving an imprinted gene through several generations and by people of different sex will reveal a parent-of-origin effect. The mutation will be inconsequential when transmitted by the parent who is silencing the gene, i.e. the child is unaffected.

However, when the same mutant gene is transmitted by a person of the other sex and becomes the 'active' allele, the child will be affected, because the allele from the other parent is normally silenced. Syndromes due to *de novo* **microdeletions** can also be informative, because the parental origin of the deleted chromosome can be determined by polymorphic DNA markers. If an imprinted locus is deleted, the deletion will be inconsequential (with respect to that locus) if it occurs on one parental chromosome, but cause the disorder if it involves the other parental chromosome. As a consequence, in clinical practice the syndrome will always be associated with microdeletions of one parental type. The third situation involves a recently recognized chromosomal aberration, uniparental disomy. If indeed a gene is silenced when transmitted by one parent, then if *both* chromosomes come from the parent of that sex, there will be no active alleles and the child should be affected. Uniparental disomy, namely, both chromosomes of a normal looking pair coming from the same parent, can arise following the loss of one chromosome from a trisomic conceptus.

The one condition that shows all the above types of evidence for genomic imprinting is the Angelman syndrome (AS). This is a disorder associated with mental retardation, absent speech, jerky ataxic movements, fits, a low laughter threshold and subtle but characteristic facial features. Large pedigrees exist where a mutation in the AS locus has been transmitted by males to their daughters with no ill effect, but when these daughters have children, 50 per cent suffer AS. Microdeletions within the q11–13 region of chromosome 15 are found in about 75 per cent of sporadic cases of AS and without exception, all have arisen in the *maternal* 15. Finally, about 3 per cent of cases have shown uniparental *paternal* disomy (with no chromosome 15 from the mother but two from the father), confirming that the AS locus is silenced by an imprint during spermatogenesis. It happens that genomic imprinting also occurs in the Prader–Willi syndrome (hypotonia, mental retardation, short stature, hypogenitalism, obesity and hyperphagia). At the Prader–Willi locus (very close to, but distinct from AS at 15q12) it is the maternally transmitted allele that is silenced, in contrast to AS. The Beckwith–Weidemann locus (11p15.5) where it seems that it is the paternally transmitted allele that is silenced, provides another example. There is some evidence that a parent-of-origin effect (possibly genomic imprinting) modifies the inheritance of atopic asthma.

# Mitochondrial gene defects

Mitochondria contain their own genetic material; between two and ten copies of a double-stranded, circular DNA molecule that is 16 569 base pairs in length. The mitochondrial chromosome encodes 13 subunits of the mitochondrial respiratory chain and oxidative phosphorylation system, as well as the mitochondria's own translational machinery, there being two ribosomal RNA and 22 transfer RNA (tRNA) genes. An increasing number of diseases (typically variable multiorgan energy failure over time) are being recognized as due to mitochondrial mutations.

A mature ovum has about 2000 mitochondria, but during the passage from one generation to the next the number of mitochondria in the germ cell lineage is thought to go through a 'bottleneck' of less than 10

mitochondria. Whilst both eggs and sperm have mitochondria, none is transferred with the sperm pronucleus at fertilization, so mitochondrial inheritance is exclusively maternal. What is true of normal mitochondria is true of mutant mitochondria, and exclusive maternal transmission characterizes those diseases due to mutation in the mitochondrial chromosome. The mitochondria accumulate mutations at a relatively fast rate and, due to the 'bottleneck' effect, some offspring of a woman carrying one or a few mutant mitochondria can end up with the majority, even all, of their mitochondria of the mutant variety. A mutation or polymorphism that is present in all copies of the mitochondrial chromosome is said to be homoplasmic, whilst the term heteroplasmy refers to a mixture of mutant and normal mitochondrial chromosomes. The proportion of mutant mitochondria in any particular tissue can account for much of the variable expression seen within and between families, but not all. The point mutation at base-pair position 3243 in the tRNA leucine gene, present in the family with diabetes mellitus and deafness depicted in Fig. 7.7, is more typically found in patients with myopathy, encephalopathy, lactic acidosis and stroke-like episodes (MELAS). Clearly, additional genetic variation in the nuclear or mitochondrial genome, plus environmental factors over time, must be influencing which tissues are most affected and therefore with

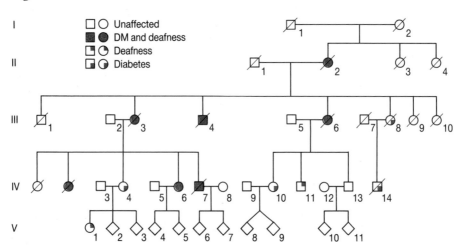

**Figure 7.7** Diabetes mellitus (DM) and deafness due to a mutation in the mitochondrial genome that is only transmitted through the female line but affects both sexes. Circle = female. Square = male. Oblique line = deceased. Completely blue solid symbols = diabetes mellitus and deafness. Upper right quarter blue = deafness. Lower right quarter blue = diabetes mellitus.

what symptoms the patient first presents.

Perhaps the best known mitochondrially inherited disorder is Leber's hereditary optic neuropathy (LHON), which gives rise to acute or subacute blindness affecting males more commonly than females. There is some evidence that interaction with a regular X-linked poly-morphic gene is necessary. Like nuclear-encoded genetic disease, mitochondrially inherited disorders also show genetic heterogeneity. There are now several high-risk, intermediate and low-risk 'LHON' mutations affecting respiratory complexes I, II and IV. Some patients have combinations of 'LHON' mutations.

# MULTIFACTORIAL INHERITANCE

Common disorders often show a familial tendency and if we are to understand their pathogenesis fully and devise preventive measures it will be helpful to know which genes predispose or protect the individual.

The correlation between the height of parents and their children's eventual height is clear for all to see. The inheritance of quantitative characters, like height, has been the subject of careful study for over a century, and it can be shown that the correlation between various relatives can be explained on the basis of many genes each of small effect segregating in a normal Mendelian fashion (i.e. obeying the same rules described so far in this chapter).

It has been thought that a similar mechanism of polygenic inheritance might produce an underlying 'distribution of susceptibility' with those individuals beyond a particular threshold being affected by a common malformation or later onset disorder. Whilst this may indeed be the basis for some disorders, it is equally possible that the inherited tendency observed can be accounted for by just one or a few susceptibility genes of major effect with other genetic modifiers being only minor influences. Those cases or families where this is so are likely to have their genetic susceptibility elucidated first, and this is beginning to happen. For example, a proportion of patients with congenital heart defects only are now known to have submicroscopic deletions at 22q11.2, the region that is deleted in those with the Di George and velo-cardio-facial syndromes.

Overall, the genetic contribution to the cause of common congenital malformations like spina bifida, cleft lip ± palate or congenital heart disease appears to be on the basis of several genes each having a positive or negative effect on the susceptibility of the fetus to the malformation.

First-degree relatives (brothers and sisters or children) of an affected person have a considerable risk of being affected, but this increased risk diminishes rapidly when one moves to second-degree relatives (nephews, nieces and grandchildren) and is almost back to the general population incidence for third-degree relatives (cousins). This general point about multifactorial inheritance is illustrated by cleft lip ± palate which has an incidence of about 1 per 1000 live births in Britain. In first-degree relatives of an affected case the incidence is about 40 per 1000, but falls to 7 per 1000 for second-degree relatives and 2–3 per 1000 for third-degree relatives. When a couple has had two affected children, the risk to a further child is higher, about 14 per cent. In reality, of course, the risk has been the same for each pregnancy; what has increased is our information about how susceptible the children of this couple are to the malformation. It must be emphasized that largely unknown environmental factors also play an important part in the cause of these common malformations, and 'preventative measures' around the time of conception and in early pregnancy might be possible in the future. There is evidence that maternal folic acid supplementation is associated with a reduction in the recurrence risk for spina bifida and anencephaly.

Many common disorders of adult life, such as diabetes mellitus, arterial hypertension, epilepsy or schizophrenia, have a significant genetic component with close relatives having an increased risk of developing the disease. However, it is becoming clear that there are probably several causes of these conditions, some largely environmental, some genetic, whilst others are multifactorial, involving both the action of several genes and environmental factors.

Type 1 or insulin-dependent diabetes mellitus appears to be usually the result of virus-triggered autoimmune destruction of the β-islet cells in genetically susceptible individuals. The main susceptibility gene(s) are located on chromosome 6 within or close to the HLA gene complex. Much of this genetic susceptibility is dependent on the absence of aspartic acid at residue 57 of the DQβ chain. Overall a sibling of an index case has a risk of about 5–6 per cent of developing diabetes mellitus by the age of 16 years. However, if the sibling has inherited the same two number 6 chromosomes as the index case (that is, they are HLA identical), the risk is much higher, perhaps 30 per cent by the age of 30; and it is correspondingly very low if the sibling has no chromosome 6 in common with the index case. It should be stressed that the HLA region gene(s) only account for about half the inherited susceptibility and studies in a good mouse model suggest several other susceptibility loci.

Type 2 or maturity-onset diabetes shows close to 100 per cent concordance in monozygotic twins (compared with just under 60 per cent concordance in monozygotic twins where one has type 1 diabetes), indicating almost complete genetic determination. Obesity clearly contributes in some way; and if the index case with type 2 diabetes mellitus is obese, the risk to a non-obese sibling is about 5 per cent whilst with a non-obese index case the risk to an obese sibling is about 25 per cent.

There is slow progress in defining susceptibility genes. It is now clear that mutations in the mitochondrial genome can cause familial adult-onset diabetes mellitus (± deafness) which is associated with relative β-cell failure. Maturity-onset diabetes of the young (MODY) has been shown to be due to mutations in the glucokinase gene (7p) in some families.

## CHROMOSOME ABNORMALITIES

Chromosome abnormalities fall into two broad categories: disorders of chromosome number, and rearrangements or changes in chromosome structure. The overall incidence in live births is about 5–6 per 1000, and it is estimated that about 50 per cent of early spontaneous abortions are chromosomally abnormal, and of 1000 recognized pregnancies there are about 75 fetal or neonatal deaths due to chromosome abnormalities, the great majority arising as new mutations in the ovum, sperm or early zygote.

## Disorders of chromosome number

During meiosis, the reduction division that leads to the ovum and sperm having a single, haploid, set of chromosomes, homologous chromosomes pair up before moving apart to the opposite poles of the dividing cell. Failure of the pair to associate in the first place, or failure to dissociate, can lead to an ovum or sperm with an extra chromosome, or one missing. The term non-dysjunction, which assumes the latter mechanism, is often used for this error of chromosome segregation. The causes of non-dysjunction are largely unknown, but the chance of it having occurred in the ovum increases with age. The resulting fetus will either have three copies of a particular chromosome (trisomy) or only one (monosomy). In practice the trisomies are the most important, monosomies in general being non-viable.

In some individuals the non-dysjunction occurs after zygote formation, and in this case there are two cell lines each with a different chromosome complement. Such cases are called mosaics. Overall, mosaics tend to manifest fewer abnormalities of development than the full tri-somy, although this is not necessarily so and prediction of the clinical outcome when mosaicism is found on a prenatal test is not possible.

As mentioned earlier, a trisomic conceptus may lose one of the three chromosomes in the cell line that forms the baby, resulting in uniparental disomy in some instances.

## ANOMALIES OF SEX CHROMOSOME NUMBER

Trisomies involving the X or Y chromosome are relatively common and lead to surprisingly minor physical abnormalities considering the size of the X chromosome and the many genes it carries. The explanation resides in the phenomenon of X chromosome inactivation described earlier. Only one X chromosome remains active in any one cell beyond an early stage of development, and the inactive X chromosome becomes the X chromatin body (formerly known as the Barr body) which is visible close to the nuclear membrane in a proportion of cell nuclei in females. XXX females have two X-chromatin bodies in their cell nuclei, and the much rarer XXXX females have three X-chromatin bodies.

About 1 in 700 newborn males has the chromosome complement 47XXY, is X-chromatin positive, and has the clinical picture of Klinefelter's syndrome. Twenty per cent of Klinefelters are mosaics (e.g. 47XXY/46XY etc.). Those affected are outwardly nearly normal males, but the testes are always small after puberty with complete, or almost complete, azoospermia. In 30 per cent there is enlargement of the breasts, termed gynaecomastia, and concern about this, or infertility, are common ways for these patients to present. About 50 per cent have delayed language development, and although the IQ is below 90 in 30 per cent, only a few have an IQ below 80.

About 1 in 1000 newborn females has the chromosome complement 47XXX. Although disturbances of menstruation and fertility are common, many are essentially normal, fertile females. About 50 per cent have delayed language development and the IQ is below 70 in 15 per cent. Theoretically a proportion of their ova would carry two X chromosomes, leading to XXX or XXY offspring. This event has been observed, but there is probably selection against the abnormal ova.

With the relatively high incidence of 47XXY and 47XXX newborns, one would expect the complementary product of the non-dysjunction, the 45X individual, to be common. It probably is at the time of conception, but about 98 per cent are lost as early abortions and only about 1 in 10000 female births has the 45X chromosome complement with the associated clinical picture of Turner's syndrome. Affected females are short and fail to menstruate, their ovaries being replaced by streaks of connective tissue. There are often associated physical abnormalities, such as neck webbing, renal malformations, deafness and coarctation of the aorta, but intelligence is usually normal. Twenty per cent with Turner's syndrome have an isochromosome X, where a maldivision around the centromere has led to two long arms and no short arm.

The XYY complement is found in about 1 in 700 newborn males. Usually tall (at least 180 cm) and fertile, the great majority remain undiagnosed leading normal lives. There is language development delay in 30 per cent and the IQ is below 90 in 30 per cent with few below IQ 80. Some with mental retardation have antisocial behaviour leading to an overrepresentation in institutions for dangerous mentally ill subjects.

## DOWN'S SYNDROME DUE TO PRIMARY TRISOMY 21

Down's syndrome, always due to an extra chromosome 21, is the commonest viable autosomal trisomy, presumably because of the small size of the chromosome involved. Overall about 96 per cent are due to a primary non-dysjunction, and over 90 per cent involve errors in the formation of the ovum rather than the sperm. In the other 4 per cent the extra chromosome 21 is attached to another chromosome and will be discussed in the next section. The incidence of Down's syndrome increases from about 1 in 1200 in mothers under 30 years to about 1 in 100 at the age of 40 years, and at present accounts for about a third of all cases of severe mental handicap at school age.

# Chromosomal translocations and other structural abnormalities

With the change from simple staining (Fig. 7.5) to banding of chromosomes (Fig. 7.1) it became possible to identify individual chromosomes and parts of chromosomes, and to describe regions and bands (Fig. 7.8). This allowed more accurate description of translocations and structural changes like small deletions. The condensed chromosomes in Fig. 7.5 show the two chromatids and centromeres where they are joined. These are less obvious in the longer chromosomes analysed earlier in cell division (Fig. 7.1). It is now possible to hybridize fluorescently labelled DNA probes directly to the kind of metaphase spreads shown in Figs 7.1 and 7.5 and see where they 'light up'. This technique goes by the acronym FISH, fluorescent *in situ* (suppression) hybridization and can be used two ways. By using a mixture of many probes specific for a particular chromosome, the whole of both chromosomes of the pair can be 'painted' with a specific fluorochrome. Other chromosomes can be painted with fluorochromes giving different colours. Chromosome painting is very helpful for revealing the chromosomal origin of fragments attached to other chromosomes or lying free. It also helps to resolve the nature of complex translocations, important in both general clinical genetics as well as cancer cytogenetics. An alternative approach is use of a gene- or marker-specific probe to determine its rough location on the chromosome and its relationship to other sequences. Not only is this a very powerful way to map newly cloned cDNAs, but it can be used in clinical practice to look for the deletion or relocation of known genes, or parts of large genes.

An internationally agreed shorthand for describing a karyotype is as follows: 'p' indicates the short arm, 'q' the long arm, and 't' a translocation. The total chromosome count is written first followed by the sex chromosome complement. A gain or loss of a whole chromosome is indicated by '+' or '−' before the number of the chromosome involved; for exam-

ple, 47XX + 21 = female Down's. A balanced reciprocal translocation between 1 and 3 would be written 46XXt(1; 3)(q32; q25), the position of the break points being described by arm, region and band for 1 and 3, respectively.

A **reciprocal translocation** occurs when two different chromosomes break simultaneously and a portion of one joins up with a portion of the other, and vice versa. Such a person has 46 chromosomes but part of two chromosomes, say

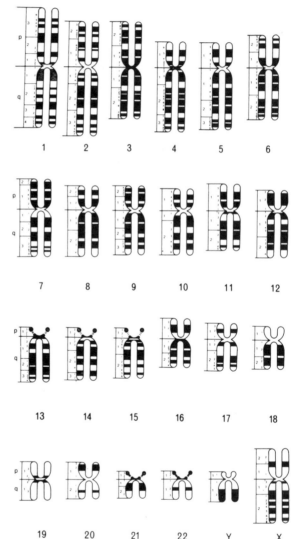

**Figure 7.8** Ideogram of the human chromosomes showing the banding pattern that allows each one to be identified. Chromosomes are analysed during division and each chromosome is shown divided into two daughter chromatids but attached at the centromere. Chromosomes 13, 14, 15, 21 and 22 are termed acrocentric, with only ribosomal genes encoded on the short arms.

a number 1 and a number 3, have been re-arranged. There is no loss of genetic material and the carrier of this balanced reciprocal translocation is healthy. However, trouble can occur at meiosis, for normally just one of each homologous pair is passed on by the ovum or sperm. If the normal chromosome 1 and the normal chromosome 3 are passed on, a child with a normal chromosome complement will result. If the chromosome 1 carrying a bit of 3 and the chromosome 3 carrying a bit of 1 are passed on, a healthy child with a balanced translocation, like the parent, will result. However, if either of the other two combinations are passed on the child will have an unbalanced translocation and development can be severely disturbed. Risks vary with the particular translocation involved. A male or female carrier of a balanced reciprocal translocation ascertained because of an abnormal child has about a 20 per cent chance of a subsequent child having an unbalanced translocation. The risk is about 5 per cent if the carrier was picked up in some other way.

## TRANSLOCATION DOWN'S SYNDROME

We have seen that primary non-dysjunction is the main cause of Down's syndrome and increases with maternal age. However, in about 8–10 per cent of the subjects with Down's syndrome born to mothers under 30 years, the extra 21 chromosome is attached by its short arm to the short arm of another acrocentric chromosome (13–15 or 21–22), usually chromosome 14. This type of fusion of two acrocentric chromosomes is termed a **Robertsonian translocation**. Thus the Down's syndrome child has 46 chromosomes, but one in fact is a composite chromosome $14^{21}$.

In about a third of cases one or other parent carries the $14^{21}$ Robertsonian translocation. However, they have only 45 chromosomes, including a normal 14, a normal 21 and the composite $14^{21}$; and since they have the right amount of chromosome material they are healthy. The short arm material can be lost without ill effect. Again the problems arise at meiosis, when the 14, the 21 and the $14^{21}$ chromosomes have to associate together and then segregate. Normal ova or sperm can be formed leading to normal offspring. The ova or sperm may carry the composite $14^{21}$ without the other 21 or 14, and produce healthy offspring carrying the translocation. Finally, both the composite $14^{21}$ and the other 21 may pass into the ovum or sperm and a child with Down's syndrome will result. There is selection against the unbalanced gametes and a woman carrying a $14^{21}$ translocation has a risk of about 1 in 8 of producing a child with Down's syndrome, whilst for a man the risk is about 1 in 50.

# *Microdeletion syndromes*

An increasing number of disorders, usually sporadic but not always, are being shown to be due to microdeletions. Table 7.4 gives some selected examples from the autosomes, where the characteristic combination of features had been recognized as a clinically recognizable syndrome before the microdeletions underlying the majority of cases was defined. In some there is direct proof of the different features being due to deletion of distinct neighbouring genes; in the combination of Wilms' tumour, aniridia, genitourinary abnormalities and mental retardation (WAGR) the Wilms' tumour (WT1) gene and the aniridia (AN1) gene are quite separate. These deletions are often on the limit of resolution using traditional cytogenetics, and although they were first detected by this method, DNA hybridization techniques using CA repeat polymorphisms or FISH are needed for reliable detection.

# *T*HE USE OF DNA ANALYSIS IN CLINICAL PRACTICE

## *Mutation detection and the polymerase chain reaction*

Mutation detection will eventually become the mainstay of the diagnosis of all Mendelian disorders, whichever clinical specialist is involved, and also contribute significantly to the diagnostic workup of most cancers and many other multifactorial diseases. If the past is anything to go by, it will take some time before clinicians appreciate that diagnostic classification by mutation, whilst not the whole story, will be the best starting point from which to consider prognosis, patient treatment and care, and counselling to the family. The next few years will see the development of large-scale, automated mutation detection methods. Clinical acumen will,

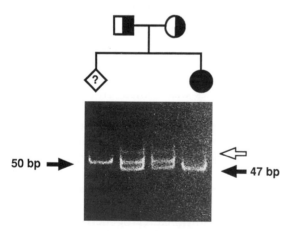

**Figure 7.9** Pedigree showing a female with cystic fibrosis, her carrier parents, and a fetus undergoing prenatal diagnosis. Below each individual in the pedigree is the DNA track showing the normal 50 base pair DNA fragment and/or the 47 base pair fragment, due to deletion of codon 508. The open arrow shows a faint band in the heterozygotes due to a pairing between the 50 base pair and 47 base pair DNA strands (heteroduplex) which travels more slowly in the polyacrylamide gel. The fragments are generated by the polymerase chain reaction (PCR) using primers that flank codon 508 and are just stained with ethidium bromide.

in part, be judged by the ability to predict at which gene locus the mutation will be found. This revolution in the diagnosis of genetic disease stems from the development of the polymerase chain reaction (PCR). This is an *in vitro* technique for replicating a known target section of DNA from the patient's total DNA, thereby simplifying analysis.

The polymerase chain reaction allows the clinical molecular geneticists to generate millions of copies of the target DNA sequence of interest in a matter of hours (page 33). The quantity of PCR product can be so great that it can be visualized directly after simple staining with ethidium bromide, and so mutation detection becomes a matter of detection of PCR products that differ in size, or presence, depending on the existence or not of a specific mutation in the initial DNA. The simplest system is illustrated (Fig. 7.9) by detection of the three nucleotide deletion at codon 508 of the CFTR gene; the commonest mutation in cystic fibrosis. Primers either side of codon 508 generate a 50 bp PCR product from a normal gene, but a 47 bp product from a mutant gene. Other mutation detection strategies have one of the primers hybridizing to the precise site of the mutation. If the mutant sequence is present, PCR amplification takes place and a product will be detected, but not if the sequence is normal. The result is confirmed by a second test using a different primer set that works with the normal sequence but not the mutant one. These and some other systems detect *known* mutations. Searching for unknown single nucleotide mutations in the exons and exon/intron boundaries of specific genes requires other approaches that can indicate the existence of some sequence difference from normal. The precise nature of the change can then be established by DNA sequencing.

Whilst rapid technical progress in mutation detection can be expected, there are still a large number of situations where families wish to have genetic predictions made even though mutation detection has not proved possible. Much can be offered if the gene locus involved, or the chromosomal region, is known.

# Gene tracking

Fortunately for the families with inherited disorders where the gene involved or exact mutation is unknown, there is an alternative approach called gene tracking. Rather than define the DNA defect within the gene, one tracks the inheritance of the particular region of chromosomal DNA that includes the gene locus. β-Thalassaemia always involves the β-globin gene locus, which is situated on the short arm of chromosome 11. A homozygous affected child has inherited two number 11 chromosomes from his parents (each carrying some form of β-thalassaemia mutation); so if these two chromosomes can be distinguished from the parents' other two number 11 chromosomes, then transmission of the β-thalassaemia genes can be predicted in a future fetus. What are required are common genetic markers closely linked to the disease gene locus. Naturally occurring variations in DNA sequence are exploited as DNA markers for chromosomal bands or specific gene loci.

# Restriction fragment length polymorphism

Only a very small percentage of total genomic DNA is actually coding sequence for proteins. The non-coding regions that flank genes, the intergenic DNA and to some extent the intervening sequences, are less conserved during evolution and point mutations are tolerated and become established in populations. About 1 in 200 nucleotide bases differ between the chromosome pair. A number of these DNA sequence polymorphisms involve the recognition sequence of four or six bases of a particular restriction enzyme, and this results, on digestion, in different size restriction fragments from each of the homologous chromosome pairs. Restriction enzymes are naturally occurring enzymes from bacteria that cut DNA at only very specific sites. Thus a restriction fragment length polymorphism (RFLP) is a relatively common change in

DNA sequence that either destroys or creates a restriction enzyme recognition site, or alters the distance between two sites. In anyone who is heterozygous for an RFLP one restriction band pattern corresponds to the other chromosome of the pair. This allows one to track the transmission of a single chromosome region through a family, and to see if a particular monogenic disease coinherits with the polymorphic site; in other words, perform classical linkage studies. Once linkage is proven or if a gene-specific probe is used, genetic prediction (prenatal diagnosis or carrier detection) becomes possible in many families (Fig. 7.10).

In recent years, gene tracking has been enhanced by the detection of an abundant class of

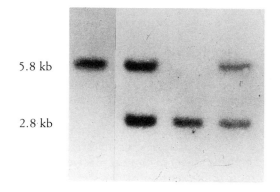

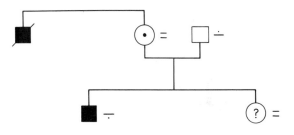

**Figure 7.10** Autoradiograph of DNA tracks from four family members digested with restriction enzyme Bgl II, and hybridized with probe DX13 that is closely linked to haemophilia A. The restriction fragment length polymorphism (RFLP) is represented by the polymorphic bands 5.8 kb and 2.8 kb. It will be seen that the 5.8 kb appears to be coinheriting with the haemophilia mutation and the sister has inherited this band from her mother and the 2.8 kb band from her father. Barring an error due to recombination, she is therefore a carrier.

DNA sequence polymorphisms, dinucleotide (CA) or tetranucleotide repeats, that can be used as markers. The variable number of these repeat sequences results in the two chromosomes of the pair usually having a different repeat sequence length, which is reflected in the size of the PCR product generated from each chromosome. To distinguish the two chromosomes in key family members in this way is one of the requirements for gene tracking, and the new markers have gone some way to overcoming this limitation in the application of gene tracking. Another limitation is the need to obtain blood or other samples for DNA extraction from other family members. In the family analysis depicted in Fig.

7.10, lack of DNA from either the father or affected brother would prevent a carrier prediction being made. A third limitation of gene tracking is the difficulty that arises when the stated father turns out not to be the biological father. Finally, even when using a polymorphism within the disease gene itself as a marker, there is the small chance that a recombination between the marker and the mutation will result in a wrong prediction. Despite these limitations when compared to mutation detection gene tracking has the huge advantage of being independent of the particular type of mutation in that family. All that is required is to know which gene locus is involved.

# MOLECULAR GENETICS OF MULTIFACTORIAL DISEASES

DNA analysis is already established as a clinical service in relation to genetic counselling for Mendelian disorders, providing much needed carrier detection, first trimester prenatal diagnosis and presymptomatic diagnosis. With perhaps the exception of cancers and infectious diseases, molecular genetic investigation is not yet a routine aspect of clinical practice where the common multifactorial diseases are concerned. A huge amount of biologically significant variation in important genes has been discovered, but the role of this variation in health and disease is yet to be determined. A combination of case control and longitudinal studies will be needed before the relevant information is available. It is essential to remember that from an evolutionary point of view, it is genotypes conferring resistance to disease or environmental stresses that are likely to be overrepresented in subsequent generations, despite medicine's legitimate focus on disease susceptibility. It is also important to remember that environmental selective pressures can change much more rapidly than the genetic makeup of the population in response; variation found in genes today may be the result of selective pressures long since past.

It has been known for many years that 5–10 per cent of Europeans are 'poor metabolizers' of debrisoquine and many other drugs because of a recessively inherited defect in one of the

cytochrome P450 enzymes (now known to be gene CYP2D6). It is becoming clear that these enzymes have endogenous substrates, suggesting roles beyond detoxification of noxious substances, and recently it has been shown that mutations in the CYP2D6 gene are unduly common in Parkinson's disease. However, more studies are needed before this information can be sensibly incorporated into the prognosis and treatment plans of individual patients. Much of our understanding of the genetic influences in the common diseases is in a similar or even more rudimentary state, despite some success in defining the molecular pathology in a small subset of families whose disorder falls within the broad disease category, for example, low density lipoprotein (LDL) receptor mutations in familial hypercholesterolaemia as part of 'coronary artery disease'.

There are two approaches to defining the susceptibility genes; either by asking with genetic linkage studies 'Which bit of DNA do affected sibling pairs share in common more often than expected by chance?', or by defining the genes involved in the rarer Mendelian examples of the disorder and then searching for mutations in these 'candidate' genes in the common form of the disease. The latter approach has been very successful in elucidating the role of somatic mutations in some common cancers, notably colorectal cancers, which evolve from small benign adenomas to larger malignant carcinomas over the course of several decades.

The story of mapping the gene involved in autosomal dominant familial adenomatous polyposis (FAP), in which colorectal cancer develops in early adult life, began with the discovery of polyposis coli in a multihandicapped individual with a visible deletion of part of chromosome 5q. The absence of a gene in that region was predisposing to adenomatous polyp formation, suggesting that it normally functioned as a **tumour suppressor gene**. Using this mapping clue, linkage studies in FAP families quickly confirmed linkage of the mutant gene to 5q21 and eventually using physical mapping methods with yeast artificial chromosomes (YACs) and exploiting submicroscopic deletions in key patients, the adenomatous polyposis coli (APC) gene was identified. Constitutional (germline) mutations in the APC gene have been demonstrated in hundreds of unrelated FAP patients worldwide, with most causing truncation of the protein product. It is this germline mutation that is transmitted in an autosomal dominant fashion, but this represents only the first step in the multistep path to colon cancer; it is a predisposition that is inherited. Additional (somatic) mutations in the APC gene on the other chromosome 5 have been found in the tumour tissue itself, indicating that it is complete absence of the APC protein in a cell that encourages clonal proliferation. This 'recessive' nature of the mutation at the cell level is a common finding with inherited cancer syndromes involving tumour suppressor genes and is in line with the 'two hit' hypothesis; the first hit is inherited, the second acquired as a somatic mutation. The second hit can be a gross chromosomal event within the cell such as non-dysjunction which eliminates the normal gene/chromosome, leading to what is called allele loss or loss of heterozygosity.

Naturally, somatic mutations in the APC gene were next sought in the tumour tissue of common sporadic colorectal cancers and adenomas. Mutations were found in the majority, often involving the APC gene on both chromosomes 5 with allele loss in about a third. Importantly, the proportion of mutant APC genes was the same in the very early adenomas as in the late malignant carcinomas, suggesting that APC mutation is the key first step. Evidence to date points to the following next steps, although not necessarily in this order. Progression to cancer is often associated additionally with DNA hypomethylation, point mutations in the *ras* family of oncogenes (50 per cent), allele loss at the DCC locus on 18q (50–70 per cent), 17p allele loss (75 per cent) and various other late events.

To this list must be added missense mutations in the p53 gene, the product of which seems to act as a transcriptional regulator of important growth inhibitory genes. p53 mutations, which may significantly disrupt total p53 activity even in the heterozygous state, are found frequently in many different cancers and point to a common key mechanism which prevents malignant proliferation in cells stressed by genetic or other damage. In summary, it seems that much of the neoplastic process is mediated through two types of mutations; those causing loss of function of growth inhibitory genes (tumour suppressor genes), and those causing activation or enhanced unregulatable function of a gene involved in cell division (so-called **cellular oncogenes**). Milder types of these mutations may exist as genetic polymorphisms and underlie differences in specific cancer risk between families or populations, but much more genetic epidemiology will be necessary to elucidate this and the interacting environmental influences such as smoking.

The structure or activity of cellular oncogenes may be altered by chromosomal translocations, and in this respect the association of a malignancy with a specific translocation is interesting. For example, patients with chronic myeloid leukaemia have a specific chromosome abnormality called the Philadelphia (Ph[1]) chromosome, which usually results from a translocation between chromosomes 9 and 22 with breakpoints at 9q34 and 22q11. This translocation involves the movement of an oncogene, *c-abl*, which is normally situated on chromosome 9. The breakpoint of this deletion has been analysed in detail. It turns out that it involves the juxtaposition of a region of chromosome 22 to sequences near the 5′ end of *c-abl*. The region on chromosome 22 has been called *bcr* (breakpoint–cluster region). The translocation creates a fused *bcr–abl* gene which, after some different splicing of the RNA, generates a novel protein with transforming activity. In Burkitt's lymphoma the cancer cells have specific chromosome changes: 90 per cent of patients have an 8/14 translocation, while others have 8/2 or 8/22 translocations. Chromosomes 14, 2 and 22 carry the genes encoding the immunoglobulin heavy chain, and $\varkappa$ and $\lambda$ light chains respectively. The cellular oncogene *c-myc* is located on chromosome 8. It turns out that the breakpoint of all three translocations is at the site of the *c-myc* gene. Thus the important regulatory gene is transposed directly into regions of the genome which are undergoing major rearrangements during B-cell maturation.

# GENETIC COUNSELLING AND PRENATAL DIAGNOSIS

The object of genetic counselling is to provide information on the risk to offspring, at a time appropriate to the options available for modifying the outcome, and to put the risk into perspective. The object is **not** to reduce the birth incidence of genetic disease, although this may be a **consequence** of genetic counselling. What action is taken in the light of the information provided is up to the person or couple concerned. It is important to remember that risk has two elements: the chance of happening and the extent of the damage or burden. The former should be assessed as accurately as possible. Perception of the latter can have a large subjective component, much influenced by personal experience and beliefs. If the couple do not regard the genetic condition as any burden at all, then even the use of the word risk (rather than chance) may seem inappropriate to them and interpreted as 'directive'.

The great majority of people seeking genetic counselling are couples who have had a child with an abnormality and want to know the chance of further children being affected. The first responsibility is to give them as reliable an estimate of the chance as possible, and put it into perspective. In any random pregnancy the chance of any serious error of development is about 1 in 40 and this is a useful yardstick for the couple in assessing the degree of risk. Whether or not to go ahead with planning further children is clearly, in the end, the couple's own decision. The clinical geneticist should discuss the various options available, including prenatal diagnosis followed by selective abortion of an affected fetus. There are some couples who will not entertain an abortion on any grounds, but there are many who see this as a way of having a healthy family. Most prenatal tests are specific, and for this reason it must be clear for what particular abnormality the fetus is at risk. In metabolic genetic disorders a precise biochemical diagnosis on the affected relative is essential before embarking on prenatal diagnosis. It is also essential to know which gene locus is involved if using gene tracking by DNA analysis.

**Amniocentesis** is done at about 16 weeks gestation, and ultrasound examination is an integral part of the process and is increasingly used to detect anatomical defects. Amniotic fluid contains cells of fetal origin and these can be cultured for chromosome, biochemical or DNA analysis. Sometimes the amniotic fluid can be used directly, for example, when measuring the α-fetoprotein (AFP) level for the detection of open spina bifida. **Chorionic villus sampling** has largely replaced amniocentesis in high-risk situations. It can be offered from 9 weeks of pregnancy and yields cellular material that can be used for chromosome or DNA analysis or metabolic studies.

In addition to prenatal diagnosis in specific families at risk, there are now prenatal screening procedures that are available in many centres to women who wish to have them. Pregnant women of 38 years and over or those shown to have a high chance of carrying a Down's fetus based on maternal serum markers such as a low AFP can be offered mid-trimester amniocentesis for chromosomal prenatal diagnosis for the exclusion of Down's syndrome. Spina bifida and anencephaly are relatively common congenital malformations in Britain, and a woman carrying an affected fetus tends to have a higher than normal serum AFP level. Taken at 16–17 weeks gestation, the maternal serum level can be used to define an 'at risk' group, who can then be offered the definitive prenatal diagnostic tests, measurement of amniotic AFP, detection of a specific neural cholinesterase in amniotic fluid and careful ultrasound examination. Detailed ultrasound examination of the fetus at 18 weeks, the anomaly scan, is increasingly offered as a screening procedure for gross structural abnormalities. The difficulties arise when minor 'abnormalities' of uncertain clinical significance for the baby are also disclosed.

# GENETIC SCREENING AND THE USE OF GENETIC INFORMATION

The above examples of anomaly scans and prenatal screening for Down's syndrome or neural tube defects in the fetus are already highlighting the ethical and other difficulties that arise in moving from genetic services for families who seek help because of a (perceived) high genetic risk, to offering screening tests to whole populations. Some of the problems arise from the lack of accurate knowledge about the long-term impact of having a screening test. This ranges from being frightened into a decision to abort a fetus because of the inability of doctors to reassure the mother about the significance of an ultrasound finding, to persistent fears about the baby's wellbeing after the 'false alarm' of being screen positive, but definitive test negative.

Population screening for heterozygotes of certain autosomal recessive diseases in selected populations is already underway in many countries. These screening programmes include β-thalassaemia, sickle cell and Tay–Sachs disease. Pilot studies of screening for cystic fibrosis carriers are underway. When and where should these programmes operate: in the antenatal clinic, in general practice, in schools or even added to the neonatal Guthrie-card screening programme? Should screening be offered only to couples and not individuals? How will the success or otherwise of these programmes be assessed by the health authorities – by cost effectiveness in terms of affected fetuses aborted, by some measure of reproductive choice, or by the number of healthy children born to couples facing a high genetic risk?

The above, together with presymptomatic testing for disorders such as Huntington's disease, are just some of the immediate difficult issues raised by our increasing ability to determine genetic information. Disclosure of information to insurance companies or a requirement for employees to be screened for a genetic susceptibility to a known workplace hazard raise further ethical issues. Genetics is not only an integral part of modern medicine, but a legitimate concern of our whole society.

# Clinical Immunology

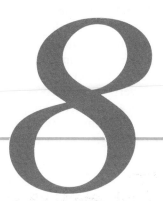

8

# INTRODUCTION

**Immunity** means to make safe or secure (*Oxford English Dictionary*) and, in terms of medicine, it usually refers to the state of being resistant to infection. **Immunology** as a subject emerged from the observation that individuals who had a particular infection, became resistant to that infection. However, we now appreciate that those very same processes which make us immune are important in pathological processes such as autoimmunity, immunodeficiency and hypersensitivity. Many diseases of importance to clinicians have an immunological basis and their diagnosis and treatment depend on understanding the immunological processes involved. These are becoming better defined with increasing knowledge of the way in which the immune system functions, particularly due to the input from molecular biology. The results of the increased knowledge are already being seen, for example, in the use of monoclonal antibodies in the diagnosis and treatment of certain diseases.

# THE IMMUNE SYSTEM

The majority of infections in a normal individual are of limited duration because the immune system fights the disease process. The means by which the immunity is effected is divided into the innate and adaptive (or acquired) immune systems. Both use cells and soluble molecules, distributed about the body, to bring about immunity.

## The innate immune system

The innate immune system consists of physical barriers, biochemical and genetic factors and cells which work together to protect an individual from infection (Fig. 8.1). Genetically there are clearly differences between species and individuals in their susceptibility to infection. Many physical and chemical factors also prevent micro-organisms gaining access to our bodies. Skin forms a protective and usually impervious layer; only when it is breached by wounding such as by cutting or burning do we become vulnerable to infection [1] ia this route. In the trachea there are cilia which constantly beat upwards to sweep micro-organisms away from the lungs; when their beating is compromised chest infections are more likely. Exterior biochemical defences are various and include sebaceous gland secretions, mucus and lysozyme in tears.

Once micro-organisms have gained access to tissues there are cells and chemicals to limit infection. Ingested micro-organisms are exposed to the acid secretions of the stomach, and the normal gut flora establish a hostile and competitive environment which prevents infection. Interior biochemical defences include interferon, which provides a defence against viruses, the acute phase proteins and the complement cascade. The last is a series of 20 proteins found in serum which become activated in a stepwise fashion. Some micro-organisms are able to activate the complement cascade by what is known as the alternative pathway. Complement also interacts with antibodies generated in the adaptive immune system activating it by what is known as the classical pathway (see later and Fig. 8.9, page 92).

The cells involved in innate immunity include the **natural killer (NK) cells** and those cells which are phagocytic, i.e. the mononuclear phagocytes (macrophages and monocytes) and the polymorphonuclear leukocytes (PMNs). Natural killer cells are a type of lymphocyte sometimes referred to as the large granular

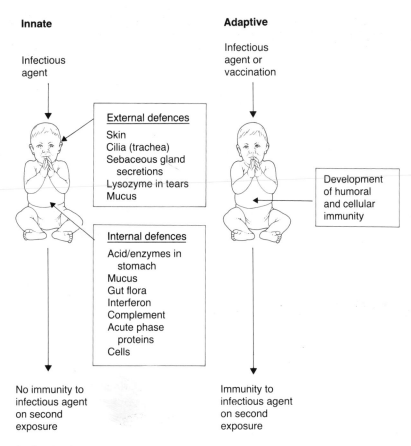

**Figure 8.1** Innate and adaptive immune responses.

lymphocyte. They are able to recognize cell surface changes on tumour cells and virally infected cells and are able to kill them, i.e. they are cytotoxic.

The role of the **phagocytes** is to engulf particles, including micro-organisms such as bacteria, and destroy them. Destruction is achieved by a combination of acid pH, oxygen metabolites, such as hydrogen peroxide and superoxide, and a number of cytotoxic proteins. Bone-marrow derived monocytes and PMNs can migrate from the blood to sites of infection where they are able to phagocytose and thus restrict the infective process. The life of a PMN is short, while monocytes live longer and can become resident macrophages, for example, alveolar macrophages of the lung, Kupffer cells of the liver, microglial cells of the brain and mesangial cells of the kidney, and can continue their functions of phagocytosis and destruction at sites of strategic importance. Macrophages have a number of important functions,

many of which are associated with their ability, much enhanced when activated, to secrete a large number of proteins, including cytokines (Table 8.1).

# The adaptive immune system

In contrast to innate immunity, adaptive immunity leads to resistance to infection on second exposure to the same micro-organism (Fig. 8.1). The process of **vaccination** illustrates a number of features of the adaptive immune system. In the UK most infants receive triple vaccination in the first years of life. This provides protection against diphtheria, tetanus and whooping cough. The injections protect children for life against these three infections providing there is

**Table 8.1** Some important cytokines and their activities.

| Cytokine | Abbreviation | Activity |
| --- | --- | --- |
| Interleukin-1 | IL-1 | Released by many cells. Stimulates proliferation of T- and B-lymphocytes. Many inflammatory activities |
| Interleukin-2 | IL-2 | Released by T-lymphocytes. Stimulates growth of T- (and B-) lymphocytes. Activates natural killer cells |
| Interleukin-3 | IL-3 | Stimulates growth of haematopoietic progenitor cells |
| Interleukin-4 | IL-4 | Released by T-lymphocytes. Growth factor and regulator of isotype switching for B-lymphocytes |
| Interleukin-5 | IL-5 | Released by lymphocytes. Stimulates activation and proliferation of B-lymphocytes. Eosinophil growth factor |
| Interleukin-6 | IL-6 | Released by many cells. Induces B-lymphocyte differentiation and release of acute phase reactants by hepatocytes. Many inflammatory activities |
| Interleukin-7 | IL-7 | Released by stromal cells. Growth factor for early T- and B-lymphocytes |
| Interleukin-8 | IL-8 | Released by mononuclear phagocytes. Chemotactic for polymorphonuclear leukocytes (PMNs) and T-lymphocytes |
| Interleukin-10 | IL-10 | Released by T- and B-cells and macrophages. Inhibits the release of some cytokines by some T-cells |
| Granulocyte colony-stimulating factor | G-CSF | Stimulates growth and differentiation of PMN progenitors. Activates mature PMNs |
| Macrophage colony-stimulating factor | M-CSF | Stimulates growth and differentiation of macrophage progenitors. Activates mature macrophages |
| Granulocyte macrophage colony-stimulating factor | GM-CSF | Stimulates growth and differentiation of myeloid progenitors. Activates mature PMNs and macrophages |
| Tumour necrosis factor-$\alpha$ | TNF$\alpha$ | Released principally from macrophages. Many inflammatory activities |
| Interferons-$\alpha$, -$\beta$ and -$\gamma$ | IFN-$\alpha$, -$\beta$ and -$\gamma$ | Antiviral activity. Activates leukocytes ($\gamma$) |

appropriate boosting. That such a process does not provide any protection against other infections, for example, measles, illustrates an important feature of the immune system, namely, **specificity**. The fact that immunity lasts a long time illustrates the second important feature, **immunological memory**. By vaccination the child has been exposed to an innocuous form of the infectious agent in such a way that when that child encounters the infection subsequently its body is able to respond immediately and be protected, even if that encounter is some years later. In a similar fashion to vaccination, natural infection leads to protection which is both specific and long lasting.

There are two phases to the adaptive immune response. The first, sometimes called the afferent arm of the immune response, is concerned with the recognition of something as foreign. Molecules recognized by the immune system are referred to as **antigens** and the function of the immune system is to recognize antigens on pathogenic micro-organisms. Since most micro-organisms are made up of a large variety of different molecules they present a variety of different antigenic determinants to the immune system, each determinant being referred to as an **antigenic epitope**.

The cells which are able to recognize antigens specifically and which are able to 'remember' that they have done so, are the lymphocytes, which are subdivided into two types, **B- and T-lymphocytes**. The importance of lymphocytes is reflected in their number; there are approximately $2 \times 10^{12}$ lymphocytes in an adult human making up about 2 per cent of the total cells in the body. Lymphocytes arise from progenitor cells which have migrated to what are called the primary lymphoid organs, namely, the thymus, the fetal liver and the bone marrow. Within these organs the cells develop and mature. Cells then emerge from the thymus as mature T-lymphocytes whereas mature B-lymphocytes emerge from the bone marrow. These cells then migrate to secondary lymphoid organs such as the spleen, tonsils, Peyer's patches and lymph nodes and other lymphoid tissue dispersed throughout the body. However, they are not sessile for long since they are able to circulate and recirculate around the body via the lymph and blood and then return to the lymphoid tissue. Within lymphoid tissue cells populate specific areas which consist either mostly of T-lymphocytes or mostly of B-lymphocytes.

In the second phase of the immune response, lymphocytes which have recognized antigen respond to eliminate it by what is sometimes referred to as the efferent arm of the immune response. The two major types of lymphocytes (T and B) effect elimination of antigens in two ways. The first way (**cellular immunity**) is largely directed against micro-organisms whose life-cycle is predominantly intracellular, for example, viruses, intracellular bacteria and protozoa, and is effected by T-lymphocytes. The second way (**humoral immunity**) is directed against extracellular micro-organisms, for example, bacteria, and is effected by the proteins which are immunoglobulins and which are known as antibodies. Most immune responses to any micro-organism are a mixture of both types of response although one may be more effective than the other in eliminating infection.

Both afferent and efferent responses occur by cooperation between lymphocytes themselves and lymphocytes and other cell types and by the release of soluble proteins called **cytokines** from a wide variety of cells (Table 8.1).

# CLASSIFYING CELLS OF THE IMMUNE SYSTEM

In many situations in clinical immunology it is necessary to identify the cells participating in an immune reaction. In tissue specimens from organs or from blood, examination of the cells present and evaluation of how they vary from normality can provide valuable insights into a disease process or progression. In humans, where blood is the most convenient tissue for access, studying the numbers and types of cells has been very informative, for example, in human immunodeficiency virus (HIV) disease where measurement of T-cell subpopulations has provided a method of monitoring disease progression (see over).

It is convenient then that cell types, and subpopulations of cell types, differ in their expression of cell surface proteins. The cell surface proteins are classified by **cluster designation** (CD) number (Table 8.2). Their presence on the surface of cells is usually detected with monoclonal antibodies.

It is also convenient that the expression of different CD antigens may indicate functionally distinct populations of cells. Accordingly all T-lymphocytes have CD3 and some of these have CD4 and some CD8. CD4 and CD8 lymphocytes have distinct functions (see below). Thus CD4 lymphocytes are referred to as T-helper cells and CD8 as cytotoxic/suppressor cells. In human blood around 75 per cent of all lymphocytes express CD3 and are thus T-cells. Around 45 per cent of lymphocytes express CD4 (together with CD3) and 35 per cent CD8 (together with CD3). Individual T-cells in blood do not usually express both CD4 and CD8 together. Around 15 per cent of the remaining lymphocytes are B-cells expressing CD20 and the rest express neither T- nor B-cell surface proteins and are called null cells.

**Table 8.2** Some important CD* molecules.

| CD molecule | Distribution |
| --- | --- |
| CD2 | All T-lymphocytes and thymocytes |
| CD3 | All T-lymphocytes and some thymocytes |
| CD4 | Subpopulation of T-lymphocytes (T-helpers), macrophages and dendritic cells |
| CD8 | Subpopulation of T-lymphocytes (T-cytotoxic/suppressors) |
| CD14 | Monocytes |
| CD15 | Granulocytes |
| CD20 | B-lymphocytes |
| CD25 | Activated T- and B-lymphocytes and macrophages (interleukin-2 receptor) |

*CD = cluster designation, the number is used to indicate a specific molecule on a cell surface which is recognized by a group of monoclonal antibodies.

# RECOGNITION OF ANTIGEN

Lymphocytes recognize antigenic epitopes by receptors which are specific for each epitope. Both B- and T-lymphocytes have such receptors on their surface but the structure of the receptors differs for the two types of cells (Fig. 8.2). In the case of T-lymphocytes the receptor is known as the T-cell receptor, or TCR, and consists of two polypeptide chains (usually $\alpha$ and $\beta$) which are linked by a disulphide bond and anchored in the cell membrane. In the case of B-lymphocytes the receptor is membrane-bound (surface) immunoglobulin (SIg).

During the early development of an animal, T- and B-lymphocytes are generated which are able to recognize all sorts of different antigenic epitopes, even though they have not actually seen them before; these are therefore called naive lymphocytes (Fig. 8.3). Thus, we are born with the capability to recognize all the antigens we are likely to encounter later in life. When an antigen first enters the body a lymphocyte with the appropriate receptor for the antigenic epitope binds to it and the resulting interaction leads to division of that lymphocyte (**primary response**). Repeated division leads to the formation of a clone of lymphocytes all able to recognize the same antigen and all bearing the same antigen receptor. These cells either deal with that antigen (**effector cells**) by the means described below, or become **memory cells** which remain in the circulation until such times as they are required. If the antigen is encountered on a second occasion the memory cells, now more numerous than the original antigen-recognizing lymphocyte, again respond to the antigen by clonal expansion and give rise to more effector cells and more memory cells (**secondary response**). By these means lymphocytes recognize and respond to antigenic epitopes specifically and their continued presence forms the basis of immunological memory. The cellular expansion ensures that the secondary response is more vigorous than the primary response.

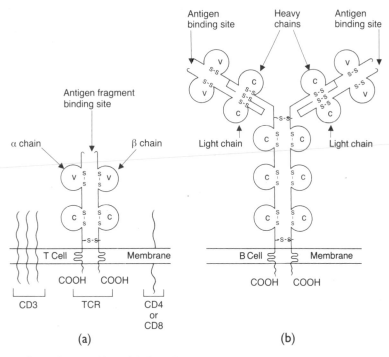

**Figure 8.2** Receptors for antigen on T- and B-lymphocytes. CD = cluster designation. TCR = T-cell receptor.

The antigenic structures seen by T- and B-lymphocytes differ. Thus B-lymphocytes recognize antigens which are in solution or on the surface of cells and which are in their native configuration. The affinity of antigen for its receptor will depend on the shape of the antibody combining site which is complementary for the shape of the antigen. Antibody recognition thus tends to be of tertiary structures. In contrast, T-lymphocytes see antigen which has been fragmented within cells and which is located at the surface of cells where it is bound to the products of the major histocompatibility complex (MHC).

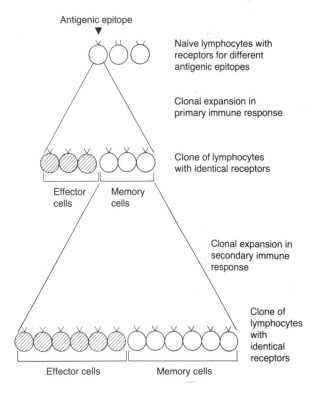

**Figure 8.3** The cellular basis for recognition, specificity and memory.

# *T*HE MAJOR HISTOCOMPATIBILITY COMPLEX

The major histocompatibility complex, known as the **human leukocyte antigen (HLA)** system in humans, is a series of linked genes located on chromosome 6 (Fig. 8.4). The MHC is divided into subregions which encode proteins referred to as class I, class II and class III proteins. The class I proteins are encoded by the HLA-A, HLA-B and HLA-C loci and the class II proteins are encoded by the HLA-D locus which is further subdivided into DP, DQ and DR. Class III proteins include the complement components C4a and C4b, factor B and C2, the two genes for cytochrome P450 21-hydrolase (21-OHA and 21-OHB), the cytokines tumour necrosis factor α and β, as well as many other proteins yet to be identified. The class I and class II proteins are cell surface proteins which are important in cell–cell recognition and are also the targets of the immune response in graft rejection. They differ in two ways: their structure and their cell surface distribution.

Class I proteins consist of a single transmembrane polypeptide folded into three extra-cellular loops or domains referred to as $\alpha_1$, $\alpha_2$ and $\alpha_3$ and a single intracellular domain (Fig. 8.4). The domains are held by disulphide bonds and the polypeptide is glycosylated. The transmembrane polypeptide is always associated with another polypeptide known as $\beta_2$ microglobulin which is not encoded within the MHC but on chromosome 15. The two proteins assemble within the cell and are transported to the cell surface together to form the class I cell surface proteins. Class I proteins are expressed on all nucleated cells of the body.

Class II MHC proteins consist of two transmembrane proteins, the α and β chains, folded into two domains each. The structure is held together with disulphide bonds and is glycosylated (Fig. 8.4). These molecules are only normally expressed on some nucleated cells such as mononuclear phagocytes, dendritic cells and B-lymphocytes which are collectively referred to as **antigen-presenting cells (APCs)**.

In molecular terms the overall secondary structure of class I HLA antigens is very similar.

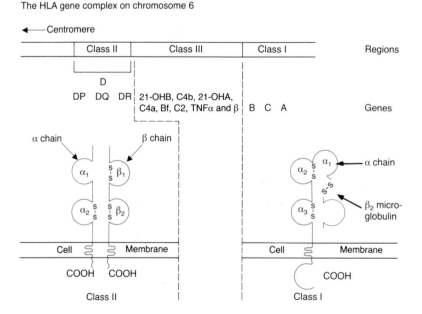

**Figure 8.4** The human major histocompatibility complex (MHC). HLA = human leukocyte antigen. TNF = tumour necrosis factor.

When the primary structures of all HLA-A proteins are examined they are found to be largely similar (and all HLA-B antigens are similar etc.). However, there are parts of the molecule which vary much more frequently between individuals. These are located in the $\alpha_1$ and $\alpha_2$ domains of class I proteins and the $\alpha_1$ and $\beta_1$ domains of class II proteins. There are thus many variants of the structure of HLA-A, -B, -C and -D antigens which occur with an appreciable frequency within the population; the MHC is said to be a highly polymorphic molecule.

Another important feature of MHC expression is that the MHC proteins are expressed codominantly on all cells meaning that the genetic information which is inherited from both parents is expressed. Thus, all nucleated cells have two (maternal and paternal) polymorphic variants of HLA-A, -B and -C (six proteins in all) and all APCs have these together with the maternal and paternal HLA-D proteins. This means that each individual expresses a number of HLA proteins and because of that, and because of polymorphism, it is unlikely that any individual will be like any other unrelated individual. These features are of importance because the rejection of grafts arises because of differences between individuals in HLA types (see below). However, graft implantation has no natural counterpart, apart from pregnancy in which half the MHC (the paternal half) is foreign to the mother. The biological importance of the MHC arises from its role in intercellular communication.

## THE FUNCTION OF THE MAJOR HISTOCOMPATIBILITY COMPLEX; ANTIGEN PROCESSING AND PRESENTATION

Antigens are processed within cells to fragments which are transported to the cell surface bound to class I and class II MHC antigens for presentation to T-lymphocytes (Fig. 8.5). Recognition of foreign antigen by T-lymphocytes only occurs when these cells see foreign antigen together with self MHC. The recognition occurs by the T-cell receptor. The processing pathways differ within the cell for antigens which are derived endogenously, as in the case of viral antigens expressed in virally infected cells, and those which are derived exogenously by phagocytosis or pinocytosis. Endogenous antigens are processed in such a way that a fragment of the antigen, about eight amino acids in length, becomes bound to class I MHC proteins. The antigen is bound to a groove formed by the $\alpha_1$ and $\alpha_2$ domains. This complex on the surface of a cell is recognized by the T-cell receptors of T-lymphocytes which express the CD8 cell surface protein.

Antigens which are exogenous to the cell are taken up by pinocytosis or phagocytosis and are broken down within the lysosomal compartment of the cell into fragments. Peptides of around 12 amino acids then become associated with a groove formed by the $\alpha_1$ and $\beta_1$ domains of class II MHC antigens. This complex on the surface of a cell is recognized by the T-cell receptors of T-lymphocytes which express the CD4 cell surface protein.

The importance of the MHC in antigen recognition has generated interest in the associations between certain MHC types and disease (Table 8.3). For example, HLA-B27 is found in 8 per cent of Caucasians, but 90 per cent of Caucasian patients with ankylosing spondylitis are found to have HLA-B27. Thus, there is an association between having the disease and having a particular HLA type; this is often calculated as the relative risk (RR). The higher the value of RR the closer is the association. Associations have not only been found for a number of diseases, but also for rate of progression of diseases and therapeutic responses.

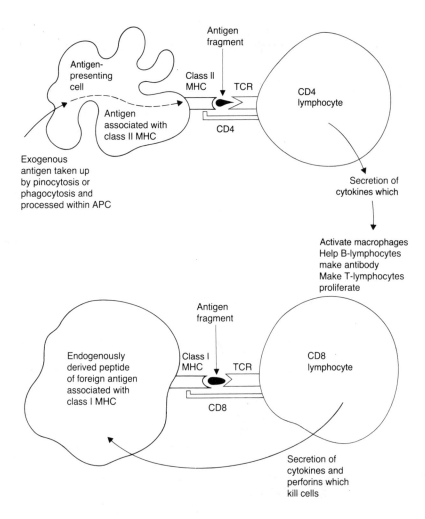

**Figure 8.5** Processing and presentation of antigen to T-lymphocytes. MHC = major histocompatibility complex. APC = antigen-presenting cell. TCR = T-cell receptor. CD = cluster designation.

**Table 8.3** Some disease associations of human leukocyte antigens (HLA) in European Caucasians.

| Disease | Antigen | Frequency (%) | | Relative risk |
|---------|---------|---------------|---------|---------------|
| | | Controls | Patients | |
| Ankylosing spondylitis | B27 | 8 | 90 | 87.8 |
| Reiter's disease | B27 | 9 | 80 | 35.9 |
| Rheumatoid arthritis | DRW4 | 31 | 64 | 4.0 |
| Addison's disease | DW3 | 21 | 70 | 8.8 |
| Myasthenia gravis | B8 | 16 | 39 | 3.4 |
| | DRW3 | 17 | 40 | 3.0 |
| Coeliac disease | B8 | 20 | 67 | 8.6 |
| | DW3 | 27 | 96 | 73.0 |
| Chronic active hepatitis | B8 | 16 | 36 | 9.2 |
| | DRW3 | 7 | 79 | 4.6 |

# FUNCTIONS OF T-LYMPHOCYTES

There are two major types of T-lymphocytes with differing functions (Table 8.4). Those which express the CD8 cell surface protein are principally cytotoxic cells capable of killing cells by recognizing the antigen/class I MHC complex. Killing is accomplished by the release of cytotoxic substances (cytokines and perforins). Some of the CD8 cells may also have a suppressive function and for this reason CD8 expressing T-lymphocytes are sometimes called cytotoxic/suppressor cells.

T-lymphocytes which express the CD4 cell surface protein have a number of functions which arise from their capacity to secrete polypeptides known as cytokines (Table 8.1) which influence the behaviour of other cells; for this reason CD4-expressing cells are sometimes referred to as helper cells. CD4 cells secrete cytokines which help B-lymphocytes to make antibody to T-dependent antigens, cytokines which make macrophages 'angry' and able to kill

**Table 8.4** Functions of T-lymphocyte subpopulations.

| Lymphocyte | Cell surface proteins | Functions |
|---|---|---|
| Helper | CD4, CD3 | Helps B-cells make antibody to T-dependent antigens |
| | | Synthesize cytokines with a variety of immunoregulatory functions |
| Suppressor/ cytotoxic | CD8, CD3 | Kills virally infected cells |

effectively and cytokines which make T-lymphocytes divide. CD4 cells are thus crucial to the adequate functioning of the immune system.

# FUNCTIONS OF B-LYMPHOCYTES

The function of B-lymphocytes is to respond to antigen and to become plasma cells which secrete antibody. Antibodies are generated in response to two types of antigen. Most antibodies can only be made with the cooperation of T-lymphocytes and are called T-dependent antigens (Fig. 8.6). Cooperation takes the form of both cell–cell contact and cytokine release. A minority of antibodies are generated in the absence of T-lymphocytes and the antigens which do this are said to be T independent. These antigens are mostly made up of repeated subunits such as those found on the surface of certain bacteria, for example, pneumococcal polysaccharide. Stimulation of B-lymphocytes with T-independent antigens results in little generation of memory B-cells and the generation of immunoglobulin M (IgM) antibodies.

# STRUCTURE AND FUNCTION OF ANTIBODIES

Antibodies belong to the group of proteins known as **immunoglobulins** (Igs). Each antibody molecule consists of one or more basic units. Each unit consists of two identical heavy (H) chains and two identical light (L) chains (Fig. 8.7). In any antibody molecule the light chains are one of two types, $\varkappa$ or $\lambda$. Together, the H and L chains form a Y-shaped structure which has flexibility at the junction of the three arms (the hinge region). The molecules are bifunctional

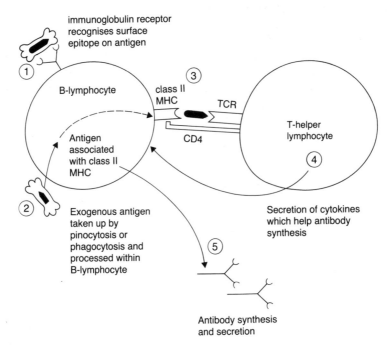

**Figure 8.6** Cooperation between T- and B-lymphocytes. 1. Antigenic epitopes are recognized by B-lymphocyte antigen receptors (surface immunoglobulin). 2. The same complex antigen is taken up by B-lymphocyte and degraded to peptides. 3. Peptide presented together with class II major histocompatibility complex (MHC) to the T-lymphocyte receptor (TCR). 4. T-lymphocyte secretes cytokines which help B-lymphocyte make antibody. 5. B-lymphocyte becomes plasma cell which synthesizes antibody with specificity for antigenic epitope recognized by surface immunoglobulin. CD = cluster designation.

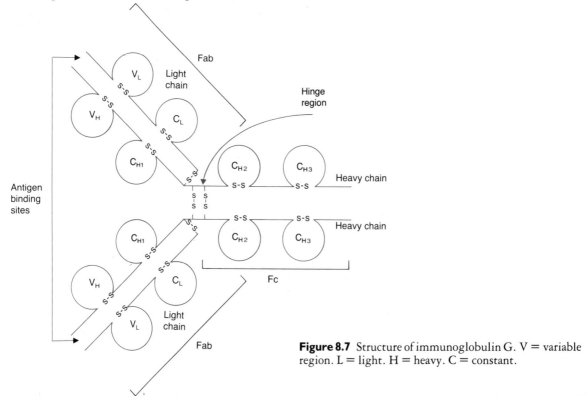

**Figure 8.7** Structure of immunoglobulin G. V = variable region. L = light. H = heavy. C = constant.

with two F(ab) portions which bind to antigen and an Fc portion which interacts with cells of the immune system or with complement.

Antibodies, the T-cell receptor (TCR), CD4 and CD8 and several other cell surface proteins important in immunological interactions are made up of domains of similar overall structure and are members of a group of similar proteins known as the immunoglobulin supergene family. When the primary structures of different antibodies are compared, they are found to consist of several domains which do not vary greatly between the different antibodies. These form the constant, or C, region of the molecule. However, domains in the F(ab) region differ greatly between different antibody molecules and are said to be variable or V regions. Antibodies with different variable region sequences combine with different antigens. The variations in the variable domain, particularly in its most variable part, known as the hypervariable regions, are called **idiotypes**.

It is the hypervariable regions of the V domains which are directly concerned with binding antigen. The complementarity determining regions, or CDRs, of which there are three which are non-contiguous, are found in each of the heavy and light chains and make up the antigen-binding site, the hypervariable region. The antigen-binding site is thus a small region in the F(ab) portion which can bind an antigenic epitope of complementary shape. Most usually this shape would represent a three-dimensional structure on the surface of complex antigen. Since antigens can have many epitopes it is not surprising that we can make many different antibodies: in fact it has been estimated that we can make tens of millions of antibodies each with different specificities for the different antigens we may encounter during our lives.

Antibodies do not directly damage antigens. The binding of an antigen to an antibody forms an immune complex which results in the destruction of antigens in a number of ways (Fig. 8.8). Although antibodies may bind directly to antigens to neutralize them as, for example, in the removal of bacterial toxins, more often they achieve their effect by cross-linking antigen receptors for the Fc portion of immunoglobulin which are found on the surface of phagocytic cells. This process encourages the phagocytic cell to engulf the complex of antigen and antibody and destroy it. The antibody is said to have opsonized the antigen. The process of antigen binding to antibody may lead to activation of the complement pathway by the classical pathway leading to inflammation and phagocytosis. Finally, the antibody may bind to an antigen on the surface of a cell or a parasite and make it susceptible to attack and killing by a cell which has an Fc receptor in a process called antibody-dependent cellular cytotoxicity (ADCC).

There are five types, or classes, of immunoglobulin molecule: IgG, IgM, IgA, IgD and IgE. Each has a different structure and different functions. The class of an immunoglobulin is determined by its heavy chain type (Table 8.5). The different heavy chains are called isotypes.

**Table 8.5** Immunoglobulin classes.

| Class | Molecular weight | Heavy chain | Distribution % intravascular pool | Serum concentration (g/l) |
|-------|------------------|-------------|-----------------------------------|---------------------------|
| IgG*  | 150000 | $\gamma$ | 70–75 | 7–19 |
| IgA†  | 160000 | $\alpha$ | 15–20 | 3.0 |
| IgM   | 900000 | $\mu$ | 10 | 0.5–2 |
| IgD   | 180000 | $\delta$ | 1 | 0.03 |
| IgE   | 190000 | $\varepsilon$ | Trace | 17–450 ng/ml |

*There are four subclasses of IgG (IgG1, IgG2, IgG3 and IgG4) which differ slightly in structure and function.
†There are two subclasses of IgA (IgA1 and IgA2).

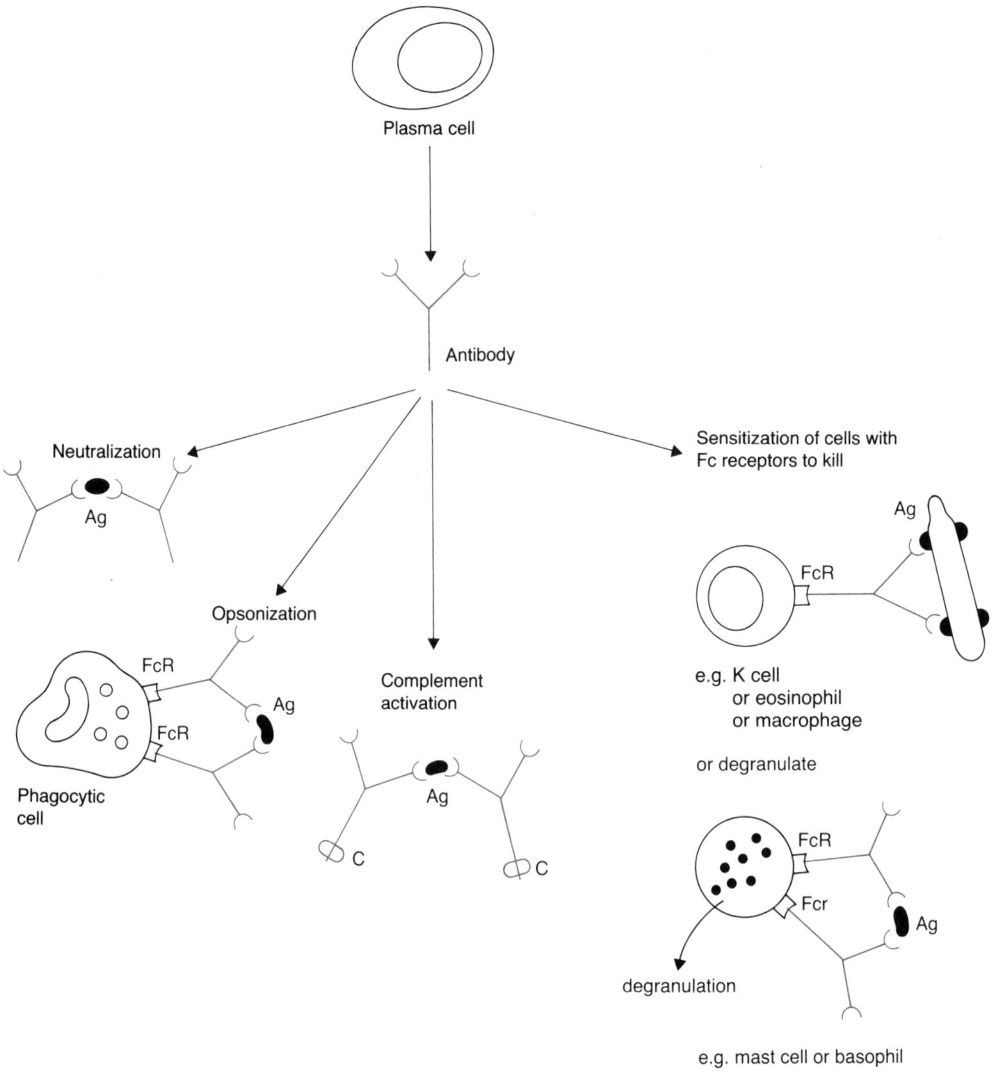

**Figure 8.8** Functions of antibodies. Ag = antigen. FcR = Fc receptor. C = complement.

In health the amounts of the immunoglobulin classes present in serum fall within a normal range (Table 8.5). IgG predominates and IgA and IgM are readily detectable by immuno-electrophoresis. However, IgD and IgE are present in very small amounts and are only detectable by very sensitive methods such as radioimmunoassay. Deviations from the normal range can indicate malfunction within the immune system.

## *IgG*

IgG is the major immunoglobulin in normal serum accounting for 70–75 per cent of the immunoglobulin pool. It diffuses easily into extravascular spaces, is the major antibody in secondary antibody responses and exclusively neutralizes bacterial toxins. It is a powerful opsonin and fixes complement ($IgG_1$ and $IgG_2$). IgG is the only immunoglobulin which crosses the placenta and therefore transfers passive immunity from mother to baby providing protection until it is catabolized, which may be as long as 18 months *post-partum*.

# IgA

IgA makes up about 15–20 per cent of the immunoglobulin pool, where more than 80 per cent occurs as four chain monomers and the rest are found as dimers and sometimes trimers. It is the major immunoglobulin class in body secretions such as saliva, tears, intestinal and respiratory secretions and colostrum. In secretions IgA is mostly dimeric. It is held in a dimer by a joining (J) chain and is associated with the secretory component synthesized by epithelial cells. It provides an immunological barrier on exposed mucosal surfaces where it prevents entry of micro-organisms.

# IgM

IgM accounts for around 10 per cent of the immunoglobulin pool in serum. It has a pentameric structure being made up of five monomers of immunoglobulin held together by a protein chain known as the J chain. Because IgM has a large number of antigen binding sites it is capable of binding with great strength to antigens and is important in agglutination and complement activation. Because of its size IgM is largely confined to the bloodstream. IgM is the predominant antibody in early (primary) immune responses. It is the first antibody made by the fetus and high IgM levels in a newborn baby may be indicative of interuterine infection.

# IgD

IgD makes up only 1 per cent of serum immunoglobulin but is present in large quantities on the surface of circulating B-lymphocytes. Its precise function is not well known but it is thought to be important in the differentiation of B-cells.

# IgE

IgE comprises only 0.004 per cent of the serum pool of immunoglobulin. However, it is found bound to the surface of basophils and mast cells. It may be important in protective immunity against helminthic worms and is found elevated in the circulation in some parasitic infections. It is important in diseases associated with immediate hypersensitivity such as asthma and hay fever (see below).

# THE COMPLEMENT SYSTEM

The complement system is a cascade of about twenty proteins analogous to the coagulation system. There are two major pathways for the cascade: the classical and alternative pathways (Fig. 8.9). Antigen–antibody complexes activate the classical pathway and this is the major pathway of complement activation. The alternative pathway is triggered by substances such as lipopolysaccharide in the cell walls of Gram-negative micro-organisms and is an important component of innate immunity.

The consequences of complement activation are opsonization, cell activation and lysis. These various functions are achieved by complement components derived during the development of the cascade. Components split off during this process including C3b which, like specific antibody, can act as an opsonin. Thus, if a micro-organism becomes coated with complement components it can be readily taken up by phagocytes with appropriate receptors. C3a and C5a cause release of inflammatory mediators

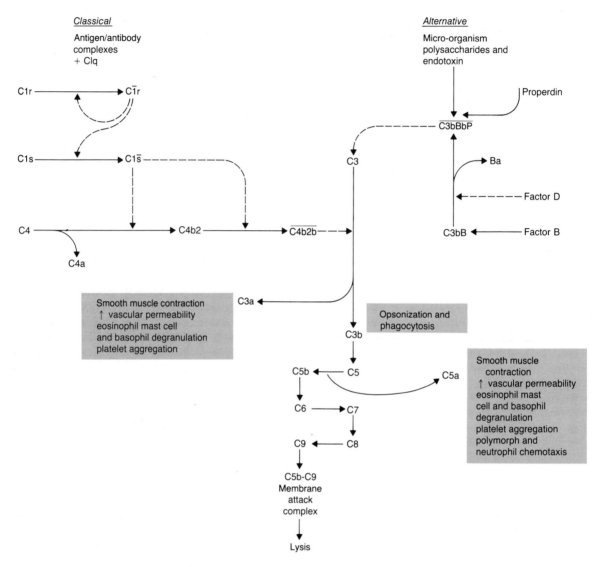

**Figure 8.9** The complement pathways. Components are numbered from C1 to C9. Bars, e.g. C̄1̄r indicate enzymatically active form of precursors and the dotted line enzymatic activity. Small cleavage fragments are denoted by 'a' and large cleavage fragments by 'b'.

from basophils and mast cells, and smooth muscle contraction and increased vascular permeability. C3b activates phagocytes and NK cells and C5a is chemotactic for polymorphs and macrophages. The final complex of C5b to C9 [the membrane attack complex (MAC)] forms pores in cells to which it attaches leading to disruption and lysis of the cells. Normally the disrupted cells are bacteria. However, such disruptive mechanisms may be turned against self in autoimmunity.

# *I*MMUNOPATHOLOGY

There are three major ways in which the immune system is involved in immunopathological disease.

1 There may be a failure to produce an adequate immune response in which case the individual may be said to be immunodeficient. This immunodeficiency may be an inherited failure of part of the immune system in which case it is genetic immunodeficiency. Alternatively, and more commonly, the immunodeficiency is acquired.
2 There may be an overactive immune response which produces more damage than it prevents. These types of responses are usually referred to as hypersensitivity reactions.
3 There may be recognition of inappropriate antigens resulting in autoimmunity.

# *Immunodeficiency*

Immunodeficiency arises when one or more parts of the immune system fail to work properly. The most obvious manifestation of immunodeficiency is infection, often with microorganisms which are rarely a problem to the normal healthy individual. The type of infections which affect an immunodeficient individual are sometimes a key to the underlying problem. Thus we have learnt a great deal about the immune system from observing the very rare congenital immunodeficiencies such as Bruton's syndrome (X-linked agammaglobulinaemia), in which children are born with few B-lymphocytes and are thus unable to make antibodies, and Di George syndrome, in which children are born with a complete or partial absence of a thymus and thus have no, or few, T-cells. Consistent with the roles of B- and T-lymphocytes, patients with Bruton's syndrome suffer from recurrent bacterial infections, particularly respiratory tract infections, leading to pneumonia, and patients with Di George syndrome suffer from severe fungal and viral infections as well as bacterial infections.

In addition to these very rare examples of immunodeficiency there are several other primary deficiency diseases which affect the immune system not only arising from absence or malfunction of T- and B-lymphocytes but also the phagocytic cells and the complement system (Table 8.6).

In terms of patient numbers acquired or secondary immunodeficiency is far more important than primary immunodeficiency. This category includes not only patients who have acquired immune deficiency syndrome (AIDS) but also those who are immunodeficient because they have other diseases, because of the treatment they are receiving, or because they suffer from malnutrition (Table 8.7). In these cases immunodeficiency may be transient and life-threatening infections may be prevented by removing or treating the insult that caused the immunodeficiency.

## AIDS AND HIV INFECTION

The acquired immune deficiency syndrome (AIDS) is the final outcome of infection with the human immunodeficiency virus (HIV) of which there are two types: HIV-1 which is now found in almost every country of the world and HIV-2 which is found in West Africa and is spreading to other global locations. The virus is transmitted sexually, by blood or transplacentally and infects CD4-expressing cells which are principally but not exclusively T-lymphocytes (Table 8.2). It infects these cells because the CD4 cell surface antigen is the cell receptor for viral attachment and entry. Of those individuals who have become infected a substantial proportion have not shown the signs of immunodeficiency disease in the ten years of follow-up which has been possible so far. AIDS is the final outcome of a long period of viral infection and manifests itself as infection with opportunistic pathogens of a type that reflect an underlying cell-mediated immune deficiency and/or the development of opportunistic tumours such as Kaposi's sarcoma.

The body mounts an immune response

**Table 8.6** Primary immunodeficiency diseases.

| System affected | Name | Clinical effect |
|---|---|---|
| Antibody | X-linked hypogammaglobulinaemia (Bruton's syndrome) | Bacterial infection |
| | Transient hypogammaglobulinaemia of infancy | Bacterial infection |
| | Selective IgA deficiency | Gut infections and allergy |
| | Selective IgM deficiency | Septicaemia |
| T-cells | Congenital thymic aplasia (Di George syndrome) | Viral infection |
| | PNP deficiency | Viral infection |
| | ADA deficiency | Viral infection |
| Antibody and T-cells | Severe combined | Various childhood infections |
| (Combined immunodeficiencies) | Nezelof's syndrome | Virus and bacterial |
| | Ataxia telangiectasia | Viral infection |
| | Wiskott–Aldrich syndrome | Viral infection eczema and thrombocytopenia |
| Phagocytes | Chronic granulomatous disease | Abcesses and granulomata |
| | Chediak–Higashi syndrome | Pneumonia |
| | Myeloperoxidase deficiency | Systemic candidiasis and pneumonia |
| | Job's syndrome | Abscesses |
| Complement | C1, 2 or 4 deficiency | Immune complex disease |
| | C3 or C3b inhibitor deficiency | Infection |
| | C5, 6, 7, 8 or 9 deficiency | Neisserial infection |
| Other | Opsonization defects | Bacterial infection |
| | CD11/CD18 deficiencies | Bacterial infection |

PNP = purine nucleoside phosphorylase. ADA = adenosine deaminase.

against the virus with a variety of antibodies, and circulating T-lymphocytes which recognize HIV viral antigens. However, these responses are insufficient to contain the virus which replicates inside cells. By a combination of the lytic effects of the virus itself and the destruction of infected cells by the immune response there is a steady and relentless reduction in the number of CD4-positive T-lymphocytes as the disease progresses. The virus also directly affects the

**Table 8.7** Causes of secondary immunodeficiency.

| Category of cause | Examples | |
|---|---|---|
| Disease | Malignancy: | Hodgkin's disease Myeloma, chronic lymphocytic leukaemia Advanced tumours |
| | Nephrotic syndromes | |
| | Infection: | Measles Cytomegalovirus Infectious mononucleosis Human immunodeficiency virus |
| | Some autoimmune diseases | |
| Treatment | Splenectomy Cyclophosphamide Azathioprine Cyclosporin A Steroids X-irradiation | |
| Other | Malnutrition: | General Ion deficiencies (Zn, Mn) |

**Table 8.8** Effects of human immunodeficiency virus (HIV) on the immune system.

| Cells affected | Way affected | Effect seen |
|---|---|---|
| T-lymphocytes | ↓ CD4 lymphocytes | Lack of DTH to recall antigens ↓ Proliferation ↓ Cytokine release ↓ Cytotoxic response |
| Antigen-presenting cells | | ↓ Antigen presentation ↓ Intracellular killing |
| B-cells | Polyclonal activation | ↑ IgE ↑ IgG$_1$, IgG$_3$, IgA ↓ IgG$_2$, IgG$_4$ ↑ Immune complexes |
| Natural killer cells | | ↓ Killing |

DTH = delayed type hypersensitivity. ↓ = decrease.
↑ = increase.

function of other CD4-positive cells (macrophages and dendritic cells) and indirectly affects the functions of other cells of the immune system which depend on CD4-positive cells. Thus the effects of this virus on the immune system are many (Table 8.8). As a consequence of cellular destruction and malfunction there is immunodeficiency and thus inability to restrict infection by micro-organisms and the growth of tumours.

Evidence of HIV infection in an individual is obtained by the demonstration of antibody in the blood of suspect cases. However, negative results may be obtained in patients in the very early stages of infection and positive results may be obtained in uninfected babies who have obtained antibodies from their infected mothers by transplacental passage of the antibody. In these cases isolation of the virus is needed to settle whether the patient is infected. Disease progression can then be monitored by the presence of viral antigens in blood, skin and lymphocyte tests and most importantly the proportions and absolute numbers of CD4-positive lymphocytes in the blood.

Current strategies for treatment involve the use of antiretroviral therapy together with treatment and prophylaxis for opportunistic infections and tumours. In the long term it is hoped that it will be possible to develop a vaccine not only to offer protection to the uninfected but also to restrict disease progression in those already infected.

# Hypersensitivity

The term hypersensitivity was introduced to describe an exaggerated and inappropriate form of abnormal adaptive immune response which is itself destructive. It is usual to classify hypersensitivity reactions into four types, sometimes referred to as types I, II, III and IV. The first three types involve antibody and the final type T-lymphocytes and macrophages (Fig. 8.10).

*Immediate or anaphylactic (type I) hypersensitivity*

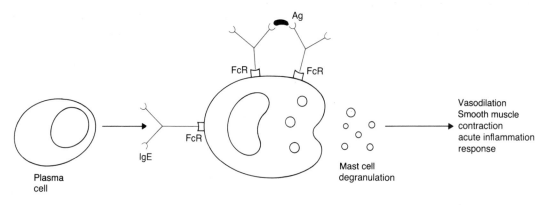

*Antibody-mediated cytotoxicity (type II)*

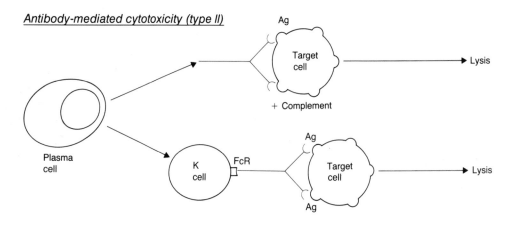

*Immune complex (type III)*

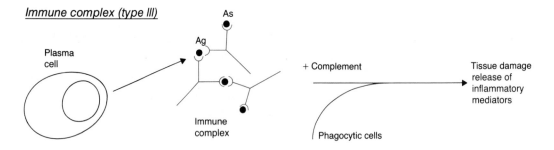

*Delayed or cell-mediated (type IV) hypersensitivity*

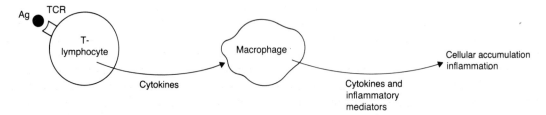

**Figure 8.10** Hypersensitivity reactions. FcR = Fc receptor. Ag = antigen. TCR = T-lymphocyte receptor.

## IMMEDIATE OR ANAPHYLACTIC (TYPE I) HYPERSENSITIVITY

This reaction is the basis of extrinsic asthma, eczema, urticaria, hay fever and anaphylaxis. It is sometimes referred to as either type I or immediate hypersensitivity because of the speed with which it occurs, usually within minutes of exposure to antigen. The capacity to respond to certain antigens, referred to in this context as allergens, is commonly called allergy. The term **atopy** is used to describe the tendency of more than 15 per cent of the population to suffer from allergic disease.

Reactions occur because IgE antibody, which is cytophilic and binds to the surface of mast cells and basophils, binds to allergen and this leads to the release of mediators from the cells. These mediators which include preformed mediators such as histamine, proteolytic enzymes, heparin, chemotactic factors and newly synthesized mediators, such as prostaglandins, thromboxanes, slow-reacting substance A (SRS-A) and the leukotrienes, have profound pharmacological effects. They lead to smooth muscle contraction, vasodilation and increased vascular permeability, oedema and infiltration of phagocytes.

Symptoms occur according to the target organ exposed to the allergen. Common antigens are derived from cat saliva, house dust mite, grass, flower and tree pollens and certain foods such as eggs and cow's milk which particularly affect young children. Therapy usually involves drugs which prevent mast cell degranulation or which are non-specifically anti-inflammatory and, where it is possible, avoidance of allergens.

## ANTIBODY-MEDIATED CYTOTOXICITY (TYPE II)

This reaction is mediated by IgG or IgM antibodies formed against the surface of cells. Their binding to cells results in cell lysis, either as a result of cross-linking of Fc receptors and cell activation or as a result of complement activation. This type of reaction is important in autoimmune diseases such as Goodpasture's syndrome and pemphigoid, transfusion reactions and haemolytic disease of the newborn and in transplantations (hyperacute graft rejection).

## IMMUNE COMPLEX (TYPE III)

This reaction is mediated by antibodies which become complexed with soluble antigen. The formation of immune complexes is a perfectly normal part of an immune response; complexes are normally cleared by the monocyte–macrophage system. However, in type III reactions the complexes persist and become tissue damaging. Such reactions may accompany persistent infection as occurs in viral hepatitis or staphylococcal infective endocarditis when the antibodies are directed at microbial antigens and the immune complexes are lodged in the infected organ and often in addition in the kidney. Alternatively, they may accompany autoimmune diseases such as systemic lupus erythematosus (SLE). Here the antigens are the patient's own tissue and the complexes are lodged in the kidney, joints, arteries and skin. Finally, antibodies may form to extrinsic antigens from the environment as in farmer's lung and pigeon fancier's disease. The pathology that follows immune complex deposition depends on where the immune complexes are located and their size. Lodged complexes cause complement activation and attract phagocytic cells that attempt to clear them. The result is an inflammatory process which is tissue damaging.

## DELAYED OR CELL-MEDIATED (TYPE IV) HYPERSENSITIVITY

This type of hypersensitivity results from the consequences of immune T-lymphocytes interacting with antigen. The classical manifestation of this response is the tuberculin skin reaction seen following Heaf or Mantoux testing used to check previous exposure to *Mycobacterium tuberculosis*. The reaction is called delayed because injection of antigen into a sensitized individual results in an indurated and erythematous reaction peaking 24 to 48 hours later. Clinically, the manifestations of this hypersensitivity are the granulomatous reaction (seen in such diseases as leprosy and tuberculosis) and in contact sensitivity to such agents as nickel and chromate. The mechanisms involved, as in the normal T-lymphocyte response, include release of cytokines which then activate macrophages.

# *Autoimmunity*

The ways in which lymphocytes of the immune system recognize foreign antigens are described above. This in simple terms rests on the fact that lymphocytes exist which are capable of recognizing the variety of shapes provided by extrinsic antigens. Clearly the body must learn to recognize and differentiate those shapes and structures which are extrinsic and potentially harmful from those which are intrinsic, part of oneself and not harmful. The ability not to interact with oneself is called **tolerance** and there are a number of means by which the body limits self reactivity. These include deletion of self-reactive clones during lymphocyte development, inability of such clones to recognize antigen (clonal anergy), the presence of cells which suppress lymphocyte activation (T-suppressor cells) and the anatomical restriction of some antigens which prevents them coming into contact with lymphocytes. It is therefore held that in the normal individual reactivity against self either fails to occur or if it does it is suppressed.

In autoimmunity it is held that tolerance is broken, allowing clones of B- and T-lymphocytes to emerge which interact with self antigens. It is important to realize that these autoimmune reactions may not necessarily be causally related to the presence of autoimmune disease. A disease process may lead to the release of tissue antigens to which there is then an immune response. Autoimmune reactions may thus accompany specific diseases rather than cause them.

Evidence that autoimmunity can lead to human disease comes from neonatal thyrotoxicosis and myasthenia gravis. In thyrotoxicosis antibodies are directed at the thyroid-stimulating hormone (TSH) receptors and are therefore called thyroid-stimulating immunoglobulin. In myasthenia gravis antibodies develop to the acetylcholine receptor. In both these diseases affected mothers can pass the IgG antibodies to the fetus transplacentally with the result that the child is born with clinical manifestations of the disease. These disappear either following treatment or when the maternal IgG is catabolized.

Autoimmune diseases represent a spectrum from those which are organ specific to those which are non-organ specific (Table 8.9). At one end is Hashimoto's thyroiditis in which antibodies are directed against only thyroid tissue

**Table 8.9** Important autoimmune diseases.

| Type | Example | Organs affected |
|------|---------|-----------------|
| Organ specific | Hashimoto's thyroiditis | Thyroid |
| | Graves' disease | Thyroid |
| | Atrophic gastritis | Stomach |
| | Pernicious anaemia | Stomach |
| | Chronic active hepatitis | Liver |
| | Primary biliary cirrhosis | Liver |
| | Addison's disease | Adrenal |
| | Type I diabetes mellitus | Pancreas |
| | Myasthenia gravis | Nerve/muscle |
| | Goodpasture's syndrome | Kidney/lung |
| | Sjögren's syndrome | Salivary gland, eye, joints |
| Non-organ specific | Rheumatoid arthritis | |
| | Polymyositis | Joints, lung, |
| | Scleroderma | blood, skin |
| | Systemic lupus erythematosus | and kidney |

and at the other end is systemic lupus erythematosus (SLE) in which antibodies are found to a variety of antigens distributed throughout the body. In between lie many diseases with antibodies showing more or less organ specificity.

The fact that autoantibodies are found in a number of diseases is exploited by immunology laboratories for diagnosis. Autoimmune serology is used to assist in the diagnosis of a number of diseases even though the relationship between the presence of those antibodies and the pathology of the disease is not obvious. Thus, antimitochondrial antibodies are found in 95 per cent of cases of primary biliary cirrhosis and antinuclear antibodies are found in 95 per cent of cases of SLE.

# Transplantation

One of the achievements of modern medicine is the replacement of a diseased organ with a healthy one, either from a live related donor or from a cadaver. Success of the transplant depends on prevention of its rejection by the immune system of the host. The immune response involves both T-lymphocytes and antibodies and is predominantly directed against the HLA antigens on the cells of the graft with the result that those cells and hence the graft are destroyed. The principal mechanism of rejection depends on the organ and how well vascularized

it is, and thus how easily antibodies and T-lymphocytes can gain access.

Prevention of rejection requires that the donor and recipient share as many HLA antigens as possible and this is achieved by tissue-typing potential donors and matching that to the tissue type of known recipients. It also requires that a recipient does not have preformed antibodies to HLA antigens prior to transplantation (a process called cross-matching). Finally, it usually involves administering immunosuppressive drugs to the recipient to prevent the development of sensitization to donor HLA antigens. Sufficient immunosuppressive drugs must be given so that rejection is prevented without making the recipient so immunosuppressed that they become infected. Cyclosporin A, which acts selectively by suppressing activated T-lymphocytes, is widely used along with corticosteroids and antiproliferative agents like azathioprine. Monoclonal antibodies to molecules found on all T-lymphocytes, such as those against CD3, are increasingly being used to suppress acute rejection episodes.

In bone marrow grafts a different form of rejection complicates the process. Bone marrow grafts are used in patients whose own bone marrow has been destroyed by drugs and/or irradiation because of leukaemias or whose own bone marrow is deficient. The new bone marrow will give rise to lymphocytes which may reject the host if there are HLA incompatibilities, a condition known as **graft-versus-host disease** (GVHD). It is also treated with immunosuppressive therapy (see page 629).

## *F*UTURE DIRECTIONS

Immunological techniques and approaches are contributing more and more to the practice of clinical medicine. Not only does this expertise contribute to diagnosis and management but also to a growing number of therapeutic strategies which are being considered and which use molecules to alter immunological reactions.

These molecules include monoclonal antibodies to cell surface proteins or to idiotypes, cytokines, peptides which can compete for binding sites on T-cell receptors and immunoglobulins. These approaches are at various stages of development but no doubt their efficacy and practicality will be tested in the next decade.

# **D**iagnostic
# Imaging

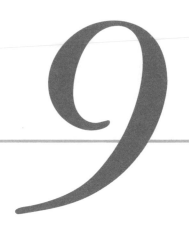

# INTRODUCTION

Diagnostic imaging began when Röntgen discovered X-rays in 1895 and for many years X-rays were the only form of imaging. Over the past 30 years, however, a range of alternative forms of imaging has been developed (Table 9.1) each with particular advantages and limitations. These developments have changed the ways we investigate clinical problems. For example, while X-rays still provide much of the imaging information in chest medicine and bone disorders, in the urinary tract the excretory urogram has been largely replaced by ultrasound. Changes of this sort come about because the newer modalities may have greater sensitivity or accuracy or may cost less or may avoid the use of radiation or be less invasive. Other forms of investigation such as endoscopy have begun to

**Table 9.1** Imaging modalities.

Conventional X-ray studies ± contrast
Digital radiography
Ultrasonic scanning (US)
Nuclear medicine (isotope scanning)
Computed tomography (CT)
Magnetic resonance imaging (MRI)

+

X-ray/US/CT-guided biopsy
Interventional radiology

compete with imaging studies such as the barium meal or barium enema. It is vital for clinicians to keep up-to-date in such matters through regular audit.

# THE USE OF IMAGING TESTS IN MEDICINE

Before discussing the various imaging modalities it is important to make some general points about the use of tests in medicine) (Table 9.2).

## Every test has limitations

Although the sensitivity and specificity of imaging tests overall is continually improving, the reliability of an individual test can vary, not only through its intrinsic capabilities but also with the patient's condition, with the skill of the operator and with the quality of equipment

**Table 9.2** Uses of diagnostic imaging tests.

1.  Screening – presymptomatic
2.  Diagnosis – symptomatic
3.  Extent of disease
4.  Monitoring progress/regression of disease
5.  Anatomical guide (biopsy, angioplasty etc.)

used. So the results of a study should always be considered with the clinical findings. If they do not make sense the problems should be discussed with the imaging department.

## Communication with imaging colleagues is important

Doctors working in imaging departments are trained to interpret the results in the light of the patient's clinical situation as described by the referring clinician. If the clinician does not crisply set the clinical scene and identify the questions to be answered, the radiologist/ nuclear physician will not review the images with such an informed eye, let alone choose the most appropriate investigation and view. This does the patient a disservice. Consultation beforehand allows the correct choice of imaging techniques and views for the clinical situation.

# There are two ways to use tests

Diagnostic tests can broadly be used either by requesting all the tests which are conceivably relevant, or by selecting appropriate tests after taking a careful history and examination.

The first mode is less intellectually demanding and is often defended as leaving no stone unturned. However, the good doctor usually picks the right stone early on: apart from being good medicine the discriminating use of diagnostic tests is important because:

1 Some tests are painful, some potentially harmful and many carry a small risk from radiation
2 Time spent on inappropriate investigations delays the correct diagnosis and treatment
3 They are expensive.

# A test should make a difference

It has been estimated that at least 20 per cent of diagnostic X-rays performed are not clinically useful in the sense that the result – positive or negative – does not alter patient management. Take, for example, a previously fit patient of 45 with acute lower back pain who has no history of trauma. A lumbar spine examination may seem appropriate but:

1 Acute disc prolapse rarely produces any change on such an examination
2 Disc narrowing and osteophytosis are common in middle-aged asymptomatic subjects
3 The vast majority of such patients improve over the next few weeks so that the X-ray alters nothing

Unless therefore the patient has a history to suggest infection or possible malignant disease, nothing is likely to show on the plain film which will indicate precisely the cause of the pain nor change the approach to treatment, which is symptomatic: should the symptoms continue or worsen, an X-ray is justified even though it may still be negative. If, however, the patient had been a 60-year-old woman there would have been the possibility of osteoporotic collapse and an X-ray would have been useful. The question 'how will the results of this test affect my management of the patient?' should be asked before requesting any tests.

# X-RAYS AND THEIR USE IN DIAGNOSIS

X-rays are part of the electromagnetic spectrum with wavelengths between $10^{-9}$ and $10^{-13}$ m. They are generated in an evacuated tube by passing electrons from a cathode on to a target anode, usually of tungsten. Gamma-rays resulting from decay of radioactive isotopes are identical in properties and behaviour to X-rays. The size of the resulting X-ray beam is controlled by lead diaphragms. The 'penetration' of the X-ray beam depends on the kilovoltage applied to the tube, commonly between 60 and 120 kV. ('Penetration' in this context means the proportion of the incident beam which emerges from the area of the patient being examined.)

X-rays have sufficient energy to pass through tissues unless they encounter its atoms. The attenuation of X-rays in tissues depends on:

1 The kV applied to the X-ray tube; higher kV means less attenuation
2 The thickness of the tissues, for example, thigh versus ankle
3 The atomic numbers of the tissue's components: lung causes little attenuation compared to bone which is said to be 'radio-opaque'

Thus the pattern of the emerging X-ray beam reflects the tissue structure in the region through which it has passed. It should be appreciated that the conventional X-ray picture is only two-dimensional while the structure which it represents is three-dimensional. Many structures have so little variation in X-ray attenuation that they are not distinguishable on an X-ray image but their attenuation, and so their radio-opacity, may be artifically altered by introducing a **contrast material**, most commonly containing barium or iodine. These agents enable structures such as the gastrointestinal tract or kidneys or blood vessels to be opacified and so show up on X-ray images.

# Air as a contrast medium

Most plain X-rays are exposed so as to show air as black, bone as white and soft tissues as shades of grey. In films of the chest inhaled air and in the abdomen swallowed air behave as contrast agents. So the normal lung pattern on a chest X-ray is produced by the lung vessels (soft tissue) surrounded by air in normal alveoli. If the air is replaced, for example, when left ventricular failure fills the alveoli with oedema fluid, the vessels cease to be visible. On a postero-anterior (PA) chest film the heart outline and diaphragm are sharply defined because X-rays are passing tangentially to their margins, outlined by air. Arising from this fact:

1 A lung abnormality, for example, pneumonia, next to the cardiac margin will cause loss of that part of the heart outline on the PA film. This can be both a pointer to the presence of an abnormality and a way of localizing it.
2 If the X-ray beam is not tangential to the interface a sharp outline is no longer seen. On a lateral chest film the heart borders are seldom visible because the tangential points are within the mediastinum.

# Hazards of radiation

When an X-ray meets an atom it will frequently hit one of its electrons and knock it out of orbit.

This results in ionization which can cause a chemical change in the cell. The vast majority of such changes are transient but permanent changes in cellular DNA can result and these are responsible for three adverse effects of radiation.

1 Tissue injury: visible signs of damage from diagnostic X-rays are almost unknown today but some degree of damage almost certainly occurs with larger doses.
2 Carcinogenesis: the occurrence of tumours and leukaemias in subjects exposed to radiation is well documented.
3 Genetic injury: X-rays can produce mutations in germ cells. The resulting abnormalities may not be evident for one or two generations.

All such harmful effects are, broadly, dose related but there is no X-ray dose which is absolutely safe in relation to carcinogenesis or genetic damage since a crucial mutation might be the result of a very small radiation dose. When the clinical indications are appropriate the small risk from diagnostic X-rays is amply justified by the resulting benefit, but no X-ray study should be requested unless there are clear indications.

All of us are, of course, exposed to naturally

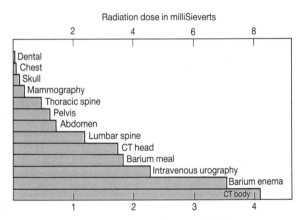

**Figure 9.1** Relative doses of some common examinations using X-rays. Note that these doses are given both in milliSieverts (mSv) and also in terms of the equivalent number of years of natural background radiation. CT = computed tomography. Reproduced with kind permission of the National Radiological Protection Board.

occurring background radiation from such sources as radon gas, γ-rays from the earth and from buildings, cosmic rays and even from some food and drink. The contribution of medical radiation to the total exposure of the population is only 14 per cent but it provides the great majority of man-made, i.e. avoidable, radiation. For individual patients undergoing multiple tests the total radiation dose can greatly exceed background levels. Figure 9.1 shows the relative dose from common X-ray procedures. The high dose from computed tomography (CT) will be noted. Radioisotope scans also give a radiation dose but in most cases this is appreciably less than from X-ray studies.

The measurement of radiation dose, given in sieverts (Sv), starts with the amount of radiation energy deposited in the tissues and then applies correction factors, partly for the type of radiation and partly the area irradiated. Some organs, for example, gonads, are much more liable to injury and so a dose there is equivalent in harmful effects to a much higher dose in, say, a limb.

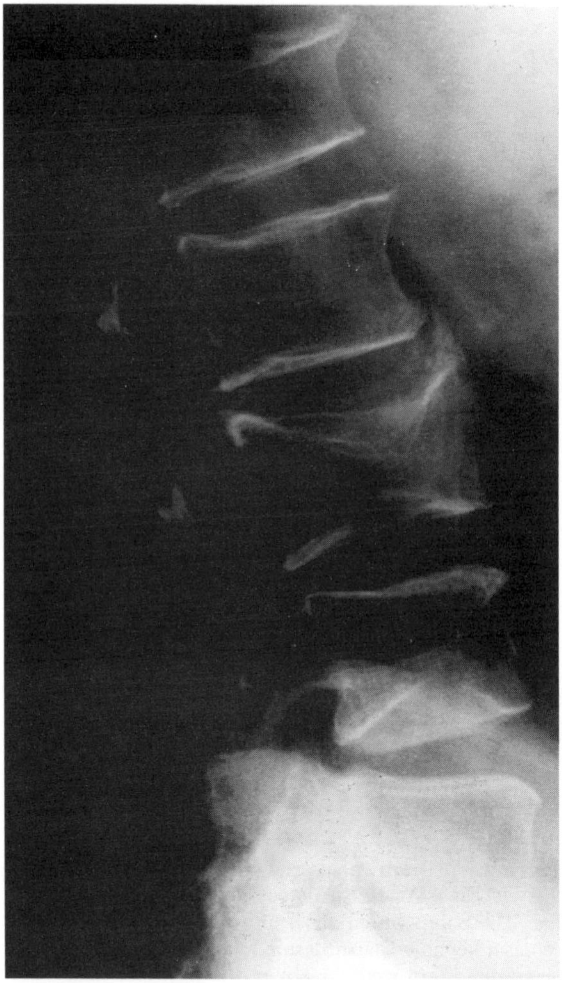

## Producing the X-ray image

The X-ray image can be moving or still. Both types currently depend on substances which

**Figure 9.2** Vertebral collapse due to osteoporosis. The body of L3 shows marked wedging with a deep impression on its upper aspect where the disc has been driven into the softened bone. There is a similar deep impression on the inferior aspect of L4 again due to bone softening from osteoporosis. L1 also shows wedging and a disc impression. The new bone reaction on the anterior aspect of L3 indicates that changes have been present for some time.

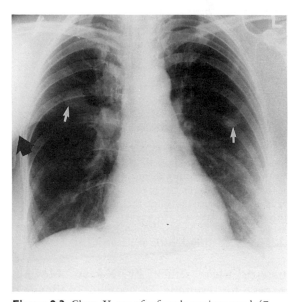

**Figure 9.3** Chest X-ray of a female patient aged 47 years. The right breast has been removed because of a carcinoma. The characteristic residual skin fold (black arrow) is seen in the axillary region with absence of the breast shadow. There are a number of densities in both lungs due to secondary deposits, for example, those marked with white arrows.

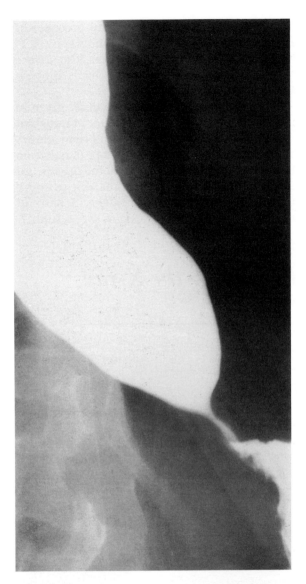

**Table 9.3** Pros, cons and limitations of X-ray studies.

**Pro**
Simple, widely available
Good detail of bone, lungs and organs outlined by contrast

**Con**
Radiation dose may be significant
Some procedures are relatively invasive

**Limitations**
Little functional information
Many areas poorly shown – brain, liver, spleen, pancreas, muscles

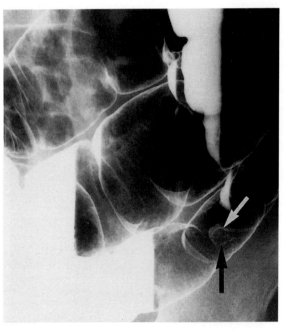

**Figure 9.4** Barium swallow in achalasia of the cardia. The patient is swallowing in the upright position and the dilated oesophagus tapers to a sharp narrowing in the lowermost portion. When the patient was examined in the supine position there was no evidence of any normal contractions in this oesophagus. The appearances are characteristic of achalasia.

**Figure 9.5** Barium enema showing a colonic polyp. This view is taken with the patient lying on the right side. The polyp which has been coated with barium is seen as a keyhole-shaped lesion hanging from the wall of the sigmoid (arrowed). A polyp this size, less than 1 cm, is almost always benign.

fluoresce when struck by X-rays. Moving images, for example, a patient swallowing barium, are shown on a TV monitor after electronic amplification of the faint fluorescent image. The process of looking at a patient in this way is called **fluoroscopy**. Still images (often referred to as 'X-rays') are currently produced on a film sandwiched in a cassette between fluores-cent 'intensifying screens'. The light from these screens produces much of the film blackening which gives the picture. Developments in digital radiography (see below) may well replace conventional radiographs over the next decade or so.

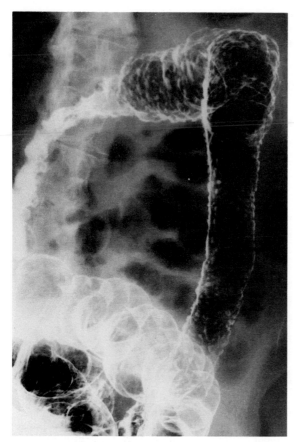

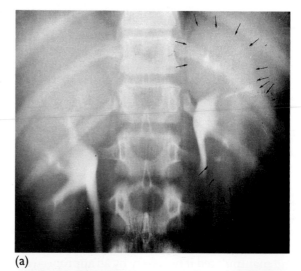

(a)

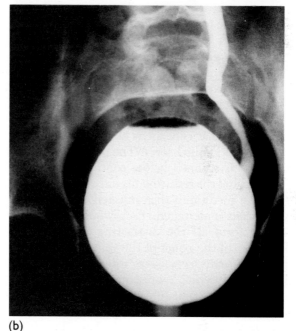

**Figure 9.6** Barium enema in ulcerative colitis. The affected area of colon shows severe irregularity of its contour due to numerous ulcers which protrude from the lumen. Where the ulcers are projected face on they are seen as small round densities within the lumen of the bowel. In this patient the changes were predominantly in the distal colon but in other cases the whole bowel may be involved.

(b)

# *When are X-rays best?*

In spite of their drawbacks X-rays are still widely used (Table 9.3). Plain X-rays, i.e. films without contrast, are useful for skeletal problems (Fig. 9.2) and for lung abnormalities (Fig. 9.3). X-rays of breast tissue (mammograms) remain the most sensitive technique for detecting early breast pathology such as cancer.

X-rays are also used widely after giving contrast media, for showing the gastrointestinal tract (Figs 9.4–9.6), the urinary tract (Fig. 9.7) and for showing arteries and veins. There are also

**Figure 9.7** Intravenous urography showing scarring in reflux nephropathy. (a) The right kidney is normal with a good thickness of parenchyma around the calices both medially and laterally. The contrast is concentrated in the collecting system within the kidney (pyelogram). The outline of the left kidney is indicated by arrows. On the lateral aspect there is a deep indentation, due to a scar, which comes very close to the laterally projecting calix. Less severe scarring is seen medially on the upper pole and on the lower pole where the parenchyma also shows thinning compared to the rest of the kidney.
(b) Micturating cystogram showing marked vesicoureteric reflux on the left as the patient voids. Reflux is a common cause of renal damage particularly in patients with urinary infection.

many examinations in which contrast media, injected locally, can outline particular organs or systems, for example, tear ducts, salivary glands, bladder and urethra, bile and pancreatic ducts, as well as sinuses and fistulae in any situation.

# Digital imaging

Conventional X-ray pictures are analog images but it is possible to scan such a grey-scale image and so to convert the film blackening at each point to a number. These readings can be stored and manipulated if necessary by an appropriately programmed computer. In practice this is seldom done to an actual film but the fluorescent image on a fluoroscopic unit can be scanned directly to give digital information which can then be manipulated by computer. Currently the most important use of this process is in **digital subtraction angiography**, more commonly called digital angiography.

Imagine that contrast is about to be injected into the abdominal aorta. The image of the area of study is scanned before contrast medium is injected and the resulting digital data are stored. Contrast medium is then injected and a series of such scans undertaken. Each would have in its analog form all the distracting densities and lucencies of the bones of the spine and of intestinal gas and feces. The information on the initial scan, which represents all these interfering shadows, can be subtracted by the computer so that each subsequent image shows the contrast without any disturbing shadows (Fig. 9.8). As a result less contrast is needed. Furthermore, because X-ray film is less sensitive than this process, X-ray dosage is reduced.

# Interventional radiology

The techniques used to visualize an organ or structure by opacification with contrast medium have been developed for therapeutic purposes (Table 9.4). For example, if angiography shows a narrowing in an iliac or renal artery, it is

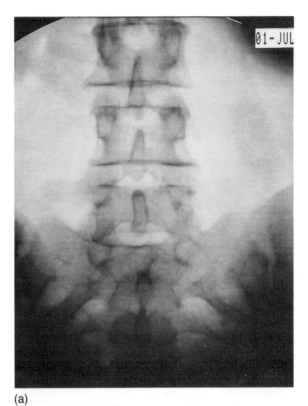

(a)

**Figure 9.8** Mechanism of digital subtraction angiography. (a) Image of the lower abdomen acquired without contrast. The information inherent in this image is recorded in digital form and stored in the computer. (b) Image of the same region after injection into the lower abdominal aorta showing the lower aorta

**Table 9.4** Interventional radiology.

**Drainage**
e.g. Abscesses
Obstructed kidneys
Cysts, e.g. pancreatic
Obstructed bile ducts

**Restoration of lumen (± use of stents)**
Angioplasty: Arteries
                 Veins
Stenting* of obstructed ureters or bile duct

**Arrest of circulation (embolization via catheter)**
Bleeding after trauma, from ulceration, tumours etc.: mainly kidneys, liver, gastrointestinal tract
Obliteration of arteriovenous malformations e.g. lungs, kidneys

*A stent is an artificial means of maintaining the patency of a vessel or duct. Most stents are plastic tubes of some form but a few are expansive, metallic mesh tubes which dilate an area and maintain the dilation.

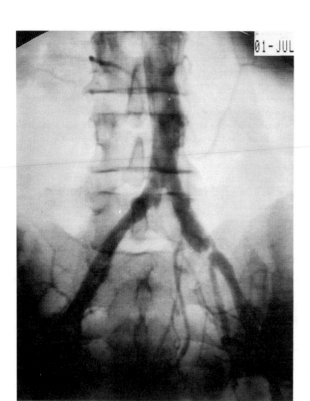

(b)

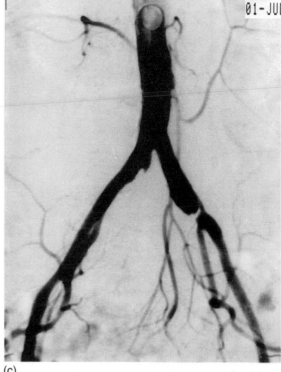

(c)

and the iliac vessels. The contrast is relatively dilute and details are difficult to see in some areas. This image is also held in digital form. (c) Digital subtraction image. The image shown in (a) has been electronically 'subtracted' from that shown in (b) leaving only the contrast images which are much more sharply defined.

The stricture in the left common iliac is now well seen. Note too the clarity of definition of small branches particularly in the inferior mesenteric artery. Reproduced courtesy of Dr J. Reidy.

possible to insert a catheter which has an inflatable balloon into the area of narrowing. The balloon is manufactured so as to inflate to a particular diameter under high pressure. It is usually possible to dilate atheromatous strictures and restore normal dimensions and flow (Fig. 9.9). Techniques of this kind (**angio-** **plasty**) can often replace surgical treatment and are usually less invasive than surgery because most use needle puncture and local anaesthetic. The techniques most commonly used are shown in Table 9.3 but new developments are constantly appearing.

# NUCLEAR MEDICINE

While X-ray examinations give good anatomical representations with little functional information, nuclear medicine is the reverse. The images are anatomically less detailed than X-rays but provide far more data on function and this complementary information is of enormous value in certain situations (Figs 9.10–9.13; Tables 9.5 and 9.6).

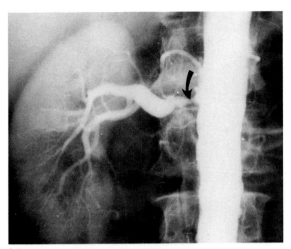

**Figure 9.9** Use of angioplasty in the treatment of arterial stenosis. (a) Aortogram of a patient with hypertension and early renal failure. The right kidney is the only functioning kidney. There is a marked narrowing close to the origin of the renal artery (curved arrow). The distal branches appear normal. (b) During angioplasty a balloon catheter has been passed through the narrowed area and the balloon inflated. The smooth contour of the balloon shows that the narrowed area has been completely dilated. (c) Aortogram following angioplasty shows that the arterial lumen has been returned almost to normal. Some further improvement may well be expected in the months which follow. Reproduced courtesy of Dr J. Reidy.

(a)    9.9(a)

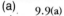

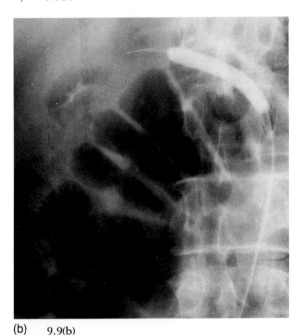

(b)    9.9(b)

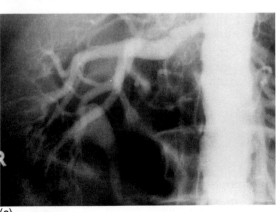

(c)    9.9(c)

**Figure 9.10** Nuclear medicine bone scan for suspected deposits in a patient with breast cancer. There is increased tracer uptake in the sternum at the site of a metastatic deposit. These changes have occurred earlier than those on the X-ray and are particularly helpful in an area which is often difficult to evaluate by X-ray. Reproduced courtesy of Professor M. Maisey.

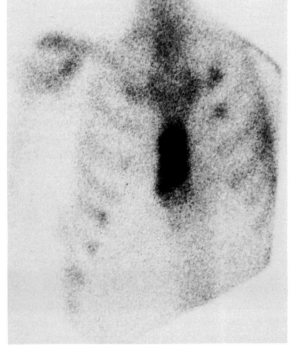

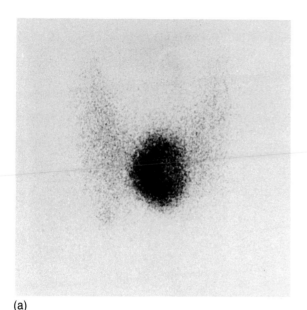

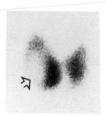

(a)                             (b)

**Figure 9.11** Nuclear medicine thyroid scans. (a) Scan showing a focus of increased tracer uptake in a nodule in the isthmus of the thyroid. The increased hormone production is causing some suppression of the rest of the gland via the thyroid-stimulating hormone mechanism. (b) Scan showing a cold nodule. There is a nodule in the right lobe of the thyroid (arrow) which does not take up tracer – a cold nodule. This corresponds to the palpable nodule found on clinical examination. Reproduced courtesy of Professor M. Maisey.

**Table 9.5** Common radionuclide investigations.

| Organ | Function | Radiopharmaceutical | Common indications |
|---|---|---|---|
| Brain | Blood–brain barrier<br>Blood flow | $^{99}Tc^m$-DTPA<br>$^{99}Tc^m$-HMPAO | Dementia; ischaemia; epilepsy |
| Lung | Perfusion<br>Ventilation | $^{99}Tc^m$-MAA<br>$^{81}Kr^m$ gas<br>$^{133}Xe$ gas | Pulmonary embolism |
| Heart | Perfusion<br>Contraction | $^{201}Tl$<br>$^{99}Tc^m$-RBC | Myocardial ischaemia<br>Left ventricular failure |
| Thyroid | Iodine metabolism | $^{99}Tc^m$-O$_4$. or $^{123/131}I$ | Hyper- and hypothyroidism |
| Liver | Kupffer cells (reticuloendothelial system)<br>Hepatocytes | $^{99}Tc^m$-colloid<br>$^{99}Tc^m$-HIDA | Cirrhosis; metastases<br>Cholecystitis |
| Kidney | Glomerular filtration rate and excretion<br>Tubular (total renal function) | $^{99}Tc^m$-DTPA<br>$^{99}Tc^m$-DMSA | Unequal sized kidneys; transplants |
| Bone | Bone metabolism | $^{99}Tc^m$-MDP | Metastases |
| Adrenal | Cortex metabolism<br>Medulla metabolism | Se-cholesterol<br>$^{131}I$-MIBG | Tumours<br>Phaeochromocytoma |
| Spleen | Reticuloendothelial function<br>Red cell sequestration | $^{99}Tc^m$-colloid<br>Denatured $^{99}Tc^m$-RBC | Trauma<br>Hypersplenism |
| White cells | Infection/inflammation | $^{111}In$-white cells | Pyrexia of unknown origin; abscess |

DTPA = diethylenetriamine pentaacetate. HMPAO = hexamethylpropyleneamine oxime. MAA = macroaggregated albumin. RBC = red blood cells. HIDA = an iminodiacetic acid derivative. DMSA = dimercaptosuccinic acid. MDP = methylene diphosphonate. MIBG = metaiodobenzylguanidine.

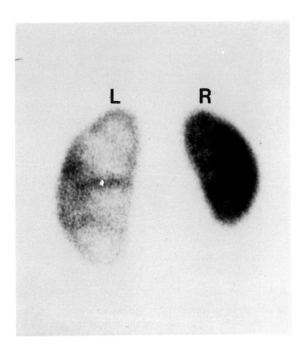

**Figure 9.12** Value of dimercaptosuccinic acid (DMSA) scan in renal obstruction. Posterior view after the kidneys have been outlined by DMSA. This allows the assessment of the amount and distribution of functioning renal parenchyma. In this case measurements showed that 34 per cent of the glomerular filtration rate (GFR) was in the obstructed left kidney. The normal right kidney shows characteristically even uptake of tracer. Reproduced courtesy of Professor M. Maisey.

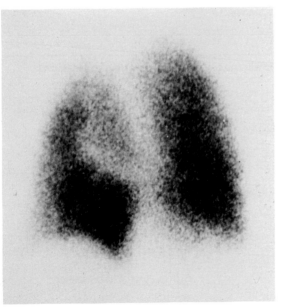

(a)

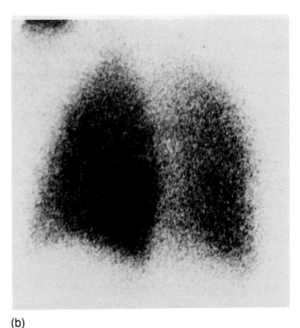

(b)

**Figure 9.13** Ventilation/perfusion scan in suspected pulmonary embolism. This patient had a normal chest X-ray. (a) The perfusion scan shows a large deficit of perfusion in the right upper lobe. (b) The ventilation scan shows normal distribution of tracer because this area is ventilated normally. This 'mismatch' is pathognomonic of pulmonary embolism. Reproduced courtesy of Professor M. Maisey.

**Table 9.6** Pros, cons and limitations of nuclear medicine.

**Pro**
Measures function
Gives quantitative data; useful for monitoring response to therapy

**Con**
Small radiation dose

**Limitations**
Restricted range of applications
Poor anatomical resolution

# Physical basis of nuclear medicine

The radioisotopes employed in diagnostic nuclear medicine are gamma emitters. They are commonly used by incorporating trace amounts in carrier compounds with physiological or pharmacological properties which carry them – and the isotope – to a particular site in the body where the amount and distribution can be measured and imaged. The ideal isotope should have a half-life about 1.5 times the duration of the procedure undertaken, should be of low toxicity and should only emit $\gamma$-rays: the energy should be in the range 100–300 keV to provide adequate tissue penetration while allowing good detection by gamma cameras. Technetium-99m ($^{99}Tc^m$), with a half-life of 6 hours, is close to this ideal and is readily incorporated in a number of carriers. It is therefore the commonest isotope in use for diagnosis. Accumulation of isotope in an organ under study may take some hours before the static images are obtained. In scans which depict functional changes, such as the excretion of $^{99}Tc^m$-labelled diethylenetriamine pentaacetate (DTPA) via the kidneys, scanning lasts for the duration of the examination; this is usually only half or an hour or so.

# Imaging with the radioisotope

When an isotope has accumulated in the appropriate site its distribution and concentration is recorded with a gamma camera. This consists of:

1  A collimator with numerous fine holes which accept only radiation coming from a particular direction so providing the spatial resolution inherent in the camera.
2  A radiation detector in the form of a sensitive sodium iodide crystal which produces light in response to incident photons. The light intensity is increased by so-called photomultipliers and converted to an electrical signal.

The relative light intensity, corresponding to the intensity of radiation across the area under examination, is analysed to provide a spatially accurate image: this is shown on a display monitor which is linked to a camera system for producing a permanent record.

# How isotopic imaging reflects functional changes

Take a patient with a known breast cancer undergoing a bone scan for possible metastases: 3 hours after injection of $^{99}Tc^m$-labelled methylene diphosphonate (MDP) images are obtained showing the skeleton. The isotope distribution represents areas of bone turnover and is even but faint in areas of normal bone. Where there is a so-called 'hot spot' (Fig. 9.10) the bone turnover is increased. This could be due to metastatic deposits, to healing fractures or to areas of degenerative osteophytosis, since in all such areas there is increased laying down of bone. Therefore, the scan is sensitive in demonstrating abnormal areas of bone but is not specific as to the cause of the abnormality although the position and pattern of functional activity can frequently allow a reasonable estimate of the most likely disease process.

# POSITRON EMISSION TOMOGRAPHY

Positron emission tomography (PET) is the technique using radionuclides which has been most recently introduced into clinical medicine. Whilst most radionuclides decay by releasing a photon (γ-ray) a few radionuclides decay by releasing a positron (positively charged electron). This positron travels only a very short distance from the site of its release (1–2 mm) before meeting an electron. When this occurs annihilation radiation is the result in which the mass of the electron and the positron is transposed into two high-energy γ-rays (511 keV) which are emitted from the body in opposite directions. These γ-rays can be detected and localized using computed tomography (CT) and magnetic resonance imaging (MRI) mathematical reconstruction techniques with a very high degree of precision using a ring of detectors around the patient. The resulting images are sectional or tomographic in type (see below). Apart from this accuracy in detection and locali-zation the other advantages of PET are the very short half-lives of most of the radionuclides and the fact that they are radionuclides of key organic elements: carbon – 20 min half-life; oxygen – 2 min half-life; nitrogen – 10 min half-life; fluorine – 2 hour half-life. These provide enormous opportunities for labelling organic compounds which is not possible with conventional radionuclides. Currently the most commonly used labelled compound is fluorine-18 deoxyglucose ($^{18}$FDG) (an analogue of glucose) which can be used for imaging substrate glucose metabolism and has diagnostic uses in the brain, the heart and for cancers. Others include water, oxygen and ammonia, and all the time other drugs and receptor agents are being prepared for clinical use. Positron emission tomography provides major new information about physiological and pharmacological pathways and processes as well as their disturbance by various disease processes.

# SECTIONAL IMAGING

Conventional X-rays and most nuclear medicine images are two-dimensional representations of solid, i.e. three-dimensional, structures. This means that a PA chest X-ray includes all the structures from the front to the back of the chest. The trained eye learns to ignore the ribs and concentrate on lung changes but even so it may be hard to see the details of an abnormality. This led to the development of **tomography** (from the Greek tomos-slice). In this technique the X-ray film is placed underneath the patient and the X-ray tube above the patient and they are linked so that they pivot about a fixed point. Then, during a relatively long exposure time, the tube and film move in opposite directions. The effect of the movement is to blur out all structures except those at the level of the pivotal point. This point can be raised or lowered, making it possible to show structures at selected levels, for example, the hilar regions or the kidneys. The tomographic effect, showing structures in particular tissue planes, usually less than a centimetre thick, can be achieved in a number of other ways. It is seen on ultrasound, CT and MRI as well as when using the specialized techniques of nuclear medicine – PET and single photon emission computed tomography (SPECT). For such techniques the terms 'tomographic', 'planar' or 'sectional' imaging are employed. The word 'scan' derives from the movement of the X-ray tube in CT scanning, the sound beam in ultrasound and the detectors in early nuclear medicine systems. It is widely used in non-X-ray imaging even if not always appropriately.

# ULTRASONIC SCANNING

Modern ultrasonic scanning uses probes containing piezoelectric crystals which generate ultrasonic pulses. The pulses are directed into the tissues and are reflected with differing intensity by the different tissue interfaces. On their return to the probe the pulses are detected and a picture is built up of the tissues in terms of their acoustic impedance. Most show variable but incomplete sound reflection and differences in texture can be shown, for example, between renal cortex and medulla. Bone and gas cause complete reflection, blocking the onward transmission of the sound waves. This is a major limitation of the technique. On the other hand clear fluid, for example, urine, causes no reflection and this makes it possible to examine the female pelvis through a full bladder and to recognize hydronephrosis or cysts in the kidneys and elsewhere.

Ultrasonography requires appreciable operative skill, partly in circumventing bowel gas or bone, for example, rib, partly in recognizing abnormalities during scanning and partly in freezing a good image for recording on film.

Images are often difficult for others to interpret because they may be derived in unfamiliar planes and also because they lack the 'context' given by bones in other types of image. Ultrasound is less effective in showing deep structures, as resolution is poorer here. Nonetheless, ultrasound now plays a major part in diagnosis and even when it does not provide the final answer it may determine the direction of subsequent investigation (Fig. 9.14 and 9.15).

The advantages of ultrasound are set out in Table 9.7. The absence of ionizing radiation has made it ideal for studying the pregnant uterus but it is also valuable for demonstrating abdominal solid organs – liver, spleen, kidneys, pancreas – and organs such as the thyroid, testis, female pelvic organs and at times the breast. It is also used in many situations to direct biopsy needles into masses or other suspicious areas.

Two examples may be given of the use of ultrasound in determining the subsequent investigation of a patient. In jaundice ultrasound can rapidly show if the bile duct is dilated. If it is, this implies an obstructive cause and the examination may also show an obstructing mass or stone. If the duct is not dilated a 'non-surgical' cause such as hepatitis is more likely.

Similarly, in renal failure the first question is whether the patient's kidneys are obstructed or not and this can be rapidly shown by ultrasound

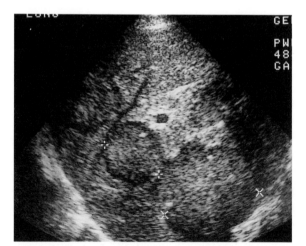

**Figure 9.14** Ultrasonic liver scan in a patient with metastatic deposits. The scan is in the longitudinal plane. The upper part of the image shows normal liver tissue. In the lower part of the picture, corresponding to the posterior part of the right lobe of the liver, there are two rounded areas which have been marked by crosses. These are metastatic deposits. Reproduced courtesy of Dr A. Saunders.

**Table 9.7** Pros, cons and limitations of diagnostic ultrasound.

**Pro**
No ionizing radiation
Quick, informative, repeatable
Good for children and pregnant women

**Con**
No known contraindications

**Limitations**
Operator dependent; impeded by bone and gas: no information on bones, lungs, gastrointestinal tract, brain (except neonates)
Poor at showing deeper tissues

(Fig. 9.15). If there is an obstruction it may be possible to show the cause such as bladder infiltration by a prostatic neoplasm. Even if the cause is not shown the direction of further investigation is clear: CT scanning of the retroperitoneum and pelvis may show obstructing nodes or other masses. If there is no evidence of hydronephrosis the renal size may be important, small kidneys suggesting chronic renal disease or enlarged polycystic kidneys may be shown. The ability to speed the diagnostic process has made ultrasound one of the most significant additions to modern diagnostic imaging.

# Flow studies

Ultrasound examinations are almost wholly concerned with anatomico-pathological changes and not with function. Newer equipment is, however, capable of registering blood flow using Doppler signals from red cells in motion. This can be used to determine flow patterns in arteries or veins but is also useful in other ways. Thus a

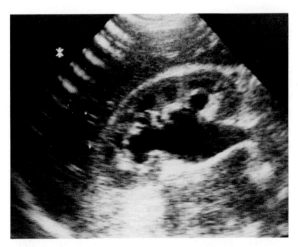

**Figure 9.15** Ultrasonic scan of an obstructed right kidney. The dark area representing the dilated calices and pelvis produces an effect very similar to that of a pyelogram (see Fig. 10.7). Reproduced courtesy of Dr A. Saunders.

mass lesion in the liver might be caused by an abscess or a tumour. Demonstration of blood flow in the mass would confirm that it was a tumour, since there are no vessels in an abscess cavity.

# COMPUTED TOMOGRAPHY

Conventional X-ray images show good detail of bones and lungs but structures with soft tissue density are almost indistinguishable. To some extent this is overcome by the use of contrast agents but organs such as the liver, spleen or pancreas, the muscles and retroperitoneal structures are poorly seen. Similarly the brain is not satisfactorily displayed even with injection of contrast agent into the cerebral arteries. The development of CT scanning by Sir Godfrey Hounsfield overcame this problem by a radically different way of using X-rays (Table 9.8).

When a narrow X-ray beam passes through body tissues the attenuation it undergoes is the summation of all the tissue densities encountered on its path. A sensitive detector placed to record the beam, coupled to the X-ray source,

**Table 9.8** Pros, cons and limitations of computed tomography.

**Pro**
High tissue discrimination: of particular value in brain, thorax, abdomen

**Con**
High radiation dose

**Limitations**
High capital cost
Almost limited to transaxial (cross-sectional) plane
Limited functional information
Some brain disorders, e.g. multiple sclerosis, are not demonstrated

will show a variation with changes in the beam direction as the beam passes through different structures. When the source (X-ray tube) and detectors are arranged so that they can rotate around the patient it becomes possible to get readings from each point on the rotation (Fig 9.16a). Figure 9.16b shows the principle by which it is possible to calculate the densities in small boxes of material from readings taken at different angles. In a CT scanner the readings are far more numerous, requiring a computer to calculate them, but the essential principle is similar. In this way the relative tissue density in all the tiny cubes of tissue in the selected cross-sectional plane of the patient can be computed. Each cube is allocated a number on a scale from −1000 to +4000 HU (Hounsfield units). These values are then displayed on a grey-scale image with bone showing white (+4000 HU), air as black (−1000 HU) and water 0 HU) at the mid-point on the scale.

# Clinical uses of computed tomography

Until the advent of MRI the CT scan was paramount in imaging the brain. It is still the main modality in neuroradiology (Fig. 9.17). In the chest and abdomen it is more often used to evaluate lesions found on other studies or to give supplementary information (Figs 9.18 and 9.19). Thus a mass in the mediastinum found on a chest X-ray may be shown either to be cystic − suggesting a developmental cyst − or it may be solid requiring needle biopsy to determine its nature. Similarly an abdominal CT scan may be undertaken on a patient with a testicular or cervical tumour or a lymphoma to determine whether or not the retroperitoneal lymph nodes are involved. Such oncological evaluation is a major source of referrals.

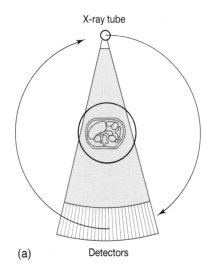

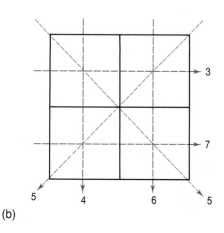

(a)   Detectors        (b)

**Figure 9.16** (a) Diagram of the essential elements in a computed tomographic (CT) scanner. An X-ray tube, emitting a fan-shaped beam of radiation rotates on a circular track around the patient. On the opposite side of the patient is a bank of radiation detectors linked to the tube. The individual detectors are usually about 1 mm wide and there are commonly 700–800. As the tube and detectors rotate round the patient readings are generated from each detector at each point of rotation. These readings are fed into a computer which is programmed to calculate the relative density of each small volume of tissue in the cross-section. The width of the radiation beam, i.e. the thickness of the 'slice', can vary from 10 mm down to 1–2 mm. Modern scanners complete a rotation in 1–2 sec and some are now able to scan continuously down the patient up to 50 cm of body length. (b) Puzzle to illustrate the principle of the CT scanner. The four squares represent adjacent volumes of tissue each with a different density. The arrows represent X-ray beams passing in different directions. The number at the end of each arrow is the sum of the densities in the two squares traversed by the arrow. Work out the number in each square (answer at the end of the chapter).

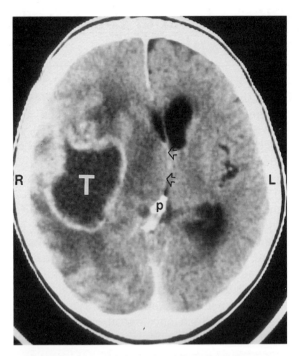

**Figure 9.17** Computed tomographic scan of the brain in a patient with a right-sided brain tumour (T) – a glioblastoma multiforme. The patient has been given a contrast agent, so increasing the density of the margins of the tumour in the right temporal region: the darker central area probably represents necrosis. The mid-line structures are displaced to the left (arrows) and there is compression of the anterior horn of the right lateral ventricle. The calcified pineal (p) is also shifted to the left. Reproduced courtesy of Dr T. Cox.

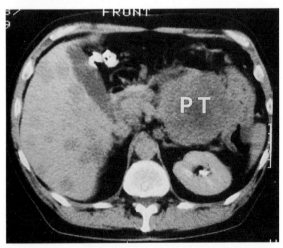

**Figure 9.18** Pancreatic carcinoma with liver metastases. Computed tomographic scan through the upper abdomen showing part of the right lobe of the liver which contains numerous dark areas indicating secondary deposits. Anterior to the left kidney there is a large rounded mass (PT) with irregular margins: this is a massive tumour in the body and tail of the pancreas. Reproduced courtesy of Dr S. Rankin.

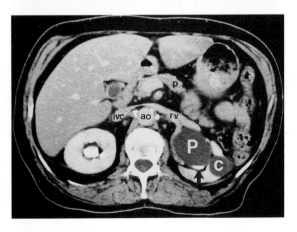

**Figure 9.19** Computed tomographic scan of upper abdomen in a patient with hydronephrosis and a renal cyst. The patient has been injected with contrast medium shortly before the scan. The vessels within the liver therefore show as whiter areas. There is also contrast medium in the aorta, inferior vena cava (ivc) and left renal vein as well as in the collecting system of the normal right kidney. On the left side there is a dilated pelvis (P) containing mainly unopacified urine with a small amount of contrast medium in the most dependent area (arrow) indicating the beginning of contrast medium excretion into this obstructed system. On the lateral aspect of the kidney there is a further area of low attenuation due to a cyst (C) in the kidney parenchyma. The anatomy is well shown with the left renal vein (rv) anterior to the dilated renal pelvis, and anterior to this the pancreas (p). The aorta (ao) is seen anterior to the spine and on its right the ivc. Reproduced courtesy of Dr S. Rankin.

# Magnetic resonance imaging

The physical basis of MRI is very complex but the more basic elements in the process may be explained as follows: charged atomic nuclei spin on their axes and in doing so behave like tiny magnets, responding to a strong magnetic field. While spinning they 'precess' about their axis of spin just as a top wobbles while it spins. The frequency of precession varies with the atom. In MRI spinning hydrogen nuclei (protons) are selected for study because of their abundance in the tissues, particularly in water and fat.

In addition to responding to a magnetic field protons can also be influenced by radiofrequency (RF) energy but only if it has the same frequency as their frequency of precession. Under these circumstances the protons will absorb energy and may be deflected, changing their orientation.

If the protons are randomly orientated such a deflection is not significant. But in MRI the patient lies within a massive tubular magnet whose field strength is usually between 0.25 and 1.5 Tesla (a Tesla being about 20 000 times the earth's magnetic field). The strength of the field is varied slightly along its length to provide a gradient which is sufficient to allow localization of signals to a particular part of the patient. Within this powerful magnetic field a small proportion of protons align to the field, still precessing. Radiofrequency coils which are placed inside the magnet and close to the patient are made to emit brief but intense pulses of appropriate frequency. This causes the protons to twist, usually through 90°, against the continuing effect of the magnetic field. As the pulse ends the protons revert to their original orientation and when this happens the energy released causes an RF signal which is detected by the coil. The speed with which protons return to their original orientation varies with the tissue in which they are sited. This gives the basis for an image in which the different degrees of recovery of individual protons is shown on a grey scale (T1 image). A second source of image information is the degree of dephasing among the protons at the different sites (T2). This yields images with different characteristics and is particularly sensitive to changes in water so that areas of pathological change are made more conspicuous.

In both types of image, moving blood does not show a signal because the protons move during the period of the RF pulse and recovery and this leads to a so-called signal void. In conclusion of this brief account of MRI it may be mentioned that certain substances, for example, gadolinium DTPA, behave as 'paramagnetic' contrast agents. This allows the demonstration of vascularized structures, for example, it may show brain tumour separate from surrounding oedema.

## Clinical value of magnetic resonance imaging

The discriminating capability of MRI is currently most striking in areas where there is little respiratory or cardiac movement such as the brain (Fig. 9.20), spinal cord (Fig. 9.21) and joints (Table 9.9). The ability to show lesions

**Table 9.9** Pros, cons and limitations of magnetic resonance imaging.

**Pro**
Sensitive to a wide range of tissue disturbances including plaques of multiple sclerosis
Able to demonstrate structures/disorders in multiple planes
Non-invasive: no ionizing radiation
Some blood flow information

**Con**
Danger if ferrous materials in the magnetic field
Contraindicated when a pacemaker is present or when aneurysm clips have been used or after metal injury to the eye

**Limitations**
High capital cost
Claustrophobia
Movement may degrade the image

such as the demyelination of multiple sclerosis (Fig. 9.20) is only a small part of its value in the brain where the ability to show structures free from bony artefacts is particularly valuable for internal auditory canals and posterior fossa tumours. In addition, the capacity to show structures in three planes is often a major advantage relative to CT especially for planning surgery and radiotherapy. This is because it is possible to demonstrate the extent of a lesion graphically, for example, how far a renal carcinoma extends into the liver or the inferior vena cava. As MRI scanners become able to acquire data more rapidly the value of abdominal and thoracic scans will increase further. It will also be possible to achieve greater patient throughput so reducing the cost of individual scans. Interestingly, although cortical bone does not itself produce any signal, the changes in adjacent structures/tissues such as bone marrow, articular cartilage, muscle etc. make it possible to detect fractures and to evaluate intra-articular pathology such as meniscal tears in the knee.

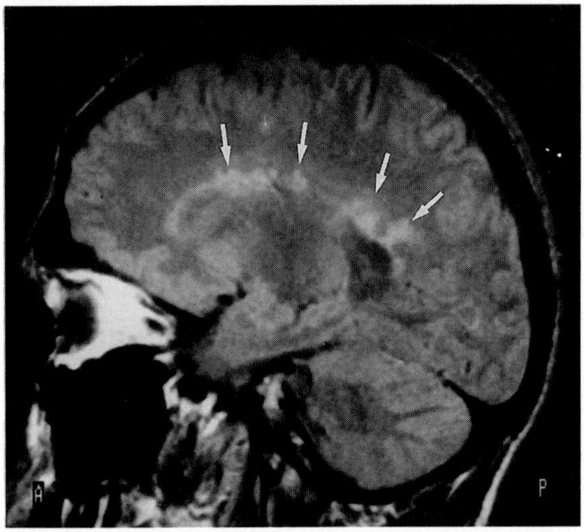

**Figure 9.20** Magnetic resonance imaging of the brain in multiple sclerosis. A sagittal image just lateral to the mid-line showing the structures of the cerebral and cerebellar hemispheres. Part of the eye is visualized anteriorly. In the pericallosal region there are a number of white areas (arrows) with the characteristic distribution seen in multiple sclerosis. Reproduced courtesy of Dr J. Bingham.

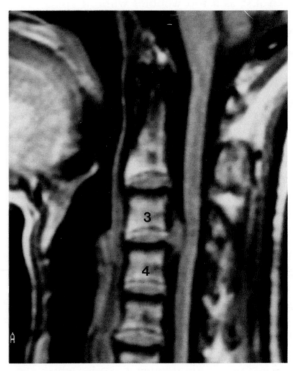

**Figure 9.21** Magnetic resonance imaging of the spine. A sagittal image of the cervical spine and spinal cord in a patient with a disc protrusion. The disc at C3/C4 protrudes posteriorly causing an anterior impression on the spinal cord. Reproduced courtesy of Dr J. Bingham.

*Answer to the puzzle in Fig. 9.16b*
The answer to the CT diagram in Fig. 9.16b is:

| 1 | 2 |
|---|---|
| 3 | 4 |

# Oncology

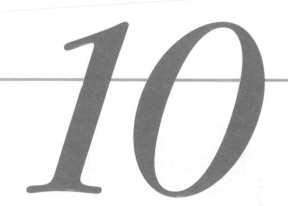

**10**

# *I*NTRODUCTION

Twenty-five per cent of all deaths are from cancer and in the UK, an estimated one in three people will develop cancer during their lifetime, with 70 per cent of all cancers developing over the age of 60.

Only a few tumour types are responsible for more than half of all new cases, with lung cancer accounting for 16 per cent, colon and rectum 11 per cent, skin excluding melanoma 11 per cent, breast cancer (almost entirely in women) 10 per cent and stomach 5 per cent. The incidence of the leading malignancies for men and women in the UK are set out in Table 10.1.

In terms of mortality Britain has the unenviable position of leading the world in terms of deaths from breast cancer and Scotland has the highest rate of death from lung cancer. The ten most frequent causes of cancer death for men and women are set out in Table 10.2. Lung cancer alone causes 25 per cent of all *cancer* deaths (6 per cent of *all* deaths), in addition colon and rectal cancer account for 12 per cent, breast cancer 9 per cent (20 per cent of female cancer deaths) and stomach cancer 7 per cent of all cancer deaths.

Thirty per cent of all cancer deaths have been attributed to tobacco smoking (a proportion of lung, mouth, pharynx, larynx, oesophagus, bladder, pancreas and kidney).

Epidemiological studies have established the association between a number of environmental factors and the incidences of different types of cancer. The association is strong with regard to smoking and lung cancer and between sunlight and melanoma. Less clear is why there is an eight-fold variation in incidence rates worldwide in breast cancer. Japanese women have low breast cancer rates but the second and subsequent generations of those who migrate to the USA have the same high rates as their host population. (Standard mortality rates 5.8 versus 22.1.) This suggests that social and environmental factors have an impact over and above genetic factors.

In classical multistage models for carcinogenesis the various stages of cancer development can be described as initiation, promotion and progression. In initiation a few cells are exposed to a threshold level of carcinogen and are primed to become cancer cells. Promotion occurs after further exposure to the carcinogen or to a promoting agent. Eventually in the later stages the tumour can progress to a more malignant pheno-

**Table 10.1** New cases of malignancy in the UK in 1985.

|  | Male | | | Female | | |
|---|---|---|---|---|---|---|
|  | **Number** | **%** | **Rank** | **Number** | **%** | **Rank** |
| All (253 111) | 119 961 | 100 |  | 133 150 |  |  |
| Lung | 29 340 | 24 | 1 | 11 490 | 9 | 3 |
| Breast | 199 | – | 27 | 25 140 | 19 | 1 |
| Skin | 14 320 | 12 | 2 | 12 620 | 9 | 2 |
| Prostate | 10 820 | 9 | 3 | – | – | – |
| Colon | 7490 | 6 | 6 | 9230 | 7 | 4 |
| Ovary | – | – | – | 5020 | 5 | 5 |
| Bladder | 7760 | 6 | 4 | 2999 | 2 | 11 |
| Stomach | 7450 | 6 | 5 | 4860 | 4 | 6 |
| Cervix | – | – | – | 4500 | 3 | 8 |
| Rectum | 5890 | 5 | 7 | 4640 | 3 | 7 |
| Uterus | – | – | – | 3770 | 3 | 9 |
| Pancreas | 3180 | 3 | 8 | 3240 | 2 | 10 |
| Oesophagus | 2760 | 2 | 9 | 2075 | 1 | 14 |
| Non-Hodgkin's lymphoma | 2670 | 2 | 10 | 2458 | 1 | 12 |

**Table 10.2** UK top 13 cancer deaths in 1988.

| | Male | | Female | |
|---|---|---|---|---|
| | **Number** | **%** | **Number** | **%** |
| All neoplasms | 84 640 | | 77 920 | |
| Lung | 27 970 | 33 | 12 260 | 16 |
| Breast | 81 | – | 15 300 | 20 |
| Prostate | 8230 | 10 | – | – |
| Colon | 5860 | 7 | 7110 | 9 |
| Stomach | 6320 | 7 | 4290 | 6 |
| Ovary | – | – | 4280 | 5 |
| Bladder | 3670 | 4 | 1693 | – |
| Pancreas | 3280 | 4 | 3510 | 5 |
| Rectum | 3570 | 4 | 2920 | 4 |
| Oesophagus | 3360 | 4 | 2230 | 4 |
| Non-Hodgkin's lymphoma | 2035 | 3 | 1886 | 2 |
| Cervix | – | – | 2170 | 2 |
| Brain | 1660 | 2 | 1280 | 1 |

type. Uncontrolled proliferation is an important event in the oncogenic cascade and genes are implicated in the control of cell proliferation, for example, **oncogenes** and **tumour suppressor genes**. Such proliferation not only increases the chances of acquiring more genetic damage but is also essential for the expansion of an aggressive subclone of cells. To possess metastatic potential a cell has to be able to invade the surrounding tissue, spread via the lymphatics and/or the bloodstream, leave that system, that is extravasate, and then multiply at secondary sites. Genes involved in cell attachment, motility and proteolytic degradation of the extracellular matrix are likely to be important in this process.

It is this ability of the cells of a cancer to spread and form new foci of growth that represents its most malignant characteristic and is responsible for the majority of cancer deaths. The site of such metastasis will relate to both haemodynamic factors and the selective growth of cells in certain organs. Whilst lung, liver, lymph nodes and brain are the most common sites of spread, the lesser more specific sites led Paget in 1889 to propose the 'soil and seed' hypothesis that differing tumour cell/host organ interactions could occur which were more or less favourable for metastatic development.

The identification of the genetic steps associated with the onset and progression of cancer is now the focus of molecular oncological research.

# ONCOGENES, TUMOUR FORMATION AND PROGRESSION

Oncogenes have been traditionally defined as genes able to confer on cells the property of unregulated growth. Oncogenes are derived from 'proto-oncogenes', their genetic counterparts which are found normally in all mammalian cells and generally play a role in the normal process of cell growth and differentiation. When proto-oncogenes undergo alteration their function may change from the normal control of growth and differentiation to the promotion of neoplastic development. This was originally assessed on the basis of their ability to induce transformation to a malignant phenotype in tissue culture or tumour 'genecity' when cells expressing those genes were introduced into animals. All species have numerous genes (oncogenes) which may be homologous to transforming oncogenes carried by specific RNA retroviruses. Some human tumours have mutations in these oncogenes which may have led to their activation. Such genes appear to be probable candidates for direct-acting germ line mutations predisposing to malignancy, however there is no evidence for germ line mutations in oncogenes.

Examples of oncogenes include *rasH* (Harvey ras) and *myc*. The *rasH* oncogene was originally cloned from a cell line derived from a human bladder carcinoma. This oncogene is very similar to the transformintg gene of the murine retrovirus, the Harvey sarcoma virus. The cellular oncogene and the retroviral transforming gene (*V-rasH*) are both closely related to a normal cellular gene the *C-rasH* proto-oncogene. The cellular proto-oncogene becomes the oncogene via the acquisition of any of several well-defined point mutations in its coding regions. In mouse embryo cell lines transformation with the *rasH* oncogene can induce those cells to metastasize. Further investigations in transfected cell lines confirmed that *rasH* did have significant effects on the properties of tumour progression. Furthermore, such cells acquired great irradiation and chemotherapy resistance.

The genetic changes associated with malignancy can not only lead to increased activity of a protein that can have a positive effect on the unrestrained growth of cells – oncogenes, but can lead to a decreased activity of a protein whose role is to restrain growth. These genes, several of which have been identified, are called tumour suppressor genes. It is becoming increasingly apparent that loss of tumour suppressor genes is widespread. The initial observation by Knudson concerned retinoblastoma. He postulated that in both familial (developing at a median age of 14 months, bilateral and frequently familial) and sporadic (developing at a median age of 2.5 years, no family history) cases single tumour cells carried two genetic changes which had to occur for malignant growth to begin. It subsequently became apparent that the mutations proposed were two copies of a genetic abnormality on chromosome 13, the Rb gene. These mutations *inactivated* the Rb gene cells by deletion from the chromosome or by more subtle mutations resulting in alteration of a small number of DNA bases. Its inactivation plays a part in osteosarcomas, small cell lung cancer, and some bladder and breast carcinomas. The p53 gene is another gene that in some circumstances can negatively regulate the cell cycle. Initially found in cells transformed by the simian tumour virus as the p53 protein (molecular weight 53 kD) it was classified as a tumour antigen but complementary DNA p53 clones turned out to be mutant forms of p53, able to act in a dominant negative fashion, binding to 'wild' or natural p53 protein, thereby releasing growth inhibitory signals. Normal cells may shut down their proliferation in a number of ways. Tumour suppressor genes (and their encoded protein) are part of the machinery enabling the cell to stop proliferating. Their neturalization by a genetic mutation removes this brake, interfering with the normal differentiation of the cells and their planned senescence and death (apoptosis). A study of families with the Li-Franmeni syndrome where high rates of cancer in a variety of organs are present has shown a mutant allele of the p53 suppressor gene. Its presence is closely linked to cancer susceptibility in individual family members.

Mutations in oncogenes appear to be restricted to somatic cells. Many mutations result in instability of the genome and lead indirectly to a high degree of risk. An example of this is the autosomal recessive disease xeroderma pigmentosum, sufferers of which have a well-documented defect in their ability to repair DNA damage caused by ultraviolet light and some chemical agents. This defect leads to a high incidence of various types of skin cancer, presumably as a failure to repair lesions caused by the ultraviolet components of sunlight. Chronic myeloid leukaemia (CML) was the first malignancy in which a reproducible chromosomal abnormality was described. The leukaemic cells contain a unique small chromosome called the Philadelphia chromosome (Ph), an abnormality of chromosome 22 derived from a reciprocal translocation between chromosomes 22 and 9. This leads to an alteration of the *abl* oncogene. The *abl* gene moves from chromosome 9 to 22 and the *sis* gene from 22 to 9. The translocation results in the production of an abnormal form of the *abl* protein.

In Burkitt's lymphoma, the common translocations involving chromosome 8 and chromosomes 2, 14, or 22 result in the relocation of the *myc* oncogenes near to genes which code for a constant region of the immunoglobulin heavy chain gene on chromosome 14.

Little information is available about chromosomal abnormalities in solid tumours although there are known abnormalities in subsets of ovarian tumours (translocation of 6:14), meningiomas (single chromosome 22), some small cell lung cancer tumours and neuroblastomas.

Dominantly inherited cancers are known and include retinoblastoma, adenopolyposis of colon and rectum, Wilm's tumour, basal cell naevus syndrome, neurofibromatosis, multiple endocrine adenomatosis syndrome and neuroblastoma. In these tumours a precise chromosomal location has been established for genes where mutation leads to malignancy. It is likely that other tumours, indeed most cancers, will probably have an inherited subgroup and further studies will reveal this.

# *T*HE MALIGNANT CELL

Normal tissue may be classified into cells which are constantly 'renewing' their population, for instance, bone marrow and the intestinal mucosa, those that 'proliferate' slowly but may repair in response to injury, for example, lung and liver, and those that are 'static', for example, nerve and muscle. The renewing tissues represent cells produced by differentiation and cell division from a small number of stem cells. In response to various signals, these stem cells proliferate with expansion of the population and production of numerous differentiated cells. The cell renewal system is under control so the loss of mature functional cells is balanced by production of new cells. Stem cells therefore have to generate a large family of descendants which will perform the function of the tissue and they must also demonstrate the property of self-renewal so that their own numbers are not depleted in the process. Tissues with self-renewal capacity may undergo expansion either with (**metaplasia**) or without (**hypoplasia**) changes in the proportion of differentiated cells. An example of this might be the endometrium in response to hormonal changes during the menstrual cycle and in the skin condition psoriasis. These benign processes are reversible. When neoplastic change occurs the response is permanent and inherited by subsequent generations of cells. Tumour growth is therefore related to changes in the control of cell proliferation and differentiation which can be inherited.

Tumours grow because they contain a population of cells which is expanding as a result of cell division and they differ from normal tissue because that population of tumour cells fails to respond effectively to the natural control mechanisms maintaining the appropriate number of cells in the renewal tissue.

Experimental evidence from stem cell assays does support in some tumours a possible monoclonal origin. Particular examples cited include multiple myeloma, chronic lymphatic leukaemia, non-Hodgkin lymphomas and T-cell lymphomas. However, the evidence in solid tumours is still limited.

Tumour cells with a high rate of mutation, and the selection of mutant subclones with a growth advantage, may lead to the progression of tumours with more malignant properties. The growth of cells in tissue culture certainly depends on the presence of growth factors and recent experiments have linked the properties of growth factors with those of oncogenes and suggested a relationship between malignancy and many mechanisms which control cell proliferation in normal tissues. Epidermal growth factor (EGF) for instance has homology with the product of the *V-erb-B* oncogene, platelet-derived growth factor (PDGF and PDGF-like peptides) has structural homology to the product of the *V-cis* oncogene of the simian sarcoma virus, transforming growth factor-alpha is structurally related to EGF and can compete with it as an agonist for the receptor.

A human solid tumour cannot be detected when it is a single cell, indeed after 30 doublings when it will weigh approximately 1 g and contains $10^9$ cells it is the smallest clinically detectable mass. After a further three doublings, it will be some 10 g in size and contain $10^{10}$ cells and is usually detectable, certainly within lung tissue. After seven further doublings the tumour would weigh approximately 1 kg and contain $10^{12}$ cells which is estimated to be the maximum mass of a malignant tumour compatible with life.

Tumour growth has been determined by serial measurements and is said to be exponential when the rate of cell production and cell loss are proportional to the number of cells present in the population. Such growth often leads to the false impression that the rate of tumour growth is accelerating, however three volume doublings will increase a tumour from 0.1 to 1 cm in size and similarly from 5 to 10 cm in size in the same period of time.

The aggressiveness of a given tumour type is frequently reflected in the 5-year survival rate. Primary liver cancer (hepatoma), oesophageal, gastric and lung cancer are all considered to be very aggressive with an overall 5-year survival rate below 20 per cent. Survival is not only a reflection of the aggression (growth fraction) of the tumour but also depends on which particular organ is affected. Liver and brain metastases have a poor prognosis on the whole. It must be remembered however that 5-year survival rates do not necessarily reflect curability (Table 10.3). The most common forms of cancer amongst men (prostatic cancer) and women (breast cancer) are both characterized by a high overall 5-year survival rate of 72 and 62 per cent, respectively, even in cases in which patients present with distant metastases (30 and 19 per cent, respectively). Such tumours once they have metastasized are controllable rather than curable.

# PRINCIPLES OF MANAGEMENT

At the time of first referral to a department of oncology the majority of patients will have a previous diagnosis of cancer, however a small but increasing proportion of patients are being referred for assessment before formal diagnosis.

Twenty-five per cent of the population will die of cancer or with cancer and it is very important that at the time of the first assessment clear communication is established as to what is suspected, routine procedures that will need to be completed, and as to how the results of tests and investigations will be discussed. An open and honest appraisal of the situation, and an understanding of the worries of the patient and their family can do much to help at that difficult time.

**Table 10.3** Percentage of patients alive 5 years from registration in the UK.

| 50% or more | 10–49% | Less than 10% |
|---|---|---|
| Bladder | Bone | Gall bladder (F) |
| Breast | Brain | Liver |
| Cervix | Colon | Lung |
| Connective tissue | Kidney | Oesophagus |
| Eye | Gall bladder (M) | Pancreas |
| Hodgkin's disease | Leukaemia (all types) | Pleura |
| Larynx | Mouth | Stomach |
| Melanoma | Multiple myeloma | |
| Placenta | Non-Hodgkin's lymphoma | |
| Prostate | Ovary | |
| Skin | Pharynx | |
| Thyroid | Rectum | |
| Testis | Small intestine | |
| Uterus | | |

# Investigations, staging and prognosis

It cannot be stressed too much that all investigations should be *relevant* to the clinical situation of that particular patient. This will require an immediate assessment as to the patient's general condition which can be reflected numerically as a performance score (Table 10.4), age, other general medical problems, the nature of the tumour and the clinical evidence of metastasis. If the liver is clearly enlarged with features typical of metastasis and deranged liver function tests, it would usually be unnecessary to perform liver ultrasound or computed tomography (CT) to assess it. Similarly, scanning of the thorax would usually be irrelevant if there are multiple metastases on a plain chest X-ray film.

Staging investigations are used to assess the primary tumour and the local and distant metastases where (1) there are relevant treatment options and (2) the general medical situation makes such an assessment pertinent in guiding further treatment or prognosis.

The conventional method of staging assesses the tumour (T), lymph node metastasis (N) and evidence of metastasis beyond local lymph nodes and to other organs (M) (the TNM system). **The 'TNM' system** has proved widely applicable in guiding prognosis in the majority of solid tumours but is not relevant to lymphomas or leukaemias where separate staging annotations are used. In carcinoma of the colon Duke's staging is commonly reported according to the depth of invasion, nodal involvement, trans-colonic spread and distant metastasis (A, B, C and D).

An example of the TNM staging system for lung cancer is set out in Table 10.5.

**Table 10.4** Performance score.

**Karnofsky performance scale**

| Able to carry on normal activity; no special care is needed | 100 | Normal; no complaints; no evidence of disease |
| | 90 | Able to carry on normal activity; minor signs or symptoms of disease |
| | 80 | Normal activity with effort; some signs or symptoms of disease |
| Unable to work; able to live at home and care for most personal needs; a varying amount of assistance is needed | 70 | Cares for self; unable to carry on normal activity; or to do active work |
| | 60 | Requires occasional assistance but is able to care for most of own needs |
| | 50 | Requires considerable assistance and frequent medical care |
| Unable to care for self; requires equivalent of institution or hospital care; disease may be progressing rapidly | 40 | Disabled; requires special care and assistance |
| | 30 | Severely disabled; hospitalization is indicated although death not imminent |
| | 20 | Very sick; hospitalization necessary; active supportive treatment is necessary |
| | 10 | Moribund; fatal processes progressing rapidly |
| | 0 | Dead |

**Table 10.5** TNM staging system: lung cancer stage and prognosis.*

**Tumour (T)**

| TX | Occult carcinoma (malignant cells in sputum or bronchial washings, but tumour not visualized by imaging studies or bronchoscopy) |
| T1 | Tumour $\leq$3 cm in greatest diameter, surrounded by lung or visceral pleura, but not proximal to a lobar bronchus on bronchoscopy |
| T2 | Tumour >3 cm in diameter, or with involvement of main bronchus at least 2 cm distal to carina, visceral pleural invasion, or associated atelectasis or obstructive pneumonitis extending to the hilar region but not involving the entire lung |
| T3 | Tumour invading chest wall, diaphragm, mediastinal pleura, or parietal pericardium; or tumour in main bronchus within 2 cm of but not invading the carina; or atelectasis or obstructive pneumonitis of entire lung |
| T4 | Tumour invading mediastinum, heart, great vessels, trachea, oesophagus, vertebral body, or carina; or ipsilateral malignant pleural effusion |

**Nodes (N)**

| N0 | No regional lymph-node metastases |
| N1 | Metastases to ipsilateral peribronchial or hilar nodes |
| N2 | Metastases to ipsilateral mediastinal or subcarinal nodes |
| N3 | Metastases to contralateral mediastinal or hilar nodes or to any scalene or supraclavicular nodes |

**Distant metastases (M)**

| M0 | No distant metastases |
| M1 | Distant metastases |

| **Stages** | | **5-year survival** |
|---|---|---|
| Occult | TXN0M0 | |
| Stage I | T1–2N0M0 ⎱ | |
| Stage II | T1–2N1M0 ⎰ | 40% |
| Stage IIIa | T3N0–1M0 ⎱ | |
| | T1–3N2M0 ⎰ | |
| Stage IIIb | T4N0–2M0 ⎱ | 4–8% |
| | T1–4N3M0 ⎰ | |
| Stage IV | TX–4N0–3M1 | <1% |

*Modified from Beahrs et al.

## THE PRIMARY TUMOUR (T STAGING)

The size and position of the tumour are assessed in association with its attachments. Overall T stage gives an indication as to whether or not a primary tumour is resectable but such assessment has to take place in the light of the further staging of nodes and distant organs.

## NODAL ASSESSMENT (N)

The relevance of local nodal involvement compared to more distant nodal involvement is assessed. This will need interpreting according to the primary tumour site, ipsilateral local nodes being acceptable in, for instance, primary lung tumour where they can be resected along with the tumour, however fixed nodes or more distant nodes would clearly carry a graver prognosis and would render surgery inappropriate.

## METASTASIS (M)

The site, number and size of metastases are relevant to guiding prognosis and the presence of metastases usually renders radical surgery with curative intent inappropriate.

## STAGING TECHNIQUES

The assessment of the primary tumour and its local lymph nodes where relevant has become increasingly sophisticated and accurate with the introduction of the imaging techniques, ultrasound, computed axial tomographic scanning and magnetic resonance imaging (MRI). In addition the new techniques such as positron emission tomography (PET) are being introduced. In nuclear medicine the basic techniques are being rapidly widened with the development of further isotope linkages for both diagnosis and treatment. An example of this is the use of $^{125}$I-metaiodo *bis*-guanidine ($^{125}$I-MIBG) in the diagnosis and treatment of adrenal tumours. The majority of patients will have as their initial investigations a chest X-ray and routine haematological and biochemical evaluations.

The haematological investigations may reveal anaemia, the presence or absence of iron deficiency, the presence of abnormal cells or a shift of the film to more primitive cells suggesting the possibility of marrow invasion, a raised sedimentation rate etc. The routine biochemical tests should include measurement of liver function, of lactic dehydrogenase (a surprisingly useful tumour marker), of renal function and of serum calcium and phosphate. The use of tumour markers, for example, $\alpha$-fetoprotein (AFP) and the $\beta$ subunit of human chorionic gonadotrophin ($\beta$HCG) in the diagnosis and follow-up of germ cell tumours, CA125 in the follow-up of patients with ovarian cancer, CA19-9 in colon cancer and carcinoembryonic antigen (CEA) in many tumours are helpful and at the time of presentation, if abnormal, they can prevent irrelevant investigation.

## DIAGNOSTIC ULTRASOUND

Ultrasound offers a non-invasive method of assessment and in experienced hands can offer considerable information concerning anatomical structures such as the thyroid, breast, liver, spleen, kidneys, lymph nodes and pelvis. It can be used both as the primary method of assessment and also to assess response to treatment. Such comparisons are very useful indeed but are not always completely reproducible between operators.

## COMPUTED TOMOGRAPHY

Computed tomographic scanning revolutionized the non-invasive investigation techniques and remains complementary to the later introduction of magnetic resonance imaging and positron emission scanning. It is able to assess the resectability of primary tumours, and the presence of secondaries in other organs and nodes. Imaging has had a major impact on diagnosis and staging, replacing many 'diagnostic' thoracotomies and laparotomies, whilst encouraging therapeutic surgery. Nevertheless, the clinical situation always needs interpreting in the light of all these studies and if there is any doubt the potentially curative operation should be attempted.

## MAGNETIC RESONANCE IMAGING

This is of particular importance in imaging the central nervous system and the spinal cord. It is also proving very helpful in the assessment of bone and bone marrow disease. It gives good definition of anatomical structures. It offers additional information to the CT scan.

## CHOICE OF IMAGING MODALITY

The imaging department should be consulted on the best approach to assessing difficult situations. The techniques now available are numerous. 'Cost' and 'relevance' are very important factors and *appropriate* use of any particular imaging technique will help in preventing long waiting times.

## RADIOLOGICALLY GUIDED BIOPSY

Increasing use is being made of the departments of radiology to perform guided biopsies of liver, lung nodules, bone, adrenal glands etc. Such biopsies can take place under fluoroscopic, CT or ultrasound guidance.

# Investigations and treatment options

The curability of a tumour will depend on the tumour type, its position, the presence or absence of metastasis and the general condition of the patient taking into account past medical history, age etc. Extensive investigations for metastases from an adenocarcinoma of unknown primary will be irrelevant and are seldom helpful. One must exclude a thyroid primary, in women breast carcinoma and in men prostatic cancer. For all these there are specific treatment possibilities. In the general screen for an adenocarcinoma of unknown primary extensive CT scanning and barium studies will usually prove unhelpful.

## THE CANCER CLINIC

The treatment of cancer requires an interdisciplinary approach with close cooperation between surgeon, radiation oncologist, medical oncologist and clinical haematologist. These units must integrate closely with the family practitioner and, where relevant, the department of social services, home care services and hospice teams are also necessary for optimum management.

Traditionally, surgeons have been the first to treat the cancer patient, however, new treatment approaches have created important roles for the radiotherapist and medical oncologist in their primary management.

## MULTIDISCIPLINARY CLINICS

In an ideal situation the multidisciplinary clinic focussed on tumour type will give the optimal service. Such clinics need not be needlessly protracted but notes can be reviewed, staging investigations planned, relevant biopsies obtained and pathology reviewed. The array of alternatives for the treatment of cancer is constantly expanding as new chemotherapeutic, biological and physical therapies become available to treat with both palliative and (it is to be hoped) curative intent.

Where possible, existing standard treatment strategies should be used. Where relevant, clinical trials, both local and national, should be entered into. Such trials inevitably generate work and especially paper work but are essential for the continuing audit of results and for the development of new appropriately based treatments. Such clinical trials will of necessity have the approval of the local Research Ethics Committees and will be performed to the guidelines laid down in good clinical practice. All relevant information must be provided.

The welfare of the patient is the predominant issue and the basis for the trial must be carefully set out and appropriate informed consent obtained.

## DRUGS IN CANCER TREATMENT

In some disseminated cancers chemotherapy and combination chemotherapy have proved curative. The MOPP combination of mustine, vincristine, procarbazine and prednisolone in the treatment of Hodgkin's disease saw an immediate major improvement in the survival of these patients such that in stage III or IV disease it is now expected that a cure rate of 50 per cent or greater will be achieved, with an overall 5-year survival rate of 67 per cent. Similar cure rates are achievable in diffuse high-grade non-Hodgkin's lymphoma (stage III or IV), in childhood acute lymphocytic leukaemia, Burkitt's lymphoma, Wilms' tumour and childhood sarcomas. In testicular carcinoma stage III and IV a 75 per cent or greater cure rate will be achieved and in gestational choriocarcinoma greater than 90 per cent. Five-year survival rates for a number of tumours are set out in Table 10.3.

The cure rate for the majority of metastatic solid tumours is less but significant achievements are being made in the palliation of many tumours with chemotherapy and a careful assessment has to be made of the benefits of response and the negative effects of treatment toxicity, time spent in hospital etc. Examples of significant palliation include the treatment of ovarian carcinoma, small cell lung cancer and gastric cancer.

Combination chemotherapy with curative intent is now used for (1) **remission induction**, (2) **consolidation therapy** (maintenance therapy) and (3) in the **adjuvant** setting in patients who have had primary tumours resected and who are at risk of a recurrence. Adjuvant chemotherapy regimens have significantly extended the survival of patients with breast cancer and osteosarcoma. Neoadjuvant chemotherapy has been used to reduce the bulk of primary tumours before surgical resection or irradiation in head and neck, breast and cervical cancers.

The design of drug treatment regimens is based on a number of considerations, the most important of which is prior knowledge of the responsiveness of such tumours to specific drugs. This knowledge will have been acquired through clinical trials both non-randomized (early phase II trials) and randomized trials (phase III and IV). In planning such regimens cell kinetic, pharmacokinetic and biochemical considerations will be taken into account.

## CHEMOTHERAPY, CELLULAR KINETICS AND DRUG RESISTANCE

The cell cycle is depicted in Fig. 10.1. Immediately after cell division (M) there is a period when little appears to happen. This is called the $G_1$ phase. Cells which are not dividing at all may

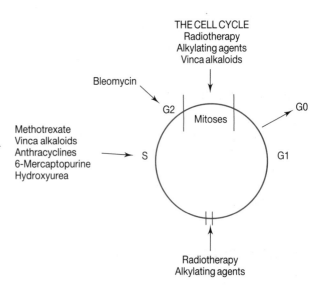

**Figure 10.1** Mitosis, prophase, metaphase, anaphase, telophase: pairs of chromosomes separate. Cell division: G0 = resting phase; G1 = early growth phase: S = DNA synthesis – chromosome material doubled; G2 = later growth phase – premitosis phase.

enter a resting phase during $G_1$ which is termed $G_0$. Following this there is a period in which DNA synthesis takes place during which time the DNA content of the cell is doubled. This is called the S-phase. Following this there is another period termed $G_2$ before mitosis takes place and actually leads to cell division. Experimental evidence shows that the antimetabolites exert lethal toxicity only to cells which are synthesizing DNA whereas cyclophosphamide and doxorubicin have maximum toxicity at this point (S) but have some activity during other phases of the cycle. The vinca alkyloids, vincristine and vinblastine, are known to disrupt formation of the mitotic spindle leading to arrest of cells in mitosis, however, they also exert their lethal effect when cells are in the S-phase when formation of the mitotic spindle is initiated. Many alkylating agents, for example, cyclophosphamide, ifosfamide, melphalan and nitrogen mustard, have a similar phase activity to that of radiation therapy, with two peaks of maximum lethal activity, one at the $G_2$–M phase and one near the $G_1$–S phase boundary. Bleomycin acts mainly in the $G_2$ phase and mitosis, while cisplatin may have greatest activity in some cells in the $G_1$ phase. The nitrosureas (best considered an alkylating agent) also have an activity on resting cells.

Drugs such as methotrexate or vincristine are called *phase-specific* drugs. A drug such as an alkylating agent which acts by cross-cycle linking the DNA can do so at any phase of the cell cycle although the damage will only become apparent during the replication of the DNA. Drugs like this are called *cycle specific*. Their action is more dose dependent but not so much affected by the schedule of administration.

## Cellular kinetics

The fractional cell kill hypothesis has been defined experimentally. This states that a given drug concentration applied for a defined time would kill a constant fraction of the cell population independent of the absolute numbers of cells, therefore each treatment cycle kills a specific fraction of the remaining cells.

In practical terms, by the time a tumour is clinically recognized it will contain a high fraction of non-dividing ($G_0$) to dividing cells, due to many factors including the effect on growth of poor vascularity (the tumour has outgrown its blood supply), hypoxia, competition for nutrients and other unidentified factors. An initially slowly responding tumour may become more responsive to therapy as reduction in cell numbers produced by surgery, radiotherapy or the anticancer agents stimulate the slowly dividing cells into more rapid cell division where they will become increasingly susceptible to treatment.

Counterbalancing the above effects is the demonstration that human tumours are composed of cell types with differing biochemical, morphological and drug response characteristics. This heterogenicity presumably results from mutation of the original tumour line and accounts for the development of resistant tumour cells during relapse of formally sensitive tumours. There is a high likelihood of the presence of drug-resistant mutants at the time of clinical presentation. Such a model would lead to the suggestion that the earliest possible use of non-cross-resistant drugs is essential so that double mutants cannot be selected by sequential chemotherapy. The corollary would be that doses of drugs should be administered as frequently as possible to achieve maximum cell kill of both sensitive and moderately resistant cells.

## Drug resistance

The development of multidrug resistance does occur and considerable work is taking place in overcoming such mechanisms. The P170 membrane glycoprotein which mediates the eflux of vinca alkyloids, anthracyclines, actinomycin-D and epipodophylotoxin has been identified. Resistance appears to be due to decreased intracellular drug levels and this action can be reversed experimentally by the use of calcium channel blockers. A further important cause of multiple drug resistance is mediated by altered drug binding to topoisomerase-II, an enzyme believed to promote DNA strand breaks in the presence of anthracyclines, podophylotoxins etc. Other mechanisms of resistance include, with the alkylating agents, an increase in the proficiency of repair of DNA; with the antimetabolites an increase in levels of target enzymes causing a decrease in drug activation and increase in drug degradation.

## Drug intensity

Dose intensity is important to attain maximum drug kill. This is usually expressed as $mg/m^2$ of drug administered/unit time (usually per week). What is clear is that if the patient requires treatment then the correct dose should be delivered on time. The reasons for any dose modification should be noted and should fall within clear guidelines. All drug combination regimens require dose adjustments when compared to a drug used as a single agent and such compromises in dose have to be appropriate. Dose reductions for toxicity have to be built into schedules and less frequently dose escalations are also included.

The conventional routine protocol demands combination chemotherapy given on a fixed schedule, however, an alternative to this policy is the concept of alternating regimens with non-cross-resistant groups of maintenance therapy after induction of remission. This has proved successful in preventing relapse in childhood acute lymphoblastic leukaemia but maintenance therapy has not improved survival in the majority of solid tumours.

## *Dose escalation, bone marrow transplantation and support*

Dose escalation can be performed where the predicted toxicities can be overcome. Where bone marrow toxicity is the predominant problem this can be ameliorated by bone marrow support programmes. Marrow stem cells are harvested prior to the intensive treatment and reinfused intravenously following the clearance of the cytotoxic agent. Bone marrow support can be from the same patient (autologous) or, as used in leukaemic patients, from a matched donor (allogenic).

The development of **haematopoietic growth factors** is significantly changing clinical practice. Following the observation almost 25 years ago that colonies containing mature neutrophils would develop when haematopoietic cells were immobilized in a soft gel matrix and provided with media conditioned by the growth of non-haematopoietic cells, considerable effort went into isolating and characterizing the factors involved. Recombinant DNA technology has now allowed the isolation of the genes coding for the colony-stimulating factors (CSFs) and the production of large amounts of protein using bacterial, yeast and mammalian cell systems. Granulocyte colony-stimulating factor (G-CSF), macrophage colony-stimulating factor (M-CSF), granulocyte macrophage colony-stimulating factor (GM-CSF) and interleukin-3 (multi CSF) have been developed in addition to the established erythropoietin. These allow the amelioration of neutropenia and the use of priming doses with or without chemotherapy has lead to the technique of peripheral stem cell harvesting, whereby stem cells are harvested from peripheral blood and can be reinfused in a similar way to bone marrow reinfusion. Current studies are also demonstrating a faster engraftment for patients supported with peripheral blood stem cells when compared to bone marrow stem cells, and of course the physical discomfort of bone marrow harvesting is avoided.

## TOXICITY OF CHEMOTHERAPY

In the past there have been horrific accounts of the toxicity of chemotherapy such that patients have refused treatment in a potentially curative situation.

The side effects will be considered in general although the potential severity of the problem will vary from drug schedule to drug schedule. Individual drugs have specific toxicities but the majority will have some effect on nausea and vomiting, alopecia, mucositis and malaise.

## *The side effects of cytotoxic chemotherapy*

The nature of these agents is to have a profound effect on the proliferating cancer cell and not surprisingly there is also a marked effect on normal tissues. The general side effects include nausea and vomiting, mucositis, alopecia and malaise. More specific side effects will be discussed under the individual groups of agents.

## *Nausea and vomiting*

Table 10.6 sets out the cytotoxics in order of their association with vomiting. Vomiting may be shortly after the delivery of the cytotoxic or may be delayed. Delay may be 6–8 hours in the case of cyclophosphamide and sometimes may be experienced some days later as a recall phenomenon (particularly with *cis*-platinum). If vomiting is not controlled then 'anticipatory'

**Table 10.6** Cytotoxic drugs in the order of their association with vomiting.

| Chemotherapeutic agent | Emetogenicity |
|---|---|
| Cisplatin | Most emetogenic |
| Dacarbazine | |
| Dactinomycin | |
| Cyclophosphamide | |
| Lomustine | |
| Carboplatin | |
| Doxorubicin | |
| Daunorubicin | to |
| Cytarabine | |
| Procarbazine | |
| Etoposide | |
| Mitomycin-C | |
| 5-Fluorouracil | |
| Hydroxyurea | |
| Bleomycin | |
| Vinblastine | |
| Vincristine | |
| Chlorambucil | Least emetogenic |

nausea and vomiting can occur, for instance on the way to hospital or clinic making treatment less and less tolerable.

For many patients prolonged nausea is a more troublesome side effect than acute vomiting.

In the past, the antiemetics commonly used were metoclopramide (Maxolon), domperidone (Motilium) and corticosteroids. There is no doubt that the addition of corticosteroids to the standard antiemetics did lead to a substantial improvement. The recent development of the histamine type III receptor agonists ($HT_3$ receptor blockers) ondansetron and granisetron have led to a substantial improvement in the tolerability of many chemotherapy regimens. Previously some blockade of these receptors within the gut could take place with very high doses of metoclopramide although with the risk of developing extrapyramidal side effects. The $HT_3$ antagonists have proved very able in controlling the nausea and vomiting of intermediate and severely emetogenic protocols. Combinations with corticosteroids are impressive and they are equally effective on the emesis of radiotherapy.

## Alopecia

Hair loss (scalp, eyebrows, eye lashes, beard) is a significant morbidity associated with some chemotherapeutic regimens. The hair loss of the anthracycline group may be ameliorated by scalp cooling which allows the first pass effect of the drug to bypass the hair follicles in the cooled area by contraction of the blood supply. For alkylating agents, for instance cyclophosphamide and ifosfamide and for etoposide, the half-life of the respective drugs makes this inappropriate. In combination chemotherapy regimens therefore scalp cooling is not appropriate or satisfactory.

Where alopecia is likely appropriate advice must be given to the patient and a wig service provided. It is very debilitating at a time when the patient feels very vulnerable.

## Malaise

Chemotherapy undoubtedly is associated with tiredness. This can be lessened by careful control of nausea and vomiting and the judicious use of corticosteroids during the immediate post-treatment period. Patients must be advised to live within their energy level and will need more rest than before treatment.

## Mucositis

The development of a sore mouth and change in taste is frequent with cytotoxics. The taste may be particularly associated with drugs which are excreted in the saliva. The whole of the gastro-intestinal tract is at risk of mucositis. Rhinorrhoea is also frequently seen.

## Specific side effects

The vinca alkyloids are associated with a largely sensory peripheral neuropathy which may be marked. The dose must be attenuated or stopped where appropriate. Cisplatin is also associated with neuropathy both in terms of the 8th cranial nerve (high tone hearing loss) and a sensory and motor peripheral neuropathy. Appropriate dose reductions and curtailment need to be practiced.

Bleomycin is associated with pulmonary fibrosis. The anthracyclines are associated with cardiotoxicity. Alkylating agent metabolites may be associated with chemical cystitis which can be severe.

Many agents are vesicant if the intravenous cannula is insecurely placed. Chemical burns will result from their extravasation and this is particularly reviewed under the specific drugs involved, for example, anthracyclines and vinca alkaloids.

## THE DRUGS AVAILABLE

Table 10.7 shows the anticancer drugs in common usage.

## Alkylators

The use of nitrogen mustard, the original alkylating agent, is now largely confined to the treatment of Hodgkin's disease as part of the MOPP protocol. Chlorambucil is often substituted for this. Melphalan has a more profound effect on the stem cell and may be used in bone marrow conditioning programmes prior to bone marrow transplantation and is also used in the treatment of haematopoietic tumours. The alkylators cyclophosphamide and ifosfamide are converted by the liver into active metabolites and have activity against a wide variety of tumours. Ifosfamide appears to have greater activity against testicular cancer and soft tissue sarcomas. Melphalan has been widely used in the treatment of ovarian carcinoma, multiple myeloma and breast carcinoma. Chlorambucil is most widely used in the treatment of chronic lymphatic leukaemia, lymphomas and ovarian carcinoma. The usual dose-limiting toxicity of alkylating agents is bone marrow suppression with degree, time course and cellular pattern varying from alkylator to alkylator. They are toxic to gonadal function and careful consideration must be given to alternative treatments in young patients. They are associated with lung fibrosis and may sensitize the lung to subsequent radiotherapy leading to radiation fibrosis. Cyclophosphamide and ifosfamide are also associated with haemorrhagic cystitis largely due to the excretion of the metabolite acrolein. This effect is ameliorated by the sulphhydral donating compound mercaptoethane sulphonate (mesna) which can be given orally or intravenously. Alopecia is dose and schedule dependent.

The late development of second malignancies may be seen particularly in the development of acute leukaemia.

**Table 10.7** Anticancer drugs.

| Alkylating agents | Intercalating agents |
|---|---|
| Nitrogen mustard | Doxorubicin (Adriamycin) |
| Melphalan | Daunorubicin |
| Chlorambucil | Epirubicin |
| Cyclophosphamide | Mitoxantrone |
| Ifosfamide | |
| Bisulphan | **Nitrosoureas** |
| | CCNU |
| **Platinum compounds** | BCNU |
| Cisplatin | TCNU |
| Carboplatin | |
| | **Miscellaneous** |
| **Antimetabolites** | Dacarbazine |
| Methotrexate | Procarbazine |
| 5-fluorouracil | Hexamethylmelamine |
| 6-mercaptopurine | Bleomycin |
| 6-thioguanine | |
| Cytosine arabinoside | **Podophyllotoxins** |
| | Etoposide |
| **Spindle poisons** | Teniposide |
| Vincristine | |
| Vinblastine | |
| Vindesine | |
| Taxol | |
| Navelbine | |

## Anthracyclines

The anthracyclines are second only in their spectrum of activity to the alkylating agents. They are commonly used in the combination chemotherapy of epithelial tumours, for example, breast and lung cancer, the lymphomas, leukaemias, myeloma and sarcomas.

If they extravasate from the intravenous cannula all members of the group are vesicants, however this is less with epirubicin. Care must be taken in preventing this problem and with siting of the cannula away from joints. If extravasation does occur the severe local injury can continue to progress over weeks or months as the drug has been shown to bind locally to tissues. Skin grafting is not successful unless preceded by extensive excision of the involved tissue, however, debridement should be undertaken with extreme caution in the initial phases of extravasation injury. A wide range of treatments have been used immediately after extravasation including ice, steroids and bicarbonate. Most recently the substance DMH3, a powerful reductant, has proved useful.

Cardiotoxicity particularly in children is seen as both an acute and chronic toxicity. A range of arrhythmias including heart block, pericarditis, myocarditis and an accumulative cardiotoxicity can be seen in young and old. The risk of cardiotoxicity is minor at a total dose of doxorubicin below 350 mg or daunomycin below 700 mg. Above these doses the risk steadily accelerates. For epirubicin the accumulative doses are higher. Recent work suggests that the cardiotoxic risk is a function of peak drug level and not of area under the curve and appropriate alterations in schedule can be helpful. The development of the investigational agent ICRF 187 has dramatically reduced the cardiotoxicity in one series of patients treated for breast cancer although with some potentiation of the toxicity on bone marrow.

## Vinca alkyloids, antimetabolites and platinums

The spindle poisons, vincristine, vinblastine and vindesine and the newer agent navelbine, are derived from the periwinkle plant. The older agents are associated with peripheral neuropathy, the first symptom of which is paraesthesiae of the fingers or toes. The vinca alkaloids are associated with tissue destruction if the drug extravasates during treatment and great care must be taken to prevent this.

Methotrexate acts by depleting the cell of tetrahydrofolic acid and its action may be readily reversed by the administration of folinic acid which replenishes the tetrahydrofolate pool. Very high doses can therefore be used where necessary and normal tissues protected by folinic acid rescue.

5-Fluorouracil features widely in the treatment of gastrointestinal tumours and is part of the classic CMF regimen for the treatment of breast cancer (cyclophosphamide, methotrexate, 5-fluorouracil). An understanding of its pharmacology has lead to its use by continuous infusion rather than by short bolus treatment and also to prolonging its activity by means of pharmacological manipulation with folinic acid and with methotrexate.

The platinum compounds have exceptional activity in testicular and ovarian cancer and also have a wide spectrum of activity. Cisplatin is associated with severe nausea and vomiting although this can be controlled by the 5-hydroxytryptamine type III receptor blockers. Renal toxicity can be severe and pre- and post-hydration are essential to ameliorate this. Glomerular filtration rate should be decided prior to each dose which is adjusted accordingly. High tone hearing loss and indeed sensory neuroal deafness can occur, as can sensory—motor peripheral neuropathy. Renal tubular damage may lead to profound magnesium loss. It is not particularly marrow suppressive. The side effects of carboplatin are much reduced although it is more myelosuppressant.

The podophylotoxins, etoposide and teniposide, have shown excellent activity in the treatment of testicular cancers, lymphomas and lung cancer. The side effects are myelosuppression and hair loss.

Dacarbazine causes little myelosuppression but may cause marked nausea and vomiting. It is predominantly used in the treatment of Hodgkin's disease and melanoma. Procarbazine where antitumour action is via decarboxylation is also a weak monoaminoxidase inhibitor and side effects may include an adverse reaction to alcohol. It is used in the treatment of Hodgkin's disease. Bleomycin has activity in testicular tumours and squamous carcinomas. It is associated with pulmonary fibrosis, fevers, rigors, hair loss and pain at the injection site.

## THE ENDOCRINE THERAPIES

Oestrogens have been known to play an important role as promotors of human breast tumours for more than 60 years. Breast cancers depend on these hormones as a key growth factor and may either recruit circulating (endocrine or paracrine) oestrogens or produce oestrogens themselves (autocrine production). Autocrine oestrogen accounts for a substantial proportion of the required oestrogens in most but not all breast tumours. The oestrogens bind to cytoplasmic proteins, the oestrogen receptors (ERs). In the cell nucleus the complex activates genes which promote cell division. The oestrogen dependence of breast tumours calls for an antagonistic endocrine therapy. Such an approach is possible by (1) blocking the hormonal cascade at the pituitary level, (2) blocking the conversion of precursors into oestrogens, and (3) blocking oestrogen effects at the target organs.

Before the menopause the main source of oestrogen is the ovaries where luteinizing hormone stimulates the theca cell resulting in the production of progesterone and androgen precursors of the oestrogen. In the ovarian granulosa cell these precursors are then converted into oestrogen by aromatization via the aromatase enzymes and stimulated by follicle-stimulating hormone. Negative feedback mechanisms between ovary, pituitary and hypothalamus regulate gonadotrophin levels. After the menopause the ovaries stop producing oestrogens and the negative feedback ceases therefore luteinizing hormone, follicle-stimulating hormone and adrenocorticotrophin (ACTH) levels rise as do the oestrogen precursor levels. Oestrogens are then produced in peripheral tissues, especially in fat and muscle tissue by aromatization of androstene dione and peripheral aromatase activity is enhanced.

The anti-oestrogen tamoxifen has become a standard first-line hormonal therapy for both premenopausal and postmenopausal metastatic breast cancer and is now used also as part of adjuvant therapy for both groups. It and its related compounds have multiple actions competing with oestrodiol for binding to oestrogen receptors and promoting a tight association between the receptor and the nuclear component. There is also evidence of distant tamoxifen cytoplasmic binding sites that do not bind oestrogens. It appears to block the cells in the mid-$G_1$ phase, that is, it is a cell-cycle phase-specific cytostatic and cytotoxic agent. It also stimulates the production of tumour growth factor-beta (TGF-$\beta$). It has minimal long-term toxicities although it is associated with amenorrhoea and hot flushes due to its anti-oestrogenic effects, nausea with occasional vomiting, hypercalcaemia (in patients with bone metastases, 'flare reaction'), with possibly an increase in ovarian cysts. Overall, its safety profile is excellent with very occasional reports of changing liver function tests and thrombophlebitis, and there is continuing evaluation as to whether it causes depletion of bone mineral content in the long term.

### The aromatase inhibitors

Oestrogens are produced in the ovaries and are also derived by aromatization of circulating adrenal androgens in peripheral tissues such as fat, muscle, and liver and breast tumours.

Aminoglutethamide, an inhibitor of cholesterol conversion to pregnenolone, together with dexamethasone has been used as a medical 'adrenalectomy'. The major action of the drug is blockade of peripheral aromatization. It achieves this action by binding to the aromatase enzyme (type 1 reaction) and also by interfering with a broad spectrum of steroid hydroxylators by binding to cytochrome P450 (type 2). Aromatase inhibitors are capable of both significantly lowering the level of circulating oestrogen and blocking autocrine oestrogen production by the tumour.

Responses in metastatic breast cancer have been observed in approximately 40 per cent of women. The side effects of aminoglutethamide include lethargy in about 40 per cent and ataxia in 10 per cent. These soporific side effects usually resolve after about 6 weeks of treatment. A maculopapular skin rash appears in about one-third of patients and may well resolve spontaneously. Dizziness, leg cramps, facial

fullness, weight gain and nausea are also seen. Thrombocytopenia is the most common haematological side effect, usually within 3 to 7 weeks of starting therapy. There have been case reports of deaths due to septicaemia and marrow aplasia. White cell and platelet counts should be checked at weeks 4, 8 and 12 after starting therapy.

New aromatase inhibitors such as 4-hydroxy-androstene dione (4-OHA) have been developed which are not only highly potent but also highly specific and hence very well tolerated. They have no oestrogen agonistic effects and no cross-resistance with anti-oestrogen. It is possible that in some premenopausal women the combination of gonadotrophin-releasing hormone analogues with an aromatase inhibitor may be superior to such analogues alone.

### Progesterones

Medroxyprogesterone acetate is commonly used for treating breast and endometrial carcinoma. Its mechanism is unknown but hypotheses include a direct cytotoxic effect, associated changes in hormone level (gonadotrophins, cortisol, DHE and oestrodiol), a decrease of oestrogen receptors, its androgenic properties, the production of growth inhibitory factors and the inhibition of induced protein.

Toxicity includes a major increase in appetite and weight gain with or without fluid retention, mild hypertension, the possibility of congestive heart failure, fatigue, rash, oedema, sweating and diabetes. In women there may be vaginal spotting, amenorrhoea and changes in menstrual flow with hot flushes and in men impotence, hot flushes, headache, insomnia, nausea and phlebitis. Central nervous system effects, cholestatic jaundice, alopecia, acne, hirsuitism and thromboembolic disorders are all seen. Certainly caution should be used in patients with conditions that could be aggravated by fluid retention or with a history of thromboembolism.

## RADIOTHERAPY

The main action of radiation therapy is damage to DNA through the production of reactive radicals, the effect is greatest on rapidly dividing cells. When therapeutic radiation is given the fields of radiation and the doses are carefully controlled. The radiation field is planned on the basis of clinical examination and imaging techniques, the radiosensitivity of the tumour and the normal tissues in the radiation beam. Because of the position of most tumours some normal tissue will be in the field.

The most sensitive normal tissues are those with quickly dividing stem cells, for example, the bone marrow, gut mucosa and skin. Bone marrow suppression, diarrhoea, malabsorption, erythema and hair loss may result from irradiation. Other tissues with slower cell turnover can be affected by ischaemia secondary to damage to blood vessels by irradiation, for example, lung and brain. More general effects of nausea, vomiting and systemic upset are not prominent.

Tumours also vary in their radiosensitivity. Lymphoma, seminoma, Wilm's tumour and myeloma are relatively sensitive, others such as melanoma and osteosarcoma are resistant. The radiation dose is usually most effective and least toxic when given in multiple fractions. In some circumstances the radioactive source is placed in a tumour or body cavity to emit radiation locally (**brachytherapy**). An example of this technique is the use of the isotope $^{137}$Cs in carcinoma of the cervix. Isotopes which are preferentially taken up by certain organs can be used to deliver radiation selectively, for example, $^{131}$I in carcinoma of the thyroid. In addition, $^{131}$I may be used to damage non-neoplastic thyroid tissue in the treatment of hyperthyroidism (page 520).

The total absorbed radiation dose is measured in gray (Gy) where one gray is one joule of energy per kg of tissue (previous units were rads, 1 Gy = 100 rad).

# GENERAL MANAGEMENT

Most patients with cancer are told of the diagnosis. This is particularly important when decisions on the treatment to be used are being made. Although the outlook of different cancers varies enormously and other diseases may have equivalent prognoses the diagnosis of cancer produces a considerable impact on patients and their families. Communication of the diagnosis and support of the patient and family require sympathy, time, expertise and a coordinated approach from the whole medical team. The patient must be given a chance to absorb the information and to come back with further questions. Trained counsellors play an important role in most oncology units and some have a psychiatrist attached. When no further attempts at curative treatment are planned more time needs to be given to the patient to talk about their condition and any fears for the future. Most fears about intractable terminal pain and distress can be allayed.

Weight loss is prominent in many cancer patients because of loss of appetite, local tumour growth (e.g. stomach cancer) and the effects of treatment. High calorie oral supplements may help to maintain nutrition during radiotherapy or chemotherapy and may speed recovery.

Coordinated support is essential during active treatment and when no cure is available. Palliative treatment is usually possible. This may involve the treatment of nausea or breathlessness but most often relates to pain relief which could be local radiotherapy, nerve block or analgesia. The hospice movement in the UK has contributed a great deal to rational pain relief in cancer stressing the need for adequate regular analgesia anticipating pain rather than reacting to it. In this way pain can be adequately controlled in the great majority of patients. Symptom control nurses play an important role in the management of patients at home, and hospices are available in most areas with staff trained in the care of terminally ill patients. The psychological and spiritual needs of the patient will also need careful attention.

Most patients with cancer will die of their disease despite treatment but their family may need continued support after the death. Bereavement counselling can be very helpful.

# ADJUVANT CHEMOTHERAPY

The use of systemic chemotherapy for the control of metastatic disease is well known. Chemotherapy used to treat patients who have undergone complete resection of a cancer with no evidence of residual disease is more difficult. The benefits of such 'prophylactic' chemotherapy has to be balanced against the toxicity.

Controlled clinical trials in breast cancer suggested that significant benefits could be attained and this has recently been confirmed by an overview (meta) analysis. A review of all available randomized trials which began before 1985, in the treatment of early breast cancer with adjuvant tamoxifen, cytotoxic chemotherapy, radiotherapy or ovarian ablation included approximately 40000 women in 100 randomized trials. With early breast cancer the overall reduction in the odds of death during the first 5 years was 16 per cent for tamoxifen versus no tamoxifen with a $P$ value less than 0.00001 and 11 per cent for chemotherapy versus no chemotherapy with a $P$ value of 0.0003. It should be stressed that this is an actual reduction in mortality. What is clear from this and subsequent analysis is that six cycles of adjuvant chemotherapy is as good as treatment of any longer duration. The way forward is open for combinations of hormone therapy and chemotherapy.

The need for adjuvant therapy also arises in soft tissue sarcoma, osteogenic sarcoma, Duke's B and C colon cancer and various solid tumours of childhood. In these tumours adjuvant chemotherapy appears to be of use in stages of growth when tumour burden is least, whereas in advanced disease chemotherapy is seldom curative. Further large randomized studies are needed in many tumour types to define this role.

# *Conclusion*

This chapter has by design limited discussion of the place of surgery and radiotherapy in the treatment of cancer. Medical oncology is part of a multidisciplinary approach to the treatment of tumours and of prime importance is the appropriate use of surgery and radiotherapy. For localized tumours, for example, colorectal, gastro-oesophageal, head and neck, breast cancer and sarcomas the results of surgery and/or radiotherapy are outstanding. The treatment of cancer is, however, a multidisciplinary process and medical oncologists, surgeons and radiotherapy oncologists must work closely in collaboration. The use of postoperative adjuvant chemotherapy and radiotherapy have built on the results of surgery alone and are essential in the treatment of many tumours. This integration will be discussed in the following chapters. Particular relevance to this integrated approach is seen in the treatment of breast cancer where surgeon, medical oncologist and radiation oncologist work closely together in the treatment of primary disease to allow, where possible, less aggressive surgery to give equivalent or better results than mastectomy alone. Determination of nodal status, endocrine status (pre- or postmenopausal) and receptor status of the tumour itself (oestrogen and progesterone receptors), the size of the tumour and the grade of the tumour will all help to define a treatment strategy which is appropriate for a particular patient.

There have been many developments in the treatment of cancer over the last decade but the opening of the next decade is even more exciting. New chemotherapeutic drugs are becoming available, both less toxic analogues of previously known drugs and the development of agents with novel modes of action. Examples of these are taxol and taxotere which are both derived from the Pacific yew tree whose mode of action is on the mitotic spindle where inhibition of assembly causes mitotic arrest. The overcoming of tumour resistance by action on topoizomerase two is a real possibility. An understanding of the molecular basis of the oncogenic process may allow specific correction of defects and correction of risk factors, inherited or acquired, and may lower the incidence of cancer. Smoking must be actively discouraged by social and fiscal methods and the dramatic rise in melanoma halted by care in exposure of the susceptible to the sun.

The developments of the growth factor, erythropoeitin, granulocyte colony-stimulating factor (G-CSF), granulocyte monocytic colony-growth factor (GM-CSF), and multigrowth factor (interleukin-6, IL-6) (M-CSF) will all help lessen the toxicity of current treatment and their use in bone marrow and stem cell support programmes will allow intensified treatment to be given more safely.

Perhaps, the most glittering prize of all will be the molecular manipulation of the tumour cell with perhaps correction of oncogene and suppressor activity fundamentally altering the ability of the tumour cell to grow, invade and metastasize.

# Disorders of the Cardiovascular System

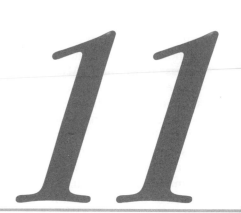

**11**

# INTRODUCTION

During this century the pattern of cardio-vascular disease in the industrialized world has changed considerably. Syphilitic and tuber-culous involvement of the cardiovascular system is now rare, and the incidence of rheumatic disease is declining. Myocardial and conducting tissue disease, on the other hand, are being diagnosed more frequently and the importance of arterial hypertension is well recognized. Nevertheless, it is coronary artery disease that has emerged as the major cardiovascular disorder of the present era. Indeed, this 'modern epidemic' has long been the single most common cause of premature death in Europe and North America. Coupled with the long-standing observations that smoking, obesity and hyper-tension are linked to coronary artery disease comes the new knowledge of a genetic pre-disposition to the development of atheroma.

Although the development of angioplasty and coronary artery bypass grafting are successful in relieving the symptoms and increasing life expectation when appropriately used in coronary artery disease these methods are treating only the end of the chain of aetiological factors. The basic aetiology of atheroma remains unknown, and so fundamental treatment is still elusive. This is not to gainsay the success that community-based programmes of sensible diet, exercise and reducing smoking can have in reducing the frequency of this condition. An even more challenging area of prevention is to reduce the development of coronary artery disease in third world countries in which the incidence of this disease is rising due to smoking and the adaptation of western-type diets.

Major recent advances in the investigation and management of heart disease include tech-niques of imaging and assessing cardiac function by echocardiography and radionuclides, and the successful development of heart transplantation, mainly by improvements in immunosuppres-sion, so that length and quality of survival following this operation are now acceptable.

# SYMPTOMS OF HEART DISEASE

## Chest pain

Common cardiovascular causes of chest pain are myocardial ischaemia, pericarditis and aortic dissection.

### MYOCARDIAL ISCHAEMIA

This results from an imbalance between myocar-dial oxygen supply and demand and produces pain called **angina** (Table 11.1). Angina is usually a symptom of coronary artery disease which impedes myocardial oxygen supply. The history is diagnostic if the location of the pain, its character, its relation to exertion and its duration are typical. The patient describes retro-

**Table 11.1** Causes of angina.

### Impaired myocardial oxygen supply
Coronary artery disease
  Atherosclerosis
  Arteritis in connective tissue disorders
Coronary artery spasm
Congenital coronary artery disease
  Arteriovenous fistula
  Anomalous origin from pulmonary artery
Severe anaemia

### Increased myocardial oxygen demand
Left ventricular hypertrophy
  Hypertension
  Aortic valve disease
  Hypertrophic cardiomyopathy
  Thyrotoxicosis
Tachyarrhythmias

sternal pain which may radiate into the arms, the throat or the jaw. It has a constricting character, is provoked by exertion and relieved in a few minutes by rest. When coronary occlusion produces myocardial infarction the pain is similar in location and character but is usually more severe and more prolonged, often lasting for hours.

## PERICARDITIS

This also causes central chest pain which is sharp in character and aggravated by deep inspiration, cough or movement. The pain may be relieved by sitting up. It may last several days.

## AORTIC DISSECTION

This produces tearing pain in either the front or the back of the chest. The onset is abrupt, unlike the crescendo quality of ischaemic cardiac pain.

# Dyspnoea

Dyspnoea is an abnormal awareness of breathing occurring either at rest or at an unexpectedly low level of exertion. Left heart failure is the major cardiac cause but mechanisms are complex. In acute pulmonary oedema and **orthopnoea**, dyspnoea is due mainly to the elevated left atrial pressure that characterizes left heart failure (page 160). This produces a corresponding elevation of the pulmonary capillary pressure and increases transudation into the lungs, which become oedematous and stiff. The extra effort required to ventilate the stiff lungs causes dyspnoea. In exertional dyspnoea, however, other mechanisms apart from changes in left atrial pressure are also important (see below).

## EXERTIONAL DYSPNOEA

This is the most troublesome symptom in heart failure. Exercise causes a sharp increase in left atrial pressure and this contributes to the pathogenesis of dyspnoea by causing pulmonary congestion (see above). However, the severity of dyspnoea does not correlate closely with exer-

tional left atrial pressure and other factors must therefore be important. These include respiratory muscle fatigue and the stimulation of peripheral chemoreceptors by exertional acidosis. As left heart failure worsens exercise tolerance deteriorates. In advanced disease the patient is dyspnoeic at rest.

## ORTHOPNOEA

Lying flat causes a steep rise in left atrial pressure in patients with heart failure, resulting in pulmonary congestion and severe dyspnoea. To obtain uninterrupted sleep extra pillows are required, and in advanced disease the patient may choose to sleep sitting in a chair.

## PAROXYSMAL NOCTURNAL DYSPNOEA

Frank pulmonary oedema on lying flat wakens the patient from sleep with distressing dyspnoea and fear of imminent death. The symptoms are corrected by sitting or standing upright which allows gravitational pooling of blood to lower the left atrial pressure.

# Fatigue

Exertional fatigue is an important symptom of heart failure and is particularly troublesome towards the end of the day. It is caused partly by deconditioning and muscular atrophy through lack of use but also by inadequate oxygen delivery to exercising muscle, reflecting impaired cardiac output.

# Palpitation

Awareness of the heart beat is common during exertion or heightened emotion. Under other circumstances it is often symptomatic of cardiac arrhythmia. A description of the rate and rhythm of the palpitation is essential. The pause or the forceful beat that follows an ectopic beat may be noticed by introspective individuals but does not necessarily signify important disease. Rapid irregular palpitation is typical of atrial fibrillation. Rapid regular palpitation occurs in atrial, junctional and ventricular tachyarrhythmias.

# Dizziness and syncope

Cardiovascular disorders produce dizziness and syncope by transient hypotension resulting in abrupt cerebral hypoperfusion. Recovery is usually rapid, unlike other common causes of syncope (e.g. stroke, epilepsy, overdose).

## POSTURAL HYPOTENSION

Syncope on standing upright reflects inadequate baroreceptor-mediated vasoconstriction. It is common in the elderly. Abrupt reductions in blood pressure and cerebral perfusion cause the patient to fall to the ground, whereupon the condition corrects itself.

## VASOVAGAL SYNCOPE

Autonomic overactivity in response to emotional or painful stimuli causes vasodilation and inappropriate slowing of the pulse. These combine to reduce blood pressure and cerebral perfusion. Recovery is rapid if the patient lies down.

## CAROTID SINUS SYNCOPE

Exaggerated vagal discharge following external stimulation of the carotid sinus (e.g. a tight shirt collar) causes reflex vasodilation and slowing of the pulse. These combine to reduce blood pressure and cerebral perfusion.

## VALVAR OBSTRUCTION

Fixed valvar obstruction in aortic stenosis may prevent a normal rise in cardiac output during exertion, such that the physiological vasodilation that occurs in exercising muscle produces abrupt reduction in blood pressure and cerebral perfusion, resulting in syncope. Intermittent obstruction of the mitral valve by left atrial tumours (usually myxoma) may also cause syncopal episodes.

## STOKES–ADAMS ATTACKS

These are caused by self-limiting episodes of asystole or rapid tachyarrhythmias (including ventricular fibrillation). The loss of cardiac output causes syncope and striking pallor. Following restoration of normal rhythm recovery is rapid and is associated with flushing of the skin as flow through the dilated cutaneous bed is re-established.

# SIGNS OF HEART DISEASE

# Oedema

Oedema which pits on digital pressure is a cardinal feature of congestive heart failure. It is caused by salt and water retention by the kidney. Two mechanisms are responsible:

1 Reduced sodium delivery to the nephron. This is caused by reduced glomerular filtration caused by constriction of the preglomerular arterioles in response to sympathetic activation and angiotensin II production.

2 Increased sodium reabsorption from the nephron. This is the more important mechanism. It occurs particularly in the proximal tubule early in heart failure but, as failure worsens, renin angiotensin activation stimulates aldosterone release which increases sodium reabsorption in the distal nephron.

Salt and water retention expands plasma volume and increases the capillary hydrostatic pressure. Hydrostatic forces driving fluid out of the capillary exceed osmotic forces reabsorbing it, so that oedema fluid accumulates in the interstitial space. The effect of gravity on capillary hydrostatic pressure ensures that oedema is most prominent around the ankles in the ambulant patient and over the sacrum in the bedridden patient. In advanced heart failure oedema may involve the legs, genitalia and trunk. Transudation into the peritoneal cavity (ascites) and the pleural and pericardial spaces may also occur.

# Cyanosis

Cyanosis is a blue discolouration of the skin and mucous membranes caused by increased concentration of reduced haemoglobin in the superficial blood vessels.

## PERIPHERAL CYANOSIS

This may result when cutaneous vasoconstriction slows the blood flow and increases oxygen extraction in the skin and the lips. It is physiological during cold exposure. It also occurs in heart failure when reduced cardiac output produces reflex cutaneous vasoconstriction most easily seen in the fingers. In mitral stenosis, cyanosis over the malar area produces the characteristic mitral facies.

## CENTRAL CYANOSIS

This results from the reduced arterial oxygen saturation caused by cardiac or pulmonary disease and can be detected when there is more than 2 g of desaturated haemoglobin. It affects not only the skin and the lips but also the mucous membranes of the mouth. Cardiac causes include pulmonary oedema (which prevents adequate oxygenation of the blood) and congenital heart disease. Congenital defects associated with central cyanosis include those in which desaturated venous blood bypasses the lungs by right-to-left ('reversed') shunting through septal defects or a patent ductus arteriosus (e.g. Fallot's tetralogy, Eisenmenger's syndrome).

# Coldness of the extremities

In patients with heart disease this is an important sign of reduced cardiac output. It is caused by reflex vasoconstriction of the cutaneous bed. Measurement of skin temperature provides a useful indirect means of monitoring cardiac output in patients with heart failure undergoing treatment in the coronary care unit.

# Clubbing of the fingers and toes

In congenital cyanotic heart disease clubbing is not present at birth but develops during infancy and may become very marked. Another cardiac cause of clubbing is infective endocarditis.

# Arterial pulse and blood pressure

The arterial pulses should be palpated for evaluation of rate, rhythm, character and symmetry.

## RATE AND RHYTHM

By convention, both rate and rhythm are assessed by palpation of the right radial pulse. If this is not palpable the carotid pulse should be felt instead. Rate, expressed in beats per minute, is measured by counting over a timed period of 15 seconds. Normal sinus rhythm is regular but in young patients may show phasic variation in rate during respiration (**sinus arrhythmia**). An irregular rhythm usually indicates atrial fibrillation but may also be caused by frequent ectopic beats. In patients with atrial fibrillation the rate should be measured by auscultation at the cardiac apex because beats that follow very short diastolic intervals may create a 'pulse-deficit' by not generating sufficient pressure to be palpable at the radial artery.

## CHARACTER

This is defined by the volume and waveform of the pulse and should be evaluated at the right carotid artery, i.e. the pulse closest to the heart and least subject to damping and distortion in the arterial tree. Pulse volume provides a crude indication of stroke volume, being small in heart failure and large in aortic regurgitation. The waveform of the pulse is of greater diagnostic importance. Aortic stenosis produces a slowly rising carotid pulse; in aortic regurgitation, on the other hand, the large stroke volume vigorously ejected produces a rapidly rising carotid pulse which collapses in early diastole

owing to back flow through the aortic valve. In mixed aortic valve disease a **bisferiens pulse** with two systolic peaks is occasionally found. **Pulsus alternans** – alternating high and low systolic peaks – occurs in severe left ventricular failure but the mechanism is unknown. **Pulsus paradoxus** – an inspiratory decline in systolic pressure greater than 10 mm Hg – occurs in cardiac tamponade and, less frequently, in constrictive pericarditis and obstructive pulmonary disease. It represents an exaggeration of the normal inspiratory decline in systolic pressure and is not, therefore, truly paradoxical.

## SYMMETRY

Symmetry of the radial, brachial, carotid, femoral, popliteal and pedal pulses should be confirmed. An absent pulse indicates an obstruction more proximally in the arterial tree, caused usually by atherosclerosis or thromboembolism. Coarctation of the aorta causes symmetrical reduction and delay of the femoral pulses compared with the radial pulses.

# MEASUREMENT OF BLOOD PRESSURE

Blood pressure is measured indirectly by sphygmomanometry. Supine and erect measurements should be obtained to provide an assessment of baroreceptor function. A cuff (at least 40 per cent of the arm's circumference) is attached to a mercury or aneroid manometer and inflated around the extended arm. Auscultation over the brachial artery reveals five phases of **Korotkoff sounds** as the cuff is deflated:

| | |
|---|---|
| Phase 2 and 3 | The first appearance of the sounds marking systolic pressure |
| Phases 2 and 3 | Increasingly loud sounds |
| Phase 4 | Abrupt muffling of the sounds |
| Phase 5 | Disappearance of the sounds |

Phase 5 provides a better measure of diastolic blood pressure than phase 4, not only because it corresponds more closely with directly measured

diastolic pressure, but also because its identification is less subjective. Nevertheless, in those conditions where Korotkoff sounds remain audible despite complete deflation of the cuff (aortic regurgitation, arteriovenous fistula, pregnancy) phase 4 must be used for the diastolic measurement.

# Jugular venous pulse

Fluctuations in right atrial pressure during the cardiac cycle generate a pulse which is transmitted backwards into the jugular veins. It is best examined while the patient reclines at 45°. If the right atrial pressure is very low, however, visualization of the jugular venous pulse may require a smaller reclining angle. Alternatively, manual pressure over the upper abdomen may be used to produce a transient increase in venous return to the heart which elevates the jugular venous pulse (hepatojugular reflex).

## JUGULAR VENOUS PRESSURE

The normal upper limit is 4 cm vertically above the sternal angle. This is about 9 cm above the right atrium and corresponds to a pressure of 6 mm Hg. Elevation of the jugular venous pressure indicates elevation of the right atrial pressure unless the superior vena cava is obstructed, producing engorgement of the neck

**Table 11.2** Causes of elevated jugular venous pressure.

Congestive heart failure
Cor pulmonale
Pulmonary embolism
Right ventricular infarction
Tricuspid valve disease
Tamponade
Constrictive pericarditis
Hypertrophic/restrictive cardiomyopathy
Superior vena cava obstruction
Iatrogenic fluid overload, particularly in surgical and renal patients

veins (Table 11.2). During inspiration the pressure within the chest falls. This allows an increase in venous return to the right heart and thus a fall in the jugular venous pressure. In constrictive pericarditis, and less commonly in tamponade, inspiration produces a paradoxical rise in the jugular venous pressure (**Kussmaul's sign**) because the increased venous return cannot be accommodated within the constricted right side of the heart.

## WAVEFORM OF JUGULAR VENOUS PULSE

The jugular venous pulse has a flickering character caused by 'a' and 'v' waves separated by 'x' and 'y' descents. The 'a' wave produced by atrial systole precedes tricuspid valve closure. It is followed by the 'x' descent (marking descent of the tricuspid valve ring) which is interrupted by the diminutive 'c' wave as the tricuspid valve closes. Atrial pressure then rises again, producing the 'v' wave as the atrium fills passively during ventricular systole. The decline in atrial pressure as the tricuspid valve opens to allow ventricular filling produces the 'y' descent. Important abnormalities of the pattern of deflections are shown in Fig. 11.1.

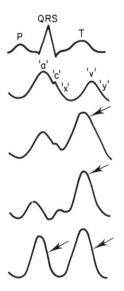

ECG. Electrical events precede mechanical events. Thus the P wave and QRS complex of the ECG precede the "a" and "v" waves, respectively, of the JVP.

NORMAL JVP. The "a" wave is usually the most prominent deflection. The "x" descent is interrupted by the small "c" wave marking tricuspid valve closure.

GIANT "V" WAVE ( Arrowed ). This is an important sign of tricuspid regurgitation. The regurgitant jet produces pulsatile systolic waves in the JVP.

CANNON "a" WAVE ( Arrowed ). This is caused by atrial systole against a closed tricuspid valve It occurs when the atrial and ventricular rhythms are dissociated ( e.g. complete heart block ) and marks coincident atrial and ventricular systole.

PROMINENT "x" and "y" DESCENTS ( Arrowed ). These occur in constrictive pericarditis and give the JVP an unusually dynamic appearance. In tamponade only the "x" descent is exaggerated.

**Figure 11.1** Waveform of the jugular venous pulse.

# EXAMINATION OF THE HEART

## Inspection

Chest wall deformities such as pectus excavatum should be noted because these may compress the heart and displace the apex, giving a spurious impression of cardiac enlargement. Large ventricular or aortic aneurysms may cause visible pulsations. Vena caval obstruction is associated with prominent venous collaterals on the chest wall. Prominent venous collaterals around the shoulder occur in axillary or subclavian vein obstruction.

## Palpation

The location of the apical impulse inferior or lateral to the fifth intercostal space or the midclavicular line, respectively, usually indicates cardiac enlargement. Palpable third and fourth heart sounds give the apical impulse a double thrust. In the past, considerable importance has been attached to the character of the apical impulse ('thrusting' in aortic valve disease, 'tapping' in mitral stenosis) but this is of very limited value in differential diagnosis.

Left ventricular aneurysms can sometimes be palpated medial to the cardiac apex. Right ventricular enlargement produces a systolic thrust in the left parasternal area. The turbulent flow responsible for heart murmurs may produce palpable vibrations ('thrills') on the chest wall, particularly in aortic stenosis, ventricular septal defect and patent ductus arteriosus.

## Auscultation

The diaphragm and bell of the stethoscope permit appreciation of high- and low-pitched sounds, respectively. The apex, lower left sternal edge, upper left sternal edge and upper right sternal edge should be auscultated in turn. These locations correspond to the mitral, tricuspid, pulmonary and aortic areas, respectively, and loosely identify sites at which sounds and murmurs arising from the four valves are best heard.

### FIRST SOUND (S1)

This corresponds to mitral and tricuspid valve closure at the onset of systole. It is accentuated in mitral stenosis because prolonged diastolic filling through the narrowed valve ensures that the leaflets are widely separated at the onset of systole. Thus valve closure generates unusually vigorous vibrations. In advanced mitral stenosis the valve is rigid and immobile and S1 becomes soft again.

### SECOND SOUND (S2)

This corresponds to aortic and pulmonary valve closure following ventricular ejection. S2 is single during expiration. Inspiration, however, causes physiological splitting into aortic followed by pulmonary components because increased venous return to the right side of the heart delays pulmonary valve closure. Important abnormalities of S2 are illustrated in Fig. 11.2.

### THIRD AND FOURTH SOUNDS (S3, S4)

These low-frequency sounds occur early and late in diastole, respectively. When present they give a characteristic 'gallop' to the cardiac rhythm. Both sounds are best heard with the bell of the stethoscope at the cardiac apex. They are caused by abrupt tensing of the ventricular walls following rapid diastolic filling. Rapid filling occurs early in diastole (S3) following atrioventricular valve opening and again late in diastole (S4) due to atrial contraction. S3 is physiological in children and young adults but usually disappears after the age of 40. It also occurs in high-output states caused by anaemia, fever, pregnancy and thyrotoxicosis. After the age of 40, S3 is nearly always pathological, usually indicating left ventricular failure or, less commonly, mitral regurgitation or constrictive pericarditis. S4 is sometimes physiological in the elderly. More commonly, however, it is pathological and occurs when vigorous atrial contraction late in diastole is required to augment filling of a hypertrophied, non-compliant ventricle (e.g. hypertension, aortic stenosis, hypertrophic cardiomyopathy).

## SYSTOLIC CLICKS AND OPENING SNAPS

Valve opening, unlike valve closure, is normally silent. In aortic stenosis, however, valve opening produces a click in early systole which precedes the ejection murmur. The click is only audible if the valve cusps are pliant and non-calcified and is particularly prominent in the congenitally bicuspid valve. A click later in systole suggests mitral valve prolapse, particularly when followed by a murmur. In mitral stenosis, elevated left atrial pressure causes forceful opening of the thickened valve leaflets. This generates a snap early in diastole which precedes the mid-diastolic murmur.

## HEART MURMURS

These are caused by turbulent flow within the heart and great vessels and may indicate valve disease. Heart murmurs – defined by loudness, quality, location, radiation and timing – may be depicted graphically (Fig. 11.3).

The loudness of a murmur reflects the degree of turbulence. This relates to the volume and velocity of flow and not the severity of the cardiac lesion. Loudness is graded on a scale of 1 (barely audible) to 6 (audible even without application of the stethoscope to the chest wall). The quality of a murmur relates to its frequency and is best described as low, medium or high pitched. The location of a murmur on the chest wall depends on its site of origin and has led to the description of four valve areas (see above). Some murmurs radiate, depending on the velocity and direction of blood flow. The high-velocity systolic flow in aortic stenosis and mitral regurgitation, for example, is directed towards the neck and the axilla, respectively. The high-velocity diastolic flow in aortic regurgitation is directed towards the left sternal edge. Murmurs are timed according to the phase of systole or diastole during which they are audible (e.g. mid-systolic, pan-systolic, early diastolic).

Murmurs may occur without underlying heart disease. 'Innocent' murmurs of this type are common in children. In adults they usually reflect hyperkinetic circulation in conditions such as anaemia, fever, pregnancy and thyrotoxicosis, which lead to turbulent flow in the aortic or pulmonary outflow tracts. They also occur quite commonly in hypertension. Innocent murmurs are always mid-systolic in timing, are rarely louder than grade 3, may vary with posture and are not associated with other signs of heart disease.

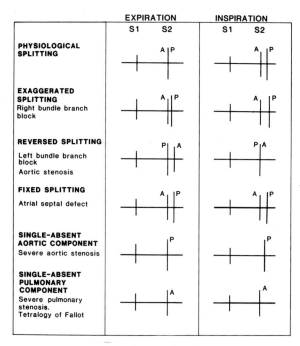

**Figure 11.2** Splitting of the second heart sound. The vertical lines representing S1 and S2 divide the horizontal line into systolic and diastolic intervals. Because auscultation is at the pulmonary area the pulmonary component of S2 is slightly louder than the aortic component (A); both components are louder than S1. This information is conveyed by the vertical heights of the lines. Additional sounds and murmurs may be superimposed on this basic format as illustrated in Fig. 11.3.

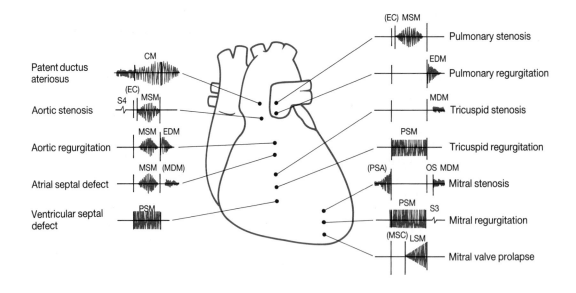

**Figure 11.3** Heart murmurs. EC = ejection click. OS = opening snap. MSM = mid-systolic murmur. LSM = late systolic murmur. MDM = mid-diastolic murmur. S3 = third heart sound. S4 = fourth heart sound. MSC = mid-systolic click. CM = continuous murmur. PSM = pansystolic murmur. EDM = early diastolic murmur. PSA = presystolic accentuation. Parentheses indicate that the finding is variable and not always present.

## FRICTION RUBS AND VENOUS HUMS

A friction rub occurs in pericarditis. It is a high-pitched scratching noise audible during any part of the cardiac cycle and over any part of the left precordium. A continuous venous hum at the base of the heart reflects hyperkinetic jugular venous flow. it is particularly common in infants and usually disappears on lying flat.

# CARDIAC INVESTIGATION

# The electrocardiogram

The electrocardiogram (ECG) records the electrical activity of the heart at the skin surface. A good-quality 12-lead ECG is essential for the evaluation of every cardiac patient.

## GENERATION OF ELECTRICAL ACTIVITY

The wave of depolarization that spreads through the heart during each cardiac cycle has vector properties defined by its direction and magnitude. The net direction of the wave changes continuously during each cardiac cycle and the ECG deflections change accordingly, being positive as the wave approaches the recording electrode and negative as it moves away. Electrodes orientated along the axis of the wave record larger deflections than those orientated at right angles to it. Nevertheless, the size of the deflections is determined principally by the magnitude of the wave, which is a function of muscle mass. Thus the ECG deflection produced by depolarization of the atria (P wave) is smaller than that produced by the depolarization of the more muscular ventricles (QRS complex). Ventricular repolarization produces the T wave.

## INSCRIPTION OF THE QRS COMPLEX

The ventricular depolarization vector can be resolved into two components:

1 Septal depolarization which spreads from left to right across the septum.
2 Ventricular free wall depolarization which spreads from endocardium to epicardium.

Left ventricular depolarization dominates the second vector component, the resultant direction of which is from right to left. Thus electrodes orientated to the left ventricle record a small negative deflection (Q wave) as the septal depolarization vector moves away, followed by a large positive deflection (R wave) as the ventricular depolarization vector approaches. The sequence of deflections for electrodes orientated towards the right ventricle is in the opposite direction (Fig. 11.4).

Any positive deflection is termed an R wave. A negative deflection before the R wave is termed a Q wave (this must be the first deflection of the complex), while a negative deflection following the R wave is termed an S wave.

## ELECTRICAL AXIS

Because the mean direction of the ventricular depolarization vector (the electrical axis) shows a wide range of normality, there is a corresponding variation in QRS patterns consistent with a normal ECG. Thus correct interpretation of the ECG must take account of the electrical axis. The frontal plane axis is determined by identifying the limb lead in which the net QRS deflection (positive and negative) is least pronounced. This lead must be at right angles to the frontal plane electrical axis which is defined using an arbitrary hexaxial reference system (Fig. 11.5).

## NORMAL 12-LEAD ECG

This is illustrated in Fig. 11.6. Leads I to III are the standard bipolar leads, which each measure the potential difference between two limbs:

Lead I      Left arm to right arm
Lead II     Left leg to right arm
Lead III    Left leg to left arm

The remaining leads are unipolar connected to a limb (aVR to aVF) or to the chest wall (V1 to V6). Because the orientation of each lead to the wave of depolarization is different, the direction and magnitude of ECG deflections is also different in each lead. Nevertheless, the sequence of deflections (P wave, QRS complex, T wave) is identical. In some patients a small U wave can be seen following the T wave. Its orientation (positive or negative) is the same as the T wave but its cause is unknown.

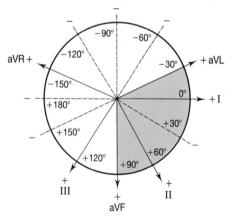

**Figure 11.5** Frontal plane electrical axis. This hexaxial reference system identifies the orientation of each of the standard limb leads to the heart. When the mean frontal QRS axis is directed towards lead I, it is arbitrarily defined as 0°: the maximal positive deflection is in lead I and the equiphasic deflection is in lead aVF. Axis shifts are ascribed, a negative sign if directed leftwards and a positive sign if directed rightwards. Axes between −30° and +90° within the shaded area of the figure, are normal axes less than −30° (left axis deviation) or greater than +90° (right axis deviation) are abnormal.

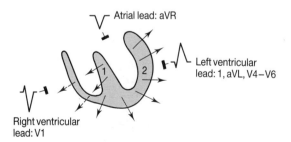

**Figure 11.4** Inscription of the QRS complex. The septal depolarization vector (1) produces the initial deflection of the QRS complex. The ventricular free-wall depolarization vector (2) produces the second deflection which is usually more pronounced. Lead aVR is orientated towards the cavity of the left ventricle and records an entirely negative deflection.

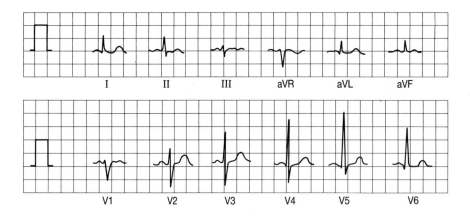

**Figure 11.6** Standard 12-lead electrocardiogram. This is a normal recording. The QRS deflections are equiphasic in lead III. This is at right angles to lead aVR (see Fig. 11.5) which is dominantly negative. The frontal plane QRS axis is, therefore, +30°. The square wave calibration signal is 1 mV.

# Analysis of the electrocardiogram

## HEART RATE

The ECG is usually recorded at a paper speed of 25 mm/s. Thus each large square (5 mm) represents 0.20 s. The heart rate (beats/min) is conveniently calculated by counting the number of large squares between consecutive R waves and dividing this into 300.

## RHYTHM

In normal sinus rhythm, P waves precede each QRS complex and the rhythm is regular. Absence of P waves and an irregular rhythm indicate atrial fibrillation.

## ELECTRICAL AXIS

Evaluation of the frontal plane QRS axis is described above.

## P WAVE MORPHOLOGY

The duration should not exceed 0.10 s. Broad, notched P waves (P mitrale) indicate left atrial dilation caused usually by mitral valve disease or left ventricular failure. Tall, peaked P waves

(P pulmonale) indicate right atrial enlargement caused usually by pulmonary hypertension and right ventricular failure.

## PR INTERVAL

The normal duration is 0.12 to 0.20 s measured from the onset of the P wave to the first deflec-

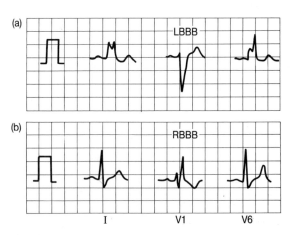

**Figure 11.7** Bundle branch block. (a) Left bundle branch block. The entire sequence of ventricular depolarization is abnormal, resulting in a broad QRS complex with large slurred or notched R waves in I and V6. (b) Right bundle branch block. Right ventricular depolarization is delayed, resulting in a broad QRS complex with an rSR' pattern in V1 and prominent S waves in I and V6.

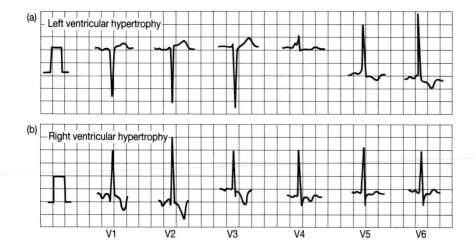

**Figure 11.8** Ventricular hypertrophy. (a) Left ventricular hypertrophy. The QRS voltage deflections are exaggerated such that the sum of S and R waves in V1 and V6, respectively, exceeds 35 mm. T wave inversion in V5 and V6 indicates left ventricular 'strain'. (b) Right ventricular hypertrophy. Prominent R waves in V1 and V2 associated with T wave inversion are shown.

tion of the QRS complex. Prolongation indicates delayed atrioventricular conduction (heart block). Shortening indicates rapid conduction through an accessory pathway bypassing the atrioventricular node (Wolff–Parkinson–White syndrome).

## QRS MORPHOLOGY

The duration should not exceed 0.12 s. Prolongation indicates slow ventricular depolarization due to bundle branch block (Fig. 11.7), pre-excitation (Wolff–Parkinson–White syndrome), ventricular tachycardia or hypokalaemia.

Exaggerated QRS deflections indicate ventricular hypertrophy (Fig. 11.8). Voltage criteria for left ventricular hypertrophy are fulfilled when the sum of the S and R wave deflections in leads V1 and V6, respectively, exceeds 35 mm (3.5 mV). Right ventricular hypertrophy causes tall R waves in right ventricular leads (V1 and V2). Diminished QRS deflections occur in myxoedema and also when pericardial effusion or obesity insulate the heart. The presence of pathological Q waves (duration greater than 0.04 s) should be noted because this usually indicates previous myocardial infarction.

## ST SEGMENT MORPHOLOGY

Minor ST elevation reflecting early repolarization may occur as a normal variant (Fig. 11.9) particularly in patients of African or West Indian origin. Pathological elevation (>2.0 mm above the isoelectric line) occurs in acute

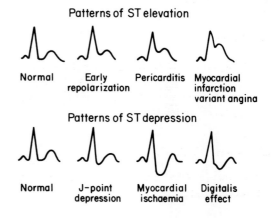

**Figure 11.9** ST segment morphology: common causes of ST segment elevation and depression. Note that depression of the J point (junction between the QRS complex and ST segment) is physiological during exertion and does not signify myocardial ischaemia. Planar depression of the ST segment, on the other hand, is strongly suggestive of myocardial ischaemia.

myocardial infarction, variant angina and pericarditis. Horizontal ST depression indicates myocardial ischaemia. Other important causes of ST depression are digitalis therapy and hypokalaemia.

## T WAVE MORPHOLOGY

The orientation of the T wave should be directionally similar to the QRS complex. Thus T wave inversion is normal in leads with dominantly negative QRS complexes (aVR, V1, and sometimes lead III). Pathological T wave inversion occurs as a non-specific response to various stimuli (e.g. viral infection, hypothermia). More important causes of T wave inversion are ventricular hypertrophy, myocardial ischaemia and myocardial infarction. Exaggerated peaking of the T wave is the earliest ECG change in acute myocardial infarction. It also occurs in hyperkalaemia.

# The chest X-ray

Good-quality posteroanterior (PA) and lateral chest X-rays are of considerable value in the assessment of the cardiac patient (Fig. 11.10).

## CARDIAC SILHOUETTE

Although the PA chest X-ray exhibits a wide range of normality, the transverse diameter of the heart should not exceed 50 per cent that of the chest. Cardiac enlargement is caused either by dilation of the cardiac chambers or pericardial effusion. Myocardial hypertrophy rarely affects heart size.

### Ventricular dilation

The PA chest X-ray does not reliably distinguish left from right ventricular dilation. The lateral chest X-ray is more helpful. Thus dilation of the posteriorly located left ventricle encroaches on the retrocardiac space, while dilation of the anteriorly located right ventricle encroaches on the retrosternal space.

### Atrial dilation

Right atrial dilation is usually due to right ventricular failure but occurs as an isolated finding in tricuspid stenosis and Ebstein's anomaly. It produces cardiac enlargement without specific radiographic signs.

Left atrial dilation occurs in left ventricular

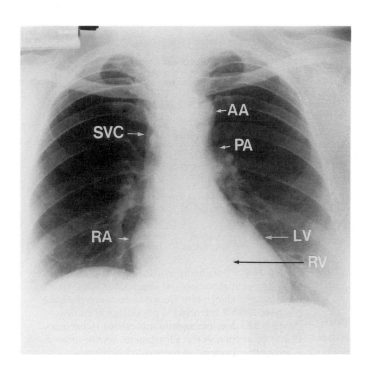

**Figure 11.10** Normal chest X-ray. The standard posteroanterior projection is shown. Note that the heart is not enlarged (cardiothoracic ratio <50 per cent) and the lung fields are clear. SVC = superior vena cava. RA = right atrium. AA = aortic arch. LV = left ventricle. PA = pulmonary artery. RV = right ventricle.

failure and mitral valve disease (Fig. 11.11). Radiographic signs are:

1 Flattening and later bulging of the left heart border below the main pulmonary artery.
2 Elevation of the left main bronchus, with widening of the carina.
3 Appearance of the medial border of the left atrium behind the right side of the heart (double-density sign).

## Vascular dilation

Aortic dilation caused by aneurysm or dissection may produce widening of the entire upper mediastinum. Localized dilation of the proximal aorta occurs in aortic valve disease and produces a prominence in the right upper mediastinum. Dilation of the main pulmonary artery occurs in pulmonary hypertension and pulmonary stenosis and produces a prominence below the aortic knuckle.

## Intracardiac calcification

Because the radiodensity of cardiac tissue is similar to that of blood, intracardiac structures can rarely be identified unless they are calcified. Valvar, pericardial or myocardial calcification may occur and usually indicate important disease of these structures. Calcification is best appreciated on a penetrated lateral chest X-ray.

## LUNG FIELDS

Common lung field abnormalities in cardiovascular disease are caused either by altered pulmonary flow or increased left atrial pressure.

## Altered pulmonary flow

Increments in pulmonary flow sufficient to cause radiographic abnormalities are caused by left-to-right intracardiac shunts (e.g. atrial septal defect, ventricular septal defect, patent ductus arteriosus). Prominence of the vascular markings give the lung fields a plethoric appearance. Reductions in pulmonary flow, on the other hand, cause reduced vascular markings. This may be regional (e.g. pulmonary embolism) or global (e.g. severe pulmonary hypertension).

## Increased left atrial pressure

This occurs in mitral stenosis and left ventricular failure and produces corresponding rises in pulmonary venous and pulmonary capillary pressures. Prominence of the upper lobe veins is an early radiographic finding. As the left atrial and pulmonary capillary pressures rise above 18 mm Hg, transudation into the lung produces interstitial pulmonary oedema, characterized by prominence of the interlobular septa, particularly at the lung bases (**Kerley B lines**). Further elevation of pressure leads to alveolar

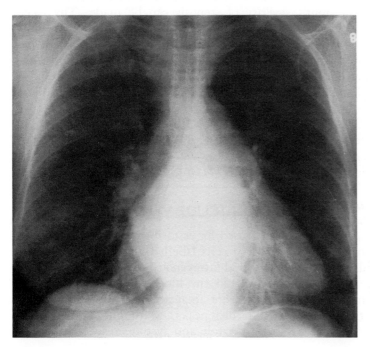

**Figure 11.11** Left atrial dilation. This is a penetrated PA chest X-ray in a patient with mitral stenosis. The dilated, posteriorly located left atrium is clearly visible. Note flattening of the left heart border, widening of the carina and the double-density sign at the right heart border.

pulmonary oedema characterized by perihilar 'bat's wing' shadowing.

# The computed tomogram

Computed tomography (CT) measures the differential attenuation of X-rays after they traverse body tissues. A sensor rotates about the chest and utilizes attenuation measurements to construct a two-dimensional, cross-sectional image. The modern generation of ultrafast scanners with image acquisition times of less than a second can provide very high resolution cardiac images in both static and video modes. At present, however, cardiac applications of CT scanning are limited to diagnosis of aortic dissection, cardiac tumours and pericardial thickening in constrictive disease.

# The echocardiogram

Echocardiography is the most versatile and widely applicable imaging technique in clinical cardiology. Reflected ultrasound provides a high-resolution dynamic image of the four cardiac chambers and the myocardial, valvar and pericardial structures. Thus dilation and hypertrophy of the cardiac chambers can be identified and quantified and ventricular contractile dysfunction is readily appreciated. Echocardiography plays an important role in the diagnosis of valvar heart disease and is the most sensitive technique available for diagnosis of pericardial effusion. Other clinical applications include the detection of vegetations in endocarditis, thrombus and intracardiac tumours.

Complete echocardiographic examination requires M-mode and two-dimensional studies (Fig. 11.12). The M-mode study provides a unidimensional 'ice-pick' view through the heart, but continuous recording adds a time dimension for appreciation of the dynamic component of the image. The two-dimensional study provides more detailed structural and dynamic information.

Recently available is the transoesophageal echocardiogram in which the transducer is mounted on a probe and positioned in the oesophagus, directly behind the heart. This provides better quality images because there are no intervening ribs and the probe is closely applied to the posterior aspect of the heart. It is particularly useful for imaging the left atrium, aorta and prosthetic heart valves.

# Doppler echocardiography

This non-invasive technique is now widely used for grading the severity of stenotic and regurgitant valve lesions and for localizing intracardiac shunts through septal defects. According to the Doppler principle, when an ultrasound beam is directed towards the bloodstream the frequency of the ultrasound reflected from the blood cells is altered. The frequency shift – or Doppler effect – is related to the direction and velocity of flow. Thus in valvar regurgitation the retrograde flow that occurs after valve closure is readily detected. In valvar stenosis the velocity of flow across the valve can be measured. Because the peak velocity (as opposed to volume) of flow is directly related to the degree of stenosis, an evaluation of the severity of stenosis can be made. The recent introduction of colour-flow mapping simplifies the interpretation of Doppler imaging. It permits construction of a colour-coded map which can be superimposed on the standard two-dimensional echocardiogram to relate alterations in flow with structural abnormalities.

# Radionuclide imaging

## RADIONUCLIDE VENTRICULOGRAPHY

This is used for assessment of ventricular function. Red cells labelled with technetium-99m are injected intravenously and allowed to equilibrate within the blood pool. The ventricular chambers are imaged with a gamma camera which records peaks and troughs of radioactivity during diastole and systole, respectively. This

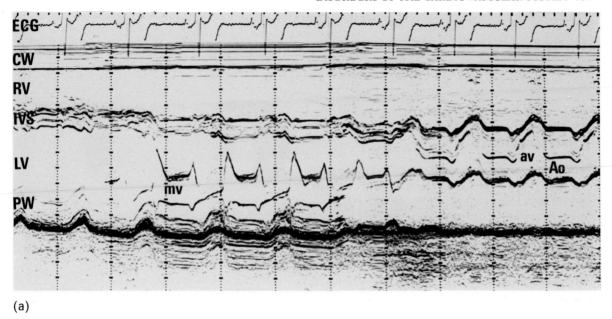

(a)

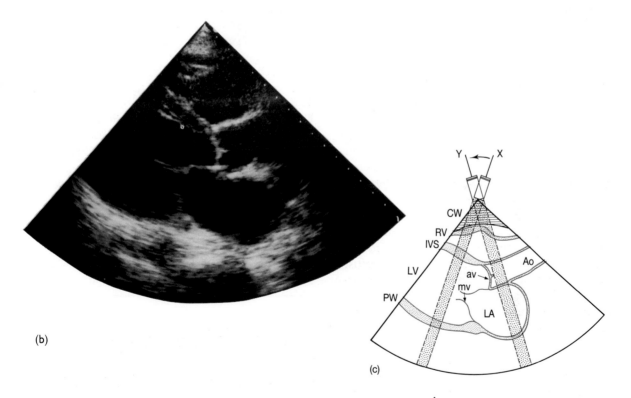

(b)

(c)

**Figure 11.12** Normal echocardiograms. (a) M-mode recording; angulation of the ultrasound beam from X to Y (see line drawing in part 'c') permits sequential examination of the right ventricle and the left-side cardiac chambers and heart valves. By convention the anteriorly located ('right-sided') cardiac structures are displayed towards the top of the echocardiogram, and the posteriorly located ('left-sided') structures are displayed below. The dense dots are a scale: 1 cm vertically, 1 s horizontally. (b) Two-dimensional recording: interpretation of the echocardiogram is provided by the line drawing, and the dots are a 1 cm scale. (c) Schematic diagram of 'b'. CW = chest wall. IVS = interventricular septum. PW = posterior wall of the left ventricle. RV = right ventricle. LV = left ventricle. Ao = aorta. av = aortic valve. mv = mitral valve. LA = left atrium.

permits construction of a dynamic ventriculogram which may be used to examine ventricular wall motion and chamber dimensions (Fig. 11.13).

## MYOCARDIAL PERFUSION SCINTIGRAPHY

This is used for diagnosis of coronary artery disease. The patient is exercised and, after an intravenous injection of thallium-201, is imaged under a gamma camera. In normal subjects, thallium-201 is distributed homogeneously throughout the myocardium according to coronary flow, but in coronary artery disease regional impairment of flow produces scintigraphic perfusion defects. Repeat imaging after 2–4 hours permits reassessment of scintigraphic defects, those that disappear (reversible defects) indicating areas of exercise-induced ischaemia, those that persist (fixed defects) indicating infarcted myocardium.

# Pulmonary scintigraphy (lung scan)

This is used for diagnosis of pulmonary embolism. Albumin microspheres labelled with technetium-99m are injected intravenously and become trapped within the pulmonary capillaries. Imaging with a gamma camera provides a perfusion scintigram. The normal perfusion scintigram shows homogeneous distribution of radioactivity throughout both lung fields, but following thromboembolism regional impairment of pulmonary flow produces one or several scintigraphic perfusion defects. The appearance, however, is non-specific and occurs in other pulmonary disorders. Simultaneous ventilation scintigraphy enhances specificity. Inhaled xenon-133 is normally distributed homogeneously throughout the alveoli. In pulmonary embolism (unlike other pulmonary disorders) the distribution remains homogeneous. Thus the finding of scintigraphic perfusion defects not 'matched' by ventilation defects is highly specific for pulmonary embolism.

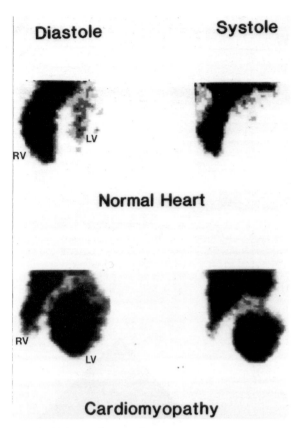

**Figure 11.13** Radionuclide ventriculography. The right (RV) and left (LV) ventricles are clearly visible. Note that in the normal heart the left ventricular cavity is small and during systole contracts vigorously. In cardiomyopathy, the left ventricle is considerably dilated and there is global impairment of contractile function.

# Magnetic resonance imaging

Magnetic resonance imaging (MRI) is a new non-invasive imaging technique which requires the patient to lie in a strong, artificially graded, magnetic field. Exposure to pulsed radiowaves causes the hydrogen protons of fat and water to resonate at different frequencies in different parts of the imaging zone. Analysis of the emitted frequencies permits construction of very high resolution tomographic images of the heart (Fig. 11.14). The role of MRI in clinical cardiology has yet to be defined but potential applications include identification of histological and

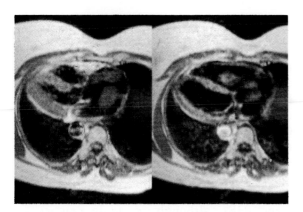

**Figure 11.14** Magnetic resonance imaging: left atrial myxoma. This high resolution image shows a lobulated myxoma (a benign tumour) in the left atrium. During diastole (right frame) one lobe prolapses through the mitral valve.

metabolic cardiac disorders, and assessment of myocardial perfusion using paramagnetic contrast agents.

# Cardiac catheterization

Catheters introduced into an artery or vein may be directed into the left or right sides of the heart, respectively. Originally developed for diagnostic purposes (intracardiac pressure measurement and angiography), catheter techniques are now being used increasingly for the interventional management of cardiovascular disease.

## INTRACARDIAC PRESSURE MEASUREMENT (Fig. 11.15)

The fluid-filled catheter is attached to a pressure transducer. Right-sided pressures are conveniently measured with the balloon-tipped Swan Ganz catheter. With the balloon inflated in a central vein, the catheter is flow-guided through the right side of the heart into the pulmonary artery. If the balloon is wedged in an arterial branch the pressure recorded at the tip is an indirect measure of left atrial pressure transmitted retrogradely through the pulmonary veins and capillaries. Pulmonary wedge pressure measurement is widely used in the intensive care unit to monitor left atrial pressure in patients with left ventricular failure. Although right heart catheterization may be performed at the bedside, left heart procedures require the special facilities of a catheterization laboratory. Left ventricular pressure is measured by passing an arterial catheter retrogradely through the aortic valve.

## CARDIAC ANGIOGRAPHY

This is performed in the catheterization laboratory. Contrast material is injected into the area of interest during radiographic recording on cine or video film.

### Left ventricular angiography

Contrast medium injected into the left ventricle demonstrates contractile function and chamber dimensions and also permits evaluation of mitral valve function. The normal mitral valve prevents backflow of contrast medium, but in mitral regurgitation opacification of the left atrium occurs.

### Aortic root angiography

Contrast medium injected into the aortic root demonstrates the anatomy of the ascending aorta and permits evaluation of aortic valve function. The normal aortic valve prevents backflow of contrast medium, but in aortic regurgitation opacification of the left ventricle occurs.

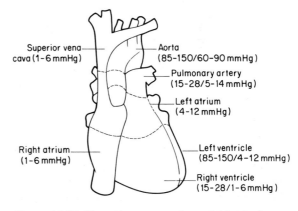

**Figure 11.15** Normal pressure values within the heart and great vessels.

## Coronary arteriography

This requires selective injection of contrast medium into the left and right coronary arteries. Intraluminal filling defects or arterial occlusions indicate coronary artery disease, which is nearly always due to atherosclerosis.

## Pulmonary angiography

Contrast medium injection into the main pulmonary artery produces opacification of the arterial branches throughout both lung fields. Intraluminal filling defects and vessel cutoffs usually indicate pulmonary thromboembolism.

## INTERVENTIONAL CATHETERIZATION

This has extended the role of the cardiologist into areas that were once exclusively surgical.

The earliest example was insertion of electrode-tipped catheters for pacing patients with bradyarrhythmias (page 205) but the interventional management of arrhythmias has now expanded to include electrical and radio-frequency ablation of conducting tissue with catheters placed strategically within the heart (page 216). Balloon angioplasty is a catheter technique used widely for the treatment of coronary artery disease (page 172) and balloon valvuloplasty has found application in paediatric cardiology for treatment of pulmonary stenosis (page 238), although in adult practice its application is more limited. The insertion of catheter-mounted obstructors for closing patent ductus arteriosus is reducing the requirement for surgery in young children (page 238).

# Clinical Problems

## Heart Failure

Heart failure is a syndrome in which a cardiac disorder produces inadequate cardiac output for the perfusion requirements of metabolizing tissues. It usually implies a disturbance of ventricular function. The major determinants of ventricular function are (Fig. 11.16):

1. Contractility: the force and velocity of contraction, independent of loading conditions. It is not amenable to direct measurement.
2. Preload: the passive stretch (or tension) of the ventricular myocardium at end diastole. Because tension is largely pressure dependent, preload is conveniently measured by ventricular end-diastolic pressure or atrial pressure (ventricular 'filling pressures').
3. Afterload: systolic wall tension developed by the ventricle to expel blood against vascular resistance. It is conveniently measured by arterial pressure.

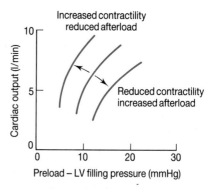

**Figure 11.16** Determinants of left ventricular function. The curvilinear relation between preload (mean left atrial pressure or left ventricular end-diastolic pressure) and cardiac output was described by Starling in 1918. It provides a useful means of evaluating left ventricular function. Changes in contractility and afterload influence ventricular function independently of preload. Thus at a given preload changes in contractility result in changes in cardiac output in the same direction while changes in afterload result in changes in cardiac output in the opposite direction.

Although diastolic wall tension (preload) and systolic wall tension (afterload) are conveniently measured by atrial and arterial pressures, respectively, the contribution that ventricular volume makes to wall tension should not be overlooked. This is defined by the law of Laplace:

$$\text{Ventricular wall tension} \times \text{ventricular radius} = \text{ventricular pressure}$$

Thus as the failing heart dilates, wall tension increases and both preload and afterload rise independently of atrial and arterial pressures.

## AETIOLOGY

### Low-output failure

Cardiac disorders produce low-output failure by restriction of ventricular filling, excessive ventricular loading or impairment of contractile function (Table 11.3).

Restriction of ventricular filling reduces preload, which depresses cardiac output. There is no intrinsic impairment of ventricular contractile function.

Excessive ventricular loading may be caused by either pressure or volume which exert their major influence on afterload and preload, respectively. It is important to distinguish between the effects of acute and chronic loading. In acute pressure loading (e.g. accelerated hypertension, pulmonary embolism) ventricular failure is caused by the abrupt increase in afterload which depresses cardiac output. Acute volume loading (e.g. acute valvar regurgitation) overwhelms the Starling reserve of the ventricle. In chronic pressure or volume loading, however, compen-

**Table 11.3** Causes of heart failure.

| Ventricular pathophysiology | Clinical examples | Ventricle predominantly affected | | |
|---|---|---|---|---|
| | | Left | Right | Both |
| Restricted filling | Mitral stenosis | × | | |
| | Tricuspid stenosis | | × | |
| | Constrictive pericarditis | | × | |
| | Tamponade | | × | |
| | Restrictive cardiomyopathy | | | × |
| | Hypertrophic cardiomyopathy | × | | |
| Pressure loading | Hypertension | × | | |
| | Aortic stenosis | × | | |
| | Coarctation of the aorta | × | | |
| | Pulmonary vascular disease | | × | |
| | Pulmonary embolism | | × | |
| | Pulmonary stenosis | | × | |
| Volume loading | Mitral regurgitation | × | | |
| | Aortic regurgitation | × | | |
| | Pulmonary regurgitation | | × | |
| | Tricuspid regurgitation | | × | |
| | Ventricular septal defect | × | | |
| | Patent ductus arteriosus | × | | |
| Contractile impairment | Coronary artery disease | × | | |
| | Dilated cardiomyopathy | | | × |
| | Myocarditis | | | × |
| Arrhythmia | Severe bradycardia | | | × |
| | Severe tachycardia | | | × |

satory mechanisms (see below) protect against heart failure for a variable (often prolonged) period before ventricular contractile impairment supervenes.

Ventricular contractile impairment is the major cause of low-output failure. It occurs in myocardial infarction, cardiomyopathy and in the end-stage of chronic pressure and volume loading. Once established, ventricular contractile impairment is often irreversible.

## High-output failure

Occasionally the perfusion requirements of the body cannot be met despite considerable increments in cardiac output above the normal range. The principal causes of high-output failure are:

1 Increased metabolic rate, e.g. thyrotoxicosis
2 Reduced oxygen-carrying capacity of the blood, e.g. anaemia, severe lung disease
3 Arteriovenous shunting which reduces the fraction of cardiac output delivered to the metabolizing tissues, e.g. arteriovenous fistula or malformation, beri-beri (page 00), Paget's disease (page 00).

In all these conditions the volume imposed by chronically elevated cardiac output eventually leads to biventricular failure.

## PATHOPHYSIOLOGY

Compensatory mechanisms in heart failure are directed at maintaining cardiac output despite abnormal loading or contractile impairment (Fig. 11.17).

## Neurohumoral activation

Increased sympathetic activity helps to maintain cardiac output by increasing heart rate and contractility. It also constricts the venous capacitance vessels, which redistributes flow centrally and improves cardiac output by increasing preload. Activation of the renin–angiotensin system in response to reduced renal perfusion increases angiotensin II synthesis and stimulates aldosterone release. Aldosterone stimulates salt and water retention which expands plasma volume and further increases preload and cardiac output. However, as fluid retention increases, pulmonary congestion and peripheral oedema develop. Moreover, the vasoconstrictor effects of both sympathetic stimulation and angiotensin II increase afterload which helps maintain blood pressure but also causes left ventricular function to deteriorate. Thus the compensatory effects of neurohumoral activation in heart failure are limited and ultimately contribute to a vicious cycle of clinical deterioration.

## Cardiac dilation and hypertrophy

Dilation is most marked in the volume-loaded ventricle and is caused by central redistribution of flow and salt and water retention which combine to increase ventricular filling pressures. Hypertrophy, on the other hand, is most marked in the pressure-loaded ventricle. Although ventricular dilation and hypertrophy increase diastolic wall tension (preload) and systolic thrust, respectively, they also increase systolic wall tension (afterload) and ultimately contribute to a vicious cycle of clinical deterioration.

Thus all the compensatory mechanisms in heart failure are of limited potential and, although they can often maintain haemodynamic stability for prolonged periods, in the long term they are often unable to prevent decompensation from occurring.

## CLINICAL FEATURES

Manifestations of left and right heart failure are conveniently considered separately. Nevertheless, they often occur together, resulting in congestive heart failure.

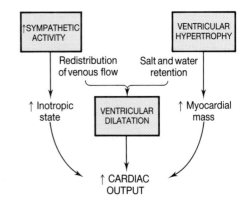

**Figure 11.17** Compensatory physiology in heart failure. If these physiological responses are inadequate, heart failure develops.

## Chronic left heart failure

This is usually the result of left ventricular failure, but in mitral stenosis it occurs without intrinsic impairment of left ventricular contractile function. Symptoms include exercise-related dyspnoea, orthopnoea and paroxysmal nocturnal dyspnoea (page 143). Fatigue is usually attributed to inadequate cardiac output. Signs of low cardiac output and reflex sympathetic stimulation include tachycardia, cool skin and peripheral cyanosis. Inspiratory crackles (page 276) are heard at the lung bases. A third heart sound occurs except in mitral stenosis, where the narrowed valve orifice prevents rapid ventricular filling (page 194). In severe failure, left ventricular dilation may stretch the mitral valve ring and papillary muscles, producing 'functional' regurgitation manifested by a pansystolic apical murmur. Pulsus alternans may also be present in severe failure (page 146).

## Acute left heart failure

This is a medical emergency usually caused by myocardial infarction. Other causes include acute aortic and mitral regurgitation. Fulminant myocarditis and mitral stenosis may also present acutely. Pulmonary oedema and systemic hypoperfusion are invariable. The patient becomes abruptly dyspnoeic and in severe cases may cough up pink, frothy oedema fluid. Signs of pulmonary oedema (late inspiratory crackles at the lung bases, central cyanosis) are commonly associated with hypotension and signs of peripheral hypoperfusion (cold extremities, mental clouding and a falling urine output). For a fuller discussion see page 178.

## Chronic right heart failure

This is usually the result of chronically elevated pulmonary artery pressure in patients with either left heart failure or obstructive pulmonary disease. In these cases dyspnoea is always prominent. In other cases of right heart failure the effects of low cardiac output, elevated right atrial pressure and salt and water retention dominate the clinical picture. Fatigue, abdominal discomfort and loss of appetite are the principal symptoms. Examination reveals an elevated jugular venous pulse – often with a giant 'V' wave if right ventricular dilation has stretched the tricuspid valve ring and caused 'functional' tricuspid regurgitation. Peripheral oedema may be severe and commonly involves the abdominal viscera, particularly the liver which is responsible for the abdominal discomfort. In advanced cases hepatic dysfunction results in jaundice and impaired protein synthesis. Hypoalbuminaemia reduces plasma osmolality which exacerbates oedema and contributes to the development of ascites.

## Acute right heart failure

This is a medical emergency seen in massive pulmonary embolism and, less commonly, in right ventricular infarction. Signs are those of critically reduced cardiac output and include cool skin, systemic hypotension and peripheral cyanosis. Variable elevation of the jugular venous pulse is usually present (page 147).

## INVESTIGATIONS

Electrocardiographic abnormalities in heart failure are often non-specific and may be limited to T wave changes only. The chest X-ray shows cardiac enlargement, and in left-sided failure this is commonly associated with pulmonary venous dilation or pulmonary oedema.

The echocardiogram is potentially diagnostic of many of the common causes of heart failure. Left ventricular dilation and regional contractile impairment indicate ischaemic disease, while four-chamber dilation and global contractile impairment indicate cardiomyopathy. Heart failure caused by valvar disease is readily apparent.

Cardiac catheterization is rarely necessary for diagnostic purposes, but in patients with surgically correctable lesions (e.g. valvar disease, ventricular aneurysm) the surgeon usually requires precise definition of the lesion with haemodynamic measurements and angiography.

## DIAGNOSIS

The diagnosis of heart failure relies chiefly on the clinical history, examination and the chest X-ray. The cause may also be evident or may require further investigation.

## COMPLICATIONS

### Cardiac arrhythmias

Atrial fibrillation is common in heart failure and often poorly tolerated. Ventricular arrhythmias, however, are more sinister and if sustained cause abrupt clinical deterioration or sudden death.

### Deep venous thrombosis

This is the result of sluggish flow in the deep veins of the legs and pelvis. Pulmonary thromboembolism is a common cause of death in patients with heart failure.

### Intracardiac thrombosis

Thrombosis within the dilated cardiac chambers predisposes to systemic and pulmonary thromboembolism, particularly in patients with atrial fibrillation who require prophylactic anticoagulation.

### Renal failure

The kidney is particularly sensitive to the effects of hypoperfusion, and worsening renal failure commonly accompanies the progression of heart failure.

### Hepatic failure

Hepatic congestion causes jaundice and elevation of liver enzymes. This is usually reversible, but in long-standing right heart failure cardiac cirrhosis develops, characterized by centrilobular necrosis and fibrosis.

### Bronchopneumonia

Chronic pulmonary congestion in left heart failure predisposes to chest infection. Bronchopneumonia is a common cause of death.

## TREATMENT OF CONGESTIVE HEART FAILURE

The primary goal of treatment is to identify and correct the underlying cause. In practice this goal cannot always be achieved and once ventricular contractile impairment is established treatment is directed towards controlling symptoms and slowing the progression of disease.

### Correction of aggravating factors

Cardiac arrhythmias, hypertension and severe anaemia exacerbate heart failure and should be corrected. Salt and water retention in heart failure provides a rationale for limiting salt intake, but the availability of potent diuretics usually makes this unnecessary.

### Medical therapy (Table 11.4)

Diuretics and angiotensin-converting enzyme inhibitors are first-line treatment in congestive heart failure. Other vasodilators and inotropic agents are of less value.

#### Diuretics

Diuretics promote salt and water excretion. This lowers atrial pressures and corrects pulmonary and systemic congestion. The associated reduction in body weight provides a useful clinical yardstick for assessing the efficacy of treatment. Diuretics do not improve ventricular function. Indeed, by reducing preload they tend to have the reverse effect, and overdiuresis must therefore be avoided.

Thiazides increase sodium excretion in the distal renal tubule. They are mild diuretics and, in severe heart failure, the more potent loop diuretics are necessary. These inhibit sodium reabsorption in the ascending loop of Henle, effectively removing the osmotic gradient in the renal medulla and preventing concentration of the urine.

#### Angiotensin–converting enzyme inhibitors

Angiotensin-converting enzyme (ACE) inhibitors block the conversion of angiotensin I to angiotensin II. Removal of angiotensin II has two important effects. It produces vasodilation, which increases cardiac output by reducing blood pressure and afterload. It also removes the major stimulus for aldosterone secretion, enhancing the renal excretion of salt and water. Thus, by increasing cardiac output and promoting salt and water excretion, ACE inhibitors improve both peripheral perfusion and the congestive manifestations of heart failure. These drugs have made a major impact on the management of heart failure because they not only correct symptoms but can also improve long-term prognosis although the mechanism of this

**Table 11.4** Drugs for the treatment of congestive heart failure.

| Drug | Dose | Adverse effects | Interactions |
|---|---|---|---|
| **Thiazide diuretics** | | | |
| Bendrofluazide | 2.5–10 mg orally daily | Hypokalaemia; uric acid retention with gout; | Causes lithium retention; diuresis reduced by NSAIDs |
| Cyclopenthiazide | 250 µg–1.0 mg orally daily | diminishing glucose tolerance rarely with diabetic-like state | |
| Metolazone | 2.5–5.0 mg daily (provides very potent diuresis when used in conjunction with loop diuretics) | | |
| **Loop diuretics** | | | |
| Frusemide | 40–200 mg orally daily | As for thiazides; high dose i.v. frusemide can cause deafness | As for thiazides; also they enhance the nephrotoxicity of aminoglycosides |
| Bumetanide | 500 µg–5.0 mg orally daily | Muscle pain | |

Both groups of diuretics cause hypokalaemia. Risk factors are high dose, poor diet, concurrent potassium-losing drugs (e.g. steroids). Enhanced toxicity of digitalis results. At-risk patients should be given either supplementary potassium (25–50 mmol daily as a slow-release preparation) or simultaneously a potassium-sparing diuretic, which is probably more effective.

| Drug | Dose | Adverse effects | Interactions |
|---|---|---|---|
| **Potassium-sparing diuretics** | | | |
| Amiloride | 5–10 mg daily | Hyperkalaemia in poor renal function and diabetes; combined with thiazide it can also cause sodium deficiency | All potassium-sparing diuretics can cause hyperkalaemia if combined with ACE inhibitors or with supplementary potassium |
| Triamterene | 50 mg daily | Hyperkalaemia as above; GI tract upsets | |
| Spironolactone | 50–100 mg daily Takes 2–3 days to work | Hyperkalaemia as above; gynaecomastia; menstrual upsets; nausea | |

A number of fixed-dose preparations containing a thiazide and a potassium-sparing diuretic are available; they are useful if compliance is a problem but do not allow flexibility in dose.

| Drug | Dose | Adverse effects | Interactions |
|---|---|---|---|
| **ACE inhibitors** | | | |
| Captopril Enalapril Lisinopril Quinopril | Start with a low dose because of risk of hypotension, especially if the patient is on a diuretic. Captopril: 6.25 mg and increase if necessary to 25 mg three times daily Enalapril: 2.5 mg daily increased to 10–20 mg daily | Hypotension; hyperkalaemia (care in renal failure). Captopril (only in high dose); proteinuria (test urine monthly). Leukopenia, especially in immuno-suppressed, or SLE (blood counts for first three months) Transient taste disturbances Cough | Hypotension with other blood pressure-lowering drugs, especially diuretics; hyperkalaemia with potassium-sparing diuretics |
| **Vasodilators** | | | |
| Isosorbide mononitrate | 40–80 mg daily | Headache; flushing; hypotension | |

NSAIDs = non-steroidal anti-inflammatory drugs. ACE = angiotensin-converting enzyme. SLE = systemic lupus erythematosus.

beneficial effect is not known. Nevertheless, they are the only drugs available which produce a substantial improvement in prognosis and are recommended in all patients in whom left ventricular impairment and fluid retention are sufficiently severe to require diuretic therapy. Recent evidence suggests that even in the absence of symptoms, patients with left ventricular impairment can benefit prognostically from treatment with ACE inhibitors.

### Vasodilators

Drugs with venodilator (e.g. nitrates), arteriolar dilator (e.g. hydralazine) or both properties (e.g. prazosin) have been widely used in the treatment of heart failure. Venodilation causes pooling of blood in the capacitance vessels, which reduces venous return to the heart and lowers atrial pressures (preload). Arteriolar dilation improves cardiac output by reducing the blood pressure (afterload). The combination of these effects has the potential to improve both pulmonary congestion and peripheral perfusion, respectively. While there is no doubt about the acute benefits of vasodilator therapy (see below), efficacy is often short-lived so that not all patients experience long-term symptomatic improvement.

### Inotropic agents

Digitalis is the only orally active inotropic drug currently licensed for the treatment of congestive heart failure. By inhibiting membrane-bound sodium–potassium adenosine triphosphatase (ATPase) it increases the availability of intracellular calcium to the myocardial contractile proteins and strengthens the force of contraction. The therapeutic range is narrow and the risk of side effects demands careful therapeutic monitoring. The inotropic properties are slight and for the patient in sinus rhythm, digitalis is usually only recommended if their symptoms remain despite treatment with diuretics and ACE inhibitors. For the patient in atrial fibrillation, however, digitalis is the drug of choice for slowing atrioventricular conduction and controlling the ventricular rate (page 211).

## Surgical therapy

Heart failure caused by valve disease, left ventricular aneurysm or certain congenital defects is potentially correctable by surgery, but in the majority of patients with congestive heart failure, **heart transplantation** is the only surgical option. This is only appropriate in patients with advanced left ventricular contractile impairment resistant to all medical therapy. The risk of perioperative death is small compared with the hazards of organ rejection and immunosuppressive agents. These hazards are greatest during the first year following surgery, but thereafter the threat of accelerated coronary atherosclerosis (the cause of which is unknown) becomes increasingly important. Nevertheless, owing largely to advances in the early recognition and treatment of rejection, results of heart transplantation have improved rapidly and there is now a 70–80 per cent 2-year survival.

## TREATMENT OF ACUTE LEFT VENTRICULAR FAILURE

### General measures

The patient should be nursed sitting up. Correction of cardiac arrhythmias and hypertension is essential. Treatment of hypoxaemia is directed at maintaining an arterial oxygen tension of more than 9.0 kPa.

### Medical therapy (Table 11.5)

#### Opiates and diuretics

These are first-line agents. Intravenous morphine relieves dyspnoea by a combination of venodilation, respiratory suppression and relief of anxiety. Intravenous frusemide usually initiates a prompt diuresis. Nevertheless, because diuretic activity depends largely on adequate renal perfusion, frusemide is less helpful in severe low-output states.

#### Vasodilators and inotropes

If opiates and diuretics are not rapidly effective, vasodilator or inotropic therapy should be started. These drugs should be given by infusion into a central vein with the dual aim of reducing the left atrial pressure and increasing cardiac output. If possible the indirect left atrial pressure (wedge pressure) should be monitored

**Table 11.5** Drugs for treatment of acute left ventricular failure.

| Drug | Dose | Adverse effects |
|---|---|---|
| **Opiate** | | |
| Morphine | 5–10 mg i.v. bolus | Vomiting (combine with prochlorperazine |
| Diamorphine | 2.5–5 mg i.v. bolus | 12.5 mg i.v.); care in obstructive airways disease (use half dose) |
| **Diuretics** | | |
| Frusemide | 40–80 mg i.v. | See Table 11.4 |
| Bumetanide | 1–2 mg i.v. | |
| **Vasodilators** | | |
| Glyceryl trinitrate | Infusion, starting with 1.5 µg/min and increasing as required; max. 200 µg/min | Headache; flushing; hypotension; tachycardia |
| Sodium nitroprusside | Infusion, starting with 15 µg/min and increasing as required; max. 200 µg/min | 5% glucose must be used for infusion solution; protect from light; headaches; nausea; retrosternal pain |
| **Inotropes** | | |
| Dopamine | Infusion for renal vasodilatation 2.5 µg/kg/min; | Dopamine can cause intense vasoconstriction at high doses. Both drugs |
| Dobutamine | Infusion 5–20 µg/kg/min | may provoke tachyarrhythmias, nausea, vomiting and headache |

Low-dose dopamine may be combined with dobutamine to raise cardiac output and improve renal perfusion.

using a Swan Ganz catheter (page 159). At a level of 15–20 mm Hg pulmonary oedema begins to clear, but further reductions should be avoided because the reduction in preload lowers cardiac output. Cardiac output is best monitored indirectly by measurement of urine flow and skin temperature.

Glyceryl trinitrate and sodium nitroprusside are widely used vasodilators. Glyceryl trinitrate is predominantly a venodilator, but sodium nitroprusside has a more balanced effect, dilating both veins and arterioles. The venodilator property of both agents reduces the venous return to the heart and lowers the left atrial pressure. The arteriolar–dilator property of sodium nitroprusside, however, ensures that this agent produces greater increments in cardiac output by lowering the blood pressure and afterload. Systolic blood pressure must not be allowed to fall below 90 mm Hg because of the risk to vital organ perfusion. Indeed, in patients who are already hypotensive, vasodilators are usually contraindicated.

Dobutamine and dopamine are inotropic agents with sympathomimetic activity. Stimulation of cardiac β-adrenoceptors enhances contractility and cardiac output. Dopamine (unlike dobutamine) also exhibits important peripheral vascular effects. Low doses (up to 5 µg/kg/min) selectively dilate the renal arterioles and improve renal perfusion. Higher doses, however, produce widespread α-adrenoceptor-mediated arteriolar constriction. This improves the blood pressure but further depresses left ventricular function by increasing afterload. Thus dopamine is best used at low doses for its renal action. Dobutamine, on the other hand, does not share the peripheral vascular effects of dopamine and produces dose-related increments in cardiac output. Combination therapy with dobutamine and low-dose dopamine can be particularly beneficial for improving both cardiac output and renal perfusion.

Inotropic agents rarely produce significant reductions in left atrial (pulmonary wedge) pressure. Thus simultaneous treatment with diuretics and vasodilators is often necessary for correction of pulmonary oedema.

## *Surgical therapy*

Surgery is potentially life-saving when an acute mechanical lesion produces left ventricular failure without substantial myocardial damage. Thus infective endocarditis complicated by left ventricular failure is usually an indication for urgent valve replacement. Similarly, papillary muscle or septal rupture following myocardial infarction usually requires prompt surgical correction.

## PROGNOSIS

Heart failure that is the result of a surgically correctable lesion often has an excellent prognosis following definitive treatment. The majority of patients, however, have irreversible ventricular dysfunction. In these patients prognosis is less good and largely dependent on the degree of ventricular dysfunction. In the most severe cases 3-year survival is less than 20 per cent. Treatment with angiotensin-converting enzyme inhibitors improves prognosis, as does heart transplantation.

# SHOCK

Shock is a syndrome of critically impaired vital organ perfusion which, if not rapidly corrected, leads to irreversible cellular injury with multiple organ failure and death. It is usually caused by severe heart failure (cardiogenic shock), hypovolaemia or septicaemia. The pathogenesis is complex and poorly understood, involving a combination of haemodynamic and toxic factors. Widespread capillary damage characterizes the syndrome and intensifies the perfusion deficit. The myocardial perfusion deficit establishes a vicious cycle of worsening contractile function and end-organ damage. Renal failure occurs early but can be treated by dialysis. Cardiopulmonary failure, on the other hand, is less amenable to treatment. Pulmonary oedema is often 'non-cardiac' in origin and results from pulmonary capillary damage which permits transudation into the lung (adult respiratory distress syndrome). Heart failure may respond temporarily to inotropic therapy but the prognosis is very poor with mortality greater than 80 per cent. A more detailed account of shock is given on page 249.

# CORONARY ARTERY DISEASE

## AETIOLOGY

Coronary artery disease is nearly always caused by atherosclerosis. Indeed the two terms are often used synonymously. Other causes of coronary artery disease are rare (Table 11.6).

The cause of atherosclerotic coronary artery disease is unknown. Epidemiological evidence points to a complex interaction of genetic and environmental influences. Although the cause is unknown a number of risk factors have been identified (Table 11.7). The cumulative effect of multiple risk factors produces an exponential rise in the incidence of future coronary events.

Nevertheless, it is important to emphasize that risk factors, although associated with coronary artery disease, are not essential for its development.

## PATHOLOGY

The disease usually occurs in the proximal 6 cm of the coronary arteries with relative sparing of the smaller distal vessels. It is characterized pathologically by the atherosclerotic plaque, a focal proliferation of smooth muscle cells, collagen and cholesterol esters lying within the

**Table 11.6** Causes of coronary artery disease.

Atherosclerosis
Arteritis
    Systemic lupus erythematosus
    Vasculitis
    Rheumatoid arthritis
    Ankylosing spondylitis
    Syphilis
    Takayasu disease
Embolism
    Infective endocarditis
    Left atrial/ventricular thrombus
    Left atrial/ventricular tumour
    Prosthetic valve thrombus
    Complication of cardiac catheterization
Coronary mural thickening
    Amyloidosis
    Radiation therapy
    Hurler's disease
    Pseudoxanthoma elasticum
Other causes of coronary luminal narrowing
    Aortic dissection
    Coronary spasm
Congenital coronary artery disease
    Anomalous origin from pulmonary artery
    Arteriovenous fistula

intimal and medial layers of the arterial wall. As the plaque increases in size it may ulcerate, providing a focus for platelet deposition and thrombosis.

## Clinicopathological correlates

Coronary atherosclerosis is often asymptomatic. The development of symptoms is closely related to the pathology of the atherosclerotic plaque. Four symptom complexes are recognized, each associated with characteristic coronary pathology.

### Stable angina

This is associated with a smooth, endothelialized coronary plaque causing coronary stenosis. Stenosis greater than 70 per cent of the coronary luminal diameter may restrict flow to the extent that myocardial oxygen supply fails to meet demand. This produces myocardial ischaemia, experienced by the patient as angina.

### Variant angina

This unusual condition is caused by unprovoked increments in coronary tone (spasm) that

**Table 11.7** Risk factors for coronary artery disease.

**Potentially reversible**

| | |
|---|---|
| Tobacco smoking | Risk rises in proportion to the amount of tobacco smoked |
| Hypertension | Risk rises in proportion to the level of systolic and diastolic blood pressure |
| Hyperlipidaemia | Hypercholesterolaemia is the major risk factor, but hypertriglyceridaemia may be important in women Elevation of low-density lipoproteins increases the risk considerably. High density lipoproteins, however, are protective |
| Lipoprotein (a) | Blood concentrations above 0.3 g/l are associated with an increased risk. There is no effective treatment |
| Obesity | The increased risk is due largely to associated hypertension, hypercholesterolaemia and diabetes |
| Physical inactivity | This increases risk, probably through adverse effects on blood lipids and blood pressure |
| Diet | Although a high-cholesterol diet and excessive alcohol and coffee consumption have all been associated with increased risk, the evidence is inconclusive |

**Irreversible**

| | |
|---|---|
| Family history | Although family history is an independent risk factor, genetic predisposition to hypertension, hypercholesterolaemia and diabetes contributes to the familial incidence of coronary artery disease |
| Advanced age | Risk rises progressively with age |
| Male sex | Risk is low in young women, but after the menopause it increases and comes to equal that of men |
| Diabetes mellitus | This increases the risk in both men and women |
| Personality type | Although the type A personality (chronic sense of time urgency) has been associated with an increased risk compared with the more placid type B personality, the evidence remains inconclusive |

restricts coronary flow sufficiently to cause angina. Although variant angina is usually associated with underlying coronary atherosclerosis, the coronary arteries are normal in 30 per cent of cases.

### Unstable angina

This is provoked by the abrupt rupture of an atheromatous plaque, providing a focus for platelet deposition and thrombosis. In unstable angina the thrombus is subocclusive but causes intense myocardial ischaemia.

### Myocardial infarction

The pathological process is identical to unstable angina, except that the thrombus completely occludes the coronary artery resulting in infarction of the myocardium subtended by the occluded vessel.

# Stable angina

## CLINICAL FEATURES

Angina is experienced as a retrosternal constricting discomfort that may radiate down either arm and into the throat or jaw. Typically, the pain is provoked by exertion and relieved within 2 to 10 minutes by rest. Heightened emotion and sexual intercourse may also provoke angina. Symptoms are usually worse after a heavy meal and in cold weather. Surprisingly the severity of symptoms is not closely related to the extent of coronary artery disease. Indeed extensive disease is sometimes entirely asymptomatic ('silent' myocardial ischaemia), although the risk of myocardial infarction and death remains significant.

The examination is usually normal. Nevertheless, elevated blood pressure and evidence of other major risk factors – including hypercholesterolaemia and diabetes – should be noted. Patients with signs of peripheral vascular disease (absent pulses, arterial bruits) usually have associated coronary artery involvement.

## DIAGNOSIS

A careful history provides the most useful diagnostic information. Thus in the patient with typical symptoms the probability of coronary artery disease is high, exceeding 90 per cent when the patient is male and aged over 40.

### Exercise testing

Although the resting ECG and thallium-201 perfusion scan are often normal in the patient with angina, exercise-induced myocardial ischaemia may provoke symptoms associated with downward displacement of the ST segment and scintigraphic perfusion defects, respectively. Similarly, exercise-induced abnormalities of left ventricular wall motion may be detected on the radionuclide ventriculogram. These abnormalities reverse during rest and are highly suggestive of coronary artery disease. Nevertheless, exercise testing is imperfect and may give false positive results, particularly in asymptomatic patients and in young women with atypical symptoms. In older patients with more typical symptoms, however, a positive exercise test points strongly to the presence of coronary artery disease.

### Coronary arteriography

This is the definitive diagnostic test for coronary artery disease (page 160). It is usually reserved for patients being considered for coronary artery bypass grafting or angioplasty. Other indications are shown in Table 11.8.

## DIFFERENTIAL DIAGNOSIS

### Neuromuscular disorders

Chest wall pain from the costochondral junctions or the muscular insertions on to the ribs and sternum is common. The pain is usually

**Table 11.8** Indications for coronary arteriography.

Severe angina unresponsive to medical treatment
Angina in patients under 50
Unstable angina
Myocardial infarction in patients under 50
Angina or a positive exercise test following myocardial infarction
Cardiac arrhythmias when there is clinical suspicion of underlying coronary artery disease
Preoperatively in patients requiring valve surgery when an age >50 or angina suggest a high probability of associated coronary artery disease

sharp and localized and may be provoked by coughing or isometric stress such as pushing or pulling. The affected area is often tender to palpation.

## Oesophagitis and oesophageal spasm

Oesophageal pain due to acid reflux is retrosternal but may be distinguished from angina by its burning quality and its provocation by stooping or lying flat, particularly after a meal. Antacids often provide effective relief. Oesophageal spasm may be more difficult to distinguish from angina because the pain is retrosternal and may be relieved by glyceryl trinitrate. Nevertheless, the pain is often protracted and unrelated to exertion.

## Psychological disorders

Neurotic anxiety that focusses on the heart is common and disabling. Symptoms, however, are rarely typical of angina. Stabbing pains in the left side of the chest are a common complaint and may be associated with hyperventilation. Time spent discussing the problem with the patient is more productive than extensive investigation, which only serves to reinforce fixed notions of underlying heart disease.

## COMPLICATIONS

Angina is a symptom and does not itself produce complications. However, these patients are at risk of all the other manifestations of coronary artery disease, such as infarction, arrhythmias, heart failure and sudden death.

## TREATMENT

### General measures

Severe anaemia, hypertension and thyrotoxicosis exacerbate angina and require treatment. Correction of major reversible risk factors is essential because, in the case of cigarette smoking and hypercholesterolaemia, this has been shown unequivocally to have a beneficial effect on the natural history of coronary disease. Treatment of hypertension probably yields similar benefits, although the evidence is less convincing; nevertheless, there is no doubt that it improves angina by reducing ventricular wall tension and myocardial oxygen demand.

## Drug therapy (Table 11.9)

Drugs used to treat angina improve the myocardial oxygen supply–demand imbalance. The only important mechanism for improving oxygen supply is coronary vasodilation. Reductions in oxygen demand, however, may be achieved by reducing heart rate, contractility or left ventricular wall tension (reflected by blood pressure). Nitrates and $\beta$-blockers are usually used as first-line agents in the treatment of angina, but if symptoms remain troublesome a calcium antagonist can be added.

### Nitrates

The vasodilator action of these drugs improves coronary flow and, more importantly, reduces ventricular wall tension by lowering the blood pressure. Sublingual glyceryl trinitrate by tablet or spray is rapidly absorbed through the buccal mucosa. Relief of angina occurs within about 2 minutes. The drug can also be used prophylactically to prevent angina during vigorous exertion. A glyceryl trinitrate patch for

**Table 11.9** Drugs used to treat angina.

| Drugs | Dose |
|---|---|
| **Nitrates** | |
| Glyceryl trinitrate | |
| Sublingual tablet | 0.5 mg as required |
| Aerosol spray | 0.4–0.8 mg as required |
| Cutaneous patch | 25–50 mg daily (only 5–10 mg absorbed) |
| Isosorbide mononitrate | 20 mg twice daily |
| **β-Blockers** | |
| Non-selective | |
| Propranolol* | 40–80 mg three times daily |
| Cardioselective | |
| Metoprolol* | 50–100 mg three times daily |
| Atenolol | 50–100 mg once or twice daily |
| Bisoprolol | 5–10 mg once daily |
| **Calcium antagonists** | |
| Nifedipine* | 5–10 mg three times daily |
| Verapamil* | 40–80 mg three times daily |
| Diltiazem* | 60–120 mg three times daily |
| Amlodipine | 5–10 mg once daily |

*Slow-release preparations are available for once or twice daily administration.

percutaneous absorption provides a sustained anti-anginal effect in some patients, but tolerance is common unless the patch is removed intermittently to provide a 'nitrate-free interval' at least once every 24 hours.

Long-term nitrates for regular oral administration are widely used. Isosorbide dinitrate undergoes considerable first-pass metabolism in the liver, but isosorbide mononitrate does not and is the preferred agent in a twice-daily regimen. Side effects of nitrates relate to vasodilation and include postural dizziness and headache.

### β-Blockers

These drugs slow the heart rate and reduce contractility and wall tension. A wide variety of different agents are available all with similar anti-anginal efficacy. In general, long-acting drugs such as atenolol are preferred for once- or twice-daily administration. Additional advantages of atenolol are its cardioselectivity and its lipid insolubility, which ensures it does not enter the brain. β-Blockers, even cardioselective agents, should not be used in patients with a history of asthma because they can precipitate severe attacks of bronchospasm. They should also be avoided in heart failure because of their negative inotropic action.

### Calcium antagonists

Like nitrates these drugs are vasodilators and improve the myocardial oxygen balance by their effect on coronary flow and blood pressure. They also cause variable reductions in contractility, particularly diltiazem and verapamil which should be avoided in severe heart failure. Side effects include facial flushing, headache and postural dizziness. Mild ankle oedema may also occur but its cause is unclear.

## Myocardial revascularization procedures

### Coronary artery bypass grafting

In patients with proximal coronary artery stenoses or occlusions (demonstrated by arteriography), saphenous vein grafts applied to the ascending aorta may be inserted into the coronary arteries distal to the diseased segments. Alternatively the internal mammary artery can be mobilized and used to bypass the diseased segments. These procedures correct myocardial perfusion and provide significant relief from angina in over 80 per cent of cases. The principal indication for bypass grafting is angina that cannot be controlled by medical therapy. Nevertheless, because surgery improves long-term survival in patients with left main stem or multivessel coronary artery disease, coronary arteriography is now recommended in all symptomatic patients aged under 50 (Table 11.8). This permits identification of those in whom surgery offers prognostic benefit.

### Coronary angioplasty

Coronary angioplasty (Fig. 11.18) is being used increasingly for myocardial revascularization. A catheter with a terminal balloon is introduced percutaneously and positioned across the stenosed coronary arterial segment. Inflation of the balloon dilates the stenosis and restores normal coronary flow. Results are best in patients with a proximal stenosis in only a single major vessel, although multivessel disease may also be treated in this way. Coronary angioplasty provides effective relief of angina, but early recurrence occurs in about 20 per cent of cases. Effects on prognosis are unknown.

## PROGNOSIS

Mortality from coronary artery disease has declined in recent years, particularly in the USA. There has probably been a similar decline in the incidence of coronary artery disease. The reasons for this are not known. Nevertheless, the changing natural history of the disease makes prognosis difficult to assess. In the patient with angina, symptoms may remain stable over several years or may even improve as collateral vessels open up. More commonly, however, there is a gradual deterioration with an annual mortality of about 4 per cent. Prognosis is improved by coronary artery bypass grafting in patients with left main or multivessel disease. Low-dose aspirin therapy (150–300 mg daily), stopping cigarette smoking and correcting hypercholesterolaemia also improve prognosis.

# Variant angina

This relatively unusual anginal syndrome was first described by Prinzmetal. It is characterized

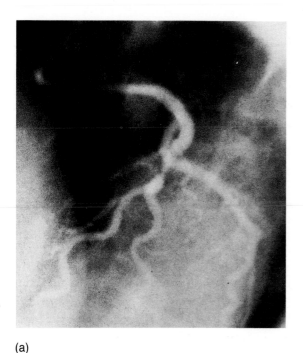

(a)

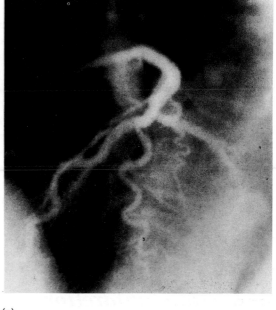

(c)

(b)

**Figure 11.18** Coronary angioplasty. (a) Before angioplasty: there is a tight stenosis in the left anterior descending coronary artery. (b) During angioplasty: the angioplasty balloon has been positioned across the stenosis and inflated. (c) After angioplasty: the stenosis has been successfully dilated and the artery is now widely patent.

by unprovoked episodes of chest pain which may be associated with ST segment elevation on the ECG. Coronary atherosclerosis is present in 70 per cent of cases, but in the remainder the coronary arteries appear normal at arteriography. An exaggerated increase in coronary arterial tone (spasm) has been demonstrated in these patients during attacks of angina. The spasm is usually focal in distribution, involving the proximal segment of a major coronary artery. Even in the absence of atherosclerosis, spasm can restrict coronary flow sufficiently to produce myocardial ischaemia. These patients are at risk of cardiac arrhythmias, and in prolonged attacks of spasm myocardial infarction may occur. Calcium antagonists prevent spasm and are the treatment of choice. Nitrates are also beneficial, but β-blockers are of less value and may be detrimental if unopposed α-adrenergic stimulation further increases coronary tone.

## Unstable angina

Unstable angina may be defined as recurrent episodes of angina occurring on minimal exertion or at rest. Attacks of pain are often associated with reversible ST segment depression on the ECG. The patients usually have critical coronary stenoses with subocclusive thrombus, and are at risk of progression to coronary occlusion with myocardial infarction or death. Treatment is with bed-rest and sedation. Glyceryl trinitrate infusion supplemented with oral β-blockers will often control symptoms. The antithrombotic effects of heparin infusion and low-dose aspirin (150–300 mg daily) protect against thrombotic coronary occlusion and have been shown to improve prognosis. Cardiac catheterization with a view to myocardial revascularization is recommended in all patients under 50 and also patients whose symptoms remain unstable despite treatment.

# Myocardial infarction

Myocardial infarction is responsible for 160000 deaths annually in the UK and for 35 per cent of all deaths in the western world. Fifty per cent of the deaths occur in the first few hours after the onset of symptoms.

## CLINICAL FEATURES

Myocardial infarction usually presents with unprovoked chest pain which is similar in quality to angina but more severe and more prolonged. Autonomic responses produce anxiety, sweating and occasionally vomiting. Examination reveals tachycardia but in other respects may be normal. Nevertheless, signs of myocardial damage, including a palpable dyskinetic impulse over the left precordium and a fourth heart sound, are often present. Low-grade fever is common during the first 3 days. In an estimated 5–10 per cent of cases myocardial infarction is asymptomatic, particularly in diabetics and the elderly.

## DIAGNOSIS

### Electrocardiogram

This is the most useful diagnostic test. Peaking of the T wave followed by ST segment elevation occur during the first hour of pain (Fig. 11.19). Reciprocal ST depression may be seen in the opposite ECG leads. Usually a pathological Q wave (page 153) occurs during the following 24 hours and thereafter persists indefinitely. The ST segment returns to the isoelectric line within 2–3 days and T wave inversion may occur. Occasionally T wave inversion is the only ECG change and is usually attributed to limited subendocardial infarction if other criteria for infarction are fulfilled.

The ECG is a valuable indicator of infarct location. Changes in leads II, III and aVf indicate inferior infarction, while changes in leads V1 to V6 indicate anteroseptal (V1 to V3) or anterolateral (V4 to V6) infarction. When the infarct is located posteriorly ECG changes may be difficult to detect, but dominant R waves in leads V1 and V2 often develop.

### Serum enzymes

Following myocardial infarction enzymes are released into the circulation by the necrosing myocytes (Fig. 11.20).

Creatine phosphokinase is the most useful enzyme for diagnostic purposes. Serum levels peak within 24 hours. The enzyme is also found in skeletal muscle. Thus false positive results may occur following intramuscular injections or external cardiac massage. Creatine phosphokinase isoenzymes can be used to differentiate skeletal and cardiac muscle damage.

Glutamic oxaloacetic transaminase peaks later but remains elevated for about a week. Its diagnostic value is limited by lack of specificity. Thus disease of the liver, kidney and brain may all give false positive results.

Lactic dehydrogenase peaks late but remains elevated for up to 2 weeks. It is also found in red cells, and traumatic venesection may give false positive results.

## DIFFERENTIAL DIAGNOSIS

Unstable angina, pericarditis, aortic dissection and pulmonary embolism are important causes of chest pain which may also be associated with ECG changes. All are discussed elsewhere in this chapter.

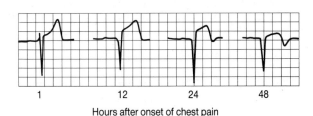

**Figure 11.19** Electrocardiogram (ECG) in acute myocardial infarction. This is lead V2 and shows the typical evolution of changes. Peaking of the T wave and elevation of the ST segment occur during the first hour. Thereafter a Q wave develops and usually persists indefinitely. As the ST segment returns to the isoelectric line, T wave inversion may occur. Thrombolytic therapy accelerates the evolution of ECG changes if successful reperfusion of the infarct-related artery occurs.

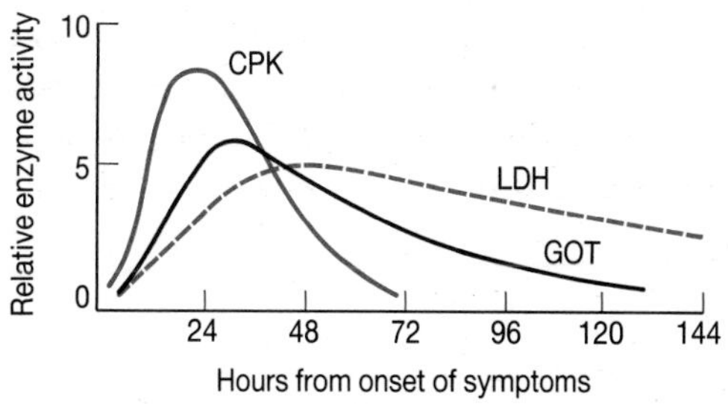

**Figure 11.20** Enzyme release in acute myocardial infarction. These are time–activity curves for creatine phosphokinase (CPK), glutamic oxaloacetic transaminase (GOT) and lactic dehydrogenase (LDH). Serum enzyme activity is expressed as multiples of the upper reference limit.

## COMPLICATIONS

### Cardiac arrhythmias

Following myocardial infarction, arrhythmia provocation is enhanced by autonomic responses, metabolic abnormalities (particularly hypokalaemia and hypoxaemia), continuing myocardial ischaemia and drug actions. Management of the arrhythmia must include correction of these provocative factors as well as specific anti-arrhythmic therapy.

#### Atrial arrhythmias

Atrial fibrillation is a common and usually self-limiting arrhythmia in the early hours following myocardial infarction. Paroxysmal attacks may be suppressed with amiodarone, but sustained atrial fibrillation may require direct current shock if it produces heart failure or angina.

#### Ventricular arrhythmias

Ventricular premature beats occur in nearly all patients after myocardial infarction. Certain patterns (including very frequent beats or very early 'R on T' beats) have been identified as predictors of ventricular fibrillation. Nevertheless, the logic of treating these 'warning' arrhythmias with lignocaine infusion is now in doubt because there is little evidence that it reduces the incidence of ventricular fibrillation and no evidence that it improves prognosis in patients admitted into the coronary care unit.

#### Idioventricular rhythm

Accelerated idioventricular rhythm (rate 60–120 beats/min) commonly complicates acute myocardial infarction, but is rare in other contexts. The accelerated ventricular ectopic focus is usually in continuous competition with the sinus node such that the idioventricular rhythm is typically intermittent, alternating with episodes of sinus rhythm (Fig. 11.21). Treatment is unnecessary.

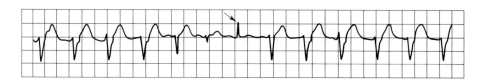

**Figure 11.21** Accelerated idioventricular rhythm. The broad-complex idioventricular rhythm is interrupted by 'fusion' beats (part sinus and part ventricular in origin) and a single sinus beat (arrowed).

## Tachycardia

Ventricular tachycardia (rate >120 beats/min) always requires prompt treatment. Paroxysmal attacks may be suppressed with lignocaine bolus followed by infusion (Table 11.10), but sustained attacks require direct current cardio-version.

## Ventricular fibrillation

Ventricular fibrillation requires urgent direct current cardioversion to prevent death. It usually occurs as a 'primary' electrical pheno-menon in the early hours after myocardial infarc-tion, emphasizing the importance of rapid access to resuscitation facilities following the onset of chest pain (Fig. 11.22). Ventricular fibrillation sometimes occurs late after myocardial infarc-tion when it is usually 'secondary' to extensive myocardial damage. If resuscitation is success-ful, long-term anti-arrhythmic therapy is neces-sary because secondary ventricular fibrillation predicts a high incidence of sudden death following hospital discharge.

## Heart block

Myocardial infarction may damage the special-ized conducting tissues. If this causes (or threatens to cause) an excessively slow heart rate, temporary pacemaker therapy may be necessary to maintain cardiac output and prevent asystole (Table 11.11). The prognostic implications of heart block in myocardial infarction are shown in Table 11.12.

## Atrioventricular block

This is usually a complication of inferior infarc-tion and is caused by inflammation and oedema around the atrioventricular node. In third-degree (complete) atrioventricular block a junc-tional escape rhythm usually takes over with a reliable rate of 40–60 beats/min (Fig. 11.23). In most cases this is sufficient to maintain normal cardiac output. Complete recovery of atrio-ventricular conduction nearly always occurs within 2 weeks. If the junctional escape rhythm is very slow it will often respond to intravenous atropine (0.6 mg). Indications for pacemaker

**Table 11.10** Vaughan-Williams classification of anti-arrhythmic drugs.

| | Acute intravenous therapy | | | |
|---|---|---|---|---|
| | Bolus* (mg) | Infusion (mg/min) | Chronic oral therapy daily dose (mg) | Therapeutic blood levels (mg/l) |
| **Class I (depress the rapid influx of sodium ion that initiates the action potential)** | | | | |
| A (prolong the Q–T interval) | | | | |
| Quinidine | † | † | 1000 | 2.0–5.0 |
| Disopyramide | 100–150 | 0.5 | 300–800 | 2.0–5.0 |
| B (shorten the Q–T interval) | | | | |
| Lignocaine | 50–200 | 1.0–4.0 | † | 2.0–5.0 |
| Mexiletine | 125–250 | 0.5–1.0 | 600–1000 | 0.75–2.0 |
| C (Q–T interval unaffected) | | | | |
| Flecainide | 100–150 | 0.25 | 200–400 | 0.4–1.0 |
| Propafenone | † | † | 450–1200 | – |
| **Class II (β-blockers, protective against excessive adrenergic stimulation)** | | | | |
| Atenolol | 5–10 | † | 50–100 | 0.1–1.0 |
| **Class III (prolong the action potential, increasing the refractory period of conducting tissue)** | | | | |
| Amiodarone | 300–900 | 0.5–1.0 | 200–400 | 0.6–2.5 |
| Bretylium | 500–1000 | 0.5–2.1 | † | – |
| Sotalol | 20–60 | † | 120–240 | – |
| **Class IV (calcium blockers, decrease depolarization and slow atrioventricular conduction)** | | | | |
| Verapamil | 5–10 | 0.05–0.1 | 120–240 | 0.1–0.2 |

*Bolus injections should always be given slowly over at least 5 minutes. The injection may be repeated after 15 minutes if the desired effects are not achieved. †Not available.

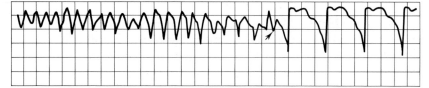

**Figure 11.22** Primary ventricular fibrillation. The electrocardiogram shows changes of acute myocardial infarction with sinus tachycardia and ST segment elevation. A very early premature beat (arrowed) triggers ventricular fibrillation.

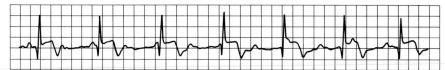

**Figure 11.23** Third-degree (complete) heart block in inferior myocardial infarction. Block is at the atrioventricular node and has caused dissociation of the atrial and ventricular rhythms. Thus the P waves and the QRS complexes are completely independent of one another. Because the 'escape' rhythm is junctional in origin, the QRS complexes are narrow and the rate is well maintained. The monitoring lead is III and shows a Q wave with ST segment elevation.

**Table 11.11** Indications for temporary pacing in acute myocardial infarction.

Third-degree (complete) atrioventricular block complicating inferior myocardial infarction and any of the following:

    (a) Rate less than 40 beats/min, unresponsive to atropine
    (b) Heart failure
    (c) Unreliable escape rhythm
    (d) Bradycardia-dependent ventricular arrhythmias which require suppression

All cases of third-degree (complete) or Mobitz type II second-degree atrioventricular block complicating anterior myocardial infarction

Bifascicular heart block

therapy are shown in Table 11.11. When atrioventricular block complicates anterior myocardial infarction, this usually implies extensive left ventricular injury with damage to both left and right bundle branches. Ventricular escape rhythms are always slow and unreliable, and whether the block is complete or intermittent (Mobitz type II, page 207) pacemaker therapy is indicated.

*Bundle branch block*
Isolated left or right bundle branch block is an adverse prognostic sign but requires no specific treatment. Left or right axis deviation (hemiblock) in myocardial infarction often indicates damage to the anterior or posterior fascicle of the

**Table 11.12** Acute atrioventricular block in myocardial infarction.

| Conduction defect | Incidence (%) | Risk of progression to third-degree block (%) | Mortality (%) |
|---|---|---|---|
| None | 70 | 6 | 15 |
| First-degree block | 5 | 6 | 15 |
| Second-degree block | | | |
|   Mobitz type I | 5 | 7 | 15 |
|   Mobitz type II | 1 | 70 | 50 |
| Third-degree block | 7 | – | 25 |
| Left anterior hemiblock | 5 | 3 | 27 |
| Left posterior hemiblock | 1 | 0 | 42 |
| Right bundle branch block | 2 | 43 | 46 |
| Left bundle branch block | 5 | 20 | 44 |
| Bifascicular block | 5 | 46 | 45 |

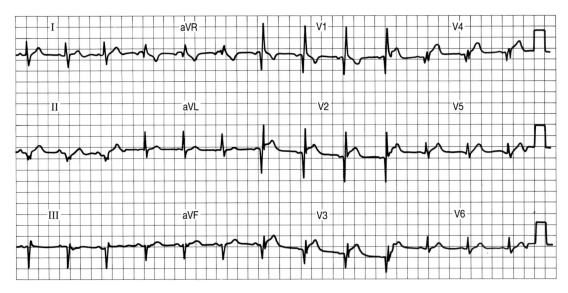

**Figure 11.24** Bifascicular block complicating acute myocardial infarction. Note the pathological Q waves and ST elevation in leads V1 to V4 indicating anterior infarction. The QRS complexes are broad due to right bundle branch block (large R wave in V1 with late S waves in I and V6) and there is marked left axis deviation (−90°) indicating left anterior hemiblock. Thus atrioventricular conduction is dependent on the posterior division of the left bundle branch and the risk of complete heart block is high.

left bundle, respectively. When hemiblock is associated with right bundle branch block ('**bifascicular block**'), atrioventricular conduction is dependent upon the remaining fascicle of the left bundle (Fig. 11.24). The risk of complete heart block developing is considerable and prophylactic pacing should be undertaken.

## Left ventricular failure

This affects about 33 per cent of all patients with myocardial infarction and is the principal cause of death following admission to the coronary care unit. Because right ventricular damage is rarely severe, left ventricular failure usually dominates the clinical picture. The severity of failure is closely related to infarct size; when about 40 per cent of the left ventricle is damaged cardiogenic shock occurs (pages 168 and 249). The principal clinical manifestations of left ventricular failure are pulmonary oedema and peripheral hypoperfusion, caused by elevated left atrial pressure and reduced cardiac output, respectively. Four subsets of patients have been identified based on these clinical manifestations

and defined by a cardiac output of 3.5 l/min and a left atrial (pulmonary artery wedge) pressure of 18 mm Hg (Fig. 11.25):

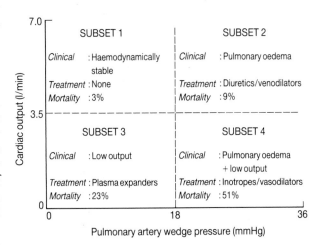

**Figure 11.25** Haemodynamic subsets in acute myocardial infarction. The subset divisions are defined by the intersection of a pulmonary artery wedge pressure of 18 mm Hg and a cardiac output of 3.5 l/min. The clinical, therapeutic and prognostic correlates of subset classification are illustrated.

Subset 1:  Well-preserved left ventricular function requiring no specific therapy.

Subset 2:  Pulmonary oedema with well-maintained cardiac output. Treatment with morphine and diuretics is usually effective.

Subset 3:  Critical reduction in cardiac output without pulmonary oedema. Oliguria and hypotension are corrected by infusion of a plasma volume expander (e.g. plasma, blood) which increases cardiac output by the Starling mechanism. Careful monitoring of pulmonary artery wedge pressure is essential to prevent overloading the circulation. Pulmonary oedema develops if the wedge pressure rises above 18 mm Hg.

Subset 4:  Low cardiac output and pulmonary oedema occur together. Treatment must be directed towards improving left ventricular function with vasodilators or inotropes. These drugs should be given by controlled intravenous infusion to reduce pulmonary artery wedge pressure and improve cardiac output. Responses are best monitored with a Swan Ganz catheter.

Subset classification provides not only a useful basis for therapeutic decision making but also a means of predicting prognosis. Thus mortality rises from less than 5 per cent in subset 1 to greater than 50 per cent in subset 4.

## Right ventricular failure

Occasionally, inferior myocardial infarction is associated with extensive right ventricular damage and leads to right ventricular failure with elevation of the right atrial and jugular venous pressures. From the clinical point of view, low cardiac output is the principal problem, and a useful improvement can often be achieved by further increasing the right atrial pressure with infusions of plasma volume expander. This increases the right ventricular output by the Starling mechanism. Monitoring

of pulmonary capillary wedge pressure is a sensible precaution during the infusion in order to guard against pulmonary oedema.

## Myocardial rupture

This usually occurs during the first 10 days following myocardial infarction. When it involves the free wall of the ventricle it causes severe tamponade, which is usually fatal. Rupture of a papillary muscle or the interventricular septum both cause circulatory collapse with a pansystolic murmur. Doppler echocardiography is diagnostic by demonstrating the severe mitral regurgitant flow in papillary muscle rupture or the left-to-right flow across the defect in ventricular septal rupture. In most cases, however, urgent cardiac catheterization is required to define the lesion and to assess the potential for surgical correction.

## Pericarditis and Dressler's syndrome

Pericarditis during the first 3 days after myocardial infarction is a direct consequence of the underlying muscle damage and usually resolves rapidly. Pericarditis which presents later may indicate Dressler's syndrome, particularly when associated with fever, pericarditic chest pain and an alevated erythrocyte sedimentation rate. Dressler's syndrome is probably an autoimmune phenomenon. It is self-limiting, but anti-inflammatory analgesics (e.g. aspirin) provide effective symptomatic relief. Occasionally corticosteroids are necessary. Relapses up to 2 years after myocardial infarction may occur.

## Thromboembolism

Deep venous thrombosis and intracardiac mural thrombosis (overlying the infarcted ventricular myocardium) are potential sources of pulmonary and systemic thromboembolism, respectively. Heparin therapy reduces the risk of these complications.

## Ventricular aneurysm

If scar formation is inadequate following myocardial infarction, a thin-walled left ventricular aneurysm may develop. This is often associated with persistent ST segment elevation on the ECG. Ventricular aneurysm predisposes to arrhythmias, heart failure and thromboembolism and may require surgical excision.

## TREATMENT

The main aims of treatment are to correct symptoms, especially chest pain, and prevent death. Myocardial infarction has an estimated 35–40 per cent mortality. About half these deaths occur within 2 hours of the onset of chest pain, before arrival at hospital, and in most cases are the result of ventricular fibrillation, although myocardial rupture also contributes. In hospital, however, lethal arrhythmias can be corrected by defibrillation and the most important cause of death is left ventricular failure due to extensive infarction. Patients with large infarcts are also at risk of death in the year following hospital discharge. Thus, significant reductions in mortality from acute myocardial infarction can be achieved by ensuring early access to a defibrillator and by intervention with specific drugs to prevent myocardial rupture and reduce infarct size.

### General measures

Early access to a defibrillator in order to prevent death from ventricular fibrillation requires prompt hospital admission. The patient should be placed in the coronary care unit and attached to an ECG monitor. An intravenous line should be established. Pain relief and sedation are of overriding importance. Intravenous diamorphine (2.5–5.0 mg) is the drug of choice for both purposes, and should be repeated as necessary. Drug-induced nausea and vomiting are reduced by intravenous prochlorperazine (25–50 mg). Anticoagulation with heparin is recommended, not only as an adjunct to thrombolytic therapy (see below), but also to guard against thromboembolism by preventing deep venous and mural thrombosis. If the early course is uncomplicated the patient may be transferred to the general ward after 24 hours. Mobilization is started after 3 days with a view to discharge after 7–10 days.

### Treatment to prevent myocardial rupture

Intravenous β-blockers (metoprolol or atenolol, 5 mg) reduce hospital mortality by about 15 per cent, probably by protecting against myocardial rupture. Treatment should be reserved for hypertensive patients (systolic pressure >160 mm Hg) who are at special risk, but is contraindicated in patients with asthma, severe bradycardia or left ventricular failure.

### Treatment to reduce infarct size

Following thrombotic coronary occlusion, the full extent of myocardial damage may take 6 hours or more to develop. Treatment with thrombolytic drugs within this period can dissolve the thrombus in 50–70 per cent of cases, leading to recanalization of the occluded artery, reperfusion of the jeopardized myocardium, and reduction in infarct size (Fig. 11.26). Early treatment reduces hospital mortality by up to 50 per cent, but some benefit can still be demonstrated in patients treated within 24 hours. Aspirin also reduces mortality, probably because its effects on platelet function favour coronary patency. Current recommendations are for intravenous infusion of streptokinase (1.5 million units over 1 hour) and oral aspirin (150 mg) to be given as soon as possible after admission to all patients who present within 12 hours of the onset of chest pain. Concurrent heparin infusion (1000 units/hour) may help maintain coronary patency after successful thrombolysis and is usually continued until the patient starts to mobilize, with maintenance aspirin treatment thereafter. Contraindications to thrombolytic therapy include active peptic ulceration, prolonged resuscitation, and surgery or cerebrovascular accident (CVA) within the previous 4 weeks.

Streptokinase is antigenic and elicits an antibody response which, in the event of re-exposure to the drug, neutralizes its thrombolytic activity and predisposes to anaphylaxis. Thus the 5 per cent of patients who experience recurrent myocardial infarction within a year of receiving streptokinase should be treated with alteplase, an alternative, more expensive but equally effective thrombolytic agent that is not antigenic because it is synthesized by recombinant DNA technology to resemble the tissue plasminogen activator normally secreted by human endothelial cells.

Magnesium may also reduce hospital mortality although further studies are needed to determine whether its use in combination with thrombolytic therapy should be adopted as standard practice.

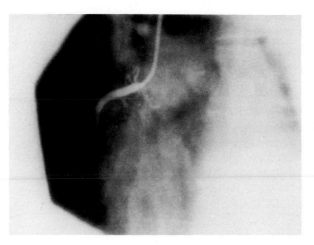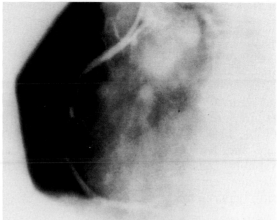

**Figure 11.26** Thrombolytic therapy in acute myocardial infarction. The panel on the left shows the right coronary arteriogram in a patient with inferior myocardial infarction. The artery is occluded near its origin. The panel on the right shows the arteriogram following streptokinase therapy. The artery is now recanalized but there is a tight residual stenosis. Further management must include measures to prevent re-occlusion such as anticoagulant therapy or revascularization (angioplasty, bypass surgery).

## Rehabilitation

Formal rehabilitation programmes are available in some centres, most offering simple health education and a few providing supervised physical training in addition. Advice suitable for all patients should include a graded return to activity within the limits of their exercise tolerance. They should be strongly advised to stop smoking and to reduce their weight to the ideal level for their height and age. They should not drive for 2 months. Normal sexual activity can be resumed after a month provided exercise tolerance is satisfactory. Patients may require advice about their future occupation. They should usually be able to return to work in 8–12 weeks and thereafter should be encouraged to lead as full and as normal a life as possible.

## Secondary prevention

In the year that follows myocardial infarction there is a significant risk of recurrent infarction or sudden death. Measures of proven value for reducing that risk are stopping cigarette smoking, and treatment with β-blockers. There is also increasing evidence that daily aspirin is beneficial, and treatment to lower blood cholesterol in patients with hypercholesterolaemia. Recently treatment with angiotensin-converting enzyme inhibitors has been shown to protect against worsening heart failure and death in patients with left ventricular impairment following acute myocardial infarction.

Recurrent infarction is more common following successful thrombolytic therapy because of the risk of coronary re-occlusion. Daily aspirin may reduce that risk but there is no clear evidence that revascularization by angioplasty or surgery is helpful. This is usually reserved for patients with continuing chest pain or evidence of residual ischaemia during exercise stress testing. Thus all patients with uncomplicated infarction should undergo stress testing before discharge. Those who develop ST depression suggestive of ischaemia (page 170) or ventricular arrhythmias require referral for cardiac catheterization with a view to revascularization. Despite continuing enthusiasm for this relatively simple method of selecting and treating 'high-risk' patients, convincing evidence for its efficacy in terms of improving long-term prognosis has not been forthcoming.

## PROGNOSIS

Myocardial infarction is fatal in about 40 per cent of cases: 20 per cent within 6 hours of the attack before hospital admission, 10–15 per cent in hospital, and 10 per cent during the first year after discharge. The prehospital mortality is due to primary ventricular fibrillation in the majority of cases. Primary ventricular fibrillation, however, does not necessarily reflect extensive myocardial damage, and prognosis following resuscitation is similar to that of other early survivors.

Hospital mortality is closely related to infarct size. When infarction is sufficiently extensive to cause severe heart failure, mortality exceeds 50 per cent. Other factors, apart from overt heart failure, are also predictive of a poor prognosis (Table 11.13). With the exception of advanced age and female sex, however, these are all variably related to extensive myocardial damage, emphasizing the important relationship between infarct size and prognosis.

**Table 11.13** Adverse prognostic factors in myocardial infarction.

Advanced age
Female sex
Anterior transmural infarction
Bundle branch block and advanced atrioventricular block
Heart failure
Systolic hypotension
Complex ventricular arrhythmias occurring greater than 24 hours after the onset of symptoms
History of previous myocardial infarction
Diabetes mellitus

# CARDIOMYOPATHY

The cardiomyopathies are a group of chronic heart muscle disorders of unknown cause classified into dilated, hypertrophic and restrictive types. This definition excludes those specific heart muscle disorders that are secondary to coronary artery disease, valvar disease, hypertension and other systemic disorders.

## Dilated cardiomyopathy

### AETIOLOGY

The cause of dilated cardiomyopathy is by definition unknown. There is some evidence for an infectious–autoimmune aetiology related to viral myocarditis, but this is unproven.

### PATHOLOGY AND PATHOPHYSIOLOGY

Dilated cardiomyopathy is characterized by progressive dilation, hypertrophy and fibrosis of all the cardiac chambers. Contractile function is severely impaired. Atrial fibrillation commonly supervenes and stretching of the atrioventricular valve rings can lead to functional mitral and tricuspid incompetence. These complications produce additional impairment of ventricular function.

### CLINICAL FEATURES

Dilated cardiomyopathy often remains asymptomatic in its early stages, but with progression of the disease, symptoms and signs of congestive heart failure develop (page 162).

### DIAGNOSIS

The chest X-ray shows cardiac enlargement with dilated upper lobe veins and, in advanced cases, pulmonary oedema. The echocardiogram shows four-chamber dilation and global left ventricular contractile impairment (Fig. 11.27). Doppler studies often reveal mitral and tricuspid regurgitation even if these are not evident clinically.

### DIFFERENTIAL DIAGNOSIS

This includes all those conditions listed in Table 11.14 that cause specific heart muscle disease. Coronary artery disease is suggested by a history of angina or myocardial infarction associated with pathological Q waves on the ECG. Valvar disease is confirmed by echocardiography. Hypertensive and alcoholic heart disease are sometimes impossible to distinguish from dilated cardiomyopathy. Nevertheless, a careful history often provides the aetiological diagnosis, and the examination may reveal non-cardiac manifestations of hypertensive or alcoholic end-

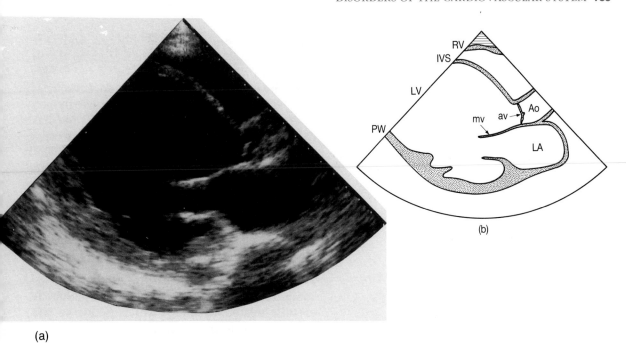

(a)

(b)

**Figure 11.27** (a,b) Echocardiogram in dilated cardiomyopathy. Two-dimensional recording showing enormous dilation of the left ventricle (compare with Fig. 11.12b).

organ damage. Viral myocarditis is usually a subclinical complication of upper respiratory infection, but occasionally it causes severe heart failure and mimics dilated cardiomyopathy. Complete recovery, however, can be expected in most cases of viral myocarditis. Doxorubicin, a widely used antineoplastic agent, causes dose-related myocardial toxicity. The risk is particularly high once a cumulative dose of $550\,mg/m^2$ has been exceeded. Once heart failure is established the condition is similar to dilated cardiomyopathy but progresses more rapidly.

## COMPLICATIONS

Cardiac arrhythmias are common in dilated cardiomyopathy, particularly atrial fibrillation and ventricular extrasystoles. More complex ventricular arrhythmias (ventricular tachycardia and fibrillation) are a cause of sudden death. Systemic and pulmonary thromboembolism is common, particularly in patients with atrial fibrillation.

## TREATMENT

Dilated cardiomyopathy should be managed in the same way as other causes of congestive heart failure with diuretics and angiotensin-converting enzyme inhibitors. Patients in atrial fibrillation require digoxin to control the ventricular rate and anticoagulation with warfarin to protect against thromboembolism.

## PROGNOSIS

This depends on the severity of left ventricular dysfunction. Once symptoms of heart failure develop the average 5-year survival is less than 50 per cent. Angiotensin-converting enzyme inhibitors are helpful, but in patients with end-stage disease heart transplantation is the only treatment likely to be of long-term benefit (page 166).

# Hypertrophic cardiomyopathy

## AETIOLOGY

Hypertrophic cardiomyopathy shows an autosomal dominant pattern of inheritance but it occurs sporadically in about half of all cases.

**Table 11.14** Causes of specific heart muscle disease.

**Cardiovascular**
Coronary artery disease
Chronic valvar disease
Hypertension

**Infective**
Viral (e.g. Coxsackie A and B)
Influenza, varicella, mumps
Herpes simplex
Protozoal (e.g. trypanosomiasis–Chagas' disease)

**Metabolic**
Thiamine deficiency (beriberi)
Kwashiorkor

**Endocrine**
Thyrotoxicosis
Myxoedema
Diabetes mellitus

**Toxic**
Alcohol
Doxorubicin
Cobalt

**Connective tissue disease**
Vasculitis
Systemic lupus erythematosus

**Neuromuscular disease**
Muscular dystrophy
Friedreich's ataxia

**Infiltrative**
Amyloidosis
Haemochromatosis
Sarcoidosis
Neoplastic

**Miscellaneous**
Post-partum cardiomyopathy

## PATHOLOGY

Hypertrophic cardiomyopathy is characterized anatomically by ventricular hypertrophy usually with disproportionate involvement of the interventricular septum. Histologically there is disarray and disorganization of the cardiac myocytes.

The physiological disorder is one of impaired diastolic relaxation. Systolic contraction is normal and often hyperdynamic. The hypertrophied ventricle is stiff (non-compliant) and adequate filling demands high end-diastolic pressure. Atrial contraction provides an important boost to ventricular filling, and the development of atrial fibrillation often results in abrupt clinical deterioration.

In the past considerable importance has been attached to the pressure gradient which can often be demonstrated in the left ventricular outflow tract beneath the aortic valve. However, the pressure gradient does not always reflect significant obstruction to flow and appears to have little influence on symptoms and prognosis in patients with hypertrophic cardiomyopathy.

## CLINICAL FEATURES

Hypertrophic cardiomyopathy is often asymptomatic. The most common complaint is exercise-related dyspnoea which is due to the elevated left atrial pressure required to fill the stiff, non-compliant ventricle. In advanced cases frank congestive heart failure occasionally develops. Angina, due to the excessive oxygen demand of the hypertrophied ventricle, may also be troublesome.

Examination reveals a 'jerky' carotid pulse owing to vigorous left ventricular ejection in early systole. The apical impulse is prominent and often has a double thrust caused by a palpable fourth heart sound. Auscultatory features include the fourth heart sound and a mid-systolic ejection murmur at the aortic area caused by turbulent flow in the left ventricular outflow tract. Mitral regurgitation affects nearly half of all cases and when present produces an apical pansystolic murmur.

## DIAGNOSIS

The ECG shows left ventricular hypertrophy. This is confirmed by the echocardiogram which usually shows disproportionate involvement of the interventricular septum (Fig. 11.28). Other echocardiographic findings are systolic anterior motion of the mitral valve and early closure of the aortic valve. When the diagnosis remains unclear, cardiac catheterization can be performed for measurement of the pressure gradient in the left ventricular outflow tract and angiographic demonstration of the abnormal left ventricular contraction pattern.

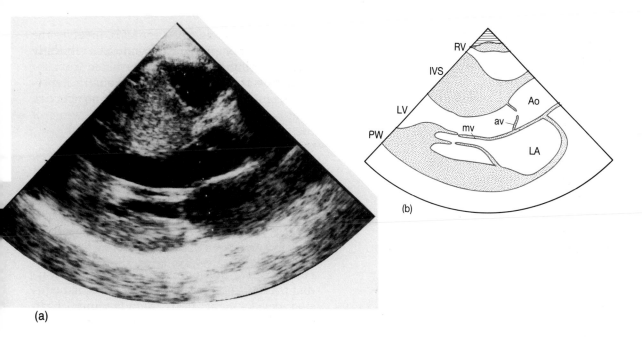

(a)

(b)

**Figure 11.28** (a,b) Echocardiogram in hypertrophic cardiomyopathy. Two-dimensional recording showing massive left ventricular hypertrophy predominantly affecting the interventricular septum (compare with Fig. 11.12b).

## DIFFERENTIAL DIAGNOSIS

Hypertension and aortic stenosis both produce left ventricular hypertrophy and share many of the clinical and ECG features of hypertrophic cardiomyopathy. Nevertheless, the elevated blood pressure and slow rising pulse which, respectively, characterize these conditions help in making the correct differential diagnosis. Moreover, in both conditions the echocardiogram shows concentric left ventricular hypertrophy without other features of hypertrophic cardiomyopathy; the valvar abnormality in aortic stenosis is readily apparent.

Hypertrophic cardiomyopathy must also be differentiated from coronary artery disease. This may require coronary arteriography in patients with angina.

## COMPLICATIONS

Cardiac arrhythmias are the major complication. Atrial fibrillation causes abrupt clinical deterioration (pages 184 and 211). More sinister, however, are ventricular arrhythmias which produce dizziness and syncope (Stokes–Adams attacks) and are portents of sudden death.

## TREATMENT

No drugs affect the progression of disease in hypertrophic cardiomyopathy. Treatment is aimed at correcting symptoms and preventing sudden death. β-Blockers control angina and also produce a variable improvement in ventricular diastolic relaxation. This reduces the left atrial pressure and improves dyspnoea. All patients should undergo ambulatory ECG monitoring (page 211). If ventricular arrhythmias are detected amiodarone is the drug of choice because it may prevent sudden death. Screening of family members and genetic counselling should be undertaken, as with other inherited disorders.

# *Restrictive cardiomyopathy*

Restrictive cardiomyopathy is characterized by endomyocardial fibrosis with progressive obliteration of the ventricular cavities. Systolic function is normal but diastolic relaxation is restricted. Restrictive cardiomyopathy is rare in the UK and nearly always associated with cryptogenic hypereosinophilia (page 623). Presentation is with congestive heart failure. Steroids or cytotoxic agents lower the eosinophil count and may halt the progression of disease.

Primary amyloidosis commonly involves the heart and may produce a syndrome clinically and physiologically indistinguishable from restrictive cardiomyopathy, although hypereosinophilia is not present. There is no effective treatment and death occurs within 2 years of presentation.

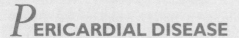

# PERICARDIAL DISEASE

## Acute pericarditis

### AETIOLOGY

Causes of pericarditis are listed in Table 11.15. Viral infection probably accounts for the majority of cases, including many of those idiopathic cases in which a specific cause cannot be positively identified.

### PATHOLOGY

Pathological features are those of any acute inflammatory process. An inflammatory exudate commonly occurs resulting in pericardial effusion.

### CLINICAL FEATURES

Central chest pain is the predominant symptom and may be associated with fever. The pain is

**Table 11.15** Causes of acute pericarditis.

Idiopathic
Infective
   Viral (Coxsackie B, influenza, *Herpes simplex*)
   Bacterial (*Staphylococcus aureus, Mycobacterium tuberculosis*)
Connective tissue disease
   Systemic lupus erythematosus
   Rheumatoid arthritis
   Vasculitis
Uraemia
Malignancy (e.g. breast, lung, lymphoma, leukaemia)
Radiation therapy
Acute myocardial infarction
Post myocardial infarction/cardiotomy (Dressler's syndrome)

typically sharp in quality and is aggravated by deep inspiration, coughing and changes in posture. Auscultation usually reveals a pericardial friction rub (page 150). If pericardial effusion develops the heart sounds diminish in intensity but the friction rub does not necessarily disappear.

### DIAGNOSIS

The ECG shows widespread ST segment elevation. The ST segments are concave upwards (unlike myocardial infarction) and return towards baseline as the pericardial inflammation subsides.

The aetiological diagnosis in viral pericarditis requires demonstration of elevated serum viral antibody titres with return towards normal during convalescence. In connective tissue disorders (page 571) there is usually evidence of multisystem disease, and specific serology, including rheumatoid or antinuclear factors, may be positive. When the aetiological diagnosis is obscure pericardial fluid (if present) should be aspirated for bacteriological, cytological and serological examination (Table 11.15).

### DIFFERENTIAL DIAGNOSIS

Important differential diagnoses are myocardial infarction and pleurisy, although it should be appreciated that both conditions may themselves be associated with pericarditis. The quality of pericarditic pain, the failure of Q waves to develop on the ECG and the absence of significant serum enzyme changes effectively exclude myocardial infarction. Pleuritic pain is similar to pericarditic pain but its location is usually different, and a pleural rub is often audible over the painful area.

## COMPLICATIONS

The major complication of pericarditis is pericardial effusion which may cause tamponade. Pericarditis can also progress to pericardial constriction. Atrial arrhythmias are common but rarely troublesome.

## TREATMENT

Anti-inflammatory analgesics (e.g. aspirin) are effective for controlling chest pain. In viral pericarditis no other treatment is necessary. Bacterial pericarditis requires vigorous antibiotic therapy.

Pericarditis may be a recurrent illness particularly in Dressler's syndrome, connective tissue disorders and idiopathic disease. When recurrence is frequent, low-dose corticosteroid therapy (prednisolone, 5–10 mg daily) offers effective prophylaxis.

## PROGNOSIS

Pericarditis is usually a benign disorder and the prognosis depends on the underlying cause. Nevertheless, the development of tamponade or pericardial constriction may be fatal if not corrected.

# Cardiac tamponade

## AETIOLOGY

In the UK the principal causes of cardiac tamponade are haemopericardium following heart surgery and pericardial effusion complicating neoplastic disease. Nevertheless, almost any other cause of pericardial haemorrhage or effusion may cause tamponade, depending principally on the rate of fluid accumulation within the pericardial sac.

## PATHOPHYSIOLOGY

Gradual accumulation of fluid permits progressive stretching of the pericardial sac such that a substantial effusion may develop without significant elevation of intrapericardial pressure. Rapid accumulations, on the other hand, cause elevation of pressure within the pericardial sac, which leads to tamponade. This tends to constrict the heart and impede diastolic relaxation. Adequate ventricular filling depends on the diastolic pressures in both ventricles rising to equilibrate with the intrapericardial pressure. As tamponade worsens, progressive increments in ventricular filling pressures become inadequate to maintain cardiac output.

## CLINICAL FEATURES

Presentation is abrupt following pericardial haemorrhage but it is usually more gradual in patients with pericardial effusion. Shortness of breath and fatigue are the principal complaints. Examination reveals tachycardia, elevated jugular venous pressure with a prominent 'x' descent, hypotension and signs of reduced cardiac output or cardiogenic shock. Pulsus paradoxus (page 146) is invariable, and in some patients Kussmaul's sign is also present (page 147). The heart sounds are faint and a pericardial friction rub may be audible.

## DIAGNOSIS

The chest X-ray shows globular cardiac enlargement. The ECG shows diminished voltage deflections which may be associated with electrical alternans (Fig. 11.29). Echocardiography confirms pericardial effusion.

## DIFFERENTIAL DIAGNOSIS

Tamponade must be differentiated from other causes of low cardiac output and shock, including myocardial infarction, pulmonary embolism and septicaemia. The differential diagnosis is not difficult if pulsus paradoxus and pericardial effusion can be demonstrated.

## TREATMENT

Tamponade requires urgent pericardiocentesis in order to decompress the heart. A needle is introduced into the angle between the xiphisternum and the left costal margin and advanced

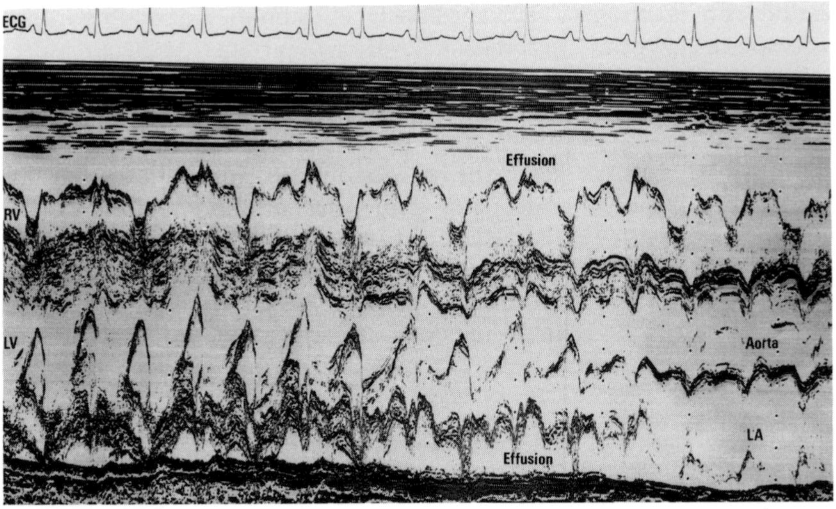

**Figure 11.29**
Electrocardiogram (ECG) and echocardiogram in pericardial effusion. This M-mode echocardiogram shows a pericardial effusion evidenced by the echo-free space in front of and behind the heart (compare with Fig. 11.12a). The movement of the heart within the effusion is unrestricted resulting in beat-to-beat variation in the electrical axis of the ECG (electrical alternans).

beneath the costal margin towards the left shoulder. Following entry into the pericardial sac, the effusion is aspirated. Further treatment is directed at the underlying cause.

## PROGNOSIS

Cardiac tamponade is potentially lethal, but following pericardiocentesis the prognosis depends on the underlying cause of the fluid accumulation.

# Constrictive pericarditis

## AETIOLOGY

Constrictive pericarditis is no longer common in the UK owing largely to the decline in incidence of tuberculosis. Most cases are now idiopathic in origin.

## PATHOPHYSIOLOGY

Fibrosis and shrinkage of the pericardial sac impedes diastolic relaxation of the ventricles and prevents adequate filling. Thus abnormal physiology in constrictive pericarditis is very similar to that seen in tamponade (page 187).

## CLINICAL FEATURES

Constrictive pericarditis is a chronic wasting illness. Although symptoms and signs of low cardiac output are usually present, the consequences of elevated right atrial pressure and salt and water retention dominate the clinical picture. The appearances are those of severe right heart failure with elevation of the jugular venous pressure, hepatomegaly, ascites and peripheral oedema. Kussmaul's sign (page 147) is always positive, but pulsus paradoxus is seen less commonly. Auscultation reveals an early third heart sound (pericardial 'knock').

## DIAGNOSIS

The ECG shows diminished voltage deflections. The chest X-ray is often normal but may show pericardial calcification, particularly in tuberculous disease. Cardiac catheterization confirms elevation of the left and right atrial pressures, which equalize with loss of the normal differential. The ventricular diastolic pressure signal shows a characteristic dip and plateau configuration (the 'square-root' sign).

## DIFFERENTIAL DIAGNOSIS

This includes all other causes of right heart failure. Cirrhosis of the liver must also enter the differential diagnosis. In most cases of right heart failure the heart is enlarged and right ventricular dilation can be demonstrated by echocardiography. Moreover, in the majority of cases associated pulmonary disease or left heart failure is evident. Cirrhosis of the liver produces ascites and debility but does not share the cardiovascular manifestations of constrictive pericarditis.

## TREATMENT

Diuretics control salt and water overload, but pericardiectomy is the treatment of choice. The procedure is technically demanding but if successful the results are excellent.

# *R*HEUMATIC FEVER

Rheumatic fever remains a major health problem in many parts of the world. In developed countries, however, its incidence has declined dramatically in the last 50 years although recent reports of regional outbreaks indicate that there are no grounds for complacency.

## AETIOLOGY

A small proportion (less than 1 per cent) of patients with group A haemolytic streptococcal pharyngitis develop rheumatic fever 2 or 3 weeks later. The disease occurs most commonly between the ages of 5 and 15 years. The precise pathogenic role of the Streptococcus is unknown but an autoimmune process is suggested by the latency period between throat infection and development of rheumatic fever and the immunological cross-reaction between streptococcal antigens and myocardial sarcolemma.

The tendency of rheumatic fever to be familial and the high incidence of recurrence after an initial attack indicate heightened susceptibility in certain individuals, possibly due to genetic predisposition. Nevertheless, the major factors predisposing to the disease are crowding and social deprivation which encourage spread of the Streptococcus. Improvements in housing and welfare have undoubtedly played the major role in reducing the incidence of rheumatic fever throughout the developed world. Other contributory factors have been the availability of penicillin and the changing virulence of the Streptococcus itself.

## PATHOLOGY

Myocarditis and transient pericarditis occur commonly but are rarely severe. Endocarditis is the major cardiac lesion. Inflammation of the valve cusps is associated with verrucous nodules along the lines of valve closure. This may cause severe valve damage acutely, but more commonly valve function is little affected in this phase of illness. During healing, however, progressive scarring of the valve may lead to chronic rheumatic heart disease (see below).

## CLINICAL FEATURES

Fever and arthralgia are often the only symptoms. These may be attributed to a simple viral infection which is soon forgotten by the patient.

### *Carditis*

This affects about 50 per cent of cases. It may cause severe heart failure and death, although usually it produces no symptoms at all. Tachycardia, gallop rhythm and a soft ejection murmur at the aortic area are typically present, but in children these findings are non-specific manifestations of any feverish illness. Thus a diagnosis of rheumatic carditis should not be made unless there is clear evidence of valvar involvement. The apical pansystolic murmur of mitral regurgitation is the most constant finding. A mid-diastolic murmur at the same location also indicates mitral disease. The early diastolic murmur of aortic regurgitation occurs less commonly.

### *Non-cardiac disease*

Polyarthritis usually affects the large joints of the extremities. A migratory pattern is characteristic and as one joint recovers another becomes involved. Cutaneous involvement is characterized by small painless nodules and erythema marginatum – an evanescent rash which occurs on the trunk but never on the face. Chorea (Sydenham's chorea, St Vitus' dance) often occurs several months after the initiating streptococcal pharyngitis. Severity is variable, ranging from occasional involuntary movements to violent jerking movements of the entire body. These systemic manifestations are also thought to be caused by immune cross-reactivity between streptococcal and tissue antigens.

## DIAGNOSIS

If recent streptococcal throat infection can be confirmed by demonstration of elevated serum antistreptolysin O titre, Jones' criteria may be used for diagnosis of rheumatic fever (Table 11.16). The presence of two major criteria, or one major and two minor criteria, indicates a high probability of rheumatic fever.

**Table 11.16** Jones' criteria for the diagnosis of rheumatic fever.

| Major criteria | Minor criteria |
| --- | --- |
| Carditis | Fever |
| Polyarthritis | Arthralgia |
| Erythema marginatum | Previous rheumatic fever |
| Chorea | Elevated erythrocyte sedimentation rate |
| Subcutaneous nodules | Prolonged P–R intervals |

## DIFFERENTIAL DIAGNOSIS

Differential diagnoses include other causes of childhood arthritis, bacterial endocarditis and viral pericarditis. Still's disease, the major cause of childhood arthritis, runs a chronic course and other criteria for rheumatic fever are not present. When bacterial endocarditis is suspected, positive blood cultures and other signs should be sought. Simple viral pericarditis is never associated with valvar disease, unlike rheumatic pericarditis in which valvar involvement and heart murmurs are always present.

## TREATMENT

In patients with a streptococcal throat infection, amoxycillin (250 mg three times daily) is effec-

tive in preventing rheumatic fever. In established rheumatic fever no specific treatment affects the course of the illness. Bed-rest is usually recommended and a course of penicillin should be given to eradicate residual streptococcal infection. Aspirin, starting at 100 mg/kg/day, is highly effective for treating fever and arthritis. Steroids are equally effective and are sometimes preferred in patients with carditis, although there is no evidence that they prevent chronic valvar damage. Following rheumatic fever, phenoxymethylpenicillin (125 mg orally twice daily) should be given to guard against recurrent attacks and continued up to the age of 25.

## PROGNOSIS

Acute rheumatic fever usually subsides within 6 weeks but intractable carditis or chorea may last up to 6 months. Recurrent attacks are common, and in patients with carditis these exacerbate cardiac damage and increase susceptibility to heart failure and death. In most cases, however, heart failure is delayed until the development of chronic rheumatic heart disease several years later. Chorea and arthritis rarely produce chronic sequelae.

### Chronic rheumatic heart disease

Following an attack (or recurrent attacks) of rheumatic fever, cardiac function usually returns to normal. During healing of the inflamed valves, however, progressive scarring may lead to chronic rheumatic heart disease 15 to 20 years later. Adhesion of the valve commissures and shrinkage of the cusps and subvalvar apparatus produce variable stenosis and regurgitation. Valvar calcification exacerbates the process. By the age of 30 many patients have had their first attack of congestive heart failure, which is often precipitated by the onset of atrial fibrillation or by the stress of pregnancy.

The mitral valve is most commonly affected in chronic rheumatic heart disease, and may be associated with aortic valve involvement. Isolated rheumatic disease of the aortic valve, however, is unusual in the UK and disease of the right-sided heart valves is rarely seen.

# *I*NFECTIVE ENDOCARDITIS

Infective endocarditis usually involves the heart valves but may also affect other congenital or acquired cardiac defects. Infection of the endothelial lining of arterial aneurysms or arteriovenous fistulae, though rare, produces a similar illness.

## AETIOLOGY

Endocarditis is now seen increasingly in the elderly, unlike 50 years ago when it was more common in young adults. *Streptococcus viridans* is the most common infecting organism. It is a normal commensal of the upper respiratory tract and produces a chronic, subacute illness. Other more virulent organisms, notably *Staphylococcus aureus*, produce a rapidly progressive acute illness (Table 11.17).

Endocarditis may affect healthy patients with entirely normal hearts. Nevertheless, patients at greater risk are those with pre-existing valvar disease. Other high-risk groups are shown in Table 11.18. The left-sided heart valves, ventricular septal defects, and patent ductus arteriosus are the most common sites of infection. Right-sided endocarditis is rare, usually affecting main-lining drug addicts.

The source of infection cannot usually be identified. *Streptococcus viridans* bacteraemia is almost invariable during dental surgery, but fewer than 15 per cent of patients with endocarditis give a history of recent dental treatment. Instrumentation of the genitourinary and gastrointestinal tracts also causes bacteraemia but is not often implicated in the development of endocarditis.

## PATHOLOGY

Endocarditis leads to aggregation of fibrin, platelets and other blood products at the site of infection. This produces a vegetation which is relatively avascular and tends to isolate the infective organism from host defences and antimicrobial agents. Valve destruction produces worsening regurgitation and commonly leads to heart failure. In endocarditis caused by *Staph. aureus*, valve destruction is rapid and local abscess formation commonly occurs. In less aggressive infections (e.g. from *Str. viridans*) the progression of disease is slower and large craggy vegetations develop which are prone to embolism. The chronic infection may lead to immune complex disease with vasculitic involvement of kidneys, joints and skin.

**Table 11.17** Organisms implicated in endocarditis.

| Organism | Typical source of infection | First choice antibiotics (pending sensitivity studies) |
|---|---|---|
| Streptococcus viridans | Upper respiratory tract | Benzylpenicillin, gentamicin |
| Streptococcus faecalis | Bowel and urogenital tract | Ampicillin, gentamicin |
| Anaerobic streptococcus | Bowel | Ampicillin, gentamicin |
| Staphylococcus epidermidis | Skin | Flucloxacillin, gentamicin |
| Fungi: Candida, Histoplasmosis | Skin and mucous membranes | Amphotericin B*, 5-fluorocytosine* |
| Coxiella burnetti | Complication of Q fever | Chloramphenicol*, tetracycline* |
| Chlamydia psittaci | Contact with infected birds | Tetracycline* and erythromycin |
| **Acute disease** | | |
| Staphylococcus aureus | Skin | Flucloxacillin, gentamicin |
| Streptococcus pneumoniae | Complication of pneumonia | Benzylpenicillin, gentamicin |
| Neisseria gonorrhoeae | Venereal | Benzylpenicillin, gentamicin |

*These drugs are not cidal and valve replacement is nearly always necessary to eradicate infection.

**Table 11.18** Groups at increased risk of endocarditis.

The elderly (>60 years)
Patients with intrinsic cardiovascular disease; high-risk lesions are:
    Ventricular septal defect
    Aortic regurgitation
    Mitral regurgitation
    Aortic stenosis
    Patient ductus arteriosus
    Coarctation of the aorta
Patients with valve prostheses, tissue grafts and other intracardiac foreign material
Main-lining drug addicts (right-sided valvar endocarditis occurs relatively commonly in this group)
Immunosuppressed patients

## CLINICAL FEATURES

In staphylococcal endocarditis, presentation is commonly with septicaemia, severe valvar regurgitation and circulatory collapse. In the more common streptococcal endocarditis, the onset is more insidious, with influenza-like symptoms including fever, night sweats, arthralgia and fatigue. Petechial haemorrhages in the skin and under the nails ('splinter' haemorrhages) are a common but non-specific finding. Valvar endocarditis causes regurgitant murmurs (typically aortic or mitral) owing to destruction of the valve leaflets. Other 'classical' manifestations of endocarditis, including Osler's nodes (tender erythematous nodules in the pulps of the fingers), Roth's spots in the retina (small haemorrhages with a white centre), clubbing of the fingers and splenomegaly are now rarely seen. By contrast a growing proportion of patients may have an atypical illness with fever and weight loss but no systemic signs and even no murmurs. This is particularly so in the elderly and patients with prosthetic valves.

## DIAGNOSIS

Endocarditis should be considered in every patient with fever and a heart murmur or pyrexia of unknown origin. Laboratory findings include leukocytosis, normochromic, normocytic anaemia and elevation of the erythrocyte sedimentation rate. Analysis of the urine commonly reveals haematuria. Blood cultures are usually positive and at least three specimens should be obtained in the first 24 hours before antibiotic treatment is started. Culture-negative endocarditis is caused by pretreatment with antibiotics, inadequate blood sampling or infection with unusual micro-organisms. The echocardiogram identifies underlying valvar disease and vegetations may also be seen if large enough.

## DIFFERENTIAL DIAGNOSIS

Infective endocarditis must be distinguished from the other main causes of fever and heart murmurs which are rheumatic fever and connective tissue disorders such as systemic lupus erythematosus. Particular difficulty arises in patients with pre-existing valvar disease who develop an associated trivial infection (e.g. viral pharyngitis). Nevertheless, if recovery is not rapid, investigation to exclude endocarditis is essential.

## COMPLICATIONS

### Heart failure

This is the major complication of endocarditis and the usual cause of death.

### Immune complex disease

Vasculitic rash and arthritis with red, tender joints occasionally occur. More important, however, is glomerulonephritis which may progress to intractable renal failure (page 439).

### Embolism

Vegetations may embolize peripherally, threatening limbs or major organs. Metastatic abscesses are not uncommon, particularly in the spleen or brain. Coronary embolism with myocardial infarction is seen occasionally.

### Heart block

Abscess formation in the aortic valve ring may cause heart block by damaging the conducting tissue in the interventricular septum.

### Mycotic aneurysm

Aneurysms may develop locally in the sinuses of Valsalva or elsewhere in the circulation. They result from embolic occlusion of the vasa vasorum and may be infected or sterile. Rupture can occur during the acute phase of the illness or at any time following its eradication.

## TREATMENT

This must not be delayed beyond the time necessary to obtain three blood specimens for culture. Bactericidal antibiotic therapy should then be started and continued for at least 4 weeks. For the first 2 weeks combination therapy with two antibiotics is recommended. These should be given intravenously using a central line. Thereafter the course may be completed using a single antibiotic given orally. Because streptococcal infection accounts for over 70 per cent of cases, initial treatment should be with benzylpenicillin (12 mega units daily) and low-dose gentamicin (titrated against blood levels) which enhances penicillin activity. When the results of blood cultures become available different antibiotics may be necessary depending on the organism grown.

Valve replacement may be necessary in endocarditis, but ideally this should be delayed until antibiotic therapy has resolved the infection. Nevertheless, urgent surgical intervention during the acute phase of the illness is necessary if heart failure develops; any delay often results in the death of the patient. Other relative indications for early surgery are conduction defects, recurrent embolism, fungal endocarditis and resistant infection, particularly in prosthetic valve endocarditis.

### Prophylaxis

Antibiotic prophylaxis to prevent bacteraemia during dental surgery and other non-sterile invasive procedures is required in all patients with valve disease and other cardiac defects. A single 3 g oral dose of amoxycillin should be given 1 hour before dental work (scaling, filling, extraction) or other instrumentation of the upper respiratory tract (e.g. bronchoscopy). Erythromycin (1.5 g) or clindamycin (600 mg) can be used in penicillin-sensitive patients. Instrumentation or surgery of the gastrointestinal or genitourinary tracts only requires prophylactic antibiotic cover (amoxycillin, 3 g, and gentamicin, 120 mg) in patients with a prosthetic heart valve or a history of previous endocarditis.

## PROGNOSIS

With the introduction of penicillin nearly 50 years ago, mortality in endocarditis fell from 100 per cent to about 30 per cent. It has remained at that level since that time. The continuing high mortality is the result of multiple factors, including the emergence of antibiotic-resistant organisms, the difficulty of treating infection on prosthetic heart valves, the widespread use of immunosuppressive therapy, the worsening problem of intravenous drug abuse, and the older more debilitated age group now at risk. The major impediment to effective treatment, however, is delayed diagnosis. The insidious onset of endocarditis often causes it to be overlooked until it is too late to save the patient. This is a particular problem in the elderly who may present with non-specific features.

# VALVAR HEART DISEASE

The heart valves direct the cardiac output forwards into the pulmonary and systemic circulations without impeding the flow. Valvar dysfunction is the result of incompetence or stenosis which produce backward flow (regurgitation) or impeded flow, respectively. Regurgitant valve lesions volume-load the ventricles, while stenotic lesions of the ventricular outflow valves (aortic and pulmonary) pressure-load the ventricles. Stenotic lesions of the ventricular in-flow valves (mitral and tricuspid), on the other hand, impede filling and reduce preload. Abnormal loading has the potential to cause heart failure, but this may be delayed by the effects of compensatory mechanisms (page 162), particularly in chronic valve disease.

The important role of echocardiography in the diagnosis of valve disease has already been emphasized. Used in conjunction with Doppler studies the pressure gradient across the stenosed valve and the regurgitant flow through an incompetent valve can be quantified. Indeed, in patients with valve disease, cardiac catheterization is rarely necessary for diagnostic purposes, although it is often requested by the surgeon for precise documentation of the valve lesion and angiographic examination of the coronary arteries. In patients with coronary disease, by-pass grafting can be performed at the same time as valve replacement.

Surgery has revolutionized the management of valvar heart disease and can produce complete haemodynamic correction. The timing of valve surgery is important because if it is delayed until ventricular dysfunction (or, in the case of mitral disease, pulmonary hypertension) becomes irreversible the risks are greater and the results less satisfactory. In mitral stenosis dilation of the valve (valvotomy) is effective if the valve is competent and not calcified. Regurgitant lesions of the mitral and tricuspid valves can sometimes be corrected by repair procedures. In most cases of valve disease, however, surgical correction requires replacement of the valve with a tissue graft or prosthesis. Porcine xenografts have been widely used because, unlike prostheses, they are not thrombogenic and do not expose the patient to the inconvenience and risk of long-term anticoagulant therapy. Nevertheless, tissue grafts are prone to calcification and failure within 7 years and for this reason prostheses are often preferred. Prostheses are usually ball and cage or tilting disc mechanisms. Both types are reliable but tilting discs present less obstruction to flow. Long-term anticoagulant therapy is essential following insertion of a prosthetic valve.

It is convenient to consider each of the important valve lesions separately. It must be recognized, however, that an individual valve may be both regurgitant and stenosed. Moreover, disease involving more than one valve is not uncommon, particularly in rheumatic disease and endocarditis. Multivalvar disease increases the haemodynamic burden on the heart and often leads to heart failure earlier than disease affecting a single valve.

# Mitral stenosis

## AETIOLOGY

Mitral stenosis is nearly always rheumatic in origin, although fewer than 50 per cent of cases give a clear history of previous rheumatic fever. Rarely mitral stenosis may occur as a congenital defect.

## PATHOLOGY AND PATHOPHYSIOLOGY

In mitral stenosis the valve commissures are fused and the leaflets are thickened and often calcified. Adequate filling of the left ventricle is impaired, and the left atrial pressure rises producing a diastolic pressure gradient across the valve (Fig. 11.30). Left ventricular contraction is unaffected but, because filling is impeded, adequate cardiac output cannot be maintained, particularly during exercise. As the pressure rises in the left atrium it dilates and is prone to fibrillate. This compromises left ventricular filling still further, partly because of the rapid heart rate which reduces diastolic filling time, and partly because of the loss of atrial systole.

The elevated left atrial pressure produces pulmonary congestion and pulmonary hypertension which in turn leads to right ventricular failure. In advanced mitral stenosis, irreversible pulmonary hypertension may develop.

## CLINICAL FEATURES

Mitral stenosis produces orthopnoea and exertional fatigue and dyspnoea in the same way as other causes of left heart failure. In advanced disease life-threatening attacks of acute pulmonary oedema occur. Chronic pulmonary congestion may produce cough and haemoptysis and predisposes to winter bronchitis. The onset of atrial fibrillation is often associated with abrupt clinical deterioration. A similar deterioration may occur during pregnancy owing to the increase in circulating volume and increased cardiac output.

Cyanotic discoloration of the cheeks produces the typical mitral facies (malar flush). Atrial

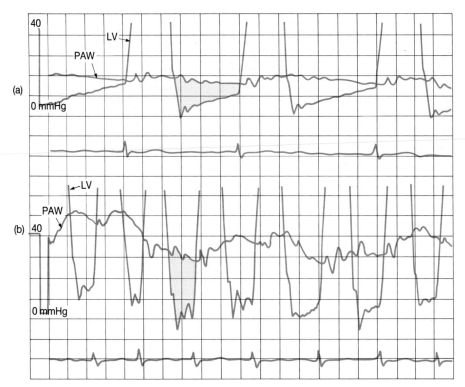

**Figure 11.30** Cardiac catheterization in mitral stenosis. (a) Recording made at rest. The heart rate is slow and the diastolic pressure gradient (shaded area) is trivial. (b) Recording made during exertion. This produced tachycardia and a steep rise in left atrial pressure. The diastolic pressure gradient (shaded area) is now substantial. The ECG shows atrial fibrillation. LV = left ventricular pressure signal. PAW = pulmonary artery wedge pressure signal.

fibrillation results in an irregular pulse. The apex beat is often described as having a 'tapping' character, but this is now regarded as a very subjective finding of little clinical value. Auscultation at the cardiac apex reveals a loud first sound and an opening snap in early diastole followed by a low-pitched mid-diastolic murmur. Presystolic accentuation of the murmur occurs only in sinus rhythm. In advanced mitral stenosis the loud first sound and the opening snap become less prominent, and the opening snap moves closer to the second heart sound as left atrial pressure rises.

The development of right ventricular failure produces elevation of the jugular venous pulse and peripheral oedema. The dilated right ventricle displaces the apical impulse towards the left axilla and causes a left parasternal systolic thrust. Prominence of the pulmonary component of the second heart sound reflects pulmonary hypertension.

## DIAGNOSIS

The ECG shows P mitrale when the patient is in sinus rhythm (page 152). Atrial fibrillation, however, is more common. Signs of right ventricular hypertrophy may be present in advanced disease. The chest X-ray shows left atrial enlargement often with a normal heart size (Fig. 11.11, page 155). Prominence of the upper lobe veins is almost invariable; pulmonary oedema may also occur. Calcification of the mitral valve or left atrial wall is sometimes seen on penetrated lateral films.

The echocardiogram is diagnostic and shows thickening and rigidity of the mitral valve leaflets associated with dilation of the left atrium (Fig. 11.31). The right-sided cardiac chambers may also be dilated. Doppler studies permit quantification of the pressure gradient across the valve. This may be confirmed by cardiac catheterization (Fig. 11.30).

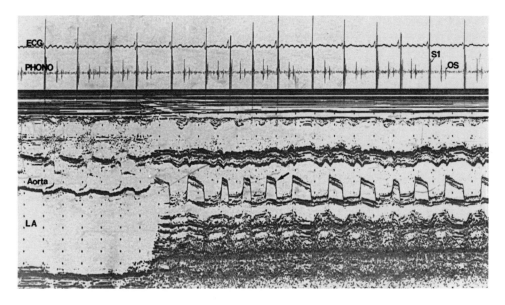

**Figure 11.31** Echocardiogram in mitral stenosis. This M-mode recording shows thickening and rigidity of the mitral valve (arrowed). The left atrium (LA) is considerably dilated (compare with Fig. 11.12a, page 157). The phonocardiogram shows a loud first heart sound (S1) followed by a normal second heart sound. The opening snap (OS) in early diastole has also been recorded. The ECG shows atrial fibrillation.

## DIFFERENTIAL DIAGNOSIS

Mitral stenosis must be differentiated from other conditions in which dyspnoea is associated with added diastolic sounds. Left ventricular failure produces similar symptoms and the unwary may mistake the third heart sound for a mid-diastolic murmur. A mid-diastolic apical murmur also occurs in severe aortic regurgitation owing to preclosure of the mitral valve (Austin–Flint murmur). Perhaps the most important differential diagnosis is left atrial myxoma (page 226). This is difficult to distinguish from mitral stenosis on clinical grounds but the echocardiogram is diagnostic.

## COMPLICATIONS

### Atrial arrhythmias

Atrial fibrillation nearly always develops in long-standing mitral stenosis.

### Thromboembolism

Haemostasis in the dilated left atrium predisposes to thrombosis, particularly following the onset of atrial fibrillation. The risk of systemic embolism to the brain or elsewhere is reduced by prophylactic anticoagulation with warfarin.

### Pulmonary vascular disease

Pulmonary hypertension is an inevitable consequence of elevated left atrial pressure but is usually corrected by mitral valve replacement. Occasionally, however, in long-standing mitral stenosis, pulmonary hypertension is irreversible because of the development of obliterative pulmonary vascular disease.

### Endocarditis

This rarely occurs in pure mitral stenosis unassociated with mitral regurgitation. Nevertheless, antibiotic prophylaxis prior to dental surgery should always be given (page 193).

### Chest infection

Chronic pulmonary congestion predisposes to chest infections which are a common cause of death in mitral stenosis.

## TREATMENT

Diuretics produce effective symptomatic relief by correcting pulmonary and systemic congestion. Following the onset of atrial fibrillation, digoxin should be prescribed to control the ventricular rate, and anticoagulation with warfarin is mandatory to protect against thromboembolism.

Indications for surgery are dyspnoea unresponsive to medical treatment and right ventricular failure. Valvotomy is the procedure of choice, but if the valve is calcified or regurgitant it must be replaced with a tissue graft or prosthesis.

The recent development of mitral balloon valvuloplasty avoids the need for surgery in some patients with competent, non-calcified valves. The balloon catheter is advanced from the femoral vein into the right atrium and thence into the left atrium by trans-septal puncture. The balloon is then positioned across the mitral valve and inflated. This dilates the stenosed valve orifice and can produce sustained benefit, unlike aortic balloon valvuloplasty for aortic stenosis (see below) in which any improvement is nearly always temporary.

## PROGNOSIS

Following rheumatic carditis in childhood, symptomatic mitral stenosis may take up to 20 years to develop, though pregnancy or the development of atrial fibrillation may prompt an earlier presentation. Once symptoms are established progressive deterioration often leads to death within 5 to 10 years unless surgery is performed. Death may be the result of pulmonary oedema, chest infection, endocarditis or thromboembolism.

# Mitral regurgitation

## AETIOLOGY

Mitral regurgitation has many causes, the majority of which relate to acquired disease of the valve leaflets or subvalvar apparatus (Table 11.19).

## Mitral valve prolapse

This is a common and usually asymptomatic condition in which one (or both) of the mitral valve leaflets bulges backwards into the left atrium during systole. This produces mitral regurgitation in some but not all cases. Only rarely is the mitral regurgitation severe. Mitral valve prolapse affects about 5 per cent of the population and is particularly common in young women. Most cases are idiopathic but it may also be associated with a variety of cardiac and systemic disorders, including rheumatic and ischaemic heart disease and Marfan's syndrome. Chest pain and cardiac arrhythmias may occur, particularly ventricular extrasystoles and supraventricular tachycardias. Auscultation typically reveals a mid-systolic click which is followed by a murmur in patients with mitral regurgitation. Definitive diagnosis requires echocardiography which identifies the prolapsing leaflet. Antibiotic prophylaxis against endocarditis is only required in those patients in whom the systolic click is followed by a murmur, indicating mitral regurgitation.

## Chordal rupture

This is usually idiopathic in origin but may also occur in endocarditis or rheumatic disease. It usually produces acute mitral regurgitation and may present abruptly with pulmonary oedema.

## Papillary muscle disease

Myocardial ischaemia can cause dysfunction of the papillary muscles with variable mitral regurgitation. Papillary muscle rupture complicating myocardial infarction always produces torrential mitral regurgitation and pulmonary oedema requiring urgent valve replacement.

**Table 11.19** Causes of mitral regurgitation.

**Valve leaflet disease***
Mitral valve prolapse
Rheumatic disease
Infective endocarditis†

**Subvalvar disease***
Chordal rupture†
Papillary muscle dysfunction
Papillary muscle rupture†

**Dilating left ventricular disease**
'Functional' mitral regurgitation

---

*Note that the subclassification into valve leaflet and subvalvar disease is to some extent artificial because all the causes of valve leaflet disease are usually associated with subvalvar dysfunction.
†These disorders produce acute mitral regurgitation.

## PATHOPHYSIOLOGY

Mitral regurgitation volume-loads the left ventricle leading to compensatory dilation and hypertrophy. The increase in left atrial pressure and volume causes pulmonary congestion. The dilated left atrium is prone to fibrillate.

## CLINICAL FEATURES

Mitral regurgitation is usually asymptomatic until the left ventricle begins to fail. In acute mitral regurgitation this occurs abruptly but in chronic disease it may take several years. Symptoms including orthopnoea and exercise-related fatigue and dyspnoea are the same as occur in other causes of left heart failure. Severe pulmonary hypertension is unusual in mitral regurgitation and for this reason features of right ventricular failure are rarely prominent.

The pulse is often irregular owing to atrial fibrillation. The cardiac apex is displaced, reflecting cardiac enlargement. Auscultation at the apex reveals a pansystolic murmur which radiates into the left axilla. A third heart sound is often present owing to rapid filling from the volume-loaded left atrium.

## DIAGNOSIS

The ECG shows P mitrale if the patient is in sinus rhythm (page 152). The chest X-ray shows cardiac enlargement, left atrial dilation and prominence of the upper lobe veins. The echocardiogram confirms dilation of the left-sided chambers which is associated with worsening contractile impairment as the left ventricle fails. Diagnostic abnormalities of the valve itself occur when the leaflets are diseased. In subvalvar disease, however, the echocardiogram may show an apparently normal valve. Doppler studies identify the regurgitant jet in the left atrium. The diagnosis is confirmed by left ventricular angiography which documents the severity of mitral regurgitation and left ventricular contractile impairment.

## DIFFERENTIAL DIAGNOSIS

Mitral regurgitation must be distinguished from other causes of a pansystolic murmur, particularly tricuspid regurgitation and ventricular septal defect. In both conditions, however, the murmur is loudest at the left sternal edge and does not radiate into the axilla.

## COMPLICATIONS

Patients with mitral regurgitation are prone to thromboembolism from the dilated left atrium, particularly following the development of atrial fibrillation. The risk of endocarditis is considerable and antibiotic prophylaxis is required prior to dental surgery (page 193). Nevertheless, the major complication of mitral regurgitation relates to left ventricular volume overload which may lead eventually to irreversible impairment of contractile function.

## TREATMENT

Diuretics are often sufficient to control dyspnoea in mitral regurgitation. The development of atrial fibrillation requires digitalis to control the ventricular rate and anticoagulation with warfarin. Vasodilators such as angiotensin-converting enzyme inhibitors act by lowering peripheral vascular resistance; forward flow into the aorta increases, reducing the volume of blood that regurgitates backwards through the mitral valve.

If symptoms cannot be controlled by medical measures, mitral valve replacement should be considered. If surgery is delayed unnecessarily, irreversible deterioration in left ventricular contractile function occurs. In acute mitral regurgitation diuretics and vasodilators are helpful, but early valve replacement is often necessary.

## PROGNOSIS

Chronic mitral regurgitation is only slowly progressive and is compatible with a normal life-span. Nevertheless, if the volume-loaded left ventricle develops contractile failure the prognosis is considerably worse and death usually occurs within 5 to 10 years.

# *Aortic stenosis*

## AETIOLOGY

In the UK aortic stenosis is usually caused by calcification of the valve leaflets. This is a slowly progressive, degenerative process. When it affects a previously normal valve it rarely presents before the age of 60. When it affects a congenitally bicuspid valve, on the other hand, presentation in middle age is more common. Rheumatic aortic stenosis is now relatively unusual and rarely occurs without associated mitral disease. All the important causes of aortic stenosis are also causes of aortic regurgitation. Thus a combination of both defects commonly occurs in the same patient.

## PATHOPHYSIOLOGY

Aortic stenosis obstructs left ventricular outflow. A systolic pressure gradient is produced across the valve, and this increased load leads to left ventricle hypertrophy. The hypertrophied ventricle is stiff and non-compliant so that adequate filling depends on a high diastolic pressure. Atrial contraction provides an important boost to ventricular filling, and the development of atrial fibrillation often produces clinical deterioration. As aortic stenosis worsens, irreversible impairment of left ventricular contractile function eventually occurs. Forward flow across the valve can no longer be maintained and the heart dilates, leading to frank left ventricular failure.

## CLINICAL FEATURES

Elevation of the left atrial pressure produces exertional dyspnoea, which is particularly severe following the onset of left ventricular failure. Other major symptoms include angina (caused by the exaggerated oxygen demands of the hypertrophied left ventricle) and syncope. Syncope typically occurs during exertion because flow through the stenosed aortic valve cannot increase sufficiently to maintain blood pressure in the face of vasodilation in exercising skeletal muscle (pages 144 and 161). Vasodilator drugs can produce hypotension and syncope by the same mechanism and should be avoided in aortic stenosis. Syncope may also result from paroxysmal ventricular arrhythmias (Stokes—Adams attacks).

The carotid pulse has a slow upstroke. Left ventricular hypertrophy does not always displace the apex beat, which is thrusting in character and may have a double impulse owing to a palpable fourth heart sound. A systolic thrill is often palpable over the aortic area and the carotid arteries. Auscultation reveals a medium-pitched mid-systolic murmur which is loudest at the aortic area and radiates into the neck. It is preceded by an ejection click if the valve cusps are pliant and not heavily calcified. A fourth heart sound and reversed splitting of the second heart sound are usually present although the aortic component of the second sound becomes softer or inaudible as stenosis becomes more severe.

## DIAGNOSIS

The ECG shows left ventricular hypertrophy (Fig. 11.8, page 153). The chest X-ray shows a normal heart size unless there is left ventricular failure or associated aortic regurgitation. Post-stenotic dilation of the ascending aorta is usually evident (Fig. 11.32) and the penetrated lateral film may reveal valvar calcification. The echocardiogram shows a thickened, rigid aortic valve and symmetrical left ventricular hypertrophy. Doppler studies may be used to quantify the valve gradient.

Cardiac catheterization permits direct measurement of the pressure gradient across the aortic valve (Fig. 11.33). Angiographic assessment of left ventricular contractile function can also be obtained. Because angina is common in aortic stenosis, coronary arteriography is essential before valve replacement to rule out associated coronary artery disease.

## DIFFERENTIAL DIAGNOSIS

Hypertrophic cardiomyopathy and hypertension are both associated with left ventricular hypertrophy and have many of the clinical features of aortic stenosis. These include angina, mid-systolic murmur and the fourth heart sound.

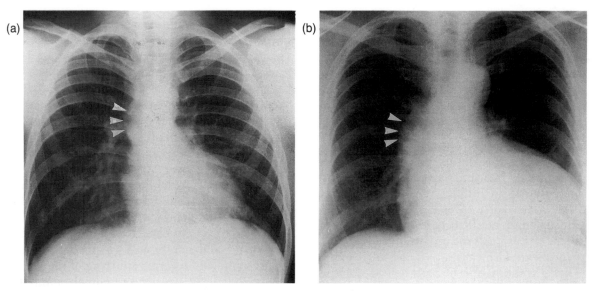

**Figure 11.32** Chest X-ray in aortic valve disease. Aortic valve disease produces dilation of the ascending aorta (arrowed). (a) In aortic stenosis, the heart size is normal because the pressure-loaded left ventricle hypertrophies but does not dilate until failure supervenes. (b) In aortic regurgitation, volume-loading produces a variable degree of left ventricular dilation.

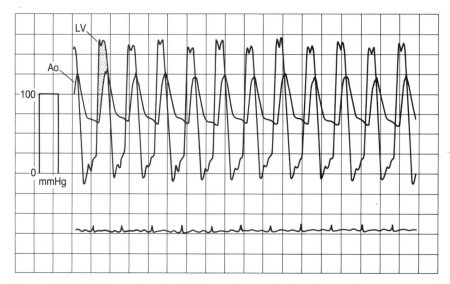

**Figure 11.33** Cardiac catheterization in aortic stenosis. Aortic stenosis causes a systolic pressure gradient across the aortic valve (shaded area) such that left ventricular pressure is higher than the aortic pressure. LV = left ventricular pressure signal. Ao = aortic pressure signal.

Moreover, ECG abnormalities in both conditions are similar to those in aortic stenosis. Nevertheless, in neither hypertrophic cardiomyopathy nor hypertension is the carotid pulse slow rising, nor does the echocardiogram show a thickened aortic valve.

Innocent mid-systolic murmurs should not be confused with aortic stenosis. They may occur in healthy individuals but are more common in conditions such as anaemia, fever, thyrotoxicosis and pregnancy. The hyperdynamic circulation characteristic of these conditions increases the velocity of ejection sufficiently to produce turbulence across the aortic and pulmonary valves. Innocent murmurs are usually soft, are always mid-systolic in timing and are never associated with a slow-rising carotid pulse.

## COMPLICATIONS

### Left ventricular failure

The chronic pressure load may eventually lead to irreversible left ventricular contractile impairment.

### Endocarditis

This is an ever-present risk in aortic stenosis. Antibiotic prophylaxis prior to dental surgery and other non-sterile invasive procedures is essential.

### Arrhythmias

Atrial fibrillation is not uncommon in aortic stenosis and often produces clinical deterioration. More important are ventricular arrhythmias which are a cause of syncope and sudden death.

### Heart block

This is an occasional complication of calcific aortic stenosis and results from calcific destruction of the conducting tissue in the adjacent part of the interventricular septum.

## TREATMENT

Aortic stenosis that is subcritical requires no specific treatment while it remains asymptomatic. The development of symptoms, however, is an indication for valve replacement. Other indications for valve replacement are left ventricular contractile impairment and critical aortic stenosis (peak systolic pressure gradient above 50 mm Hg) even in the absence of symptoms. Catheter balloon valvuloplasty may be possible in patients unfit for surgery. The balloon is positioned across the aortic valve and dilated in order to relieve the stenosis. However, this technique has not found wide application because the results are often poor and restenosis within a few months commonly occurs.

## PROGNOSIS

Aortic stenosis is often well tolerated but following the development of symptoms death occurs within 3 to 5 years. The outlook is worse in patients with left ventricular failure. Valve replacement improves both symptoms and prognosis in patients with aortic stenosis.

# Aortic regurgitation

## AETIOLOGY

Aortic regurgitation may be caused either by disease of the valve cusps or by aortic root disease which leads to dilation of the valve ring (Table 11.20).

## PATHOPHYSIOLOGY

Aortic regurgitation volume-loads the left ventricle. When this occurs acutely it may cause severe decompensation by overwhelming the Starling reserve of the ventricle. In chronic aortic regurgitation, however, left ventricular dilation and hypertrophy compensate for the volume-load. The regurgitation of blood through the aortic valve increases diastolic filling and produces vigorous ventricular contraction by the Starling mechanism. This maintains forward cardiac output despite regurgitation through the aortic valve. These compensatory mechanisms, however, have limited potential and contractile function may eventually deteriorate, leading to left ventricular failure.

**Table 11.20** Causes of aortic regurgitation.

**Valve leaflet disease**
Congenital bicuspid valve
Calcific disease
Rheumatic disease
Infective endocarditis*

**Aortic root dilating disease**
Marfan's syndrome
Ankylosing spondylitis
Syphilis
Hypertension
Aortic dissection*
Aortic root aneurysm
Deceleration injury*

*These disorders produce acute aortic regurgitation. In the remainder the course is chronic.

## CLINICAL FEATURES

Acute aortic regurgitation may present dramatically with pulmonary oedema and low-output failure. Chronic aortic regurgitation, however, often remains asymptomatic for several years until the development of exertional fatigue and dyspnoea marks the onset of left ventricular failure. Angina may also occur owing to the increased oxygen requirements of the dilated, hypertrophied ventricle. The carotid pulse is visible in the neck (Corrigan's pulse). It has a rapid upstroke and collapses in early diastole owing to regurgitation of blood into the left ventricle. The pulse pressure is widened, with exaggeration of the systolic peak and the diastolic nadir. The radial pulse is still sometimes described as being a 'water-hammer' pulse named after a Victorian toy. The apex beat is displaced towards the left axilla and has a prominent impulse. Auscultation reveals a high-pitched early diastolic murmur which is often louder at the left sternal edge than the aortic area. A mid-systolic ejection murmur is commonly present: it reflects the increased volume and velocity of flow across the aortic valve and does not necessarily indicate associated aortic stenosis. In severe disease the regurgitant jet causes preclosure of the anterior leaflet of the mitral valve and results in an apical mid-diastolic (Austin Flint) murmur.

## DIAGNOSIS

The ECG shows evidence of left ventricular hypertrophy (Fig. 11.8, page 153). The chest X-ray shows an enlarged heart and dilation of the ascending aorta (Fig. 11.32). Penetrated lateral films may reveal calcification of the aortic valve. The echocardiogram shows an abnormal aortic valve only if the cusps are diseased. In aortic root disease the valve itself appears normal although the aorta is dilated. The regurgitant jet produces fine vibrations on the anterior leaflet of the mitral valve which are often visible on the M-mode recording. The left ventricle shows variable dilation and vigorous contractile function until this deteriorates in end-stage disease. Doppler studies identify the regurgitant jet. Left ventricular and aortic root angiography permit direct assessment of contractile function and the severity of aortic regurgitation, respectively.

## DIFFERENTIAL DIAGNOSIS

Aortic regurgitation must be distinguished from other conditions with an early diastolic murmur. Pulmonary regurgitation is relatively unusual and is nearly always associated with evidence of severe pulmonary hypertension (page 163). In patent ductus arteriosus the murmur is continuous, but loudest at end-systole/early diastole. The pulse pressure is usually widened and confusion with aortic regurgitation, therefore, is not uncommon.

## COMPLICATIONS

Irreversible left ventricular contractile impairment and endocarditis are the major complications of aortic regurgitation. Antibiotic prophylaxis prior to dental surgery is essential (page 193).

## TREATMENT

In acute aortic regurgitation associated with left ventricular failure, valve replacement should not be delayed. In chronic aortic regurgitation treatment is less urgent because symptoms are rarely obtrusive until the onset of left ventricular failure. Mild shortness of breath may respond to diuretic therapy. Vasodilators (e.g. hydralazine, angiotensin-converting enzyme inhibitors) are often useful, because reductions in peripheral vascular resistance increase forward flow and reduce regurgitation through the valve. When aortic regurgitation becomes significantly symptomatic valve replacement is usually indicated, particularly when symptoms are associated with echocardiographic evidence of left ventricular contractile impairment. If surgery is delayed contractile impairment becomes irreversible and the results of valve replacement are less satisfactory.

## PROGNOSIS

Mild aortic regurgitation is compatible with a normal life-span. In more severe cases left ventricular failure develops, and thereafter prognosis is poor and similar to that of other causes of left ventricular failure. Timely valve replacement that anticipates deterioration in ventricular function improves the prognosis considerably.

# Tricuspid valve disease

## TRICUSPID STENOSIS

Tricuspid stenosis is almost invariably rheumatic and is usually associated with mitral valve disease. Indeed, symptoms of mitral valve disease usually dominate the clinical picture. Severe tricuspid stenosis, however, may produce right heart failure characterized by fatigue, elevation of jugular venous pulse and peripheral oedema. A low-pitched mid-diastolic murmur, augmented during inspiration, is audible at the lower left sternal edge. These findings, associated with echocardiographic evidence of tricuspid valve thickening and right atrial dilation, are diagnostic. Surgery is indicated only when right heart failure is severe.

## TRICUSPID REGURGITATION

Tricuspid regurgitation is the most common right-sided valve lesion. It is usually 'functional', caused by stretching of the tricuspid valve ring in patients with advanced right ventricular failure. Other causes, including rheumatic disease, infective endocarditis, Ebstein's anomaly and carcinoid syndrome, are rare.

Tricuspid regurgitation volume-loads the right ventricle and may lead to (or, more commonly, exacerbate) right heart failure. The regurgitant jet produces systolic waves in the jugular veins, called giant 'V' waves. Sometimes systolic expansion of an enlarged liver can also be detected. Auscultation reveals a pansystolic murmur at the lower left sternal edge. Confirmation of tricuspid regurgitation is provided by Doppler echocardiography which demonstrates the regurgitant jet in the right atrium.

Tricuspid regurgitation is often well tolerated. Diuretics control peripheral oedema and reduce right ventricular volume, which improves functional regurgitation. Tricuspid valve surgery is only rarely necessary.

# Pulmonary valve disease

Rheumatic disease of the pulmonary valve is rare. Endocarditis occurs occasionally, usually in main-lining drug addicts. The most common pulmonary valve defects are congenital stenosis (page 238) and regurgitation secondary to pulmonary hypertension. Pulmonary regurgitation produces a high-pitched early diastolic murmur at the upper left sternal edge (Graham Steell murmur) very similar to that of aortic regurgitation. Nevertheless, signs of pulmonary hypertension are usually prominent (page 163) and the carotid pulse is normal. Pulmonary regurgitation is well tolerated and produces negligible haemodynamic embarrassment. The prognosis is determined by the severity of the associated pulmonary hypertension.

## CONDUCTING TISSUE DISEASE

Synchronized contraction of the four cardiac chambers is dependent upon the organized spread of a wave of depolarization through the heart. All cardiac cells will depolarize in response to a stimulus of sufficient magnitude. Only the specialized conducting tissues, however, will depolarize spontaneously. This property – called automaticity – is essential to the pacemaker function of the sinus node, the conducting tissue with the highest intrinsic firing rate. The impulse generated by the sinus node first triggers atrial depolarization and then spreads through the atrioventricular node into the His-Purkinje tissue, triggering ventricular depolarization. The atrioventricular node provides the only pathway connecting the atria and the ventricles. The remainder of the atrioventricular ring tissue is electrically inert. Impulse conduction through the atrioventricular node is slow; this ensures that ventricular filling is complete before the onset of systole and that the ventricles will not respond to excessively rapid atrial rates.

# Sinoatrial disease ('sick sinus syndrome')

## AETIOLOGY

Causes of sinoatrial disease are shown in Table 11.21. The most common cause is idiopathic fibrosis, a disease of the elderly which may affect the conducting tissue anywhere in the heart.

## PATHOLOGY

The spontaneous discharge of the normal sinus node is influenced by a variety of neurohumoral factors, particularly vagal and sympathetic activity which slow and quicken the heart rate, respectively. A rate of 35–40 beats/min is normal during sleep, but this may rise to 200 beats/min during exertion. The rate of sinus node discharge is also influenced by age and slows progressively after the age of 60.

Sinus node discharge is not itself visible on the surface ECG, but the atrial depolarization it triggers produces the P wave. Sinus node discharge may be suppressed by drugs and disease or it may be blocked and fail to activate atrial depolarization. Under these circumstances

**Table 11.21** Causes of sinoatrial disease.

**Acute**
Myocardial infarction
Drugs (e.g. β-blockers, digitalis)
Hypothermia
Atrial surgery

**Chronic**
Idiopathic fibrotic disease
Congenital heart disease
Ischaemic heart disease
Amyloid

the pacemaker function can be assumed by foci lower in the atrium, the atrioventricular node or the His-Purkinje conducting tissue in the ventricles. The intrinsic rate of these 'escape' pacemaker foci is slower than the normal sinus rate.

## CLINICAL FEATURES

Sinoatrial disease is commonly asymptomatic. Dizzy attacks or blackouts may occur, caused by extreme bradycardia or prolonged sinus pauses without an adequate escape rhythm. Generally speaking pauses of greater than 4 s are necessary to produce symptoms. Additional complaints may include exertional fatigue or dyspnoea due to failure of physiological increments in heart rate (chronotropic incompetence). Palpitations also occur, caused by premature beats or paroxysmal tachyarrhythmias (see below).

## DIAGNOSIS

In common with all other cardiac arrhythmias, electrocardiographic documentation of sinoatrial disease is a prerequisite of accurate diagnosis. Although the resting ECG may be helpful, the disorder often occurs intermittently, in which case continuous in-hospital or ambulatory ECG monitoring is necessary (page 211).

### Sinus bradycardia (less than 50 beats/min)

This is physiological during sleep and in trained athletes but in other circumstances often reflects sinoatrial disease, particularly when the heart rate fails to increase normally with exercise.

### Sinoatrial block

If the sinus impulse is blocked and fails to trigger atrial depolarization, a pause occurs in the ECG. No P wave is seen during the pause owing to the absence of atrial depolarization. The electrically 'silent' sinus discharge, however, continues uninterrupted. Thus the pause is always a precise multiple of preceding P–P intervals. Sinoatrial block that cannot be abolished by atropine-induced vagal inhibition usually indicates sinoatrial disease, particularly with pauses longer than 2 s.

## *Sinus arrest* (Fig. 11.34)

Failure of sinus node discharge produces a pause on the ECG that bears no relation to the preceding P–P interval. Pauses longer than 2 s are usually pathological. Prolonged pauses are often terminated by an escape beat from a 'junctional' focus in the bundle of His.

## *Bradycardia–tachycardia syndrome*

In this syndrome atrial bradycardias are interspersed by paroxysmal tachyarrhythmias, usually atrial fibrillation. Nevertheless, it is the bradycardia that usually causes symptoms, particularly dizzy attacks and blackouts.

## DIFFERENTIAL DIAGNOSIS

Sinoatrial disease must be distinguished from other cardiac and non-cardiac causes of dizzy attacks and syncope (page 144).

## COMPLICATIONS

### *Tachyarrhythmias*

Paroxysmal atrial arrhythmias occur in the bradycardia–tachycardia syndrome (see above). Ventricular arrhythmias may also occur if there is associated His-Purkinje disease.

### *Thromboembolism*

Systemic embolism from the left atrium occasionally occurs in the bradycardia–tachycardia syndrome.

## TREATMENT

Asymptomatic patients require no treatment, although drugs such as β-blockers which suppress the sinus node should be avoided. In patients with symptomatic bradycardias and sinus pauses, however, pacemaker therapy is indicated (page 208). Atrial pacing (AAI) is the method of choice but in patients with associated atrioventricular conducting disease a dual demand (DDD) unit should be used (Table 11.22). This maintains the heart rate, preventing syncopal episodes and improving exercise tolerance.

Troublesome tachycardias in the bradycardia–tachycardia syndrome require antiarrhythmic drug therapy. Drugs of this type often exacerbate sinus node dysfunction, and a pacemaker is usually necessary to protect against severe bradycardia. Anticoagulation with warfarin is recommended in the bradycardia–tachycardia syndrome in order to protect against thromboembolism.

## PROGNOSIS

The prognosis in sinoatrial disease depends mainly on the underlying cause and the thromboembolic risk. In idiopathic fibrosis of conducting tissue, for example, the outlook is good. Dizzy attacks and syncopal episodes are inconvenient but not directly life-threatening.

**Table 11.22** Methods of pacing: three-letter code.

| Chamber paced | Chamber sensed | Response to sensing |
|---|---|---|
| O = None | O = None | O = None |
| A = Atrium | A = Atrium | T = Triggered |
| V = Ventricle | V = Ventricle | I = Inhibited |
| D = Dual (A+V) | D = Dual (A+V) | D = Dual (T+I) |

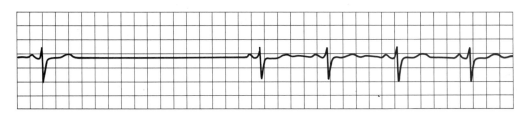

**Figure 11.34** Sinus arrest. After the first sinus beat there is a long pause before sinus rhythm re-establishes itself.

# *Atrioventricular block*

## AETIOLOGY

Myocardial infarction is the commonest cause of acute atrioventricular block (Table 11.23). Chronic atrioventricular block in the UK is usually due to idiopathic fibrosis of the bundle branches, particularly in the elderly, although ischaemic disease is more common in middle-aged patients. Chagas' disease in Central and South America, however, is probably the commonest cause of atrioventricular block worldwide.

## PATHOPHYSIOLOGY

In atrioventricular block, conduction is delayed or completely interrupted, either in the atrioventricular node or in the bundle branches. When conduction is merely delayed (e.g. first-degree atrioventricular block, bundle branch block) the heart rate is unaffected. When conduction is completely interrupted, however, the heart rate may slow sufficiently to produce symptoms. In second-degree atrioventricular block, failure of conduction is, by definition, intermittent, and if sufficient sinus impulses are conducted to maintain an adequate ventricular rate symptoms may be avoided. In third-degree atrioventricular block there is complete failure of conduction and continuing ventricular activity depends on the emergence of an escape rhythm. If the block is within the atrioventricular node the escape rhythm usually arises from a focus just below the node in the bundle of His (junctional escape) and is often fast enough to

**Table 11.23** Causes of atrioventricular heart block.

### Acute
Myocardial infarction
Drugs (e.g. β-blockers, verapamil, digitalis, adenosine)
Surgical or catheter ablation of the His bundle

### Chronic
Idiopathic fibrosis of both bundle branches
Ischaemic heart disease
Congenital heart disease
Calcific aortic valve disease
Chagas' disease
Infiltrative disease (amyloid, haemochromatosis)
Granulomatous disease (sarcoid, tuberculosis)

prevent symptoms. If both bundle branches are blocked, however, the escape rhythm must arise from a focus lower in the ventricles. Ventricular escape rhythms of this type are nearly always associated with symptoms because they are not only very slow but also unreliable, and may stop altogether producing prolonged asystole.

## CLINICAL FEATURES

### *First-degree atrioventricular block*

This is an electrocardiographic diagnosis and produces no symptoms or signs.

### *Second-degree atrioventricular block*

Intermittent failure of atrioventricular conduction rarely produces symptoms unless the heart rate is very slow. On examination, occasional dropped beats may be detected, but diagnosis is effectively impossible without an ECG.

### *Third-degree (complete) atrioventricular block*

The ventricular escape rhythm is often slow and does not speed up significantly during exercise. Exertional fatigue is always troublesome, and frank congestive heart failure may occur if the rate is very slow, particularly when there is associated valvar or myocardial disease. Moreover, if the escape rhythm is unreliable, intermittent periods of asystole produce dizzy attacks or syncope.

Examination reveals a slow regular pulse, usually about 40 beats/min. The atrial and ventricular rhythms are 'dissociated'. Signs of dissociation include intermittent cannon 'a' waves in the jugular venous pulse (Fig. 11.1, page 147), and beat-to-beat variation in the intensity of the first heart sound. These signs, however, are not present if the atria are fibrillating.

## DIAGNOSIS

Definitive diagnosis of heart block depends upon electrocardiographic documentation of the rhythm. If the disorder is intermittent this may require in-hospital or ambulatory ECG monitoring (page 210).

### *First-degree atrioventricular block*

Delayed atrioventricular conduction causes prolongation of the P–R interval ($>0.20$ s).

Ventricular depolarization occurs rapidly by normal His-Purkinje pathways and the QRS complex is usually narrow.

## Second-degree atrioventricular block

### Mobitz type I (Wenckebach)

This (Fig. 11.35) occurs commonly in inferior myocardial infarction, successive sinus beats find the atrioventricular node increasingly refractory until failure of conduction occurs. The delay permits recovery of nodal function and the process may then repeat itself. The ECG shows progressive prolongation of the P–R interval, culminating in a dropped beat. Block is within the atrioventricular node itself and ventricular depolarization occurs rapidly by normal pathways. Thus the QRS complex is usually narrow.

### Mobitz type II

This (Fig. 11.36) always indicates advanced conducting tissue disease affecting the bundle branches. The ECG typically shows a normal P–R interval in conducted beats with bundle branch block, intermittent block in the other bundle branch resulting in complete failure of atrioventricular conduction and dropped beats.

## Third-degree (complete) atrioventricular block

The atrial and ventricular rhythms are 'dissociated' because none of the atrial impulses is conducted. Thus the ECG shows regular P waves (unless the atrium is fibrillating) and regular but slower QRS complexes occurring independently of each other. When block is within the atrioventricular node (e.g. inferior myocardial infarction, congenital atrioventricular block) a junctional escape rhythm with a reliable rate (40–60 beats/min) takes over (Fig. 11.23, page 177). Ventricular depolarization occurs rapidly by normal pathways, producing a narrow QRS complex. However, when block is within the bundle branches (e.g. idiopathic fibrosis) there is always extensive conducting tissue disease. The ventricular escape rhythm is slow and unreliable, with a broad QRS complex (Fig. 11.37).

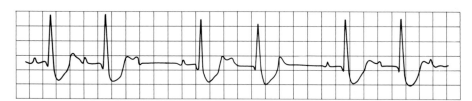

**Figure 11.35** Mobitz type I second-degree atrioventricular block. Three Wenckebach cycles are shown, during each of which gradual prolongation of the P–R interval culminates in a non-conducted impulse.

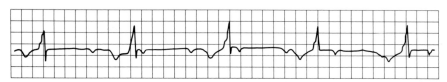

**Figure 11.36** Mobitz type II second-degree block. Alternate P waves are not conducted (2:1 block). Note that the PR interval of the conducted beats is normal and that the QRS complex is broad with a bundle branch block pattern – both typical features of Mobitz type II block.

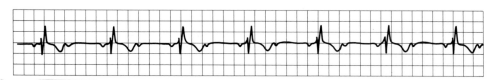

**Figure 11.37** Third-degree (complete) atrioventricular block. The patient has idiopathic fibrosis of both bundle branches. Note the dissociated atrial and ventricular rhythm and the slow ventricular escape rhythms with a broad QRS complex (compare with Fig. 11.23, page 177).

## *Right bundle branch block*

See Fig. 11.7, page 153. This may be a congenital defect but is more commonly the result of organic conducting tissue disease. Right ventricular depolarization is delayed, resulting in a broad QRS complex with an rSR pattern in lead V1 and prominent S waves in leads 1 and V6.

## *Left bundle branch block*

See Fig. 11.7, page 153. This always indicates organic conducting tissue disease. The entire sequence of ventricular depolarization is abnormal, resulting in a broad QRS complex with large slurred or notched R waves in leads 1 and V6.

## TREATMENT

The treatment of acute atrioventricular block complicating myocardial infarction has already been discussed (page 176). In chronic atrioventricular block, treatment is necessary only in Mobitz type II second-degree block and third-degree (complete) block. In both conditions there is always the risk of prolonged asystole and sudden death. Thus pacemaker therapy is mandatory.

### *Pacemaker therapy*

A pacemaker wire with two terminal electrodes (cathode at the tip and anode about 1 cm proximally) is introduced into a central vein and directed into the apex of the right ventricle. The wire is attached to a pulse generator for delivery of electrical pulses which depolarize the ventricles and stimulate systolic contraction. Temporary pacing using an external power source is appropriate when the need for rate control is likely to be short-lived (e.g. heart block in inferior myocardial infarction) or as a prelude to permanent pacing in patients with severe bradycardias. Permanent pacing is required for symptomatic sinoatrial disease (page 204) and for all patients with chronic Mobitz type II or complete atrioventricular block. The generator powered by lithium batteries (life 7–10 years) is implanted subcutaneously, usually in the infraclavicular pectoral position.

An international three letter code describes the various methods of pacing (Table 11.23).

Atrial pacing (AAI) is the method of choice in symptomatic sinoatrial disease. The pacing wire is positioned in the right atrial appendage. Spontaneous atrial contractions inhibit the pacemaker such that pacing only occurs during atrial stand-still to prevent prolonged asystolic pauses. In patients with associated atrioventricular block, AAI pacing cannot be used and dual chamber pacing (DDD) should be substituted (see below).

Ventricular pacing (VVI) with a right ventricular pacing wire is used for temporary pacing in acute myocardial infarction or other emergencies. It is still widely used in chronic Mobitz type II or complete atrioventricular block although it is no longer the method of choice for most cases. Spontaneous ventricular beats are sensed and inhibit the pacemaker which is only activated when the rate falls below a preselected rate. If the pacemaker is prophylactic against occasional asystolic pauses a slow rate (perhaps 50/min) is sufficient to guard against syncopal attacks but in complete atrioventricular block a faster rate is necessary.

Although VVI pacing is relatively simple, it has important disadvantages because it fails to maintain the normal conducting sequence (atrial followed by ventricular contraction) and does not permit heart rate to increase during exercise. Dual chamber (DDD) pacemakers are therefore preferable for most patients with chronic Mobitz type II or complete atrioventricular block. The pulse generator is attached to two wires, one positioned in the right atrium and the other in the right ventricle. Reductions in atrial rate caused by sinus arrest or bradycardia are sensed by the atrial pacer which is then activated to maintain the rate above a preselected level. So long as the atrial beats (spontaneous or paced) are conducted promptly to the ventricle, initiating depolarization, the ventricular pacer remains inhibited. However, if ventricular depolarization fails to occur the ventricle is paced. Thus neither, either or both chambers of the heart may be paced with this form of pacemaker. If atrioventricular block is present, but the sinus node is functioning normally with a physiological response to exercise, the ventricular rate will follow the atrial rate during exercise in a synchronized manner. DDD pacing, therefore, is rate *responsive* because it re-establishes atrioventricular synchrony and allows the sinus node to control the heart rate.

Patients in whom the atrium is fibrillating cannot benefit from DDD pacing and VVI pacing must be used in chronic Mobitz type II or complete atrioventricular block. However, rate responsiveness can be achieved by using pacemakers which sense the physical vibration and muscle noise that occurs during exercise and respond with a graded increase in pacing rate.

## PROGNOSIS

First-degree and Mobitz type I second-degree atrioventricular block pose no direct threat to the patient, and the prognosis is therefore determined by the cause of the underlying conducting tissue disorder. The same is true of isolated left or right bundle branch block. Mobitz type II second-degree block and third-degree atrioventricular block always carry the risk of prolonged asystole and sudden death. Nevertheless, following pacemaker insertion this risk is effectively abolished and prognosis then relates to the underlying conducting tissue disorder. In idiopathic fibrosis of the conducting system, for example, the prognosis is excellent. In ischaemic disease, on the other hand, the prognosis is much worse.

# Tachyarrhythmias

## AETIOLOGY

Many factors may predispose to the development of tachyarrhythmias. These include both cardiac and non-cardiac disorders and the effects of drug toxicity (Table 11.24).

## PATHOLOGY

The principal mechanisms involved in the pathogenesis of tachyarrhythmias are enhanced automaticity and re-entry.

## *Enhanced automaticity*

Automaticity – spontaneous depolarization – is a property common to all the specialized conducting tissues within the heart (page 203). The automatic discharge of the sinus node, however, normally proceeds at a faster rate than the remainder of the conducting tissue which is, therefore, continuously suppressed. Nevertheless, a variety of stimuli (e.g. trauma, ischaemia, drug toxicity) can enhance the automaticity of an ectopic atrial or ventricular focus, allowing it to depolarize more rapidly than the sinus node. This produces a premature beat. Repeated automatic discharge from an ectopic focus of this type at a rate in excess of the sinus node can take over the pacemaker function and result in sustained atrial or ventricular tachyarrhythmias.

**Table 11.24** Causes of atrial (A), junctional (J), and ventricular (V) arrhythmias.

| Cause | Arrhythmia |
|---|---|
| **Cardiac disorders** | |
| Coronary artery disease | A and V |
| Pericardial disease | A |
| Cardiomyopathy | A and V |
| Mitral valve prolapse | A and V |
| Mitral stenosis/regurgitation | A |
| Aortic stenosis/regurgitation | V |
| Pre-excitation syndromes | A and J |
| Long QT syndrome | V |
| Chagas' disease | V |
| Cardiac trauma | A and V |
| **Non-cardiac disorders** | |
| Thyrotoxicosis | A |
| Phaeochromocytoma | V |
| Dystrophia myotonica | A and V |
| Hypothermia | A and V |
| Hypokalaemia | A and V |
| Hypomagnesaemia | A and V |
| Hyperkalaemia | V |
| Hypoxaemia | A and V |
| Acidosis | A and V |
| **Drug toxicity** | |
| Caffeine | A and V |
| Alcohol | A |
| Aminophylline | A and V |
| Tricyclic antidepressants | A and V |
| Sympathomimetic amines | A and V |
| Anaesthetic agents | A and V |
| Digitalis | A and V |

## Re-entry

The basic requirements for re-entry are two or more non-homogeneous conducting pathways with different electrical characteristics. A typical re-entry circuit (Fig. 11.38) is seen in the **Wolff–Parkinson–White syndrome** involving the atrioventricular node (slow conductor) and an accessory atrioventricular pathway (fast conductor). An atrial premature beat A finds the accessory pathway refractory at point B but conducts slowly through the atrioventricular node. Rapid ventricular depolarization occurs by His-Purkinje pathways activating cells immediately distal to the accessory pathway at point C. By this time the accessory pathway is no longer refractory and conducts the impulse retrogradely into the atria completing the re-entry circuit and initiating self-sustaining tachycardia. The anatomical distribution of the re-entry circuit is large in Wolff–Parkinson–White syndrome, but when re-entry occurs within the atria or ventricles it is much smaller, often consisting of only a few myocardial cells, which together constitute a microcircuit with slow- and fast-conducting limbs.

## CLINICAL FEATURES

All tachyarrhythmias may be entirely asymptomatic. Generally speaking symptoms are determined by the ventricular rate and the presence and severity of underlying heart disease.

Palpitation is the most common symptom caused by tachyarrhythmias. Nevertheless, isolated premature beats usually pass unnoticed, although the patient is occasionally aware of the pause or the forceful beat that follows. Paroxysmal tachycardias may also pass unnoticed, particularly if the attacks are short. More commonly, however, the patient will notice the abrupt onset and termination of the attack. Sustained tachyarrhythmias usually produce rapid palpitation which is irregular in atrial fibrillation.

Angina may occur if the rapid ventricular rate causes myocardial oxygen demand to exceed supply. Although angina is particularly troublesome in patients with coronary artery disease, it sometimes occurs in patients with normal coronary arteries if the rate of the tachycardia is very fast.

Tachyarrhythmias may present with dyspnoea due to heart failure particularly in patients with associated left ventricular or valvar disease. Tachyarrhythmias are an important treatable cause of heart failure.

Syncopal episodes (**Stokes–Adams attacks**) occur when paroxysmal tachyarrhythmias produce abrupt reductions in blood pressure and cerebral perfusion (page 144). Paroxysmal ventricular arrhythmias are usually responsible and if sustained may cause death. Sudden death is an inevitable consequence of sustained ventricular fibrillation.

## ARRHYTHMIA DETECTION AND DIAGNOSIS

Electrocardiographic documentation of the arrhythmia should be obtained prior to instituting treatment. In patients with sustained arrhythmias a 12-lead recording at rest is usually diagnostic but a long continuous recording of the lead showing the clearest P wave (if present) should also be obtained. In patients with paroxysmal arrhythmias special techniques may be required for electrocardiographic documentation.

### In-hospital ECG monitoring

Patients who have had out-of-hospital cardiac arrest or severe, arrhythmia-induced heart failure should undergo ECG monitoring in hospital under the continuous surveillance of trained staff.

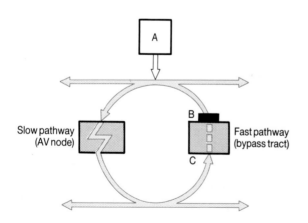

**Figure 11.38** A model of re-entry involving the atrioventricular (AV) node and a fast-conducting nodal bypass tract (see text for discussion).

## Ambulatory ECG monitoring

Patients with intermittent palpitation or dizzy attacks should have a continuous 24-hour ECG recording while engaging in normal day-to-day activities. Portable cassette recorders are available for this purpose. Analysis of the tape often identifies the cardiac arrhythmias, particularly if symptoms were experienced during the recording.

## Patient-activated ECG recording

For patients with very infrequent symptoms, the detection rate with 24-hour ambulatory monitoring is low and patient-activated recorders are therefore more useful. When symptoms occur the patient applies the recorder to the chest wall and may then transmit the ECG by telephone to the hospital for scrutiny by the physician.

## Exercise testing

The ECG recorded during exercise may be helpful when there is a history of exertional palpitation. Arrhythmias provoked by ischaemia or increased sympathetic activity are more likely to be detected during exercise.

## Programmed cardiac stimulation

This technique requires cardiac catheterization with electrode catheters. Premature stimuli are introduced into the atria or ventricles with a view to stimulating re-entry arrhythmias. In the normal heart sustained arrhythmias of this type are rarely provoked by premature stimuli. Thus arrhythmia provocation during programmed stimulation is usually diagnostic, particularly when the arrhythmias reproduce symptoms. The test can be repeated after administration of anti-arrhythmic drugs to test the efficacy of treatment.

## ATRIAL ARRHYTHMIAS

In this chapter the term supraventricular tachycardia is used to describe all tachy-arrhythmias originating from the atria or the atrioventricular junction, not just atrioventricular junctional re-entry tachycardia.

## Atrial premature beats

These rarely indicate heart disease. They often occur spontaneously but may be provoked by toxic stimuli such as caffeine, alcohol and cigarette smoking. They are caused by the premature discharge of an atrial ectopic focus and an early and often bizarre P wave is essential for the diagnosis. The premature impulse enters and depolarizes the sinus node such that a partially compensatory pause occurs before the next sinus beat during resetting of the sinus node. No treatment is necessary.

## Atrial fibrillation

See Fig. 11.31, page 196. This is common in ischaemic heart disease, mitral valve disease, thyrotoxicosis and left ventricular failure. It also occurs after major surgery and in response to various toxic stimuli, particularly alcohol. Atrial activity is chaotic and mechanically ineffective. P waves are therefore absent and are replaced by irregular fibrillatory waves (rate: 400–600 beats/min). The long refractory period of the atrioventricular node ensures that only some of the atrial impulses are conducted to produce an irregular ventricular rate of 130–200 beats/min. If the atrioventricular node is diseased the ventricular rate is slower, but in the presence of a rapidly conducting accessory pathway in Wolff–Parkinson–White syndrome dangerous ventricular rates above 300 beats/min may occur (page 213). Treatment is directed at either converting the arrhythmia to sinus rhythm (flecainide, amiodarone, direct current shock) or controlling the ventricular response with drugs that slow conduction through the atrioventricular node (digitalis, β-blockers, verapamil).

It is now well established that atrial fibrillation increases the risk of thromboembolism, predisposing to stroke, peripheral ischaemia and visceral infarction. The risk is greatest for patients with rheumatic mitral valve disease but even in patients with non-rheumatic disease the incidence of thromboembolic stroke is increased significantly, particularly in the elderly and in patients with underlying organic heart disease. For this reason anticoagulation with warfarin is now recommended in atrial fibrillation although in patients under 50 without evidence of organic heart disease, low-dose aspirin is a reasonable alternative.

### Atrial flutter

This (Fig. 11.39) is less common than atrial fibrillation but occurs under exactly similar circumstances. Re-entry mechanisms produce an atrial rate close to 300 beats/min. The normal atrioventricular node conducts with 2:1 block giving a ventricular rate of 150 beats/min. Higher degrees of block may reflect intrinsic disease of the atrioventricular node, but the conduction ratio is nearly always multiples of two (i.e. 4:1 or 6:1). The ECG characteristically shows sawtooth flutter waves which are most clearly seen when block is increased by carotid sinus pressure. Atrial flutter is an unstable rhythm which usually converts spontaneously to sinus rhythm or atrial fibrillation. Specific treatment to restore sinus rhythm requires flecainide, amiodarone, antitachycardia atrial pacing or direct current shock. Satisfactory control of the ventricular rate can usually be achieved with drugs that slow conduction through the atrioventricular node (see above).

## JUNCTIONAL ARRHYTHMIAS

These are often called supraventricular tachycardias (SVTs) and are usually paroxysmal without obvious cardiac or extrinsic causes. They are re-entry arrhythmias caused either by an abnormal pathway between the atrium and the atrioventricular node (atrionodal pathway) or an accessory atrioventricular pathway (bundle of Kent) as seen in Wolff–Parkinson–White syndrome.

### Atrioventricular junctional re-entry tachycardia (AVJRT)

The abnormal atrionodal pathway provides the basis for a small re-entry circuit (see above). In sinus rhythm, the electrocardiogram is usually normal although occasionally the P–R interval is short (Lown–Ganong–Levine syndrome). During tachycardia, the rate is 150–250 beats/min. Ventricular depolarization usually occurs by normal His-Purkinje pathways, producing a narrow QRS complex which confirms the supraventricular origin of the arrhythmia. Rate-related or pre-existing bundle branch block, on the other hand, produces broad ventricular complexes difficult to distinguish from ventricular tachycardia (Fig. 11.40). The arrhythmia is usually self-limiting but will sometimes respond to carotid sinus pressure. If this fails intravenous verapamil or adenosine are usually effective by blocking the re-entry circuit within the atrioventricular node. Antitachycardia pacing or DC cardioversion may also be used. More patients are now being treated by catheter ablation to destroy the abnormal atrio-nodal pathway and avoid the need for long-term drug therapy (see below).

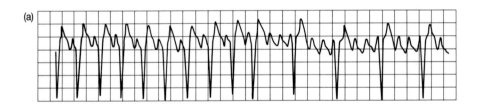

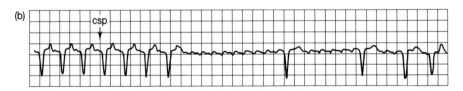

**Figure 11.39** Atrial flutter. (a) Typical sawtooth flutter waves are seen. Atrioventricular (AV) conduction is initially with 2:1 block but later changes spontaneously to 4:1 block. (b) Flutter waves are less obvious until the application of carotid sinus pressure (csp) exacerbates AV block and reveals the underlying atrial rhythm.

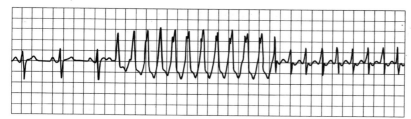

**Figure 11.40** Atrioventricular junctional re-entry tachycardia (AVJRT). Sinus rhythm is terminated by the onset of a broad complex tachycardia. Although this resembles ventricular tachycardia, the QRS complexes become abruptly narrow confirming the supraventricular origin of the arrhythmia. Thus the broad QRS complexes must have been caused by bundle branch block.

## Wolff–Parkinson–White syndrome

This congenital disorder affecting 0.12 per cent of the population is caused by an accessory pathway (bundle of Kent) between the atria and ventricles. During sinus rhythm, atrial impulses conduct more rapidly through the accessory pathway than the atrioventricular node such that the initial phase of ventricular depolarization occurs early (pre-excitation) and spreads slowly through the ventricles by abnormal pathways. This produces a short P–R interval and slurring of the initial QRS deflection (delta wave) (Fig. 11.41). The remainder of the ventricular depolarization, however, is rapid because the delayed arrival of the impulse conducted through the atrioventricular node rapidly completes ventricular depolarization by normal His-Purkinje pathways. Cardiac arrhythmias affect about 60 per cent of patients with Wolff–Parkinson–White syndrome and are usually re-entrant (rate 150–250 beats/min) triggered by an atrial premature beat (Fig. 11.38). In most patients the re-entry arrhythmia is 'orthodromic' with anterograde conduction through the atrioventricular node (producing a narrow QRS complex without pre-excitation) and retrograde conduction through the accessory pathway.

Occasionally the re-entry circuit is in the opposite direction ('antidromic') producing a very broad, pre-excited tachycardia. Treatment of these re-entry tachycardias is the same as for AVJRT.

Patients with Wolff–Parkinson–White syndrome are more prone to atrial fibrillation than the general population. If the accessory pathway is able to conduct the fibrillatory impulses rapidly to the ventricles it may result in ventricular fibrillation and sudden death. Digoxin (and to a lesser extent verapamil) should be avoided because it shortens the refractory period of the accessory pathway and can heighten the risk. Patients with dangerous accessory pathways of this type require ablation of the pathway either surgically or, preferably, by catheter techniques. Ablation therapy is also being used increasingly in patients with frequent re-entry arrhythmias which, though not dangerous, are often very troublesome.

## VENTRICULAR ARRHYTHMIAS

### Ventricular premature beats

These may occur in normal individuals in response to toxic stimuli such as caffeine or sympathomimetic drugs. They are caused by the premature discharge of a ventricular ectopic focus which produces an early and broad QRS complex. The premature impulse may be conducted backwards into the atria, producing a retrograde P wave, but penetration of the sinus node is rare. Thus resetting of the sinus node does not usually occur and there is a fully compensatory pause before the next sinus beat. If ventricular premature beats cause troublesome symptoms they may be suppressed by a variety of

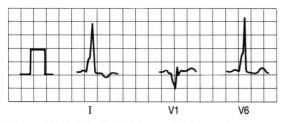

**Figure 11.41** Wolff–Parkinson–White syndrome: ECG. The short P–R interval and the slurred initial deflection (delta wave) or the QRS complex are clearly seen.

anti-arrhythmic drugs. However, treatment is never indicated on prognostic grounds because all anti-arrhythmic drugs have pro-arrhythmic side effects and may, unpredictably, induce more dangerous ventricular arrhythmias.

## Accelerated idioventricular rhythm

This nearly always occurs as a complication of acute myocardial infarction and is discussed on page 175 and see Fig. 11.21.

## Ventricular tachycardia

This is always pathological (Fig. 11.42). It is defined as three or more consecutive ventricular beats at a rate above 120/min. Ventricular depolarization inevitably occurs slowly by abnormal pathways producing a broad QRS complex. This distinguishes it from most atrial and junctional tachycardias which have a narrow QRS complex although differential diagnosis may be more difficult for atrial or junctional tachycardias with a broad QRS complex caused by rate-related or pre-existing bundle branch block (Fig. 11.40). Nevertheless, ventricular tachycardia can usually be identified by careful scrutiny of the 12 lead ECG (Fig. 11.42): findings that support the diagnosis include:

1 Very broad QRS complex (>140 ms)
2 Extreme left or right axis deviation
3 Atrioventricular dissociation evidenced by P waves, at a slower rate than the QRS complexes, 'marching through' the tachycardia (Fig. 11.43)
4 Ventricular capture and/or fusion beats, in which the dissociated atrial rhythm penetrates the ventricle by conduction through the atrioventricular node and interrupts the tachycardia, producing either a normal ventricular complex (capture) or a broad hybrid complex (fusion) that is part sinus and part ventricular in origin (Fig. 11.44)
5 Concordance of the QRS deflexions in V1 to V6, either all positive or all negative
6 Configurational features of the QRS complex, including an RSr′ complex in V1 and a QS complex in V6
7 **Torsades de pointes** (Fig. 11.45) – changing wavefronts are particularly characteristic of the ventricular tachycardia that complicates long QT syndrome, often resulting in sudden death. The syndrome may be inherited as an autosomal dominant (Romano–Ward syndrome) or as an autosomal recessive (Lange–Nielsen syndrome) trait when it is associated with congenital deafness.

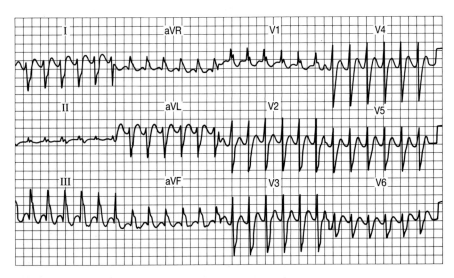

**Figure 11.42** Ventricular tachycardia: 12 lead ECG. The following features confirm that this broad complex tachycardia is ventricular in origin: very broad QRS complex (>140 ms); extreme right axis deviation; atrioventricular dissociation – note the dissociated P waves seen clearly in leads II, III, aVF and V1; and RSr′ complex in V1.

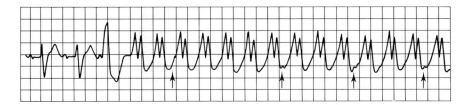

**Figure 11.43** Ventricular tachycardia: atrioventricular (AV) dissociation. P waves (arrowed) are seen 'marching through' the broad-complex tachycardia. Atrioventricular dissociation confirms the ventricular origin of the arrhythmia.

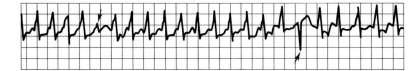

**Figure 11.44** Ventricular tachycardia: fusion and capture beats. The tachycardia is interrupted first by a fusion beat and later by a capture beat (both arrowed) confirming its ventricular origin.

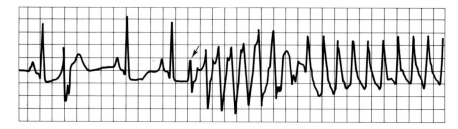

**Figure 11.45** Ventricular tachycardia: torsades de pointes. An early ventricular premature beat occurs after the first sinus beat (note the long Q–T interval). This recurs (arrowed) after the fourth complex and initiates a broad-complex tachycardia. The changing wavefronts (torsades de pointes) of the arrhythmia confirm its ventricular origin.

Ventricular tachycardia nearly always requires urgent treatment, either with intravenous anti-arrhythmic drugs (lignocaine, disopyramide, amiodarone), antitachycardia pacing or, most effectively, direct current shock. In patients with paroxysmal attacks, appropriate suppressive therapy must be instituted.

### Ventricular fibrillation

This occurs most commonly in severe myocardial ischaemia either with or without frank infarction. It is a completely disorganized arrhythmia characterized by irregular fibrillatory waves with no discernible QRS complexes (Fig. 11.22). There is no effective cardiac output and death is inevitable unless resuscitation with direct current cardioversion is instituted rapidly.

### TREATMENT

The usual aims of treatment are to suppress paroxysmal arrhythmias and to convert established arrhythmias to sinus rhythm. In patients with atrial arrhythmias (particularly atrial fibrillation) in whom these aims cannot be fulfilled, treatment is directed at controlling the rate of the ventricular response. Electrocardiographic documentation of the arrhythmia is essential before starting treatment. In the patient with a relatively benign atrial or junctional arrhythmia treatment is usually chosen empirically, with more sophisticated testing reserved for cases refractory to this approach. However, in the patient with a dangerous Wolff–Parkinson–White syndrome or ventricular tachycardia, there is no role for empirical measures, and treatment must be guided by appropriate tests to confirm its efficacy. This will usually involve provocative testing to ensure effective suppression of the arrhythmia. In all cases, other cardiac or non-cardiac disorders must be treated, particularly myocardial ischaemia, heart failure, metabolic and electrolyte disturbance and drug intoxication.

## General measures

A number of factors are known to predispose to cardiac arrhythmias (Table 11.24) and where possible these should receive specific treatment.

## Non-pharmacological therapy

### Carotid sinus pressure/Valsalva
The reflex vagotonic response to these manoeuvres slows conduction through the atrioventricular node and may terminate some junctional re-entry arrhythmias.

### Antitachycardia pacing
Re-entry arrhythmias are amenable to treatment of this type using either a temporary or permanent antitachycardia pacemaker. The pacemaker senses the abrupt increase in heart rate at the onset of the arrhythmia and delivers strategically timed electrical stimuli in order to break the re-entry circuit and permit return to normal conduction. Permanent antitachycardia pacing is now rarely used, however, because catheter ablation techniques have rendered it almost redundant.

### Catheter ablation
Electrode ablation catheters attached to an energy source may be placed strategically within the heart and used to cause selective damage to the conducting system. Direct current electrical energy from a defibrillator, or radiofrequency energy (similar to surgical diathermy) are used most commonly. The technique was used originally for ablation of the atrioventricular node in patients with troublesome atrial arrhythmias (particularly atrial fibrillation) resistant to conventional drug therapy. It results in complete atrioventricular block which prevents conduction of the arrhythmia to the ventricles. Following the procedure, permanent ventricular pacing is required.

The role of catheter ablation has been extended and its major application is now for the ablation of atrionodal and accessory pathways to correct troublesome re-entry arrhythmias in patients with Wolff–Parkinson–White syndrome and other junctional arrhythmias.

### Arrhythmia surgery
Current indications for arrhythmia surgery are the Wolff–Parkinson–White syndrome for destruction of the accessory pathway when catheter ablation has failed, and life-threatening ventricular arrhythmias that are resistant to drug therapy. Most ventricular arrhythmias originate from the endocardial surface of the heart and limited endocardial resection, leaving the rest of the ventricular muscle intact, is often sufficient to prevent further attacks.

### Direct current shock
Electrode paddles placed against the chest wall permit delivery of a high-energy direct current shock across the heart. General anaesthesia is necessary if the patient is conscious. This technique corrects the majority of acute-onset atrial and ventricular tachyarrhythmias by depolarizing the heart and allowing the sinus node to re-establish itself. The rapid, almost instantaneous response makes this the treatment of choice in emergency management.

### Implantable cardioverter defibrillator
This device is indicated in patients with paroxysmal, life-threatening, drug-resistant, ventricular arrhythmias that cannot be treated by ablation or arrhythmia surgery. Until recently, implantation required a thoracotomy but defibrillator coil electrodes are now available for transvenous insertion.

The defibrillator itself (about the size of a pack of cards) is implanted in the abdomen beneath the rectus muscle and automatically delivers a direct current shock in the event of ventricular tachycardia or fibrillation. The number of shocks that can be delivered is limited by the battery life of the defibrillator but most devices now have antitachycardia pacing capability and only use shocks if this fails to terminate the arrhythmia.

## Drug therapy
Table 11.10 (page 176) shows the Vaughan-Williams classification of anti-arrhythmic drugs. Because all these drugs have 'pro-

arrhythmic' side effects that may paradoxically exacerbate cardiac arrhythmias, they must be used cautiously. Electrocardiographic documentation of the arrhythmia is essential before starting treatment in order that the appropriate agent may be selected. The therapeutic range for most drugs is narrow and regular measurements of plasma concentrations should be made if possible in order to avoid toxic side effects. Careful electrocardiographic monitoring of the response to treatment is important, and if the arrhythmia persists despite therapeutic plasma concentrations an alternative drug should be substituted. A partial response might justify combination with a second agent, but regimens of this type should if possible be avoided because of the risk of drug interactions and exaggerated side effects. Class III and class IA drugs, for example, both prolong the Q–T interval and their combination can provoke severe ventricular arrhythmias. Class II and class IV drugs both slow conduction through the atrioventricular node and should not usually be taken together because of the risk of complete atrioventricular block.

## Class I drugs

These drugs stabilize irritable foci within the conducting tissue by depressing the rapid influx of sodium ion that initiates the action potential. Effects on repolarization are variable and provide the basis for a subclassification into groups A, B and C which prolong, shorten and have little effect on the Q–T interval, respectively.

Disopyramide is the most widely used class IA drug and is effective against atrial and ventricular arrhythmias. It is negatively inotropic and must be used with caution in heart failure. Anticholinergic properties help maintain the sinus rate (by blocking vagal activity) but may lead to a dry mouth and to urinary retention in the elderly.

Lignocaine is the most widely used class IB drug. It suppresses ventricular arrhythmias and is particularly useful in myocardial infarction (page 176). It is ineffective against atrial arrhythmias. Parenteral administration is always necessary because of gastrointestinal side effects and first-pass metabolism in the liver. It can be given as an initial bolus of 50–100 mg followed by an infusion of 4.0 mg/min which is

gradually reduced and should not normally be continued for more than 48 hours. Important side effects include bradycardia, hypotension, drowsiness and convulsions, particularly if the drug is given too rapidly. Mexiletine is in all respects similar to lignocaine except that it may be given orally and is suitable therefore for outpatient use, although nausea may be a problem.

Flecainide and propafenone are potent class IC drugs that are effective against atrial, junctional and ventricular arrhythmias. Both are moderately negatively inotropic and pro-arrhythmic side effects are well documented.

## Class II drugs

These are the β-blockers which protect the heart against excessive adrenergic stimulation. They are useful in combination with digoxin for controlling the ventricular rate in atrial fibrillation but their anti-arrhythmic effects are generally weak except in thyrotoxicosis. They are occasionally useful in junctional arrhythmias although large doses are necessary which are often not tolerated. They also have a special role for long-term therapy after myocardial infarction when they increase the fibrillation threshold and reduce the incidence of arrhythmic death. Propranolol is usually chosen for intravenous use, but for long-term oral use there is little to choose between β-blockers in terms of their anti-arrhythmic efficacy.

Side-effects are described on page 172 and 224.

## Class III drugs

These drugs prolong the duration of the action potential, increasing the effective refractory period throughout the conducting system. Amiodarone is the most important drug in this class, although sotalol, a β-blocker, also has mild class III activity. Amiodarone is available for oral and parenteral use and is effective against a wide range of atrial and ventricular arrhythmias. Therapeutic plasma concentrations may take a week or more to achieve during oral administration; and because the half-life is very long activity persists for up to 4 weeks following discontinuation of the drug. It is usual, therefore, to start treatment with 200 mg three times daily for 1 week, then reduce the dose to the minimum necessary. The drug is more rapidly effective following intravenous loading, but occasionally causes profound hypotension and bradycardia. Chronic therapy has been associated with a variety of side effects, including photosensitivity rashes, skin discolouration, pulmonary fibrosis, and liver and thyroid dysfunction (either hypothyroidism or, less commonly, hyperthyroidism).

## Class IV drugs

These drugs are calcium antagonists. Verapamil has been the most important drug in this class although diltiazam is also useful. Selective blockade of the slow calcium channel decreases depolarization and slows conduction through the atrioventricular node. Thus class IV drugs have an important role for controlling the ventricular rate in atrial fibrillation, often in combination with digoxin. Given intravenously they are useful for terminating junctional arrhythmias, and they can also be used prophylactically, although in Wolff–Parkinson–White syndrome they shorten the refractory period of the accessory pathway, and can increase the ventricular rate in atrial fibrillation. Verapamil and diltiazem are negatively inotropic and should be used with caution in heart failure. Intravenous verapamil is contraindicated in patients taking β-blockers since it may cause intractable heart block.

## Digitalis

Digoxin, the most commonly used cardiac glycoside, defies classification by Vaughan-Williams' criteria. In addition to its mild positive inotropic properties the drug slows conduction through the atrioventricular node by a direct effect on depolarization and by its vagotonic action. In atrial fibrillation it is the drug of choice for slowing the ventricular rate but is only rarely useful for prophylaxis against paroxysmal attacks. It has almost no other role for the treatment of arrhythmias. Digoxin can be given by slow intravenous infusion for loading purposes (500 μg followed after an hour by a further 250 μg), but is most commonly used orally (125–500 μg daily, depending on the clinical response). The therapeutic range is narrow and dose increases may need to be titrated against plasma concentrations. It is excreted by the kidneys, and in patients with renal failure the dose must be reduced. Other factors which increase the risk of digoxin toxicity include old age, hypokalaemia and hypomagnesaemia. Important side effects are loss of appetite, nausea, vomiting, visual disturbances and bradyarrhythmias. Digoxin may also cause a variety of tachyarrhythmias by enhancing automaticity. Digoxin therapy produces important ECG changes including prolongation of the P–R interval, and sagging of the ST segment with T wave inversion. These abnormalities do not necessarily indicate toxicity.

## Adenosine

Adenosine is a new drug which, like digoxin, defies classification by Vaughan-Williams' criteria. Its short half-life of <10 s requires it to be given by rapid intravenous injection. It is a potent atrioventricular nodal blocker and a dose of 0.1 or 0.2 mg/kg will nearly always terminate junctional arrhythmias; even if complete atrioventricular block occurs its short half-life ensures almost immediate recovery. Other side effects (flushing, nausea, hypotension) are similarly evanescent. Thus adenosine is safe and is particularly useful in the critically ill, haemodynamically compromised patient, although in other situations intravenous verapamil remains the drug of first choice for terminating junctional arrhythmias.

# Cardiac arrest

## AETIOLOGY

Cardiac arrest is usually caused by ventricular fibrillation or asystole but may also be caused by rapid ventricular tachycardia. These arrhythmias are usually the result of severe myocardial ischaemia or infarction but may also complicate hypoxia, electrolyte imbalance and a variety of drug interventions. Autonomic reflexes in response to endotracheal intubation or urethral catheterization occasionally cause cardiac arrest.

## CLINICAL FEATURES

In cardiac arrest, there is no effective cardiac output. The diagnosis is made clinically by loss of the arterial pulse followed rapidly by unconsciousness, apnoea and dilation of the pupils.

Irreversible brain damage usually occurs if the circulation is not re-established within 4 minutes, though factors such as hypothermia may prolong this time.

## TREATMENT

A firm thump over the sternum occasionally converts ventricular tachycardia or fibrillation to sinus rhythm; if this fails, full cardiopulmonary resuscitation should be instituted. The patient is placed supine on a firm surface with the neck extended. The airway must be cleared, and positive pressure ventilation and external cardiac massage can then be started. These should be continued uninterrupted until adequate spontaneous circulatory and respiratory function are restored. All drugs during resuscitation should be given into a central vein but if this is impossible double doses of adrenaline, lignocaine and atropine can be given by the endotracheal tube. Acidosis commonly develops in a prolonged resuscitation and may be corrected by intravenous sodium bicarbonate (50 ml of an 8.3 per cent solution), though ideally requirements should be titrated against arterial gas analysis.

### Positive pressure ventilation

The lungs should be inflated between 10 and 12 times per minute. Adequate oxygenation of the blood can usually be achieved by hand ventilation, using a face mask, or by mouth-to-mouth techniques. Endotracheal intubation, however, should not be delayed because this not only improves alveolar ventilation but also protects the airway against regurgitated gastric contents.

### External cardiac massage

This is applied by sharp compression of the lower end of the sternum about 60 times per minute. As soon as possible, the patient should be attached to an electrocardiogram monitor in order to determine the cardiac rhythm. Further management is directed at restoring an effective spontaneous cardiac output.

### Ventricular fibrillation

This is treated with direct current shock using 200 joules first which, if unsuccessful, may be repeated once before resorting to 360 joules.

Patients resistant to cardioversion should be given adrenaline (1 mg) before trying again, with repeat injections every 5 minutes as necessary. This produces a coarser fibrillatory pattern that is often more susceptible to cardioversion. Anti-arrhythmic drugs such as lignocaine (100 mg given slowly intravenously) make resistant ventricular fibrillation more responsive to direct current cardioversion.

### Asystole

Successful treatment is difficult. Inotropic drive is provided by adrenaline (1 mg) repeated every 5 minutes as necessary. Patients unresponsive to the first dose of adrenaline should be given atropine (2 mg). If asystole persists it is always worth trying direct current shock. When available, external or transoesophageal pacing may help, or a pacemaker catheter can be introduced into the right ventricle. A paced rhythm can usually be established by these means, but electromechanical dissociation often prevents restoration of effective cardiac output. Calcium chloride (5 ml in 10% solution) should only be used if the patient is hyperkalaemic, hypocalcaemic or known to be on calcium antagonists.

If these measures succeed in restoring spontaneous circulatory function, further management is directed towards the maintenance of a stable cardiac rhythm and oxygenation of the blood. Prophylactic anti-arrhythmic drugs are usually necessary and many patients require mechanical ventilation.

## PROGNOSIS

Following resuscitation, prognosis depends upon the cause of arrest and the resultant ischaemic cerebral damage. Prompt resuscitation prevents neurological sequelae and in those cases caused by drugs and other toxic insults, life expectancy may be normal. In the majority of cases, however, cardiac arrest reflects severe underlying heart disease and prognosis is usually poor. An important exception is primary ventricular fibrillation in acute myocardial infarction, when prognosis following resuscitation is only a little worse than for other survivors.

# HYPERTENSION

Hypertension is abnormal elevation of the arterial blood pressure. It is an important and potentially treatable cause of cardiovascular disease and death. Abnormal elevation of blood pressure implies a level above which the risk of morbid complications rises substantially. This level, however, is impossible to define because the risk of complications rises in approximately linear relation to both systolic and diastolic measurements. Moreover, the influence of blood pressure on morbid cardiovascular events is modified importantly by other factors such as age, race and sex, with young black males being at greatest risk. Attempts to define limits of normality are further confounded by the diurnal variability of blood pressure, with peak levels occurring early in the day and trough levels at night. Superimposed on this diurnal rhythm are the effects of exertion and anxiety, both of which increase blood pressure substantially. Blood pressure also shows long-term variability and in western societies rises progressively with age, men on average having higher levels than women.

For all these reasons any definition of hypertension must inevitably be arbitrary. For practical purposes, however, hypertension in adults may be defined as follows (the diastolic level representing disappearance of sounds; see page 146):

| | |
|---|---|
| Mild | 140/90–160/100 mm Hg |
| Moderate | 160/100–180/120 mm Hg |
| Severe | >180/120 mm Hg |

## AETIOLOGY

Blood pressure is determined by cardiac output and systemic vascular resistance. Hypertension is nearly always the result of increased systemic vascular resistance caused by arteriolar constriction. In the majority of patients no specific aetiological factor can be identified. Essential hypertension of this type must be distinguished from secondary hypertension in which a specific cause can be identified.

## Essential hypertension

This accounts for 95 per cent of all cases. The cause is by definition unknown, but evidence points to an interaction between hereditary and environmental factors. A hereditary influence must account in part for the familial incidence of essential hypertension. Abnormal membrane handling of sodium has often been demonstrated but its aetiological significance is unclear. Increases in circulating catecholamines and activation of the renin–angiotensin system occur in individual cases but are often not present. Environmental factors that have been associated with hypertension include obesity and several studies have shown a close positive correlation between body fat and blood pressure. Specific dietary factors have been more difficult to identify but recent work has shown an important relation with both salt and alcohol consumption. Thus, an increase in sodium intake of 100 mmol/24 hours is associated with an average rise in blood pressure ranging from 5 mm Hg at age 15–19 years to 10 mm Hg at age 60–69. Excessive alcohol consumption also has an adverse effect on blood pressure, systolic blood pressure being almost 10 mm Hg higher in men drinking six to eight units daily than in abstainers. Importantly, reductions in salt or alcohol consumption cause parallel reductions in the blood pressure. The role of stress and other psychosocial factors is difficult to define. Acute stress produces a physiological rise in blood pressure which may be sustained if the stress becomes chronic. Thus job loss, bereavement, divorce and similar events are all associated with a greater than expected incidence of hypertension.

## Secondary hypertension

In most cases, secondary hypertension is the result of renal disease or hormonal disorders (Table 11.25). Renal causes include both vascular and parenchymal disease, and in both cases activation of the renin–angiotensin system accounts at least in part for the elevation of blood pressure (page 162). Hormonal disorders are responsible for hypertension in primary

**Table 11.25** Causes of secondary hypertension.

___

**Renal parenchymal disease**
Glomerulonephritis
Pyelonephritis
Polycystic disease
Diabetic nephropathy
Connective tissue disease
Hydronephrosis

**Renal artery stenosis**
Atherosclerosis
Fibromuscular hyperplasia
Congenital

**Endocrine disease**
Adrenal cortex (Cushing's syndrome, Conn's syndrome)
Adrenal medulla (phaeochromocytoma)
Acromegaly
Iatrogenic (contraceptive pill, corticosteroids, sympathomimetic agents)

**Miscellaneous**
Coarctation of the aorta
Pregnancy (pre-eclampsia, eclampsia)
Acute porphyria
Increased intracranial pressure

___

aldosteronism and Cushing's syndrome, owing to excessive mineralocorticoid activity, and in phaeochromocytoma owing to the effects of adrenal catecholamines (page 538). The most common hormonal cause of hypertension, however, is the oral contraceptive which almost invariably produces an increase in blood pressure. Nevertheless, the increase is usually small and reverses promptly on stopping the drug. Activation of the renin–angiotensin system is probably responsible.

## PATHOLOGY

Hypertension is usually the result of peripheral arteriolar constriction. In the early stages this is reversible, but in the long term irreversible fibrinoid necrosis develops in the arteriolar wall. Hypertension is an important risk factor for atherosclerosis (page 169).

### The heart

Hypertension leads to left ventricular hypertrophy which compensates for the increase in afterload (page 162). In long-standing disease, however, irreversible deterioration in left ventricular contractile function may develop, leading to heart failure. The reduction in cardiac output often normalizes the blood pressure and the condition may be clinically indistinguishable from dilated cardiomyopathy. The development of left ventricular hypertrophy and heart failure can be prevented by starting antihypertensive therapy early in the course of the illness.

Hypertension is also a major risk factor for coronary artery disease and predisposes to myocardial ischaemia and sudden death. Evidence is now available suggesting that correction of hypertension reduces the risk.

### The brain

Accelerated atherosclerosis and microaneurysms are the principal cerebral consequence of hypertension. Both predispose to stroke by causing cerebral infarction and cerebral haemorrhage, respectively. Treatment of hypertension substantially lowers the risk of stroke.

### The kidney

Vascular changes in the renal arterioles and glomerular tufts decrease the glomerular filtration rate and produce tubular dysfunction. Proteinuria and haematuria occur and a vicious cycle of worsening renal function and increasing hypertension may develop. This may be prevented by starting antihypertensive therapy early in the course of the illness.

## CLINICAL FEATURES

Uncomplicated hypertension is usually asymptomatic. Contrary to popular belief the incidence of headache and epistaxis is not significantly increased and the onset of symptoms usually signals the development of major complications. Angina due to coronary atherosclerosis, left ventricular hypertrophy or a combination of the two is common, and in end-stage disease symptoms of heart failure occur. Retinal haemorrhage and exudates produce blurring of vision, while cerebrovascular disease may lead to transient ischaemic episodes or major stroke.

Examination confirms elevated blood pressure. The cardiac apex is not usually displaced, but it may have a thrusting quality and a double impulse due to a palpable fourth heart sound. Auscultation confirms the fourth sound and reveals accentuation of the aortic component of the second sound. An innocent mid-systolic murmur at the aortic area is not uncommon owing to forceful ejection by the hypertrophied left ventricle. Occasionally aortic dilation leads to the development of mild aortic regurgitation, evidenced by an early diastolic murmur at the left sternal edge.

Examination of the optic fundus permits direct inspection of the small blood vessels. Four grades of hypertensive retinopathy are recognized:

Grade I    Narrowing and increased tortuosity of the retinal arteries and increased light reflection from the arteries (silver wiring)

Grade II   Accentuation of the arterial changes and apparent narrowing (nipping) of the retinal veins at arteriovenous crossings

Grade III  Vascular changes associated with haemorrhage and exudates

Grade IV   Previous grades with papilloedema

Grades I and II are not specific for hypertension as they can occur in the elderly, but grades III and IV are pathognomonic of hypertensive retinal damage.

## DIAGNOSIS

Hypertension is diagnosed by sphygmomanometry (page 146). Blood pressure may show considerable variation in an individual; if it is found to be elevated, further measurements should be taken after a brief rest period and again at a subsequent clinic visit before committing the patient to life-long antihypertensive treatment. If the diagnosis is confirmed further investigation is directed at determining the aetiological diagnosis and assessing end-organ damage.

### Aetiological diagnosis

Because the large majority of patients have essential hypertension, a routine search for unusual causes is unnecessary. Special investigations to screen for secondary hypertension are indicated when the clinical findings are suggestive of a treatable underlying cause (e.g. ultrasound and arteriography for renal artery stenosis; urinary vanillyl mandelic acid for phaeochromocytoma). The threshold for undertaking special investigations of this type should be low for hypertensives under 35 years old, particularly when there is no family history of hypertension because in this group the incidence of secondary hypertension is higher.

### Assessment of end-organ damage

Routine cardiac investigations should include an ECG and chest X-ray for assessment of left ventricular hypertrophy and failure. Renal status is evaluated by analysis of the urine for blood and protein and measurement of blood levels of urea and creatinine. A serum potassium level is needed as a baseline prior to starting diuretic therapy. This also provides a simple screen for primary aldosteronism.

## COMPLICATIONS

The major complications of hypertension are heart disease, stroke, retinal damage and renal failure.

## TREATMENT

Only a small minority of patients have hypertension that is amenable to surgical correction. They include those with adrenal disease, unilateral renal disease and coarctation. The remainder require medical management.

### Aims of treatment

Treatment is aimed at lowering the blood pressure with a view to reducing the incidence of major complications. The efficacy of treatment for preventing stroke is well established, but reductions in the incidence of myocardial infarction have been more difficult to demonstrate. Nevertheless, the overall mortality of treated hypertensives is lower than for those who receive no treatment.

### Who to treat?

Patients with mild hypertension (up to 160/100 mm Hg) do not require treatment because it produces no appreciable benefit in terms of long-term morbidity and mortality. The benefit of treating moderate and severe hypertension is, however, well established.

There is no evidence that different treatment policies are required in particular racial, sex or age groups. Although the elderly (>70 years) are often less able to tolerate antihypertensive drugs they are most at risk of stroke and benefit from treatment as much, if not more, than younger hypertensives.

## General measures

Hypertension is not a medical emergency and in many cases can be improved (or even corrected) without drug treatment. Women on the contraceptive pill should, where possible, use an alternative method of contraception. The obese patient should be encouraged to lose weight because this often produces a significant reduction in blood pressure. Moderation of alcohol consumption is beneficial, particularly in the heavy drinker. Patients should be advised not to add extra salt to their food. Relief of stress, though difficult to achieve, is beneficial in some patients. A variety of relaxation and meditation techniques have been shown to lower blood pressure, at least in the short term. Undoubtedly the most important general measure, however, is the avoidance or correction of other risk factors for arterial disease, particularly smoking and hypercholesterolaemia. In the majority of clinical trials, smoking has emerged as a more important predictor of both myocardial infarction and stroke than a moderate increase in blood pressure.

## Drug therapy

In hypertension, treatment must usually continue indefinitely. Thus the acceptability of treatment in terms of dosage frequency and side-effects must always be a major consideration. Indeed, poor compliance with the treatment regimen is the usual reason for inadequate control of blood pressure. From the wide range of drugs available (Table 11.26), five groups of agents come closest to fulfilling the combined requirement for antihypertensive efficacy and patient acceptability.

### Diuretics

Salt and water excretion lower blood pressure by reducing plasma volume and cardiac output. Nevertheless, these changes are short lived and the mechanisms responsible for the long-term antihypertensive efficacy of diuretics are unknown. Although thiazides and loop diuretics are equally effective, thiazides are usually preferred because they produce a less vigorous diuresis. If hypokalaemia develops then they should be used in combination with potassium-sparing diuretics. Impotence may affect up to 15 per cent of patients treated with thiazide diuretics which are best avoided in younger sexually active patients. Thiazides cause modest elevations of blood sugar and triglycerides and there is a theoretical risk of long-term cardiovascular complications in young patients. At present, however, there is no evidence that the metabolic side effects of thiazides increase cardiovascular morbidity.

### β-Blockers

These drugs tend to lower cardiac output by their effect on heart rate and contractility, and also inhibit sympathetically mediated renin release from the kidney which reduces angiotensin II synthesis. Nevertheless, it is unlikely that these properties account fully for the antihypertensive efficacy of β-blockers, the mechanism of which remains uncertain.

β-Blockers may be used as monotherapy but are particularly useful in combination with thiazides or calcium antagonists both of which tend to increase renin release – an unwanted effect which is modified by β-blockers. In addition, β-blockers prevent reflex tachycardia caused by the vasodilator effects of calcium antagonists and α-blockers. The choice of β-blocker depends principally on patient acceptability, atenolol usually being preferred because it is long-acting, cardioselective and does not cross the blood–brain barrier. β-Blockers may cause a small rise in blood cholesterol, although whether this affects the risk of developing arterial disease is not known.

### Calcium antagonists

These drugs relax vascular smooth muscle, producing arteriolar dilation, and are effective in all degrees of hypertension. Nifedipine is best given in combination with a β-blocker to prevent reflex tachycardia. Verapamil and diltiazem cause less reflex tachycardia and can be used as single therapy. Although these drugs are

**Table 11.26** Drugs commonly used to treat hypertension.

| Drug | Dose | Adverse effects | Interactions |
|------|------|-----------------|--------------|
| **Thiazide diuretics** | | | |
| Bendrofluazide | 2.5 mg once daily | See Table 11.4 | ·See Table 11.4 |
| **β-Blockers** | | | |
| Atenolol | Start with 50 mg once daily; increase if necessary to 100 mg daily | Precipitation of asthma, and cardiac failure<br>Lack of energy, cold hands; bradycardia; depression and nightmares (especially propranolol) and impotence<br>Retained in renal failure | Don't combine with intravenous verapamil (page 218) Action increased by cimetidine (metroprolol) Action decreased by some NSAIDs<br>Antagonizes the effects of theophylline |
| **Angiotensin-converting enzyme inhibitors** | | | |
| Captopril | 12.5 mg twice daily; increase if necessary to 50 mg twice daily | See Table 11.4 | See Table 11.4 |
| Enalapril | 5.0 mg once daily; increase if necessary | | |
| **Calcium antagonists** | | | |
| Nifedipine | 10–20 mg three times daily | Headaches; flushing; ankle swelling; | |
| Amlodipine | 5–10 mg daily | | |
| Diltiazem | 60 mg three times daily | | |
| Verapamil | 40–80 mg three times daily | Constipation; flushing; headaches; negative inotrope effect | |
| **α-Blockers** | | | |
| Prazosin | Initial dose 0.5 mg before retiring because of postural hypotension on first dose; thereafter 1.0 mg three times daily; increased as necessary | Drowsiness; headache; constipation; postural hypotension | Action reversed by some NSAIDs |
| Doxazosin | Initial dose 1 mg before retiring; thereafter 1 mg daily; increase as necessary | Postural hypotension; headache | |

NSAIDs = non-steroidal anti-inflammatory drugs.

relatively short-acting and require to be given three times daily, slow-release preparations are now available for twice daily dosage which improves patient compliance. Long-acting calcium antagonists, such as amlodipine, for once daily administration may have a particularly useful role for the long-term management of hypertension.

*Angiotensin-converting enzyme inhibitors*
These drugs produce arteriolar dilation by blocking the synthesis of angiotensin II, a potent vasoconstrictor. They are effective in all degrees of hypertension and are now being used increasingly because side effects are rarely troublesome and quality of life is often well preserved. Impotence and drowsiness, in

particular, seldom occur with angiotensin-converting enzyme inhibitors. These drugs do not have adverse effects on lipid profiles and in many cases cause small reductions in blood cholesterol, though whether this protects against arterial disease during long-term treatment is unknown. A wide variety of different agents are now available but long-acting drugs for once daily administration (e.g. enalapril, lisinopril) are usually preferred.

### α-Blockers

Prazosin, a postsynaptic α-adrenoceptor blocker, has been widely used in the past but doxazosin, a longer acting drug for once daily administration, has now largely replaced it in the treatment of hypertension. Doxazosin is effective and well tolerated and, like angiotensin-converting enzyme inhibitors, may cause concomitant small reductions in blood cholesterol levels. Side effects related to vasodilation (headache, dizziness) are rarely troublesome and, like angiotensin-converting enzyme inhibitors, the incidence of impotence is low.

### Choice of drugs

The choice of treatment should be tailored to the individual. In young patients an angiotensin converting enzyme inhibitor or α-blocker is often preferred because side effects are rarely obtrusive and impotence, in particular, is seldom a problem. In addition these drugs do not have unfavourable effects on glucose or lipid metabolism and, on theoretical grounds, may protect against development of arterial disease in later life. The elderly are sometimes unwilling to take vasodilators because of postural hypotension and often find diuretics more acceptable. β-Blockers have a useful role in patients with exaggerated tachycardia or an anxiety component to their hypertension, while for many patients calcium antagonists are the best tolerated and most effective drugs. β-Blockers may exacerbate peripheral vascular disease. In renal impairment atenolol may accumulate and should be replaced by shorter acting β-blockers. If a single agent provides inadequate blood pressure control a second one can be added. Persistent hypertension requires the addition of a third agent and in the most severe cases, four or more different drugs may be necessary.

## PROGNOSIS

The prognosis is determined by the extent of associated cardiac, cerebral and renal disease. It relates principally to the duration of hypertension and its severity. Thus by detecting hypertension at an early stage and treating it effectively the prognosis can be improved. Prognosis is also affected by the age, race and sex of the patient, with young black men being at greatest risk of premature death. The interaction of other cardiovascular risk factors, particularly cigarette smoking, increases the risk considerably.

# Accelerated hypertension

This occurs in both essential and secondary hypertension and is characterized by severe elevation of the blood pressure (often above 200/140 mm Hg) and grade IV retinopathy, sometimes associated with encephalopathy characterized by headache, nausea, clouding of consciousness and convulsions. The marked increase in afterload may cause left ventricular failure and pulmonary oedema. Impairment of renal function usually occurs and if treatment is not instituted rapidly oliguric renal failure develops.

Accelerated hypertension is a medical emergency. Treatment is aimed at reducing the diastolic blood pressure to between 90 and 110 mm Hg. Blood pressure reduction should be smooth and controlled because there is risk of cerebral infarction if it drops abruptly to very low levels. For this reason bolus injections of diazoxide or hydralazine are no longer recommended because the blood pressure response is unpredictable and difficult to control. A graded reduction in blood pressure can be achieved by intravenous infusions of nitroprusside or labetalol. Nitroprusside infusion should start at 25 μg/min with small increments every 15 minutes until the desired response is achieved. Labetalol infusion should start at 1 mg/min with increments every 30 minutes. Because labetalol is a β-blocker as well as an α-blocker, it should be used cautiously in severe left ventricular failure. Following control of the blood pressure oral treatment should be prescribed to prevent recurrence of the hypertensive crisis.

# CARDIAC TUMOURS

## Primary tumours

Primary cardiac tumours (Table 11.27) are rare. The histologically benign myxoma accounts for at least half of all cases. Myxomas usually arise in the left atrium but may also be found in the other cardiac chambers. Typically the tumour is pedunculated and attached to the interatrial septum such that it prolapses into the mitral valve orifice during diastole. This impedes diastolic filling of the left ventricle and produces symptoms similar to those of mitral stenosis. Dyspnoea, however, is often episodic and provoked by changes in posture which encourage gravitational prolapse of the tumour into the mitral valve. On examination there is a low-pitched noise in mid-diastole (tumour 'plop') probably caused by the myxoma striking the left ventricular wall. This may be intermittent but can be mistaken for the mid-diastolic murmur of mitral stenosis. Other symptoms and signs of myxoma include fever, weight loss and clubbing but these are unusual. The erythrocyte sedimentation rate may be raised and systemic thromboembolism is common. Sudden death may occur if the tumour causes unrelieved obstruction of the mitral valve. In the past left atrial myxoma was usually misdiagnosed as mitral stenosis, but the echocardiogram and other imaging techniques now permit visualization of the tumour and rule out mitral valve disease. Treatment is by surgical excision of the tumour.

**Table 11.27** Classification of primary cardiac tumours.

| Benign | Malignant |
| --- | --- |
| Myxoma | Angiosarcoma |
| Lipoma | Rhabdomyosarcoma |
| Rhabdomyoma | Fibrosarcoma |
| Fibroma | |

## Metastatic tumours

Metastases account for the majority of cardiac tumours and usually originate from the breast or lung. Although any part of the heart may be involved, the pericardium is most commonly affected and presents with pericardial effusion and tamponade. Invasion of the conducting tissue may produce heart block. Occasionally extensive myocardial involvement or valvar obstruction leads to heart failure.

## Carcinoid syndrome

Carcinoid tumours in the appendix and other parts of the small bowel secrete kinin peptides and serotonin which are largely inactivated in the liver. Following metastasis to the liver, however, the systemic circulation is no longer protected from these substances which are responsible for the characteristic clinical features of carcinoid syndrome. These include diarrhoea, bronchospasm, flushing attacks and telangiectasia. Cardiac manifestations are the result of toxic damage to the tricuspid or pulmonary valves. Variable regurgitation or stenosis often develops. Left-sided valvar disease is rare but is occasionally seen in patients with pulmonary metastases.

# THE PULMONARY CIRCULATION

## Pulmonary embolism

This is described on page 305.

## Pulmonary heart disease

### AETIOLOGY

Pulmonary heart disease is usually called cor pulmonale. In the UK chronic obstructive pulmonary disease is the leading cause. Other causes are shown in Table 11.28.

### PATHOLOGY

Pulmonary heart disease is the result of chronic pulmonary hypertension caused by obliteration of the pulmonary vascular bed and hypoxic pulmonary arteriolar constriction. The right ventricle compensates by progressive hypertrophy but dilation and contractile failure eventually supervene.

### CLINICAL FEATURES AND TREATMENT

These are described on page 288.

**Table 11.28** Causes of pulmonary heart disease.

**Obstructive airways disease**
Bronchitis
Emphysema
Asthma

**Parenchymal lung disease**
Sarcoidosis
Pneumoconiosis
Bronchiectasis

**Neuromuscular and chest wall disease**
Poliomyelitis
Kyphoscoliosis

**Impaired respiratory drive**
Respiratory centre abnormalities
Sleep apnoea syndrome

**Pulmonary vascular disease**
Primary pulmonary hypertension
Chronic pulmonary embolism
Eisenmenger's syndrome

# PERIPHERAL VASCULAR DISEASE

## Aortic aneurysm

### AETIOLOGY

Aortic aneurysm is nearly always the result of atherosclerosis. Other causes include syphilis, Marfan's syndrome and idiopathic cystic medial necrosis.

### PATHOLOGY

The wall tension in a blood vessel is determined by the product of intravascular pressure and diameter (law of Laplace). The aorta is the largest artery in the body and its walls, therefore, are under considerable tension. Disease of the aortic wall causes destruction of the elastic fibres in the media which allows the vessel to dilate. The dilation itself increases wall tension and a vicious cycle of worsening dilation and increasing wall tension becomes established.

Most aortic aneurysms are fusiform, involving the total circumference of a segment of the vessel wall. Occasionally they are saccular and consist of an out-pouching of the vessel wall. Aneurysms occur most commonly in the abdominal aorta below the renal arteries, although any other part of the aorta may be affected.

## CLINICAL FEATURES

Aortic aneurysms are usually asymptomatic. Local pressure may cause pain in the lumbar or thoracic spine depending on the location of the aneurysm. Rupture causes more severe pain and commonly leads to hypovolaemic shock and death.

Abdominal aortic aneurysms produce a pulsatile mass in the abdomen. A bruit is often audible owing to turbulent flow through the aneurysm. Thoracic aneurysms usually produce no physical signs unless they involve the aortic root, when the early diastolic murmur of aortic regurgitation may be audible.

## DIAGNOSIS

A plain chest or abdominal X-ray is often diagnostic, particularly when the aneurysm is calcified. Ultrasound studies are also useful, but computed tomography provides definitive diagnostic information. Angiography is usually required before surgery but is not necessary for diagnostic purposes.

## DIFFERENTIAL DIAGNOSIS

Abdominal aneurysms must be distinguished from other abdominal masses, particularly those which overlie the aorta and transmit pulsation. Nevertheless, only aortic aneurysms are expansile. Thoracic aneurysms must be distinguished from other causes of a mediastinal mass, particularly carcinoma.

## COMPLICATIONS

### Thromboembolism

Thrombosis within the aneurysm predisposes to thromboembolism.

### Infection

Aortic aneurysms may become infected and produce a syndrome almost identical to endocarditis, though heart murmurs are not present.

### Aortic regurgitation

Aneurysmal involvement of the aortic valve ring is not uncommon in Marfan's syndrome and causes aortic regurgitation.

### Rupture

Aneurysmal rupture is a surgical emergency which is often fatal.

## TREATMENT

Blood pressure control is important and β blockade delays the progress of aneurysm formation. Surgical resection is indicated when symptoms or complications (e.g. aortic regurgitation) cannot be controlled, or when rupture threatens. Aneurysms of the abdominal aorta are most prone to rupture and when greater than 6 cm in diameter require prompt surgical resection.

## PROGNOSIS

Atherosclerotic aortic aneurysms are often associated with advanced coronary artery disease. Indeed, myocardial infarction is the usual cause of death. Five-year survival is less than 50 per cent.

# Aortic dissection

## AETIOLOGY

Like aortic aneurysm, dissection is caused by disease of the aortic media, usually atherosclerosis. The majority of patients are hypertensive, particularly when the dissection arises in the aortic arch.

## PATHOLOGY

The development of a tear in the aortic intima causes the high-pressure aortic blood to create a false lumen for a variable distance through the diseased media. The tear is usually in the proximal part of the aorta just above the sinus of Valsalva, but in about 25 per cent of cases it is distal and located within the aortic arch. The dissection can partially or completely occlude any of the branch arteries arising from the aorta and, if proximal, may disrupt the aortic valve ring producing aortic regurgitation. The false lumen may rupture externally (particularly into the pericardial or left pleural spaces) or may re-enter the true lumen of the aorta more distally.

## CLINICAL FEATURES

Presentation is with the abrupt onset of severe tearing pain in the front or the back of the chest. Examination may reveal absent pulses caused by side branch occlusions. The blood pressure is often elevated but in the event of rupture may be very low owing to hypovolaemia or tamponade. The early diastolic murmur of aortic regurgitation is commonly present in proximal dissections.

## DIAGNOSIS

Electrocardiographic changes are non-specific but may show acute infarction if the dissection occludes the coronary ostium. The chest X-ray shows dilation of the aorta, often with widening of the entire mediastinum. External rupture into the pericardial or pleural spaces causes cardiac enlargement or left pleural effusion, respectively. The echocardiogram often demonstrates the false lumen in proximal dissections and may also show pericardial haematoma and signs of aortic regurgitation; the transoesophageal technique (page 156) is particularly useful for imaging the ascending and arch aorta. More useful information, however, is provided by computed tomography which reliably demonstrates the true and false aortic lumens separated by an intimal flap. When the diagnosis is in doubt urgent aortic root angiography is required to define the origin and the extent of the false lumen (Fig. 11.46).

## DIFFERENTIAL DIAGNOSIS

Differential diagnosis is from other causes of acute chest pain, including myocardial infarction, pericarditis, pulmonary embolism and pneumothorax.

## COMPLICATIONS

### Branch artery occlusion

This may cause myocardial infarction, stroke, intestinal infarction, renal failure or limb ischaemia. If both vertebral arteries are occluded paraplegia occurs.

### Aortic regurgitation

Disruption of the aortic valve ring may demand valve replacement during surgical repair of the dissection.

### Rupture

Rupture into the pericardial sac causes severe tamponade. Rupture into the pleural or peritoneal spaces may lead to hypovolaemic shock.

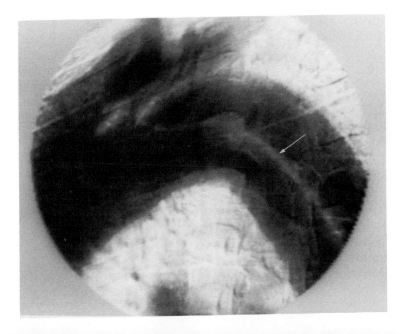

**Figure 11.46** Aortic dissection: angiography. This digital subtraction angiogram of the aortic arch shows abrupt widening of the aorta after the left subclavian branch. The intimal flap (arrowed) dividing the true and the false lumens is clearly seen.

## TREATMENT

The first step is to relieve pain, which usually requires diamorphine (2.5–5 mg i.v.). In proximal dissection, expeditious surgical repair improves the prognosis and is the treatment of choice. In uncomplicated distal dissection, surgery has not been shown to affect the prognosis, but strict control of the blood pressure is essential. β-Blockers are drugs of first choice because they reduce the pulse pressure as well as lowering the blood pressure.

## PROGNOSIS

Untreated proximal dissection is usually fatal within 3 weeks of presentation. Patients with distal dissection fare little better, though lowering the blood pressure helps prevent rupture and may permit longer survival.

# Acute limb ischaemia

## AETIOLOGY

Acute limb ischaemia is usually caused by embolic, thrombotic or traumatic arterial occlusion. Emboli usually originate from the left side of the heart in conditions such as mitral valve disease, cardiomyopathy, myocardial infarction and endocarditis. Thrombosis is usually the result of advanced atherosclerosis or local trauma.

## PATHOLOGY

Acute arterial occlusion provides no time for the development of collateral supply to the threatened limb. Profound ischaemia is therefore inevitable. This causes severe cell swelling and leads to irreversible damage within 6 hours. Muscle swelling in the anterior compartment of the leg, the compartment syndrome, may exacerbate tissue damage by compressing muscular arterioles. Decompression by fasciotomy may prevent ongoing tissue damage following surgical revascularization of the leg.

## CLINICAL FEATURES

Acute arterial occlusion causes the abrupt onset of pain in the distal part of the limb, which thereafter becomes pale and cold. No pulses are palpable beyond the occlusion. Later the pain becomes less severe, but within 6 hours irreversible ischaemic damage develops.

## DIAGNOSIS

Diagnosis is by clinical criteria. Arteriography is unnecessary and needlessly delays definitive treatment.

## TREATMENT

Urgent surgery is necessary if the limb is to be salvaged. Embolectomy may be performed under local anaesthesia. In the patient with thrombotic occlusion of diffusely atherosclerotic vessels, emergency surgery to bypass the obstruction may be necessary. Fasciotomy to relieve compression in the anterior compartment of the leg is sometimes helpful (see above).

If embolectomy fails, treatment is directed at preserving flow to the limb, which should be elevated to prevent swelling. Vasodilators such as nifedipine are usually prescribed, though their efficacy is unproven. Heparin and dextran infusions prevent extension of thrombosis within the limb. Infusion of streptokinase directly into the femoral artery may stimulate thrombolysis and restore flow.

## PROGNOSIS

Acute arterial occlusion in the lower limb nearly always progresses to gangrene and requires amputation if flow is not restored soon enough. In the arm, gangrene is rare but ischaemic (Volkmann's) contracture renders the limb useless.

# Chronic limb ischaemia

## AETIOLOGY

Chronic limb ischaemia is nearly always the result of atherosclerosis. Risk factors are the same as for coronary artery disease. Thus men over 50 are most frequently affected, particularly if there is associated cigarette smoking, hyperlipidaemia or hypertension. Diabetic patients are also at increased risk.

## PATHOLOGY

The atherosclerotic plaque which characterizes the condition enlarges and causes arterial stenosis which may proceed to thrombotic occlusion. This impairs distal perfusion of the limb. The lesions are found mainly in the large and medium-sized arteries, particularly the aorta and iliofemoral vessels. The upper limb is rarely affected. Diabetics are prone to more extensive disease, often with small vessel involvement.

## CLINICAL FEATURES

Clinical features are largely dependent on the site of the obstruction. Two syndromes can be defined.

### Femoropopliteal obstruction

This is the more common syndrome. The femoropopliteal disease results in intermittent claudication – a cramp-like pain felt in the calf which is brought on by walking and relieved by rest. As the disease advances, exercise capacity becomes progressively more limited until eventually rest pain occurs. Rest pain is usually felt in the feet and is most troublesome at night when it prevents sleep. Some relief is obtained by hanging the legs over the edge of the bed. On examination popliteal and pedal pulses are either reduced or absent. Arterial bruits may be audible over the femoral pulses. The skin of the legs is typically shiny and hairless. In severe ischaemia, areas of gangrene may develop. This often follows trauma, particularly around the nail bed and over the heels. In the most advanced cases, gangrene may extend to involve the whole foot and the leg.

### Aortoiliac obstruction

The main obstruction is in the lower aorta at its bifurcation and in the iliac arteries. Calf claudication is an early symptom but the pain spreads to the thighs and buttocks. This may be associated with impotence (Leriche syndrome). On examination the femoral pulses are reduced or absent, often with wasting of the buttock and thigh muscles. Auscultation over the lower abdomen and femoral pulses may reveal arterial bruits.

## DIAGNOSIS

The diagnosis is usually clear on the basis of the history and examination, particularly when there are absent pulses in the leg. Doppler studies permit flow measurements in the leg at rest and during exercise. This quantifies the perfusion deficit. If surgical treatment is contemplated arteriography is essential to define the location and the extent of disease.

## DIFFERENTIAL DIAGNOSIS

The chronically ischaemic limb must be distinguished from other causes of exercise-related pain in the legs, particularly musculoskeletal disorders and nerve root irritation in the lumbosacral spine.

## COMPLICATIONS

Ischaemic ulcers and gangrene are the major complications. Ulcers often develop in response to minor trauma. Healing is always slow. Gangrene is the result of severe ischaemia and may require amputation of the limb. Diabetic patients are particularly at risk of these serious complications.

## TREATMENT

### General measures

Exercise is helpful because it encourages collateral flow and may improve symptoms. Trauma to the feet (e.g. ill-fitting shoes) should be avoided and a chiropodist should help with care of the toe-nails. The bed at night should not be excessively warm because cutaneous vasodilation diverts flow away from muscle and exacerbates rest pain. Cigarette smoking must be strongly discouraged: it accelerates disease progression and produces vasoconstriction, which further reduces blood flow.

### Specific therapy

Vasodilator drugs are of no value. Improved blood flow to the ischaemic limb can only be achieved by sympathectomy, angioplasty or by-pass surgery. Most patients with intermittent claudication, however, never need surgical therapy.

Lumbar sympathectomy causes arteriolar dilation and improves perfusion of the ischaemic limb. It is not helpful in intermittent claudication but relieves rest pain in about 50 per cent of cases. Nevertheless, early recurrence of symptoms is common. Angioplasty is only feasible in patients with isolated iliofemoral stenoses. The role of lasers in iliofemoral occlusions is under investigation. Bypass surgery corrects peripheral ischaemia in most cases. Results are better in patients with aortoiliac disease than those with more distal disease. In patients with severe rest pain or gangrene, amputation may be necessary.

### PROGNOSIS

Prognosis is poor in patients with symptomatic peripheral vascular disease, with a 5-year survival of less than 50 per cent. Myocardial infarction is the usual cause of death because nearly all these patients have associated coronary artery disease.

# Buerger's disease

This is a rare condition occurring almost exclusively in men between the ages of 20 and 40 years. It is always associated with heavy cigarette smoking. The lesions occur principally in the small arteries of the feet (less commonly the hands) and lead to progressive arterial obliteration. Severe claudication often involving the instep is characteristic. Examination reveals absent foot pulses with normal femoral and popliteal pulses. Effective treatment is difficult. Abstinence from smoking is essential. Lumbar sympathectomy may help, but amputation is often necessary.

# Raynaud's syndrome

Raynaud's syndrome is caused by spasm of the digital arteries in response to cold exposure. It is usually idiopathic and develops during adolescence, more commonly in women. Occasionally the syndrome is secondary to some other disorder (Table 11.29). This should be suspected when the onset is later in life, particularly in men, and when the digital involvement is either unilateral or asymmetrical.

**Table 11.29** Causes of Raynaud's syndrome.

| |
|---|
| Idiopathic |
| Connective tissue disease (scleroderma, systemic lupus erythematosus) |
| Thoracic outlet syndrome (cervical rib) |
| Occupational (use of vibrating tools) |
| Drugs (β-blockers) |

Cold exposure typically causes a triphasic colour response. Profound blanching of the fingers and hands (the hallmark of Raynaud's syndrome) is followed by cyanotic mottling. During recovery the hands become pink and warm. The toes and even the nose may also be affected. In long-standing disease trophic changes in the fingertips occur, sometimes progressing to frank gangrene.

Treatment is by avoiding cold exposure. Underlying causes, if present, should be corrected. Vasodilator drugs such as nifedipine may be helpful. Sympathectomy is beneficial in some cases but early relapse is common.

# Deep venous thrombosis

### AETIOLOGY

Prolonged immobility in bed is the usual cause of thrombosis in the deep veins of the legs and pelvis. This affects up to 35 per cent of patients following major surgery – particularly in those who have undergone abdominal and hip operations. Other risk factors for deep venous thrombosis are shown in Table 11.30. Upper limb venous thrombosis is less common but may occur after trauma to the axillary vein or in

**Table 11.30** Risk factors for deep venous thrombosis.

---

Immobility, particularly following hip and abdominal surgery

Venous stasis in legs (varicose veins, vena caval compression, e.g. gravid uterus, bony fracture of legs)

Heart disease (myocardial infarction, heart failure)

Endocrine/metabolic factors (diabetes, obesity, contraceptive pill, *post-partum* period)

Malignant disease, particular pancreatic and bronchial carcinoma

Miscellaneous (polycythaemia, Behçet's disease)

---

association with indwelling catheters, pacemaker wires or external compression.

## PATHOLOGY

Thrombosis is usually in the iliac, femoral or calf veins. In about 10 per cent of cases a portion of thrombus may break off and cause pulmonary embolism (page 305). This is unlikely if thrombosis is confined to the calf veins but becomes more likely with extension to the iliofemoral veins.

## CLINICAL FEATURES

Symptoms and signs of deep venous thrombosis in the legs are variable and non-diagnostic. Pain and swelling of the calf occasionally occurs, but many cases are clinically silent. Confirmation of the diagnosis requires special investigations.

## DIAGNOSIS

### Doppler ultrasound

This detects reductions in blood flow velocity caused by thrombosis in the iliofemoral veins. It is of no value for detecting thrombosis in the smaller veins of the calf.

### Venography

This provides definitive evidence of deep venous thrombosis. Following injection of contrast medium into a vein in the foot, radiographic imaging of the leg and pelvis identifies venous filling defects caused by thrombosis.

## DIFFERENTIAL DIAGNOSIS

Deep venous thrombosis is usually unilateral and must be distinguished from other causes of a swollen leg, including trauma and infection. In patients with arthritis of the knee, rupture of a Baker's cyst into the calf is commonly mistaken for deep venous thrombosis. Bilateral deep venous thromboses must be distinguished from cardiac oedema, dependent oedema of the elderly and lymphoedema.

## COMPLICATIONS

Pulmonary embolism (page 305) is the most important complication of deep venous thrombosis and is a major cause of in-hospital morbidity and mortality. Embolism is less common with upper limb thrombosis. Thrombotic damage to the veins and their valves may compromise venous drainage and lead to chronic elevation of venous pressure around the ankles. This produces the post-thrombotic syndrome characterized by varicose veins and trophic skin changes, including pigmentation (haemosiderosis) and ulceration of the skin around the ankles.

## TREATMENT

### Prophylaxis

Patients at risk of deep venous thrombosis may be given prophylactic heparin. This is now regular practice following myocardial infarction and also in patients undergoing major surgery. Subcutaneous heparin, 5000 units 8-hourly, is effective and in surgical patients should start preoperatively.

### Specific therapy

In established deep venous thrombosis, anticoagulation should begin with intravenous heparin followed by oral anticoagulation with warfarin (page 305). In patients with recurrent pulmonary embolism, life-long anticoagulation is sometimes necessary.

Thrombolytic agents (e.g. streptokinase) effectively lyse fresh venous thromboses but their role, if any, in the management of this condition is not yet defined.

## PROGNOSIS

Complete resolution of deep venous thrombosis usually occurs following anticoagulation and mobilization. In the absence of pulmonary embolism, therefore, the prognosis is good unless there is underlying malignant disease or other serious systemic disorders.

# Superficial thrombophlebitis

This is an acute inflammatory process involving superficial veins in the arms or legs. The aetiology is often obscure, although it may occur as a complication of varicose veins. In hospital practice it is commonly associated with indwelling venous cannulae when infection or local irritation by parenterally administered drugs are the likely causes. The thrombosed vein may be palpated as a cord. It is tender and the overlying skin is erythematous. The risk of pulmonary embolism is negligible. It may be associated with an underlying adenocarcinoma (e.g. pancreas, stomach). Treatment is directed at

reducing inflammation by elevating the limb and prescribing anti-inflammatory analgesics.

# Lymphoedema

Inadequate drainage of lymph from the extremities leads to its accumulation in the interstitium. This produces lymphoedema. Lymphoedema may be congenital but more commonly it is the result of lymphatic obstruction by organisms (e.g. *Wuchereria bancrofti*), trauma (e.g. burns, irradiation, surgery) or malignancy. Essential lymphoedema of unknown cause (Milroy's disease) appears at puberty and mainly affects women. The yellow-nail syndrome is an unusual association of thick yellow nails, lymphoedema, pleural effusions and bronchiectasis.

The affected limb becomes progressively more oedematous and in chronic cases the skin becomes coarse and discoloured. The oedema is characteristically non-pitting, in contrast to cardiac oedema. Response to diuretics is poor. Surgical excision of oedematous tissue is reserved for the most severe, disfiguring cases.

# CONGENITAL HEART DISEASE

Cardiac defects are the most common of all serious congenital abnormalities. About 0.8 per cent of babies born alive have congenital heart disease, a figure that excludes non-stenotic bicuspid aortic valve and mitral valve prolapse. Untreated, the mortality is high, and by the age of 5 years 70 per cent of affected children are dead. Those who survive have less severe cardiac lesions but few live beyond the age of 40. Congenital defects in which survival to adulthood is common are shown in Table 11.31.

## AETIOLOGY

Genetic factors can be identified in less than 1 per cent of cases (Table 11.32). These include cardiac disorders which occur in congenital

**Table 11.31** Congenital heart defects in which survival to adulthood is common.

Bicuspid aortic valve
Pulmonary stenosis
Coarctation of the aorta
Atrial septal defect (secundum)
Patent ductus arteriosus
Tetralogy of Fallot
Complete heart block

syndromes, those associated with recognizable chromosomal abnormalities (e.g. Down's syndrome, Turner's syndrome) and single-gene disorders which account for the familial incidence of certain defects. In most cases, however, the relatives of patients with congenital heart

**Table 11.32** Aetiology of congenital heart disease.

**Genetic factors**

1. *Chromosomal abnormalities*

| | |
|---|---|
| Trisomy 21 (Down's syndrome) | ASD, VSD, Fallot's tetralogy |
| XO (Turner's syndrome) | VSD, PDA, pulmonary stenosis |
| XXXY | PDA, ASD |

2. *Single-gene disorders*

| | |
|---|---|
| Autosomal dominant | ASD (secundum), hypertrophic cardiomyopathy, mitral valve prolapse |
| Autosomal recessive | ASD (primum) |

3. *Congenital syndromes*
   Autosomal dominant

| | |
|---|---|
| Marfan | Aortic and mitral regurgitation |
| Leopard | Pulmonary stenosis, hypertrophic cardiomyopathy |
| Holt–Oram | ASD, VSD |
| Romano–Ward | Prolonged Q–T interval |

   Autosomal recessive

| | |
|---|---|
| Osteogenesis imperfecta | Aortic regurgitation |
| Pseudoxanthoma elasticum | Mitral regurgitation |
| Lawrence–Moon–Biedl | VSD |

**Environmental factors**

1. *Viral infection*

| | |
|---|---|
| Rubella | PDA, pulmonary stenosis, ASD |

2. *Drugs*

| | |
|---|---|
| Alcohol | ASD, PDA |
| Trimethadone | Complete transposition, Fallot's tetralogy |
| Lithium | Ebstein's anomaly, ASD |
| Amphetamines | VSD, PDA, complete transposition |

ASD = atrial septal defect. PDA = patent ductus arteriosus. VSD = ventricular septal defect.

disease have only a slightly increased risk of being affected. Indeed, concordance for congenital cardiac defects is unusual in monozygotic twins. Thus environmental factors are likely to play an important role either directly or through interaction with genetic predisposition. Environmental factors known to influence the development of the heart during early pregnancy include maternal rubella and certain drugs.

# *Intracardiac shunts*

## ATRIAL SEPTAL DEFECT

### *Pathology*

Communications between the atria may be caused by sinus venosus defects high in the septum or 'primum' defects low in the septum. These are commonly associated with anomalous pulmonary venous drainage and mitral valve abnormalities, respectively. However, the most common atrial septal defect is the 'secundum' defect of the oval fossa. Blood shunts preferentially from the left atrium through the right side of the heart into the low-resistance pulmonary circulation. The chronic increase in pulmonary flow may cause irreversible obliterative disease of the pulmonary arterioles during adulthood. Rising pulmonary vascular resistance causes pulmonary hypertension and right ventricular hypertrophy. This leads to progressive reductions in both cardiac output and left-to-right shunting. Eventually the pressures in the pulmonary and systematic circulations equilibrate and shunting becomes negligible or reversed (**Eisenmenger's syndrome**).

### *Clinical features*

Atrial septal defect is usually asymptomatic until the chronic increase in pulmonary flow leads to pulmonary hypertension during adulthood. This causes fatigue and dyspnoea owing to reductions in cardiac output. Symptoms are exacerbated by atrial fibrillation, which may precipitate right ventricular failure. Physical signs are fixed splitting of the second heart sound and a mid-systolic murmur at the pulmonary area owing to increased flow through the valve. When the shunt is large a mid-diastolic tricuspid flow murmur may also be present. The primum type of defect is often associated with an apical pansystolic murmur and other signs of mitral regurgitation.

In those patients who develop severe pulmonary hypertension and shunt reversal (Eisenmenger's syndrome), central cyanosis occurs owing to mixing of venous and arterial blood in the left atrium. This is associated with digital clubbing, polycythaemia and signs of pulmonary hypertension (page 163).

The defect in the atrial septum provides the potential for 'paradoxical' thromboembolism in which thrombus from the deep veins of the leg or the right atrial cavity embolizes through the defect into the systemic circulation where it may cause stroke, visceral infarction or limb ischaemia. Infective endocarditis is rare in atrial septal defect, though patients with a primum defect are prone to infection of the mitral valve.

## Diagnosis

The ECG shows left axis deviation in primum atrial septal defect, but in the more common secundum defect the axis is normal or to the right and may be associated with right bundle branch block. The chest X-ray shows cardiac enlargement with dilation of the proximal pulmonary arteries and plethoric lung fields reflecting increased pulmonary flow. The echocardiogram shows dilation of the right-sided cardiac chambers and Doppler studies are diagnostic if the abnormal flow across the atrial septum can be detected. Cardiac catheterization confirms the diagnosis. Serial measurements of oxygen saturation in the vena cava, right atrium, right ventricle and pulmonary artery show an abrupt 'step-up' at right atrial level owing to shunting of oxygenated blood through the defect. The catheter can be directed across the defect into the left atrium. Measurements of pulmonary and systemic flow using the Fick principle permit quantification of the shunt ratio. When a high oxygen saturation is found in the superior vena cava, or when the catheter enters a pulmonary vein directly from the right atrium, a sinus venosus defect with anomalous pulmonary drainage is likely.

## Treatment

Surgical correction of atrial septal defect is recommended in all patients with a pulmonary-to-systemic flow ratio in excess of 2:1. Whether this policy protects against the development of Eisenmenger's syndrome is now uncertain. In established Eisenmenger's syndrome, pulmonary hypertension is irreversible and closure of the defect is, therefore, unhelpful. Total heart and lung transplantation is the only surgical option.

## Prognosis

Untreated, atrial septal defect rarely permits survival beyond the age of 60.

# VENTRICULAR SEPTAL DEFECT

## Pathology

Ventricular septal defect is the most common congenital cardiac anomaly. It usually occurs in the perimembranous part of the septum. Blood shunts preferentially from left to right into the low-resistance pulmonary circulation. About 40 per cent of defects close spontaneously in early childhood, but in those that remain patent the chronic increase in pulmonary flow predisposes to obliterative pulmonary vascular disease and Eisenmenger's syndrome.

## Clinical features

If the shunt is large, heart failure occurs in infancy. Smaller shunts often remain asymptomatic until adulthood when fatigue and shortness of breath are common. These symptoms are accentuated by the development of obliterative pulmonary vascular disease. Examination reveals cardiac enlargement with a prominent left ventricular impulse. A systolic thrill over the lower left sternal edge can often be felt in association with a pansystolic murmur at the same location.

Patients with ventricular septal defect are always at risk of endocarditis, and antibiotic prophylaxis is essential.

## Diagnosis

The ECG and chest X-ray may be normal if the defect is small. Larger defects produce left ventricular hypertrophy and cardiomegaly with pulmonary plethora caused by increased pulmonary flow. The echocardiogram may permit the defect to be imaged but Doppler studies are diagnostic if the abnormal flow across the septum can be detected. Cardiac catheterization confirms the diagnosis. There is a step-up in oxygen saturation at right ventricular level, and left ventricular angiography produces prompt opacification of the right ventricle through the defect.

## Differential diagnosis

Differential diagnosis is from other causes of a pansystolic murmur. In mitral regurgitation the murmur is apical and radiates into the axilla. In tricuspid regurgitation the location of the murmur at the lower left sternal edge is similar to ventricular septal defect, but the murmur is accentuated by inspiration and giant V waves are visible in the jugular venous pulse (page 147).

## Treatment

Ventricular septal defect requires urgent repair if it causes heart failure in infancy. In asymptomatic cases conservative management is usually appropriate; but if signs of pulmonary hypertension develop during follow-up, cardiac catheterization is required with a view to closure of the defect. In established Eisenmenger's syndrome closure of the defect is unhelpful and total heart and lung transplantation is the only surgical option.

## Prognosis

When spontaneous closure of ventricular septal defect occurs in childhood, life expectancy is normal. Persistent small defects (maladie de Roger) are consistent with a normal life-span. Larger defects may produce heart failure and death in infancy or lead to Eisenmenger's syndrome in later life.

# PATENT DUCTUS ARTERIOSUS

## Pathology

The ductus arteriosus joins the main pulmonary trunk to the aorta. In the fetus gas exchange takes place at the placenta. Saturated vena cava blood from the placenta passes through the right side of the heart and shunts through the ductus arteriosus into the low-resistance systemic circulation, bypassing the high-resistance pulmonary bed. At birth the lungs take over the role of gas exchange. Systemic resistance rises with loss of the placental circuit and pulmonary resistance falls owing to inflation of the lungs. Flow through the ductus arteriosus therefore diminishes and the effects of local prostaglandins stimulate its closure.

In the premature infant persistent patency of the ductus arteriosus is common because normal mechanisms for its closure are not developed. At full-term relative hypoxaemia (high-altitude, pulmonary disease, cyanotic heart disease) delays normal closure. In other cases a patent ductus arteriosus is properly regarded as a congenital defect. It occurs more commonly in females. Blood shunts from left to right across the patent ductus arteriosus into the low-resistance pulmonary bed. This increases the pulmonary flow and volume-loads the left side of the heart. If the shunt is large, obliterative pulmonary vascular disease and Eisenmenger's syndrome may develop.

## Clinical features

The chronic volume-load may lead to left ventricular failure which, in the premature infant, exacerbates respiratory distress caused by hyaline membrane disease. In the full-term infant, left ventricular failure may also occur, but in many cases the condition remains asymptomatic. Examination reveals a collapsing carotid pulse owing to diastolic shunting through the ductus. The cardinal physical sign, however, is a continuous 'machinery' murmur at the upper left sternal edge caused by turbulent flow through the ductus which occurs throughout the cardiac cycle. The murmur is loudest at end-systole and early diastole.

## Diagnosis

The chest X-ray is usually normal but may show cardiac enlargement and pulmonary plethora if the shunt is large. In adults, calcification of the ductus arteriosus may be visible. Doppler studies are potentially diagnostic. Cardiac catheterization confirms the diagnosis.

## Complications

When the shunt is large, a patent ductus arteriosus may cause left ventricular failure or obliterative pulmonary vascular disease, leading to Eisenmenger's syndrome. The risk of endocarditis is considerable.

## Treatment

Patent ductus arteriosus always requires closure regardless of the size of the shunt. It is a low-risk procedure and guards against the development of complications, particularly endocarditis. In the premature infant cyclo-oxygenase inhibitors (e.g. indomethacin) may be effective, but in older children surgical closure is required. Recently catheterization techniques have been developed which permit closure of the ductus by a synthetic obstructor. This avoids the small risk of surgery.

## Prognosis

The natural history of patent ductus arteriosus is variable. If the shunt is large the risk of life-threatening complications is considerable. Endocarditis is an ever-present risk regardless of the size of the shunt. Nevertheless, patients with a very small defect may have a normal life-span.

# Obstructive valvar and vascular lesions

## AORTIC STENOSIS

Congenital aortic stenosis is caused by commissural fusion which results most commonly in a bicuspid valve. Associated anomalies may include patent ductus arteriosus and coarctation of the aorta. Bicuspid aortic valve may present in infancy with left ventricular failure due to outflow obstruction. More commonly, however, significant valvar stenosis does not occur until adulthood when the cusps calcify (page 199). On examination the carotid pulse may be slow rising, depending on the degree of valvar stenosis. An ejection click followed by a mid-systolic murmur is audible at the aortic area. Heart failure in infancy requires surgery (usually valvotomy), but asymptomatic cases without significant valvar stenosis require no specific treatment apart from antibiotic prophylaxis to protect against endocarditis.

In a minority of cases the obstruction is subvalvar caused by a muscular band or diaphragm. Clinical manifestations are very similar to valvar stenosis. Supravalvar aortic stenosis occurs at the superior margin of the sinuses of Valsalva above the coronary arteries. It is commonly associated with idiopathic hypercalcaemia, mental retardation and characteristic elfin-like facies.

## PULMONARY STENOSIS

This is one of the most common congenital cardiac anomalies. The right ventricular outflow obstruction produces a pressure gradient across the valve and variable right ventricular hypertrophy. Auscultation reveals an ejection click at the pulmonary area followed by a mid-systolic murmur. Mild-to-moderate pulmonary stenosis (peak systolic valve gradient less than 70 mm Hg) is only rarely symptomatic and is consistent with a normal life-span. In more severe cases, right ventricular failure may occur and valvotomy is required to relieve the outflow obstruction. Effective relief of outflow obstruction may also be achieved by balloon dilation of the pulmonary valve during cardiac catheterization, which avoids the risks of surgery.

## TETRALOGY OF FALLOT

### Pathology

The tetralogy consists of subvalvar pulmonary outflow obstruction, ventricular septal defect, overriding of the aorta and right ventricular hypertrophy. Depending largely on the severity of the right ventricular outflow obstruction, desaturated blood shunts from right to left across the ventricular septal defect. In severe outflow obstruction the shunt is large and cyanosis severe. In mild outflow obstruction, on the other hand, pulmonary flow may be close to normal and shunting is negligible – 'acyanotic Fallot's'. Nevertheless, even in acyanotic Fallot's, the outflow obstruction is often progressive and cyanosis usually develops during early childhood.

### Clinical features

Tetralogy of Fallot is the most common cardiac cause of central cyanosis after the first year of life. When pulmonary outflow obstruction is very severe and shunting considerable, the volume-loaded left ventricle fails in infancy. Unprovoked attacks of intense cyanosis may occur leading to syncope, convulsions or death. In less severe cases important symptoms do not occur until later, when the child is troubled by exertional dyspnoea and may squat to relieve symptoms. Squatting improves arterial oxygen saturation by increasing systemic vascular resistance, thereby reducing the shunt through the ventricular septal defect. Examination reveals central cyanosis and clubbing. Physical development is often impaired, though mental development is usually normal. A mid-systolic ejection murmur is audible at the pulmonary area, but the pulmonary component of the second heart sound is absent. A left parasternal systolic thrust due to right ventricular hypertrophy is usually present.

## Diagnosis

The ECG shows variable right ventricular hypertrophy depending on the degree of outflow obstruction. The chest X-ray shows a boot-shaped heart with a deep concavity of the left heart border due to a diminutive pulmonary artery. The echocardiogram is diagnostic if the ventricular septal defect and overriding aorta are imaged. The diagnosis is confirmed by cardiac catheterization.

## Differential diagnosis

Tetralogy of Fallot can usually be distinguished from other cardiac causes of central cyanosis (Table 11.33) on the basis of the echocardiographic findings. In the adult, Eisen-menger's syndrome is the major differential diagnosis. Both conditions are associated with central cyanosis, clubbing and heart murmurs. Nevertheless, the pulmonary component of the second heart sound which is loud in Eisenmenger's syndrome is absent in tetralogy of Fallot.

## Complications

In severe cases the right-to-left shunt can cause left ventricular failure in infancy. In children and adults, on the other hand, right ventricular failure is more common owing to chronic outflow obstruction. Other complications include cardiac arrhythmias and endocarditis.

## Treatment

Treatment is by total correction of the abnormality, which involves closure of the ventricular septal defect and relief of pulmonary outflow obstruction. In infants, however, palliative procedures are usually performed pending total correction later in life. These procedures are directed at improving the pulmonary flow by creating an anastomosis between the ascending aorta and the pulmonary artery (Waterston shunt) or the subclavian artery and the pulmonary artery (Blalock shunt).

## Prognosis

Death in infancy may occur if right ventricular outflow obstruction is very severe. Less severe disease permits survival into adulthood but few patients live beyond the age of 40. In infants cyanotic attacks are the major cause of death, but in children and adults right ventricular failure, arrhythmias and endocarditis are more important.

**Table 11.33** Causes of central cyanosis in congenital heart disease.

**Plethoric lung fields**
Transposition of great arteries
Total anomalous pulmonary drainage
Common atrium
Hypoplastic left heart syndrome
Common arterial trunk

**Oligaemic lung fields**
Tricuspid atresia
Severe pulmonary stenosis
Severe Fallot's tetralogy
Eisenmenger's syndrome

## COARCTATION OF THE AORTA

### Pathology

Coarctation is a localized fibrotic narrowing of the aorta which arises in association with the ductus arteriosus just beyond the origin of the left subclavian artery. It occurs more commonly in males and may be associated with bicuspid aortic valve, berry aneurysm or gonadal dysgenesis (Turner's syndrome).

If coarctation is severe and obstruction to aortic flow complete, left ventricular failure occurs in infancy. More commonly, however, the obstruction is partial and heart failure is avoided by the development of compensatory left ventricular hypertrophy and collateral flow around the coarctation.

## Clinical features

Coarctation is usually asymptomatic if heart failure in infancy does not occur. On examination the femoral pulses are delayed and diminished compared with the radial pulses (radiofemoral delay). The blood pressure in the arms is elevated but in the legs it is normal or low. Left ventricular hypertrophy produces a prominent apical impulse and a fourth heart sound. A systolic murmur is almost invariable from turbulent flow through the coarctation and collateral vessels. The murmur is often louder over the back of the chest and may be continuous if the collateral circulation is extensive. In adults with coarctation the shoulders and arms are often noticably better developed than the lower extremities.

## Diagnosis

The ECG shows left ventricular hypertrophy depending on the severity of hypertension. The chest X-ray characteristically shows notching on the underside of the ribs owing to erosion by dilated interocostal collateral arteries (Fig. 11.47). Angiography confirms the diagnosis.

## Differential diagnosis

Other obstructive lesions of the aorta also cause diminished or absent femoral pulses. The most important of these is advanced atherosclerosis. Nevertheless, patients with atherosclerosis are usually elderly and complain of intermittent claudication, which is not a feature of coarctation.

## Complications

The principal complications are those of sustained hypertension in the upper half of the body. This produces left ventricular failure and predisposes to stroke and aortic dissection. Patients with coarctation are also prone to subarachnoid haemorrhage (due to ruptured berry aneurysm), endocarditis and arrhythmias.

## Treatment

Treatment is by resection of the coarctation and end-to-end anastomosis of the aorta. This should be performed electively in childhood when relief of aortic obstruction corrects hypertension and removes the risk of left ventricular failure and stroke. Later in life hypertension may become irreversible.

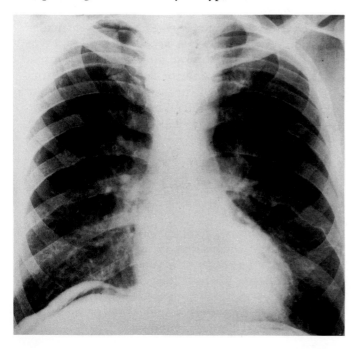

**Figure 11.47** Coarctation: PA chest X-ray. Notching of the inferior margins of the ribs is shown. The air under the diaphragm was the result of recent abdominal surgery.

## Complications

Complications of coarctation rarely permit survival beyond the age of 40 unless surgical correction is undertaken.

## CONGENITAL HEART BLOCK

Congenital complete heart block may not present until adolescence or early adult life. Treatment is by implantation of a permanent pacemaker.

# PREGNANCY

Pregnancy causes an increase in plasma volume which by the third trimester may be 50 per cent greater than prepregnancy levels. This is associated with a fall in plasma osmotic pressure which predisposes to oedema even in the absence of pre-eclampsia. Oedema is usually mild and tends to affect the lower limbs where venous pressure is high owing to compression of the pelvic veins by the uterus. Elevated venous pressure is also an important factor in the development of varicose veins and haemorrhoids, which are commonly seen during pregnancy.

In pregnancy the skin is warm and often flushed because of peripheral vasodilation. The pulse rate is increased and may have a collapsing quality. During the third trimester the pregnant uterus may cause upward displacement of the diaphragm. This compresses the heart such that the apex beat becomes palpable in the fourth intercostal space in the anterior axillary line. Auscultation during this period commonly reveals an 'innocent' ejection murmur at the base of the heart and a third heart sound – both manifestations of the hyperdynamic circulation.

The ECG and chest X-ray are usually normal, but late in pregnancy may show changes reflecting cardiac compression. These include a degree of left axis deviation and apparent radiological cardiac enlargement. Atrial and ventricular premature beats are frequently found.

## Heart disease in pregnancy

Flow murmurs, added heart sounds, peripheral oedema and minor ECG and chest X-ray abnormalities often give rise to a spurious impression of heart disease in the pregnant woman. In such cases the echocardiogram provides a safe and useful means of ruling out valvar and myocardial disorders.

Valvar and myocardial disease typically present during the third trimester or at the time of delivery when increments in plasma volume and cardiac output are at their peak. Mitral stenosis in particular is poorly tolerated and there is a considerable risk of pulmonary oedema. It is best treated by valvotomy before the onset of labour, but if valvar calcification or regurgitation contraindicate this procedure, medical management is preferable to valve replacement. Although mild bacteraemia is common during vaginal delivery, the risk of endocarditis in women with valvar disease is negligible and antibiotic prophylaxis (intravenous gentamicin and amoxycillin) is required only for complicated instrumented deliveries and for all women with prosthetic heart valves or a history of previous endocarditis.

Dilated cardiomyopathy that presents 3 months before or after labour has been named peripartum cardiomyopathy. This appears to be a specific entity related to pregnancy and is particularly common in women of West African origin. Nevertheless, it remains unclear whether peripartum cardiomyopathy represents the direct effects of pregnancy on a previously normal heart or merely a deterioration in a pre-existing cardiomyopathy.

# Intensive Care

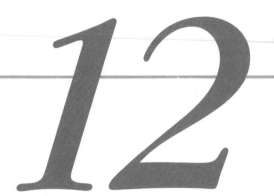

12

# INTRODUCTION

Admission to an intensive care unit (ICU) implies that a patient has a severe and deteriorating or unstable condition requiring regular observation, monitoring and intervention. Many of the underlying conditions resulting in the patient's critical illness are described elsewhere in this book. Intensive care units are areas in which sophisticated monitoring equipment is available as well as skilled trained nursing and medical care. This concentrated deployment of expensive and skilled resources has been shown to improve the management of critically ill patients and allows for the provision of organ support techniques, such as mechanical ventilation and renal replacement therapy. This chapter deals with a number of important general areas of intensive care common to many of these critically ill patients.

# MONITORING IN THE INTENSIVE CARE UNIT

To the uninitiated observer the intensive care unit presents a bewildering array of technology and personnel surrounding the critically ill patient. In order to provide optimal care for critically ill patients both monitoring and observation of the patients is necessary, hence the high nurse-to-patient ratio and technological equipment. This section briefly outlines some of the principal measures and observations made routinely in ICU. To monitor and observe patients successfully it is necessary not only to understand the basic principles of measurements but also the limitations of those measurements.

## Vital signs and routine intensive care unit observations

The basic observation of vital signs, heart rate, blood pressure and respiratory rate are recorded hourly as a minimum, although measurements are usually more frequent and may be continuous. Heart rate, for example, is usually recorded as a continuous electrocardiographic (ECG) trace from one of the standard leads. Other observations of organ function include the continuous and discreet measures shown in Table 12.1.

## Haemodynamic monitoring

Three types of haemodynamic monitoring are frequently used in the ICU: ECG, blood pressure and central venous pressure. In addition, measurements from a thermistor-tipped pulmonary artery flotation catheter (the Swan–Ganz catheter), are often required in the critically ill. Invasive techniques are indicated when treatment based on simpler clinical findings is not effective and the benefits are likely to outweigh the risks involved. Such examples are hypotension that is not responsive to simple treatment and acute respiratory failure requiring mechanical ventilation.

Haemodynamic monitoring over time is used as a guide to the progress of patients. Fluid therapy and the use of vasoactive agents are judged on the basis of the values and the clinical picture.

**Table 12.1** Observations of organ function in the intensive care unit.

| System | Continuous measures | Discreet measures |
|---|---|---|
| General | Temperature – core/peripheral, fluid balance | |
| Respiratory | Saturation, $FiO_2$, ventilator observations | Blood gases, oxygen transport |
| Cardiac | Central venous pressure, pulmonary artery occlusion pressure | Cardiac output |
| Renal | Urine output, fluid balance | Blood and urine urea, creatinine concentration |
| Liver | Few except signs of fulminant hepatic failure | Liver function tests, prothrombin time and serum albumin |
| Gut | Nasogastric aspirate, diarrhoea | Abdominal girth, bowel habit, tonometry |
| Skin | Pressure areas, ischaemia | |
| Neurological | Level of consciousness including Glasgow Coma Scale | |

Continuous = hourly or more frequently if required.
Discreet = Six hourly to daily. $FiO_2$ = inspired oxygen concentration.

# Arterial monitoring

Blood pressure (systolic, diastolic and mean) can be measured non-invasively using the familiar mercury manometer. Arterial catheters allow continuous blood pressure monitoring and repeated blood sampling, for blood gas and other analysis. These benefits often outweigh the risks of infection and distal ischaemia. The preferred sites are the radial or dorsalis pedis artery which carry the least risk of distal ischaemia, but the femoral, brachial and axillary arteries are also used. The arterial catheter is connected by fluid-filled low compliance tubing to a pressure transducer and the hydrostatic reference zero is usually taken as the level of the patient's right atrium.

# Central venous pressure

Jugular venous pressure and peripheral oedema can be assessed clinically and, with fluid balance and daily weight, may guide fluid therapy. More satisfactory monitoring is achieved by using central venous catheters, usually via cannulation of the internal jugular or subclavian veins to measure the central venous pressure (CVP) in the superior vena cava (SVC). Central vein access also permits venous blood sampling and administration of intravenous fluids and medication.

In critically ill patients alterations in the tone of venous capacitance vessels can maintain the CVP in the presence of a reduced blood volume but, in general, the CVP is a fair guide to the combination of blood volume and right ventricular function.

# Pulmonary artery pressures

A standard balloon-tipped, flow-directed catheter allows full right heart catheterization at the bedside with continuous measurement of pulmonary artery pressures and intermittent measurement of pulmonary artery occlusion pressure, mixed venous saturation and cardiac output (Fig. 12.1). Right heart catheterization allows pressures and oxygen saturations in the superior vena cava, right atrium, right ventricle and pulmonary artery to be measured. The waveform should be displayed continuously to ensure that there is no pulmonary artery obstruction or rupture.

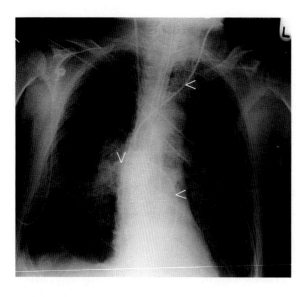

**Figure 12.1** A chest X-ray of a man with a pulmonary artery line seen in the right pulmonary artery (arrowed). An endotracheal tube and a central venous catheter are also present.

The **pulmonary artery occlusion pressure** (PAOP) is the best routinely available measure of left ventricular preload. The catheter used has a small balloon at its tip. When the balloon is inflated a small branch of the pulmonary artery is occluded and the distal tip of the catheter beyond the balloon is in a continuous column of fluid with the left heart. In the absence of obstruction the mean PAOP in end expiration approximates to the left ventricular end-diastolic pressure (Fig. 12.2).

**Mixed venous oxygen saturation** ($SvO_2$) can be sampled intermittently by taking blood samples from a catheter placed in the right atrium or ventricle. It reflects the balance of oxygen delivered to and extracted from the tissues. This can provide important information on the adequacy of oxygen delivery from the heart to the systemic circulation.

In many forms of shock it is difficult to predict the cardiac output and pulmonary artery pressure, and in half of these patients therapy

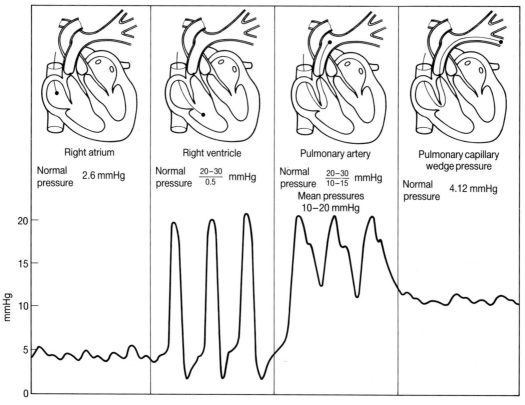

**Figure 12.2** Traces of the pressure waveforms obtained when a pulmonary artery catheter passes through a right atrium and ventricle and out into the pulmonary artery where it is wedged in a small vessel.

will be changed as a result of pulmonary artery catheterization. In myocardial infarction, pulmonary artery catheterization before inotropic therapy is unlikely to contribute any more than the clinical assessment of pulmonary artery pressure and cardiac output. The complications of invasive pressure monitoring are shown in Table 12.2. In addition technical problems such as inaccurate placement of the catheter or a blocked cannula can result in aberrant results and inappropriate therapy unless good sense and clinical judgment are maintained.

# Cardiac output

Cardiac output (C.O.) is the volume of blood ejected from the heart each minute. It is useful to consider C.O. per m² of body area – the cardiac index. The normal range for the cardiac index is 3–4 l/min/m². Cardiac output is dependent on stroke volume and heart rate.

Heart rate is under the influence of the auto nomic nerves and adrenal catecholamines. Bradycardia (<60 beats/min) does not necessarily cause a drop in C.O. if the heart can compensate with an increase in stroke volume but if the heart cannot alter stroke volume to compensate then C.O. falls. Tachycardia (>110 beats/min) often increases C.O. but may cause C.O. to decline, when diastole is shortened and ventricular filling is decreased. Arrythmias may also alter the time

**Table 12.2** Complications of invasive pressure monitoring.

| Manoeuvre | Complication |
| --- | --- |
| Insertion of cannula | Pneumothorax<br>Haemorrhage<br>Arterial puncture |
| Presence of cannula | Infection<br>Fracture embolization |
| Pulmonary artery cannula *in situ* | Arrhythmias<br>Trauma to valves<br>Prolonged occlusion leading<br>to infarction |

of ventricular filling and may decrease cardiac output.

Stroke volume is the volume of blood ejected from the ventricles during a single contraction. The stroke volume index (SVI), the cardiac index divided by heart rate (normal SVI = 45–85 ml/m²) corrects for body surface area. Stroke volume is dependent on preload, contractility and afterload.

## PRELOAD

In 1914 Starling found that up to a critical limit, the strength of contraction of myocardial muscle fibre was directly related to the amount of stretch on the fibre before contraction; i.e. as the end-diastolic fibre length increases, so does the cardiac output. Preload is closely related to the end diastolic volume. If the ventricle is overstretched, excessive dilation and thinning of the myocardium may cause stroke volume to fall.

## MYOCARDIAL CONTRACTILITY

The strength of cardiac contraction is influenced by:

1 Sympathetic nerve stimulation: the 'flight–fight' response
2 Positive and negative inotropes (page 255)
3 Coronary blood flow
4 Damaged myocardium
5 Physiological depressants: hypoxia, acidosis

## AFTERLOAD

Afterload is the resistance that has to be overcome in order for ventricular ejection to occur. Factors that influence this are tension in the ventricular wall and vascular resistance. The vascular resistance is determined by:

1 Elasticity (compliance) and size (radius) of the vessels
2 Viscosity of the blood
3 Change in pressure from one end of the vessel to the other

The radius of the vessels is the greatest determinant of peripheral resistance to blood flow.

It is important to remember that although vasodilator therapy decreases the afterload and therefore decreases the energy demands on the heart, it also increases the size of the 'vascular container'. This can result in a reduction in the amount of blood returning to the heart (venous return) and preload is decreased. Conversely, when the volume in the ventricle is more than the ventricles are able to pump effectively, decreasing the preload can unload the ventricles and improve cardiac output. If the venous return is decreased too much, the stretch on the ventricles will be inadequate and cardiac output will fall.

## MEASURING CARDIAC OUTPUT

Cardiac output measurements can be made by thermodilution. Sterile cold saline is injected into the right atrium and the temperature change is detected by a thermistor bead just behind the balloon of the catheter. The cardiac monitor should be watched during studies because arrhythmias change cardiac output. The cardiac output is calculated by dividing the product of the injectate volume and the temperature difference between body and injectate by the integral of the difference between body and pulmonary artery temperature over time. Measurements are generally performed in triplicate at random throughout the respiratory cycle and the results averaged.

# Respiratory monitoring

Respiratory problems are not confined to those with primary respiratory pathology but can occur in all severely ill patients, for example, multiple injuries, septicaemia. Clinical observation and monitoring are needed to detect acute changes in vital signs, developing or worsening of cyanosis, chest movement, air entry and synchronization with the ventilator. Ventilator system alarms help manage inflation pressure, frequency, expired minute volume and tidal volume, inspired oxygen ($FiO_2$) and inspired gas temperature. The possibility of ventilator disconnection or mechanical failure should always be borne in mind and a manual method of ventilation should always be present at the bedside.

## RESPIRATORY OBSERVATIONS

### Respiratory rate and rhythm

The rate, depth and rhythm of breathing are controlled by the respiratory centre in the pons and medulla of the brain stem. Increase in carbon dioxide ($CO_2$), metabolic rate, hypoxaemia and acidosis stimulate both rate and depth of breathing. Rapid shallow breathing is usually associated with pleuritic chest pain or abdominal distension or phrenic nerve damage. Neurological problems can alter the pattern of breathing producing yawns, sighs, irregularity and apnoea.

A variety of devices exists for measuring volumes and flow. These measurements are done regularly on asthmatic patients, or those with neurological disorders such as Guillian-Barré syndrome or myasthenia gravis.

### Chest wall and abdominal movement

Visual inspection of movement of the chest wall and abdomen offers valuable information. Asymmetric movement of the hemithoraces may suggest collapse of one lung, intubation of a main bronchus or pneumothorax. Paradoxical inward abdominal movement on inspiration can suggest inspiratory muscle fatigue.

### Heart rate and rhythm

Hypoxaemia stimulates the sympathetic nervous system causing a reflex increase in heart rate. Atrial arrhythmias and premature ventricular contraction are also seen with chronic respiratory disease.

### Skin

Cold and sweaty skin is often present in respiratory distress. Carbon dioxide retention may be suspected if the patient is vasodilated and cyanosis indicates hypoxia.

### Conscious level and behaviour

Depending on the degree of hypoxia there may be a decrease in awareness, inappropriate responses or restlessness. Patients who have respiratory distress may be unable to speak and be physically exhausted.

### Auscultation of the lungs

Auscultation of the lungs is done to assess air entry to the lung. Unilateral decrease or absent breath sounds occur when one of the following exists:

1  Accidental movement of an endotracheal tube into a main bronchus
2  Unilateral airway obstruction
3  Pneumothorax/haemothorax/pleural effusion

### Pulse oximetry

Oximetry is a non-invasive technique used for measuring oxygen saturation of haemoglobin in the blood. Oximeters are only accurate when peripheral blood flow is adequate and there is no excess pigment such as biluribin in the skin and blood.

## MONITORING OF OXYGENATION

Adequate oxygenation requires adequate perfusion and so cardiac output is a major determinant of oxygen delivery. What is delivered (and where) is also important. An arterial oxygen pressure ($PaO_2$) of less than 8 kPa or saturation of less than 90 per cent is associated with an unacceptably low arterial oxygen content. Common causes are:

1  Pre-existing lung disease
2  Pulmonary oedema due to left ventricular failure
3  Non-cardiogenic pulmonary oedema
4  Pulmonary infection
5  Pulmonary embolism

Oxygenation may be inadequate because of anaemia as the arterial oxygen content depends on the quantity of haemoglobin as well as the arterial saturation and $PaO_2$. Moreover, shifts in the oxygen–haemoglobin dissociation curve also affect the availability of oxygen for the tissues. In shock the curve moves to the right allowing more oxygen to be delivered to the tissues at any given $PaO_2$. The other two principal determinants of the oxygen–haemoglobin dissociation curve are pH and temperature. Acidosis and hyperthermia shift the curve to the right, whilst alkalosis and hypothermia shift the curve to the left although in the case of hypothermia the reduction in oxygen consumption may outweigh the reduction in oxygen delivery. The arterial pH should be maintained between 7.26 and 7.36.

The amount of oxygen available to respiring tissues is the product of the cardiac output and the arterial oxygen content and so changes in cardiac output are a major determinant of oxygen delivery.

Acid–base status (page 509), blood lactate (page 512) and changes in oxygen consumption in relation to oxygen delivery all give useful information about the state of tissue oxygenation. Tissue hypoxia cannot be diagnosed by blood gas analysis alone, these other measures provide additional information that helps us to assess whether oxygen in the arterial blood is delivered to the respiring tissues.

# Clinical Problems

# SHOCK

Shock is manifest when perfusion of vital tissues becomes inadequate and cellular hypoxia develops as a result of acute circulatory failure. The circulation can deteriorate in many different ways with inadequate or inappropriately distributed blood flow. Reversal requires both a diagnosis and knowledge of the adjustments most likely to produce optimal performance of the circulation in those circumstances. The central therapeutic aim is the maintenance of an adequate delivery of oxygen to respiring cells.

# Causes

1 An acute reduction in circulating blood volume (**hypovolaemic shock**)
2 An acute deterioration of myocardial function (**cardiogenic shock**)
3 Blood flow obstruction within the heart and lungs (**obstructive shock**)
4 Peripheral vascular abnormalities – principally a maldistribution of blood flow with vasodilation increasing the vascular volume (**distributive shock**). This maldistributive type of shock, typified by septic shock, commonly occurs with a normal or raised cardiac output.

Hypovolaemia, absolute or relative, is common to all forms of shock.

# Clinical assessment

The first parameter to assess in shock should be the intravascular volume status. The assessment should include pulse rate and character, jugular venous pulse pressure and waveform, blood pressure and the presence of a postural drop in blood pressure, urine output, skin turgor and the presence of peripheral oedema together with a thorough review of fluid balance and weight charts to estimate fluid and electrolyte depletion. The response to an intravenous fluid challenge allows an important dynamic observation of clinical signs, and in the case of hypovolaemic shock following surgery rapid fluid resuscitation may be sufficient alone to avoid further problems.

Clinical assessment of cardiac output includes measurement of core and peripheral temperature, pulse rate character, the state of the peripheral vasculature, mean arterial pressure (page 244) and urine output. Paradoxically, C.O. may be high in some forms of shock, for example, septic shock (page 253).

The correlation between these clinical signs of volume status and cardiac output with the adequacy of tissue oxygenation as judged by haemodynamic and oxygen transport data is poor. The resolution of clinical signs can lag considerably behind the resolution of circulatory failure. Moreover, investigations such as blood gas analysis and blood lactate measurements may reveal tissue hypoxia with a metabolic acidosis that is not obvious on clinical examination alone.

Clinically obvious shock is generally severe and an emergency. Rapid assessment of the clinical situation and simple investigations – electrocardiogram and blood gas analysis – will allow an initial working diagnosis. In many cases this will be sufficient to guide the initial choice of treatment. After this preliminary resuscitation further conventional clinical evaluation can be performed which, together with an assessment of the haemodynamic response to treatment, will allow a more precise diagnosis and management plan to be made.

The classification of shock is shown in Table 12.3.

# Hypovolaemic shock

This is the commonest form of shock. It results from loss of extracellular fluid (ECF), blood or other fluids, with a resulting low blood volume and inadequate ventricular filling and stroke volume. Shock results from the low cardiac output. It is characterized by tachycardia, hypotension, cold and pale peripheries ('cold shock'), rapid respiration and sweating. The patient may be thirsty, listless and very apprehensive with restlessness or alternatively torpor. Multiple compensatory reactions occur in order to defend the ECF volume:

1 There is increased sympathetic output causing the reflex tachycardia and vasoconstriction (most marked in skin and viscera) in order to maintain blood volume. A rapid thready pulse with cold pale clammy skin may be seen. Blood pressure may be maintained despite up to a 25 per cent loss in circulating volume in a young person then, as cardiac output declines, further hypotension develops. Autoregulation of blood flow preferentially spares the myocardium and brain as coronary arteries dilate with increased myocardial metabolism.

**Table 12.3** Classification of shock.

| Type of shock | Cause | Examples |
|---|---|---|
| Hypovolaemic | Haemorrhage, fluid depletion | Trauma |
| Cardiogenic | Myocardial: | Infarction |
| | | Cardiomyopathy |
| | Mechanical: | Mitral regurgitation |
| | | Ventricular septal defect |
| | | Aortic stenosis |
| | Arrhythmias | Ventricular tachycardia |
| Extracardiac obstructive shock | Pericardial tamponade | |
| | Constrictive pericarditis | |
| | Pulmonary embolism (large) | |
| | Severe pulmonary hypertension: | Primary |
| | | Eisenmenger's syndrome |
| Distributive shock | Septic shock | |
| | Drugs and toxins | Overdose |
| | Anaphylaxis | |

2 There is reduced glomerular filtration with sodium retention. Clearance of nitrogenous waste substances is reduced and if the hypotension is prolonged then acute renal failure may supervene upon the oliguria (page 428).
3 There are increased circulating catecholamines and angiotensin II, vasopressin, adrenocorticotrophin (ACTH) and aldosterone.

## CAUSES

Common causes are haemorrhage, gastrointestinal fluid loss (for example, vomiting, diarrhoea), burns or dehydration. During haemorrhage the haematocrit may not fall for several hours after the onset of bleeding when plasma volume will be restored by renal salt and water retention by the kidneys and a shift of interstitial fluid into the circulation.

Gastrointestinal fluid loss sufficient to cause shock is most common in babies and the elderly. Plasma loss from burn surfaces leads to haemoconcentration and hypovolaemia.

Metabolic disorders such as adrenal insufficiency and diabetic ketoacidosis are all characterized by ECF loss which can be sufficient to cause cardiovascular collapse secondary to the loss in plasma volume.

Specific therapy in hypovolaemic shock is aimed at removing or reducing ECF loss and appropriate volume replacement.

# Cardiogenic shock

Depressed cardiac performance results in low cardiac output and then hypotension. For cardiogenic shock to develop more than 40 per cent of the left ventricular myocardium must be damaged following infarction. It carries a grave prognosis with an in-hospital mortality of 80–90 per cent.

## CAUSES

The most frequent cause is myocardial infarction reducing left ventricular contractility and producing pump failure. Other causes of cardiogenic shock such as ventricular septal rupture after infarction, acute valvar regurgitation and myocarditis also result in a sudden fall in cardiac output.

## CLINICAL FEATURES

The reduction in cardiac output leads to a rise in left ventricular filling pressures, and back pressure into the pulmonary circulation may produce pulmonary oedema. The patient is cold and clammy, often with a raised jugular venous pressure, crackles at the lung bases and oliguria. Arterial hypoxaemia due to pulmonary oedema may be a major component of the hypoxic state. Cardiac signs may be minimal but there may be pulsus alternans (page 146), a gallop rhythm (page 148) or signs of acute mitral regurgitation or ventricular septal rupture after infarction.

Therapy is directed at reducing ischaemia and restoring perfusion in the heart muscle. Myocardial preservation might include the use of simple measures such as oxygen and nitrate therapy, or more complicated interventions such as intra-aortic balloon pumps (IABP) to reduce cardiac work and augment coronary perfusion. Cardiogenic shock for mechanical reasons (e.g. acute mitral regurgitation) requires surgical correction where possible. Measures to reduce infarct size such as thrombolytic therapy reduce the risk of cardiogenic shock.

Rhythm is important in determining cardiac output and tachycardias and bradycardias need to be corrected. For example, the conversion of atrial fibrillation to sinus rhythm with restoration of atrial transport may be critical.

# Extracardiac obstructive shock

## PERICARDIAL TAMPONADE

Pericardial tamponade, in which fluid in the pericardium prevents ventricular filling, is the best example of extracardiac obstructive shock (page 187). The ventricle is unable to fill in diastole, limiting the stroke volume and thus cardiac output. Pericardial tamponade may be recognized from its clinical manifestations: pulsus paradoxus, hypotension, distended neck veins with Kussmaul's sign and characteristic ECG and echocardiography appearances (page 188).

## MASSIVE PULMONARY EMBOLISM

Mechanical obstruction of pulmonary vessels (page 305) causes a rise in pulmonary vascular resistance and vasospasm due to the release of vasoactive mediators. Increased right ventricular load results in right ventricular failure with a raised central venous pressure and reduced venous return with shock. A patient who survives will be hypoxic, tachypnoeic and tachycardiac. The ECG shows signs of right heart strain. Radioisotope scans will show a reduction in perfusion with preserved ventilation in the affected area of lung. Pulmonary angiography may be needed if there is still doubt or if thrombolytic therapy is contemplated. Doppler ultrasound of veins in the pelvis and legs may show a source of emboli. Therapy is aimed at maintaining a pressure gradient for venous return, i.e. fluid loading and pressor inotropic agents. Anticoagulation reduces the risk of further emboli. When large emboli compromise cardiac output thrombolytic therapy and surgical embolectomy may be considered.

# Distributive shock

This is characterized by decreased peripheral vascular resistance.

Septic shock is one of the commonest causes of death in the ICU, with a mortality of 30–75 per cent. It is more frequent in the host who is immunosuppressed for whatever reason: for example, age, steroids and/or immunosuppressive drugs, surgery, drug abuse (including alcohol), malnutrition, chronic disease.

Shock is most frequently due to Gram-negative organisms but a similar clinical picture is seen with Gram-positive bacteria, fungi, rickettsia and virus infections.

In septic shock bacterial toxins (endotoxin in Gram-negative infections) cause vasodilation by activation of an inflammatory response. This comprises complement, kinin and coagulation systems, neutrophils and macrophages. In addition sepsis depresses the myocardium and increases capillary permeability, so there is loss of plasma volume into the tissues and a reduction in blood volume.

In early septic shock vasodilation, arteriovenous shunting, increased capillary permeability and defective tissue oxygen utilization are present. Cardiac output is high and peripheral vascular resistance is low before hypotension supervenes. If therapy is not rapidly instituted then cardiac output will fall as a result of the relative hypovolaemia and there will be severe hypotension, oligoanuria and peripheral vasoconstriction with a low output state that carries a very grave prognosis.

## SPECIFIC MANAGEMENT

### Infection

The most important and effective treatment is to identify and eradicate infection.

### Corticosteroids

There is no evidence that steroids improve outcome. Indeed, they may reduce the chances of long-term survival by increasing the incidence of secondary infection and acute renal failure.

### Immunotherapy

Trials are in progress with monoclonal antibodies directed against endotoxin and other mediators of inflammation.

# Anaphylactic shock

Anaphylactic shock is caused by a rapidly developing allergic reaction (page 97). The antigen–antibody reaction causes massive histamine release, with widespread dilation of arterioles and capillaries, and increased capillary permeability. The vasodilation results in a reduced venous return due to the relative hypovolaemia, and there is right ventricular failure secondary to pulmonary hypertension.

The clinical consequences are increased vascular permeability, bronchospasm, soft tissue swelling compromising the upper airway, pulmonary hypertension, platelet aggregation and systemic hypotension. There is wheeze, itch, tongue swelling, nausea, vomiting, abdominal pain, altered mental state and loss of consciousness.

## TREATMENT

Specific treatment is the removal of the inciting substance, airway protection and oxygen supplementation, and administration of adrenaline and antihistamine. Fluid replacement is important and glucocorticoids may be given.

# The multisystem effects of shock

Shock is multisystem in its effect and all organ systems are affected, precipitating reversible and later refractory organ failure. The most effective form of prevention is the prompt identification and treatment of the initiating cause of shock, so minimizing the haemodynamic disturbance.

## REFRACTORY SHOCK

When shock of any cause persists for some hours it becomes less responsive to vasopressors and myocardial function remains depressed even with a normal blood volume. There is reduced capillary perfusion leading to hypoxic tissue damage and extravasation of blood through the injured capillary walls.

If shock persists there is accumulation of metabolic products including $CO_2$ and lactic acid. Vasoactive substances relax precapillary sphincters whilst postcapillary venules which are more sensitive to hypoxia remain constricted. The capillary bed pools blood, and fluid enters the extravascular space with interstitial oedema, haemoconcentration and increased viscosity.

Refractory shock has multisystemic effects. The splanchnic circulation where vasoconstriction and reduced perfusion is most marked in haemorrhagic shock, for example, is particularly sensitive. There is evidence that as a result of the hypoxic damage the barriers to the entry of bacteria into the circulation from the intestinal tract break down.

Severe cerebral ischaemia will result in depression of the vasomotor and cardiac areas of the brain, with slowing of the heart rate and vasodilation. Blood pressure drops further reducing cerebral perfusion.

In severe shock coronary blood flow is reduced by hypotension and tachycardia even though coronary vessels are dilated. This results in myocardial depression that exacerbates the shock and acidosis. If prolonged then myocardial depression persists in spite of restoration of blood volume.

Intravascular coagulation may be triggered by substances released by damaged cells and activated white cells and platelets, a condition known as disseminated intravascular coagulation (DIC, page 645). Reduced flow with increased blood viscosity makes the blood highly coagulable. Systemic activation of the clotting cascades and platelet aggregation with clot formation occurs in the capillary bed. Consumption of clotting factors and platelets leads to bleeding problems.

The pulmonary circulation also suffers an acute lung injury which results in acute hypoxaemic respiratory failure: so-called 'shock lung' (sometimes called adult respiratory distress syndrome, page 261).

Prolonged shock can become irreversible. Myocardial function is impaired. A metabolic acidosis develops as anaerobic metabolism produces more lactic acid and the liver and renal clearance of lactate declines.

# Therapy

Each type of shock requires specific therapy aimed at the underlying pathology. The foundations of successful management must be the diagnosis and treatment of the underlying cause. As listed above these causes are diverse and many are dealt with elsewhere in this book. What follows is a description of the principles of treatment of cellular hypoxia from all causes.

Unless shock is rapidly reversed by the initial resuscitative efforts then the patient should be transferred to the intensive care unit for continued management with the aid of invasive haemodynamic monitoring.

The goals of shock therapy are:

1 To maintain blood flow to organs.
2 To maintain a mean arterial pressure that will ensure adequate perfusion of vital organs.
3 To prevent the development of lactic acidosis (page 512).

Many intensive care physicians resuscitate patients in shock not to normal values but to the hyperdynamic state which is seen in survivors of shock. In figures these goals of resuscation are:

| | |
|---|---|
| Cardiac index | 4.5 l/min/m$^2$ (50 per cent greater than normal) |
| Oxygen delivery | 600 ml/min/m$^2$ (20 per cent greater than normal) |
| Blood volume | 3.2 l/m$^2$ (male), 2.8 l/m$^2$ (female) (500 ml greater than normal) |

These supranormal values allow for the additional metabolic demands of shock and there is some evidence that the use of these targets in the treatment of critically ill patients may improve survival.

## VOLUME THERAPY

As previously pointed out, all shocked patients are relatively or absolutely hypovolaemic and the cornerstone of treatment is to establish an adequate cardiac filling.

The objectives of fluid therapy are (1) to replace body fluid and (2) to increase preload and cardiac output to increase oxygen delivery. The type of fluid used in replacement depends on the loss, and so may be blood, colloid or crystalloid. Replacement of blood losses with blood products and extravascular fluid with salt-replete fluids is desirable. Water loss with hypernatraemia and haemoconcentration needs dextrose solutions (i.e. no salt) or half normal saline replacement.

The aim is to achieve an appropriate blood volume by using 100–200 ml boluses of fluid to raise the PAOP in ventilated patients to 12–18 mm Hg with the optimization of cardiac output as shown by the failure of additional boluses of fluid to increase the cardiac output further.

It is important to individualize fluid loading with incremental doses and serial measurements of right and left ventricular filling pressure and stroke work, and cardiac output. A patient with septic shock may gain no benefit from a PAOP of greater than 14 mm Hg, but a patient with chronic left ventricular failure may on occasion need a PAOP of 25 mm Hg.

Once any hypovolaemia has been corrected patients with persistent features of shock may be categorized into those with an inadequate cardiac output and impaired tissue perfusion (hypodynamic shock) or those where a high cardiac output with peripheral maldistribution of blood flow results in impaired tissue perfusion.

## INOTROPE THERAPY

Inotropes are used when, despite appropriate fluid therapy, circulatory failure persists. They are used to increase myocardial contractility which involves increased myocardial oxygen consumption. All inotropes have some peripheral vascular effects. An ideal inotropic agent will not increase heart rate but will maintain diastolic blood pressure and improve mean arterial pressure and cardiac output so that improved tissue perfusion will reverse metabolic acidosis, increase overall oxygen delivery and maintain an adequate urine output. There is no such ideal inotrope (see Table 12.4), and each patient needs careful judgement taking into account the underlying disease process, haemodynamic status and the actions of available inotropes.

### Catecholamines

Table 12.4 lists the principal catecholamines. All act on adrenergic receptors: $\alpha$-receptor agonists vasoconstrict most systemic vascular beds and cause some increased myocardial contractility; $\beta_1$-receptor stimulation results in increased heart rate, atrioventricular conduction and myocardial contractility; $\beta_2$-receptors mediate peripheral vasodilation in some beds such as the skeletal muscle.

**Noradrenaline** is used when a rapid increase in pressure is required to avoid critical myocardial or cerebral ischaemia and can be used in septic shock to increase vascular resistance and promote urine flow.

**Adrenaline** increases heart rate and myocardial contractility together with vasoconstriction in most vascular beds at higher doses. At lower doses the $\beta_1$ effect will dilate coronary and skeletal muscle vasculature and may redistribute blood away from the splanchnic circulation.

**Dobutamine** increases myocardial contractility with only moderate effects on heart rate. Its $\beta_2$ action stimulates peripheral vasodilation which causes hypotension in hypovolaemia, when the increase in cardiac output is insufficient to overcome the vasodilation. It is used in congestive cardiac failure and in combination with other agents when there is excessive peripheral vasoconstriction.

**Dopamine** is a metabolic precursor of noradrenaline. At low dose its dopaminergic action predominates with renal vasodilation which is said to increase urine flow, but this effect is more probably due to the inhibition of tubular sodium reabsorption. At doses above 2–3 µg/kg/min there is increased contractility and heart rate with an increase in cardiac output. As the dose is increased further, the alpha effects become more marked with an increase in blood pressure

**Table 12.4** The effects of inotropic agents on myocardium and peripheral vasculature.

| Inotrope | Myocardium | | Peripheral vascular | | |
| --- | --- | --- | --- | --- | --- |
| | Rate | Contraction | Constriction | Dilation | Renal blood flow |
| Adrenaline | +++ | +++ | +++ | ++ | – |
| Dobutamine | + | +++ | – | +++ | – |
| Dopamine (low dose) | + | + | – | ++ | +++ |
| Dopamine (high dose) | ++ | ++ | +++ | – | – |
| Isoprenaline | +++ | ++ | – | +++ | – |
| Noradrenaline | + | + | +++ | – | – |

*The peripheral vascular effects are mediated through $\alpha$-adrenergic receptors for constriction, $\beta$-receptors for dilation and dopamine receptors in the renal circulation. The balance of receptor stimulation determines the overall effect of an inotrope.

and redistribution of blood to the heart and brain.

**Isoprenaline** increases heart rate and contractility and hence cardiac output, but it markedly increases myocardial oxygen consumption without improving oxygen supply. Its vasodilator action leads to a fall in blood pressure and it has marked arrhythmogenic side effects.

## Other inotropes

### Digoxin

Digoxin improves myocardial contractility, may increase peripheral resistance and has specific effects on heart rate and conduction. Some clinicians use digoxin for left ventricular failure with cardiomegaly that is refractory to diuretics and vasodilator therapy, but its use for this purpose

in the acute management of shock is controversial since in the presence of increased sympathetic activity the positive inotropic effect is poor and there is a large potential for toxicity.

### Phosphodiesterase inhibitors

Catecholamines act via intracellular second messengers. Cyclic AMP is one of these second messengers and it is broken down by the enzyme phosphodiesterase. Methylxanthines such as theophylline are phosphodiesterase inhibitors and are in high dose positively inotropic. Newer agents such as milrinone selectively and potently inhibit the cAMP myocardial-specific phosphodiesterase and can produce marked increases in cardiac output with substantial reductions in CVP and PAOP as well as peripheral vascular resistance.

# ACUTE RESPIRATORY FAILURE AND ARTIFICIAL VENTILATION

Respiratory support is a major part of intensive care. Artificial ventilation may be required because the patient is unable to maintain an adequate airway, but in general it is needed for respiratory failure because there is, or threatens to be, a failure of pulmonary gas exchange resulting in hypoxaemia (which may be taken as an arterial oxygen tension $PaO_2$ of less than 8 kPa). The lungs have a large functional capacity, so there must be considerable lung injury before gas exchange fails. Once this degree of injury has occurred however small changes in lung function can cause a rapid worsening of pulmonary gas exchange.

Respiratory failure is characterized by a low $PaO_2$ and is divided into two types according to the $PaCO_2$ level. In hypoxaemic respiratory failure (type 1) $PaO_2$ is low and the $PaCO_2$ is normal or low. Hypoxaemia here is due to a failure of gas diffusion, a mismatch of ventilation and perfusion (V/Q mismatch) or a right-to-left shunt. Common causes are pulmonary oedema, pneumonia, pulmonary embolus, the 'adult respiratory distress syndrome', fibrosing alveolitis and other chronic destructive lung pathology. In type 2 respiratory failure the $PaO_2$

is low and the $PaCO_2$ is high ($>6.5$ kPa) with inadequate alveolar ventilation. Alveolar hypoventilation may be due to diminished respiratory effort, failure to compensate for increased $CO_2$ production, or inability to meet an increase in the work of breathing caused by airflow obstruction, stiff lungs or chest wall which are often combined with V/Q mismatch. Common causes are chronic bronchitis and emphysema, chest wall abnormalities, respiratory muscle weakness and respiratory centre depression.

## CLINICAL ASSESSMENT

The most sensitive indicator of increasing respiratory difficulty is the respiratory rate. The pattern of breathing also indicates the degree of respiratory difficulty. The depth of ventilation, the use of the accessory muscles of respiration and ability to speak all provide information about the work of breathing, and when assessed in the light of general physique and underlying disease may give some guidance to the respiratory reserve.

Acute deterioration in respiratory function is

associated with increasing sympathetic activity and the patient may develop a tachycardia and become sweaty. Tachypnoea with a rise in minute volume may, in early respiratory failure, result in a mild respiratory alkalosis, with a low $PaCO_2$. If the patient is hypoxic there may be cyanosis. Signs of $CO_2$ retention with drowsiness will develop early in those whose primary problem is alveolar hypoventilation, but in those with hypoxic respiratory failure it is a late event associated with exhaustion.

Measurement of respiratory function may help to define the problem further in many of these situations. The measurement of vital capacity (VC) is useful in neuromuscular respiratory failure where it declines as weakness increases. A VC of less than a litre is generally associated with an inability to cough with sufficient force to protect the airway. However, arterial blood gas analysis is the most routine measure of respiratory distress despite its limitations. The $PaCO_2$ is dependent on alveolar ventilation in steady-state conditions and therefore can be used in judging the adequacy of ventilation but there can be severe respiratory distress with normal or even reduced $PaCO_2$, for example, in asthma. The measurement of the $PaO_2$ alone gives little useful information about pulmonary gas exchange since it may be reduced by a gas exchange problem or by reduced ventilation. The oxygen content of the blood is mainly dependent on the amount of saturated haemoglobin while cardiac output and the state of the peripheral circulation are key determinants in the delivery of oxygen to cells.

## MANAGEMENT OF ACUTE RESPIRATORY FAILURE

The cornerstones of management are supplemental oxygen, control of secretions, treatment of pulmonary infection, control of bronchospasm and limiting pulmonary oedema.

### Oxygen therapy

Oxygen is the first-line treatment for the relief of hypoxia. As gas exchange deteriorates with increasing respiratory failure the difference between inspired and arterial oxygen tension widens (the alveolar–arterial (A–a) gradient) indicating failure of gas exchange through diffusion failure or ventilation/perfusion (V/Q) mismatch. Inspired oxygen alone will not alter V/Q mismatch as the shunt remains unaltered and hypoxia is only improved by the degree to which mixed venous oxygen tension ($PvO_2$) is increased. This small benefit may be critical.

Supplemental oxygen can normally be administered by a simple face mask which will deliver an inspired oxygen concentration ($FiO_2$) of about 35 to 55 per cent at oxygen flow rates of 6 to 10 l/min or by nasal cannulae. Higher levels of $FiO_2$ necessitate endotracheal intubation and supported ventilation.

One of the commonest causes of acute respiratory failure occurs in patients with chronic bronchitis and emphysema who develop an episode of worsening airflow obstruction or reduced respiratory reserve in a postoperative period. Here 24 or 28 per cent oxygen should be given by a mask that delivers a fixed concentration as they may be dependent on their hypoxic drive (page 287).

A hypoxic patient with a low cardiac output, cold extremities, clammy skin and poor pulses, needs a high inspired oxygen concentration as part of their resuscitation in order to reverse their critically low oxygen delivery.

### Control of secretions

Marked improvement in oxygenation can be achieved by effective coughing which should be encouraged in alert and cooperative patients. Physiotherapy can be beneficial in the clearance of secretions, although care must be taken not to aggravate exhaustion. Endotracheal intubation and bronchoscopy may be required in those unable to cooperate with physiotherapy owing to drowsiness from hypercarbia, exhaustion or hypoxia.

### Reversible airway obstruction

Many patients with acute respiratory failure of whatever cause have a degree of reversible airway obstruction, and bronchodilators may not only reduce the effort of breathing, but also improve the ability to cough and cooperate with physiotherapy. In addition to nebulized $\beta_2$ agonists (salbutamol or terbutaline), inhaled ipratropium bromide may have an additional benefit.

## Pulmonary infection

In the patient admitted from the community with pneumonia or acute on chronic respiratory failure, an appropriate antibiotic is often given after bacterial cultures are taken but before the results are known, on a 'best guess' basis. In the absence of a clinically overt infection antibiotics should not be given routinely. Cultures should be taken to allow an appropriate drug to be chosen if infection develops.

## Corticosteroids

Corticosteroids are an important part of the management of acute asthma and can be useful in exacerbations of chronic airway obstruction. In patients failing to improve on standard management, steroids need to be considered in the light of their potential complications of gastrointestinal haemorrhage and secondary infection from immunosuppression. The role of steroid therapy in 'acute respiratory distress syndrome' is controversial.

## Respiratory stimulants

The value of these agents is controversial in acute respiratory failure. Doxapram, the most widely used agent acts on peripheral chemoreceptors at conventional doses but at higher doses has a central effect as well. An obtunded patient with a slow and irregular respiratory rate and hypercapnia may respond better to intubation and ventilation.

# The role of mechanical ventilation

Artificial ventilation is a powerful tool in the management of acute respiratory failure, *but* it is not a treatment of the underlying cause. The use of artificial ventilation in patients in whom the aetiology of respiratory failure is irreversible may prolong survival but will not alter the eventual outcome.

The purposes of respiratory support are to maintain gas exchange, to remove $CO_2$ by adjusting ventilation volumes as required, to relieve exhaustion and if possible to improve oxygenation. There are a number of circumstances in which it is possible to provide ventilatory support without endotracheal intubation, for example, in left ventricular failure by using continuous positive airways pressure (CPAP) to relieve afterload or in chronic respiratory muscle weakness by using intermittent negative pressure ventilation (INPV).

## INDICATIONS FOR MECHANICAL VENTILATION

All the causes already listed of both hypoxaemic (type 1) or ventilatory (type 2) respiratory failure may require respiratory support when all other appropriate methods have been applied, arterial blood gas tensions are inadequate or worsening and/or the respiratory effort is causing exhaustion. In addition mechanical ventilation may be required in cases of trauma, cardiac arrest, inhalational injury or postoperatively.

## Trauma

### Chest injuries

Multiple rib fractures can impair ventilatory capacity because a portion of the chest wall loses continuity with the rest of the rib cage. This portion, known as a 'flail' segment, moves inwards (paradoxical respiration) on inspiration so reducing ventilation.

### Head injury

In head injury and cerebral hypoxia there is a substantial risk of cerebral oedema. There is some evidence to suggest that hyperventilation to reduce the $PaCO_2$ to 4.0 kPa will prevent late oedema formation in the first 12 hours after injury by reducing cerebral blood flow. In severe head injury or following neurosurgery it can sometimes be helpful to keep patients sedated in order to prevent sudden rises in intracranial pressure, although sedation will mask changes in neurological status.

### Burns and/or multiple trauma

Sepsis, haemorrhage, mechanical impairment and fat embolism all lead to respiratory failure (page 256). The metabolic response to injury leads to an increase in $CO_2$ production necessitating an increase in alveolar ventilation. When there is little respiratory reserve because of acute or chronic lung disease this increased requirement may precipitate $CO_2$ retention and respiratory failure. Prophylactic positive pressure ventilation (page 260) may ameliorate the degree of acute respiratory failure often seen in these patients.

## Postoperative ventilation

Here the objective is to maintain optimal postoperative oxygenation during the early recovery period following major cardiothoracic, neurosurgical, upper abdominal and vascular surgery. There are often subsidiary reasons for prolonging ventilation, for example, to minimize postoperative cerebral oedema, or to allow the correction of metabolic abnormalities such as hypothermia.

## Cardiac arrest (page 218)

## ENDOTRACHEAL INTUBATION

Endotracheal intubation is necessary when the patient is unable to protect his own airway, which can be endangered by an altered level of consciousness, inadequate bulbar function or an inability to cough and/or control respiratory secretions. Intubation of patients who are critically ill is hazardous and should only be undertaken in a considered manner by experienced personnel. Early identification of the patient in need of intubation and ventilation, as detailed above, will often allow the avoidance of emergency intubation and its attendant hazards.

Tracheal intubation may be by the orotracheal or nasotracheal route, and in some situations directly by tracheostomy. An endotracheal tube has a cuff which is inflated to low pressure with air to produce a seal which prevents leak of air on positive pressure ventilation and aspiration into the lungs.

Endotracheal tubes are usually used for up to 2 weeks. Traditional teaching is that a tracheostomy should then be performed since prolonged endotracheal intubation carries the risk of damage to the tracheal wall or larynx. At tracheostomy a tube is inserted directly into the trachea through the anterior tracheal wall. A tracheostomy is better tolerated, allows easier

airway aspiration and no sedation is needed. It allows intermittent ventilation to rebuild respiratory muscle strength after prolonged ventilation. A tracheostomy carries the small risk of haemorrhage or subsequent tracheal stenosis at the site. When ventilation is not necessary and the track is well defined a speaking tube can be inserted. This does not completely occlude the trachea and allows air on expiration to pass up through the vocal cords.

# Patterns of ventilation

Modern ICU ventilators allow a wide range of ventilatory characteristics to be manipulated, i.e. respiratory rate, tidal volume, relative duration of inspiration and expiration ($FiO_2$), pattern of gas flow in inspiration and the pressure to which lung deflates in expiration. Various degrees of respiratory support are possible.

## Intermittent positive pressure ventilation (IPPV) or controlled mandatory ventilation (CMV)

Here the patient's entire ventilatory requirements are provided by mechanical ventilation and gas is delivered through an endotracheal or tracheostomy tube.

## Intermittent negative pressure ventilation

Here negative intrathoracic pressure is provided by force applied externally through the thoraco-abdominal wall. 'Tank' ventilators were once widely used for the treatment of ventilatory failure in polio, and other long-term ventilation for neuromuscular and musculoskeletal chronic respiratory failure. The 'tank' ventilators encased the whole patient, an alternative is the cuirass that encases just the thorax.

## Intermittent mandatory ventilation (IMV)

This is a partial support mode in which spontaneous breathing is augmented by additional mechanically imposed breaths. The ventilator rate and tidal volume are usually set so that a predetermined minute ventilation is achieved.

In its most widely used form, synchronized IMV (or SIMV) the mandatory breaths are timed to coincide with the patient's own respiratory efforts.

### Assisted ventilation or pressure support

In response to the patient's own inspiratory effort a preset positive pressure is applied to the airway, to augment the patient's own breath.

### Continuous positive airways pressure (CPAP)

This achieves a positive end-expiratory airway pressure for spontaneously breathing patients via a tightly fitting face mask or endotracheal tube with a preset oxygen concentration.

# Management of mechanical ventilatory support

## RESPIRATORY RATE AND TIDAL VOLUME

Gas exchange is generally more efficient with a fairly slow rate (12–14 breaths/min) and a generous tidal volume of 7–10 ml/kg so minute volume (the product of tidal volume and respiratory rate) is the same or a little greater than normal (100–120 ml/kg/min).

## INSPIRATORY: EXPIRATORY RATIO

Prolonging the inspiratory phase gives a better distribution of gas in the lungs. But it also increases the intrathoracic pressure and predisposes to air trapping. In most situations a 1:2 ratio is satisfactory with a short end-inspiratory pause (10 per cent).

## INSPIRED OXYGEN CONCENTRATION

A moderate increase in $FiO_2$ is usual even in normal lungs to offset hypoxaemia resulting from atelectasis produced by changes in mechanical properties of the lungs and gravitational redistribution of pulmonary blood flow. In most situations the $FiO_2$ is set to obtain a $PaO_2$ of 10–12 kPa, so that oxygen saturation is well in excess of 90 per cent.

## EXPIRATION

This occurs passively in mechanical ventilation. Lungs deflate to atmospheric pressure or to a predetermined pressure positive to the atmosphere: positive end-expiratory pressure (PEEP). Positive end-expiratory pressure re-expands underventilated parts of the lung, and if airway closure is contributing to hypoxaemia PEEP's effect of inflating the lungs to a greater functional residual capacity is of benefit.

## CLINICAL ASPECTS

Ventilated patients require constant clinical observation and monitoring to detect acute changes in vital signs, colour, chest movement, air entry and synchronization with the ventilator. Ventilator system alarms help manage inflation pressure, frequency, expired minute volume and tidal volume, $FiO_2$ and inspired gas temperature.

Sedation and opiate analgesics are given to enable the patient to tolerate the endotracheal tube and synchronize with the ventilator. The increased use of spontaneous breathing modes has greatly reduced the requirements for sedation in modern ICUs and ventilated patients should always be spoken to as if they were fully awake and alert.

Chest physiotherapy with endotracheal aspiration of the airway helps prevent airways plugging and collapse. Regular turning of the patient helps with the drainage of airway secretions by gravity as well as assisting in the care of pressure areas.

Humidification and gas-warming are essential in all forms of mechanical ventilation.

# Adverse effects of mechanical ventilation

Increased intrathoracic pressure impedes cardiac filling and lowers cardiac output, particularly in the presence of hypovolaemia or impaired autonomic reflexes. High airway pressures may result in mechanical damage such as pneumothorax. Secondary pulmonary infection is an ominous complication of long-term ventilation.

### Oxygen toxicity

A high $FiO_2$, paradoxically, may be dangerous. It can damage the alveolar wall and reduce gas transfer but it is often difficult to separate this effect from the underlying disease.

*(Tension pneumothorax)* (See page 322.)

# Weaning from the ventilator

Although IPPV should not be unnecessarily prolonged, premature weaning may result in failure and loss of patient morale. Before weaning one must ask the following questions:

- Is lung function adequate as assessed by blood gases and minute volume?
- Can the patient sustain the work of breathing, i.e. are the lungs too stiff (low compliance), is airflow obstruction too great, can the chest wall move adequately (muscle weakness, pain, abdominal distension)?
- Is the patient awake?

In adult respiratory distress syndrome ('ARDS') ventilation is usually required for at least 6 days. Time is needed for surfactant to regenerate and prevent atelectasis.

Wasting and weakness of respiratory muscles occurs with prolonged ventilation and hypercatabolic states. Therefore, spontaneous respiration usually has to be resumed gradually.

# ADULT RESPIRATORY DISTRESS SYNDROME

Adult respiratory distress syndrome was first described in 1967. It is a clinical syndrome, characterized by the following:

- Marked respiratory distress (with tachypnoea)
- Chest X-ray showing diffuse pulmonary infiltration
- Reduced pulmonary compliance (compliance is measured as the increase in lung volume per unit of inflation pressure; when compliance falls the lungs become more difficult to ventilate)
- Increase in alveolar–arterial oxygen difference

The abnormalities are associated with increased pulmonary capillary permeability and non-cardiogenic pulmonary oedema which is the characteristic feature of ARDS. Major risk factors are sepsis, aspiration of gastrointestinal contents, lung contusion, hypovolaemia and multiple fractures. The mortality rate is 40–67 per cent with a higher mortality rate in older patients.

The diagnosis of ARDS is mainly clinical and the criteria for diagnosis include:

- History of precipitating condition (e.g. sepsis)
- Hypoxia ($PaO_2$ <8 kPa with $FiO_2$ >40 per cent)
- Radiological evidence of bilateral pulmonary infiltrates
- Pulmonary artery occlusion pressure <18 mm Hg
- Reduced thoracic compliance (<30 ml/cm $H_2O$)

## PATHOPHYSIOLOGY

Evidence suggests that an 'insult' such as sepsis, aspiration or hypovolaemic shock can activate the complement and coagulation cascades causing the formation of platelet and protein microaggregates in the circulation which lodge in the pulmonary capillaries. Cytokines such as tumour necrosis factor are released into the circulation activating inflammatory cells such as neutrophils. Neutrophils then attach to the endothelial cells and release oxygen-derived free radicals and proteolytic enzymes.

Free radicals are toxic to a wide variety of cells

including endothelial cells, causing cell dysfunction and necrosis either directly or by blocking normal inhibitors of proteolytic enzymes. The actions of free radicals are normally limited by an antioxidant defence system and damage only occurs when there is increased generation of free radicals (e.g. from the activation of neutrophils, radiation or toxins) or when antioxidant defences are decreased. Release of proteolytic enzyme increases protein permeability at the capillary–alveolar barrier and causes pulmonary oedema. Deficiency of surfactant can increase surface tension and thereby promote atelectasis and pulmonary oedema.

Defective surfactant activity may result from washout or dilution after lung fluid accumulation, and protein denaturation by oxygen free radicals.

## MANAGEMENT

Treatment is supportive and aims to maintain oxygen delivery to all organ systems. Fluid overload must be avoided and diuretics may be needed to maintain appropriate fluid balance. Vasodilators have been used to reduce pulmonary hypertension. Numerous attempts have been made to reduce the inflammatory component in the lungs. Corticosteroids have not proved useful. Current pharmacological interventions under assessment include nitric oxide to reduce pulmonary artery pressure and improve gas exchange, anti-endotoxin antibodies in sepsis and specific anti-inflammatory agents such as leukocyte adhesion molecule antibodies. So far none of these have shown enough evidence of effectiveness to become routine therapy.

# CRITERIA FOR ADMISSION TO THE INTENSIVE CARE UNIT

Intensive care is an expensive part of modern medicine. The ratio of nurses and doctors to patients is high, the equipment and drugs used are expensive and the volume of investigations is great. It needs to be used appropriately to obtain the best value from the investment. This means that admission criteria should seek to select patients who need the care and are likely to benefit from it. Patients who can just as well be cared for on a normal ward with fewer staff should not be admitted, nor should those who have no chance of survival. Alternative options such as supplementary nursing on routine wards, extended care wards with extra nursing and equipment need to be considered.

Various scoring systems have been developed in order to audit the effectiveness of intensive care.

A common system is the Acute Physiology and Chronic Health Evaluation (APACHE) system, others include the Simplified Acute Physiology Score (SAPS) and Therapeutic Intervention Scoring Systems (TISS). The APACHE and SAPS systems measure severity of illness on the first day of admission to the ICU. Both systems include measurement of a number of physiological variables such as heart rate, blood pressure, oxygenation and renal function. In addition, the scores also weight for age, type of patient (for example, elective or emergency surgical) and the APACHE system gives a scoring of chronic ill health and diagnostic category. Both systems may be used to assess the expected mortality in groups of ICU patients. However, these scores cannot be used to replace clinical judgement in decisions about the admission of individual patients to intensive care and continuation of active treatment.

# BRAIN DEATH

When patients are thought to have suffered irreversible brain damage with loss of the capacity for consciousness and irreversible loss of the ability to breathe then brain death has occurred. If termination of ventilatory support or use of organs for transplantation is being considered then the formal criteria for brain death are applied. Great care must be taken to exclude certain causes of coma which can fulfil the criteria for brain death when the patient's condition is at its most severe, but from which recovery can occur. They are:

1 Drugs, poisons (especially sedatives, neuro-muscular blockers). If they have been given then adequate time for elimination must be allowed.
2 Hypothermia (body temperature below 35 °C).
3 Metabolic or endocrine causes of coma, for example, hypoglycaemia.

Tests for brain death must be done by two doctors of senior status, at least 6 hours after the onset of coma, on two separate occasions. The time interval between tests is not regulated provided the preconditions have been met.

The criteria to be assessed are:

1 Pupils fixed and unresponsive to light
2 Absent corneal reflexes
3 Absent oculocephalic movements (i.e. doll's eye movements positive, moving with the rotated head, not retaining fixation and Caloric testing negative (with ice-cold water)
4 No cranial nerve motor responses (e.g. grimacing to facial pain)
5 No respiration although a $PaCO_2$ >6.7 kPa (with oxygenation maintained using 6 l/min oxygen down the endotracheal tube)

Because an electroencephalogram (EEG) reflects function of the cerebral cortex and not the brain stem it is not used for the diagnosis of brain stem death in the UK.

The underlying cause is usually evident, if no obvious cause is apparent then diagnoses such as drug overdose must be considered and a longer time left for recovery.

When patients die on ICU the possibility of donation of their organs for transplantation should always be borne in mind. Transplant coordinators and teams are available to give advice on possible transplantation and communication with relatives. This is sometimes a difficult problem for inexperienced doctors to raise but many families are keen for organs to be put to such good use once they have appreciated that their relative is not going to survive.

# PERSISTENT VEGETATIVE STATE

In this condition the brain stem retains some activity such as breathing but there is no recognizable cortical activity. Little recovery is likely beyond the first few weeks but survival for some years is quite possible with nutritional support and nursing care. Such patients have functional decortication and do not respond to any external stimulus in a meaningful fashion. Reflex responses in the limbs remain.

Usually breathing is spontaneous in the persistent vegetative state. Enteral feeding will often have been started early in the course of the problem and decisions may have to be made about the long-term future of such care. All decisions should be discussed with the relatives and action planned in response to all the information. All discussions and intentions should be clearly documented in the notes.

Any significant recovery is extremely unlikely after 12 months of the vegetative state. There have been suggestions and legal judgement that in some patients withdrawal of nutrition and hydration may be appropriate although this will lead to certain death.

# **D**isorders of the Respiratory System

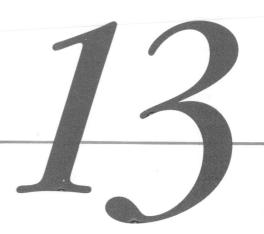

13

# INTRODUCTION

Respiratory disorders make up a large part of the workload of general medicine. Over 20 per cent of admissions to medical wards are for respiratory problems and similar proportions of primary care consultations.

Advances in imaging are improving our diagnostic ability in lung disease. Computed tomographic scanners are more sophisticated than they used to be, providing more detailed views of lung tissue and mediastinum. Magnetic resonance imaging and positron emission tomography are promising techniques which have yet to define their roles in lung disorders.

Advances in molecular biology and immunology have increased our knowledge of the inflammatory processes in asthma and infiltrative lung disorders.

Many challenges remain. The prevalence and severity of asthma are increasing. While suppressive treatment has improved, curative treatment has proved elusive. Carcinoma of the bronchus will remain a common problem while smoking continues. In pulmonary infections the many manifestations of acquired immune deficiency syndrome (AIDS) have brought new problems over the last 10 years and the spectre of multiply resistant tuberculosis is a frightening prospect for the future.

# STRUCTURE AND FUNCTION

Respiration involves the exchange of oxygen and carbon dioxide between the environment and the blood. These processes involve:

- Diffusion of gases between alveolar gas and blood in the pulmonary capillaries
- Carriage of blood containing the gases to and from the alveoli

The ventilation of alveoli and their perfusion must be matched to allow optimal gas exchange.

The lung is involved in functions other than gas exchange. Some are related to ventilation:

- Conditioning the inspired air by warming and humidifying it
- A defence system involving anatomical barriers, mucociliary clearance, cough, biochemical and immunological processes

There are also metabolic functions; the pulmonary capillary endothelial cells have remarkable activity. Substances such as angiotensin I, bradykinin and prostaglandin E are almost completely inactivated by a single passage through the pulmonary circulation.

## Structure

The upper airway passages of the nose, mouth and pharynx are important parts of the respiratory tract. Abnormalities in this area may influence respiration (see obstructive sleep apnoea, page 289). The lungs weigh around 1 kg, of which nearly 50 per cent is blood. The trachea has a cross-sectional area of 2.5 cm$^2$ and begins the branching process of the airways at the carina. Cartilaginous bronchi lead to membranous bronchioles ($\geq 1$ mm in diameter) and on to gas exchange ducts (respiratory bronchioles and alveolar ducts). The cross-sectional area of the airways reaches 11–12 000 cm$^2$ at the alveolar ducts.

This vast increase in cross-sectional area as the airways divide has a number of consequences. The airflow slows towards the periphery of the bronchial tree to end as diffusion. A great deal of damage can occur in the terminal airways before they limit airflow significantly or produce respiratory symptoms.

The alveolocapillary membrane allows gases

to equilibrate in the 0.5–1.0 s that blood spends in a capillary since it is only 0.2 μm thick with a total surface area of about 70 m². The process of oxygen transfer relies on available haemoglobin within the capillary blood. Anaemia will reduce oxygen carriage by the blood.

The pulmonary circulation brings carbon dioxide to the lungs and oxygenated blood leaves in the pulmonary veins. The pulmonary arterial system is a low pressure system (about 25/8 mm Hg). There is a gradient of flow across the lung according to gravity. In the upright position blood flow at the base of the lung exceeds that at the apex. The gradient for ventilation is similar but less marked giving higher ventilation/perfusion ratios at the apex than at the base of the lung. The lung tissue itself down to the terminal bronchioles is supplied by the bronchial circulation which branches off the descending aorta or the intercostals. Some of the bronchial venous blood drains into the azygos and hemi-azygos veins but some reaches pulmonary venules to bring a small amount of desaturated blood into the systemic circulation.

There is an extensive lymphatic system in the lungs draining into hilar lymph nodes and then mediastinal lymph nodes and central lymphatic channels.

Smooth muscle in the airway wall is supplied by the vagus nerve and there are receptors for circulating catecholamines. The sympathetic nerve supply is mainly to vascular smooth muscle with some innervation of airway glands. There are non-cholinergic, non-adrenergic pathways which may be important in control of airway calibre and other airway functions. Sensory fibres are of myelinated and unmyelinated forms. There are two myelinated types, the slowly adapting stretch receptors and the rapidly adapting irritant receptors found in the larger airways. The un-myelinated slowly conducting C fibres are mainly further out in the airways and are the most numerous type of sensory fibres.

# Ventilation

A rhythmic discharge of neurones, largely in the medulla, generates a pattern of breathing which is influenced by receptors in the medulla, carotid bodies, chest wall and lungs. In addition there is a conscious cortical influence on respiration.

Normal ventilation consists of a tidal volume of around 500 ml with a frequency of 14–20 per minute. Anatomic dead space of conducting airways makes up 150 ml leaving an alveolar ventilation of around 5 l/min at rest.

The lung volumes are conventionally divided as shown in Fig. 13.1. The volumes within the range of the vital capacity can all be measured by simple spirometry. The residual volume (RV) after full expiration cannot. Measurement of RV and therefore functional residual capacity (FRC) and total lung capacity (TLC) can be done by one of three techniques:

1 Radiographic – this is not suitable for repetition
2 Helium dilution – this measures accessible gas, for example, it would not include 'trapped' air in a cyst which did not ventilate (Fig. 13.2)
3 Body plethysmography – this relies on an adaptation of Boyle's law measuring pressure and volume changes in an enclosed box. All gas subject to intrathoracic pressures will be included (Fig. 13.3)

Most disorders of ventilatory function of the lung can be divided into those with reduced maximal airflow, i.e. obstructive problems, and those with reduced volumes, i.e. restrictive problems. Obstruction can be caused by a reduction in elastic recoil pressure (the floppy lungs of emphysema) as well as by structural narrowing of the airways or constriction of bronchial

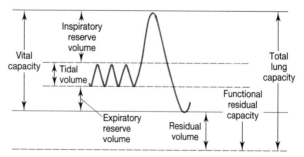

**Figure 13.1** Divisions of lung volumes. The subject has taken three tidal breaths followed by a full inspiration and maximal expiration. The measurements labelled on the left can be obtained by simple spirometry.

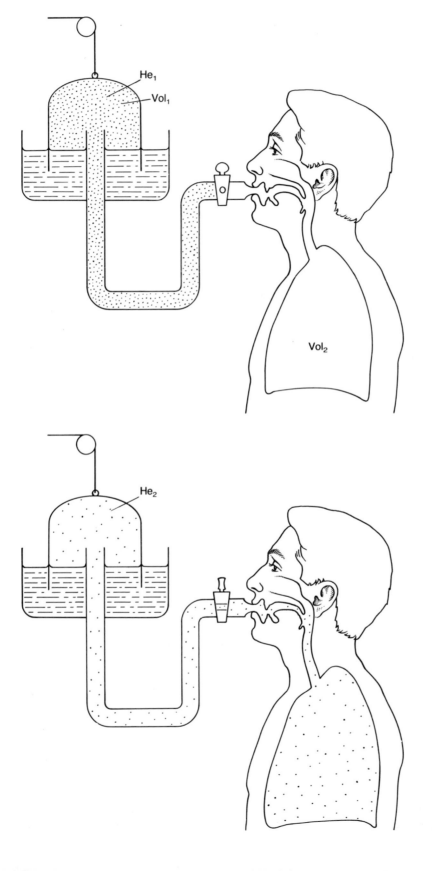

**Figure 13.2** Helium dilution technique for measurement of lung volumes. The subject breathes until equilibrium is achieved (shown by a stable helium concentration). Carbon dioxide is absorbed and oxygen added to maintain a constant overall volume. $He_1$ = initial helium concentration. $He_2$ = final helium concentration. $Vol_1$ = apparatus volume. $Vol_2$ = lung volume + mouthpiece etc. $He_1 \times Vol_1 = He_2 \times (Vol_1 + Vol_2)$.

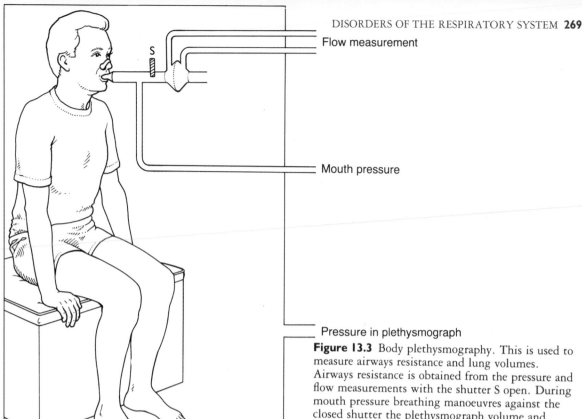

Flow measurement

Mouth pressure

Pressure in plethysmograph

**Figure 13.3** Body plethysmography. This is used to measure airways resistance and lung volumes. Airways resistance is obtained from the pressure and flow measurements with the shutter S open. During mouth pressure breathing manoeuvres against the closed shutter the plethysmograph volume and pressures are used to estimate lung volume.

smooth muscle. Restrictive problems may be related to the lungs themselves, poorly compliant or stiff lungs, or to abnormalities in the chest wall and musculature which limit expansion.

# Lung function testing

Lung function tests can point towards a diagnosis but only in combination with the rest of the clinical information. The tests are more useful in establishing the degree of abnormality. Repeated measurements at short intervals (e.g. for asthma or muscle weakness) or longer intervals (e.g. for pulmonary fibrosis, chronic bronchitis or emphysema) can be used to monitor the progress of a disorder and its treatment.

Measurements of expiratory airflow are the most common objective test of respiratory function. A forced maximal expiration (Fig. 13.4) provides the conventional measurements of forced expiratory volume in 1 s ($FEV_1$) and forced vital capacity (FVC). The ratio of the two ($FEV_1/FVC$ = forced expiratory ratio or FER) is low in obstructive lung disease (normal FER varies with age, below 70 years an FER<70 per cent is reduced). In restrictive problems both $FEV_1$ and FVC are reduced and the FER is normal or high. The simplest measurement of obstruction is the peak expiratory flow rate (PEFR). It is the maximal slope of the spirometry curve but is measured by simple meters (Fig. 13.5) which should be used as part of the regular care of asthmatic patients.

The information in the spirometry (volume—time) trace can also be displayed as flow plotted

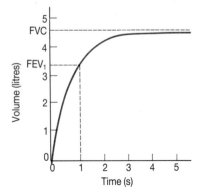

**Figure 13.4** Spirometry trace. $FEV_1$ = forced expiratory volume in 1 s. FVC = forced vital capacity.

against volume and the same parameters can be measured during maximal inspiration (Fig. 13.6). If this is combined with a measurement of lung volume (page 267) then the flow–volume curve can be placed at absolute lung volume and changes in degree of inflation shown in addition to flow and volume. The envelope of the curve cannot be exceeded however the manoeuvre is performed, i.e. the flow at each point is maximal flow at that lung volume.

The advantage of the flow–volume loop is that changes in flows at low lung volumes (the bottom 50 per cent of the vital capacity) may reflect abnormalities in small airways which do not affect $FEV_1$ and FVC in the early stages. Various typical patterns of abnormality can be recognized from the shape of the loop (Fig. 13.6).

# Gas transfer

Gas transfer is a guide to the ability of the lung to transfer oxygen from the air to the blood. Carbon monoxide is used as a substitute for oxygen since it simplifies the test. The subject takes a deep inspiration of a gas mixture containing a low concentration of carbon monoxide and helium. This is held in the lungs for 10 s and then breathed out. The reduction in the concentration of helium comes from dilution with gas in the lungs (page 268) and the reduction in carbon monoxide comes from dilution and transfer into the pulmonary capillaries. The gas transfer can be expressed as a total gas transfer for the lungs (TLCO) or as transfer per unit accessible lung volume (KCO = TLCO ÷ alveolar volume from helium dilution). Causes of change in gas transfer are shown in Table 13.1.

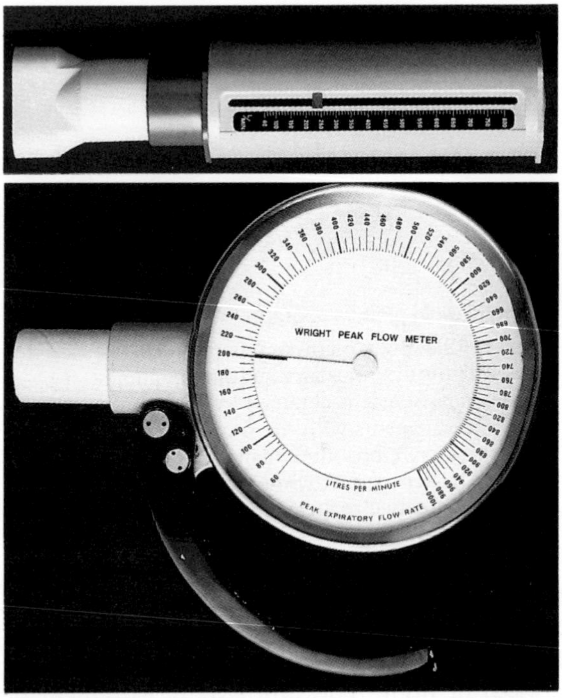

**Figure 13.5** (a) A portable peak flow meter suitable for home monitoring in asthma. (b) A Wright peak flow meter.

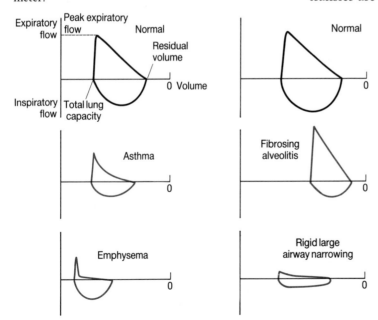

**Figure 13.6** Typical flow–volume curves in normal subjects and obstructive and restrictive abnormalities.

**Table 13.1** Causes of changes in gas transfer (TLCO).

| Causes of reduced gas transfer | Causes of increased gas transfer |
| --- | --- |
| Low accessible lung volume | Polycythaemia (correction can be applied) |
| Low haemoglobin (correction factor can be applied) | Left-to-right intracardiac shunt (increasing pulmonary blood flow) |
| Reduced alveolocapillary membrane (emphysema) | |
| Obliterated pulmonary vessels (pulmonary vascular disease) | Increased pulmonary venous pressure increasing capillary bed (early left heart failure, decreases later as alveolar flooding occurs) |
| Obliterated vessels + impaired diffusion (interstitial lung disease, e.g. fibrosing alveolitis) | |
| (n.b. KCO is also low except in a low accessible lung volume) | Free haemoglobin in alveoli (pulmonary haemorrhage, after 24–48 hours haemoglobin denatures and transfer factor drops) |
| | Asthma |

# $A$RTERIAL BLOOD GASES AND PH

Respiratory failure is defined in terms of the arterial blood gases. When the oxygen is the important factor the oxygen saturation of haemoglobin can be estimated non-invasively with a pulse oximeter. This is a very useful technique in anaesthesia, intensive care, sleep studies, bronchoscopy and in general clinical use. However, the shape of the oxygen saturation curve needs to be remembered when interpreting the values (Fig. 13.7).

The normal level of *arterial* $PO_2$ is 11.3–13.3 kPa (85–100 mmHg). It falls with age by around 1 kPa every 30 years so that a $PaO_2$ of 9.5 kPa would be within the expected range by the age of 80 years. The causes of a low $PaO_2$ are listed in Table 13.2. Tissue hypoxia may occur despite a normal $PaO_2$ if the haemoglobin is low, perfusion reduced or tissue enzymes are disturbed (e.g. in cyanide poisoning).

*Cyanosis* occurs when there is more than 2 g desaturated haemoglobin (85 per cent saturation with a normal haemoglobin level). Severe hypoxia leads to confusion but this is a late sign.

The normal *arterial* $PCO_2$ (arterial $CO_2$ tension) is 4.6–6.0 kPa (35–45 mmHg) and it

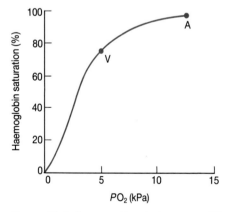

**Figure 13.7** Oxygen dissociation curve. The curve is moved to the right (less affinity for oxygen) by increases in temperature, $PCO_2$, hydrogen ion concentration and 2,3-diphosphoglycerate (2,3-DPG). 2,3-DPG increases in chronic hypoxia and falls in stored blood. Typical venous blood (V) and arterial blood (A) levels are indicated.

**Table 13.2** Causes of a low $PaO_2$. Respiratory quotient is the ratio of $CO_2$ produced to oxygen consumed in metabolism (usually around 0.8).

1 Hypoventilation (alveolar air equation shows that a rise in carbon dioxide must reduce alveolar $PO_2$

$$\text{Alveolar } PO_2 = \text{Inspired } PO_2 - \frac{\text{Alveolar } PCO_2}{\text{Respiratory quotient}})$$

2 Right-to-left shunts (the only cause of hypoxia not substantially corrected by high inspired oxygen concentrations)

3 Ventilation/perfusion (V/Q) mismatch (well-ventilated alveoli cannot compensate for poorly ventilated alveoli and the mixed blood has a low $PO_2$)

4 Impaired diffusion (in fibrosing lung conditions the low $PaO_2$ is a mixture of this and V/Q mismatch)

5 Low inspired oxygen (high altitude)

depends upon alveolar ventilation and $CO_2$ production:

$$PaCO_2 = k \times \frac{CO_2 \text{ production}}{\text{Alveolar ventilation}}$$

Therefore, hyperventilation will reduce $PaCO_2$ and may be voluntary or as part of disorders such as asthma, pulmonary embolism or pneumonia. A raised $PaCO_2$ from hypoventilation occurs when there is central respiratory depression (e.g. caused by sedatives) or a reduced response of the respiratory system to the central output (e.g. because of weak muscles, kyphoscoliosis, severe restrictive or obstructive defect). In chronic obstructive lung disease $PaCO_2$ may rise because of a combination of reduced central sensitivity to $CO_2$, small tidal volumes which ventilate dead space rather than the alveoli and severe airflow obstruction.

A large rise in $PaCO_2$ produces headache and drowsiness but these are late, unreliable signs and measurement of blood gases is essential to quantify disturbances in $PaO_2$ and $PaCO_2$.

Normal *arterial pH* at rest is 7.38–7.42 ($H^+$ concentration 35–45 nmol/l). Disturbances in pH occur in four situations (Table 13.3).

**Table 13.3** Abnormal acid–base states (see page 509).

| | | |
|---|---|---|
| 1 | Metabolic acidosis | Low pH, low $HCO_3$ with compensation by increased ventilation to reduce $PaCO_2$ |
| 2 | Metabolic alkalosis | High pH, raised $HCO_3$. There may be a mild degree of hypoventilation increasing $PaCO_2$ |
| 3 | Respiratory acidosis | Acute rise in $PaCO_2$ with reduction in pH: chronic $HCO_3$ rises and the pH returns to normal with high $PaCO_2$ and $HCO_3$ |
| 4 | Respiratory alkalosis | Low $PaCO_2$ and high pH with a reduction in $HCO_3$ |

# $S$YMPTOMS OF RESPIRATORY DISEASE

## *Cough*

Cough is a very common symptom which is experienced by everybody at some time. The major sites of stimulation for the cough reflex are the larynx and the major airways down to the segmental bronchi of each lobe. Other sites, even the external auditory meatus, can cause cough but they are much less common. Cough consists of a deep inspiration, a build up of pressure against a closed glottis which then suddenly opens. The expiratory airflow, just below peak flow shears mucus off the walls of the large airways.

Although it is a common symptom it may be an early sign of serious disease. Stimulation of irritant receptors in the airways may come from mucus, cigarette smoke and other irritants or from abnormalities in the wall itself. Wall abnormalities may be the inflammatory change of asthma or tumours in the bronchial mucosa. Laryngeal irritation may arise from a postnasal drip in sinusitis or from oesophageal reflex.

Cough may produce its own complications. Cough syncope can occur when the reduction of venous return from high intrathoracic pressures results in momentary loss of consciousness because of the reduced cardiac output.

## *Sputum*

Coughing is only able to clear the larger airways, the smaller airways rely on mucociliary clearance. Cilia transport mucus to the large airways and up to the larynx. The normal daily mucus production is around 100 ml but this passes over the larynx to be swallowed and not perceived. When the volume is larger, the mucus more sticky or the ciliary escalator fails then it is coughed up.

Patients should be asked about sputum volume, colour and quality. Any available sputum should be inspected. A simple increase in mucus production leads to clear, mucoid sputum. Degenerating white cells in the sputum make it yellow or green; this usually implies infection but may occur with the eosinophilic sputum of asthma. Asthmatic patients may expectorate firm plugs in their sputum. These plugs have been blocking airways in the lung and may be complete casts of the airways especially when asthma is complicated by a sensitivity to the Aspergillus fungus in allergic bronchopulmonary aspergillosis (page 280).

Blood in the sputum, *haemoptysis*, is usually a dramatic symptom for patients. Haemoptysis can generally be differentiated from haematemesis (vomiting blood) by careful questioning, including the appearance of sputum before and after the main occurrence of the blood. Small amounts of blood streaking in the sputum are most often caused by chronic bronchitis but haemoptysis should always be taken seriously since it may be the first sign of an underlying tumour. In pneumonia degenerating red cells may produce a rusty coloured sputum. In left heart failure severe pulmonary oedema may result in frothy pink sputum. When conditions such as pulmonary infarction result in haemoptysis the sputum is usually all blood rather than mixed with mucus.

# Breathlessness

Breathlessness is an unpleasant sensation related to the effort involved in breathing. It may be normal on vigorous exercise but it is abnormal when it occurs at rest or with less exercise than expected for the patient's age, weight and level of fitness. A precise history is important in the symptom of breathlessness, it should be quantified in relation to everyday tasks familiar to the patient, for example, walking on the flat or upstairs. Variation should be sought over time (asthma) or with position (lying flat in pulmonary oedema or diaphragmatic weakness).

Breathlessness in hyperventilation often has characteristic features such as the lightheadedness or paraesthesiae of hypocapnia and the sensation of being unable to fill the lungs satisfactorily.

# Wheeze

Expiratory wheezing may be a symptom volunteered by asthmatics when it may be related to specific exposures. Wheezing in inspiration and expiration may signify an upper airway narrowing. Patients often need a precise explanation of what is meant by the term wheezing.

# Chest pain

The lung itself does not contain pain receptors so lung conditions are painless unless they involve surrounding structures. Pleural inflammation stimulates receptors in the parietal pleura. *Pleuritic pain* occurs when the pleural surfaces move over each other during coughing, breathing or movement. Irritation of the diaphragmatic pleura gives pain referred to the tip of the shoulder. *Chest wall pain* is worse on movement and may come from the ribs or intercostal muscles. Coxsackie B virus may cause local pain and tenderness in the chest wall muscles (Bornholm's disease). Pain in the costal cartilages, especially the second cartilage, may occur in costochondritis (Tietze's syndrome). Pain localized to a dermatome may occur before the rash of herpes zoster infection (shingles). Central chest pain may be found with inflammatory conditions of the mediastinum. Usually this is a dull pain, poorly localized in the centre of the chest but in situations such as oesophageal rupture it may be very severe.

The differential diagnosis of central chest pain includes angina, dissecting aortic aneurysm and oesophagitis but the differentiation can usually be made on a clearly taken history.

# Other points in the history

Various other areas of the history are very important in lung disease. Family history provides important information in asthma and rarer conditions such as antiprotease deficiency emphysema and cystic fibrosis. A detailed occupational history should always be taken. Other risk factors such as smoking, foreign travel and exposure to pets at home need to be assessed.

## EXAMINATION OF THE RESPIRATORY SYSTEM

The assessment of a patient with lung disease relies on a combination of history, physical examination, radiology and other investigations. The advent of new imaging and laboratory techniques does not diminish the importance of an accurate history and examination.

The respiratory system is examined as part of the overall evaluation but in this section features with particular reference to the chest will be singled out.

# Examination of the hands

## CLUBBING OF THE FINGERS

Clubbing of the fingers is a long established sign relevant to pulmonary disease. There are many causes of clubbing of the fingers (Table 13.4). Common abnormalities relevant to the respiratory system are carcinoma of the lung, diffuse pulmonary fibrosis and any cause of pus in the chest: empyema, lung abscess or bronchiectasis.

## HYPERTROPHIC PULMONARY OSTEOARTHROPATHY

Hypertrophic pulmonary osteoarthropathy is a painful condition occurring near the ends of the long bones. Bleeding occurs under the periosteum with new bone formation. Hypertrophic pulmonary osteoarthropathy occurs in association with clubbing, usually carcinoma of the bronchus, less often with the other causes of clubbing. As with clubbing the mechanism is unknown. It can be detected as duplication of the periosteum on X-ray or as increased activity on bone scan.

## CYANOSIS

Cyanosis is seen in the fingers when there is central cyanosis or when peripheral blood flow is very sluggish leading to increased oxygen extraction. Central cyanosis is seen in the tongue and the lips and shows that blood leaving the left side of the heart contains more than 2 g of desaturated haemoglobin. This occurs when lung disease interferes with oxygenation or when a right-to-left shunt allows some blood to bypass the lungs altogether. Detection of a small degree of cyanosis requires careful observation and good lighting.

## PULSUS PARADOXUS

During inspiration venous return to the right side of the heart is increased but pulmonary blood volume is also higher decreasing return to

**Table 13.4** Causes of clubbing of the fingers.

| Respiratory conditions | Other causes |
| --- | --- |
| Carcinoma of the lung | Cyanotic congenital heart disease |
| Fibrosing alveolitis | |
| Bronchiectasis | Bacterial endocarditis |
| Lung abscess | Atrial myxoma |
| Empyema | Cirrhosis (especially alcoholic) |
| Pleural fibroma | |
| Benign lung tumours | Inflammatory bowel disease |
| Secondary lung tumours | |

the left side of the heart. Systolic blood pressure, therefore, falls slightly on inspiration. In some situations this fall is exaggerated; above 10 mm Hg can be considered abnormal and is described as pulsus paradoxus. This can be measured by slowly reducing the pressure in the sphygmomanometer cuff while listening for the systolic sounds over the brachial artery. They will appear first in expiration and later throughout the respiratory cycle. The difference between the two levels is the degree of paradox.

Pulsus paradoxus is seen when pericardial effusions or constrictive pericarditis limit cardiac filling (cardiac tamponade) and in acute asthma when there is overinflation of the lungs and large pressure changes within the thorax during respiration. Paradox does not always occur in severe asthma but when it is present it is monitored as a guide to progress.

## JUGULAR VENOUS PRESSURE

The jugular venous pressure measures the filling pressure in the right atrium and also reflects intrathoracic pressure. The level of jugular venous pulsation is raised in right heart failure. In the presence of airflow obstruction the pressure swings within the thorax make it more difficult to determine the true level of the jugular pressure, particularly when the respiratory rate is high. The other usual sign of right heart failure is peripheral oedema. This may occur in chronic bronchitis and emphysema through fluid retention and raised pulmonary pressures.

When the superior vena cava is obstructed the jugular venous pressure is raised but the upper level cannot be seen and there is no pulsation. The usual cause is malignant nodes or infiltration in the mediastinum. Other mediastinal processes such as lymphoma, thymoma, aortic aneurysm, tuberculosis, mediastinal fibrosis and vena caval thrombosis are much less common.

## *Examination of the chest*

The first things to observe in examination of the chest are the shape and breathing pattern. In airflow obstruction the chest becomes over-inflated or 'barrel-shaped' with a large antero-posterior diameter. Abnormalities such as kyphoscoliosis can be important in restriction of lung expansion.

The respiratory rate should be measured without altering the pattern of breathing. This may be done while feeling the pulse or examining the hands with the patient lying quietly in bed. The muscles used in respiration should be noted. When the diaphragm is not working the abdomen will move in rather than out with each breath. Accessory muscles, such as the sterno-mastoids, contract during inspiration when respiratory effort is increased. When the lungs are stiff (e.g. because of fibrosis) the breathing will be rapid and shallow while airflow obstruction usually leads to a long expiratory phase.

## MEDIASTINUM

The position of the mediastinum is assessed from the position of the apex beat and the trachea. The direction the trachea is taking in the mediastinum needs careful detection. It is best done with the patient sitting up, looking straight forward. The position of the lower mediastinum is taken from the apex beat although this may be displaced by cardiac changes as well as lung disease. The distance from the cricoid cartilage to the suprasternal notch should be more than 4 cm and is reduced when the chest is over-inflated.

## MOVEMENT

The symmetry and degree of chest wall movement are estimated by placing the hands with the fingers spread over upper and lower chest wall, front and back. Total expansion can also be measured from full expiration to full inspiration with a tape measure. The symmetry of movement is often seen well by watching quiet respiration from the foot of the bed with the chest uncovered.

## PERCUSSION

Percussion should be performed down both sides of the chest and laterally. The two sides are compared. When the site being percussed does not overlie air-containing lung the percussion note will be altered. Consolidated or collapsed lung is dull to percussion but not so markedly dull as fluid in a pleural effusion. A pneumothorax may increase the percussion note. Percussion may be used to elicit the position and movement of the diaphragm and the extent of cardiac dullness.

## VOICE SOUNDS

Speech sounds generated at the larynx are transmitted to the periphery but filtered by the air-containing lung. A residual vibration is palpable as tactile vocal fremitus (TVF) or audible through the stethoscope as conducted voice sounds. Increased air or a separation of the pleural surfaces reduces the transmission while consolidated lung is a better conductor of the central sounds so TVF and conducted voice sounds are increased and whispered speech may also be audible (whispering pectoriloquy).

## AUSCULTATION

The normal breath sounds heard with the stethoscope are the remnants of sounds generated in the larger airways and filtered by the air-containing lung. They are reduced when local ventilation is lower except when underlying solid lung with open airways is able to conduct the sound better than usual (consolidation). This results in **bronchial breathing** with a prolonged expiratory phase and a gap between inspiration and expiration.

The two main types of added sounds which may be heard are crackles and wheezes. A number of names have been used but it is best to stick to these simple terms. **Wheezes** are continuous sounds produced by the vibration of the walls of a narrowed airway. Usually multiple wheezes are heard on expiration but in the presence of large airway narrowing there may be a single wheeze.

**Crackles** are interrupted sounds caused by the snapping open of airways. They occur at the end of inspiration in fibrosing alveolitis and in pulmonary oedema. In chronic bronchitis and emphysema they are heard early in inspiration. The crackles of bronchiectasis are coarser, localized to the area of abnormality and occur at any time during inspiration.

Other added sounds may be heard during the respiratory cycle. Squeaking sounds may occur in bronchiolitis and when there is pleural inflammation pleural rubs occur as superficial creaking or grating noises.

# INVESTIGATION OF THE RESPIRATORY SYSTEM

## *Imaging*

The chest X-ray is a fundamental investigation in respiratory disease. It is complementary to a good history and examination for pulmonary disorders. Experience allows pattern recognition of abnormalities on the chest X-ray. This experience is gained by careful systematic examination of many cases. This should take in the technical aspects, lung fields, cardiac outline, mediastinal structures, pleura, bones and soft tissue (Table 13.5). The structures outlined in the normal posteroanterior and lateral chest X-rays are shown in Fig. 13.8.

The contrast between air and tissue is important in many aspects of chest X-ray interpretation. It helps to place abnormalities anatomically, for example, shadowing in the anteriorly placed middle lobe or lingula obscures the heart border while shadowing in the posteriorly placed lower lobes leaves the heart border outlined by adjacent air-containing lung. Air in the bronchi is evident when surrounding lung is involved in an alveolar filling process, for example, consolidation in pneumonia.

Computed tomography (CT) of the chest has become an essential element in the investigation of respiratory disease (page 116). Within the lung parenchyma it provides information on the extent and position of lesions, for example,

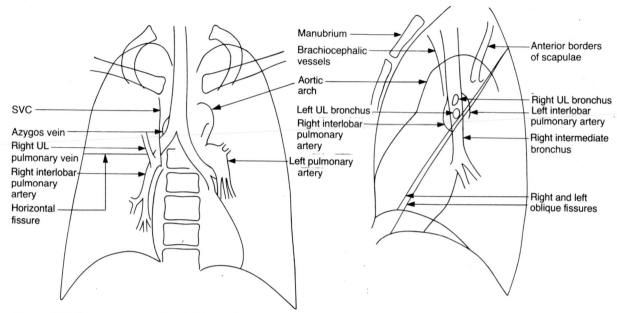

**Figure 13.8** Structures normally visible on the posteroanterior and lateral chest X-rays. SVC = superior vena cava. UL = upper lobe.

**Table 13.5** Areas to be considered in the interpretation of the chest X-ray.

| Posteroanterior view | Lateral view |
| --- | --- |
| 1 Name, date | 1 Name, date |
| 2 Technical aspects (penetration, centering) | 2 Penetration |
| 3 Lung fields | 3 Lung fields |
| 4 Pulmonary vessels, hila | 4 Retrosternal area |
| 5 Costophrenic, cardiophrenic angles | 5 Retrocardiac area |
| 6 Horizontal fissure | 6 Fissures |
| 7 Trachea, carina | 7 Heart |
| 8 Aorta | 8 Aorta |
| 9 Diaphragms | 9 Trachea |
| 10 Pleura | 10 Hila |
| 11 Bones | 11 Bones |
| 12 Soft tissues including neck, subdiaphragmatic areas | 12 Soft tissues |

carcinoma of the bronchus, the extent of emphysema and the presence of calcification within solid lesions. Thin cuts of the lung tissue are useful in the assessment of bronchiectasis and fibrosis. In addition it provides a way of looking more closely at mediastinal and pleural structures. In order to assess mediastinal structures, CT scans after injection of intravenous contrast medium may be helpful. In carcinoma of the bronchus extension of thoracic CT scans down to the liver and adrenals is often used to look for metastases in the staging process.

Magnetic resonance imaging (MRI) is less widely available and its role in the investigation of respiratory disease is not yet established as firmly as CT scanning.

Nuclear medicine techniques are used for lung scanning. This is most often used as perfusion and ventilation scans in the investigation of pulmonary embolism. Loss of perfusion to a segment with maintained perfusion is very suspicious of embolism. Conditions such as pneumonia or effusion produce an area of reduced ventilation and perfusion. However, where there is significant parenchymal lung disease both ventilation and perfusion scans are often abnormal in a patchy fashion and the diagnosis of pulmonary embolism is much more difficult.

# Bronchoscopy and lung biopsy

**Fibreoptic bronchoscopy** is usually performed under local anaesthetic and sedation if necessary. It allows inspection of the bronchial tree and can be used to obtain material from the distal areas of the lung. Fibreoptic bronchoscopy also has some therapeutic uses. The most frequent indication is the inspection of the airways for evidence of bronchial carcinoma, biopsy and assessment of operability. Lesions visible on the X-ray but not through the bronchoscope can be biopsied under X-ray control by transbronchial biopsy through the bronchoscope. Transbronchial biopsy can also be used to obtain material in diffuse lung disease such as sarcoidosis or infection. The cellular content of the alveoli can be sampled by washing out the airspaces in an alveolar lavage. This is useful in diffuse lung disease and in infections particularly *Pneumocystis carinii* infection in immunosuppressed patients.

Rigid bronchoscopy has been in use for much longer than fibreoptic techniques. It usually requires a general anaesthetic. It retains a usefulness in removal of foreign bodies and with substantial haemoptysis when vision and suction of the fibreoptic instrument are inadequate.

Therapeutic bronchoscopy is related mainly to clearing of the airways. This may be necessary when there is mucus plugging with infection, particularly in the intensive care unit. Endoscopic laser techniques can be used to provide temporary relief from obstruction by tumour. Newer techniques of intrabronchial radiotherapy require placement via the bronchoscope.

# Mediastinoscopy

This technique is used to sample glands in the upper mediastinum for diagnosis or for assessment of operability in bronchial carcinomas. This involves a small incision in the suprasternal notch. In the left side of the mediastinum a more extensive procedure of anterior mediastinotomy may be necessary through the site of the second costal cartilage.

# Pleural aspiration

Pleural aspiration is often necessary to sample fluid in the pleural space. Usually the site can be chosen from the X-ray and clinical examination but if the volume of fluid is small ultrasound guidance may be advisable. The parietal pleura can be sampled by blind biopsy when there is fluid present. In **thoracoscopy** a telescope or a bronchoscope is inserted into the pleural space between the ribs, this allows direct inspection and biopsy of the pleura. Video endoscopic techniques allow lung biopsy or stapling of bullae through the thoracoscope.

# Needle biopsy

Needle aspiration and biopsy is a useful technique for sampling intrapulmonary lesions. When they are close to the pleura a core of tissue may be obtained for histology but deeper in the lung substance a smaller gauge needle is necessary providing a cytological specimen for diagnosis. The risk of pneumothorax is around 20 per cent but intercostal drainage is necessary in less than 10 per cent of cases.

# Open lung biopsy

When a larger piece of lung tissue is needed then open lung biopsy will be required. This involves a small submammary incision and is used most often for diffuse lung disease where other biopsy methods produce too small a sample.

# *Clinical Problems*

## CONDITIONS WHICH CAUSE AIRFLOW OBSTRUCTION

Airflow obstruction can occur at any level in the bronchial tree. In the upper airway it is at the level of the larynx, trachea or major bronchi. Such obstructions are most often caused by tumours, damage to the airway wall or arteritic/granulomatous conditions such as Wegener's granulomatosis (page 319). Acute obstruction can occur from inhalation of a foreign body or from laryngeal swelling in anaphylaxis. In children and occasionally in adults epiglottitis may cause obstruction. Obstruction at a pharyngeal level may occur during sleep in a sleep apnoea syndromes (page 289).

More often obstruction reflects widespread airway narrowing. This situation is usually caused by asthma or chronic bronchitis and emphysema.

# *Asthma*

## DEFINITION

Asthma is a condition in which there is widespread narrowing of intrathoracic airways which changes in severity with time or as a result of treatment. The characteristic of asthma is that the airways are hypersensitive. They respond by narrowing to a wide variety of stimuli. This can be demonstrated in the laboratory using non-specific stimuli such as methacholine, histamine or cold air. Allergic triggers also cause airway narrowing and a response to an allergen may leave the airways more reactive to non-specific stimuli for days afterwards. In some asthmatics who develop problems later in life it may be difficult to identify specific provoking factors other than respiratory infections.

## EPIDEMIOLOGY

Asthma is a common condition affecting around 10 per cent of children and 6 per cent of adults in the UK. There is an underlying genetic predisposition to atopic conditions; allergic rhinitis, eczema and asthma. This then requires further environmental factors to make it clinically manifest.

Around 2000 people die of asthma every year in the UK. In most countries asthma seems to be increasing both in prevalence and in severity. This is seen particularly in association with migration from underdeveloped areas to urban environments. Various explanations related to high allergen levels in indoor environments, high dietary sodium and pollution have been proposed.

## PATHOPHYSIOLOGY

Hyperresponsiveness of the bronchi may be related to inflammation in the walls. This inflammation involves oedema and a cellular infiltrate (Fig. 13.9). Together with smooth

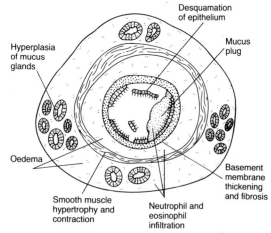

**Figure 13.9** Pathological changes which cause narrowing in asthmatic airways.

muscle contraction and mucus production it is responsible for the airflow obstruction which occurs in asthma.

The cells in the airway walls are responsible for the inflammatory changes. Mast cells, eosinophils and neutrophils can release preformed mediators such as histamine, neutrophil chemotactic factor and platelet-activating factor (PAF). They can also produce new mediators by metabolism of arachidonic acid from the cell membranes. Arachidonic acid can be metabolized to produce prostaglandins or leukotrienes. These are capable of producing direct changes on the smooth muscle and the airway wall and acting as chemotactic factors for further cell infiltration.

The cells in the airway wall can be stimulated by immunological stimuli but also by physical stimuli such as the drying and cooling of the airway wall which occurs on exercise.

There is a close interrelationship with the nerve supply to the wall. The smooth muscle has $B_2$ adrenergic receptors but not a direct sympathetic nerve supply. However, there are parasympathetic nerves which constrict the muscle and a non-adrenergic, non-cholinergic system.

When an asthma attack is fatal, at *post-mortem* the airways are occluded by plugs of sticky mucus. The airway wall is oedematous and inflamed and the surface epithelium may be lost or disrupted. Even in mild asthma when there are few if any clinical manifestations bronchial wall biopsies show that a degree of inflammation remains leaving a vulnerability to future problems.

## CLINICAL FEATURES

The main clinical manifestations of asthma are wheeze, shortness of breath and cough. In some circumstances cough may be the only symptom, it is likely to be worst at night or on exposure to cold air or exercise.

Asthma most often comes on in childhood and has identifiable causes. In most cases it is intermittent with periods of relative or complete freedom. Precipitating causes should be identified from the history so that they can be avoided when possible. When asthma develops in adults precipitating causes other than upper respiratory tract infections may be less obvious. Some asthma is caused by exposure at work and this

should always be carefully sought by enquiring about chemicals, dusts and animals at work.

The degree of airflow obstruction in asthma varies throughout the day. It is typically at its worst at 2 to 4 a.m. and at its best in the afternoon. Questions about disturbance of sleep are important in the assessment of asthmatic patients.

In chronic or intermittent asthma the severity is assessed in terms of the disturbance to normal routine, the degree of treatment which is necessary and the severity of any exacerbations.

In acute attacks of asthma it is important that the severity of the condition is carefully evaluated. Deaths in acute asthma continue to occur because the doctor or the patient has underestimated the severity of the attack. The features associated with a severe attack of asthma are shown in Table 13.6.

**Table 13.6** Features of an acute severe attack of asthma.

| |
|---|
| 1 Pulse >100 per minute |
| 2 Respiratory rate >25 per minute |
| 3 Peak flow rate <200 l/min or 40 per cent predicted or best known |
| 4 Too breathless to speak in sentences |
| 5 Cyanosis |
| 6 Lack of wheezing in the chest (airflow too low) |
| 7 Unable to walk |
| 8 Pulsus paradoxus >15 mm Hg |

Some asthmatics develop a sensitivity to a common fungus, *Aspergillus fumigatus* resulting in **allergic bronchopulmonary aspergillosis** (ABPA). This mould thrives on rotting vegetation. It causes a number of respiratory problems. In asthma this is an allergic phenomenon in which there is plugging of the airways by rubbery masses of fungal hyphae, eosinophils and inflammatory exudate. These can cause damage to the airway wall with cylindrical, proximal bronchiectasis. The rubbery, brown plugs may be coughed up. The blood shows an eosinophilia, skin tests show a reaction to Aspergillus and the X-ray may show patchy infiltration, areas of collapse or fibrosis and bronchiectasis.

Asthma is seen in the rare Churg–Strauss syndrome (allergic granulomatosis (page 320) and occurs quite frequently in cystic fibrosis (page 295).

## INVESTIGATION

The diagnosis of asthma relies on the demonstration of reversibility of airflow obstruction. The obstruction is easily measured with a peak flow meter (page 270) or by spirometry. Portable peak flow meters can be used at home for regular monitoring of asthma as well as for diagnosis. They are particularly important at times when the treatment is changed and most asthmatics should keep one at home to monitor their condition and to detect deterioration. When acute asthma attacks necessitate hospital treatment peak flow charts usually show that there has been a steady deterioration for days or weeks before the admission.

For diagnosis peak flow can be measured before and after a bronchodilator such as salbutamol. When baseline peak flow is normal recordings can be made over a few weeks at home to look for diurnal variation (Fig. 13.10) or provocation by exercise (Fig. 13.11). It is rarely necessary to use agents such as histamine and methacholine or specific allergens in clinical practice.

The blood count will often show eosinophilia except in the presence of oral steroid treatment. Skin prick tests can be used to look for IgE reactions to common allergens. They show that a subject is atopic but do not necessarily diagnose asthma or establish the importance of any particular precipitant. They should be assessed with the clinical history. IgE antibody activity against specific substances can also be measured by the radioallergosorbent test (RAST).

In acute asthma, in addition to pulse, respiratory rate, peak flow and paradoxical pulse the blood gases are usually measured and a chest X-ray taken. The blood gases breathing air show a low $PaO_2$ and generally a low $PaCO_2$. The low $PaCO_2$ is a response to hypoxia and stimuli from the lungs. When the $PaCO_2$ is normal or high this is a danger sign that the patient is tiring and that ventilatory support may be necessary soon. The chest X-ray often shows overinflation of the lungs. There may be areas of consolidation or collapse due to mucus plugging. One reason to do a chest X-ray is to rule out a pneumothorax which, although unusual, may be difficult to diagnose clinically in acute asthma.

## TREATMENT

### *General approach*

There are three main avenues of treatment in asthma. The first is to avoid the provoking agent where possible. The second is through bronchodilator drugs which reverse airway narrowing and the third is through prophylactic therapy directed at the underlying inflammation. The recognition of persistent inflammatory changes in the airway wall in asthma has brought about a change in the general approach with much earlier use of anti-inflammatory drugs rather than reliance on bronchodilators. For treatment schemes for chronic and acute severe asthma see Tables 13.7 and 13.8, respectively.

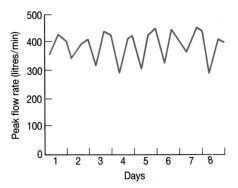

**Figure 13.10** Typical early morning dips in peak flow in an asthmatic patient.

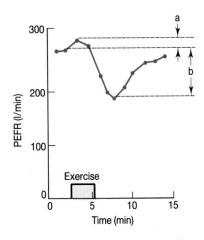

**Figure 13.11** Exercise challenge in asthma showing bronchodilation during exercise (a) followed by bronchoconstriction (b) maximal after the end of exercise. PEFR = peak expiratory flow rate.

**Table 13.7** Treatment of chronic asthma.

## 1 Look for avoidable factors
(a) Avoidable allergens
(b) Drugs – β-blockers, aspirin
(c) Occupational exposure

## 2 Bronchodilators
Salbutamol (200 μg) or terbutaline (500 μg) as necessary

## 3 Inhaled anti-inflammatory agent
If a bronchodilator is used more than once daily or symptoms occur at night, continue the bronchodilator as necessary and add:

(a) Sodium cromoglycate 5–10 mg four times daily or
(b) Inhaled corticosteroid 100–400 μg twice daily

## 4 Long-acting inhaled bronchodilator in addition to anti-inflammatory
For example, salmeterol 50 μg twice daily

## 5 High-dose inhaled steroids
For example, up to 2000 μg daily given via large volume spacer

## 6 Additional bronchodilators
(a) Ipratropium bromide 40–80 μg four times a day
(b) Slow release theophylline to obtain a blood level of 8–20 mg/l

## 7 Regular oral steroids

### Notes
1 A short course of oral steroids (30 mg daily for 2 weeks) may help to establish control.
2 With asthma under good control therapy may be reduced. In general good control should be established for 3–6 months before going back from step 3.

## Education

Asthma is a variable disease where treatment may need to be adjusted to symptoms but some drugs need to be taken regularly. Patients need to understand how to take their treatment and how to adjust it. This is helped by a simple written plan and by the regular use of a peak flow meter as a guide to severity. Acute attacks of asthma can often be prevented by adjustment of treatment at the right time. The patient must know what to do when control starts to deteriorate. Much of the treatment is given by the inhaled route, which has the advantages that the

**Table 13.8** Treatment of acute severe asthma.

## 1 Assess the severity of the attack (page 280)

## 2 Oxygen
Give at the highest concentration available. In patients with chronic airflow obstruction high concentrations may depress ventilation. Therefore, controlled concentrations (24–28 per cent) should be used in patients over 55 years when the diagnosis is uncertain

## 3 Nebulized β-agonist
This should be given immediately and repeated as necessary. This may be at 15–30 min intervals in severe cases, 2–4 hourly in milder cases with a good response. Drive the nebulizer by oxygen or give oxygen through nasal cannulae

## 4 Nebulized ipratropium bromide
This should be added to the β-agonist in the nebulizer if the response to the first β-agonist dose is not satisfactory

## 5 Steroids
These should be given in nearly all cases of severe asthma. Usually this can be oral prednisolone, 30–60 mg daily, or intravenous hydrocortisone in very severe cases

## 6 Intravenous bronchodilators
If nebulized bronchodilators are not giving satisfactory improvement intravenous salbutamol or aminophylline should be considered

## 7 Potassium
Steroids, β-agonists and increased ventilation will all tend to reduce serum potassium which should be monitored and replaced

## 8 Fluids
Often asthmatic patients in severe attacks are fluid depleted and will need intravenous replacement

## 9 Ventilation
If the blood gases deteriorate, particularly if the $PaCO_2$ is rising, and the patient is tiring a period of ventilatory support may need to be considered. When this is necessary it is important that it is predicted by careful observation rather than precipitated by a respiratory arrest

An acute attack of asthma should be regarded as a failure of routine management. The reasons for failure should be explored with the patient so that future severe attacks can be prevented. The patient will need plans for follow-up and an action plan to deal with exacerbations of asthma.

drug is given directly to the airways, the dose can be kept low and systemic effects minimized. There are many different inhaler devices and most patients can use this route efficiently once taught. Their competence with the device should be checked periodically.

## Avoidance

When a distinct provoking factor is identified it may be possible to avoid it. This applies with some animal contacts or occupational elements. Often they are such common substances in the environment, such as grass pollen or house dust mite, that avoidance is difficult. Usually the hyperresponsive airways respond to a large number of substances and avoidance of single agents is of little help. Occasionally foods or drinks may provoke asthma. These areas should always be carefully explored in the history. Elaborate exclusion diets are rarely necessary. Although exercise provokes asthma it does not subsequently increase sensitivity to other agents and should not be avoided. Exercise-induced asthma can usually be prevented by warming up beforehand or by premedication with β-agonists or sodium cromoglycate.

## Bronchodilators

There are three groups of bronchodilators used regularly in asthma:

**1 β-Agonists.** These drugs work on the $\beta_2$-adrenoreceptors on smooth muscle in the airways. *In vitro* they can be shown to have other actions on mediator release. They are the most effective bronchodilator drugs in asthma and are used by inhalation. Higher doses can be delivered by nebulizer and occasionally intravenously in acute asthma. Long-acting oral preparations are available but are rarely necessary since the development of long-acting inhaled preparations such as salmeterol. Conventional β-agonists such as salbutamol and terbutaline last from 3 to 5 hours. Salmeterol bronchodilates for over 12 hours. β-Agonists should be used as necessary to reverse airway narrowing and remove breathlessness. They can be used before exercise to prevent exercise-induced asthma. Otherwise they should not be used as regular prophylactic treatment. If bronchodilators are used more than once a day

regular treatment with prophylactic agents such as inhaled steroids should be considered.

The selective β-agonists such as salbutamol and terbutaline have few side effects when given by inhalation. The main side effect is tremor; occasionally cramps occur and vasodilation may cause a reflex tachycardia. Rarely, large doses by nebulizer or parenterally can precipitate arrhythmias or angina.

The main delivery devices for inhalation are pressurized metered dose inhalers or dry powder inhalers. Where coordination is poor dry powder devices are easier to use or metered dose inhalers can be breath-activated or combined with a large plastic chamber spacing device (Volumatic or Nebuhaler) which removes the need to coordinate inhaler activation and inspiration.

**2 Anticholinergics.** These atropine-like drugs reverse vagally induced airway narrowing. The two agents available are ipratropium bromide and oxitropium bromide which is longer acting. They are given by metered dose inhaler or by nebulizer. In asthma they are generally less effective than β-agonists but may be useful in older patients and in acute severe asthma. The onset of action is slower than β-agonists, the maximum effect taking 60 min rather than 30 min.

**3 Methylxanthines (theophylline and aminophylline).** These drugs cannot be given by inhalation. They are used orally in chronic asthma and aminophylline can be given intravenously in acute asthma. The oral route means that side effects are more troublesome. Nausea and vomiting are common and arrhythmias and fits occur at higher blood levels. Slow release preparations give more stable blood levels which need to be monitored. Theophyllines are used when asthma persists despite treatment with other bronchodilators and inhaled steroids.

## Preventative treatment

**1 Sodium cromoglycate and nedocromil sodium.** These drugs were originally thought to act by stabilization of mast cells but may well have other actions. They are most useful in younger asthmatics although nedocromil sodium may have more activity in older patients. Although they can work as single doses to prevent exercise-induced asthma, in other situations they need to be given regularly. The benefit of treatment may take weeks or months to develop.

**2 Inhaled corticosteroids.** Inhaled corticosteroids are given by metered dose, dry powder or nebulizer delivery systems. At doses below 1000 μg daily of beclomethasone dipropionate or budesonide they have few if any systemic effects. Between 1000 and 2000 μg biochemical effects on the pituitary–adrenal axis may be detectable and skin changes may occur. Local problems in the mouth with candidiasis or hoarseness can usually be avoided by spacing devices and mouth washing. These are minor problems and inhaled steroids provide excellent control without side effects for many asthmatics. The newer agent fluticasone has fewer systemic effects and may be preferable at higher doses.

**3 Oral corticosteroids.** These are often used in short courses in acute asthma or to establish good control in chronic asthma. Occasionally oral corticosteroids need to be used on a long-term basis but, because of their side effects, this should only be done when high-dose inhaled steroids and bronchodilators have failed to produce good control.

### Other measures

Other drugs such as α-blockers, antihistamines and ketotifen (with antihistamine and mast cell stabilizing properties) may have a minor effect on asthma but have little use in clinical practice. In some countries desensitization to allergens is widely used. There is some evidence of an effect in some asthmatics but such an approach is not often necessary and adverse reactions can occur. Deaths from anaphylaxis have been recorded regularly, usually when there has been a mistake in the dosing regime.

Alternative treatments such as hypnosis, homeopathy, acupuncture and yoga have shown minor effects in some trials but there is little evidence that they offer anything substantial to most patients.

### PROGNOSIS

Asthma which develops in childhood may resolve with age. Around a half of those with mild to moderate asthma at the age of 7 years are free of problems by 21 years. Boys are more likely to develop asthma in childhood but do better in adolescence so that the sex ratio is nearly equal in adults. Asthma is more likely to resolve during teenage years if it is mild in childhood. Severe childhood asthma is likely to give problems throughout life. Even if asthma resolves after childhood the underlying predisposition is likely to be present and may show itself again given the right provocation.

# Allergic rhinitis

Allergic rhinitis is characterized by nasal obstruction, rhinorrhoea and sneezing. It is often associated with conjunctival infection, tears and nasal and pharyngeal itching. It is another manifestation of an underlying atopic state and may be associated with asthma. The commonest form of allergic rhinitis is hayfever where pollens cause a seasonal problem. Grass pollens are most troublesome in June and July, while many tree pollens such as plane and birch are more prevalent in April and May. Perennial rhinitis is often related to house dust mite sensitivity.

Allergic rhinitis can be treated by antihistamines orally or by local treatment with intranasal steroids or sodium cromoglycate. Sodium cromoglycate can also be used on the conjunctiva. In seasonal rhinitis nasal steroids should be started before the expected start of symptoms.

# Chronic bronchitis and emphysema

These two conditions are considered together since they nearly always exist together. They usually have a common cause in cigarette smoking. However, there are other causes of both conditions. The airflow obstruction caused by the combination of chronic bronchitis and emphysema goes under a number of different names such as chronic obstructive airways disease (COAD), chronic obstructive lung disease (COLD) or chronic obstructive pulmonary disease (COPD).

## Chronic bronchitis

The common definition of chronic bronchitis is an epidemiological definition which requires the production of sputum on most days for 3 months of two consecutive years without a specific underlying cause such as bronchiectasis. Increased mucus production comes from enlargement of submucosal glands and increased numbers of goblet cells. Studies of cigarette smokers find that cough and sputum production are very common symptoms and may be just markers of cigarette smoking not predictive of future obstruction.

## Emphysema

The definition of emphysema is anatomical, based on enlargement of terminal airspaces with destruction of alveolar walls. It is therefore more difficult to make during life. It is divided pathologically into pan-acinar emphysema where generalized destruction occurs and centrilobular emphysema, but these may be extremes of the same condition.

## AETIOLOGY

Cigarette smoking is much the most important factor in chronic bronchitis but atmospheric pollution and occupational factors have a minor role. Cigarette smoking is also the dominant factor in emphysema.

Insight into the mechanism came through the discovery of $\alpha_1$-antiprotease ($\alpha_1$-antitrypsin) deficiency. This inherited condition of lack of the major serum antiprotease is associated with a severe form of emphysema developing in the thirties and forties in smokers and 10–20 years later in non-smokers. Proteases are thought to be able to act in an uninhibited fashion to damage the lung tissue. There are a number of genotypic variants, the most common deficiency being the homoxygous ZZ form. Altered $\alpha_1$-antiprotease is unable to leave the liver cells and

the condition is associated with liver disease in neonates and occasionally in adults. Severe deficiency occurs in around 1 in 5000 Caucasians.

The minor drop in $\alpha_1$-antiprotease in heterozygous forms may make airway disease more likely in smokers but the effects are minor. The emphysema caused by $\alpha_1$-antitrypsin deficiency occurs predominantly at the bases of the lungs rather than the apices in conventional cigarette smoke-related disease. Replacement therapy is under investigation.

These findings concentrated interest on the protease–antiprotease system. Cigarette smoke attracts neutrophils to the lungs, which release elastase. The antiproteases are partly inactivated by cigarette smoke and the change in the balance may be a factor which allows the proteases to damage the lungs and cause emphysema. The high prevalence of cigarette smoking in the UK means that these are common conditions responsible for large numbers of deaths and a great deal of morbidity and time lost from work. Significant problems only occur in a minority of smokers, 20–25 per cent. The reasons for this susceptibility of a particular group are uncertain.

In chronic bronchitis and emphysema there is inflammatory change and destruction of small airways in addition to the emphysematous change in the alveoli. Emphysema makes the lungs floppy, more compliant, and this leads to collapse of the airways in the lungs during expiration. Both these mechanisms are involved in the obstruction to airflow in this condition.

## CLINICAL FEATURES

Symptoms of cough, sputum production and wheeze are common amongst cigarette smokers within a year or two of taking up smoking. However, significant problems with breathlessness are unusual before middle age. In the susceptible group the usual rate of loss of respiratory function with age is increased. As airway obstruction develops breathlessness may be progressive although some patients fail to notice much of a problem until their lung function is quite severely disturbed. Early morning cough and sputum production is often regarded as normal by smokers and not mentioned in the history unless specifically asked for. Recurrent infective exacerbations occur and are caused by viruses or bacteria.

Eventually loss of lung tissue leads to respiratory failure (page 290). Some patients maintain their arterial oxygen level at reasonable levels by keeping up a high minute ventilation and a low $PaCO_2$. They are breathless but not cyanosed and are given the label **'pink puffers'**. Other patients have a lower $PaO_2$ and a raised $PaCO_2$ and are more likely to develop fluid retention and right heart failure through the effect of blood gas changes on fluid retention in the kidney and through pulmonary hypertension from hypoxia and loss of the pulmonary vascular bed. This group are often oedematous and cyanosed but not so breathless and are known as **'blue bloaters'**. It was taught that 'pink puffers' have mainly emphysema and 'blue bloaters' bronchitis but the evidence suggests that the two conditions are mixed in both groups.

Unlike asthma the degree of breathlessness in chronic bronchitis and emphysema is fairly constant although it will increase during infective exacerbations. In older patients it may be difficult to differentiate late onset asthma from chronic bronchitis and emphysema. Clues should be sought in the history and the investigations. However, the most important factor is to ensure that all appropriate treatment is given and this will mean making every effort to achieve all possible reversibility of airflow obstruction in all such patients.

On examination the chest is often overinflated with a large anteroposterior diameter (barrel chest) and little expansion of the rib cage on inspiration. There may be evidence of right heart failure with raised jugular venous pressure and ankle oedema. On auscultation there may be expiratory wheezing especially on forced expiration. There are often early inspiratory crackles to be heard at the lung bases. Central cyanosis may be present and in severe cases confusion or sedation from hypoxia and a coarse tremor (flap) from $CO_2$ retention.

## INVESTIGATIONS

Measurement of airflow obstruction should be part of the examination of such patients. This will show a low peak expiratory flow rate or a low

$FEV_1$ and forced expiratory ratio on spirometry. The total lung capacity and residual volume will usually be increased but the gas transfer and KCO will be reduced. The KCO is a reasonable guide to the severity of emphysema.

The blood picture may show polycythaemia related to chronic hypoxia and in $CO_2$ retention the bicarbonate level may be raised.

The chest X-ray shows large lung fields with a long thin heart (Fig. 13.12) unless cor pulmonale is developing when the heart dilates. The proximal pulmonary arteries may be large but the lung fields may show areas of loss of lung markings. In emphysema there may be evidence of large spaces or bullae with no lung markings and a thin border. The best guide to the extent of emphysema is the computed tomographic (CT) scan which will show the extent of lung destruction (Fig. 13.13). This is not necessary as a routine investigation but may be an important guide if lung surgery is being planned for bullae or an associated lung lesion.

In advanced disease weight loss is common although this may be masked by fluid retention.

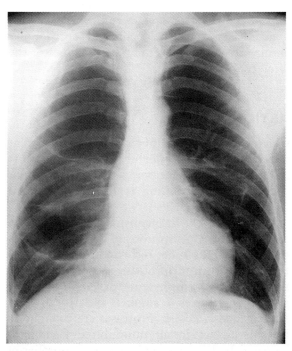

**Figure 13.12** Chest X-ray in a case of bullous emphysema. The lungs are large with reduced vascular markings and the lines in the right lung represent the edges of bullae.

## TREATMENT

### Smoking

Even though most of the damage is irreversible vigorous attempts should always be made to get patients to stop smoking. This may produce a slight improvement in lung function and stops the increased rate of decline.

### Bronchodilators

Bronchodilators should always be tried in order to relieve breathlessness. The responses should be measured by spirometry although some patients may benefit without much evidence of objective change. In older patients with chronic bronchitis and emphysema anticholinergic agents such as ipratropium bromide often have a greater effect than β-agonists. They should be given in a reasonable dose (e.g. 80 μg ipratropium three to four times daily). The patient's inhaler technique must be checked. Some severely breathless patients require regular bronchodilator treatment via a large volume spacer or a nebulizer. It has been suggested that theophylline has an extra effect improving respiratory muscle function. There is little evidence for a clinically significant effect on muscles or a bronchodilator effect above that produced by inhaled therapy.

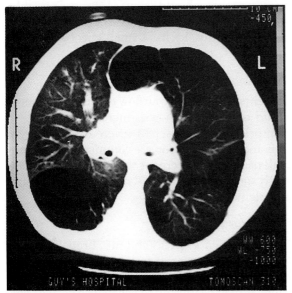

**Figure 13.13** Computed tomographic scan of the thorax in emphysema showing areas of loss of normal lung markings particularly anteriorly, laterally on the left and posteriorly on the right.

### Steroids

In patients with severe airflow obstruction a formal trial of oral corticosteroids assessed by subjective and objective measures is usually justified. A striking response is sometimes achieved. Where there are contraindications to oral steroids high-dose inhaled steroids should be assessed. If oral steroids produce an effect, an effort should be made to maintain this with inhaled steroids rather than by using long-term oral steroids. Trials are in progress to see whether inhaled steroids are able to slow the rate of decline of lung function in chronic bronchitis and emphysema. Even when oral steroids fail to have an effect in a formal trial they may still be useful in severe acute exacerbations.

### Mucolytics

In some countries mucolytics are widely used in chronic bronchitis. Some studies have suggested small effects in the reduction of exacerbations but there is little evidence that they have any worthwhile effect.

### Antibiotics

The bacteria most often responsible for exacerbations are *Streptococcus pneumoniae*, *Haemophilus influenzae* and *Moraxella catarrhalis*. They are usually sensitive to simple regimes using amoxycillin, trimethoprim or cephalosporins. Continuous antibiotics are not necessary and exacerbations should be treated as they arise. This is often best done by giving the patient antibiotics to keep at home and use when necessary. Influenza vaccination should be given in the autumn and pneumococcal vaccination considered when exacerbations are frequent.

### Oxygen

In acute exacerbations oxygen therapy must be carefully controlled. Patients who are chronically hypoxic and have $CO_2$ retention may be relying on hypoxic drive to breathe. A high concentration of inspired oxygen decreases this drive, reduces minute ventilation and allows $PaCO_2$ to rise leading to drowsiness and coma ($CO_2$ narcosis). Blood gases should be checked and if $PaCO_2$ is raised oxygen should be given in a controlled fashion with a 24 or 28 per cent mask and the gases rechecked in 30–60 minutes. The masks work on a Venturi principle to maintain their percentage at varying minute volumes. Nasal cannulae do not provide adequate control in these circumstances since reduction in minute ventilation increases the inspired oxygen concentration and makes the situation worse.

At present oxygen is the only drug to produce a sustained reduction in raised pulmonary artery pressure without systemic hypotension. Two controlled trials, one in the UK and one in North America, have shown that treatment with oxygen for more than 15 hours a day improves survival in cor pulmonale or severe blood gas disturbance. The closer the treatment is to continuous 24 hour therapy the greater the benefit. Oxygen should be delivered via an oxygen concentrator which extracts oxygen from room air by a molecular sieve. This is a cheaper and simpler option than delivery by cylinders. The current UK criteria for use of long-term oxygen treatment are shown in Table 13.9. Without oxygen 20–30 per cent of such patients survive 5 years.

Portable oxygen cylinders are available for short periods away from the home. Oxygen can be delivered in low flows by a cannula inserted through the cricothyroid membrane.

## Diuretics and vasodilators

When cor pulmonale develops diuretics will help to relieve ankle swelling and breathlessness. Too great a diuresis will decrease cardiac output. Vasodilators often have too great an effect on the systemic circulation to be useful. However, careful use of angiotensin-converting enzyme inhibitors may be helpful.

## Breathlessness

Attempts have been made to reduce ventilatory drive in pink puffers in order to relieve their breathlessness. Opiates and benzodiazepines

**Table 13.9** Criteria for the use of long-term oxygen treatment.

1 $PaO_2$ <7.3 kPa (55 mmHg) on two occasions in a stable state
2 Not smoking
3 $PaO_2$ >8 kPa on proposed oxygen therapy
4 Compliant with therapy >15 hours per day

have been used. They have not proved very useful but may be worth trying occasionally in cases of distressing breathlessness.

## Polycythaemia

Hypoxia may lead to compensatory polycythaemia. This can produce a feeling of muzziness and slowed cerebration which may be relieved by venesection. Long-term oxygen therapy stops the development of polycythaemia.

## Respiratory stimulants

In acute exacerbations doxapram may be used intravenously as a respiratory stimulant to stop respiratory depression induced by oxygen therapy. This will allow the use of a higher inspiratory oxygen concentration and raise $PaO_2$ without increasing $PaCO_2$. In the long-term various respiratory stimulants have been used. Almitrine is available in much of Europe but can cause peripheral neuropathy and is not available in the UK at present.

## Physiotherapy and rehabilitation

During acute exacerbations physiotherapy to clear secretions may be very helpful. Chronically ill patients with sputum production should be encouraged to cough effectively. It is important that patients should stay as fit as possible. General muscle training or specifically of the respiratory muscles has a small effect in increasing exercise tolerance.

## Nutrition

Patients with chronic airflow obstruction should avoid obesity which will increase oxygen consumption on exercise. In severe disease weight loss and poor nutrition are common and patients will need encouragement to keep up their intake with small but nutritious meals and appropriate supplements.

## Ventilatory support

When patients with chronic bronchitis and emphysema present in respiratory failure a difficult decision may have to be made about ventilation. It may be unkind to ventilate a patient who is a respiratory cripple and unlikely to manage subsequently without ventilatory support. However, there needs to be a very good knowledge of the patient's state over months and years before the exacerbation to be confident to with-hold ventilation in an acute situation. In the longer term some patients have been treated with ventilatory support at home by overnight ventilation via a nasal mask. The wider use of this technique is under investigation.

### Transplantation and other surgery

In emphysema with localized bullae and loss of volume in adjacent lung, surgical resection of the bullae may be helpful. In young patients with severe disease, particularly $\alpha_1$-antiprotease deficiency, lung transplantation may need to be considered.

# Sleep apnoea

In sleep apnoea breathing stops during the night in a repetitive fashion. Significant sleep apnoea probably occurs in around 1 per cent of the adult male population. There are two major forms of sleep apnoea:

1 Central sleep apnoea in which the output to the respiratory muscles stops and there is no muscle activity and no airflow.
2 Obstructive sleep apnoea in which the upper airway, usually around the back of the pharynx, collapses on inspiration and obstruction occurs until partial arousal stimulates increased respiration with opening of the pharyngeal obstruction.

A few central apnoeas are often seen in normal subjects, especially men as they get older. In order to have a significant clinical effect apnoeas or hypopnoeas must occur more than 20 times an hour throughout the night. In both forms of sleep apnoea the associated hypoxia may lead to cardiac and cerebral problems and in obstructive apnoea the disruption in the normal sleep pattern can lead to profound sleepiness during the day.

Central apnoea is associated with neurological problems and with muscular disorders.

Obstructive sleep apnoea is more likely with obesity, heavy alcohol consumption and sedative drugs. It is more common in men and is more likely with conditions which narrow the upper airway (small jaw, acromegaly etc.) or with nasal obstruction (Table 13.10).

Patients with obstructive sleep apnoea are usually loud snorers. Loud snorers without sleep apnoea have a disturbance of sleep architecture leading to daytime tiredness and snoring itself may be associated with an increased cardio-vascular and cerebrovascular morbidity and mortality as well as more frequent road traffic accidents. In obstructive sleep apnoea nocturia is common and patients may wake at night with a choking sensation. They do not feel refreshed on waking and fall asleep easily during the day. Pulmonary hypertension may develop, systemic hypertension may also be present but is probably related to the associated obesity of many of these patients.

## INVESTIGATION

A careful history from the patient and his wife will often give the diagnosis (Table 13.11). This can be further supported by recording oxygen saturation with a pulse oximeter throughout the night. This should show the typical pattern of repeated short desaturations. Where there is doubt, or in more complicated cases, a full polysomnographic sleep study should be performed recording the electroencephalogram (EEG), the electrocardiogram (ECG), oxygen saturation, airflow and chest wall movement.

## TREATMENT

Central sleep apnoea is treated by respiratory stimulants or ventilatory support at night. In

**Table 13.10** Conditions associated with sleep apnoea.

Obesity
Alcohol consumption
Sedative drugs
Nasal obstruction
Tonsillar enlargement
Small mandible
Acromegaly
Hypothyroidism
Diabetic autonomic neuropathy
Shy-Drager syndrome (autonomic neuropathy with disorder of the extrapyramidal system)
Muscle disorders (e.g. acid maltase deficiency)

**Table 13.11** Symptoms of obstructive sleep apnoea.

Daytime somnolence
Loud snoring at night (bed partner may confirm apnoeic periods with snorting commencement of breathing)
Nocturia
Choking sensation at night
Restless night
Waking unrefreshed in the morning
Morning headache
Right heart failure
Poor memory and concentration
Psychiatric changes
Dry mouth on waking

obstructive sleep apnoea obesity, alcohol, smoking and nasal obstruction should be dealt with first. In some mild cases apnoea only occurs while lying flat on the back and this may be avoided by simple devices such as a tennis ball sewn into the back of a vest. In severe cases tracheostomy was the first effective treatment. Two treatments are in current use. A continuous positive airway pressure of 5–15 cm $H_2O$ via a close fitting nasal mask is usually effective. An operation to remove the tonsils and the back of the soft palate, uvulopalatopharyngoplasty (UPPP), is very effective in relieving snoring. It reduces sleep apnoea by over 50 per cent in 60–80 per cent of patients but it is difficult to predict preoperatively who will respond.

Underlying causes are related to alterations in central drive to breathing or to narrowing of the upper airway (Table 13.10). They should be sought and treated as necessary.

# RESPIRATORY FAILURE

Respiratory failure is defined by blood gas changes. Respiratory failure is not the only cause of hypoxaemia. When there is a right-to-left shunt the $PaO_2$ will fall and if the inspired oxygen pressure is low, as at high altitude, $PaO_2$ will fall. In **type I respiratory failure** the $PaO_2$ is below 8 kPa (60 mm Hg). When in addition the $PaCO_2$ is raised to above 6.6 kPa (50 mm Hg) then effective alveolar hypoventilation is reduced and **type II respiratory failure** is present.

Respiratory failure may be acute or chronic. When type II respiratory failure is acute the bicarbonate level will not rise immediately. A chronically raised $PaCO_2$ would be expected to be associated with a raised bicarbonate level. Prolonged hypoxia may lead to compensatory polycythaemia.

Calculation of the alveolar–arterial oxygen gradient is useful in the interpretation of blood gases:

$$\text{Alveolar oxygen} = PAO_2 = PIO_2 - \frac{PACO_2}{R}$$

where $R$ is the respiratory quotient. Alveolar $PCO_2$ is taken as the same value as arterial $PCO_2$ and the inspired oxygen $PIO_2$ is known so alveolar $PO_2$ ($PAO_2$) can be calculated. If $PaO_2$ is measured at the same time then $PAO_2 - PaO_2$ (the **alveolar–arterial gradient**) can be calculated. In normal subjects this is less than 2 kPa breathing air. It rises when hypoxia is caused by gas exchange problems and not by hypoventilation.

The causes of respiratory failure are shown in Table 13.12.

**Table 13.12** Main causes of respiratory failure.

**Type I respiratory failure**
Asthma
Chronic bronchitis and emphysema
Pulmonary oedema
Fibrosing lung conditions
Pulmonary vascular obstruction

**Type II respiratory failure**
Chronic bronchitis and emphysema
Severe obstructive or restrictive lung disease
Drug-induced respiratory depression
Central respiratory depression
Neuromuscular problems affecting respiratory muscles
Thoracic cage abnormalities (e.g. kyphoscoliosis)
Hypoventilation syndromes

## CLINICAL FEATURES

Many of the clinical features of respiratory failure are not very specific. There is likely to be breathlessness and evidence of the underlying problem. Hypoxaemia causes confusion and restlessness and produces central cyanosis. Hypercapnia produces peripheral vasodilation giving warm hands with wide pulse pressure. Intracranial pressure rises and may produce papilloedema and confusion, eventually coma. There may be a flapping tremor of the outstretched hands. Signs of right-sided heart failure may be present if cor pulmonale develops.

Blood gases are likely to deteriorate further during sleep when respiratory rate and volume decrease. Recordings of overnight saturation with a pulse oximeter may be helpful in quantifying this. Nocturnal hypoventilation may lead to a morning headache or feeling of muzziness on waking.

Many of the signs are non-specific or, like cyanosis, difficult to be sure of unless very severe. Measurement of blood gases is therefore an important investigation. Where $PaCO_2$ is not raised then the situation can subsequently be followed without further arterial puncture by a pulse oximeter to measure oxygen saturation.

In neuromuscular and chest wall diseases vital capacity forms one of the best indices of progression and need for intervention. When the vital capacity falls below 1 litre blood gases should be checked and the possibility of ventilatory support considered.

## TREATMENT

Treatment is directed at the underlying condition where this is possible. If respiratory failure is still present then support with ventilation may have to be considered. This may involve agents such as doxapram to stimulate ventilation. Oxygen therapy must be carefully monitored to avoid a further rise in $PaCO_2$ in type II respiratory failure. When the patient's ventilatory efforts are not enough or exhaustion is setting in support will need to be considered. The simplest method is the use of continuous airway pressure with a tight-fitting face mask (mask CPAP = continuous positive airway pressure). The next step would be supportive ventilation by way of an endotracheal tube but this should only be used after careful consideration of the patient's normal lifestyle and limitations.

Portable devices are available to deliver pressure support through a face mask at home. Some patients have other equipment such as negative pressure devices ('iron lungs' or jackets) and phrenic pacing or rocking beds for diaphragm palsies.

For details of the use of oxygen in respiratory failure see page 257.

## INFECTIONS OF THE RESPIRATORY TRACT

## *Acute infections of the upper respiratory tract, trachea and bronchi*

Infections of the upper respiratory tract are very common particularly in the autumn and winter. They are responsible for half the time lost from work through acute illness. There is a risk of progression to lower respiratory tract infections particularly in patients with underlying lung disease.

## THE COMMON COLD (CORYZA)

The characteristic symptoms are nasal blockage, discharge and sneezing, often with a sore throat. Malaise, fever and a cough may also be present.

A number of viruses can produce these symptoms. Most common are the rhinoviruses followed by respiratory syncitial virus, parainfluenza virus, Coxsackie virus and coronaviruses. Adenoviruses and influenza viruses can produce the same symptoms although there may be more extensive respiratory tract involvement or general symptoms. In atopic individuals similar symptoms may be produced by allergic phenomena.

Colds are self-limiting and rarely last more than 10 days. Treatment with paracetamol or aspirin helps the fever and general symptoms. Sympathomimetics or anticholinergics can relieve nasal symptoms but usually no treatment is necessary. Where there is underlying lung disease such as bronchiectasis it is often worth giving a prophylactic antibiotic when a cold develops to stop progression to secondary bacterial infection of the lower respiratory tract. Sinusitis and otitis media are other possible complications.

## ACUTE PHARYNGITIS AND TONSILLITIS

Sore throats are caused by viruses in 80–90 per cent of cases. The rest are bacterial infections, usually streptococcal. Rarer causes are *Corynebacterium diphtheriae* causing diphtheria and *Borrelia vincenti*, a Gram-negative spirochaete, causing Vincent's angina in association with poor oral hygiene. Infectious mononucleosis (page 731) produces pharyngitis in 80 per cent of cases. In immunosuppressed patients and with inhaled steroid use oropharyngeal candidiasis may occur.

When streptococci are cultured or suspected antibiotic treatment with penicillin or erythromycin can be given. Candidiasis is treated with local nystatin or amphotericin or with oral fluconazole in recurrent or persistent problems such as those seen in acquired immune deficiency syndrome (AIDS) (page 300).

Local abscesses may complicate such infections. These may be in the draining lymph nodes (cervical abscess) or as a peritonsillar abscess (quinsy) or retropharyngeal abscess. Since such abscesses can compromise the airway they may need to be drained surgically. Streptococcal infection may be followed by the late sensitivity manifestations of rheumatic fever or glomerulonephritis but these are rare in most developed countries today.

## ACUTE EPIGLOTTITIS

This condition is commonest in children but can occur in adults. It is usually caused by *H. influenzae* type B. Attempts to examine the throat may induce respiratory obstruction particularly in children. Increasing numbers of *H. influenzae* produce β-lactamase and are resistant to ampicillin. Treatment should be with ceftazidime, chloramphenicol or augmentin (amoxycillin and clavulanic acid).

## SINUSITIS

In acute sinusitis bacterial infection of the sinuses occurs as a complication of a viral upper respiratory tract infection. *Str. pneumoniae* and *H. influenzae* are the commonest pathogens. In chronic sinusitis the mucosa becomes thickened and drainage is compromised. Infection also occurs when allergic rhinitis results in mucosal swelling and poor drainage. Chronic sinusitis occurs in other conditions when mucociliary clearance is impaired such as cystic fibrosis (page 295) and immotile cilia syndrome (page 293). Occasionally, dental sepsis is the source of the problem.

The maxillary and ethmoidal sinuses are most often involved. Sinus X-rays may show mucosal thickening and sinus opacification or fluid levels. Treatment of sinusitis involves antibiotics and attempts to promote drainage such as temporary use of vasoconstrictor sympathomimetic sprays or appropriate treatment of allergic rhinitis to reduce mucosal swelling. Resistant cases may require surgical drainage.

## ACUTE BRONCHITIS AND TRACHEITIS

These conditions, which cannot be satisfactorily separated clinically, often occur in association with colds or pharyngitis. The usual finding is the addition of a cough, initially dry, but often later productive. Smokers are particularly likely to suffer from acute bronchitis. Viruses or bacteria may be responsible. The tracheal and bronchial mucosa may be damaged with loss of ciliated cells interfering with mucus clearance. The damage to the respiratory epithelium may result in a persistent cough and an increase in airway reactivity (page 279) for weeks or even months afterwards.

## INFLUENZA

Within the generic types influenza A and B there are many subtypes and strains. Outbreaks occur every 1–3 years in winter. The symptoms are coryzal with generalized symptoms of malaise, fever, muscle aches, cough and headache. Symptoms last from a few days to 2 weeks.

Pneumonia may occur either as a primary influenza pneumonia or as a secondary bacterial pneumonia. There is a tendency for staphylococcal secondary infection in influenza epidemics. When patients present with a community-acquired pneumonia during an influenza epidemic it is usually wise to include antistaphylococcal antibiotics in the initial therapy before bacteriology is available. Other complications such as encephalitis and Guillain-Barré syndrome (page 692) are rare.

Paracetamol and aspirin are used for symptomatic control. Amantadine, an antiviral agent, can be used prophylactically in elderly and susceptible patients during an epidemic. Influenza vaccine should be given to such groups in the autumn.

# *Bronchiectasis*

In bronchiectasis areas of the bronchi are chronically dilated. This is associated with damage to the walls of the bronchi through local inflammatory change and destruction of muscle and elastic tissue in the wall.

## AETIOLOGY AND PATHOGENESIS

Bronchiectasis can be part of an inherited condition or acquired. It may be a widespread condition related to a generalized abnormality such as cystic fibrosis (see below) or a result of localized damage such as obstruction by a foreign body. The causes of bronchiectasis are listed in Table 13.13. In some cases large cystic spaces may form in the lung. The distribution depends upon the underlying problem. In cystic fibrosis it is often most marked in the upper lobes. In allergic bronchopulmonary aspergillosis (page 280) more proximal airways are involved.

## CLINICAL FEATURES

The common symptoms are cough and production of infected sputum. In some cases, particularly upper lobe disease where drainage is

**Table 13.13** The causes of bronchiectasis.

| **Inherited conditions** | |
| --- | --- |
| Cystic fibrosis | 1 in 1600 Caucasian births (page 295) |
| Immotile cilia syndrome | Kartagener's syndrome, associated with sinusitis, infertility in males, ectopic pregnancies in females, 50 per cent have situs inversus |
| Young's syndrome | Sinusitis, obstructive azoospermia in males, abnormally thick mucus |
| Hypogammaglobulinaemia | Seen in other immune deficiencies also |
| Sequestrated segment | Disorganized airways and poor drainage in an abnormal area of lung |
| Tracheobronchomegaly | Abnormally dilated trachea and large airways |
| **Acquired conditions** | |
| Childhood infection | Damage from measles, pneumonia or whooping cough. Occurs as part of Macleod's syndrome (Swyer–James in the USA) where infection in the very young leads to a poorly developed lung or area of lung |
| Tuberculosis | Usually upper lobe when less sputum secretion occurs because of drainage by gravity or middle lobe from lymph gland pressure on the bronchus |
| Foreign body | Especially irritant substances such as peanuts. May be no history of choking |
| Allergic bronchopulmonary aspergillosis (ABPA) | Occurs on a background history of asthma (page 280) |

good, there may be little or no sputum. Others produce large quantities of purulent sputum regularly. Haemoptysis is a fairly common complication and occasionally it may be life threatening. Shortness of breath occurs when lung destruction is widespread or where there is associated airflow obstruction with wheezing. Exacerbations occur with increased production of thick, green sputum and fever. In some patients the high persistent bacterial load and associated inflammatory change lead to progressive destruction of the airways and the lung. Such patients need to be identified and treated with vigorous antibiotic regimens. Foetor is often prominent and can lead to severe social and marital problems.

On examination there may be clubbing of the fingers. Signs of any associated medical conditions may be evident. In the chest there may be some wheezes and there are usually coarse crackles spread throughout inspiration.

Complications include progression to right heart failure when lung damage and hypoxia are severe. Other complications are spread of infection elsewhere to the pleural space in an empyema or to the brain in a cerebral abscess. Amyloidosis may occur in bronchiectasis.

## INVESTIGATION

Radiologically there may be cystic changes. The airway walls are thickened and may be seen cut across as tubular shadows or cut longitudinally as parallel 'tramlines'. The changes of bronchiectasis are best seen on CT scans (Fig. 13.14). Bronchograms (Fig. 13.15) involve the introduction of oily contrast medium into the airways. These are done much less often now that CT will show the extent of the problem, but they still produce the best definition and should be used if surgery is contemplated to demonstrate the extent of the problem.

The blood picture may show a raised white count, with an eosinophilia in ABPA. Evidence of a specific underlying cause may be sought. The sweat test identifies cystic fibrosis. In immotile cilia and Young's syndrome in males the sperm count will show abnormal and immotile sperm or absent sperm, respectively. Abnormal cilial ultrastructure and movement can be

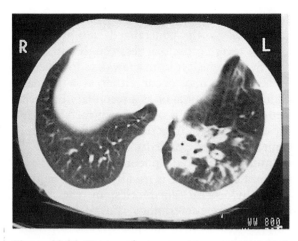

**Figure 13.14** Computed tomographic scan in a case of bronchiectasis showing dilated and thick-walled airways in the left lower lobe.

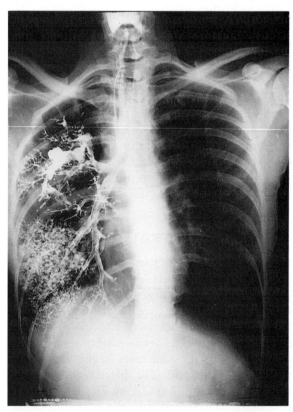

**Figure 13.15** A right bronchogram showing dilated bronchi characteristic of bronchiectasis in the right upper lobe.

seen in sperm tails or nasal mucosal biopsy.

Sputum bacteriology should be examined. The common organisms are *H. influenzae* and *Str. pneumoniae*. *Staphylococcus aureus* and

*Pseudomonas aeruginosa* may also be involved, especially in cystic fibrosis.

## TREATMENT

In general the treatment relies on physiotherapy to clear the sputum and antibiotics to reduce the infective load. Patients must be taught to perform their own physiotherapy adequately. Then those patients who produce sputum should do this once or twice daily. It can be combined with postural drainage of the affected areas. Antibiotics are used for infective exacerbations guided by the sputum sensitivity. Where there is evidence of progressive deterioration of lung function then prolonged high-dose antibiotics should be used. Nebulized antibiotics are used in cystic fibrosis and may find a place in other forms of bronchiectasis. Inhaled bronchodilators should be used for airflow obstruction. In ABPA oral corticosteroids are used to suppress the sensitivity to the fungus.

Surgery used to be performed quite regularly for bronchiectasis. However, the remaining areas of lung are usually affected and recurrent symptoms develop. Surgery is now used rarely when the bronchiectasis is limited and medical treatment fails to control the symptoms.

# Cystic fibrosis

Cystic fibrosis is an inherited disorder in which mucus-secreting glands throughout the body are affected. It is an autosomal recessive condition, 1 in 20 Caucasians carry the gene and the incidence of the homozygous state is around 1 in 1600. Heterozygous carriers are unaffected. Other groups such as Asians have a lower incidence. Great strides have been made in the genetics over the last few years after location of the abnormal gene to chromosome 7, identifying the abnormality in around 85 per cent of cases (page 60). This gene is responsible for the formation of the protein controlling chloride transport across cell membranes.

The glandular problems are related to abnormalities in chloride transport in the cell membrane through a deficiency in cystic fibrosis transmembrane conductance regulator. The diagnosis is made by the finding of high sodium and chloride in induced sweat or by measurement of potential difference across the nasal mucosa.

## CLINICAL FEATURES

There is a great variation in the clinical severity of cystic fibrosis. This variation may be related to particular genetic defects. The median survival time of cystic fibrosis patients is steadily increasing as respiratory and nutritional treatment improve. Children born now are estimated to have a median survival into the forties and this is likely to be extended by transplantation and gene therapy.

The major areas affected are the lungs and the gastrointestinal tract (Table 13.14). In the lungs bronchiectasis develops (Fig. 13.16) with *Staph. aureus* or *H. influenzae* in younger patients and a mucoid form of *P. aeruginosa* in older patients. A more damaging organism, *P. cepacia*, is associated with deterioration and can spread between patients. Bronchial reactivity (page 279) and airflow obstruction are common and Aspergillus often grows in the sputum. Sinusitis is often troublesome and clubbing usually develops.

**Table 13.14** The clinical manifestations of cystic fibrosis.

**Newborn**
Meconium ileus

**Infant**
Rectal prolapse
Failure to thrive
Recurrent chest infections

Atelectasis

**Child and young adult**
Bronchiectasis
Clubbing
Breathlessness

Pneumothorax
Haemoptysis
Nasal polyps
Malabsorption

Intestinal obstruction (meconium ileus equivalent)
Portal hypertension
Excess sodium loss in sweat
Diabetes mellitus

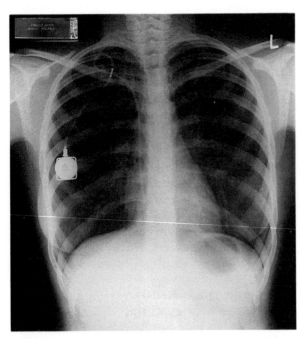

**Figure 13.16** Chest X-ray in a case of cystic fibrosis showing upper zone shadowing of bronchiectasis with a 'portacath' for access to give intravenous antibiotics.

Haemoptysis often occurs with infective exacerbations and occasionally it may be massive and life threatening. There is an increased incidence of pneumothorax.

In infants meconium ileus produces intestinal obstruction. Obstruction may also occur in adults through a mixture of thick secretions and poorly digested food. Malabsorption occurs because of the deficiency in pancreatic enzymes leading to steatorrhoea (page 333), generally poor nutrition and deficiencies of fat-soluble vitamins. Cirrhosis of the liver occurs and diabetes may develop from pancreatic damage. In very hot conditions sweating may lead to excessive salt loss.

Males are nearly always infertile.

## TREATMENT

Lung disease is treated by regular physiotherapy and by intermittent antibiotics. In patients who have been colonized by *P. aeruginosa* regular courses of antipseudomonal antibiotics three or four times a year are usually necessary. Eventually lung destruction leads to cor pulmonale.

Oxygen therapy may help and lung transplantation should be considered.

Careful attention to nutrition is important. Patients with cystic fibrosis need to take in 50 per cent more calories than normal to maintain their nutrition. High calorie supplements may help and fat-soluble vitamins should be prescribed. Pancreatic enzyme supplements allow patients to take a normal diet, restriction of fat intake makes it difficult to take in enough calories. In some patients a gastrostomy tube is necessary to boost the intake overnight.

Counselling about genetics and fertility is important for patients and families. Prenatal diagnosis of cystic fibrosis is often possible and modern techniques allow the genetic material of a fertilized embryo to be checked at the 8 cell stage before implantation. Pregnancy often leads to deterioration in the lung function of female patients although many patients have had healthy children without harm. The recent advances in the genetics of cystic fibrosis have led to trials of specific gene therapy given by inhalation.

# *Pneumonia*

Pneumonia is infection of the lung tissue itself, producing consolidation in which air in the alveoli is replaced by exudate consisting of fluid, fibrin, white cells, red cells and organisms. Pneumonia is a common cause of death from death certificate statistics. Much of this relates to a terminal illness in patients ill for other reasons. This form of pneumonia is bronchopneumonia where the infection is scattered throughout the lung. In contrast to this is lobar pneumonia where the consolidation of the lung is confined by the anatomical boundaries of the fissures.

An alternative classification which is of more practical use is:

1 Community-acquired pneumonia
2 Hospital-acquired pneumonia
3 Pneumonia in the immunocompromised host

Some other forms of pneumonia such as aspiration pneumonia and from non-infectious causes (e.g. eosinophilic pneumonia) occur less frequently.

## COMMUNITY-ACQUIRED PNEUMONIA

The distribution of the pathogens in community-acquired pneumonia varies with geography and time. The commonest pathogen is *Str. pneumoniae* which makes up 50 per cent or more of cases with an identified pathogen in most series. In most series no organism is identified in 30–40 per cent of cases. Many of these are probably *Str. pneumoniae* obscured by previous antibiotic treatment. Common pathogens are shown in Table 13.15.

**Table 13.15** Common causes of commuinity-acquired pneumonia.

| Cause | Per cent |
| --- | --- |
| Streptococcus pneumoniae | 50 |
| Mycoplasma pneumoniae | 15 |
| Viruses | 14 |
| Haemophilus influenzae | 10 |
| Legionella pneumophilia | 5 |
| Staphylococcus aureus | 4 |
| Chlamydia | 3 |

## *Investigation of community-acquired pneumonia*

There may be specific features of the clinical picture which point towards a particular organism or group of organisms. These are described below. The following investigations are useful in establishing the organism responsible.

1 Gram stain of sputum. A good specimen is necessary. This may show typical Gram-positive cocci and will then help to limit initial antibiotic therapy.
2 Sputum culture. This helps in dealing with patients who do not respond adequately to the initial choice of antibiotic.
3 Blood culture. This is positive in around 20 per cent of bacterial pneumonias. Cultures should be performed before antibiotics are started.
4 Pleural fluid. Fluid may develop as a result of inflammation in adjacent lung or as infected fluid. When response to treatment and resolution of temperature is not adequate the pleural fluid should be sampled. In early

infection a low pH or low sugar in the fluid may be suggestive before culture is available.
5 Serological tests. Such tests are useful for 'atypical pneumonias' such as Legionella and Mycoplasma. Pneumococcal antigen appears in the sputum in 80 per cent of cases, urine in 40 per cent and serum in 20 per cent.
6 Transtracheal aspiration. This can avoid oral contamination of specimens and should be considered in difficult cases. Material can also be obtained by bronchoscopic or percutaneous aspiration.

Some general principles of management apply to most pneumonias:

1 Fluids. Patients may be dry because of fever and hyperventilation.
2 Analgesia. Adequate pain relief is essential to allow the patient to breathe deeply and to cough.
3 Oxygen. This should be given freely unless there is a suggestion of underlying long-standing airflow obstruction.
4 Antibiotics. These usually have to be started blindly before any bacteriological information is available. The antibiotic should cover *Str. pneumoniae* and be broadened to cover 'atypicals' (Mycoplasma, Legionella etc.) if they are suggested by the story. In an influenza epidemic staphylococci should be covered by the addition of flucloxacillin. In mild cases amoxycillin can be used, or erythromycin in penicillin-sensitive patients. In more severe cases treatment should start with amoxycillin or cefuroxime and erythromycin. Local patterns of organisms and epidemics such as Mycoplasma should influence the choice of antibiotic.

## *Specific organisms*

### *Streptococcus pneumoniae*

*Streptococcus pneumoniae* is a gram-positive coccus with many serotypes based on variation in the polysaccharide capsule. It is most common in the winter and early spring. The onset of the condition is quite sudden although there may be a preceding sore throat or upper respiratory tract infection. The condition is usually lobar in distribution. Early features are fever, rigors, cough, tachypnoea and pleuritic chest pain. Initially there may be no sputum and the origin of the fever may be uncertain, particularly as the pain can be abdominal. Herpes simplex occurs on the lips in around one-third of cases. Red or rusty sputum may be coughed up showing the presence of red cells in the alveoli.

The typical signs of pneumonia may be present: reduced expansion, dullness to percussion, increased tactile vocal fremitus and bronchial breathing. The chest X-ray shows lobar or segmental consolidation (Fig. 13.17). Pleural effusions are common but empyemas rare.

A Gram stain of sputum with plentiful pneumococci would allow specific therapy but is only found in a minority of cases. Sputum culture is less specific since carriage in the upper airway is common. Pneumococcal antigen can be detected in blood, urine or sputum.

Where a specific diagnosis has been made treatment can be restricted to penicillin intravenously. Penicillin resistance is seen in some countries such as South Africa but has not been a significant problem in the UK.

Pneumococcal vaccine is available and should be given to those who are going to have a splenectomy or to risk groups such as those with chronic lung disease.

### Mycoplasma pneumoniae

This is the smallest free-living organism. It does not have a rigid cell wall so antibiotics such as penicillin are ineffective. Mycoplasma affects older children and young adults with epidemics every 3–4 years and a low infection rate in between. Droplet spread occurs easily in close communities.

There may be just upper respiratory symptoms without pneumonia. Ear pain is a common symptom and joint pains, muscle aches and a dry cough often precede pneumonia for days or weeks. Patchy shadowing occurs on the chest X-ray with, occasionally, pleural effusions. Cold agglutinins are found in the blood in more than 50 per cent of cases and less often produce problems with haemolytic anaemia. Unlike pneumococcal pneumonia the white count is usually normal. Cardiac, neurological and gastrointestinal manifestations are occasionally seen.

The diagnosis is made by a rise in titres of complement-fixing antibodies, cold agglutinins may help but are not specific.

Treatment is with erythromycin or tetracycline.

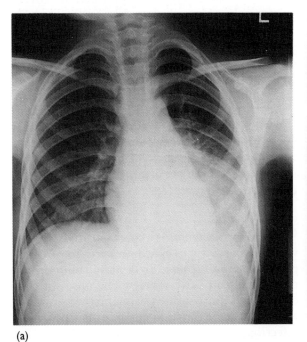

(a)

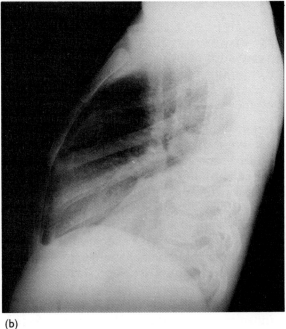

(b)

**Figure 13.17** (a) Posteroanterior and (b) lateral X-rays in a child with left lower lobe pneumonia. The consolidation is limited by the oblique fissure. In the posteroanterior view the consolidated left lower lobe obscures the left hemidiaphragm but the left heart border is still seen against the air-containing lingula.

*Viruses*

Influenza virus is the commonest respiratory virus causing pneumonia. Spontaneous antigenic change by the virus means that recurrent infections occur. The incubation period is 1–2 days. A diffuse spreading infiltrate is seen on the chest X-ray. Antiviral agents such as amantadine may have some beneficial effect and influenza vaccination is reasonably effective until mutation of the virus escapes the control. It is recommended for old people and those with an underlying respiratory disorder.

*Haemophilus influenzae*

*Haemophilus influenza* is a small Gram-negative pleomorphic bacillus of varying morphology. *Haemophilus influenzae* and *H. parainfluenzae* can cause problems. Patients with chronic lung disease often carry Haemophilus and a confident diagnosis relies on blood culture or isolation from some other tissue fluid. Amoxycillin resistance is increasing and Augmentin (amoxycillin + clavulanic acid), cefuroxime and ciprofloxacin are alternatives.

A secondary bacterial infection may occur and in some epidemics there is a particular tendency to develop staphylococcal pneumonia.

*Legionella pneumophila*

*Legionella pneumophila* was first diagnosed in 1976, but stored serum has shown cases going back 30 years earlier. It is a Gram-negative bacillus with exacting growing requirements. The organism is widespread in water and may be disseminated by droplet spread from domestic or commercial water systems.

Clinically Legionella infection may produce pneumonia (Legionnaire's disease) or a 'flu-like illness without pneumonia (Pontiac fever). Pneumonia occurs in adults often with a mild underlying susceptibility such as diabetes, immunosuppression or alcoholism. The incubation period is up to 2 weeks. The pneumonia may be very severe and associated features such as confusion, diarrhoea, abdominal pain, hepatic and renal dysfunction, low albumin, raised creatine phosphokinase (CPK) and hyponatraemia, which can occur with any pneumonia, are more common with Legionella. The X-ray pattern is variable. The diagnosis is serological or by fluorescent staining or isolation of the organism.

Treatment is with erythromycin. Alternative antibiotics which seem to be effective are rifampicin and ciprofloxacin.

*Staphylococcus aureus*

Staphylococci account for <5 per cent of community-acquired pneumonias but the illness carries a high mortality of 30 per cent or more. There is a tendency for it to occur in influenza epidemics. There is a necrotic tissue reaction which leads to cavity formation in the lung.

Treatment is with flucloxacillin together with another antistaphylococcal agent such as fusidic acid.

*Chlamydia psittaci*

Around 50 per cent of patients give a history of significant contact with birds such as parrots, budgerigars and pigeons. Chlamydia are small intracellular bacteria. There is often a history of general symptoms such as myalgia, fever and headache before the respiratory symptoms are prominent. The white count is often normal.

Treatment is with tetracycline, erythromycin, rifampicin or chloramphenicol.

*Coxiella burnetii*

Q fever can cause pneumonia. Complications include endocarditis.

Treatment is with a prolonged course of erythromycin or tetracycline.

## HOSPITAL-ACQUIRED (NOSOCOMIAL) PNEUMONIA

Nosocomial pneumonia develops in patients who are not admitted initially with chest infections. The pattern of infection is very different to that of community-acquired pneumonia (Table 13.16).

**Table 13.16** Organisms causing hospital-acquired pneumonia.

|  | Per cent |
|---|---|
| **Gram-negative bacteria** | 60 |
| Klebsiella species | |
| Pseudomonas aeruginosa | |
| Escherichia coli | |
| **Gram-positive bacteria** | |
| Staphylococcus aureus | 15 |
| Streptococcus pneumoniae | 8 |
| Anaerobes | 9 |
| Fungi | 2 |
| Others | 6 |

Ill patients in hospital, particularly in intensive care units, have their upper airway colonized by Gram-negative organisms. This makes it difficult to assess the significance of organisms in the sputum of such patients.

Klebsiella pneumonia has a tendency to cavitate and to produce enlargement of the affected lobe with bowing of the adjacent fissure.

The choice of antibiotics will depend on the typical local organisms and sensitivities. Advice should be taken from the microbiology laboratory.

## Aspiration pneumonia

Aspiration occurs as a dramatic event in some cases or as minor events in ill patients, especially those with a depressed level of consciousness and with nasogastric tubes in place. The problems with aspiration relate to obstruction by foreign material in the bronchial tree, chemical pneumonitis from the acidic fluid and infection particularly with anaerobic organisms. The severity of the problem is closely related to the degree of acidity of the aspirated fluid.

Corticosteroids are of no benefit in the management of aspiration and are probably harmful. There is no evidence that prophylactic antibiotics help although they are widely used. An alternative approach is to wait, take appropriate cultures and use antibiotics if infection is evident. Appropriate blind therapy would be amoxycillin and metronidazole.

## PNEUMONIA IN THE IMMUNOCOMPROMISED HOST

This has become a more important area with the emergence of acquired immune deficiency syndrome (AIDS). In the past iatrogenic immunosuppression after transplantation and those treated with cytotoxic drugs were the usual patients. The pattern of disease varies between these groups. In patients treated with immunosuppressants and cytotoxic drugs respiratory infections are most often caused by the usual organisms which cause pneumonia even though there is an increased incidence of unusual organisms such as fungi and viruses. In AIDS, although infections with common organisms are increased most infections are with unusual organisms particularly pneumonia caused by *Pneumocystis carinii*.

After treatment with cytotoxic or immunosuppressant drugs lung shadowing may be related to a number of different causes (Table 13.17).

In immunosuppressed patients without human immunodeficiency virus (HIV) infection who develop chest signs cultures should be taken and treatment started with broad-spectrum antibiotics. Failure of response should lead to further investigation often with bronchoscopy and alveolar lavage. Broadening of therapy with antifungal, antiviral or antituberculous therapy should be determined by the investigations, the clinical circumstances and local experience.

In AIDS first lung infections are often *P. carinii* and, if this is suspected because of a history of a week or more of dry cough, low $PaO_2$, desaturation on exercise, typical chest X-ray (Figs 13.18 and 13.19) or faster isotope transfer on diethylenetriaminepenta acetate (DTPA) scan then treatment should be started. This is usually high-dose cotrimoxazole intravenously. Around 50 per cent of patients develop adverse effects such as rashes or bone marrow depression. Intravenous pentamidine is an alternative treatment. Prophylaxis against further episodes of Pneumocystis infection will be needed subsequently with cotrimoxazole or nebulized pentamidine. Other causes of chest involvement in HIV infection are tuberculosis,

**Table 13.17** Causes of lung shadowing in patients treated with cytotoxic or immunosuppressant drugs.

A common organism which may give severe illness or respond poorly
An unusual organism (e.g. *Pneumocystis carinii*, Aspergillus, cytomegalovirus)
Toxic drug reaction (e.g. Busulphan)
Lung haemorrhage (thrombocytopenia from bone marrow suppression)
Infiltration by underlying disease (e.g. leukaemia under treatment)
Radiation fibrosis
Heart failure (overload in renal patients, cardiac toxicity)
Pulmonary embolism

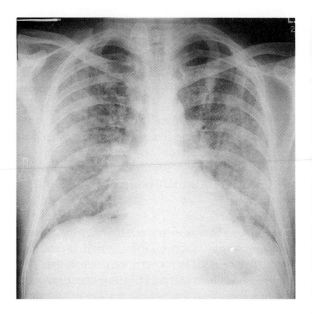

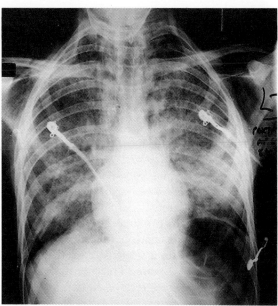

**Figure 13.18** Chest X-ray of a man with AIDS and *Pneumocystis carinii* pneumonia showing diffuse nodular shadowing throughout the lung fields.

**Figure 13.19** Chest X-ray in a severe case of *Pneumocystis carninii* pneumonia with respiratory failure. There is a small left-sided pneumothorax and surgical emphysema shown by the presence of air in the soft tissues most easily seen over the scapulae.

other mycobacteria, common bacteria, cyto-megalovirus and Kaposi's sarcoma.

# Fungal infection

Fungal infection is most often seen in immuno-suppressed patients (see above and page 762). *Aspergillus fumigatus* causes an invasive, destructive lung disease which is often fatal in such patients. In asthmatic patients a sensitivity to Aspergillus may cause problems (page 280) and Aspergillus may colonize cavities in the lung where it grows as a ball of fungus. These mycetomas or aspergillomas (Fig. 13.20) often cause haemoptysis from inflammation in the cavity wall but rarely invade lung tissue. The only successful treatment is surgical resection.

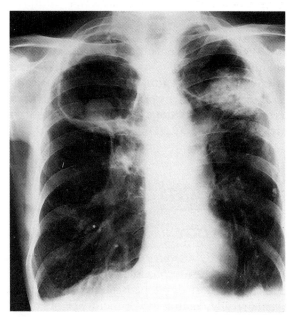

**Figure 13.20** Cavitation at both apices in a case of old tuberculosis. Mycetomas are developing in both of the cavities.

## MYCOBACTERIAL DISEASE

# Atypical mycobacteria

The main Mycobacterium causing disease in humans is *Mycobacterium tuberculosis*. Other organisms, sometimes known as atypical mycobacteria, such as *M. kansasii* and *M. xenopi* most often colonize previously damaged areas of lung. There they tend to produce gradually progressive disease. The isolation of such organisms from the sputum on a single occasion does not necessarily imply disease. Treatment should be given if there is progressive lung damage or suspicious symptoms in association with repeated isolation of the organism from the sputum. *In vitro* sensitivity testing may be unreliable in assessing which drugs to use for *M. kansasii* and *M. xenopi* which often respond to conventional antituberculous therapy.

*Mycobacterium avium intracellulare* complex (MAI/MAC) has emerged as an important pathogen in AIDS. The lung is only part of a more general involvement and MAI can often be isolated from the blood. Treatment has been tried with various regimens but toxicity is high and current treatment provides little more than temporary suppression when MAI occurs in patients with AIDS.

# Tuberculosis

## EPIDEMIOLOGY

*Mycobacterium tuberculosis* is much the most important of the mycobacteria in humans. In the UK and in most developed countries there has been a steady decline in the incidence of tuberculosis over the last century. In the last few years the incidence has been steady or beginning to rise. Many cases now are found in Asian immigrants, alcoholics and those with HIV infection. In some less developed countries tuberculosis remains a considerable problem and it is a major pathogen in HIV-infected individuals in Africa.

## PATHOLOGY

*Mycobacterium tuberculosis* grows slowly in suitable media taking 4–6 weeks before culture can be confirmed. Direct staining of smears of sputum is positive with >5000 organisms per ml but culture is usually positive with >100 per ml.

Histologically the body's reaction to the tubercle bacillus is a granulomatous inflammation involving macrophages which often fuse into giant cells. The centres of granulomas undergo caseous necrosis and healing often involves calcification.

Spread within the body may be by way of lymphatics or airways or even blood-borne spread to produce widely distributed 'miliary' lesions (Fig. 13.21) (milia = millet seeds).

## CLINICAL FEATURES

General clinical features of tuberculosis are fever, weight loss, profuse sweating at night. In

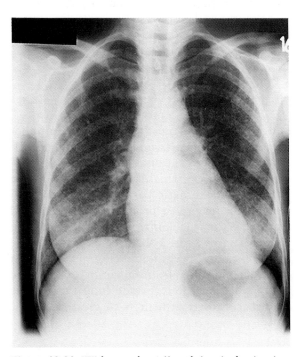

**Figure 13.21** Widespread small nodular shadowing in a woman with miliary tuberculosis.

the elderly symptoms may be just non-specific malaise. The erythrocyte sedimentation rate (ESR) is often raised and anaemia, hyponatraemia and hypercalcaemia occur in a minority of cases.

## Primary tuberculosis

The first exposure to tubercle bacilli produces a *primary* infection usually in children and young adults. Infection is by droplet spread. There is a small peripheral area of lung involvement (Ghon focus) most often in the middle or lower lobes. A granuloma forms and spread occurs to the draining hilar lymph nodes which enlarge.

These primary lesions usually heal as immunity develops over 6–12 weeks, but they may leave an area of calcification in the lung and hilar nodes. In most cases these events occur with few if any symptoms. Possible complications of the primary infection are:

1 Miliary spread to lungs, meninges etc. through erosion into a blood vessel (Fig. 13.21).
2 Local progression to produce a larger mass, a tuberculoma, or even cavitating disease
3 Bronchial compression from enlarged nodes
4 Pleural or pericardial effusion

## Post-primary tuberculosis

Organisms from the original infection can remain viable in healed lesions and cause a recurrence of the disease years later. This is most commonly pulmonary disease involving the apices of the lungs and progressing to cavitation. Untreated this may progress to a widespread tuberculous bronchopneumonia. The lung is often permanently damaged to leave fibrosed upper lobes (Fig. 13.22), bronchiectasis and cavities (Fig. 13.20).

Other organs may be involved in post-primary tuberculosis. The commonest extra-pulmonary involvement is in lymph nodes in the mediastinum and the neck. Infection in bones, kidneys and the gastrointestinal tract are less common but any organ may be involved.

Diagnosis relies on isolation of the organism or finding of the typical histology on biopsy. A positive intradermal skin test with tuberculin produces an area of induration within 72 hours (tuberculin purified protein derivative is pro-

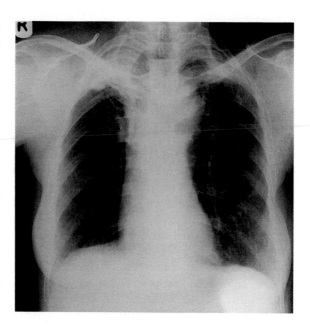

**Figure 13.22** Contraction of both upper lobes by fibrosis in a case of old healed tuberculosis. The fibrosis is greater on the right resulting in deviation of the trachea to the right side.

duced from heat-treated products of growth of the organism and given by a multipuncture Heaf gun in large vaccination programmes). A positive reaction occurs in those who have received bacille Calmette-Guérin (BCG) (page 304). Strongly positive skin reactions may help in pointing towards a diagnosis of tuberculosis but in severely ill or immunosuppressed patients the skin test may be negative. In some circumstances such as tuberculous meningitis identification of the organism may be difficult and, because of the seriousness of the disease, treatment may need to be started when there is a reasonable degree of suspicion.

## TREATMENT

Organisms may stay intracellularly or survive within macrophages. In caseating areas they divide slowly. Prolonged treatment with a number of drugs is necessary to kill organisms in all these situations and to avoid the development of resistance.

The length of regimens has come down over the last 20 years as more effective drugs have been developed. A 6 month regimen is now possible using rifampicin, isoniazid and pyrazinamide for the first 2 months. At this stage sensitivities will often be available and if the organism is sensitive and the patient is improving rifampicin and isoniazid are continued alone for the last 4 months. Details of the individual drugs are shown in Table 13.18.

The commonest cause of failure to respond is poor compliance with treatment. This may be helped by supervised twice-weekly regimens and by preparations which combine rifampicin and isoniazid. Drug resistance occurs in around 2 per cent of isolates in the UK but in larger numbers in the Far East and Africa. In the USA great problems with drug resistance are emerging, primarily in HIV-infected patients.

Extrapulmonary tuberculosis can be treated in the same way as pulmonary disease, and tuberculosis in HIV-infected patients usually responds well to the same drugs. Most patients do not need to be admitted to hospital for treatment. After about 1 week of chemotherapy they are not likely to be an infectious risk to others although this should be confirmed by sputum examination and culture if they are in close contact with vulnerable groups.

Corticosteroids provide a useful adjunct to treatment in some circumstances. They should only be started in conjunction with adequate antituberculous chemotherapy. They have been found to be useful in pleural, pericardial and meningeal disease and may be helpful in the very debilitated patient.

## PREVENTION

Tuberculosis is a notifiable disease in the UK. After notification close contacts are traced and may be investigated by chest X-ray and tuberculin test. This remains an important part of the management of tuberculosis.

In the UK a vaccine, bacille Calmette-Guérin (BCG), has been given at the age of 13 since the early 1950s. It is a live attenuated strain derived from *Mycobacterium bovis* and should not be given to immunosuppressed subjects. Infants whose parents come from high-risk areas should be vaccinated soon after birth. The BCG vaccine is 80 per cent effective in the UK in protecting against tuberculosis and severe disease is unusual after its use. In countries such as the USA where BCG is not used routinely the tuberculin test has a greater place as a diagnostic test. The reduction in tuberculosis in many developed countries has raised doubts about the cost-effectiveness of continuation of BCG vaccination. At present there are around 5000 cases of tuberculosis each year in England and Wales.

**Table 13.18** Antituberculous drugs.

| Drug | Dose/day | Adverse effects |
|---|---|---|
| Rifampicin | <50 kg:450 mg<br>>50 kg:600 mg | Orange/red colouration of urine + secretions<br>Hepatic enzyme induction (reduces anticoagulant effects, anticonvulsant levels, effectiveness of oral contraceptive etc.)<br>Hepatitis<br>Thrombocytopenia<br>Rifampicin 'flu' } with intermittent<br>Renal failure } treatment |
| Isoniazid | 300 mg | Peripheral neuropathy (pyridoxine deficiency, avoided by supplements if nutrition is poor)<br>Hepatotoxicity<br>Hypersensitivity |
| Pyrazinamide | 20–30 mg/kg | Hepatotoxicity<br>Diarrhoea, anorexia, vomiting<br>Hyperuricaemia, occasionally gout |
| Ethambutol | 15 mg/kg | Optic neuritis<br>Rashes |
| Streptomycin | 750–1000 mg i.m. | Eighth nerve toxicity |

# PULMONARY VASCULAR DISEASE

Pulmonary hypertension develops as a response to hypoxia in chronic lung disease (page 286). The other major cause of pulmonary vascular disease is pulmonary embolism. Emboli are usually detached pieces of thrombus but may consist of tumour, fat, air or injected material.

## Pulmonary thromboembolism

Thrombi can form *in situ* in the pulmonary vessels but most are emboli from the peripheral veins, mainly in the leg. There may be evidence of deep vein thrombosis but this is not necessarily clinically evident. Other less common causes of embolism include air, tumour, amniotic fluid and fat.

### CLINICAL FEATURES

The severity of pulmonary embolism is determined largely by the extent of pulmonary vascular obstruction and the associated increase in pulmonary artery pressure. The combination of chest pain, breathlessness and haemoptysis is the commonest presentation with sudden onset of the breathlessness. Pulmonary infarction occurs in around 10 per cent of cases and causes pleuritic chest pain. Haemoptysis may follow. A pleural rub may be present with tachycardia and elevated jugular venous pressure in the acute stage but there may be few if any signs. Hypoxia is usual from ventilation–perfusion mismatch and the reduction in cardiac output. In a minority of cases the ECG shows signs of right heart strain with P pulmonale, an S wave in lead I, a narrow Q in lead III with T wave inversion (SIQ3T3). The chest X-ray is usually normal but may show a small pleural effusion, small areas of collapse, consolidated lung in an infarcted area or areas of vessel loss. Lung scanning (Fig. 13.23) will show lack of perfusion with maintained ventilation (page 109). The definitive investigation is pulmonary arteriography but it is too invasive for routine use (Fig. 13.24).

Massive pulmonary embolism produces a reduction of cardiac output which may lead to death. Some patients survive with a low output and this small group may benefit from surgical

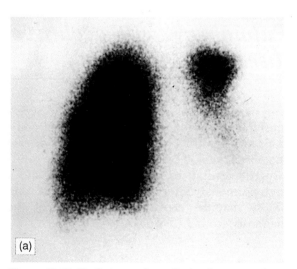
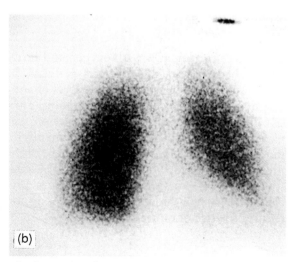

**Figure 13.23** Perfusion and ventilation lung scans in a case of pulmonary embolism. (a) The perfusion scan shows a defect in the middle and lower parts of the left lung field. (b) These areas are ventilated although the presence of the heart gives an area of decreased ventilation and perfusion medially at the left base in these anterior views.

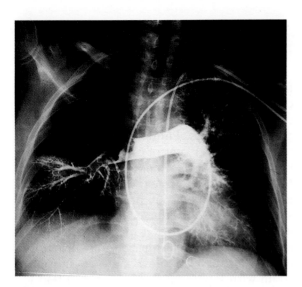

**Figure 13.24** Pulmonary arteriogram showing a pulmonary embolus in the right main pulmonary artery. The embolus prevents contrast from filling the main pulmonary artery and blocks any flow to the upper lobe.

removal of emboli or infusion of thrombolytic agents.

Individual small emboli may not cause symptoms but recurrent emboli may gradually occlude the pulmonary circulation with presentation as pulmonary hypertension and right heart failure. Signs may include a left parasternal heave, a loud pulmonary second sound, raised jugular venous pressure and tricuspid regurgitation.

### TREATMENT

Immediate treatment is with oxygen and intravenous heparin, 30–40 000 units per day, by continuous infusion, checking the level of anticoagulation with the kaolin cephalin time (KCT). After 3–4 days of anticoagulation, the patient can be transferred to warfarin, maintaining the appropriate level by measurement of the prothrombin time (PT). This should be continued for 3–6 months. Anticoagulation prevents extension of thrombus within the lung and reduces the risk of further thromboembolism. If

there is an obvious reason for the thrombosis which has now resolved the warfarin can then be stopped. In some patients there is a state of increased coagulability, for example, systemic lupus erythematosus (SLE) (page 571) and hereditary deficiencies (page 646). Anticoagulation will then need to be maintained for life.

## Primary pulmonary hypertension

This is a rare condition usually seen in young females. The clinical features are of increasing breathlessness and right heart failure. Investigations show hypoxia, reduced gas transfer and a high pulmonary artery pressure. Cardiac output is reduced in contrast to the usual situation in cor pulmonale. Recurrent pulmonary emboli must be ruled out in the diagnosis and this usually requires a pulmonary arteriogram. Even then there may be some doubt, in which case anticoagulants should be used.

Vasodilators such as hydralazine and prostacyclin have a temporary effect and heart–lung transplantation has been successful in a number of cases.

## Pulmonary veno-occlusive disease

This is rarer than primary pulmonary hypertension but the differentiation of the two conditions may be difficult. In veno-occlusive disease the obstruction is beyond the pulmonary capillary bed leading to pulmonary oedema and a high pulmonary artery wedge pressure but lung biopsy may be necessary to be sure of the diagnosis.

# LUNG TUMOURS

Carcinoma of the lung provides the commonest cause of death from malignant disease in the UK. This is the result of high levels of cigarette smoking. As these decline in developed countries rates of carcinoma of the lung will begin to fall. However, the increasing prevalence of cigarette smoking in developing countries will lead to the emergence of lung cancer in new areas. While carcinoma of the lung is the commonest lung tumour (over 90 per cent) other sorts of tumour are found within the thorax (Table 13.19).

## Benign tumours

Lipomas, fibromas, neural tumours and those from other origins can all occur within the chest but they are all rare. The commonest benign tumours are hamartomas which contain disorganized tissue derived mainly from cartilage and muscle. They are more common in males, grow slowly and rarely produce symptoms. Computed tomographic scanning or tomography may show speckled calcification within

**Table 13.19** Intrathoracic tumours.

Benign tumours
  Hamartomas
  Rare tumours of connective tissue

Carcinoid

Carcinoma of the lung
  Squamous
  Adenocarcinoma
  Large cell
  Small cell
  Alveolar cell carcinoma

Secondary tumours

Pleural tumours
  Fibroma
  Direct spread from lung cancer
  Secondary
  Malignant mesothelioma

the lesion. The common problem is differentiation from a malignant tumour. This may lead to operation when the hamartoma can usually be removed without resection of lung tissue.

## Carcinoid tumour

Carcinoid tumours make up the majority of the lesions sometimes called adenomas. This is an inappropriate term since they are malignant tumours, although usually of low grade. They often occur in young to middle-aged patients and usually present as an obstructive lesion causing segmental or lobar collapse or with haemoptysis. Most tumours are visible at bronchoscopy but may bleed excessively on biopsy. Features of the carcinoid syndrome (page 409) are rare and usually only occur after metastasis to the liver has occurred.

## Bronchial carcinoma

### AETIOLOGY

Tobacco smoke is by far the most important aetiological factor and even 'passive smoking' is associated with a slight increase in the risk. Industrial pollution probably plays a role. Occupational exposure to asbestos increases the incidence, particularly in smokers. Other occupational factors such as mining radioactive ores and working with dyes are infrequent. Adenocarcinoma of the lung is more common in smokers but the relationship is weaker than in other histological types (2:1 versus >10:1).

### PATHOLOGY

The four main types of carcinoma of the bronchus occur in the proportions shown in Table 13.20.

**Table 13.20** Pathological types of bronchial carcinoma.

|  | Per cent |
|---|---|
| Squamous | 45 |
| Adenocarcinoma | 20 |
| Small cell undifferentiated (oat cell) | 20 |
| Large cell undifferentiated | 15 |

Cell doubling times are three times faster for small cell undifferentiated tumours than for other cell types. Tumours may contain more than one cell type, particularly adenosquamous tumours. Material for cytology can be obtained from good quality sputum specimens. Biopsy specimens are obtained by bronchoscopic biopsy or by transthoracic needle biopsy.

## CLINICAL FEATURES

Bronchial carcinoma can present with general features of malignancy, local chest symptoms, evidence of local spread, metastases or non-metastatic distant manifestations.

General symptoms of malignancy are loss of appetite and weight, general tiredness and, less often, fever and anaemia.

Local chest symptoms are cough, haemoptysis and shortness of breath secondary to airway obstruction. Chest pain implies involvement of the pleura either by infection distal to obstruction or by direct invasion.

Detection of invasion locally within the chest is important since it is generally a signal of inoperability (Fig. 13.25 and Table 13.21).

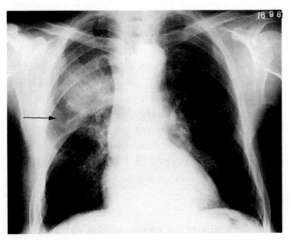

**Figure 13.25** Carcinoma of the bronchus eroding the posterior aspect of the sixth rib (arrowed) on the right side.

**Table 13.21** Structures commonly invaded locally in the chest in bronchial carcinoma.

| Structure | Effect |
|---|---|
| **Nerves** | |
| Phrenic | Raised hemidiaphragm |
| Recurrent laryngeal | Weak voice, difficulty coughing |
| Sympathetic chain | Horner's syndrome (page 665) |
| Brachial plexus (Pancoast tumour) | Pain, neurological signs in the arm |
| **Cardiovascular** | |
| Superior vena caval obstruction | Distended jugular veins, congested face |
| Pericardium | Pericarditis, arrhythmias |
| **Other structures** | |
| Oesophagus | Dysphagia |
| Chest wall | Pain |

Pleural effusions may be related to distal infection or to pleural and chest wall invasion. In the latter case they are often blood stained and malignant cells can be found on aspiration.

Distant metastases occur frequently and are often present by the time of diagnosis, particularly with small cell undifferentiated tumours. The commonest sites for metastases are local lymph nodes, liver, bone, brain, skin and adrenals. Metastases to the lymph nodes, liver and adrenals do not usually cause clinical symptoms and need to be sought specifically if surgery is contemplated. Pulmonary lymphatic obstruction by bronchial or other carcinomas can lead to severe breathlessness – lymphangitis carcinomatosa.

Non-metastatic distant manifestations are related to substances secreted by the tumour cells. Many of these are hormones and most are related to small cell undifferentiated carcinomas (Table 13.22). The commonest hormonal manifestation is the syndrome of inappropriate secretion of antidiuretic hormone (SIADH). This occurs in a variety of lung conditions including pneumonia. The serum sodium, urea and osmolarity are low while the urine osmolarity remains inappropriately high. Oedema is uncommon and the symptoms of tiredness, reduced level of consciousness and even fits are related to the hyponatraemia. Hypercalcaemia is

**Table 13.22** Non-metastatic manifestations of carcinoma of the lung.

**General**
Weight loss
Clubbing
Hypertrophic pulmonary osteoarthropathy
Anaemia
Venous thrombosis, thrombophlebitis

**Endocrine**
Syndrome of inappropriate antidiuretic hormone
  secretion
Cushing's syndrome (adrenocorticotrophic hormone
  secretion)
Gynaecomastia
Hypercalcaemia
Hyperthyroidism

**Neuromuscular**
Peripheral neuropathy
Myasthenic syndrome (Eaton–Lambert)
Cerebellar degeneration
Dermatomyositis

**Renal**
Nephrotic syndrome

most common in squamous tumours when it might be caused by bony secondaries or secretion of a factor which stimulates osteoclasts and has parathyroid-like activity.

**Clubbing** occurs in around 20 per cent of squamous carcinomas but only rarely in small cell tumours. Less common is **hypertrophic pulmonary osteoarthropathy (HPOA)** in which the periosteum is elevated and duplicated around the end of the long bones. It is a cause of severe tenderness, swelling and pain around the ankles and the wrist.

## DIAGNOSIS

The diagnosis of carcinoma of the bronchus can often be inferred from the chest X-ray especially if there is evidence of local invasion of bone or mediastinum. It is usual to confirm the diagnosis by sputum cytology or biopsy at bronchoscopy or transcutaneous needle aspiration. If metastases are already present it may be possible to biopsy these.

## TREATMENT

The main hope for cure of carcinoma of the bronchus is surgery. Complete resection of the tumour by lobectomy or pneumonectomy results in a 5-year survival rate of around 40 per cent. No other treatment approaches this success rate.

### Surgery

Only around 20 per cent of patients turn out to be suitable for surgical intervention. Surgery is contraindicated if lung function is too poor to withstand resection, local invasion of the mediastinum has occurred or distant metastases are present.

Lung function is assessed objectively (page 269) and subjectively. This must be interpreted with caution since blockage of a bronchus and collapse of a lobe or lung may have effectively removed as much lung function as the proposed surgery. Computed tomography of the thorax (page 116) allows assessment of the mediastinum and is usually taken down to include the liver and the adrenals. Computed tomography provides an anatomical not a pathological image, enlarged nodes may just show reactive changes not metastases and involved nodes are not necessarily visible on CT. Most surgeons proceed to explore the mediastinum by mediastinoscopy (page 278) if the CT scan is suspicious. Brain and bone scanning detect some metastases in the absence of symptoms but the yield is small and they are usually reserved for patients with neurological symptoms and bone pain, respectively. Positron emission tomography (PET, page 114) may turn out to have a useful role in predicting the presence of malignant change in lung nodules and lymph nodes.

Small cell tumours have usually spread by the time of diagnosis and it is unusual to be able to operate on such lesions.

When there are one or more secondary deposits in the lung from a primary tumour which can be dealt with satisfactorily then it may be appropriate to resect the secondary deposits in the lung.

### Radiotherapy

When the tumour is localized but surgery is refused or ruled out by local invasion or poor lung function then radical radiotherapy improves survival to 5 year figures of 10–15 per cent. Most often radiotherapy is used as a symptomatic treatment for haemoptysis or shortness of breath caused by bronchial obstruction. It is very useful in the management of superior vena caval obstruction and for bone pain from local invasion or secondary deposits.

### Chemotherapy

This has proved most successful for small cell carcinomas where no other treatments have been particularly effective. Benefits are greatest in relatively fit patients with disease limited to the thorax and the local lymph nodes. Some response is achieved in the majority of such patients and a few long-term survivors are obtained. Median survival is improved from 3–4 months to 9–12 months. Various chemotherapy regimens are used and updated regularly according to the results of clinical trials.

Results are much less satisfactory in non-small cell tumours. Although some regression can be achieved in 30–50 per cent, survival figures are less impressive and routine chemotherapy is not indicated outside clinical trials.

### Control of symptoms

Radiotherapy is useful for control of pain, haemoptysis, superior vena cava obstruction and breathlessness. Pain can nearly always be adequately controlled by the appropriate use of analgesics. Breathlessness may be helped by opiates. Close attention to symptom control and other needs is an essential part of the management of carcinoma of the bronchus.

# Alveolar cell carcinoma

This can be regarded as a variety of adenocarcinoma. It presents either as a single mass or as a diffuse infiltration through the lung tissue. Malignant cells grow along the walls of the alveoli and the small airways. The sexes are equally affected and smoking is not thought to be a risk factor.

The main symptom with the diffuse lesion is often breathlessness while a minority cough up large quantities of sputum each day ($>100$ ml = bronchorrhoea). The diagnosis can usually be established by sputum cytology, bronchial or transbronchial biopsy.

Localized lesions can be resected but nothing usually helps in the diffuse form.

# The solitary pulmonary nodule

A common clinical problem is the finding of a single round lesion on the chest X-ray, sometimes called a coin lesion. Previous X-rays can be invaluable in deciding on the management. The presence of calcification within a lesion suggests that it is benign (a granuloma, e.g. tuberculosis, or a hamartoma). However, malignant change can arise in or adjacent to such lesions. Calcification is best seen on CT scans which will also show up any other nodules not visible on plain films.

Lesions over 1 cm in diameter can often be sampled by percutaneous needle aspiration. A diagnosis of malignancy can be confirmed in 80–90 per cent of cases but when the lesion is benign a firm diagnosis is achieved in less than 50 per cent of cases.

If the lesion is not known to be old or calcified and the patient is over 30 years of age surgical removal is often the safest course.

# DIFFUSE LUNG DISEASE

There are many causes of diffuse infiltrative and fibrotic lung diseases. They are considered here under the headings in Table 13.23.

# Cryptogenic fibrosing alveolitis

Diffuse fibrosis throughout the lung can be the result of various insults such as radiation, cytotoxic drugs or connective tissue disorders. Cryptogenic fibrosing alveolitis (CFA) is the term used for the condition in which diffuse fibrosis is not part of some other condition and the trigger factor is unknown.

## PATHOLOGY

The condition appears to start as an inflammatory process in the alveoli with a lymphatic infiltration and an increase in connective tissue. With time the picture changes to an irreversible fibrotic appearance.

## CLINICAL FEATURES

Cryptogenic fibrosing alveolitis is twice as common in males. It may occur at any age but most often from 40 to 60 years. The original descriptions (Hamman–Rich syndrome) were of a rapidly progressive disease with death from respiratory failure in less than 6 months. The more

**Table 13.23** Diffuse and infiltrative lung disease.

Cryptogenic fibrosing alveolitis
Extrinsic allergic alveolitis
Occupational lung disease
Sarcoidosis
Drug-induced lung disease
Carcinoma (lymphangitis carcinomatosa)
Histiocytosis X
Pulmonary haemosiderosis
Connective tissue disorders
Adult respiratory distress syndrome

common picture is of a slower decline and a plateau may be reached without further progressive deterioration. Overall 5-year survival is around 50 per cent.

There is reduced lung expansion, tachypnoea and fine late inspiratory crackles at the lung bases. Clubbing occurs in 80 per cent of cases. Non-specific joint pains may be present and antinuclear factor and rheumatoid factor are common findings in the serum. These findings occur in CFA as distinct from the pulmonary fibrosis found as a complication of rheumatoid arthritis. Blood gases show hypoxia and hypocapnia and on the chest X-ray the lungs are small with fine nodular and linear shadowing most marked in the lower zones (Fig. 13.26). Overlapping shadows may eventually produce a 'honeycomb' appearance. Fine cuts on the CT scan show diffuse lung infiltration and subpleural cystic change.

There is a restrictive defect on respiratory function tests (page 269) with reduced $FEV_1$ and FVC but high FER. Total lung capacity and RV are low, as is the gas transfer and KCO.

Bronchoalveolar lavage at fibreoptic bronchoscopy (page 278) produces an abnormal differen-

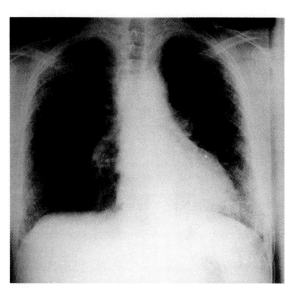

**Figure 13.26** Chest X-ray in a case of fibrosing alveolitis showing small nodular shadowing most marked in the lower zones.

tial cell count with an increase in neutrophils, lymphocytes and sometimes eosinophils. Transbronchial biopsies are often too small to give definitive information on the diagnosis or the degree of cellular infiltration. Open lung biopsy may be necessary to exclude other infiltrative processes.

## TREATMENT

Only around 20 per cent of cases have a substantial response to treatment. Response is more likely in the earlier more cellular stages. Treatment is with high doses of corticosteroids; the response rate is increased by the addition of cytotoxic agents such as cyclophosphamide. If a response occurs treatment will need to be continued for several years. In the later stages oxygen is helpful and lung transplantation has been performed successfully.

# Extrinsic allergic alveolitis

Extrinsic allergic alveolitis (EAA) is a response to inhalation of organic substances. The response relies on an IgG-mediated type III hypersensitivity reaction. A large number of types have been described, some of the commoner conditions are shown in Table 13.24.

## CLINICAL FEATURES

Exposure to antigen can produce an acute illness 6–8 hours later which is characterized by fever, cough, shortness of breath and general 'flu-like symptoms. These symptoms settle over 24–36

hours. They are associated with cellular infiltration and release of damaging enzymes such as elastase. Repeated acute exposures or prolonged lighter exposure leads to a granulomatous response which eventually produces diffuse pulmonary fibrosis. Crackles occur but often not as prominently as in CFA and clubbing occurs in the later stages of fibrosis. Unlike CFA the changes in the lungs are more marked in the upper zones. Respiratory function tests show a restrictive defect with low gas transfer.

Where the antigen has been identified serological tests are available to detect the precipitating IgG antibody in the blood. However, exposed workers may have the antibody without any evidence of the disease.

## TREATMENT

In industries where EAA occurs precautionary measures to keep down dust or breathing systems can prevent the development of the disease. When EAA has developed patients should avoid further contact with the antigen. Corticosteroids are effective in clearing the lung changes provided that fibrosis has not developed.

# Occupational lung disease

A detailed occupational history is an important part of the interview in patients with lung disease. The lungs can be involved in various ways (Table 13.25).

Only fibrotic lung disease will be dealt with in this section.

**Table 13.24** Types of extrinsic allergic alveolitis.

| Disease | Source of antigen | Test antigen |
|---------|-------------------|--------------|
| Farmer's lung | Mouldy hay, straw, grain | *Microplyspora faeni* *Thermoactinomyces vulgaris* |
| Bird fancier's lung | Excreta, bloom of pigeons, budgerigars, parrots | Avian serum |
| Bagassosis | Mouldy bagasse (sugar cane) Polyurethane foam manufacture | *Thermoactinomyces sacchari* Diisocyanates |

**Table 13.25** Types of occupational lung disorder.

Airway irritation, e.g. chlorine
Occupational asthma, e.g. platinum
Extrinsic allergic alveolitis, e.g. in farmers
Fibrotic reactions, e.g. silicosis
Granulomatous reactions, e.g. beryllium
Dust deposition without fibrosis, e.g. tin
Increased risk of malignancy, e.g. asbestos

## COAL-WORKERS' PNEUMOCONIOSIS

Inhalation of coal dust over long periods can result in three clinical problems:

1 Coal workers' pneumoconiosis (CWP)
2 Silicosis
3 Industrial bronchitis

Silicosis occurs in other industries and is described below. Coal-workers' pneumoconiosis is divided into simple and complicated forms. In simple CWP there are small rounded opacities up to 10 mm in diameter on the chest X-ray. Irregular opacities are found but may be more related to the common combination of smoking and coal working.

Complicated CWP is defined by the presence of at least one opacity greater than 1 cm in diameter together with the shadowing of simple CWP. This has been labelled **progressive massive fibrosis** (PMF) and may be associated with cavitation. Complicated CWP has three subdivisions based on opacity size (<5 cm, 5 cm–<1/3 lung, >1/3 lung field).

When CWP is extensive there is a restrictive lung defect. There may also be an obstructive element and complications from cigarette smoking. In the presence of rheumatoid arthritis large nodular shadows may occur in the lungs (**Caplan's syndrome**).

No treatment can reverse the pulmonary damage of CWP.

## SILICOSIS

Inhalation of quartz particles resulting in silicosis can occur in miners, sandblasters, quarrymen and others exposed to free silica. An acute lung reaction can occur but this is uncommon. In the commoner chronic form there is

increasing breathlessness while the chest X-ray shows fibrosis more prominent in the upper zones. There may be peripheral, linear calcification of hilar and mediastinal lymph nodes ('egg-shell' calcification). It appears that there is an increased risk of tuberculosis in silicotic lungs.

## ASBESTOS

Inhalation of asbestos produces a number of distinct problems in the lungs and pleura (Table 13.26).

**Table 13.26** Asbestos-related problems.

'Benign' asbestos plaques (Fig. 13.27)
Mesothelioma
Pulmonary fibrosis – asbestosis
Increased risk of lung carcinoma

Asbestos may be any of a group of fibrous silicates. The two most important ones are chrysotile, which makes up the majority, and crocidolite (blue asbestos) which is most often associated with mesotheliomas. Exposure is often 20–40 years before presentation. Workers in the construction industry, dockers, boilermakers and pipe laggers have often been exposed

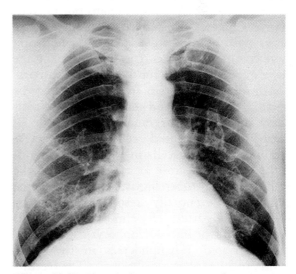

**Figure 13.27** Pleural plaques as a result of previous exposure to asbestos. The calcified plaques form irregular shapes overlying the lung fields. There may be a restrictive impairment of ventilatory function when pleural involvement is extensive.

but it will require a full occupational history covering all previous employment to be sure of the risk.

The term **asbestosis** should be limited to the condition in which widespread pulmonary fibrosis occurs in response to the inhalation of one of the fibrous silicates making up asbestos. The exposure is usually fairly extensive to produce asbestosis. This contrasts with mesothelioma where it may be less.

As pulmonary fibrosis develops there is increasing shortness of breath and tachypnoea. Clubbing, late inspiratory crackles and a troublesome cough develop. The radiological changes are most marked at the lung bases where linear and small nodular shadows may give a 'shaggy' heart border. Respiratory function changes show a restrictive defect with low gas transfer. There may be asbestos bodies (asbestos fibres with a cellular and fibrotic response) in the sputum but these can just be a marker of previous asbestos exposure.

## BERYLLIUM

Beryllium was used in the manufacture of fluorescent light tubes. Now it is limited to nuclear power, aviation and related industries. Although beryllium exposure is uncommon chronic exposure produces an interesting granulomatous reaction which mimics pulmonary sarcoidosis. The granulomas are usually limited to the lung and the liver. Large acute exposures can produce acute pneumonitis.

# $S$ARCOIDOSIS

Sarcoidosis is a multisystem condition characterized by its typical histology of non-caseating granulomas. The cause of sarcoidosis is unknown although the similarity in histology has suggested a role for mycobacteria in its initiation. The prevalence varies between communities, being considerably more common in American blacks and West Indians but uncommon in Chinese. The pattern of the disease also varies with ethnic origin, skin sarcoid being more common in blacks. It can occur at any age but is most common in the twenties and thirties.

Any organ or system in the body may be affected. Monocytes and macrophages are activated and form into granulomas made up of histiocytes (epithelioid cells). Macrophages combine into giant cells in and around granulomas. Central necrosis or caseation, as in the granulomas of tuberculosis, is rare and the granulomas eventually resolve or heal by fibrosis. The pattern of pulmonary sarcoidosis suggests that the initial lymphocytic infiltration with activated T-lymphocytes in the lungs results in a lymphocytic alveolitis. The recruitment of activated T-lymphocytes to the lungs results in a relative depletion in the peripheral blood. The common finding of a profound lymphocytic alveolitis early in the disease suggests that the aetiological agent for sarcoidosis may be inhaled.

Granulomas are found in other conditions such as extrinsic allergic alveolitis and beryllium exposure and the diagnosis of sarcoidosis relies on a combination of clinical, biochemical and histological features.

## CLINICAL FEATURES

Although sarcoidosis may involve any organs (Table 13.27) there are certain characteristic clinical patterns. There is intrathoracic involvement in around 90 per cent of patients (Table 13.28). This may involve enlargement of the hilar and mediastinal lymph nodes (Figs 13.28 and 13.29), diffuse pulmonary infiltration or a combination of the two (Fig. 13.30). Extensive pulmonary involvement leads to a restrictive defect (page 269) although occasionally endobronchial sarcoid may cause airflow obstruction. Often the radiological changes are more dramatic than the functional defect or clinical signs. Pleural involvement is much less common.

The skin is the second most common organ to be involved. **Erythema nodosum** (page 576) is the most frequent form of involvement,

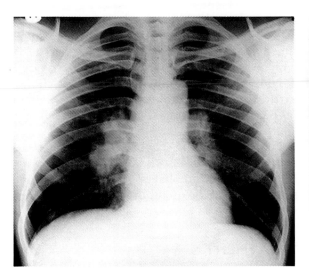

**Figure 13.28** Bilateral hilar and mediastinal lymphadenopathy in a case of sarcoidosis. The rounded masses at the hila are more marked on the right side.

**Table 13.27** Organ involvement in sarcoidosis in the UK.

| Organ | Per cent |
| --- | --- |
| Intrathoracic | 90 |
| Skin | 30 |
| Peripheral lymph nodes | 30 |
| Eyes | 20 |
| Spleen | 12 |
| Salivary glands | 10 |
| Nervous system | 5 |

**Table 13.28** Intrathoracic manifestations of sarcoidosis.

| Stage | Description | Per cent |
| --- | --- | --- |
| O | Normal | 8 |
| I | Hilar nodes | 50 |
| II | Hilar nodes + parenchyma | 30 |
| III | Parenchymal infiltration/fibrosis | 12 |

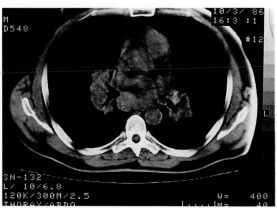

**Figure 13.29** Bilateral hilar lymphadenopathy in a case of sarcoidosis. The computed tomographic scan provides important information on abnormalities in the mediastinum and around the hila. The addition of contrast during the study helps to delineate the vasculature.

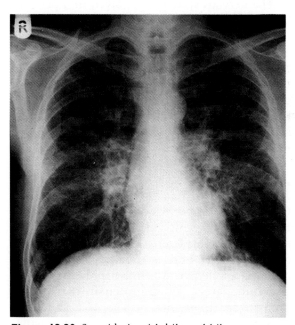

**Figure 13.30** Sacroidosis with bilateral hilar lymphadenopathy and pulmonary infiltration most marked in the mid-zones.

followed by fleshy lumps around the nose, eyes and scars, and purplish involvement of the nose (**lupus pernio**). Erythema nodosum with bilateral hilar lymphadenopathy in a young adult is a typical presentation of sarcoidosis (Lofgren's syndrome).

Eye involvement (anterior or posterior uveitis, conjunctivitis or retinitis) occurs in about 20 per cent of cases. Infiltration of the salivary and lacrimal glands can cause their enlargement with dryness of the eyes and the mouth. Facial nerve palsy may occur with salivary gland involvement. The combination of fever, parotid enlargement, uveitis and cranial nerve palsies is called Heerfordt's syndrome.

Peripheral lymph node enlargement occurs in

30 per cent of patients and splenomegaly in 10–15 per cent, both findings are commoner in blacks.

The liver usually shows granulomas on biopsy. Liver function tests are often mildly abnormal but clinically significant liver involvement is rare.

Abnormalities of calcium metabolism are common with hypercalcaemia in 5–10 per cent but hypercalciuria in 40–50 per cent. The abnormalities in calcium are related to vitamin D metabolism. Granulomas have the ability to activate 25-hydroxycholecalciferol by hydroxylation to 1, 25-dihydroxycholecalciferol.

Involvement of the heart is common on histological examination but clinical problems are less common unless granulomas impinge on the conducting system leading to arrhythmias and heart block.

The nervous system is involved in 5 per cent of cases. Many different patterns occur including peripheral nerve palsies, space-occupying cerebral lesions and meningitis.

Bone involvement produces cystic change in the bones. It occurs in less than 5 per cent of cases and is usually signalled by involvement of the overlying skin. Mild arthralgia is common but more extensive joint and muscle involvement is uncommon.

## DIAGNOSIS

Certain patterns such as erythema nodosum and bilateral hilar lymphadenopathy in a young adult may be characteristic enough to make the diagnosis. The ESR is usually raised, hypercalciuria and hypercalcaemia may help.

Serum levels of **angiotensin-converting enzyme** (ACE) are raised. The ACE is derived from endothelial cells in the pulmonary vasculature. In characteristic cases serum ACE is raised in 60–80 per cent but is less helpful in atypical sarcoidosis. Serum ACE is also raised in a minority of cases of other granulomatous and chronic inflammatory disorders. Unfortunately ACE levels have not proved as useful as was hoped in the diagnosis of sarcoidosis.

Biopsy of appropriate tissue demonstrates typical granulomas. With intrathoracic sarcoidosis transbronchial biopsies show granulomas in 80–90 per cent of patients. This may be combined with bronchoalveolar lavage (page 278) which shows an increased number of activated T-lymphocytes. Other conditions such as extrinsic allergic alveolitis may produce a similar picture. Other organs such as liver, salivary and lacrimal glands are alternative biopsy sites.

Gallium scanning (page 109) usually detects areas of active sarcoidosis. Gallium is taken up by activated macrophages. The finding is not specific but can be useful in assessing activity of sarcoidosis.

## TREATMENT

In some cases no specific treatment is necessary for sarcoidosis since spontaneous resolution occurs. Mild general symptoms, arthralgia and erythema nodosum may be helped by nonsteroidal anti-inflammatory drugs. When more specific treatment is needed steroids are the usual choice. They promote healing of granulomas and short-term resolution although their effect on the final outcome is still uncertain.

Involvement of some organs is an indication for the use of steroids (Table 13.29). In some cases local use may be satisfactory, for example, eye drops for mild anterior uveitis, local infiltration for skin involvement. Prednisolone is usually started at a dose of 30–40 mg daily. Once systemic steroids are started they are often necessary for 1–3 years in a suppressive dose of 5–15 mg daily.

Hydroxychloroquine may be useful in skin sarcoidosis and drugs such as azathioprine and methotrexate can be used to reduce the dose of corticosteroid needed in severe disease.

**Table 13.29** Situations requiring corticosteroid treatment in sarcoidosis.

Cardiac involvement
Progressive lung disease
Neurological sarcoid
Acute extensive lung infiltration + symptoms/
    respiratory function changes
Eye involvement
Hypercalcaemia

# DRUG-INDUCED LUNG DISEASE

A large number of drugs and other therapeutic agents are capable of producing adverse reactions in the lungs. Neonatal lungs are sensitive to increased levels of inspired oxygen. In adults a fraction of oxygen in inspired gas ($FIO_2$) >0.7 for >24 hours can produce lung damage and can contribute to the pathology in adult respiratory distress syndrome (ARDS, page 318).

Radiotherapy can induce damage in lung tissue which limits the amount of treatment which can be given to lung tumours. Early radiation changes are vascular damage and low pressure pulmonary oedema. Corticosteroids are useful in clearing this early response but probably do not help the more common late fibrotic response which develops over months or even years.

The most common form of drug-induced lung disease is a fibrotic reaction and the cytotoxic drugs are the most important in provoking this response (Table 13.30). Other reactions can be an eosinophilic lung infiltrate or airflow obstruction. Amiodarone (page 217) has emerged as an important agent inducing alveolar damage leading to pulmonary fibrosis.

**Table 13.30** Drug-induced lung disease.

| Drug | Response |
|---|---|
| Bleomycin, busulphan, cyclophosphamide, melphalan, chlorambucil, methotrexate, nitrogen mustard, gold, penicillamine, amiodarone | Pulmonary fibrosis |
| Nitrofurantoin, aspirin, penicillin, methotrexate, procarbazine, isoniazid sulphonamides | Eosinophilic infiltration |
| β-Blockers, aspirin and NSAIDs, penicillin | Asthma |

NSAIDs = non-steroidal anti-inflammatory drugs.

# LUNG INVOLVEMENT IN CONNECTIVE TISSUE DISORDERS

## *Rheumatoid arthritis*

The commonest lung problems in rheumatoid arthritis (Table 13.31) are pleural effusions and diffuse pulmonary fibrosis. Less common manifestations are rheumatoid nodules, diffuse small airway obstruction in an obliterative bronchiolitis and large airway obstruction from disease of the cricoarytenoid joints. Obliterative bronchiolitis appears to be more common with penicillamine treatment. Pulmonary manifestations may occasionally antedate the characteristic renal problems.

Pleural effusions are transudates. They are usually small and have a very low glucose content. Diffuse pulmonary fibrosis in association with rheumatoid arthritis has an even poorer response to treatment than CFA. Pulmonary nodules usually occur in the presence of nodules elsewhere. They are subpleural, occasionally they cavitate or erode the pleura and may be confused with primary lung cancers. Caplan's syndrome (page 313) may occur in coal workers with pneumoconiosis and rheumatoid arthritis.

**Table 13.31** Pulmonary manifestations of rheumatoid arthritis.

Pleural effusions
Fibrosing alveolitis
Pulmonary nodules
Obliterative bronchiolitis
Cricoarytenoid disease
Upper lobe fibrosis
Caplan's syndrome
Drug-induced lung disease

# Systemic lupus erythematosus

Pleurisy and pleural effusions are the most common pulmonary problems in SLE. Effusions do not have the low sugar content of rheumatoid effusions. Lupus pneumonitis produces patchy areas of consolidation which may be difficult to differentiate from associated infection. A condition of loss of lung volume (disappearing lung) may occur, sometimes in association with diaphragmatic weakness. Pulmonary emboli and thrombosis *in situ* occur in association with the clotting problems of SLE. Fibrosing alveolitis is an unusual complication of SLE.

# Other connective tissue diseases

In mixed connective tissue disease (overlap syndrome, page 579) fibrosing alveolitis is the most common problem but pleural and pulmonary vascular problems may also occur. The same problem may develop in systemic sclerosis but other complications are pulmonary hypertension, aspiration from oesophageal reflux and strictures. Ankylosing spondylitis is associated with bilateral upper lobe fibrosis. Sjögren's syndrome may be complicated by pulmonary fibrosis or small airway obstruction.

# Other pulmonary infiltrations

Diffuse pulmonary fibrosis occurs in many other conditions, including histiocytosis X, neurofibromatosis and tuberous sclerosis. In haemosiderosis, episodes of intrapulmonary haemorrhage eventually cause fibrosis. Haemosiderosis may be secondary to intrapulmonary haemorrhage or be a primary disorder in which there are haemoptyses and iron-deficiency anaemia.

# ADULT RESPIRATORY DISTRESS SYNDROME

The term adult respiratory distress syndrome (ARDS) (page 262) describes a clinical picture of hypoxaemia, diffuse pulmonary infiltrates and stiff lungs. There are many causes but haemodynamic pulmonary oedema from high left atrial pressure is excluded. In ARDS the pulmonary oedema is related to increased capillary permeability allowing fluid and protein to leak from the pulmonary circulation. If the left atrial pressure is high in addition then this will worsen the ARDS.

Predisposing causes for ARDS include shock, trauma, sepsis, aspiration, pancreatitis and uraemia. The mechanisms of damage which induce the leakiness of the pulmonary endothelium and epithelium are poorly understood. There is accumulation of leukocytes in the lung with leukotrienes, cytokines, neuropeptides and superoxides all possible contributors for the process.

## CLINICAL FEATURES

The typical pattern is the progressive development of increasing hypoxaemia, diffuse small nodular lung shadowing of an alveolar filling pattern (Fig. 13.31) with dyspnoea and increased respiratory rate. There may be inspiratory crackles on auscultation. As the lungs become stiffer and gas exchange worsens, ventilation becomes necessary and oxygenation becomes progressively more difficult.

## TREATMENT

In situations which predispose to ARDS care must be taken to avoid rises in left atrial pressure

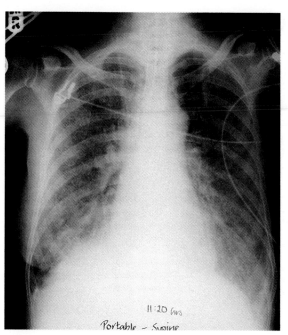

**Figure 13.31** Widespread alveolar filling in a case of adult respiratory distress syndrome requiring ventilation.

which exacerbate the problem. The left atrial pressure can be estimated by measuring the pulmonary artery wedge pressure with a balloon catheter. Oxygenation should be maintained without increasing inspired oxygen levels unnecessarily since high levels themselves can contribute to lung damage. Oxygenation is often helped by adding a positive end expiratory pressure (PEEP) to increase functional residual capacity and limit alveolar and airway collapse. This helps to maintain the compliance of the lung.

Various drugs have been used in ARDS but none have yet found an established role. Anti-inflammatory agents have not been successful; prostacyclin and nitrous oxide are under trial as pulmonary vasodilators. The figures for survival in ARDS depend on the breadth of the definition used. However, when ARDS is well established and combined with failure of at least one other major organ the mortality approaches 100 per cent.

# VASCULITIS AND RELATED CONDITIONS

## Wegener's granulomatosis

In this arteritic condition a necrotizing granulomatous arteritis in the lung and the upper respiratory tract is often associated with glomerulonephritis. Limited forms can occur with only one or two of these components. In the upper respiratory tract there may be involvement of the nose, sinuses, palate and larynx. In the lung the most common presentation is as discrete masses within the lung which cavitate and bleed. Untreated glomerulonephritis often progresses to renal failure.

The ESR is raised and antibodies against neutrophil cytoplasmic antibody (ANCA) can be detected in the serum (page 461). These findings with the typical clinical pattern provide the diagnosis. Confirmation comes from biopsy of any one of the involved sites. In the lung this often requires an open biopsy.

Treatment is with corticosteroids and cyclophosphamide. This combination produces good results in a condition which has a mortality of over 70 per cent in 1 year if untreated.

## Mid-line granuloma

This condition has also been known as Stewart's lethal mid-line granuloma. It is now thought to be a form of T-cell lymphoma. There is a progressively enlarging, destructive lesion in the mid-line of the upper respiratory tract. Local radiotherapy provides the most successful treatment.

## Vasculitis

Vasculitis (page 574) involves a widespread arteritis. Lung involvement is not a prominent feature although nodular lesions can occur.

# *Allergic granulomatosis*

This condition, also known as Churg–Strauss syndrome, is a form of vasculitis in which lung involvement is usual. Often there is a history of difficult asthma, eosinophilia is prominent and many systems are involved. The kidneys are often spared, unlike most other types of vasculitis. Pleurisy, pericarditis, neurological involvement and skin rashes are common while the most serious problem often comes from myocardial damage.

# *Goodpasture's syndrome*

In Goodpasture's syndrome an antibody against components of the basement membrane damages the alveolar wall and glomeruli in the kidney. Clinical manifestations are haemoptysis (page 273) and glomerulonephritis (page 459). The anti-basement membrane antibody can be demonstrated in the serum and the renal biopsy is typical (page 459). Treatment is by immunosuppression and plasmapheresis to remove the antibody.

# *P*LEURAL EFFUSIONS

The pleura may be inflamed and give pleuritic pain without the development of a significant effusion. This dry pleurisy occurs in many of the conditions which cause effusions and in viral infections, particularly Coxsackie B.

The pleural space is lubricated by a thin layer of pleural fluid. This fluid is in a dynamic state being absorbed through the visceral pleura. Effusions collect in the pleural space when there is a disturbance of the usual balance by increased fluid production from a local inflammatory lesion or hypoalbuminaemia or by interference with absorption by an increase in pulmonary venous pressure or lymphatic obstruction. Pleuritic pain comes from the parietal pleura and is associated with inflammation and friction between the pleural surfaces, as fluid accumulates the pain often subsides. Large effusions cause breathlessness by compression of the underlying lung.

When more than 300 ml is present the effusion may become detectable through dullness to percussion and reduced breath sounds and large effusions push the mediastinum across the midline. Typically the chest X-ray (Fig. 13.32) shows a meniscus of fluid laterally since the X-ray beam passes through a length of the thin rim of fluid. Effusions may become trapped in some areas of the pleural space if there are adhesions between visceral and parietal pleura.

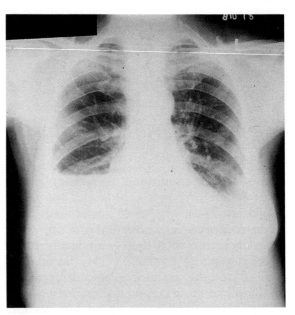

**Figure 13.32** A right-sided pleural effusion shown by the horizontal level in the right hemithorax. The left costophrenic angle is obscured by the soft tissue of the breast.

## AETIOLOGY

Effusions are broadly divided into **transudates** and **exudates** (Table 13.32) on the basis of their protein content (transudates <30 g/l) but may be lower in exudates if serum albumin is low and values are often near the borderline.

Transudates are most often caused by left heart failure (when they tend to be right sided) and hypoalbuminaemia. Other causes are shown in Table 13.32.

There are many causes of exudates (Table 13.32), the most common being infection, tumour, infarction and connective tissue disorders.

Effusions are usually investigated by aspiration of fluid. The site of aspiration may be judged by X-ray and clinical finding or by ultrasound. Aspiration is often combined with pleural biopsy particularly when tumour or tuberculosis is suspected. Fluid may be sent for biochemical, cytological and microbiological investigation (Table 13.33).

**Table 13.32** Causes of pleural effusions.

**Transudate** (protein <30 g/l)
Left heart failure
Hypoalbuminaemia
Constrictive pericarditis
Ascites or dialysis fluid from peritoneum
Meig's syndrome (ovarian tumour + right pleural effusion)
Hypothyroidism

**Exudate** (protein >30 g/l)
Infections
    Pneumonia
    Tuberculosis
    Subphrenic abscess

Malignancy
    Metastases
    Mesothelioma

Connective tissue disease etc.
    Rheumatoid arthritis
    Systemic lupus erythematosus
    Dressler's syndrome (page 179)

Other causes
    Pulmonary embolism
    Trauma
    Uraemia
    Pancreatitis
    Asbestos exposure
    Oesophageal rupture
    Familial Mediterranean fever (recurrent polyserositis)
    Yellow nail syndrome (page 234)
    Sarcoidosis

## TREATMENT

Effusions may be drained for relief of breathlessness. However, if the underlying cause is still present they often reaccumulate. If the cause cannot be dealt with (e.g. mesothelioma, secondary tumours) inflammation may be induced in the visceral and parietal pleural layers to obliterate the space in between. This can be done by surgical abrasion, iodized talc or irritant chemicals such as tetracycline. The obliteration of the pleural space produces little or no functional loss.

**Table 13.33** Investigation of a pleural effusion.

| | |
|---|---|
| Cytology | Often positive in malignant invasion |
| | Often difficult to interpret in mesothelial reactions/ mesothelioma |
| Differential cell count | (a) Lymphocytes usual in tuberculous effusions |
| | (b) Neutrophils in other infections |
| | (c) Eosinophils with blood eosinophilia, infarction, lymphoma or after blood in pleural space |
| Microbiology | Positive in empyema, often negative in tuberculosis, pleural biopsy better |
| Biochemistry | (a) Protein divides exudate from transudate (allow for low serum albumin) |
| | (b) Glucose low in infected effusion, very low in rheumatoid |
| | (c) pH low in developing empyema |
| | (d) Amylase very high in pancreatitis, high in oesophageal rupture |
| Immunological tests | (a) Antinuclear factor high in system lupus erythematosus |
| | (b) Rheumatoid factor high in rheumatoid arthritis |

# Particular forms of effusions

## HAEMOTHORAX

A collection of blood in the pleural space is most often the result of local trauma. Blood-stained pleural effusions may occur in malignant effusions and with infarction of the underlying lung. Bleeding may also occur in association with a pneumothorax from rupture of a vessel in the torn pleura. A collection of frank blood in the pleural space should be drained since it can result in a marked fibrous reaction giving pleural adhesions, restricted lung expansion and even calcification in the pleura. Drainage requires a large bore intercostal drain.

## CHYLOTHORAX

A true chylothorax implies the presence of lymph in the pleural space. This usually comes from the thoracic duct and the most common causes are trauma to the duct, including intra-thoracic surgery, or lymphomas and carcinomas which have invaded locally. Damage from radio-therapy is another possible cause. The fluid in a chylothorax contains triglycerides and chylomicrons. After trauma the fluid takes 2–10 days to collect. Management is by repeated aspiration until the defect in the thoracic duct closes or by surgical intervention to ligate the duct if this does not occur.

A chylothorax is suspected if the fluid in the pleural space is milky in appearance. A similar milky fluid is found in a **pseudochylous effusion** when the fluid does not contain chylomicrons but large amounts of cholesterol from degenerating cell walls in a chronic effusion usually caused by tuberculosis or rheumatoid arthritis.

## EMPYEMA

Infection in a pleural effusion develops into an empyema (a collection of pus in the pleural space). This may be from local spread from pneumonia or spread from infection elsewhere, introduction at aspiration or other instrumentation, oesophageal rupture or even primary empyema. Like blood the empyema is likely to produce intense local fibrosis and eventually possible calcification. Drainage of viscous pus will also need a fairly large bore intercostal drain and simultaneous antibiotic treatment. The commonest cause of primary empyema is an anaerobic organism called *Str. milleri*.

# PNEUMOTHORAX

In a pneumothorax air enters the space between the visceral and parietal pleura. The underlying lung is reduced in size. In lay terms this is often referred to as a collapsed lung but medically this term tends to be reserved for the situation where an airway is obstructed and there is absorption collapse of the distal lung. When a positive pressure builds up in the pleural space then the mediastinum is displaced to the other side, filling of the heart is impeded and cardiac output falls. This is a **tension pneumothorax** which requires urgent treatment by insertion of a needle or cannula to open the pleural space to the atmosphere and remove the positive pressure. Tension pneumothoraces can occur whatever the cause of the original pneumothorax.

## AETIOLOGY

Pneumothoraces are classified into spontaneous and traumatic types. Spontaneous pneumothoraces are further subdivided into primary and secondary. Primary spontaneous pneumothoraces are especially likely to occur in tall, thin young men. Secondary pneumothoraces occur on the background of an underlying lung disorder (Table 13.34).

## CLINICAL FEATURES

The onset of a pneumothorax is often associated with pleuritic chest pain and shortness of breath. The degree of breathlessness depends upon the

**Table 13.34** Causes of pneumothoraces.

Primary
    Enlarged apical airspaces in otherwise normal lungs

Secondary
    Chronic bronchitis and emphysema
    Pneumonia (Staphylococcal, Klebsiella, tuberculosis)
    Cystic fibrosis
    Fibrosing alveolitis
    Tumours
    Marfan's syndrome

**Traumatic**
Chest wall trauma
Barotrauma (ventilation, diving)
Biopsy of lung or pleura
Central venous cannulation

size of the pneumothorax and the state of the underlying lung.

On examination expansion is reduced on the affected side, resonance to percussion is increased, breath sounds and tactile vocal fremitus are reduced. In small left-sided pneumothoraces there may be a crunching sound in time with the heart beat.

X-rays show the line of the visceral pleura with no lung markings beyond it (Fig. 13.33). Any deviation of the mediastinum to the other side reflects positive pressure in the pleural space.

## TREATMENT

Pneumothoraces which are not causing symptoms and are less than 30 per cent down on the X-ray can be left. They will re-expand over 2–3 weeks. With mild symptoms or a larger pneumothorax the air can be aspirated from the space with a soft cannula, three-way tap and syringe. Pneumothoraces which recur after aspiration are treated by insertion of an intercostal tube connected to an underwater seal. When the lung has re-expanded and no more air is escaping

the tube should be left for 12–24 hours. If no symptoms develop and no air is bubbling out the tube can be removed and an X-ray repeated.

If air continues to bubble and the lung does not fully re-expand then a continued leak in the pleura is likely, making an open pneumothorax. This may respond to addition of suction pressure to the drainage tube. Otherwise a thoracic surgeon should be consulted since intervention may be necessary to close the leak in the pleura.

There is about a 20 per cent chance of a recurrence after a spontaneous pneumothorax. The chances are more in those who continue to smoke. After two this is up to around 50 per cent and 80 per cent after three. Therefore, after two pneumothoraces surgical intervention by pleurodesis should be considered to reduce the risk of recurrence.

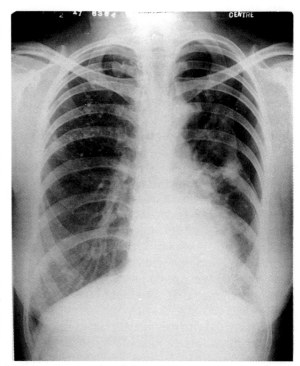

**Figure 13.33** Left-sided pneumothorax. The calcified nodular shadowing in the right upper zone represents old healed tuberculosis.

# DISORDERS OF THE MEDIASTINUM

The mediastinum lies between the lungs in the middle of the thorax bordered by the thoracic inlet above, the diaphragm below, thoracic spine behind, sternum in front and parietal pleura of the lungs on each side. The superior mediastinum is above the fourth thoracic vertebra, the lower part of the mediastinum is conventionally divided into anterior, middle and posterior portions. The superior mediastinum contains the great vessels, trachea and oesophagus, the anterior part of which can be explored by mediastinoscopy (page 278). The anterior mediastinum contains the thymus, the middle mediastinum the heart and the posterior compartment the spinal nerve roots, descending aorta and oesophagus.

## Mediastinitis

Acute inflammation of the mediastinum is most commonly caused by perforation of the oesophagus through endoscopy, swallowed bodies, surgery or vomiting. Air may be seen in the mediastinum on X-ray and may track up to the neck to be detectable in the left supraclavicular fossa. A pleural effusion often occurs and the patient is usually very ill with a fever and pain on swallowing. Surgery may be life-saving but the decision whether to operate will depend upon the underlying diagnosis and the patient's condition.

**Mediastinal fibrosis** may occur in infections such as tuberculosis or histoplasmosis. It may be idiopathic and can be associated with fibrosis elsewhere such as retroperitoneal fibrosis or sclerosing cholangitis. The usual clinical sign is superior vena caval obstruction causing distended jugular veins, swelling of the face and neck, and conjunctival oedema. Oesophageal, tracheal or pulmonary artery compression can occur. Surgical treatment or stenting of vessels can help in some cases but often little can be done for mediastinal fibrosis.

**Table 13.35** Causes of masses in the mediastinum.

**Superior mediastinum**
Retrosternal thyroid
Thymus (thymoma or cyst)
Dermoid tumour
Aortic aneurysm
Superior vena cava
Lymph nodes (usually lymphoma)

**Anterior mediastinum**
As for superior
Pericardial cyst
Diaphragmatic hernia (foramen of Morgagni)
Bronchogenic cyst

**Middle mediastinum**
Lymph nodes (usually metastases)
Bronchogenic cyst
Hiatus hernia
Oesophageal enlargement (achalasia, pouch)
Aortic aneurysm

**Posterior mediastinum**
Neurogenic tumours
Aortic aneurysm (descending)
Paravertebral abscess
Paravertebral tumour

## Mediastinal masses

These are usually considered according to their site in the mediastinum. The frequency of different lesions in series of mediastinal tumours varies according to the country of origin and the interest of the department. The commonest lesions in general experience are lymph nodes from tumours or conditions such as sarcoidosis or tuberculosis. However, these are not included in many series.

On plain X-rays it may be difficult to decide whether lesions are originating in the lung tissue or in the mediastinum. Alternative methods of imaging such as CT scanning with and without contrast medium and positron emission tomography (PET) are very helpful in defining the anatomy and likely diagnosis. Tumours in the mediastinum may be associated with distant manifestations. Thymic tumours can be found with myasthenia gravis (page 674). Thyroid and parathyroid tumours may be associated with their appropriate endocrine problems, although retrosternal goitres usually cause local pressure rather than distant hormonal effects. Paravertebral neural tumours may have a dumb-bell form with an intraspinal component which can compress the cord. The common tumours in the various mediastinal areas are shown in Table 13.35.

# Disorders of the Gastrointestinal Tract

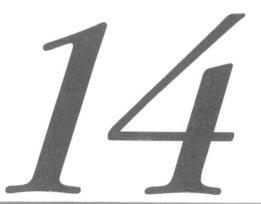

# INTRODUCTION

Alimentary disorders are important causes of illness and death. In global terms, acute diarrhoeal illnesses and hepatitis B-related liver cancer are major killers. Nearer home, peptic ulcer, gallstones and the irritable bowel syndrome cause much misery, and cancer of the gut and pancreas are leading causes of death from malignant disease.

Recent technological advances include the widespread diagnostic and therapeutic use of flexible endoscopy, ultrasound and computed tomographic (CT) scanning. There have also been important advances in medical treatment, surgical techniques and preventive medicine. Histamine 2 receptor blockers have revolutionized the treatment of peptic ulcer and the pharmacological treatment of gallstones has improved. Automatic stapling devices have facilitated cancer surgery, there are now surgical alternatives to the incontinent ileostomy and, more recently, laparoscopic surgery (e.g. cholecystectomy) is rapidly gaining popularity.

Vaccine to prevent hepatitis B is now available but has not yet been used widely. The use of oral rehydration solutions has reduced much of the morbidity and mortality from acute diarrhoeal disease in the underdeveloped world.

There are still numerous gaps in our knowledge. We do not know the cause of many common illnesses such as peptic ulcer, inflammatory bowel diseases and the major cancers of the alimentary tract. Environmental factors are probably important and are waiting to be identified. The relationship between food and gut disease provides controversy and a basis for much unorthodox medicine. There would certainly be less alimentary disease if people smoked less, drank less alcohol and ate a high fibre diet.

# SYMPTOMS OF GUT DISEASE

## Changes of appetite

Appetite is commonly lost in gut disease but this is rarely the presenting or sole feature. It is important to distinguish true **anorexia** from a reluctance to eat because food provokes distressing symptoms. Anorexia, especially for breakfast, is very common in heavy drinkers of alcohol and is often accompanied by nausea and retching. Alterations of appetite, aversion to some foods and cravings for others are well recognized in pregnancy. In older patients, carcinoma of the stomach and gastric ulcer must be excluded, if no other explanation for anorexia is apparent.

Alterations of appetite are characteristic of anorexia nervosa and may include **bulimia** (episodic overeating) in addition to self-induced vomiting and abuse of laxatives and diuretics.

Anxious and depressed patients commonly suffer marked fluctuations in appetite.

## Changes of weight

Slow loss of weight (Table 14.1) is common in many organic gut disorders and is usually due to reduced food intake, although it may be caused by loss of nutrient in the faeces in malabsorption or by increased demand for energy.

Gain in weight is uncommon in gut disease but patients with peptic ulcer may drink large amounts of milk or eat frequent snacks to relieve pain and thus put on a lot of weight.

Excess alcohol consumption is a common cause of obesity, especially in otherwise fit young men who develop the characteristic 'beer belly'.

**Table 14.1** Causes of weight loss.

Reduced food intake and/or increased physical activity

Increased metabolic requirements (e.g. hypercatabolic response to sepsis, injury, thyrotoxicosis, diabetes mellitus)

The wasting of chronic infections, inflammatory diseases and malignancy (caused by a combination of the above factors)

Loss of nutrient in faeces in malabsorption

# Oral symptoms

Patients often imagine that symptoms in the mouth (Table 14.2) indicate deep-seated and sinister abdominal disease but this is rarely true. Many patients are overanxious about coating of the tongue especially the 'black hairy tongue', for which there is usually no apparent cause. Poor dental hygiene, smoking cigarettes or a pipe and chewing tobacco often cause bad breath (halitosis) and gingivitis. Rarely, halitosis is caused by stagnation of food in a pharyngeal pouch, in the gullet in achalasia and in the stomach above pyloric obstruction.

**Table 14.2** Oral lesions which may indicate alimentary tract disease.

| Sign | Underlying disease |
| --- | --- |
| Smooth, sore tongue <br> Angular cheilosis | Nutritional deficiency <br> Oral candidiasis |
| Aphthous ulcers | Inflammatory bowel diseases <br> Coeliac disease |
| Oral candidiasis ('thrush') | Immune deficiency disorders including AIDS |
| Pigmentation around lips | Peutz–Jeghers polyposis |
| Telangiectasia (lips/face) | Hereditary haemorrhagic telangiectasia <br> Scleroderma (part of CRST* syndrome) |

CRST = calcinosis, Raynaud's phenomenon, sclerodactyly and telangiectasia.

Recurrent small, painful ulcers (**aphthae**) are very common and rarely indicate internal disease. Associations between aphthae and both coeliac disease and inflammatory bowel diseases are recognized, but investigation is only warranted if there is supporting evidence such as anaemia, weight loss or bowel disturbance.

Malnourished patients may have painful cracks at the angles of the mouth (cheilosis) and a sore, reddened smooth tongue often ascribed to specific nutritional deficiencies (Table 14.2). Similar symptoms may accompany the characteristic white buccal plaques of oral candidiasis. The sicca syndrome (dry mouth, and dry eyes) is an autoimmune disorder, affecting salivary and lacrimal glands, which may be accompanied by a polyarthritis (Sjögren's syndrome, page 561). It is found in a minority of patients with primary biliary cirrhosis (page 400). Oral Crohn's disease causes deep painful ulcers or a curious, chronic swelling of the lips.

Behcet's syndrome includes chronic, deep oral and genital ulcers and can involve many systems including the gut. The more commonly affected organs include the eye, the brain and the joints.

# Gastro-oesophageal reflux

The combination of a burning epigastric and retrosternal pain (heartburn, pyrosis) with reflux of bitter or sour gastric contents into the mouth clearly indicates the presence of gastro-oesophageal reflux. The symptoms usually occur after meals and are aggravated by stooping or lying flat. Nocturnal wakening is characteristic and the symptoms are eased by walking around and may be associated with cough or wheeze. Frequent nocturnal reflux can aggravate chronic obstructive airways disease.

In uncomplicated reflux, swallowing is usually normal, but it may be uncomfortable or even painful (odynophagia) to drink hot fluids, alcohol or citrus fruit juices.

Waterbrash is the term used for the sudden filling of the mouth with tasteless fluid (saliva) and must be distinguished from reflux of bitter gastric contents in the mouth.

# Dysphagia

This is true difficulty with swallowing as distinct from pain, discomfort or a delayed sense of block in the gullet. The difficulty is apparent during the act of swallowing and may be accompanied by regurgitation of swallowed food into the mouth, without bitter gastric contents.

The commonest causes are benign peptic stricture and carcinoma of the oesophagus or high gastric carcinoma. A preceding history of chronic gastro-oesophageal reflux would suggest the former diagnosis, but cancer may complicate chronic reflux especially if associated with extensive gastric metaplasia of the oesophageal mucosa (Barrett's oesophagus).

Rarer causes of dysphagia or odynophagia include specific infections by *Candida albicans* (thrush) and by herpes simplex virus and inflammation caused by swallowed caustics and certain drugs especially if they are retained for long periods in the gullet (e.g. slow release KCl tablets).

Chronic mechanical obstruction, most frequently caused by malignancy, produces progressive dysphagia initially for solids and later for liquids and there may be sudden complete obstruction by a bolus of food or a large tablet, requiring urgent radiological and endoscopic attention.

Disorders of motor function of the pharynx and oesophagus also cause dysphagia (Table 14.3). **Pharyngeal pouch** (Zenker's diverticulum) is probably a complication of cricopharyngeus spasm, and dysphagia may initially be relatively inapparent as food passes

**Table 14.3** Types of abnormal pharyngeal/oesophageal motility.

| | |
|---|---|
| Disorders of CNS (e.g. bulbar, pseudobulbar palsy) | |
| Cricopharyngeus spasm ± pharyngeal pouch Diffuse oesophageal spasm | Primary muscle disorder |
| Achalasia Chagas' disease | Abnormal nerve plexuses |
| Scleroderma of oesophagus | Replacement of muscle by fibrosis |

into the pouch rather than down the oesophagus (page 348). In both achalasia (page 346) and pharyngeal pouch, stagnant food may accumulate and be regurgitated hours or days after consumption, threatening the lungs if this occurs at night.

# Atypical central chest pain

Severe central chest pain, bad enough to mimic the pain of ischaemic heart disease, can be produced by diffuse oesophageal spasm, the spasm associated with so-called vigorous achalasia, bolus obstruction with food ('steakhouse coronary') and possibly by spasm secondary to gastro-oesophageal reflux. Recent studies suggest that many patients admitted to medical wards with severe central chest pain and atypical electrocardiograms (ECGs) have oesophageal rather than cardiac disorders. The increasing availability of oesophageal manometry (page 347) should help to identify these patients.

# Nausea and vomiting

These are common symptoms experienced occasionally by most people in association with acute infections or toxins with food or alcohol excess. Uncomplicated peptic ulcer may cause intermittent vomiting with temporary relief of pain, but the vomiting of ulcer or gastric cancer is usually obstructive in nature with a characteristically large volume of foul, stale food residue unaccompanied by bile (Table 14.4). Various forms

**Table 14.4** Classification of causes of vomiting.

| |
|---|
| Cerebral (e.g. migraine, raised intracranial tension) |
| Labyrinthine (e.g. travel sickness, labyrinthitis) |
| Metabolic (e.g. uraemia, hypercalcaemia) |
| Gastrointestinal (see text) |
| Psychological (see text) |

of vomiting occur in patients after peptic ulcer surgery (page 355).

Vomiting occurs in unrelieved intestinal obstruction (small or large gut) and the vomitus will be faecal in colour and smell if the site of obstruction is in the lower small intestine or beyond.

A common cause of retching and vomiting, especially in the mornings, is alcohol excess. Persistent nausea and vomiting without obvious explanations are usually psychological in origin and detailed psychiatric assessment will be required. Self-induced vomiting by finger may suggest a psychological cause, but patients with peptic ulcer and gastro-oesophageal reflux can relieve pain in this way.

# Dyspepsia/indigestion

These are vague words which describe any sort of distress caused by meals including pain, discomfort, nausea, distension, belching and heartburn. In general, patients with benign peptic ulcer (especially duodenal ulcer) feel more comfortable after meals, whereas those with most other common upper alimentary disorders feel worse. Common functional dyspeptic syndromes include a sense of bloating or distension in the epigastrium especially after fatty meals (fat intolerance) and the high colonic distension of one variant of the irritable bowel syndrome (page 373). The physiological explanations for many forms of functional dyspepsia are far from clear, but it is well established that fat delays gastric emptying and releases cholecystokinin (CCK) from the duodenal mucosa. Cholecystokinin has potent motor effects on the small and large gut and this may provide a rational explanation for the beneficial effects of a reduced fat intake in patients with these symptoms.

# Gas/wind

We all swallow air with our meals and this passes rapidly through the small intestine. Bacterial metabolism of unabsorbed food residues in the colon produces the various smells of flatus and the gases generated include methane, hydrogen, carbon dioxide, indoles and hydrogen sulphide. Belched gas (eructation) is usually odourless except when gastric contents are stagnant as in pyloric stenosis. Excessive belching is usually caused by repeated air swallowing, but is also common in patients with gastro-oesophageal reflux.

Excessive flatus is a common complaint, but is often difficult to explain. Bacterial fermentation of large amounts of dietary fibre commonly causes excess flatus and similar symptoms occur in alactasic subjects (page 342) who drink milk. Some vegetables are notorious gas producers, including beans, cabbage and sprouts, but individuals vary greatly in their responses. Increased amounts of substrate for bacterial metabolism are available in patients with malabsorption and the flatus is often particularly offensive.

Abdominal distension caused by accumulation of intestinal gas and fluid is seen in patients with intestinal obstruction. Chronic or recurrent abdominal distension and discomfort relieved by passing flatus suggests left-sided colonic pathology or the irritable bowel syndrome (page 373). Abdominal distension is often more imagined than real and can be produced voluntarily by a combination of exaggerated lumbar lordosis and diaphragmatic contraction.

# Abdominal pain

Severe abdominal pain (Table 14.5) caused by hollow organ distension is often but not always colicky in nature (i.e. it comes in waves) and makes the patient writhe or draw the knees up to the chest. It is often accompanied by vomiting and sweating. The episodes are short-lived, i.e. last for several hours only, and are either self-limiting or require relief by appropriate intervention.

Peritoneal inflammation is associated with marked tenderness and 'guarding' of the abdominal musculature. This is characteristic of a perforated viscus, when the onset is sudden and dramatic, and also accompanies the acute and

**Table 14.5** Classification of abdominal pain.

Hollow organ distension (e.g. gut, biliary, ureteric, uterine)

Peritoneal inflammation (e.g. perforated viscus, acute and chronic inflammatory diseases of gut and pelvic organs – appendicitis, diverticulitis, Crohn's disease, salpingitis)

Anterior abdominal wall problems (e.g. muscular pain, fatty hernias)

Retroperitoneal lesions (e.g. pancreatic disease)

Referred pain from spine affecting dermatomes T8–12

chronic inflammatory lesions mentioned in Table 14.5.

Most types of chronic or recurrent abdominal pain are less distinctive than these, signs may be few or absent and careful history taking is crucial. The pain of benign peptic ulcer (especially duodenal) is perhaps the most distinctive in its classic form with a periodicity over several years, i.e. prolonged periods of freedom lasting weeks or months, aggravation by hunger, relief by snacks or antacids and nocturnal wakening by well-localized epigastric pain. Radiation to the back suggests a posterior duodenal ulcer beginning to penetrate the pancreas. Unfortunately, in many patients the symptoms are less typical. The pain of gastric ulcer and carcinoma tends to be aggravated by food and is often accompanied by nausea, anorexia and loss of weight.

Colonic pain can be very distinctive, although its location may be anywhere in the abdomen. It is usually either colicky or a more continuous distension and is most commonly sited in the left iliac fossa or above the pubis. The most characteristic feature is the temporary relief by passing flatus or faeces, although occasionally defaecation may aggravate the pain. This type of pain is characteristic of the irritable bowel syndrome and of uncomplicated symptomatic diverticular disease (page 369) and the bowel habit is usually abnormal, although detailed enquiry may be required to reveal this.

Spasmodic severe rectal pain (proctalgia fugax) is felt deep in the pelvis, occurs usually at night, may be helped by firm pressure on the perineum and is usually not associated with any organic rectal or sigmoid disease. It may be provoked by sexual intercourse.

Chronic, continuous, inexorable and seemingly inexplicable abdominal pain is much less common. Organic causes include chronic pancreatitis and carcinoma of the pancreas, right-sided colon cancer, chronic intestinal ischaemia ('intestinal angina') and retroperitoneal lesions such as lymphoma and the rare fibrosis and sarcoma. In most of these patients there will be an obviously downhill course and signs will eventually develop after several months of unremitting pain.

A few patients have continuous, unexplained pain without any evidence of organic disease. They may be psychiatrically disturbed and are often very difficult to help.

Spinal pain may radiate to the abdomen if dermatomes T8–12 are affected. The pain is aggravated by certain postures, lifting and coughing and is usually associated with abnormalities on detailed spinal examination. It is not affected by eating or by defaecation. Pancreatic pain is characteristically felt in the epigastrium and spreads through to the back. Unlike lumbar pain, it is aggravated by lying flat and may be eased by sitting up and leaning forward.

Finally, mention should be made of abnormalities of the abdominal wall itself. Operation scars can produce chronic pain, which may be relieved by removing a retained suture or by injecting entrapped nerves with local anaesthetic or locally active corticosteroids (e.g. depomedrone), but this is probably uncommon. Chronic abdominal pain is often ascribed to adhesions from previous surgery, but this is very difficult to prove unless frank obstruction results from adhesive bands. Wide incisional hernias are usually painless, but epigastric herniation of fat through defects in the linea alba can cause chronic abdominal pain responsive to local injection or to surgical correction. Pain of this type is aggravated by coughing or contracting the abdominal musculature and is unaffected by food or by bowel function.

# Disturbed bowel function

Most healthy people have between three actions per day and three per week. More important than frequency is the consistency of faeces, the ease and completeness of evacuation and the ability to delay emptying until it is socially convenient. The quantity and consistency of faeces is determined mainly by the amount of fibre in the diet – that component of food that resists normal small intestinal digestion and passes into the colon where it is broken down to a variable extent by bacterial metabolism. Defaecation is also aided by physical activity, by adequate hydration and by a prompt response to the 'call to stool'. Frequent delay in responding to rectal distention results in a lessened awareness of rectal filling and gradual accumulation of faeces in the rectum.

## DIARRHOEA

Diarrhoea is best defined as an increased weight of faeces (>200 g/day), which are soft or watery in consistency. This may be difficult to establish from the history alone and inspection of the faeces is very helpful. True diarrhoea must be distinguished from faecal frequency and faecal impaction with overflow (Table 14.6). Pale, bulky, offensive stools suggest steatorrhoea (excess fat in the motion). Excess gas or fat makes faeces float and difficult to flush away. Acute episodes of watery diarrhoea are usually caused by anxiety, infections, alcohol or drugs and are self-limiting and rarely require symptomatic therapy. Diarrhoea which persists for more than two to three weeks should be investigated, although symptomatic treatment with codeine phosphate, loperamide or lomotil can be used in the meantime. These drugs should however be avoided if there is continuous abdominal pain or blood and mucus in the faeces (these symptoms should be investigated promptly).

## CONSTIPATION

Constipation is the infrequent passage of hard faecal masses with straining, difficulty and often anal pain. In the bedbound elderly and in some young children, large hard faecal masses may accumulate in the rectum with overflow and incontinence of loose faecal matter ('spurious diarrhoea'). This is due to loss of internal anal sphincter tone as a result of chronic rectal distension.

The various types of constipation are classified in Table 14.7. It is helpful to distinguish rectal constipation (i.e. the rectum is full of hard faeces on digital examination) from infrequent difficult defaecation caused by slow colonic transit and infrequent rectal filling.

Most patients with 'simple' primary constipation respond well to an increased intake of dietary fibre, provided that they obey the call to stool and allow adequate time for evacuation. The hydrophilic bulking agents (Table 14.8) are very helpful if dietary measures alone do not suffice. It is important to deal appropriately with painful anorectal disorders, although a high fibre diet and a stool softener may alleviate local symptoms considerably. Evacuant enemas may be required to initiate therapy if there is considerable faecal accumulation in the rectum. Bulking agents are not appropriate if the colon is already full of faeces even if the rectum is empty. In these patients colonic transit may be stimulated by the anthraquinone or polyphenolic

**Table 14.6** Types of diarrhoea.

**True** (increased quantity of faecal matter)
Watery diarrhoea
Steatorrhoea
Watery diarrhoea plus blood and/or mucus

**False** (normal or reduced amounts of faecal matter)
Faecal impaction with overflow
Frequency with small, bitty stools
Frequent passage of blood/mucus with little or no faeces
Passage of large volumes of mucus

**Table 14.7** Types of constipation.

Absence of primary cause, 'simple' constipation: inadequate intake of dietary fibre; dehydration; lack of exercise; failure to respond to 'call to stool'

Secondary to disease or functional disorder of colon/anus (e.g. diverticular disease, cancer, Hirschsprung's disease, painful haemorrhoids, anal fissures)

Drug-related (e.g. aluminium-based antacids, anticholinergics)

Neurological diseases affecting bowel and bladder

Metabolic diseases, especially hypothyroidism, hypercalcaemia

**Table 14.8** Classification of laxatives.

Lubricants/stool softeners (e.g. dioctyl sodium sulphosuccinate)

Bulking agents (e.g. methylcellulose, mucilagenous polysaccharides, from seeds/gums – Isogel, Fybogel)

Osmotic agents (e.g. magnesium sulphate, lactulose)

Stimulant cathartics (e.g. anthraquinones such as Senokot, bisacodyl, castor oil)

laxatives, but crampy, colonic pain is common. The continued use of the osmotic laxatives may be the only alternative in these difficult cases. Excessive or inappropriate use of laxatives will provoke large faecal losses of water and electrolytes and can lead to dehydration and hypokalaemia.

# Gastrointestinal bleeding

Acute severe upper gastrointestinal (GI) bleeding is a common and self-evident emergency which demands immediate medical attention (Table 14.9). The amount and colour of vomited blood gives little clue to the source of the bleeding. Altered blood, often described as 'coffee grounds' indicates slower bleeding with retention of blood in the stomach for several hours before vomiting. Forceful repeated vomiting of food and fluid may be followed by fresh blood from a vertical mucosal tear at the lower end of

**Table 14.9** Gastrointestinal bleeding: overall figures for the UK show the following percentage attribution of causes.

| Cause | Per cent |
|---|---|
| Duodenal ulcer | 40 |
| Gastric ulcer | 20 |
| Erosions | 15 |
| Varices | 5 |
| Mallory-Weiss | <5 |
| Carcinoma | <5 |
| Oesophagitis | <5 |
| Others/no cause | >5 |

the oesophagus ('Mallory–Weiss syndrome') but many patients with this lesion do not give a typical history.

Bleeding from all common upper GI lesions can present with melaena (black, loose, smelly faeces) in the absence of haematemesis and this is particularly likely to occur from duodenal ulcers. Bleeding from oesophageal varices, on the other hand, is usually profuse, alarming and mainly upwards. Bleeding from severe oesophagitis and gastric cancer is usually slow, chronic and occult.

Severe lower GI bleeding, sufficient to produce shock, is very much less common but can rarely complicate ulcerative colitis, diverticular disease or tumours. With the aid of arteriography of the mesenteric vessels, angiodysplasia (dilated vessels in the bowel wall) in the right colon has been recognized with increasing frequency, especially in the older age group. The colour of the blood gives a rough guide to the source because right-sided colonic bleeding is usually dark red and may be passed in clots. However, severe upper GI bleeding may be difficult to distinguish from proximal colonic bleeding at the bedside, the colour depending on the rate of loss and on the transit time through the remaining gut. The passage of more modest amounts of altered blood, associated with sudden abdominal pain in an older patient, suggests a diagnosis of vascular occlusion. Superior mesenteric arterial or venous occlusion produces severe abdominal pain and haemodyamic collapse ensues rapidly. Inferior mesenteric occlusion produces a less devastating clinical picture with reversible ischaemia or infarction of the left half of the colon ('ischaemic colitis').

Chronic occult GI blood loss is a common cause of iron deficiency anaemia and should be considered as the likeliest explanation in men and in postmenopausal women. In the older age groups it is necessary to exclude gastric and right-sided colonic cancer and important not to ascribe the bleeding to minor oesophagitis, to a duodenal ulcer with no evidence of recent bleeding, or to diverticular disease – common incidental findings in this clinical setting.

Rectal bleeding, insufficient to cause shock or anaemia, is common and usually attributable to haemorrhoids. The patient strains on hard stools and the bright red blood is on the toilet paper and on the surface of the faeces. However, the differential diagnosis must include proctitis and more sinister adenomas and cancer in the rectum and sigmoid colon. It cannot be overstressed that rectal bleeding should be investigated to exclude these lesions, especially in the over 40s and when the history is relatively short.

## PHYSICAL SIGNS OF GUT DISEASE

Physical signs are relatively few and mostly non-specific. However, much can be learnt by careful examination of the patient and a few specific diagnoses can be made on the basis of signs alone.

## State of nutrition

Observed loss of weight is an important sign in many gut disorders. In children and adolescents chronic gut disease is commonly associated with failure to gain weight and height with delayed development of secondary sex characteristics. In older girls and young women, secondary amenorrhoea usually accompanies marked loss of weight, most notably in anorexia nervosa.

Loss of subcutaneous fat is a sign of calorie (energy) deficiency and later the muscles become thin and eventually weak. Alcoholics, who derive much of their energy from alcohol and eat little protein, have thin muscles but well-preserved subcutaneous fat. Heavy drinkers, who continue to eat well, are overweight and the 'beer belly' in young men often indicates the cause of gastrointestinal complaints.

Specific nutritional deficiencies may be apparent but with the exception of anaemia and oedema, they are relatively rare even in severe chronic gut disease (Table 14.10).

Impaired nutrition is caused by neglect and poverty far more often than by chronic gut disease, especially in the older age groups. The state of the teeth should be examined because rotten teeth and badly fitting dentures make it impossible to chew food properly and food intake diminishes.

**Table 14.10** Clinical signs of specific nutritional deficiencies.

| | |
|---|---|
| Anaemia | Deficiency of Fe, folate, $B_{12}$ |
| Oedema | Protein deficiency |
| Angular cheilosis, sore tongue | Various deficiencies, including B vitamins |
| Scaly red skin | Possibly zinc or essential fatty acid deficiency |
| Bleeding gums, skin haemorrhages | Vitamic C deficiency |
| Bruising, bleeding | Vitamin K deficiency |
| Bony tenderness, proximal myopathy | Vitamin D deficiency |
| Peripheral neuropathy, ocular palsies, confusion | Vitamin $B_1$ (thiamine) deficiency |

## State of hydration

In patients with diarrhoea, vomiting and fistulous losses from the gut, dehydration and serious electrolyte deficiencies are common and readily corrected. Dehydration needing urgent correction is indicated by thirst, loss of skin turgor, dry mouth and soft eyes. In the severe cases there is hypovolaemia shown by rapid weak pulse, postural hypotension and reduced venous pressure in the neck. Severe $K^+$ deficiency causes muscle weakness and loss of tendon reflexes. Reduced plasma levels of $Ca^{2+}$ and $Mg^{2+}$ are seen infrequently in chronic gut disease but may cause muscular hyperexcitability, tetany and even convulsions, although low levels of plasma $Mg^{2+}$ can be remarkably well tolerated.

# Examination of the hands, face, neck and chest

Finger clubbing is seen in inflammatory bowel disease, especially Crohn's disease, and some other types of chronic diarrhoea. Lymphadenopathy is an important sign of metastatic malignancy especially from primary cancer of the stomach and pancreas. A particularly favoured site is behind the left sternoclavicular joint (Virchow's node).

Systemic sclerosis (page 577) is an occasional cause of dysphagia and malabsorption and would be suggested by the findings of cold hands, very tight skin over the fingers (sclerodactyly), ulcerating subcutaneous calcification (calcinosis), a small tight mouth and telangiectasia (distended capillaries) over the face and lips (often referred to as the CRST syndrome).

Rare causes of GI blood loss include **hereditary haemorrhagic telangiectasia**, with characteristic vascular abnormalities on the lips and fingers, and autosomal dominant inheritance, and the **Peutz–Jeghers syndrome** comprising small bowel polyps and a distinctive spotty pigmentation of the lips.

Examination of the mouth has already been stressed in relation to dentition and hydration and some specific oral diseases have been mentioned on page 329. Evidence of anaemia and jaundice should always be sought.

# Examination of the abdomen

Inspection may reveal obvious masses caused by tumours, inflammation (e.g. appendix mass, Crohn's disease), or huge cysts, especially arising from the ovary. A diffusely enlarged abdomen may be caused by fat, fluid, flatus, faeces or fetus and in most cases the cause is obvious. Visible peristalsis is seen if there is obstruction at the pylorus or in the lower small intestine. Large hernias will be obvious on coughing. Abdominal wall movements with respiration are absent in peritonitis and coughing aggravates the pain.

Palpation must be gentle and systematic using light touch and then deep palpation in all four quadrants. In the acute abdomen, assessment of localized tenderness and guarding of the musculature is important. Masses must be characterized in terms of size, site, consistency, fixity or movement with respiration and enlargement of liver, spleen and kidneys must be sought in all patients.

In chronic liver disease, the liver is firm and often irregular in shape, but the size can vary enormously from very small to very large. Enlargement of the spleen is common and usually indicates portal hypertension. In patients with obstructive jaundice, tense palpable enlargement of the gall bladder is usually but not always caused by malignant obstruction of the lower end of the common bile duct (Courvoisier's sign).

The hernial orifices must be examined carefully in patients with acute abdominal pain, especially if intestinal obstruction is suspected. Small hernias in the epigastrium or paraumbilical region should be sought in patients with superficial pain which is aggravated by coughing. Tenderness (and pain) will be increased if the recti abdominis are contracted by raising the head or the legs off the bed.

In males the external genitalia should be palpated because the genitalia may be small in chronic alcoholic liver disease and primary testicular tumours metastasize to abdominal lymph nodes and can cause deep abdominal or back pain.

Percussion of the abdomen is very useful in clarifying the contours of the liver and spleen, in determining the nature of suspected masses (solid or air filled), in detecting bladder enlargement and in distinguishing ascites from other causes of abdominal distension.

Auscultation is particularly useful in the acute abdomen. The ominous absence of bowel sounds betokens ileus, usually secondary to peritonitis following perforation or pancreatitis. The exaggerated, tinkling bowel sounds of intestinal obstruction are very characteristic. The gastric splash of pyloric stenosis is best heard by applying the ear to the epigastrium and gently shaking the patient's abdomen. Vascular bruits can be heard over the abdominal aorta and femoral arteries in patients with severe atheroma and an epigastric bruit accentuated by sitting up is caused by the arcuate ligament of the diaphragm compressing the coeliac artery. The clinical significance of this so-called 'coeliac axis compression syndrome' is uncertain. Some tumours, especially primary hepatocellular carcinomas, are so vascular that bruits may be heard over an hepatic mass.

# Examination of the anus and rectum

This is an essential part of the examination of all patients with bowel symptoms and lower abdominal pain. The patient is examined in the left lateral position with the legs well drawn up. The anal margin is inspected first for obvious skin disorders and for perianal tags characteristic of Crohn's disease. The patient should then strain down and this may reveal the lower part of an anal fissure, prolapsing haemorrhoids or the so-called 'descending perineum syndrome', which indicates weakness of the pelvic floor and is associated with problems of continence.

The anal canal is then examined digitally prior to deep rectal examination. An irregular painful canal usually suggests fissure or Crohn's disease if there is much induration. The consistency of any faeces present is noted and its appearance observed later when the finger is withdrawn. The finger is swept around the pelvis and will feel the sacrum posteriorly and, anteriorly, the prostate in the male and the cervix uteri in the female – an anterior bulge above the cervix may be due to a retroverted uterus. Abnormal masses within the rectum and compressing from without are noted along with any regions of particular tenderness. Pressure by the left hand above the pubis will often help to clarify the nature of a pelvic mass (bimanual examination). In the female a vaginal examination should be carried out if there appears to be a pelvic abnormality and if there are no contraindications.

Rigid sigmoidoscopy and proctoscopy are usually undertaken in the outpatient clinic in the unsedated patient, without prior bowel preparation, immediately after rectal examination. These procedures will however be described, along with other bowel investigations, in the next section.

## *I*NVESTIGATION OF PATIENTS WITH GASTROINTESTINAL DISORDERS

This will be discussed in relation to the main groups of symptoms and signs. In general symptoms which are prolonged (e.g. greater than $> 4$ weeks) unresponsive to simple therapy or recurrent and responsive to empirical treatment should all be investigated. This is especially true if there are accompanying features such as anaemia and loss of weight, or if persistent symptoms develop for the first time in the older age group ($> 50$ years).

# Investigation of dyspepsia/ abdominal pain

The most effective investigations are upper GI endoscopy and ultrasound examination of the gall bladder and pancreas, the order depending on the nature of the presentation. Barium studies of the oesophagus, stomach and duodenum and oral cholecystography still have a role and, in many hospitals, are more generally available.

### ENDOSCOPY

Upper GI endosocopy is now widely practised and many units perform $> 2000$ examinations per year. It is generally well tolerated, but most patients are given intravenous sedation and oral anaesthesia and need to recover in hospital for several hours. It is more accurate than barium meal in detecting oesophagitis, small gastric erosions, ulcers in a chronically deformed duodenal cap and recurrent ulcers after gastric surgery, and has the great advantage that biopsies and brushings for cytology can be taken from suspicious lesions. It is the investigation of choice in acute upper GI bleeding. After the patient has been resuscitated endoscopy is usually performed within the first 24 hours of admission. It is a very safe procedure, provided that the initial intubation is gentle. Difficulty may indicate cricopharyngeus spasm, a pharyngeal pouch or other high oesophageal obstruction. If these are suspected clinically, it is wise to refer the patient for a barium study first.

## BARIUM EXAMINATION

Barium examination has the great advantage that no sedation is required, it is well tolerated and the patient can leave the hospital immediately. The barium examination is better at demonstrating the initiation of swallowing, oesophageal motility and the different types of hiatal herniation (especially the rare rolling or paraoesophageal hernia). The modern double contrast technique is excellent at showing peptic ulcer, gastric cancer and even scattered small gastric ulcers. Once a duodenal cap is deformed by chronic ulceration, it is very difficult for the radiologist to demonstrate whether there is current active ulceration. It is important not to over interpret the common finding of a small sliding hiatus hernia, especially if reflux of barium into the oesophagus cannot be demonstrated using appropriate manipulation.

## ULTRASOUND

Ultrasound examination of the upper abdomen is widely performed, involves no radiation exposure and is very safe (Fig. 14.1). It shows gallstones more reliably than oral cholecystography (see below). In relation to the pancreas, ultrasound examination may be vitiated by too much gas and by obesity but it is usually an excellent way of showing cysts and pseudocysts. These can be drained using percutaneous techniques under ultrasound control for diagnostic or therapeutic purposes. Solid pancreatic masses may also be needled percutaneously under ultrasound control and material obtained for cytological or histological examination. Dilation and distortion of the duct system, features of chronic pancreatitis, are difficult to detect by ultrasound unless the changes are gross.

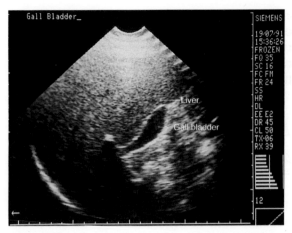

**Figure 14.1** Ultrasound scan of the normal liver and gallbladder.

## ORAL CHOLECYSTOGRAPHY

Oral cholecystography (OCG) is a simple examination and cheaper than ultrasound. It may be vitiated by poor absorption of contrast material by the gut or impaired uptake and secretion by the liver. It is useless if the patient is jaundiced. It does indicate whether the cystic duct is patent and whether any stones are radiolucent or opaque. These two points are relevant to the medical management of gallstones (page 381).

## COMPUTED TOMOGRAPHY

(CT) is particularly useful in the examination of the pancreas and other retroperitoneal structures (Fig. 14.2). It is expensive in terms of staff and equipment but is becoming more widely avail-

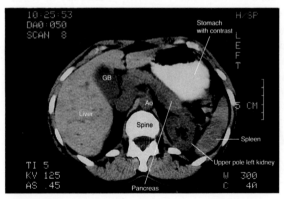

**Figure 14.2** Computed tomographic scan showing normal upper abdominal organs. GB = gall bladder. Ao = aorta.

able. It is probably superior to ultrasound in detecting solid masses in the pancreas and the changes of chronic pancreatitis, and examination is easier if the patient is relatively obese (abdominal fat produces sharp tissue planes). Suspicious pancreatic masses can be needled under CT scan control for diagnostic purposes.

## ENDOSCOPIC RETROGRADE CHOLANGIOPANCREATOGRAPHY

Using a side-viewing duodenoscope, a cannula is passed through the ampulla of Vater and contrast medium is injected into both pancreatic and bile ducts. It is technically a difficult procedure, but is becoming more generally available. It provides excellent views of the pancreatic duct system and this is valuable if surgical treatment of chronic pancreatitis is contemplated. Duodenoscopy itself will identify most cases of ampullary carcinoma of the pancreas and biopsies are easily obtained. Large carcinomas of the body and tail will usually distort the ductal anatomy, but histological material cannot be obtained. In general, ultrasound and CT scanning are better and safer than endoscopic retrograde cholangeopancreatography (ERCP) in the diagnosis of pancreatic cancer, but the final choice depends on local facilities.

# Investigation of bowel symptoms

## RIGID SIGMOIDOSCOPY AND PROCTOSCOPY

These are part of the initial examination of the patient and are undertaken (usually) without sedation or bowel cleansing. The sigmoidoscope is misnamed in the sense that it provides good views of the rectum only and examination of the sigmoid colon can be difficult and painful in perhaps 50 per cent of patients. It is helpful to see the faeces and any mucus or blood in the unprepared bowel. If bowel preparation proves necessary, it is probably better to proceed directly to flexible sigmoidoscopy if available (see

below). The normal rectal mucosa is pale pink and thin so that the submucosal vessels are easily seen. In proctitis (colitis) the mucosa becomes redder, thicker, granular and bleeds easily when gently scraped with the instrument (friability) – the blood vessels are no longer visible. Discrete ulcers are relatively uncommon but are seen in Crohn's disease (although the rectum is often 'spared') and amoebic and other specific colitides. Tumours and polyps are easily seen and mucosal biopsies taken with relative safety.

The proctoscope is a shorter, wider instrument which is designed for the examination of the anal canal itself. It is ideal for examining haemorrhoids and fissures and for injecting the former with sclerosing agents.

## FLEXIBLE SIGMOIDOSCOPY

Flexible sigmoidoscopy requires instruments of 30–60 cm in length, and the longer ones can reach the splenic flexure in most patients. The usual preparation is one or two phosphate enemas (e.g. Fletcher enemas) given a half to one hour before the procedure. Many patients will tolerate the procedure without sedation and can then leave immediately. It is very useful in patients with rectal bleeding, for the initial assessment of colonic pain and altered bowel habit, for assessing the extent of ulcerative colitis and for clarifying radiological abnormalities of the sigmoid colon seen at barium enema. Approximately 70 per cent of colonic tumours occur distal to the splenic flexure and are accessible with this instrument.

## BARIUM ENEMA AND COLONOSCOPY

Full colonic examination requires barium enema and/or colonoscopy. These are unpleasant for the patient and need meticulous bowel preparation if good views of the right half of the colon are to be obtained. It is essential in the investigation of overt lower GI bleeding and chronic occult blood loss if an adequate explanation has not been obtained by preliminary gastroscopy and flexible sigmoidoscopy. It is often required to establish the diagnosis of Crohn's disease (which frequently spares the left half of the colon) and to assess the proximal extent of ulcerative colitis (although flexible sigmoidoscopy may be adequate). It is often unrewarding in the investigation of non-descript chronic abdominal pain and watery diarrhoea, but carcinoma of the right side of the colon and proximal Crohn's colitis may have to be excluded in such patients. Diverticula are very common in older people, usually affect the sigmoid and descending colon and are often better seen by barium examination than by endoscopy. However, they may not be the cause of the patient's symptoms and should not divert attention from other more sinister possibilities.

Traditional preparation for barium enema and colonoscopy demands several days on a low residue diet and 24 hours on clear fluids only. An oral cathartic agent (e.g. Picolax or Ex-Prep) is given the evening before and on the morning of the examination. Newer large volume oral preparations (such as Golytely) can produce a clean bowel in a few hours, obviating the need for more prolonged preparations. Colonoscopy almost always requires intravenous analgesics and sedation and recovery for several hours or overnight is necessary. Barium enema is often the initial examination but, if an abnormality is found, endoscopy is usually required in order to obtain histological material or to undertake appropriate treatment, especially removal of polyps by electrocautery.

# Investigation of gastrointestinal blood loss

Overt bleeding demands endoscopic assessment, after appropriate resuscitation, if an accurate diagnosis is to be achieved. It is usual to start with upper GI endoscopy, even in the absence of haematemesis, and then to consider the colon if no abnormality is found.

Colonoscopy may be possible if the bleeding is modest, but should be avoided if there is pain or evidence of active colitis on an initial rigid sigmoidoscopy. In severe, continued lower GI bleeding, selective **visceral angiography** is required to show the site of bleeding and it may reveal a vascular tumour or malformation, such as angiodysplasia. Visceral angiography is often most helpful if bleeding is active and severe at

the time. In patients with recurrent, unexplained bleeding, it can be difficult to judge the optimum timing of the procedure. An isotopic scan, using labelled red cells, is a useful guide to the presence and approximate site of active bleeding and, if positive, can be followed immediately by angiography.

Chronic occult blood loss is a much commoner problem and is confirmed by persistently positive tests for blood in normal looking faeces. It usually demands upper GI endoscopy, barium enema or colonoscopy and small bowel radiology in that order. A useful test, in younger patients, is an isotope scan using pertechnetate which is taken up by gastric mucosa in a Meckel's diverticulum. This is a rare source of recurrent blood loss but is easily treated surgically.

# Investigation of malabsorption

Clinical suspicion may be strengthened (Table 14.11) by abnormal laboratory test results, for example, anaemia especially if macrocytic or of mixed cell type, depressed levels of serum folate and vitamin $B_{12}$, and biochemical evidence of osteomalacia or hypoalbuminaemia (although this is more commonly due to protein loss from abnormal mucosa than to malabsorption *per se*). Measurement of the fat content of faeces is unpleasant for the nursing and laboratory staff and for the patient but it is still the only direct way to document fat malabsorption and to exclude this as a cause of chronic diarrhoea. To be worthwhile, the patient must be on a known fat intake (usually 70–100 g daily) starting at least 2 days before the collection begins and all faeces passed over at least 3 days must be collected accurately.

## SMALL BOWEL BARIUM EXAMINATION

Small bowel barium examination is usually the first investigation unless there is a strong pointer to pancreatic pathology. The conventional examination is the barium meal and follow

**Table 14.11** Scheme for investigating diarrhoea/malabsorption.

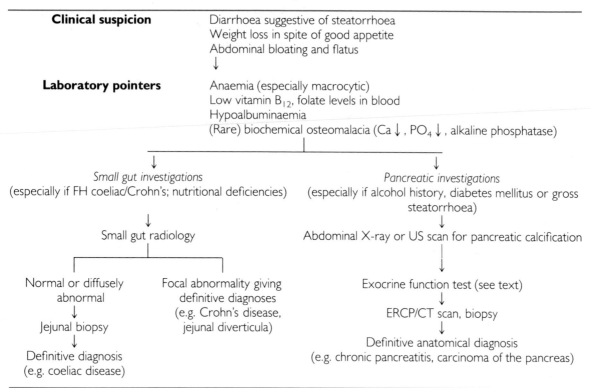

| Clinical suspicion | Diarrhoea suggestive of steatorrhoea<br>Weight loss in spite of good appetite<br>Abdominal bloating and flatus<br>↓ |
| --- | --- |
| Laboratory pointers | Anaemia (especially macrocytic)<br>Low vitamin B$_{12}$, folate levels in blood<br>Hypoalbuminaemia<br>(Rare) biochemical osteomalacia (Ca ↓ , PO$_4$ ↓ , alkaline phosphatase) |

*Small gut investigations*
(especially if FH coeliac/Crohn's; nutritional deficiencies)
↓
Small gut radiology

Normal or diffusely abnormal
↓
Jejunal biopsy
↓
Definitive diagnosis
(e.g. coeliac disease)

Focal abnormality giving definitive diagnoses
(e.g. Crohn's disease, jejunal diverticula)

*Pancreatic investigations*
(especially if alcohol history, diabetes mellitus or gross steatorrhoea)
↓
Abdominal X-ray or US scan for pancreatic calcification
↓
Exocrine function test (see text)
↓
ERCP/CT scan, biopsy
↓
Definitive anatomical diagnosis
(e.g. chronic pancreatitis, carcinoma of the pancreas)

FH = family history. ERCP = endoscopic retrograde cholangiopancreatography. CT = computed tomography. Ca = calcium. PO$_4$ = phosphate. US = ultrasound.

through, but this can be slow and tedious. It may reveal dilatation of intestinal loops and flocculation of barium, classic non-specific signs of malabsorption, or specific focal pathology such as Crohn's disease or diverticula. Better quality information, especially about focal pathology, is provided by **enteroclysis**. This involves nasoduodenal intubation and the rapid infusion of a large volume of barium and water directly into the small intestine. It is a more rapid examination, provided that the initial intubation does not take too long, but is unpleasant for the patient. Radiologists are divided about the merits of the two techniques.

## SMALL INTESTINAL MUCOSAL BIOPSY

Small intestinal mucosal biopsy is required to make a diagnosis of coeliac disease and a number of rarer causes of enteropathy such as tropical sprue etc. (page 359). It should be undertaken if the barium study shows non-specific abnormalities or, in certain circumstances, if the

study is completely normal. It can be done without preceding radiology if gut symptoms are absent but if there are strong pointers to ceoliac disease, for example, unexplained folate deficiency, Howell Jolly bodies in the red cells (page 598) or, rarely, unexplained osteomalacia (page 503). The conventional technique employs a suction biopsy capsule attached to a semistiff catheter which is passed via the mouth into the proximal jejunum under radiological control (Fig. 14.3). Useful information can be obtained from biopsies taken from the second part of the duodenum under direct vision at endoscopy. If duodenal biopsies prove difficult to interpret, then a jejunal biopsy should be obtained for clarification.

## JEJUNAL JUICE

Aspiration of jejunal juice can be undertaken at the same time as suction biopsy if a combined tube is used. The juice should be examined microscopically if giardiasis is suspected

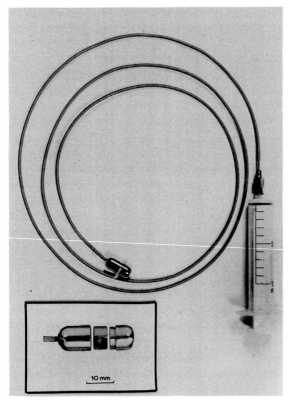

**Figure 14.3** The Watson jejunal biopsy capsule. This is mounted on a semistiff radio-opaque catheter and is advanced into the proximal jejunum under radiological control. Suction on the syringe pulls mucosa into the capsule and activates the rotating cutter (shown between the separated parts of the capsule).

(page 360). Bacterial culture using aerobic and anaerobic techniques will provide definitive evidence of overgrowth in patients with abnormally slow intestinal transit or fistulous communication between large and small bowel.

## ILEAL FUNCTION

Tests of ileal function are useful in the assessment of patients with Crohn's disease and of patients after intestinal resection. The most readily available is the Schilling test (page 606), which measures vitamin $B_{12}$ absorption in the presence of intrinsic factor. Severely impaired absorption suggests that at least 100 cm of distal ileum is diseased or has been resected (lengths of intestinal resection are notoriously difficult to assess at operation) and indicates the need for long-term vitamin $B_{12}$ replacement therapy. Vitamin $B_{12}$ absorption can however also be impaired by excessive bacterial activity in the upper small intestine.

## PANCREATIC EXOCRINE FUNCTION

Tests of pancreatic exocrine function are indicated if steatorrhoea is confirmed or obvious on clinical grounds and if the small intestine appears to be normal. Other pointers to the pancreas include heavy alcohol consumption and diabetes mellitus. The combination of steatorrhoea, diabetes and pancreatic calcification on abdominal X-ray makes formal tests of function superfluous.

The most reliable tests involve intubation of the duodenum and collection of mixed pancreatic juice and bile after a stimulus such as a mixed liquid meal (e.g. Lundh's test) or an intravenous injection or infusion of secretin and pancreozymin/cholecystokinin (CCK). The duodenal contents are assayed for output of enzymes (especially trypsin and lipase) and bicarbonate (following secretin infusion). In general, the tests based on hormone infusion are the more sensitive but are difficult to perform accurately. Lundh's test is much simpler but cruder, although it should identify patients with gross impairment of enzyme secretion.

## ASSESSMENT OF ALACTASIA

Milk intolerance attributed to reduced levels of mucosal lactase is common in many parts of the world (especially in Mediterranean countries, Africa and India) and may occur in 5 per cent of those of North European stock. A simple trial of milk exclusion may suffice but provocative tests using 25–50 g lactose are often used. In alactasic subjects, lactose produces excess gas and abdominal cramps, an increased excretion of hydrogen in the breath (which can be measured with simple portable machines) and a relatively small rise in blood glucose concentrations ($<1.1$ mmol/l). Alactasia can result from jejunal mucosal disease, especially coeliac disease, and a jejunal biopsy should be undertaken if there are any other pointers to an enteropathy.

# Clinical problems

## *D*ISORDERS OF THE OESOPHAGUS

## Gastro-oesophageal reflux

### AETIOLOGY

Reflux occurs in us all and from time to time produces mild symptoms. Frequent and prolonged reflux is the result of relative incompetence of the lower oesophageal sphincter. This is more likely to occur if the sphincter lies above the diaphragm as a consequence of sliding hiatal herniation of the upper stomach. Aggravating factors include delayed gastric emptying and oesophageal motility problems which impair the clearance of refluxed gastric contents back into the stomach.

In a **hiatal hernia** part of the stomach rises up into the thorax through the oesophageal hiatus either directly as a sliding hiatal hernia or a paraoesophageal or rolling hernia (page 348).

Symptomatic reflux is a very common problem and, in many patients, there is no obvious cause. Factors known to reduce lower oesophageal sphincter pressure include smoking, dietary fat, anticholinergic drugs and pregnancy (probably as a result of hormonal influences). Obesity and straining at stool are probable aggravating factors and may encourage hiatal herniation without directly affecting the competence of the lower oesophageal sphincter.

### PATHOLOGY

In uncomplicated reflux there may be no macroscopic or microscopic abnormality of the oesophageal mucosa. However, oesophagitis is common in patients with more severe symptoms and is usually apparent endoscopically and, if necessary, confirmed histologically. Ulceration and stricture formation are seen in the most severe cases. There is still uncertainty about the interpretation of gastric metaplasia in the lower oesophagus. Extensive upward spread of the gastric lining is easy to recognize endoscopically (**Barrett's oesophagus**) and is usually associated with chronic severe reflux. It may be associated with focal peptic ulceration and probably predisposes to the development of adenocarcinoma.

### CLINICAL FEATURES

The usual symptoms are heartburn, reflux, odynophagia and later obstructive dysphagia (pages 329–30). Less common symptoms include small haematemesis, chronic occult blood loss and cough or wheeze caused by aspiration, especially at night. Physical signs are usually absent, but the patient may become anaemic from blood loss or wasted if there is dysphagia. Rarely there are tell-tale signs of systemic sclerosis (page 577) when this causes the reflux.

### DIAGNOSIS

This can be based on history alone and investigations are only required if there is doubt or if simple therapy is ineffective. Haematemesis, anaemia and dysphagia demand investigation. The relative merits of barium studies and endoscopy were discussed on (pages 337–8). The most sensitive diagnostic method is 24 hour recording of oesophageal acidity using pH-sensitive electrodes passed transnasally. Many systems now include portable monitors for storage of data and its subsequent retrieval and analysis by computer (ambulatory pH recording).

In general, barium studies will show the propensity to reflux (hiatal hernia and reflux of barium during screening) and complications especially stricture. Endoscopy is required to assess the benign nature of a stricture and to clarify the source of bleeding.

## DIFFERENTIAL DIAGNOSIS

This is mainly from other causes of chest and epigastric pain and differentiation from cardiac pain can be especially difficult (page 330). The site of pain can cause confusion with peptic ulcer and the two problems are common enough to coexist.

## COMPLICATIONS

The serious ones are oesophageal stricture and possibly cancer, especially in relation to Barrett's oesophagus, and pulmonary aspiration.

## TREATMENT

Table 14.12 summarizes the management of gastro-oesophageal reflux. Antacids are best taken in generous doses and liquid form (10–20 ml) half to one hour after meals and before retiring. Alginate-containing preparations (Gaviscon and Gastrocote) are said to prevent reflux and provide a protective layer over the lower oesophageal mucosa.

$H_2$ receptor blockers (cimetidine, ranitidine) are effective in relieving symptoms and reducing the severity of oesophagitis and should be used if simple antacid therapy fails. The need for

**Table 14.12** Summary of medical management of gastro-oesophageal reflux.

| | |
|---|---|
| Reduce reflux | Weight reduction if obese |
| | Avoidance of straining at stool, bending at waist |
| | Elevation of head of bed (10–15 cm) |
| | Avoidance of smoking, fatty meals |
| | Avoidance of anticholinergic drugs |
| | Use of cholinergic drugs and dopamine antagonists |
| Reduce acid burden | Antacids |
| | Histamine ($H_2$) receptor blockers |
| | Omeprazole |
| Protect oesophageal mucosa | Alginate containing preparations (e.g. Gaviscon) |

their prolonged use should be regarded as a relative indication for antireflux surgery. Antacid and $H_2$ blocker therapy will be discussed in more detail on page 351.

Omeprazole is a proton-pump inhibitor which inhibits acid secretion more completely and for longer than the $H_2$ receptor blockers. It is a very effective treatment for the relief of reflux symptoms and heals severe reflux oesophagitis. It is beginning to supersede the $H_2$ receptor blockers in this context (see also page 352) and is now licensed for long-term use at a low dose (20–40 mg daily).

Metoclopramide and domperidone are dopamine antagonists, which accelerate gastric emptying and strengthen the lower oesophageal sphincter. They relieve symptoms if taken before meals and before retiring, but may cause troublesome side effects. This is especially true of the more centrally acting metoclopramide, which can cause distressing dystonias especially in older subjects.

Cisapride is a new type of drug which promotes gastric and intestinal transit and enhances the competence of the lower oesophageal sphincter. It is used similarly to the dopamine antagonists and has fewer side effects. These 'promotility' drugs are especially useful in the relief of nausea and of severe regurgitation.

### Treatment of stricture

Strictures can be dilated mechanically in a number of ways, using endoscopic or radiological techniques. At endoscopy a guidewire is passed through the stricture and the endoscope is removed. Metal 'olives', hard rubber bougies or catheter-mounted balloons can be passed along the guidewire and through the stricture, preferably under radiological control (Fig. 14.4).

In elderly or frail patients, infrequent dilation may be a satisfactory long-term treatment, but in younger fitter patients, antireflux surgery should be advised in the expectation that this will prevent continued inflammation and recurrent stricture formation.

### Surgical correction of reflux

The indications for surgery include chronic severe symptoms uncontrollable medically, the continued need for intensive medical treatment

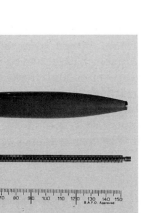

**Figure 14.4** An example of an oesophageal dilator. The semistiff dilator is attached to the flexible rod and the assembly is passed over a guidewire placed across the stricture at preliminary gastroscopy.

($H_2$ blockers or omeprazole) and the development of a stricture.

The principle of surgery is to reduce hiatal herniation, to strengthen the diaphragmatic hiatus and to reduce the risk of recurrent herniation by some form of wrap of gastric fundus around the lower oesophagus. The many procedures attest to the lack of any clear superiority of one surgical method.

The major early complications of surgery are dysphagia and the inability to belch if the gastric wrap is too tight. This can usually be managed by dilation and improves with time. Delayed recurrence of herniation and symptoms can occur, as with any form of hernia repair, and further attempts at surgery become more difficult and less likely to succeed.

## PROGNOSIS

This is good in the sense that most people respond well to medical treatment and this need not be continued indefinitely if the general measures referred to are adopted. Surgery in good hands is a very effective treatment for the minority who need it. Modern dilation techniques have improved the outlook considerably for those with strictures who are unfit for surgery. The risk of cancer seems to be very low, except perhaps in those with extensive gastric metaplasia (Barrett's oesophagus).

# Carcinoma of the oesophagus

## AETIOLOGY

There are enormous geographical variations in the incidence of oesophageal cancer and it seems certain that environmental factors are largely responsible for this. In England and Wales there are approximately 4000 new cases per year or 8 per 100 000 of the population. In most cases there is no obvious explanation or recognized predisposing cause, such as chronic reflux oesophagitis, Barrett's oesophagus, achalasia or chronic iron deficiency with oesophageal web formation (Paterson–Brown–Kelly or Plummer–Vinson syndrome).

## PATHOLOGY

The great majority of tumours arising in the mid and upper thirds of the oesophagus are squamous cell carcinomas. In the lower third, adenocarcinoma can arise from areas of gastric metaplasia but more commonly arises from the gastric fundus and spreads upwards. The tumours spread circumferentially and longitudinally and eventually invade adjacent structures especially the airways, pericardium and rarely the aorta.

## CLINICAL FEATURES

The usual symptom is remorselessly progressive obstructive dysphagia. Pain can be produced by acute bolus obstruction or by local mediastinal spread of disease. Patients rapidly lose weight and often become anaemic from blood loss (usually occult). Metastases may be palpable in the cervical glands or in the liver.

## DIAGNOSIS

This is usually strongly suspected on barium swallow and confirmed by examination of endoscopic biopsies and cytological brushings.

## DIFFERENTIAL DIAGNOSIS

This is from benign strictures, usually caused by chronic gastro-oesophageal reflux and rarely by swallowed caustics.

## COMPLICATIONS

Inanition and pulmonary aspiration are common. Obstruction of the airways, invasion of the aorta and spread into the pericardium are relatively rare. Diagnostic or therapeutic intubation procedures may be complicated by perforation and bleeding.

## TREATMENT

The only hope of cure of adenocarcinoma is radical surgery. Squamous cell carcinomas are radiosensitive and radiotherapy is usually the preferred treatment for cancers arising in the upper third of the oesophagus. However, extensive oesophageal resection is feasible and a high anastomosis between the pharynx and the gastric fundus can be created in the neck. In order to avoid fruitless surgery, it is helpful to assess operability with CT scanning to look for local nodes and invasion, and bronchoscopy to rule out invasion of the airways.

Unfortunately, most patients have inoperable tumours and, at the present time, only about 25 per cent of patients are suitable for surgical treatment. Palliation can be achieved by radiotherapy, but the morbidity is quite high. Most tumours are now treated palliatively by the insertion at endoscopy of short feeding tubes (endoprostheses) after initial dilation. Again there is appreciable morbidity because the tubes can get blocked by food boluses or become dislodged and migrate into the stomach. There is considerable current interest in the use of laser photocoagulation of tumours at endoscopy. Lasers are particularly effective if there are large soft tumour masses within the lumen and it is claimed that the quality of palliation is superior to that obtained by the placement of endoprostheses. The equipment for laser therapy is expensive and is currently only available in a few centres in the UK. There is no established chemotherapeutic programme for oesophageal cancer, although some new regimens are proving to be temporarily effective.

## PROGNOSIS

This is very poor. Patients treated palliatively rarely survive more than a few months. Mor-bidity after surgery is high and mortality rates of around 30 per cent are recorded. Individual surgeons have achieved considerably lower mortality rates and there is much to be said for treating these patients in special units. Overall long-term survival after 'curative' surgery is approximately 45 per cent at 1 year, 20 per cent at 2 years and 10 per cent at 5 years.

# Achalasia of the cardia

## AETIOLOGY

The cause of this primary neurological disturbance is unknown. A similar condition can complicate Chagas' disease (page 772), prevalent in South America, if the trypanosomal parasite damages the oesophageal nerve plexus extensively. The incidence of achalasia in the UK is approximately 1 case per 100 000 of the population per year.

## PATHOLOGY

Ganglion cells are lost from the submucosal and myenteric plexuses at the lower end of the oesophagus. Eventually there is widespread nerve damage throughout the body of the oesophagus, which becomes progressively dilated over a period of many years. Chronic oesophagitis accompanies prolonged stagnation of food in a dilated oesophagus and may account for the small long-term risk of cancer.

## CLINICAL FEATURES

There is usually a long history of variable dysphagia eventually complicated by inanition in neglected cases. Regurgitation of stagnant food may produce pulmonary complications. Episodic severe chest pain is ascribed to uncoordinated muscular activity and tends to occur in the early phase of the disease ('vigorous achalasia').

## DIAGNOSIS

Barium swallow shows a relatively normal oesophageal contour initially and the characteristic dilation and tortuosity only occur much later. Endoscopic appearances are normal in the early stages and the endoscope can usually be passed into the stomach quite easily, even though barium is held up at the tapered lower end of the oesophagus.

The abnormal motility of the oesophagus can be demonstrated by careful cine radiology while the patient swallows a bolus of food impregnated with barium. However, more accurate information is obtained by manometry, which is becoming increasingly available in specialized units. A multilumen tube assembly is passed via the nose into the stomach (this may prove to be difficult in achalasia) and then slowly withdrawn. Each lumen has an orifice through which pressures are measured and the orifices are placed 5 cm apart. In achalasia, there is a loss of coordinated peristalsis and the lower oesophageal sphincter fails to relax normally on swallowing.

## DIFFERENTIAL DIAGNOSIS

This is mainly from mechanical forms of dysphagia. Carcinoma can occasionally produce similar radiological appearance and manometry may fail if the assembly cannot be passed into the stomach. This has been called 'pseudo-achalasia'. Vigorous achalasia has to be distinguished from diffuse oesophageal spasm by manometry.

## TREATMENT

This is best achieved by the mechanical disruption of muscle fibres at the lower end of the oesophagus. This allows swallowing to occur by gravity but does not influence the disordered motor function of the oesophageal body. Heller's operation is a surgical myotomy in which the muscle is cut down to the submucosa. Various methods of forceful dilation have been devised using air, water or mercury filled balloons. There is a revival of interest in dilation techniques, which are usually employed initially and, if successful, repeated as necessary. Myotomy can be performed if dilation fails or is unacceptable to the patient.

Long-acting nitrates and nifedipine inhibit smooth muscle activity in the oesophagus and may provide some symptomatic relief, but

mechanical methods of treatment are usually required.

The major complication of successful therapy is gastro-oesophageal reflux because the sphincter is disrupted. This can be severe because oesophageal clearance of refluxed material is grossly impaired. It may be necessary to undertake antireflux surgery later.

# Diffuse oesophageal spasm

## AETIOLOGY

The cause of the disordered motility is unknown and the prevalence of this condition is uncertain.

## CLINICAL FEATURES

There is episodic severe chest pain occasionally associated with dysphagia. Conventional barium swallow and endoscopy are normal, but cine radiology of swallowing may show disordered peristalsis especially if the patient has symptoms at the time. Oesophageal manometry is abnormal and typically there is high pressure, uncoordinated, non-peristaltic activity. It may be possible to provoke this with an anticholinesterase drug, such as edrophonium, and reproduce the patient's symptoms at the same time. Normal relaxation of the lower oesophageal sphincter excludes achalasia. The main differential diagnosis is from cardiac pain, especially if there is no obvious disturbance of swallowing.

## TREATMENT

As with achalasia, long- or short-acting nitrates or nifedipine may be used to reduce muscular activity in much the same way as they are used in treating angina. For the occasional severe attack, some relief may be obtained by the sublingual application of glyceryl trinitrate in spray or tablet form or nifedipine as a crushed capsule. Response to treatment is difficult to evaluate or to predict, but most patients come to no harm especially if they are reassured that the symptom does not arise in the heart.

# Cricopharyngeus spasm and pharyngeal pouch

## AETIOLOGY

The cause of the spasm is unknown, but the pouch arises as a pulsion diverticulum through the posterior gap between the oblique fibres of the inferior constrictor muscle and the horizontal fibres of cricopharyngeus.

## CLINICAL FEATURES

There may be variable difficulty with swallowing but most food goes down the right way, while some accumulates and stagnates in the pouch, which slowly enlarges to the left of the mid-line. Pouch contents will regurgitate from time to time and this may produce cough and pulmonary aspiration. Pouches may be palpable or visible in the neck and occasionally they can reach a large size and extend down into the mediastinum.

## DIAGNOSIS

This is by barium radiology with particular emphasis on the pharyngeal phase of swallowing. Endoscopy is potentially dangerous and the diagnosis may be suggested by difficulty in passing the scope into the oesophagus. The common condition 'globus hystericus', or sense of lump in the throat, is not clearly related to and may even be relieved by swallowing. This is usually a psychological problem, and may be caused by increased tone in the cricopharyngeus muscle. However, muscular coordination during swallowing is normal.

## TREATMENT

This is surgical and it is necessary to perform a myotomy of the cricopharyngeus muscle and to excise the pouch. Occasionally myotomy alone is successful if dysphagia is the dominant symptom and if the pouch is small.

# Scleroderma of the oesophagus

This rare multisystem disorder (systemic scle-rosis) (page 577) can slowly destroy the oesophageal musculature, which is replaced by fibrous tissue. Peristalsis becomes weak and eventually disappears completely. There is dysphagia and often troublesome reflux oesophagitis, because refluxed acid is not adequately cleared. There is no specific treatment and nasogastric tube feeding may eventually be required.

# Paraoesophageal hiatal hernia (rolling)

This uncommon form of hiatal herniation (Fig. 14.5) may be a chance finding at endoscopy or on barium meal or may present acutely with severe chest pain and dysphagia if the herniated portion of stomach becomes twisted or strangulated. It is usually seen in older patients and probably does not cause chronic mild symptoms.

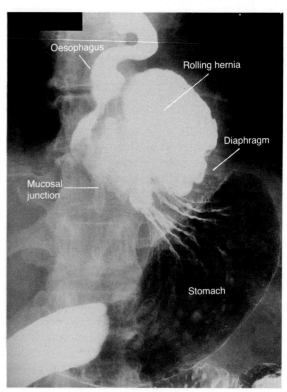

**Figure 14.5** Barium study of a mixed hiatus hernia.

## GASTRODUODENAL DISORDERS

# *Peptic ulcer*

## EPIDEMIOLOGY

There are striking geographical variations in the prevalence of peptic ulcers and in the distribution between gastric and duodenal types. In the developed world, duodenal ulcer is commoner than gastric ulcer and occurs at a younger age. Gastric ulcer becomes relatively commoner in the elderly and the use of non-steroidal anti-inflammatory drugs may account for an increasing admission rate for perforated peptic ulcer in elderly women, against a background of a sharp fall in admissions to hospital for peptic ulcer over the last 20 years. Part of this fall is due to improved medical management rather than to decreasing prevalence.

The prevalence of peptic ulcer is difficult to determine because minor digestive disturbances are not investigated and ulcers may be asymptomatic. Moreover, ulcers come and go over prolonged periods. Prevalence rates of 6 per cent for men and 2 per cent for women in the London area were obtained 20 years ago and duodenal ulcer was 2–3 times commoner than gastric ulcer. The prevalence of peptic ulcer is higher in Scotland and the north of England than in the south. Although its prevalence may be declining, peptic ulcer remains a common disease in the UK of probably diminishing severity.

## AETIOLOGY

A mucosal break in the stomach or proximal duodenum represents a temporary victory by offensive factors in gastric juice (especially acid and pepsin) over the defensive properties of the mucosa (production of mucus and antral and duodenal secretion of small amounts of bicarbonate). Reflux of duodenal contents into the stomach provides additional noxious agents (especially bile salt and pancreatic enzymes), which may be implicated in the development of gastritis and gastric ulcer. The overriding import-ance of acid is shown by the healing properties of strong antisecretory agents and the absence of peptic ulcer in patients who fail to secrete acid (e.g. pernicious anaemia). However, most patients with peptic ulcer produce amounts of acid which are within the normal range and antisecretory agents do not heal all ulcers. Acid is necessary for ulceration but impairment of mucosal resistance is clearly important, especially in patients with gastric ulcer who tend to have lower acid outputs than those with duodenal ulcer. In peptic ulcer disease, especially duodenal ulcer, the stomach is commonly colonized by a bacterium *Helicobacter pylori*, which is invariably associated with an active chronic gastritis, affecting especially the gastric antrum. It is widely speculated that *H. pylori* infection precedes the development of and indeed causes duodenal ulcer. Its eradication is associated with prolonged healing of ulcers (page 353).

Genetic and environmental factors are responsible for the development of peptic ulcers but are largely unidentified. No certain noxious agents in food have been identified and it is possible that some foods have a protective role.

Smoking cigarettes is probably an aggravating and not a causative factor and alcohol consumption has not been implicated in the pathogenesis of chronic peptic ulcer (as opposed to acute transient gastric damage).

The relationship between stressful life events and ulcer disease is unclear, but the stress of serious illness and injury is sometimes associated with acute gastric and duodenal ulceration ('stress ulcers').

## PATHOLOGY

The lesions may be superficial or deep, large or small, single or multiple, acute or chronic. Common sites of chronic single ulcers are on the lesser curve, in the antrum, pyloric channel and first part of duodenum. Multiple ulcers tend to be acute, superficial and widely scattered over the gastric mucosa. The duodenal mucosa may be diffusely inflamed with many tiny superficial ulcers (duodenitis) and this pattern may coexist with a single chronic ulcer crater. Acute, multiple ulcers are related to acute gastric injury by drugs, alcohol and perhaps stress and are clinically quite distinct from the more common chronic ulcers. Most patients have either a duodenal ulcer or gastric ulcer, but the two can coexist in which case the gastric ulcer is usually situated in or close to the pyloric channel.

The histopathological features are not in any way specific or distinctive. Chronic inflammatory changes are seen in the mucosa near gastric ulcers and various forms of intestinal metaplasia have been described. *Helicobacter pylori* can be identified in close proximity to the antral mucosa, almost universally in patients with duodenal ulcer and in 60–75 per cent of patients with gastric ulcer.

## CLINICAL FEATURES

The commonest symptom is pain and the main features have already been described (page 331). Vomiting and weight loss are common with uncomplicated gastric ulcer. The major complications include the profuse vomiting of pyloric stenosis, haematemesis and melaena and sudden perforation with peritonitis. Physical signs in the uncomplicated case are usually limited to epigastric tenderness.

## DIAGNOSIS

This depends on barium meal and/or gastroscopy as discussed on page 337. Gastric ulcers should be biopsied to exclude malignancy but this is not relevant to the management of duodenal ulcer. The differential diagnosis is wide and has been discussed in the section on investigating dyspepsia and abdominal pain (page 331). Zollinger–Ellison syndrome is described on page 356. Risk factors for developing peptic ulcer are summarized in Table 14.13.

**Table 14.13** Risk factors for peptic ulcer.

Smoking
Aspirin and/or non-steroidal anti-inflammatory drugs (NSAIDs)
Positive family history
Hypercalcaemia
Stress (difficult to define)
Corticosteroids (still some uncertainty)

## COMPLICATIONS

Acute superficial ulcers can bleed, occasionally profusely. Deep ulcers can bleed, often profusely, can perforate through the gut wall and can obstruct the pylorus or an operative stoma.

Acute upper gastrointestinal haemorrhage (Table 14.14) is a common emergency and the immediate priority is to assess the severity of blood loss, to institute appropriate resuscitative measures and then to find out the source of the bleeding. Blood transfusion is required urgently to treat shock and should be monitored by repeated measurement of central venous pressure as well as blood pressure and pulse rate. Blood should also be transfused if the haemoglobin falls below 10 g/dl or if bleeding continues. Bleeding from multiple superficial ulcers usually settles spontaneously and rarely requires surgery. Intravenous cimetidine or ranitidine and continuous alkalinization of the stomach

**Table 14.14** Emergency treatment of severe upper gastrointestinal bleeding.

Assessment of the degree of blood loss

Resuscitation with intravenous saline, followed by blood

Pulse and blood pressure monitoring

Central venous pressure monitoring (especially if frail or there is serious cardiopulmonary disease)

Nil by mouth pending decision on timing of gastroscopy

Intravenous H$_2$ receptor blockers
↓
*Endoscopy* when haemodynamically stable and within 24 hours

*Intervention*

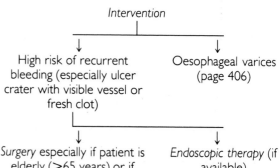

High risk of recurrent bleeding (especially ulcer crater with visible vessel or fresh clot)

Oesophageal varices (page 406)

*Surgery* especially if patient is elderly (>65 years) or if transfusion of >4 units blood and continued or recurrent bleeding

*Endoscopic therapy* (if available) e.g. laser or thermocoagulation with 2-hourly antacids may be helpful. Recurrent bleeding from a chronic ulcer crater is likely if endoscopy shows tell-tale features such as an adherent clot or the so-called 'visible vessel' – a pink or bluish bulge in the base of the crater. Such patients should be considered for emergency surgery or some form of electrocoagulation or photocoagulation therapy by laser if the facilities are available. Surgical or other intervention is probably advisable in such patients over the age of 65, unless there is a really serious contraindication, because mortality is much higher in the older age groups. However, there is still considerable debate about the wisdom and timing of surgery in this common problem and it is impossible to lay down firm rules. Relatively clear guidelines for surgery are the need to replace more than 4 units of blood and undoubted continued or recurrent bleeding, as judged by external blood loss or difficulty in maintaining the central venous pressure (CVP) (nasogastric tube aspiration is not very helpful and is best avoided). Intravenous cimetidine or ranitidine is probably of little use in stemming serious bleeding from a chronic ulcer crater but is widely prescribed.

Perforation of a deep ulcer crater usually presents with sudden severe pain and board-like abdominal rigidity. An erect chest X-ray will show free gas under the diaphragm. Treatment requires nasogastric aspiration, intravenous fluids and analgesics followed by surgery after appropriate resuscitative measures have been carried out. Perforations can close spontaneously and non-operative treatment is sometimes appropriate if there is delay in recognizing that a perforation has occurred.

Pyloric stenosis causes a characteristic form of vomiting with distinctive physical signs which have been described (page 330). The patient may be wasted if the condition has been neglected and is often dehydrated and alkalotic. The typical biochemical disturbance is a low plasma chloride, a high bicarbonate, a raised pH and somewhat raised $PCO_2$. Potassium depletion may develop as a result of excess loss in a paradoxically acid urine. Nasogastric aspiration, initially using a widebore tube and repeated lavage, will relieve gastric distress and intravenous saline supplemented by KCl will usually correct the biochemical abnormalities quite easily. Endoscopic assessment can be undertaken after lavage has cleared the stomach of gross contamination by food. Treatment is usually surgical, although rarely relatively acute ulcers with much surrounding oedema will subside rapidly with medical treatment.

## MEDICAL TREATMENT

(Table 14.15) Smoking should be prohibited because ulcers heal more slowly in smokers than in non-smokers. Sensible eating habits should be encouraged with regular meals and the avoidance of long periods without food. Symptoms may be relieved by milk and snacks, but there is no evidence that the once fashionable gastric diets (mainly steamed fish and milk) are of any real value in healing ulcers. Large volumes of milk combined with generous quantities of sodium bicarbonate or calcium carbonate were in the past responsible for hypercalcaemia and renal failure ('milk-alkali syndrome'), but this is rarely seen now with modern medical management.

### Antacids

Antacid therapy should be used first for symptomatic relief but, to be effective in healing, large volumes of a soluble preparation have to be given 1 hour after meals and on retiring (e.g. 100–200 ml daily), although smaller doses will usually provide symptomatic relief and may be taken in tablet form. There are numerous preparations and many contain several compounds

**Table 14.15** Summary of medical management of peptic ulcer.

| | |
|---|---|
| General measures | Avoidance of smoking, aspirin, non-steroidal anti-inflammatory drugs, corticosteroids; 'sensible' eating habits |
| Antacids/antisecretory agents | Histamine ($H_2$) receptor blockers Omeprazole |
| Mucosal protective agents | Sucralfate, bismuth chelate |
| Anti-Helicobacter therapy | Bismuth chelate plus 2 antibiotics (triple therapy, see text) |

in order to improve palatability and reduce the risk of complications. In general, magnesium-containing antacids produce diarrhoea and can lead to magnesium intoxication in patients with renal failure. Aluminium-containing compounds tend to produce constipation, sequester phosphate in the gut and can lead to phosphate depletion (they are used for this purpose in patients with chronic renal failure). Calcium carbonate and sodium bicarbonate are seldom used now. Some antacid mixtures contain large amounts of sodium and should be used with caution in patients with heart failure and other causes of fluid retention. In view of all these problems and the availability of more effective and acceptable drugs, antacids are seldom now the main therapy for chronic peptic ulcer, unless symptoms are mild and intermittent.

## Histamine 2 (H₂) receptor blockers

The advent of cimetidine in 1976 revolutionized the treatment of peptic ulcer. This drug and its successors provide remarkably safe, simple and effective treatment of gastric and duodenal ulcers, but they remain relatively expensive and should be used with some circumspection. It is unnecessary to demand endoscopic assessment before prescribing these drugs, but their continued use over long periods (months) or their frequent use in shorter courses should be delayed until a diagnosis has been made. One worry in the older age groups is that these drugs may mask the symptoms of gastric cancer and lead to a delay in diagnosis.

It is usual to treat symptoms for a month or so with 'full' dose, for example 800 mg cimetidine or 300 mg ranitidine in the evening. The dose can then be reduced by half to a 'maintenance' dose and this should be continued for a variable period by trial and error. Symptoms are often controlled within days and 60–80 per cent of ulcers can be expected to heal completely within 6 weeks. Up to 80–90 per cent of ulcers will heal if treatment is continued for 12 weeks, but healing rates are slower for gastric ulcer than for duodenal ulcer. Relapse rates are unfortunately high (e.g. > 50 per cent over 1 year) after the treatment is withdrawn, but not all relapses are symptomatic or necessarily harmful to the patient and symptomatic relapses can usually be controlled easily with another course of the drug.

The long-term treatment of duodenal ulcer with H₂ receptor blockers is empirical and it is doubtful whether endoscopic follow-up is of much help in management. The management of gastric ulcer is different, because endoscopic follow-up is required to ensure that the ulcer has healed and is not malignant (repeat endoscopy, biopsy and cytology at 6–8 weeks and again at 12–16 weeks if healing is slow) and also because treatment is relatively less effective and alternative drugs are more likely to be required.

The choice of H₂ blocker is determined partly by cost and partly by consideration of the potential side effects of cimetidine (Table 14.16). Ranitidine is the drug of choice for long-term use in males and for short-term use in patients taking drugs whose metabolism is impaired by cimetidine. The newer H₂ receptor blockers (nizatidine, famotidine) seem to offer no definite advantages.

**Table 14.16** Side effects of cimetidine and ranitidine.

|  | Cimetidine | Ranitidine |
|---|---|---|
| Impairs cytochrome p450 oxidase | Yes | No |
| Anti-androgenic | Yes | Probably no |
| Mental confusion | Yes | No |
| Cardiac arrhythmias | Yes | Rare, if at all |

## Omeprazole

The proton pump inhibitor, omeprazole, is a very potent antisecretory agent reducing acid output by more than 90 per cent. It heals ulcers more rapidly than H₂ receptor blockers, but relapse rates following a course of treatment are just as high. It is not yet licensed for maintenance treatment of ulcer. Its use at present is restricted to ulcers which resist conventional treatment with H₂ receptor blockers as shown endoscopically, and to the rare patient with Zollinger–Ellison syndrome (page 356). It is more widely used in the treatment of reflux oesophagitis (page 343).

## Mucosal protective agents

A number of drugs heal ulcers as effectively as H₂ receptor blockers without inhibiting acid secretion, and in various ways protect the mucosa. They can promote healing of ulcers which fail to respond adequately to $H_2$ receptor blockers, and this probably applies particularly to gastric ulcers. Their precise mode of action is uncertain. Two commonly used drugs are sucralfate (a complex of aluminium hydroxide and sulphated sucrose) and De-Nol (a potassium-citrate-bismuth chelate). Sucralfate is given twice daily over 1–2 months and the only side effect is mild constipation. De-Nol is now given in tablet form, again twice daily and colours the stools black. It should not be used in long courses for fear of bismuth accumulation and is best avoided in renal failure. There is good evidence that relapse rates after withdrawal of these drugs are less than those observed after withdrawal of $H_2$ blockers. Nevertheless they tend to be used as second-line drugs when $H_2$ blockers have failed, in spite of the fact they are somewhat cheaper.

## Triple therapy

The combination of De-Nol and antibiotics (usually amoxycillin or tetracycline and metronidazole) can eradicate *H. pylori* for weeks or months and this is associated with prolonged healing of ulcers. This 'triple therapy', which is prescribed for 2 weeks, should be tried in patients who repeatedly suffer symptomatic relapse soon after withdrawing $H_2$ receptor blockers. It may produce prolonged remission of symptoms and the course can be repeated infrequently (e.g. once or twice yearly) as required. The value of 'triple therapy' in the long-term management of peptic ulcers has not yet been established.

## Misoprostil

Misoprostil is a substituted prostaglandin which enhances mucosal cytoprotection and also inhibits gastric acid secretion weakly. It is an effective antiulcer agent but commonly produces quite severe diarrhoea. It was introduced for coprescription with non-steroidal anti-inflammatory drugs (NSAIDs) in order to prevent ulceration. It also promotes healing of ulcers which develop during NSAID therapy but in this respect it is not superior to $H_2$ receptor blockers.

Drug therapy of peptic ulceration is summarized in Table 14.17.

**Table 14.17** Summary of drugs used in treatment of peptic ulcer.

| Group | Examples | Dosage | | Side effects |
| | | Therapeutic | Maintenance | |
| --- | --- | --- | --- | --- |
| 1. Antacids | Mg containing Al containing or mixtures (e.g. Maalox) | 10–15 ml 1 hour after meals and on retiring (Symptom relief only. Healing requires larger doses) | | Diarrhoea Constipation (NB Na overload, cation toxicity in renal failure) |
| 2. Antisecretory drugs | | | | |
| (a) Histamine (H₂) receptor blockers | Cimetidine | 800 mg nocte | 400 mg nocte | Inhibits cytochrome P450 Blocks androgen receptors |
| | Ranitidine | 300 mg nocte | 150 mg nocte | Minor |
| (b) Proton pump inhibitors | Omeprazole | 20–40 mg daily | Not yet recommended | Minor |
| 3. Mucosal protective | Sucralfate | 1 g × 4 daily | 1 g × 2 daily | Constipation Al toxicity |
| | Bismuth chelate* | 120 mg × 4 daily | Not recommended | Bismuth toxicity |
| | Prostaglandin† analogues, e.g. Misoprostil | 200 mg × 4 daily | 200 mg × 2 daily‡ | Diarrhoea Abortion |

*Mg = magnesium. Al = aluminium. Na = sodium.  †Antisecretory at higher doses.
‡Especially if coprescribed with non-steroidal anti-inflammatory drugs.
Often combined with antibiotics to eradicate H. plylori (see text).

# SURGICAL MANAGEMENT OF UNCOMPLICATED PEPTIC ULCER

The relative indications are continued distressing symptoms in spite of full medical measures and the continued need to take medication if surgery can safely be offered as an alternative. Operation rates for peptic ulcer fell dramatically in the years following the introduction of cimetidine, but there is evidence of a rise again, perhaps reflecting an understandable reluctance to take medication indefinitely. Surgery tends to be offered when gastric ulcers fail to heal in a few weeks, but this reflects concern over the possibility of malignancy as well as the poorer prognosis of unhealed gastric ulcer in terms of complications.

Surgery is designed to reduce gastric acid secretion and the older operations of partial gastrectomy and vagotomy with antrectomy were undoubtedly very successful, but at the expense of sometimes distressing side effects (Fig. 14.6). Vagotomy with drainage procedures and especially highly selective vagotomy are better tolerated but have a higher rate of ulcer recurrence. A balance has to be struck between the risk of serious side effects and the risk of recurrent ulcer, but the latter is probably preferable as recurrent ulcers may respond well to modern medical treatment. Highly selective vagotomy (Fig. 14.7) is theoretically the most attractive operation for duodenal ulcers but recurrence rates as high as 20 per cent have been reported. Gastric ulcers can also be treated by this operation but there has always been reluctance to leave a gastric ulcer *in situ* (for fear of malignancy) and most surgeons still perform a limited gastrectomy with removal of the antrum and the more physiological Bilroth I anastomosis if the proximal duodenum is healthy.

Patients should reasonably expect an 85–95 per cent success rate in terms of complete or considerable relief of symptoms, but side effects may be distressing (at least temporarily) in up to 5 per cent of patients.

## *Symptoms after peptic ulcer surgery*

Vomiting may be part of the 'small stomach syndrome' with postprandial pain and fullness and early satiety (Table 14.18). This usually responds simply to reducing the size and increasing the frequency of meals. A rarer but more distressing problem is bile vomiting which occurs particularly in patients who have a gastrojejunostomy. Copious vomiting of bile rather than

**Table 14.18** Symptoms after peptic ulcer surgery.

| | |
|---|---|
| Small stomach syndrome | Early satiety, food-induced pain and vomiting |
| Rapid transit of food into intestine | Early dumping syndrome, reactive hypoglycaemia (late dumping), postvagotomy diarrhoea |
| Long-term problems | Loss of weight, anaemia (Fe, $B_{12}$ deficiency), osteomalacia |
| Reflux of bile into stomach | Bile-vomiting syndrome |
| Impaired luminal digestion | Steatorrhoea |

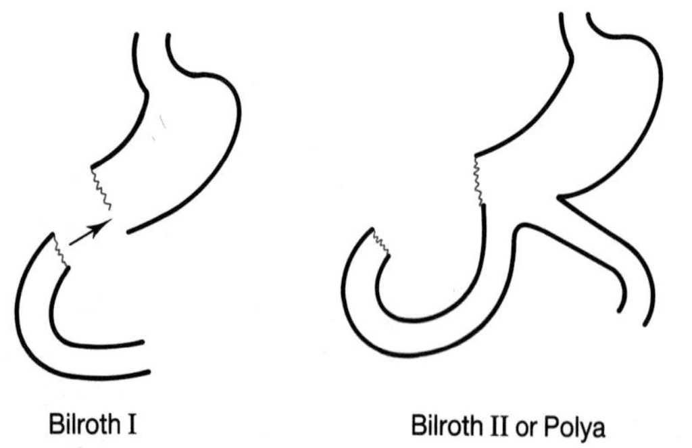

**Figure 14.6** Classical anastomoses following partial gastrectomy for gastric ulcer (Bilroth I) or duodenal ulcer (Bilroth II or Polya).

Bilroth I            Bilroth II or Polya

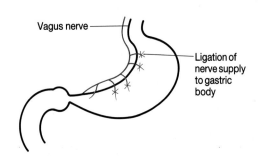

Vagus nerve

Ligation of nerve supply to gastric body

**Figure 14.7** Highly selective vagotomy which preserves gastroduodenal anatomy and antral innervation.

food occurs after meals and is ascribed to the passage of large amounts of proximal duodenal contents through the gastric remnant. It can be very difficult to control and may occasionally justify a second bile-diverting procedure (especially the *Roux-en-Y* conversion, Fig. 14.8). In well-selected patients, this can be very successful.

A change in bowel habit is common after all types of gastric surgery, but it is usually a mild increase in faecal frequency and bulk which may not be unwelcome to the patient. A modest degree of steatorrhoea is common and is not surprising in view of the gross disturbance of gastric emptying and the impaired mixing of food with pancreaticobiliary secretions. This can be helped, if necessary, by some restriction of dietary fat and occasionally by the use of pancreatic enzyme replacements (page 388).

Severe watery diarrhoea, often intermittent, is an occasional complication of truncal vagotomy and pyloroplasty and is much less of a problem after highly selective vagotomy. The mechanism is unclear, but it seems to be related in some patients to the rapid transit of intestinal contents to the colon after meals. Under these circumstances, bile salts can be swept into the colon where they exert a direct cathartic effect. In approximately 50 per cent of these patients, the diarrhoea will respond well to the bile acid binding agent cholestyramine.

The term '*dumping syndrome*' is applied to two different physiological disturbances which result from the rapid entry of gastric contents into the small intestine and the rapid absorption of carbohydrate. Early dumping occurs within 30 min of eating and is characterized by faintness, palpitations, abdominal distension and sometimes later fluid diarrhoea. Postural hypotension and temporary haemoconcentration may occur and suggest a shift of fluid from plasma into the gut lumen. Release of vasoactive compounds may also produce vasodilation. Treatment can be difficult and the usual advice is to reduce the intake of fluid with meals and to avoid sweet drinks and carbohydrate-rich foods, which would promote the osmotic attraction of fluid into the gut lumen. Late dumping consists of hypoglycaemic symptoms which develop after a delay of 1–2 hours and result from excessive insulin release in response to rapid absorption of glucose from the gut. Again a relatively low carbohydrate diet and the avoidance of sweet drinks may prevent this symptom. Agents which delay gastric emptying and retard the absorption of carbohydrate (e.g. guar gum) may help to prevent both types of dumping problem.

Loss of weight is common after gastric resection but is less marked after vagotomy. It is usually caused by reduced food intake rather than by malabsorption and the preoperative weight may never be regained. Iron deficiency anaemia is the commonest long-term nutritional deficiency seen after gastric surgery and responds well to inorganic ferrous salts. Vitamin $B_{12}$ may eventually be malabsorbed as a result of chronic inflammation of the remnant of gastric mucosa with consequent loss of the capacity to secrete intrinsic factor (IF). Osteomalacia, due to vitamin D deficiency, is an occasional consequence of gastric resection.

## PROGNOSIS

The prognosis of benign peptic ulcer disease is good in the sense that deaths are infrequent and diminishing, and modern medical treatment is effective and improving. Gastric ulceration in elderly patients taking NSAIDs has a relatively poor prognosis in that the first presentation is often a serious complication such as bleeding or perforation and emergency surgery may be required.

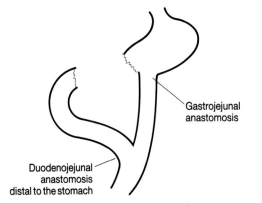

**Figure 14.8** *Roux-en-Y* procedure designed to keep bile and pancreatic juice away from the gastric remnant.

# Zollinger–Ellison syndrome (gastrinoma)

This rare condition is caused by a gastrin-producing tumour arising from islet cells of the pancreas. In over 50 per cent of cases, the tumour is malignant and can metastasize, but the natural history is a long one. Gastric secretion of acid is greatly increased and produces severe ulcer disease in stomach, duodenum and even in the jejunum. Chronic diarrhoea is common and may even be the presenting symptom. Ulcer complications are frequent and recurrent ulcer is invariable after all forms of surgery other than total gastrectomy. Very large doses of $H_2$ blockers (e.g. 2–5 g cimetidine or 1–2 g ranitidine daily) may control symptoms and reduce acid secretion. Omeprazole in large doses (e.g. 80–120 mg daily) is even more effective in controlling acid secretion and will probably supersede the $H_2$ blockers in this condition. The advent of these very powerful drugs has made total gastrectomy unnecessary in most cases.

The diagnosis is based on a raised serum gastrin in the presence of increased gastric acid secretion – a very high basal acid output ($>$ 15 mmol $H^+$/hour) is the most characteristic abnormality. It is advisable then to search for the pancreatic tumour with appropriate scanning techniques in case resection can be undertaken.

# Gastric cancer

## AETIOLOGY

Adenocarcinoma of the stomach accounts for almost 10 per cent of all cancers in the UK, although its incidence is declining. There are approximately 28 male and 19 female deaths from this cancer per 100 000 of the UK population annually. Mortality rates are lower in the USA and much higher in Japan and other parts of the Far East. It is almost certain that dietary carcinogens play a crucial role in pathogenesis.

Epidemiological evidence from Japan has implicated highly salted food as a causative factor. Genetic factors are also important as shown by studies of family history.

Certain chronic gastric lesions predispose to cancer and include the atrophy of pernicious anaemia and some types of intestinal metaplasia associated with chronic gastritis and benign gastric ulcer.

## PATHOLOGY

Adenocarcinomas arise in all parts of the stomach and are usually single, spreading lesions, which grow into the lumen, infiltrate the wall and penetrate beyond its confines. The term early gastric cancer is applied to lesions confined to the mucosa and submucosa and which, if resected, carry a remarkably good prognosis. It is clearly important to try to recognize this lesion but the clinical, radiological and even endoscopic features may be minor. Unfortunately gastric cancer is often recognized at an advanced stage when there has already been metastatic spread to local and distant lymph nodes and to the liver.

Diffuse infiltration of the stomach wall may give rise to a rigid stomach with restricted filling known as 'linitis plastica' or 'leather bottle stomach'.

## CLINICAL FEATURES

The usual symptoms are epigastric pain, nausea and anorexia in a patient over the age of 55 and the history is short. A high fundic lesion can cause obstructive dysphagia and a distal antral lesion may obstruct the pylorus and produce vomiting. Loss of weight and anaemia are common. Physical signs include wasting, palpable metastases in the neck or liver and occasionally a palpable gastric mass.

## DIAGNOSIS

This depends on barium meal and gastroscopy with biopsy and cytology. The major differential diagnosis is between a benign gastric ulcer and a flat ulcerating malignancy, and histological examination is crucial. A rarity is a gastric lymphoma, which may carry a better prognosis if treated with appropriate chemotherapy.

## COMPLICATIONS

These are bleeding and obstruction. Chronic loss of protein-rich fluid from the mucosal surface can produce marked hypoalbuminaemia and present as oedema.

## TREATMENT

The best (but small) hope of cure is radical surgical excision and this may necessitate total gastrectomy if the lesion is in the mid or upper third of the stomach. Preliminary CT scanning helps to determine operability and may reduce the need for fruitless laparotomy. If the lesion is judged to be inoperable, palliative surgery may still be worthwhile especially to bypass an obstructing antral lesion. Resection of a tumour may occasionally be justified, even if metastases are present, in order to relieve distressing gastric symptoms, anaemia or protein loss.

Non-surgical palliation is very limited in its scope. Conventional radiotherapy is ineffective, but some success has been achieved with fast neutron irradiation. There is no established chemotherapy programme, although multi-centre trials continue in many parts of the world.

## PROGNOSIS

This remains poor and patients rarely survive more than a few months unless radical resection is possible. Fewer than a third of patients are suitable for 'curative' resection and, of those, 5-year survival figures are 30 per cent less. By contrast, resection of early gastric cancer produces an 80 per cent chance of surviving 5 years or more.

# Other gastric lesions

## CHRONIC GASTRITIS

This is an endoscopic and histological diagnosis and its symptomatic significance is uncertain. It can be induced by duodenogastric reflux (e.g. postoperatively) and the excessive and continued use of alcohol, aspirin, spicy foods etc. is often implicated but without good evidence. Current interest relates to the role of infection by *H. pylori*, which is probably responsible for most cases of chronic gastritis. The main significance of chronic gastritis is its probable relation to the development of gastric ulcer and cancer.

Autoimmune destruction of the specialized gastric mucosa of the body and fundus is the basis of pernicious anaemia (page 605).

## BENIGN STOMACH TUMOURS

Benign tumours of the stomach are rare and include adenoma and leiomyoma. They are usually chance findings but may bleed and cause anaemia if the surface is ulcerated. They require removal at endoscopy or by surgery, unless they are very small, because both types can become malignant.

## MENETRIER'S DISEASE

This is a rare condition of unknown cause in which there is massive hypertrophy of the non-specialized part of the gastric epithelium. The mucosa becomes grossly folded or polypoid in appearance and histological differentiation from multiple adenomatous polyps requires deep biopsies at endoscopy. The presentation is with pain and hypoalbuminaemic oedema – it is a well-recognized cause of protein loss from the mucosa (protein-losing gastropathy). Treatment is by surgical excision, although self-limiting cases have been described. There is probably an increased risk of later adenocarcinoma.

# DISORDERS OF THE SMALL INTESTINE

## Coeliac disease (gluten sensitive enteropathy, coeliac sprue)

### AETIOLOGY

This is a diffuse enteropathy, which affects the proximal small intestine more than the distal and is caused by a sensitivity to dietary gluten. Gluten is the water-insoluble protein found in wheat, barley, rye and oats but not rice. The condition probably starts when wheat-based foods are introduced after the baby is weaned from milk. Transient sensitivity to gluten is described in infants, but in true coeliac disease the sensitivity is life long although clinical presentation can be remarkably variable and delayed. Acquired sensitivity in later life has never been described. The mechanism of gluten sensitivity remains uncertain but is thought to involve local cell-mediated immune responses in the intestinal mucosa to gluten.

The disease is far commoner in the developed world than elsewhere and the highest recorded prevalence is in the UK (1 in 2000) and in the west of Ireland (1 in 500 or even less).

Genetic factors are undoubtedly important as shown by family studies and there is a well-established association with the genetic marker HLA-B8.

### PATHOLOGY

The jejunal mucosa becomes relatively or completely flat with loss of villi, deep crypts and a marked cellular infiltrate into the lamina propria. The enterocytes (mucosal absorptive cells) are flattened, lymphocytes infiltrate the mucosal surface and there is evidence of increased mitotic activity in the crypts.

### CLINICAL FEATURES

It is now rare to see patients with severe steatorrhoea and malnutrition. However, diarrhoea and steatorrhoea may be prominent, anaemia is common and the patients are often underweight. Infants and young children are characteristically miserable and pot-bellied. Older children fail to grow normally and their development is delayed. There is a tendency for symptoms to improve in later adolescence but problems can develop again at any age.

Adults usually present with anaemia or bowel symptoms in their twenties or thirties. They tend to be thinner and shorter than the rest of their family, but may be perfectly well developed. Osteomalacia, due to vitamin D deficiency, is an unusual presentation.

### DIAGNOSIS

This depends on jejunal biopsy (page 341). Important indications for jejunal biopsy include evidence of mixed deficiency anaemia and folate depletion (page 604). Indeed the folate status (serum and red cell levels) is probably the best screening test for coeliac disease, even in the absence of overt anaemia. Hyposplenism, as shown by Howell–Jolly bodies in the red blood cells (page 598), is a well-recognized but unexplained feature of coeliac disease.

### DIFFERENTIAL DIAGNOSIS

This is from other causes of anaemia and malabsorption as discussed on page 340. Histological differentiation from other forms of enteropathy may be difficult and the biopsy may have to be repeated after periods of gluten challenge or gluten withdrawal.

### COMPLICATIONS

These tend to occur in older adults, i.e. after many years of continuous gluten exposure, and include benign ulceration, strictures and small intestinal lymphoma. There is an increased risk of adenocarcinoma of the small intestine (an otherwise rare tumour) and curiously also of carcinoma of the oesophagus. It is probable that prolonged avoidance of dietary gluten will prevent these complications.

## TREATMENT

This involves strict dietary exclusion of gluten and should ideally be encouraged for life. Many gluten-free products are available on prescription and patients can bake their own bread using gluten-free flours. The Coeliac Society provides patients with useful dietary and other advice. Anaemia should be corrected with iron and/or folate as appropriate. Vitamin $B_{12}$ deficiency is rare in coeliac disease because the lower ileum is usually not involved. Vitamin D therapy will be required for symptomatic osteomalacia.

The patients often feel better quickly (i.e. within weeks or even days) but improvement may be slow and perseverence is needed. It is important to repeat the jejunal biopsy after approximately 6 months to ensure that the histological abnormalities are improving. In most patients the mucosa will return completely to normal and this proves that the diagnosis is correct. Persistent diarrhoea may be helped in the early stages by milk exclusion, because lactase levels are often very low in the grossly abnormal mucosa (secondary hypolactasia, see page 342).

It is unusual to meet patients who fail to respond symptomatically and histologically to a gluten-free diet. In such patients it is necessary to ensure strict dietary compliance and to exclude the complications listed above by small gut radiology and, if appropriate, laparotomy. Corticosteroid therapy will produce rapid symptomatic benefit and histological improvement in coeliac disease even if the patient continues to eat gluten. It is justified if the patient is making poor progress on a gluten-free diet alone.

## PROGNOSIS

This is usually excellent if the patient adheres to the diet, but unfortunately the long-term risk of lymphoma and carcinoma remains. The magnitude of this risk is uncertain but probably less than 10 per cent.

# Dermatitis herpetiformis

This chronic, distinctive itchy rash (page 796) is closely associated with coeliac disease. Approximately 70 per cent of patients have a jejunal mucosa which is indistinguishable from that of coeliac disease. Gluten restriction will allow the mucosa to heal and the skin lesions may also improve or disappear. It is curious that overt malabsorption and anaemia are rare in these patients and many prefer to continue a normal diet because the skin lesions can usually be controlled more readily by dapsone therapy. The risk of malignancy is probably similar to that of coeliac disease.

# Tropical sprue

## AETIOLOGY

This is an enteropathy which involves the jejunum and ileum and is probably caused by abnormal bacterial colonization in the intestinal lumen. It is endemic in parts of India, the Far East and the Caribbean and can be acquired by those travelling through these areas. The term 'temperate sprue' has been applied to a similar but milder illness acquired during travel through less tropical places such as the Middle East and Northern India. Malnutrition and parasitic infestation of the small intestine can produce mucosal abnormalities leading to diarrhoea and malabsorption. This makes an exact definition of tropical sprue difficult, if not impossible, and it is unlikely that a single cause will be identified.

## PATHOLOGY

There is blunting and thickening of the villi which are usually short and irregular, but which rarely disappear completely as they do in coeliac disease. The lamina propria is heavily infiltrated with chronic inflammatory cells.

## CLINICAL FEATURES

The disease may present acutely and occur in epidemics. More commonly the illness is chronic with diarrhoea, steatorrhoea, anorexia, weakness and loss of appetite. Loss of weight and anaemia are common and folate depletion occurs in a few weeks. Diagnosis depends on jejunal biopsy and the differential diagnosis is from other forms of chronic enteropathy (page 341).

## TREATMENT

A combination of folic acid replacement and broad-spectrum antibiotics (e.g. tetracycline) is usually successful. Vitamin $B_{12}$ malabsorption occurs but deficiency is rare because of the large stores in the liver.

## PROGNOSIS

This is usually good and, in most patients returning from the tropics permanently, full recovery can be expected.

# Whipple's disease

This very rare disease is caused by a bacillus which invades the small intestine and other parts of the body (e.g. heart and brain). The intestinal mucosa is diffusely abnormal and the lamina propria is packed with large macrophages full of material which is stained by the periodic acid–Schiff reagent (PAS positive). Electron microscopy shows that this material consists of bacterial bodies. The organism has been identified as a Gram-positive actinomycete and named *Tropheryma Whippelii*.

This disease typically affects older men who present with the symptoms of chronic malabsorption and who often, in addition, have lympadenopathy and polyarthropathy. The condition, which used to be invariably fatal, does respond to protracted antibiotic therapy.

# Giardiasis

A number of chronic infections can damage the small intestine and lead to diarrhoea and malabsorption but the only one that is at all commonly seen in the western world is that caused by *Giardia lamblia*. Less common organisms are becoming increasingly recognized as causes of chronic diarrhoea and malabsorption especially in patients with impaired immunity, including acquired immune deficiency syndrome (AIDS), for example Campylobacter, Strongyloides and Cryptosporidium.

## AETIOLOGY

*Giardia lamblia* is a flagellate protozoan which infests the upper intestine and can cause variable inflammatory changes in the mucosa, occasionally as severe as that seen in coeliac disease. The encysted form is passed in the faeces. Infection is acquired from contaminated food and water and is endemic in many parts of the tropical and subtropical world and also in parts of Eastern Europe and the former Soviet Union.

## CLINICAL FEATURES

The usual symptoms of any chronic mild malabsorption are present – steatorrhoea, weight loss and usually anorexia and malaise. Diagnosis may be revealed by the presence of cysts in a faecal sample, but this is not always reliable. Aspiration of duodenal or jejunal juice is more reliable because the flagellate forms can be recognized easily by direct microscopy of suitably stained fluid. It is advisable to take a jejunal biopsy at the same time, because the organism can be identified in conventionally prepared histological sections and may also be seen by examining smears of the mucosal surface.

## TREATMENT

Metronidazole is the drug of choice and is usually given in a dose of 1200 mg daily for 7 days or 2 g daily for 3 days, but side effects are common with the higher doses. Resistance is unusual and other drugs are available including tinidazole and mepacrine.

## PROGNOSIS

Response to therapy is usually excellent but recurrent infections can occur in travellers.

Patients with immunological abnormalities, for example, congenital and acquired immunoglobulin deficiencies, are prone to recurrent episodes of infection even in the absence of foreign travel and will need repeated courses of antibiotic therapy.

# Meckel's diverticulum

This protrusion from the small intestine is a remnant of the vitellointestinal duct. Most patients with a Meckel's diverticulum have no symptoms, but it may contain gastric mucosa which can bleed. This presents as rectal bleeding. Localization of the bleeding may be difficult and the diagnosis may only become evident at laparatomy.

# Tumours of the small intestine

These are all rather rare and will not be discussed in detail. They can obstruct the lumen by intussusception and can bleed and usually require surgical resection. Benign polyps are usually hamartomatous (e.g. Peutz–Jeghers syndrome, page 329) or adenomatous and may accompany colonic polyposis (page 372). Adenocarcinoma is rare and may complicate coeliac disease (page 358) and Crohn's disease (page 362). Ileal carcinoid tumours are less rare and, although potentially malignant, have a long natural history. Their main importance is the propensity for large metastatic masses in the liver to produce the carcinoid syndrome (page 409).

The small intestine may be involved in abdominal Hodgkin's disease and non-Hodgkin's lymphoma, but the lymph nodes and spleen are the major sites of abdominal disease (page 633). Focal or diffuse intestinal lymphoma is usually a complication of coeliac disease (page 358) but does occur as a primary phenomenon especially in parts of the Middle East and North Africa where it is the commonest recognized cause of chronic malabsorption.

# Mediterranean lymphoma and α-chain disease

## AETIOLOGY

This diffuse lymphomatous process is thought to be a sequel to recurrent or chronic gut infections or infestations. It occurs in parts of the world where gut infection and malnutrition are common, but seems to be associated more with subtropical areas. Accurate figures of prevalence are not available.

## PATHOLOGY

There is diffuse mucosal and submucosal infiltration with lymphocytes, plasma cells and histocytes, and variable distortion and destruction of the villous architecture.

## CLINICAL FEATURES

There are the usual clinical features of chronic malabsorption, often with finger clubbing, loss of weight and a downhill course over several months. Laboratory tests are non-specifically abnormal, but may reveal high concentrations of isolated heavy chains of IgA in the serum. This variant is usually referred to as α-chain disease. Small bowel radiology is focally or diffusely abnormal without specific features and diagnosis is based on jejunal biopsy or on histological material obtained at laparotomy.

## TREATMENT

In the early stages broad-spectrum antibiotics may be helpful or even curative, suggesting that gut bacteria are in some way responsible for initiating the illness. Once the disease becomes established, chemotherapy is required as for other lymphomatous conditions. Surgical excision is not feasible because the disease involves much of the small intestine but radiotherapy has been used with some success in advanced disease.

## PROGNOSIS

Prognosis is generally regarded as poor even with aggressive chemotherapy, but accurate follow-up data are not available.

# Disorders of intestinal motility

Apart from the common types of 'functional' diarrhoea and abdominal pain (see irritable bowel syndrome, page 373), disorders of structure impairing motility are uncommon and include jejunal diverticulosis, scleroderma, diffuse infiltrative disorders such as amyloidosis and strictures caused by focal ischaemia as in the various forms of vasculitis. Intestinal transit can be sluggish in untreated coeliac disease (page 358) and is often abnormal in Crohn's disease (see below).

The major consequences of impaired intestinal transit are chronic pain, abdominal distension and, often, malabsorption resulting from overgrowth of colonic-type bacteria in dilated upper intestine. The diagnosis is based on small bowel radiology and treatment is often unsatisfactory. Strictures or short lengths of diseased intestine are best treated by surgical resection. If the intestine is diffusely abnormal, surgery is not feasible but treatment with broad-spectrum antibiotics is often effective and is required on an indefinite and empirical basis. Intestinal bacteria have numerous metabolic effects on food residues and can damage the intestinal mucosa. Most notably they interfere with the absorption of vitamin $B_{12}$ and deconjugate bile acids and thus impair the absorption of fats and fat-soluble vitamins.

# CHRONIC NON-SPECIFIC INFLAMMATORY BOWEL DISEASES

The above term conventionally refers to Crohn's disease and ulcerative colitis. It is convenient to consider them together because there are points of similarity although many notable differences. They are both diseases of unknown origin, mainly affect young adults, produce considerable chronic morbidity but relatively little mortality and are treated empirically with a variety of medical and surgical methods. The management of these two disorders forms a considerable part of gastroenterological practice (medical and surgical) throughout northern Europe and North America. In many other parts of the world they are considered to be uncommon or even rare.

specific mycobacterial infection in cattle is known to cause a similar chronic granulomatous disorder of the small intestine.

Although environmental factors must be of great importance, genetic factors are also important as shown by family studies and the prevalence of the histocompatibility antigen HLA-B27. There is a genetic association with both ulcerative colitis and with ankylosing spondylitis.

Prevalence rates vary in different parts of the developed world. In the UK there are 23–35 cases per 100 000 of the population with an annual incidence of new cases of 2–5 per 100 000.

## PATHOLOGY

The disease can affect all parts of the GI tract including the mouth and, very commonly, the anus. The typical lesion is focal mucosal oedema often with a cobblestone appearance accompanied by linear ulcers or fissures. More superficial aphthous ulcers may represent the first phase of the disease. There is a great tendency for abnormal intestine to adhere to other intestinal loops and to the abdominal wall. Large inflam-

# Crohn's disease

## AETIOLOGY

There have been numerous speculations about infective agents and immunological responses to food or bacterial antigens in the gut lumen. The distinctive histology has led to much interest in the possible role of atypical mycobacteria and a

matory masses are often produced and may become infected with gut organisms to produce abscesses. Fistulae commonly form between segments of small and large bowel, in the perianal region and with bladder, vagina and skin.

The commonest sites of involvement are the lower ileum and the right side of the colon. Extensive colitis is however well recognized although the rectum may be relatively spared.

Histologically there is deep submucosal, patchy chronic inflammation with relative preservation of the surface layer of mucosal cells. Granulomatous collections of lymphocytes and histiocytes, sometimes with giant cells, are the most distinctive features but are by no means always present.

## CLINICAL FEATURES

These are variable and depend on the site of involvement and the age of the patient. Abdominal pain is the most common symptom and bowel disturbance, usually with predominant diarrhoea, is usual but not invariable. Loss of weight and, in childhood failure to grow, are common features and there are often a variety of other nutritional disturbances including anaemia and hypoalbuminaemia. Physical examination may reveal abdominal masses and tell-tale signs at the anus, especially thick skin tags, induration of the anal canal, chronic anal fissure and evidence of present or past perianal sepsis.

In a minority (< 10 per cent) of cases there may be present or past evidence of various extra intestinal manifestations, including acute monoarthritis or oligoarthritis affecting major joints, acute iritis, erythema nodosum and a distinctive necrotizing lesion of the skin (usually on the legs and feet) called pyoderma gangrenosum. Sacroiliitis is occasionally evident clinically as pain and tenderness over these joints and the patient may have ankylosing spondylitis. These features are all shared with ulcerative colitis and are usually associated with extensive colonic rather than small intestinal involvement.

Small intestinal disease can present acutely with intestinal obstruction. Diffuse small intestinal disease is relatively uncommon but can produce all the features of chronic malabsorption. Small gut strictures can cause chronic partial obstruction and bacterial overgrowth in the upper small intestine.

## DIAGNOSIS

This is based on small and large gut radiology, which defines the extent of the disease and shows

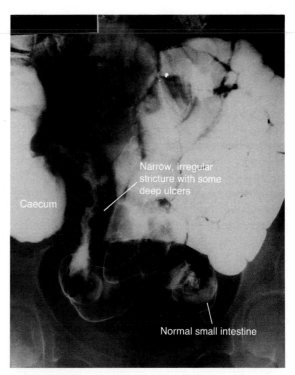

**Figure 14.9** Typical ileal Crohn's disease on barium follow-through.

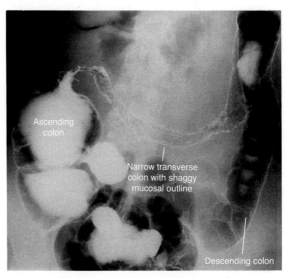

**Figure 14.10** Colonic Crohn's disease on barium enema.

the distinctive focal, ulcerating lesions, strictures and fistulae (Figs. 14.9 and 14.10). Histological diagnosis is obtained by endoscopy of the large bowel or by surgical resection, especially of focal small intestinal lesions.

## DIFFERENTIAL DIAGNOSIS

Acute ileal Crohn's disease may be confused with an acute self-limiting ileitis caused by *Yersinia enterocolitica*. This illness resembles acute appendicitis and may be strongly suspected at laparotomy if the ileum is red and thick and the regional lymph nodes are inflamed (acute mesenteric adenitis). The ileum should not be resected, although a normal appendix can be safely removed, because the disease should remit spontaneously or with appropriate antibacterial therapy (e.g. gentamicin or tetracycline). The diagnosis is usually confirmed by finding a rising titre of antibodies in the serum, although a positive faecal culture is sometimes obtained.

Extensive Crohn's colitis may be difficult to distinguish from ulcerative colitis, especially if the rectum is involved. Right-sided colitis and ileitis can be caused by *Mycobacterium tuberculosis* and this must be borne in mind in patients from the developing world and especially the Indian subcontinent. There may be evidence of pulmonary involvement on chest X-ray and characteristic histology can be obtained by endoscopic biopsy although bacteriological culture often fails. Stool examination for mycobacteria is fruitless. Diagnosis of tuberculosis commonly depends on histological examination of resected gut.

Rectal and anal disease may require differentiation from the various specific infections in this area (e.g. chlamydial proctitis, lymphogranuloma venereum and rectal schistosomiasis). However, most patients with anal fissures and perianal sepsis have no underlying chronic inflammatory bowel disease.

## COMPLICATIONS

These are numerous and include obstruction (common), abscess formation (common), fistulation to the skin, other loops of gut, bladder and vagina (relatively common), and severe bleeding (rare). Free perforation into the peritoneal cavity

is distinctly unusual. Toxic dilation of extensively diseased colon, with risk of perforation, has been described but is much less common than in ulcerative colitis.

## TREATMENT

The management of Crohn's disease is summarized in Table 14.19. Corticosteroids are the most effective medical weapon and should be used if the patient is 'toxic' (e.g. obviously unwell, and with fever, tachycardia or losing weight) and has features of active inflammatory disease (inflammatory mass, anaemia, high white blood cell count and erythrocyte sedimentation rate, active joint, skin or eye disease). In such patients it is imperative to ensure that the illness is not caused by a septic complication rather than by the primary disease itself. The diagnosis of intra-abdominal or pelvic abscess

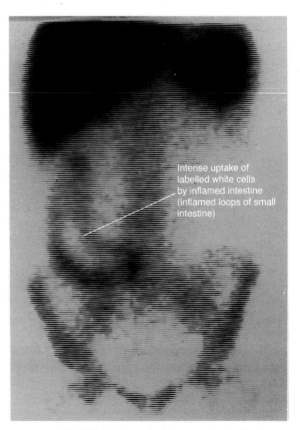

Intense uptake of labelled white cells by inflamed intestine (inflamed loops of small intestine)

**Figure 14.11** White cell scintiscan showing active inflammation in the right side of the abdomen in a patient with recurrent ileal disease after right hemicolectomy for Crohn's disease.

**Table 14.19** Summary of the management of Crohn's disease.

Nutritional support if underweight or anorexic

Correction of specific nutritional deficiencies, especially anaemia

Relief of symptoms (e.g. with analgesics, antidiarrhoeal agents)

Anti-inflammatory drugs (e.g. corticosteroids), sulphasalazine (in colonic disease), metronidazole (especially for perianal sepsis), azathioprine (especially for its 'steroid-sparing' effect)

Surgery (drainage of abscesses, relief of obstruction, resection of all or most of the disease)

can be very difficult in Crohn's disease and may be facilitated by the use of ultrasound and various isotopic techniques (e.g. the use of radio-labelled leukocytes, Fig. 14.11).

Symptoms often recur after an initially good response to a standard course of corticosteroids as the dose is reduced or after the drug is withdrawn. In these patients, continuous low-dose treatment may be required (e.g. 5–10 mg prednisolone daily or 10–20 mg on alternate days) and the effective dose may be less if simultaneous treatment with azathioprine (2 mg/kg) is given.

Sulphasalazine (as used in ulcerative colitis) is a moderately effective anti-inflammatory drug for the less ill patient with predominantly colonic disease. Metronidazole is probably as effective as sulphasalazine but is less well tolerated as long-term treatment. It has particular value in the treatment of serious perianal disease, especially if complicated by sepsis.

Surgical treatment is reserved for complications, because it is never curative. Common procedures are drainage of abscesses and resection of short segments of small intestine causing obstruction or fistulation. Defunctioning ileostomy or colostomy allows distal disease to settle and is occasionally indicated in the management of large inflammatory masses and of severe perianal disease. Gut continuity can be restored later, although disease activity is likely to increase afterwards.

Patients with complicated disease are often ill and malnourished and frequently require nutritional support in the form of sip supplements, nasogastric or intravenous feeding according to tolerance and the severity and extent of small intestinal involvement. The use of low residue liquid diets or, in very ill patients, intravenous feeding, will allow distal disease to settle with relief of symptoms and sometimes closure of fistulae.

Major colonic resection for extensive colitis, with or without ileorectal anastomosis, is justified in patients with poorly controlled symptoms and little or no small gut involvement. Ileostomy losses of fluid, electrolytes and nutrient are greater than after comparable operations for ulcerative colitis and can pose major problems of management.

Extensive small gut resection is complicated by diarrhoea, steatorrhoea and other features of malabsorption. After ileal resection, vitamin $B_{12}$ absorption is impaired and long-term replacement therapy is often required. Bile salt malabsorption produces watery diarrhoea which will usually respond to cholestyramine, 4–16 g, daily if the colon is relatively healthy.

## PROGNOSIS

There is much morbidity and most patients require some form of surgery, which may have to be repeated over the years. Nevertheless, long periods of relatively good health are possible and deaths directly attributable to Crohn's disease are infrequent. Actuarial analysis does however show that the mortality rate in patients with Crohn's disease is approximately twice that in suitably matched control subjects.

# *Ulcerative colitis*

## AETIOLOGY

This is unknown but genetic factors are involved as discussed on page 362. Many infective agents produce an acute illness morphologically indistinguishable from acute ulcerative colitis (UC) and it may be that some cases of so-called UC are in fact self-limiting specific colonic infections. However, typical UC is a chronic disease, although it is tempting to speculate that it can be initiated by specific infections.

Prevalence rates are higher than those for Crohn's disease and are relatively stable at 80–100 cases per 100 000 of the population in the UK. Annual incidence rates are 5–25 per 100 000. As with Crohn's disease, UC is seldom recognized in parts of the world where specific gut infections are very common.

## PATHOLOGY

Ulcerative colitis typically affects the rectum and spreads proximally to involve part or all of the colon. It is a diffuse, superficial inflammation which damages the mucosal cells on the surface and lining of the crypts. The disease often remains localized to the distal third of the colon or to the rectum (proctitis). In severe extensive disease, the inflammation may spread more deeply and damage or destroy parts of the muscle wall. This leads to dilation of the colon and the threat of perforation.

All these changes are non-specific and the diagnosis of UC is only established by exclusion of specific infections and by the passage of time.

In active superficial disease, ulceration is often inapparent macroscopically. In severe, chronic disease with deeper inflammation, there may be extensive areas of ulceration with islands of surviving mucosa, often heaped up into pseudopolyps.

Premalignant changes in the mucosal cells may be found in long-standing chronic, extensive disease and there is a serious risk of local and later invasive adenocarcinoma (page 371).

## CLINICAL FEATURES

The typical symptoms are bloody diarrhoea and crampy abdominal discomfort relieved by defaecation. Pain is seldom severe. In severe, acute illness the patient may rapidly become dehydrated, anaemic and weak. Marked faecal frequency, fever and tachycardia with abdominal tenderness and, sometimes, distension indicate the need for urgent admission.

Most attacks are less severe and tend to come and go without obvious explanation. There may be a precipitating factor such as stress, an infection or perhaps the use of antibiotics or analgesics. Attacks are usually brought under control or settle spontaneously within a few weeks and there may be long periods of good health.

Patients with distal UC and, especially proctitis, often have marked faecal frequency and bleeding but little faecal material is passed and hard faecal masses can accumulate in the healthy colon above (proximal constipation). The patient is seldom ill, but may become anaemic.

## DIAGNOSIS

This is usually apparent at the initial examination with the rigid sigmoidoscope. The mucosa is bright red and may be oozing blood especially if it is scraped gently with the instrument. In proctitis, healthy mucosa will be seen proximally. The lumen usually contains blood, mucopus and a variable amount and consistency of faecal material depending on the extent and severity of the disease. Luminal contents should be sampled for urgent bacteriological examination in an acute severe attack.

The extent of the disease is assessed by flexible endoscopy and barium enema as discussed on page 339 (Fig. 14.12). It is, however, dangerous and unnecessary to undertake these examinations in the acute, severe attack and the

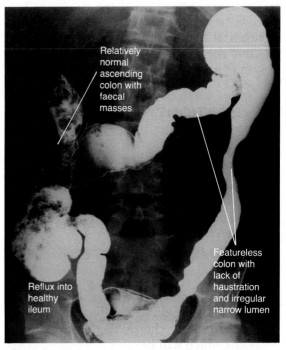

**Figure 14.12** Subtotal ulcerative colitis on barium enema.

required information can be obtained from an abdominal X-ray. This often shows the extent of disease quite clearly, indicates the presence of solid faeces and whether the colon is dilated.

## DIFFERENTIAL DIAGNOSIS

This is usually from acute colitis. Faecal material and, if present, pus must be examined bacteriologically for Salmonellae, Shigellae and Campylobacters and microscopically for *Entamoeba histolytica*. In patients recently treated with antibiotics, the faeces should also be examined for *Clostridium difficile* and its toxin, and occasionally the macroscopic appearances of **pseudomembranous colitis** will be seen, with patchy inflammation and adherent white plaques. Antibiotics commonly incriminated include lincomycin, clindamycin, ampicillin and other broad-spectrum agents.

In more chronic disease the differential diagnosis from extensive Crohn's colitis can be difficult. Proctoscopy will differentiate haemorrhoids from distal proctitis.

Rectal biopsy should be undertaken particularly in cases where the macroscopic abnormality is atypical or mild. Indeed, obvious microscopic abnormality is described in some patients with diarrhoea and normal endoscopy ('microscopic colitis'). It is not clear whether this is a variant of UC, but the symptoms may respond to anti-inflammatory drugs.

## COMPLICATIONS

The major complication of the acute, severe attack is colonic dilation followed by perforation. Profuse colonic bleeding, sufficient to produce shock, is very rare. The long-term risk of colonic cancer is mentioned on page 366. The extraintestinal manifestations of the disease, affecting especially the joints, skin and eyes have already been mentioned in relation to Crohn's disease on page 363.

Various forms of hepatobiliary disease may complicate UC and are less frequently associated with Crohn's disease. These include pericholangitis, sclerosing cholangitis and cholangiocarcinoma which will be discussed later on page 379.

## TREATMENT

Topical and systemic corticosteroids provide most effective treatment for the acute attack. Sulphasalazine is a weaker anti-inflammatory drug and is particularly indicated for the long-term prevention of acute relapses of the disease. Azathioprine is best reserved for its steroid-sparing effect, and is much less commonly required in UC than in Crohn's disease.

Supportive treatment includes the use of faecal bulking or softening agents (page 333) in patients with distal colitis and proximal constipation and the correction of iron deficiency anaemia. Antidiarrhoeal agents should be avoided in the severe, acute attack for fear of masking symptoms and, possibly, precipitating colonic dilation. Non-steroidal anti-inflammatory drugs and antibiotics can aggravate or precipitate colitis and should be used sparingly or avoided. There is no evidence that dietary factors are important but a low residue diet is usually considered prudent in patients with severe diarrhoea, whereas a high residue diet may prevent proximal constipation. Milk exclusion may help a very small minority of sufferers, but whether this relates to previously unrecognized lactase deficiency or is a true 'allergic colitis' remains unclear.

Most attacks of colitis can be handled on an outpatient basis with a course of topical steroids for disease confined to the left half of the colon or of oral prednisolone for more extensive disease. Liquid enemas of various prednisolone preparations (e.g. Predsol, Predenema) are self administered at night for a few weeks until bleeding and diarrhoea stop. A foam preparation of hydrocortisone (Colifoam) is a convenient alternative which many patients prefer. A typical course of oral prednisolone would start at around 30 mg (approximately 0.5 mg/kg) reducing by 5 mg every two weeks over the next 6–10 weeks, or faster if the symptoms are controlled rapidly. Topical and systemic steroids should be withdrawn completely if the attack is brought into complete remission as judged both by symptoms and endoscopic appearance. The minority of patients with chronic, grumbling disease may require low-dose, alternate day steroid therapy (enemas or tablets) for prolonged periods, but this is relatively uncommon and colectomy may be a preferred alternative.

Sulphasalazine is usually started during the acute attack and then continued for a prolonged period in the hope of maintaining a remission. Unfortunately, side effects are common especially with the usually recommended doses of 2–3 g daily and it is advisable to start with a lower dose. Common problems are dyspepsia (which may be averted by using an enteric-coated preparation), headache and skin rash. More severe complications include haemolytic anaemia, agranulocytosis and, rarely, widespread erythema multiforme. Reversible infertility in the male is now a well-recognized side effect. These side effects are attributed to the sulphapyridine moiety of the drug and new preparations of 5-aminosalicylic acid (e.g. mesalazine) can be prescribed to patients who are intolerant of sulphasalazine. Indeed mesalazine is beginning to supersede sulphasalazine as a first-line treatment for colitis. It is uncertain how long sulphasalazine or mesalazine should be taken after the last attack. Periods of 1–2 years are recommended and the drug should be withdrawn empirically after that. Recurrent attacks would then indicate the need for indefinite treatment.

The acute, severe attack of UC should be managed in hospital with intravenous corticosteroids in a dose of at least 60 mg daily of prednisolone or the equivalent (Table 14.20). A light diet may be taken if there are no serious abdominal signs and no evidence of colonic dilation on X-ray. However, in very ill patients it is preferable to give all the fluid and electrolyte requirements intravenously. Transfusions of blood and albumin may be needed to correct anaemia and hypoalbuminaemia, respectively. Unless the attack settles rapidly, i.e. within 2–3 days, the next step would be to start intravenous feeding using a centrally placed feeding line. Most patients will improve markedly during 5–7 days of intensive treatment of this sort, but close observation is essential and must include daily abdominal X-ray to detect colonic dilation. Failure to improve, the development of serious abdominal signs and dilation of the colon (transverse colon diameter >5.5 cm) are the usual indications for urgent colectomy. However, if the response is favourable and rapid, the patient should be able to resume normal eating and drinking after 5–7 days and

**Table 14.20** Management of a severe attack of ulcerative colitis.

| | |
|---|---|
| Criteria of severity | Liquid faeces >6 per day<br>Fever<br>Tachycardia<br>Abdominal tenderness<br>Featureless empty colon on plain X-ray |
| Treatment | Intravenous corticosteroids, e.g. prednisolone, 60 mg/day, or equivalent<br>Intravenous fluids/electrolytes<br>Intravenous albumin and/or blood according to serum albumin, haemoglobin<br>(Intravenous antibiotics only if proven infection)<br>Oral sulphasalazine or mesalazine |
| Observations | Daily abdominal X-ray to look for evidence of dilation |
| Nutrition | Oral (or nasogastric tube) unless serious abdominal signs present<br>Intravenous nutrition if abdomen very tender or colon dilating on abdominal X-ray |

prednisolone can be then given orally in a dose of 40 mg daily, reducing later to 30 mg and less according to progress.

## SURGERY

This is required for the acute, severe attack which fails to respond to the above measures and also for chronic unremitting symptoms especially if most or all of the colon is involved. A less common indication is the finding of premalignant changes in the mucosa during long-term surveillance for cancer (page 366).

Total colectomy is always required, as lesser resections are invariably followed by recurrent disease in the remaining colon. In the acutely ill patient, the rectum is left behind in order to minimize risks. In the otherwise fit patient, the colon and rectum can be removed as a one-stage panproctocolectomy bringing the ileum out to the anterior abdominal wall as a permanent ileostomy. In recent years, there has been much interest in alternatives to the conventional, incontinent ileostomy which requires a permanent bag. Those include the so-called continent ileostomy and, more recently, various forms of ileoanal anastomosis with the creation of a neo-rectum from several adjacent loops of ileum (Fig. 14.13).

Ileostomy after colectomy is usually very well tolerated once the patient learns how to use the bag and care for the skin. Specially qualified stomatherapy nurses provide invaluable care and

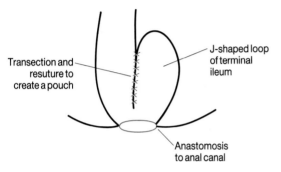

**Figure 14.13** Ileal pouch created after total colectomy for ulcerative colitis.

advice. The major risk is of salt and water depletion because relatively large volumes of fluid are lost (500–1000 ml/day). Patients should be advised to take extra water and salt in very hot weather and during temporary bouts of diarrhoea. There is a long-term risk of uric acid stones in the renal tract, because patients with ileostomies tend to pass relatively small volumes of concentrated urine.

## PROGNOSIS

This is good, provided that acute attacks are treated effectively and that colon cancer is prevented. Patients at risk of cancer are those with chronic disease affecting all or most of the colon for eight or more years, especially if symptoms have been frequent and troublesome during this period.

These patients should have annual colono-scopy with multiple biopsies. The finding of early cancer or severe dysplasia (if confirmed) should lead to total panproctocolectomy, with every hope of cure or prevention.

Long-term survival in ulcerative colitis is only slightly less than that of suitably matched controls.

# *D*ISORDERS OF THE LARGE INTESTINE

Ulcerative colitis is dealt with above (page 365).

# *Diverticular disease*

## AETIOLOGY

Diverticula (a diverticulum is a small pouch of a hollow viscus) are very common throughout the developed world in the older age groups. They are thought to result from a low fibre diet associated with slow colonic transit and high intraluminal colonic pressures. There is evidence that the disease is becoming commoner in parts of the less developed world where people have adopted the western low fibre diet. Current changes in the western diet towards more fibre

and less refined sugar may reduce the prevalence of the disease in the future.

Prevalence figures based on barium enema and necropsy vary considerably but in the western world less than 5 per cent of people aged below 40 have diverticula, whereas more than 30 per cent of those aged 60 and above are affected.

## PATHOLOGY

The disease affects the sigmoid and descending colon particularly, but all parts of the colon can be involved. The affected segments show marked hypertrophy of the circular layer of colon muscle. The pouches are formed by pulsion through tiny defects in the circular muscle, where major blood vessels penetrate, and emerge between the longitudinal taeniae on the anti-mesenteric surface of the colon.

In uncomplicated disease, no other pathological process is evident, but acute inflammation may ensue and lead to abscess formation, fistulation or free perforation. Chronic narrowing of the lumen especially of the sigmoid colon is common.

## CLINICAL FEATURES

The condition is commonly silent and is often found by chance. The most common symptoms are those of colonic pain and altered bowel habit as described on page 333. The patient tends to constipation with small, misshapen, bitty stool. There are often short episodes of diarrhoea, but prolonged painless diarrhoea should never be attributed to diverticula. Bleeding is uncommon, but rarely can be severe and demands exclusion of other pathology.

In acute diverticulitis, there is continuous pain, tenderness, fever and a mass can often be felt in the lower abdomen or pelvis. Abscess is accompanied by severe illness with a swinging pyrexia and perforation by the rapid development of peritonitis. Fistulation can present with pneumaturia, recurrent urinary infections or the passage of faeces per vagina.

## DIAGNOSIS

This is by barium enema examination (Fig. 14.14). Flexible endoscopy tends to underestimate the extent of the problem and can be difficult if the sigmoid lumen is very narrow and tortuous. In patients with acute symptoms, both procedures should be avoided for fear of aggravating the inflammation and producing a perforation. If there is marked local tenderness or a mass, an ultrasound examination will help to decide whether an abscess has formed and, in difficult cases, an isotope-labelled white cell scan may be helpful.

## DIFFERENTIAL DIAGNOSIS

The symptoms in uncomplicated disease are very similar to those of irritable bowel syndrome (page 373), but the latter is common in the under 40s and should not be diagnosed in the

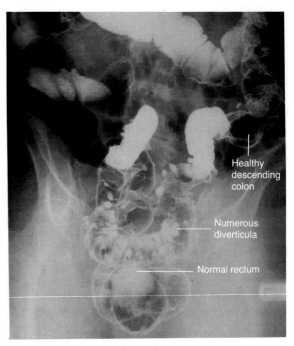

**Figure 14.14** Severe diverticulosis of the sigmoid colon.

older age group without full investigation. Localized disease especially in the sigmoid colon can coexist with adenocarcinoma or Crohn's disease. If the barium enema is at all equivocal, flexible endoscopy and biopsy should be carried out.

The common mistake is to ascribe symptoms to diverticula, when the fault lies elsewhere, simply because they are so common.

## COMPLICATIONS

These are abscess, free perforation and fistulation into neighbouring organs and onto the skin as already mentioned.

## TREATMENT

Symptomatic, uncomplicated disease usually responds to a high fibre diet supplemented if necessary by faecal bulking agents and antispasmodics as discussed on page 333, in relation to irritable bowel syndrome.

Acute diverticulitis is treated with broad-spectrum antibiotics, such as ampicillin, and will require intravenous fluids and bed rest in hospital if the patient is ill with serious abdominal signs.

Perforation is an acute emergency, which requires resuscitation, surgical drainage of the peritoneal cavity and the creation of a defunctioning colostomy. Fistula formation can only be treated by resecting the affected segment of colon and the anastomoses may require protection by a temporary defunctioning colostomy.

In general, resection of a segment of colon for diverticular disease should only be undertaken if there are or have been serious, well-documented complications. Chronic colonic pain and bowel disturbances are not usually cured by local resection.

## PROGNOSIS

This is excellent in most cases, but chronic symptoms can be difficult to treat and acute complications threaten life and may require multiple operations with all their attendant risks.

# *Adenomas and adenocarcinoma of the colon and rectum*

## AETIOLOGY

Bowel cancer is one of the commonest cancers in the developed world and the annual incidence in the UK is about 30 per 100 000 of the population.

It is thought that many cancers arise in adenomas, which can be present in the colon for years beforehand. Other precancerous lesions include chronic ulcerative colitis (page 365), familial polyposis coli (page 372), colonic schistosomiasis and possibly Crohn's colitis.

Genetic factors are undoubtedly important as shown by family clustering of early or multiple common cancers including those arising in the colon. The genetic background of familial polyposis coli has recently been clarified (page 373 and 73). In most patients, however, the genetic and environmental factors responsible are poorly defined. Dietary factors, especially fat, have been implicated by epidemiological studies. Bile salts are cocarcinogens in experimental colon cancer and have been much studied in the human disease.

## PATHOLOGY

Adenomas can arise anywhere in the colon and are frequently multiple. Probably 70 per cent arise distal to the splenic flexure. These are commonly polypoid and may have long stalks. Malignant change and invasion can be impossible to determine unless the whole adenoma is removed from its stalk. Malignant transformation is rare until they are > 2cm in diameter.

Adenocarcinoma arises more often in the left than the right half of the colon and about 50 per cent of all bowel cancers are to be found in the rectum. They are ulcerating or fungating growths which later penetrate the bowel wall, invade local structures and spread more widely. The famous Dukes' classification of tumour spread is widely used in relation to prognosis (Table 14.21). Because adenomas are often multiple, it is not uncommon for several primary adenocarcinomas to arise in one colon, both simultaneously and after an interval of many years.

## CLINICAL FEATURES

Adenomas are commonly symptomless but may ulcerate and bleed or, if large and pedunculated, can intussuscept or even appear at the anus.

Adenocarcinoma in the left side of the colon presents with blood loss (overt or occult), with altered bowel habit and with colonic or rectal pain. Right-sided cancer tends to be more silent and presents typically with iron-deficiency

**Table 14.21** Dukes' classification of large bowel cancer and 5-year survival following surgery in the UK.

|         |                                                     | Survival |
| ------- | --------------------------------------------------- | -------- |
| Stage A | No spread beyond muscularis mucosa                  | 80–95%   |
| Stage B | Spread beyond muscularis but no lymph nodes involved | 60–70%   |
| Stage C | Spread to regional lymph nodes or beyond            | 25–30%   |

anaemia and, less commonly, with chronic pain. There may be a palpable abdominal or rectal mass and the liver is commonly involved by mestastatic disease.

## DIAGNOSIS

A barium enema will usually show typical or suspicious features of cancer but the sigmoid colon can be very difficult to examine and the caecum and ascending colon are often contaminated by faeces. Endoscopic examination and biopsy are required to confirm the diagnosis, to determine the distribution of any adenomas and to exclude additional primary cancers.

## DIFFERENTIAL DIAGNOSIS

The various forms of colonic polyps are summarized below. Histological clarification is essential. Adenocarcinoma has to be distinguished from diverticular disease, in the sigmoid colon especially, and on the right side it may be mistaken for inflammatory lesions such as Crohn's disease and tuberculosis.

## COMPLICATIONS

These are obstruction, especially of the colon by left-sided cancers, and less commonly perforation, fistula formation and severe, acute bleeding. Untreated rectal cancer can penetrate widely within the pelvis invading the bladder and vagina and causing intractable pain.

## TREATMENT

Adenomas can usually be removed by electrocautery at colonoscopy if they are pedunculated and small. Larger, sessile lesions can be removed piecemeal at several sessions but much skill and care is required. It is essential to destroy the stalks and bases of larger adenomas to ensure that no malignant or premalignant tissue remains.

Adenocarcinoma is treated by wide surgical excision of bowel along with the mesenteric lymph nodes. Continuity of the bowel can often be restored at a one-stage operation, unless there has been a complication such as obstruction or perforation. Cancers in the lower half of the rectum used to be treated by total proctectomy and permanent colostomy and this may still be necessary if the lesion is very low. The newer stapling devices have enabled surgeons to perform much lower rectal anastomoses in recent years with relative ease and safety and without impairing the prognosis.

The adjuvant roles of chemotherapy and radiotherapy are difficult to define and summarize. These methods of treatment are still being assessed in multicentre clinical trials. Inoperable rectal carcinoma has a very poor outlook but useful palliation can sometimes be achieved by laser therapy at endoscopy if the facilities and skills are available. Resection should however always be undertaken if feasible, even in the presence of obvious metastases in lymph nodes or liver, because of the appalling local complications of untreated tumour.

## PROGNOSIS

The prognosis of adenomas is good provided that they are excised when still small and that the whole colon is subjected to regular and complete endoscopic surveillance (every 2–5 years).

The prognosis of adenocarcinoma depends on its spread at the time of excision and on the histological grade of malignancy. Table 14.21 shows current UK figures relating survival to the Dukes' classification.

# *Polyposis coli*

This is a confusing subject which is summarized in Table 14.22. The serious polyps are the adenomatous ones because of the high risk of cancer. The others are important to recognize because they can be confused with adenomas and give rise to unnecessary alarm. They can all bleed and, if multiple, can cause disturbance of bowel function.

Families with multiple adenomatous polyps must be screened for asymptomatic cases. Established cases should be treated by total colectomy at an early stage if cancer is to be avoided. If the rectum is not removed, endoscopic surveillance and cautery of recurrent polyps are required.

**Table 14.22** Classification of intestinal polyps.

| Type | Solitary form | Multiple form |
| --- | --- | --- |
| Neoplastic | Adenoma | Familial adenomatous polyposis coli |
| Hamartomatous | Juvenile polyps | Peutz–Jeghers syndrome (mainly small gut) |
| Inflammatory | Benign lymphoid polyps | Pseudopolyposis in colitis |

The familial adenomatous polyposis (FAP) gene has recently been assigned to the long arm of chromosome 5 (5q). DNA probing is now being used to identify members of FAP families at high and low risk of acquiring polyposis. This should facilitate family screening and only those at high risk would need to be examined sigmoidoscopically and followed up.

# Irritable bowel syndrome

Although the symptoms in irritable bowel syndrome (IBS) are mainly colonic, it should be regarded as a disorder affecting all parts of the gut. It can be defined as the association of abdominal pain with bowel disturbance in the absence of any structural disease and can thus be distinguished from other disorders of function such as non-ulcer dyspepsia, 'simple' constipation and painless chronic diarrhoea. Clearly such a definition is quite arbitrary but it is useful in practice.

## AETIOLOGY AND PREVALENCE

Studies of the 'normal' population reveal that up to 30 per cent of subjects have symptoms of this type quite frequently but most do not complain (fortunately!). In gastroenterological clinics at least 50 per cent of all new patients have no evidence of organic disease and many will be diagnosed with more or less confidence as IBS.

The cause is unknown and often assumed to be entirely psychological. Episodes can be provoked by all the usual stresses of life and a minority of patients are or will become overtly depressed. It is not uncommon for there to be many other symptoms such as migraine, vague and variable problems with breathing and swallowing, palpitations and other features of anxiety.

The possibility that symptoms are caused by intolerance of certain foods has received much recent attention. Such intolerance is unlikely to be caused by true allergy and IBS patients are not notably atopic.

Typical IBS symptoms can follow acute gut infections such as amoebic dysentry, and can coexist with those of chronic diseases, which may act as trigger factors (e.g. ulcerative colitis).

## CLINICAL FEATURES AND DIAGNOSIS

The pain can occur anywhere in the abdomen or in the flanks (Fig. 14.15). Careful history taking and inspection of the stools may be required to clarify the true nature of the bowel disturbance. Most patients present in early or middle adult life and often have a history going back to adolescence or childhood.

Examination is often negative but common findings include a thickened, tender colon in the left iliac fossa, small bitty stools on digital examination, marked spasms of the lower colon on endoscopy and excessive haustration of the left colon on barium enema. Inflation of the colon with air at endoscopy may reproduce the patient's symptoms accurately (Table 14.23).

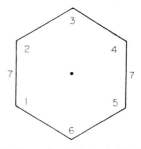

**Figure 14.15** Sites of pain in irritable bowel syndrome. Mimicry: (1) appendix, ovarian problems; (2) gallstones; (3) peptic ulcer; (4) gas in stomach; (5, commonest site) diverticular disease; (6) uterine problems; (7, flanks) lumbar, renal problems.

**Table 14.23** Positive 'signs' of irritable bowel syndrome.

Palpable, thickened colon in left iliac fossa
Fragmented, faecal pellets seen at sigmoidoscopy
Inflation of colon with air may reproduce pain
Exaggerated haustral pattern in left colon on barium
    enema

How far the patient is investigated depends on how typical the symptoms are, the patient's age and the duration of the problem. A patient presenting over the age of 40 for the first time must have at least a rigid sigmoidoscopy and barium enema. In younger patients, loss of weight or anaemia should raise the suspicion of Crohn's disease and lead to fuller investigations. It is important to remember that non-colonic symptoms are common in patients with IBS (Table 14.24).

## DIFFERENTIAL DIAGNOSIS

This is from diverticular disease and colon cancer in the older age groups and from Crohn's disease in the younger ones. The associated non-colonic symptoms shown in Table 14.24 have a wide differential diagnosis.

## COMPLICATIONS

Complications may arise as a result of over-zealous and inappropriate investigations or treatment, including the risks of unnecessary surgery. In a small minority, serious depressive

**Table 14.24** Associated non-colonic symptoms often noted in patients with irritable bowel syndrome.

Functional dyspepsias
Dyspnoea at rest, including hyperventilation
Low back pain
Menstrual disorders and dyspareunia
Micturition – frequency, hesitancy, small amounts
Migraine and 'functional' headaches

illness may be overlooked with a remote risk of suicide.

## TREATMENT

The first phase is reassurance, explanation and encouragement. It is important to come to a decision, offer a diagnosis and treat. Confidence is lost if investigations continue to be requested or if other opinions are sought.

The second phase is to try to improve bowel habit and this usually means giving advice about a high fibre diet if the patient is constipated or has the typical 'spastic' bowel habit. If this is unsuccessful, faecal bulking agents (page 333) are often helpful. Antidiarrhoeal agents should be avoided unless the patient has continuous watery diarrhoea without pain. If these measures improve bowel function but do not relieve pain, colon antispasmodics should be prescribed such as mebeverine and anticholinergic drugs (e.g. probanthine, dicyclomine). The latter however are likely to produce side effects, especially dryness of the mouth.

Most patients will respond more or less completely to these simple measures. Treatment with psychotropic drugs may be required in those who are obviously very anxious or overtly depressed. An interview with an interested pyschiatrist may be very helpful in the small minority of subjects who are extremely difficult to treat.

Exclusion diets should not be recommended unless the patient can be closely followed by a doctor or dietitian with special interest and expertise. Their use remains controversial at present.

## PROGNOSIS

Symptoms are likely to recur over many years and probably fewer than 50 per cent of sufferers ever go into complete remission. However, the majority learn to live and cope with their symptoms and few suffer from any permanent disability.

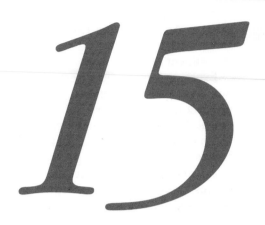

# Disorders of the Liver, Biliary System and Pancreas

# 15

# INTRODUCTION

Liver disease is common worldwide. Viral hepatitis, cirrhosis and hepatocellular carcinoma are common in the Mediterranean basin, sub-Saharan Africa and the Far East, whereas gallstones and alcoholic liver disease predominate in the affluent West.

Exocrine pancreatic disease is less frequent but pancreatic carcinoma is an increasingly important cause of mortality in the West. Pancreatic insufficiency can be caused by protein malnutrition as in India or by alcohol as in France and the USA.

Advances in endoscopic and imaging techniques have increased the diagnostic and therapeutic options in liver and pancreatic disease. The biliary tree can be investigated more easily and stones removed or strictures relieved by way of the endoscope. Advances in surgical techniques using laparoscopes are changing the approach to gallstones.

The application of advances in molecular biology has increased the ability to identify viruses causing hepatitis. This will help in understanding the epidemiology of liver disease and in the appropriate use of antiviral and immunosuppressive treatment.

# Metabolism of bilirubin

Bilirubin comes from the breakdown of haem-containing proteins and builds up when there is excess production or difficulties in elimination caused by disease of the liver cells or obstruction of the biliary system. Unbound bilirubin is taken up quickly by tissues. Most bilirubin in the blood is bound to albumin and is taken up by liver cells and made water soluble by conjugation with glucuronic acid. Then it is actively secreted into the bile and passes out through the bile ducts into the small intestine. The bilirubin is metabolized by bacteria in the gut producing urobilinogen which is water soluble and easily absorbed. After absorption most of it is taken up again by the liver while a small amount passes out in the urine.

Jaundice may be related to problems which are prehepatic, hepatic or posthepatic (Table 15.1). In haemolytic conditions producing prehepatic jaundice urinary urobilinogen is increased. Gilbert's syndrome is found in 2–4 per cent of the population. Unconjugated bilirubin is elevated in this harmless condition as transport into hepatocytes, conjugation and excretion are impaired. In posthepatic conditions soluble conjugated bilirubin darkens the urine while urobilinogen is decreased. In extrahepatic biliary obstruction the stools are pale and may be greasy and floating through fat malabsorption.

**Table 15.1** Classification of jaundice.

**Prehepatic**
Haemolysis

**Hepatic**
(a) Bilirubin transport defects, e.g. Gilbert's disease, Dubin Johnson syndrome
(b) Acute hepatocyte damage by viruses, drugs

**Posthepatic (cholestatic)**
(a) Impaired hepatocyte excretion, e.g. drugs (page 393), posthepatitis cholestasis
(b) Intrahepatic biliary disease, e.g. primary biliary cirrhosis (page 400), sclerosing cholangitis (page 382)
(c) Extrahepatic biliary obstruction by gallstones (page 379) or malignancy (page 384)

# SYMPTOMS AND SIGNS OF LIVER AND PANCREATIC DISEASE

Jaundice is a yellow discoloration of the sclera and skin occurring as a result of the accumulation of bilirubin. It is often noticed first by relatives and close associates rather than by patients. It is usually visible when the bilirubin exceeds 50 μmol/l, three times the normal level.

Fatigue is the commonest symptom of liver disease.

Pain from gallstones is felt in the right upper quadrant of the abdomen. It may also be severe with acute hepatitis or hepatic tumours. Pancreatic pain is epigastric, constant and boring through to the back, although it can be absent. It is often relieved on sitting up. In pancreatitis the pain is severe and may be associated with peritonitis.

Chronic liver disease is associated with numerous signs (Table 15.2).

**Hepatic encephalopathy** in extensive liver failure is suggested by drowsiness, hepatic breath (foetor) and a flapping tremor. Petechiae, bruising and ecchymoses are related to the clotting problems. Portal hypertension causes enlargement of the spleen and prominent collateral veins over the abdomen. Occasionally they radiate from the umbilicus to form a caput Medusae (Medusa's head).

Fluid retention causes **ascites** and, less often, pitting ankle oedema. The former causes **shifting dullness** detectable by percussing the fluid in the flanks then turning the patient on to their side and demonstrating the change in the position of the dullness to percussion. When there is a massive amount of fluid a fluid thrill can be felt by placing the flat of the hand over one flank and flicking the other, with the patient's hand in the middle to stop transmission through the anterior abdominal wall.

Hepatomegaly is an important sign. The liver edge may be felt in young, slim individuals but a tender liver is always abnormal. Enlargement of the right lobe (Riedl's lobe) is a normal variant. In chronic liver disease hypertrophy is greater in the left lobe. The upper border of the liver must be percussed to exclude a liver pushed down by lung disease. Percussion of the lower border is not so helpful since the liver is very thin anteriorly.

A palpable gallbladder in a jaundiced patient (**Courvoisier's sign**) suggests obstruction by malignancy rather than stones which would usually have resulted in a scarred and contracted gallbladder.

**Table 15.2** Stigmata (signs) of chronic liver disease.

Palmar erythema (liver palms)
Spider angiomata (naevi)
Finger clubbing
Dupuytren's contracture
Leuconychia (white nails)
Facial telangiectasia (paper money skin)
Loss of secondary sexual hair (especially axillary)
Gynaecomastia
Testicular atrophy
Parotid enlargement (alcoholic hepatitis)

# TECHNIQUES OF INVESTIGATION

Biochemical tests of liver function include the transaminases which rise predominantly in liver cell damage such as hepatitis. In obstructive conditions rises in enzymes such as alkaline phosphatase and gamma glutamyl transpeptidase are more marked (Table 15.3). Prothrombin times rise when liver damage is extensive and serum albumin reflects the synthetic activity of the liver.

The biliary tree can be visualized on an X-ray by introducing contrast medium into the biliary tree either by oral or intravenous injection (indirect) or at endoscopic retrograde cholangiopancreatography (ERCP) (see below), laparotomy or transcutaneously by inserting a needle into dilated bile ducts (direct). The indirect methods of oral cholecystography and intravenous cholangiography are done much less often than

**Table 15.3** Patterns of 'liver function test' results in jaundice.

|  | Haemolysis | Hepatitis | Cholestasis |
|---|---|---|---|
| Bilirubin |  |  |  |
| Conjugated | + | ++ | +++ |
| Unconjugated | +++ | ++ | + |
| Transaminases | N | ++++ | + |
| Alkaline phosphatase | N | + | ++++ |

they were because of the increasing expertise in invasive techniques and ultrasound.

**Ultrasound** is non-invasive and is the most useful single investigation with a high sensitivity for gallstones, hepatic cysts and tumours, ascites, dilated intrahepatic bile ducts and gallbladder stones, but it is much less good at identifying common bile duct stones. Pancreatic masses can be very difficult to detect. Obesity, previous surgery and a gassy abdomen all make ultrasound examinations more difficult. The value of an ultrasound examination depends on the skill of the examiner.

**Computed tomographic (CT) scans** are complementary to ultrasound but are much more expensive. They are more accurate in the retroperitoneal area than ultrasound. Both ultrasound and CT can be used to guide percutaneous biopsy needles or drainage catheters. Computed tomography is difficult to perform in cachectic patients or those who move.

**Radioisotope liver scans** involve the use of technetium sulphur colloid which is taken up by the Kupffer cells. In general they are less helpful than ultrasound and CT scanning, but they can show cysts, abscesses and arteriovenous malformations. Diffuse liver diseases such as cirrhosis and alcoholic hepatitis show a characteristic poor uptake of isotope.

**Percutaneous cholangiography** using 'skinny' needles is a useful diagnostic tool when intrahepatic ducts are dilated and may be used as the preliminary to therapeutic drainage or placement of a stent to overcome narrowing or obstruction of the biliary tree. It is risky when clotting is abnormal or ascites is present and difficult in the presence of non-dilated ducts.

**Endoscopic retrograde cholangiopancreatography** is the most accurate diagnostic tool in the assessment of pancreatobiliary problems and has wide therapeutic uses. It is invasive, but less so than the surgical alternatives which it can replace. The procedure involves passing a side-viewing, fibreoptic or video duodenoscope into the second part of the duodenum under mild sedation. A catheter is passed through this instrument via the ampulla of Vater into the pancreatic and biliary duct systems. Contrast medium injected via the catheter outlines stones, strictures, leaks and cysts on X-ray. A diathermy catheter can be used to perform a sphincterotomy through which stones can be crushed or removed and strictures palliated by balloon dilation or the insertion of plastic or expanding metal stents. Success of ERCP does not depend on the presence of dilated ducts. Risks of ERCP include pancreatitis and cholangitis, and of sphincterotomy, bleeding and retroperitoneal leak.

**Liver biopsy** is usually performed under local anaesthesia in the right mid-axillary line using a Tru-cut or Menghini type needle while the patient holds their breath in expiration. It is an invaluable tool in the diagnosis of cirrhosis, chronic hepatitis, and drug-induced or toxic liver disease. It is also helpful in the diagnosis of intrahepatic tumours, especially if performed under ultrasound guidance. It is dangerous if there is uncorrected coagulopathy, ascites or a very vascular tumour. Mortality is approximately 1 in 10 000.

**Pancreatic function** is tested after a meal standardized for its content (Lundh meal) or cholecystokin (CCK) injection by assessing enzyme secretion with a tube inserted orally into the second part of the duodenum. Following the stimulus, the aspirated fluid is assayed for bicarbonate, lipase and trypsin. Insufficiency suggests pancreatic disease. Various tubeless alternatives to this test have been developed, but are only useful as screening tests.

# Clinical problems

## THE BILIARY TRACT

## Gallstones

### AETIOLOGY

Most gallstones are composed of cholesterol and relatively small amounts of inorganic salts and organic debris (mucus, desquamated cells etc.) A minority (10–20 per cent) contain enough calcium salts to be opaque on an abdominal X-ray. In patients with chronic haemolytic anaemia, the main ingredient of the stones is calcium bilirubinate and they are almost black in colour.

Cholesterol stones develop when the concentration of cholesterol in gallbladder bile is high relative to the concentrations of bile acids and phospholipids, which normally keep cholesterol in solution. Bile acids are the end product of cholesterol metabolism in the liver and subtle alterations of this metabolic pathway have been demonstrated in the liver of patients with gallstones. Other mechanisms of gallstone formation such as rapid nucleation and reduced gallbladder contractility have also been implicated. Stasis and infection of gallbladder bile are usually secondary to gallstones but may encourage their further growth.

Gallstones are extremely prevalent and associated factors include being female, a positive family history, increasing age, obesity and parity. Ultrasound studies in asymptomatic subjects suggest that they occur in more than 10 per cent of women over the age of 40 and they are common incidental findings at **post-mortem**. Other risk factors include drugs, such as clofibrate and oestrogen-containing contraceptives, haemolytic anaemia and ileal resection.

### PATHOLOGY

Gallstones are formed primarily in the gallbladder, but in approximately 15 per cent of cases they migrate into the biliary tree where they can cause many complications. They rarely arise *de novo* in the bile duct unless that is chronically obstructed, as in postoperative strictures, or in the syndrome of oriental cholangiohepatitis in which very large numbers of stones may be found in the intrahepatic and extrahepatic biliary tree. Gallstones are often multiple and can reach a very large size. (Fig. 15.1).

Acute and chronic inflammatory changes in the gallbladder and biliary tree are secondary to obstruction by gallstones, often associated with secondary infection. The gallbladder wall is commonly thickened by both fibrosis and muscular hypertrophy and the mucosa can be extensively damaged or destroyed.

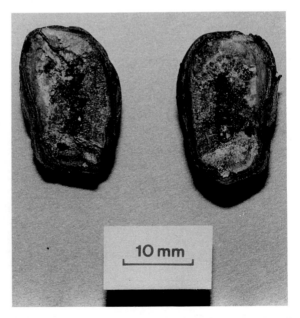

**Figure 15.1** Gallstone removed from the common bile duct.

## CLINICAL FEATURES

The typical symptom of uncomplicated stones is the pain of biliary colic (page 377). It is unwise to ascribe the common symptoms of flatulent dyspepsia and fat intolerance to stones in the absence of other evidence. Biliary colic, although commonly felt over the gallbladder, may spread across the abdomen or chest and may last intensely for hours. The essential clues are great severity and intermittent discrete attacks. Pain radiating to the back is more suggestive of stones in the bile duct (choledocholithiasis).

## COMPLICATIONS

Acute cholecystitis is associated with marked local tenderness, guarding and fever. If complicated by secondary infection with pus formation (empyema of the gall bladder) and septicaemia, the patient is very ill with high fever and marked signs over the gall bladder. Other complications are listed in Table 15.4.

## DIAGNOSIS

Diagnosis is by ultrasound or oral cholecystography (Fig. 15.2) in the uncomplicated case, as discussed on page 377. In acute cholecystitis, the cystic duct is usually obstructed and oral cholecystography will show a 'non-functioning gall bladder'. The blockage can be revealed by a gamma camera following the injection of a radiopharmaceutical such as iminodiacetic acid (HIDA), which is taken up by the liver and secreted into bile.

**Table 15.4** Complications of gallstones.

| | | |
|---|---|---|
| Acute cholecystitis Empyema of gall bladder | ± Septicaemia | superadded infection |
| Obstructive jaundice Cholangitis Acute pancreatitis | ± Septicaemia | Stone passing through the common bile duct |
| Fistula from gall bladder to intestine Obstruction of gastrointestinal tract by stone Adenocarcinoma of gall bladder | | Rare |

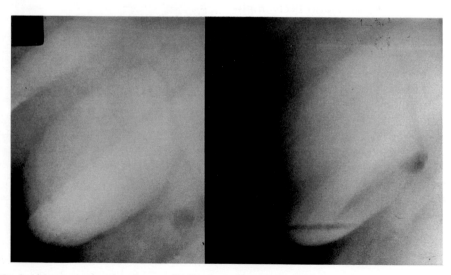

**Figure 15.2** Oral cholecystograms showing small, floating gallstones in a functioning gallbladder. These are ideal for oral dissolution therapy. Left: supine. Right: erect.

## DIFFERENTIAL DIAGNOSIS

The main conditions to be considered are peptic ulcer, perforation in the GI tract, acute hepatitis and pancreatitis.

## TREATMENT

Treatment of gallstones has undergone a revolution in recent years. Standard treatment is cholecystectomy which is increasingly being performed by the laparoscopic route. This allows a much smaller incision with a concomitant reduction in the post-operative hospital stay. In those patients who are unsuitable for or unwilling to undergo surgery many options now exist (Table 15.5). The least invasive method is oral dissolution therapy with bile acids (cheno- and ursodeoxycholic acids). The choice of technique depends on the suitability of the stones, the gallbladder and patient for the various options (as well as the patient's wishes). If the gallbladder is 'non-functioning' on oral cholecystography (blocked cystic duct), most non-operative methods of treatment will be dangerous or ineffective. Radio-opaque stones contain calcium and are not suitable for dissolution: their calcium content is best assessed by CT of the gallbladder.

Acute cholecystitis may be treated conservatively with intravenous fluids, nasogastric suction, pain relief and antibiotics followed later by elective cholecystectomy when the inflammation has settled. However, many surgeons consider that early cholecystectomy is safe and preferable. Empyema of the gallbladder demands urgent drainage, often by cholecystotomy alone in a frail, elderly patient.

**Table 15.5** Methods available for treating gallbladder stones.

| Cholecystectomy: | Standard |
|---|---|
| | Laparoscopic |
| Cholecystotomy | |
| Percutaneous cholecystolithotomy | |
| Oral dissolution therapy | |
| Dissolution by methyl tertiary butyl ether (MTBE): | |
| Percutaneous approach | |
| Endoscopic approach | |
| Extracorporeal shockwave lithotripsy with adjuvant bile acids | |
| Percutaneous rotary lithotripsy | |

At present it is not generally possible to explore the common bile duct for stones when using the laparoscopic approach but changes in the field are rapidly occurring and the ideal treatment of an individual will depend in part on local expertise. If the common bile duct is explored a 't-tube' is usually left *in situ* for some days afterwards, and before it is removed, a t-tube cholangiogram is performed to check that no residual stones are present.

Treating gallstones by the laparoscopic route, together with some of the other non-operative techniques, may leave stones within the common bile duct. These are usually treated by endoscopic sphincterotomy, performed together with ERCP just before or just after treatment of the gallbladder stones.

In some elderly individuals, treatment of the common bile duct stones alone may be sufficient. Dissolution of stones in the duct via the t-tube can occasionally be achieved but agents currently available are very slow (mono-octanoin) or potentially dangerous (methyl tertiary butyl ether, MTBE, or ethyl propionate). Retained stones may also be retrieved via the t-tube track under radiological contrast or by endoscopic control using Dormia baskets (Fig. 15.3).

Ascending cholangitis is generally considered an indication for urgent ERCP and sphincterotomy but many cases settle using the same conservative measures as for acute cholangitis, allowing sphincterotomy to be performed in a quiescent phase. Coagulopathy due to malabsorption of vitamin K with a resulting reduction in the short-lived circulating clotting factors which require this vitamin for their synthesis (II, VII, IX, X) is common in biliary obstruction. It must be corrected by parenteral vitamin K before invasive procedures are undertaken. If time is too short or there is impaired liver function, fresh frozen plasma may be used to replace the clotting factors but it has a very short effective plasma half-life.

## PROGNOSIS

The complications of gallstones are a threat to health and life especially in the elderly. However, subjects with asymptomatic stones (> 50 per cent) will probably suffer no serious

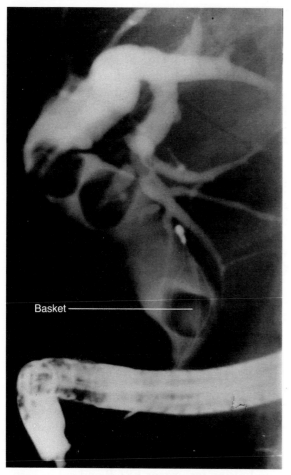

Basket

**Figure 15.3** Endoscopic retrograde cholangiopancreatography showing large common bile duct stones. One is being grasped in a Dormia basket (arrow) prior to removal.

consequences and prophylactic cholecystectomy is not recommended. Adenocarcinoma of the gallbladder has a low prevalence and is usually disregarded in considering the wisdom of cholecystectomy for stones. When it does occur, it tends to be diagnosed late and carry a poor prognosis. However, early cancer may be found incidentally at cholecystectomy for stones and the outlook is then much better.

# Sclerosing cholangitis

## AETIOLOGY

This is a rare disorder, two-thirds of cases are associated with inflammatory bowel disease in which there is a prevalence of 4–10 per cent. It may also occur in retroperitoneal fibrosis, a chronic inflammatory, fibrosing process affecting especially the retroperitoneal tissues and mediastinum. There is a male-to-female preponderance of 2:1, but autoimmune mechanisms appear important. There is a strong association with human leukocyte antigen (HLA) A1 B8 DR3 and to a lesser extent with DR2. Antibodies to biliary epithelium are commonly found.

An important cause of sclerosing cholangitis which has emerged in recent years is the acquired immunodeficiency syndrome (AIDS). In this condition there is usually an associated cytomegalovirus infection and the presentation is commonly with right upper quadrant pain.

## PATHOLOGY

There is diffuse or patchy chronic obliterative inflammation with fibrosis affecting the intrahepatic and extrahepatic biliary tree.

## CLINICAL FEATURES

Clinical features are those of chronic obstructive jaundice. In early cases there may be episodes of clinical cholangitis with long periods of apparently good health, but liver function tests are usually persistently abnormal. There may be pruritus or right upper quadrant pain in the absence of clinical jaundice.

## DIAGNOSIS

This is now made by ERCP (page 378) or other forms of direct cholangiography (Fig. 15.4). The intrahepatic biliary tree shows beading from alternate fibrosis and dilatation. The differential diagnosis is from all other types of obstructive jaundice and, if the lesion is focal, from cholangiocarcinoma which may coexist.

## COMPLICATIONS

Ascending (bacterial) cholangitis is a common problem, especially after intensive investigations such as ERCP or colonoscopy. **Cholangiocarcinoma** may occur in up to 15 per

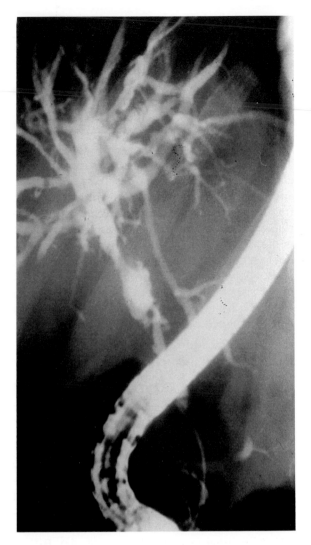

**Figure 15.4** Endoscopic retrograde cholangiopancreatography showing generalized irregularity, strictures and dilations of both intra- and extrahepatic bile ducts. This is diagnostic of sclerosing cholangitis.

cent of cases. Gallbladder carcinoma also occurs. Eventual progression to liver failure is possible.

## TREATMENT

Treatment is difficult. Corticosteroids and a variety of other agents such as penicillamine, colchicine, cyclosporin and ursodexycholic acid have been tried but none is clearly effective. Cholangitis is treated by suitable antibiotics. Symptomatic treatment includes the use of cholestyramine for itching and a low fat diet for steatorrhoea together with the appropriate use of fat-soluble vitamins as in primary biliary cirrhosis (page 400).

Dilatation of extrahepatic strictures and placement of stents at transhepatic or more usually, endoscopic, cholangiography may produce a worthwhile, and in some cases, marked benefit. Liver transplantation may be the only hope for prolonged survival in severe cases.

## PROGNOSIS

Sclerosing cholangitis is increasingly being recognized at an early stage owing to the more widespread use of ERCP in patients with inflammatory bowel disease who have persistently abnormal liver function tests. It seems that the natural history is one of very slow progression over many years, and documented remissions of over 20 years have been recorded. There is a long-term risk of cholangiocarcinoma (see below).

# Cholangiocarcinoma

## AETIOLOGY

This is a relatively rare tumour arising from the epithelium of the biliary tract. The best recognized association is with sclerosing cholangitis and inflammatory bowel disease, but it is also described in patients suffering from chronic infestation of the biliary tree with the liver fluke *Clonorchis sinensis* prevalent in the Far East.

## PATHOLOGY

The tumour grows slowly and spreads through the wall of the bile duct and to neighbouring lymph nodes, but rarely metastasizes widely.

## CLINICAL FEATURES

The patient presents with obstructive jaundice, which may be complicated by cholangitis. Diagnosis is by direct cholangiography and by obtaining material for cytology and histology. This may be possible by the transhepatic route or during ERCP, but is often only feasible at surgery.

## TREATMENT

Surgical excision is worth attempting if the lesion is in the common bile duct. A low lesion near the ampulla will require a Whipple's resection of the head of pancreas and duodenum (page 389). A high lesion arising in the hepatic ducts near the porta is very difficult to treat surgically, but may be managed by some form of dilatation and 'stenting' (i.e. placement of an internal drainage tube) using the transhepatic or endoscopic approach (Fig. 15.5). Plastic stents block after a few months and may need to be replaced several times. Expandable metal stents are an alternative but are costly.

## PROGNOSIS

Progression of the tumour is relatively slow and some patients will survive for up to 2 years even after palliative treatment alone. However, median survival times are only about 6 months and attempts at curative surgery are well worthwhile especially if the lesion is at the lower end of the common bile duct. Liver transplantation is not feasible as there is invariably rapid tumour recurrence.

# Ampullary carcinoma

This uncommon tumour occurs primarily in the elderly. It is derived from papillary epithelium and is of low malignancy, invading locally. It frequently presents with cholangitis and a fluctuating level of jaundice. Investigations often demonstrate dilated pancreatic as well as biliary duct systems. Treatment by Whipple's resection is usually curative but often not feasible in view of the age of the patient. Endoscopic procedures such as sphincterotomy or stent placement may give prolonged palliation.

# Functional disorders of the biliary tract

Intermittent abdominal pain suggesting biliary colic but with negative investigations is sometimes ascribed to disturbances of the sphincter of Oddi (biliary dyskinesia) or probably to innocent anatomical abnormalities of the gallbladder (e.g. adenomyomatosis, cholesterolosis). Biliary pressures can now be measured at ERCP and there is evidence that intermittent papillary obstruction does occur. However, dilatation of the duct and delay in emptying at ERCP may be more reliable guides to therapy. It is tempting to remove an anatomically abnormal gallbladder (without stones) or to undertake endoscopic sphincterotomy in these patients, but such treatment is often ineffective and carries its own risks. Many of these patients have the 'hepatic flexure syndrome' variant of the irritable bowel syndrome and should be treated accordingly (page 373).

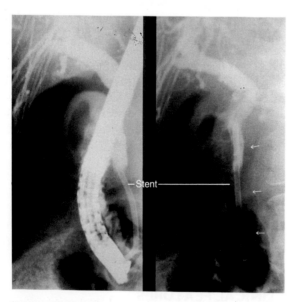

**Figure 15.5** Endoscopic retrograde cholangiopancreatography showing a tight biliary stricture which is decompressed by an endoscopically placed biliary stent or stiff tube (arrows).

# THE PANCREAS

## *Acute pancreatitis*

### AETIOLOGY

The best recognized cause is the migration of gallstones through the sphincter of Oddi, although the exact mechanism is unclear. An alcoholic binge rarely induces a first attack but can produce an acute relapse of chronic pancreatitis. The other associations in Table 15.6 are poorly understood and in 30–40 per cent of patients no clear explanation is found. Specific infections, especially with the mumps virus, are well recognized but rarely cause severe disease. Trauma is an occasional cause. A number of drugs, particularly sodium valproate, diuretics and, perhaps, corticosteroids rarely cause acute pancreatitis.

### PATHOLOGY

The pancreas is acutely inflamed and sometimes severely haemorrhagic. Full recovery of structure is possible after a moderately severe, uncomplicated attack. Typically there is widespread 'fat necrosis' of the omentum and mesentery – white plaques that are thought to be formed by the deposition of calcium salts of fatty acids, liberated by the local action of lipase.

**Table 15.6** Causes of pancreatitis.

**Gallstones**
Especially acute and recurrent acute pancreatitis

**Alcohol**
Especially chronic and chronic relapsing pancreatitis

**Other**
Virus infections, e.g. mumps
Hypertriglyceridaemia
Hypercalcaemia
Drugs, e.g. azathioprine, some diuretics,
   corticosteroids, sodium valproate
Secondary to pancreatic cancer
Trauma
Congenital malformations, e.g. reduplication cyst,
   annular pancreas
Exposure to organic solvents

In severe attacks, there can be extensive necrosis and sloughing of pancreatic tissue with secondary infection and abscess formation. Enzymes leaking into the peritoneal lesser sac and beyond may produce a chemical peritonitis with accumulation of fluid rich in pancreatic enzymes ('pancreatic ascites'). More localized leaks of pancreatic juice in and near the pancreas lead to the formation of pseudocysts which, unlike true cysts, are not lined with an epithelium but simply by adjacent tissues and later by a firm fibrous wall.

### CLINICAL FEATURES

There is usually an acute abdominal crisis of considerable severity. Typical pancreatic pain (page 377) develops often quite suddenly after a rich meal or a drinking bout and is accompanied by sweating, vomiting and later by vascular collapse and shock in a severe case.

Examination reveals marked abdominal tenderness with guarding, especially in the epigastrium, and later distension and ileus. A severe attack may be marked by bruising in the left flank. Respiratory function is commonly impaired with hypoxia and dyspnoea. Acute renal failure may complicate the illness, which then has a very grave prognosis.

### DIAGNOSIS

The cardinal investigation is the measurement of amylase or other pancreatic enzymes in the serum. Amylase levels rise rapidly in the first few hours of the attack and fall slowly over the next few days. Serum amylase is occasionally raised in diabetic ketosis and in perforated peptic ulcer, and always in uraemia, but rarely to the levels seen in acute pancreatitis. The levels may be misleadingly low in patients with acute relapses of severe chronic pancreatitis. Peritoneal lavage fluid may contain high amylase levels or blood, both suggesting pancreatitis.

Having made a diagnosis, the cause should be sought and this will include investigation of the biliary tree. In most cases this is undertaken by ultrasound and, in recurrent disease, by direct cholangiography after the attack has settled. It was previously said that ERCP should be avoided in or soon after acute pancreatitis because it may produce a recurrence or introduce infection into a pseudocyst. While such risks are present, it now appears that if ERCP is performed within 48 hours of the onset of the attack, removal of the bile duct stones by sphincterotomy will result in improved survival. Such intervention demands a high level of expertise. Endoscopic retrograde cholangio-pancreatography is useful between episodes of recurrent disease to define the anatomy of the pancreatic duct (in case surgery is required) and, particularly, to exclude and remove stones in the common bile duct.

## DIFFERENTIAL DIAGNOSIS

The main conditions to be considered are perforation and infarction of bowel in view of the severity of the clinical presentation.

## COMPLICATIONS

Pseudocysts, ascites and left pleural effusions are quite common (Table 15.7) complications of acute pancreatitis. Pancreatic necrosis and sloughing are rare. Severe bleeding can occur into the duodenum if major arteries are affected by local inflammation and necrosis. The splenic vein may become blocked and induce splenomegaly. The superior mesenteric artery may also thrombose, leading to small bowel infarction.

**Table 15.7** Complications of acute pancreatitis.

| | |
|---|---|
| Hypotension → | Renal failure |
| Septicaemia | |
| Pulmonary alveolar → | Shock lung (adult |
| damage | respiratory distress |
| Pleural effusion | syndrome, page 261) |
| Pseudocysts | |
| Pancreatic ascites | |
| Pancreatic necrosis/abscess | |
| Metabolic: Hyperglycaemia | |
| Hypocalcaemia | |
| Superior mesenteric artery/vein occlusion | |

## TREATMENT

Treatment is supportive and as yet no specific therapy has been shown to be effective. The usual measures are nasogastric suction, intravenous fluids and parenteral analgesics. Hypoxia should be looked for and treated by continuous oxygen therapy. Oral fluid and food are not allowed until pain and abdominal signs subside and gastric aspirates decline. Hypotension requires the infusion of plasma expanders and central venous pressure (CVP) monitoring. Blood transfusion may be required for anaemia secondary to extensive haemorrhage. Transient hypocalcaemia and hyperglycaemia often require correction. Antibiotics are not given routinely but will be required if features of abscess or septicaemia develop. Renal failure may require temporary haemodialysis.

Pseudocysts, ascites and abscesses should be drained and it is now usually possible to do this percutaneously under ultrasound or CT control. Surgery is usually reserved for very ill patients who have extensive pancreatic necrosis or inadequately drained abscesses. It is necessary to remove all necrotic tissue and leave wide drainage tubes in the pancreatic bed. The presence of necrosis is best assessed by contrast-enhanced CT scanning.

## PROGNOSIS

The disease carries an appreciable mortality and figures vary from 5 to 20 per cent. The course can be slow with much morbidity, but ultimately full recovery of pancreatic structure and function can occur.

Attacks may recur, especially if treatable causes such as gallstones or hypercalcaemia are ignored, but also when no obvious cause is apparent. In such cases abnormalities of the pancreatic duct may be amenable to surgical correction and should be sought by ERCP.

# Chronic pancreatitis

## AETIOLOGY

Most cases are caused by chronic, excessive alcohol consumption (Table 15.6). Uncommon causes include haemochromatosis (page 401) and hypertriglyceridaemia types I and V, and in the tropics malnutrition is thought to lead to chronic pancreatic damage. Fibrocystic disease is a cause of chronic pancreatic exocrine failure and is discussed on page 295.

## PATHOLOGY

The pancreas is irreversibly damaged with loss of exocrine and endocrine cells, disruption of the normal ductular anatomy and much fibrosis. The main ducts are irregularly dilated and contain proteinaceous plugs derived from the protein-rich exocrine secretion (Fig. 15.6). Calcification of the plugs produces radio-opaque stones and patchy calcification of the parenchyma is common, especially in alcoholics.

## CLINICAL FEATURES

Pain is the characteristic feature and it can be acute and relapsing or chronic and unremitting. The distribution of pancreatic pain was discussed on page 377. Patients with chronic pain may become addicted to strong analgesics. The disease may be silent for long periods and present with complications such as diabetes mellitus and pancreatic steatorrhoea.

Intermittent or even continuous obstructive jaundice can be produced by swelling or fibrosis of the pancreatic head (Fig. 15.7).

The many features of chronic alcohol abuse may be apparent (page 396).

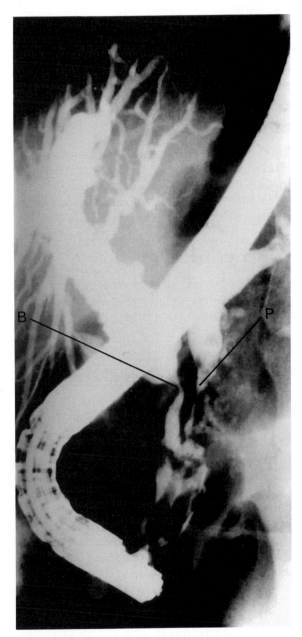

**Figure 15.7** Endoscopic retrograde cholangiopancreatography showing dilated biliary (B) and pancreatic (P) duct systems above smooth, tapering strictures as a result of chronic pancreatitis.

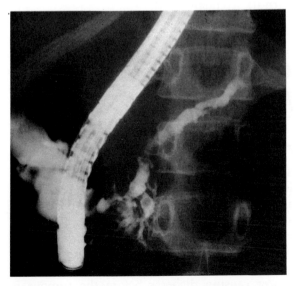

**Figure 15.6** Endoscopic retrograde cholangiopancreatography showing a dilated, irregular pancreatic duct containing filling defects (stones). This is characteristic of chronic pancreatitis.

## DIAGNOSIS

Abdominal X-ray may reveal distinctive pancreatic calcification. Pancreatic function is assessed by a glucose tolerance test and by a tube test of pancreatic exocrine secretion (page 378). Pancreatic structure is best assessed by ERCP but, as mentioned on page 378, ultrasound or CT scanning can give useful information and avoid the risks of pancreatography.

Pancreatic steatorrhoea is often gross and the faecal fat excretion can be more than ten times greater than the upper limit of normal. This is rarely seen in other forms of malabsorption.

## DIFFERENTIAL DIAGNOSIS

This is from the many other causes of chronic abdominal pain (page 331) and malabsorption (page 340). In patients with obstructive jaundice, differentiation from pancreatic cancer can be very difficult even at surgery (page 389).

## COMPLICATIONS

Complications are of endocrine and exocrine pancreatic failure and of addiction to dangerous analgesic and narcotic drugs.

## TREATMENT

The most important measure, whatever the underlying cause, is to advise complete permanent abstinence from alcohol, but compliance is often poor. Analgesics should be used sparingly and, in severe cases, percutaneous coeliac plexus block may be effective in relieving pain although it is not without risk of perforation and haemorrhage and usually only lasts for around 3 months. Further procedures are less likely to work. If pain proves intractable, ERCP may show a ductular abnormality that can be treated surgically, for example, a distended duct may be drained into a jejunal loop. Occasionally total pancreatectomy is undertaken in desperate cases, especially if function has been lost. The use of antioxidant drugs (methionine, vitamins C and E and selenium) has shown promise in one controlled trial.

Diabetes mellitus will require insulin treatment (page 476) and symptomatic steatorrhoea will respond to restriction of dietary fat and replacement of pancreatic enzymes. Enzyme therapy is difficult, however, because the various preparations available have to be taken in large doses with every meal. The enzymes are also irreversibly damaged by a gastric pH of <4 and are usually administered in the form of pH-sensitive coated microspheres which release the enzymes at the higher pH in the small intestine. An alternative is to use a histamine-2 receptor blocker or H, K ATPase blocker to raise gastric pH.

Patients often eat well and maintain their weight even if steatorrhoea is marked, unless there is much pain or overt diabetes mellitus. Reduction of fat intake alone to 40–60 g daily may be remarkably effective in relieving diarrhoea. If the appetite is poor or if there is marked loss of weight, calorie supplements will be required. Medium chain triglycerides (MCT) are absorbed in the absence of pancreatic lipase and provide a valuable source of calories. Medium chain triglycerides are available as an oil for cooking and in various powdered forms.

## PROGNOSIS

This is good in terms of survival, but severe chronic pain may require surgical intervention with its attendant risks.

# Carcinoma of the pancreas

## AETIOLOGY

This is a common cancer and the incidence is increasing. In Europe and North America there are 9–10 cases per 100 000 of the population annually.

There are no certain causes with the exception of cigarette smoking. The association with diabetes is probably related to early pancreatic cancer causing diabetes before the tumour is manifest. There are no known genetic associations but chronic pancreatitis has now been proven to be a predisposing cause.

## PATHOLOGY

The carcinoma arises from the ductular epithelium or the exocrine acini. It can occur in any part of the gland but those arising in the ampulla and head are commoner than those in the body and tail. Ampullary carcinoma arises from the mucosa which lines the short length of duct common to the biliary and pancreatic systems and spreads over an area of the duodenum around the common orifice.

The tumour spreads widely, invading local structures and metastasizing to the liver and regional lymph nodes.

## CLINICAL FEATURES

The commonest presentation is obstructive jaundice when the lesion is at the ampulla or in the head (Fig. 15.8). This tends to be steadily progressive and, although it may initially be painless, pancreatic pain eventually develops in most cases.

Cancer in the body or tail causes chronic pancreatic pain, which can defy diagnosis for months until the tumour reaches a large size.

Occasionally the tumour presents with a complication such as duodenal obstruction. Extensive pancreatic damage can lead to diabetes mellitus or steatorrhoea. Transient migratory thrombophlebitis is a rare and unexplained clinical association.

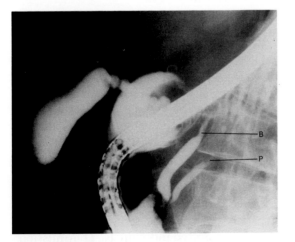

**Figure 15.8** Endoscopic retrograde cholangiopancreatography showing irregular, tapering, corresponding strictures of bile duct (B) and pancreatic duct (P) characteristic of biliary obstruction by a pancreatic cancer.

Physical examination may reveal a mass caused by a large tumour in the body or tail or an enlarged, tense gall bladder in association with obstructive jaundice (Courvoisier's sign).

## DIAGNOSIS

This is usually revealed during the investigation of jaundice or by ultrasound or CT scanning for abdominal pain. Histological confirmation is obtained percutaneously (page 378) or at surgery. Pancreatic histology can be difficult to interpret, even if obtained at surgery, because some tumours produce a lot of surrounding inflammation and fibrosis.

## DIFFERENTIAL DIAGNOSIS

This is from the many causes of abdominal pain and obstructive jaundice. The differentiation from chronic pancreatitis can prove very difficult.

## COMPLICATIONS

The main ones are obstructive jaundice, duodenal obstruction, pancreatic failure and, rarely, compression of the superior mesenteric artery with small intestinal ischaemia or infarction.

## TREATMENT

The only possibility of cure is surgical resection but this is rarely feasible except when the tumour is confined to the head or ampulla and produces jaundice relatively early. The preferred procedure is **Whipple's operation** which involves resection of the head of the pancreas and the C loop of the duodenum with gastrojejunostomy. Separate anastomoses between the bile and pancreatic ducts and a loop of jejunum are created.

Palliation of jaundice is commonly necessary and the placement of plastic or expanding metal stents using the endoscopic or transhepatic routes is now the method of choice. Sometimes surgical drainage, preferably the 'triple' bypass, choledochojejunostomy, gastrojejunostomy and jejunojejunostomy is performed, especially if there is duodenal obstruction.

For severe pancreatic pain in untreatable cancer coeliac plexus block is often very effective and it can be undertaken at surgery or percutaneously.

Radiotherapy is not used and chemotherapy has not yet found an established place in treatment, although life can be prolonged by a few weeks or months.

## PROGNOSIS

This is still very poor and few patients survive more than 6 months. Whipple's resection for ampullary carcinoma can produce a 30–40 per cent chance of surviving for 5 years, but cancer at other sites is associated with a much poorer survival rate, even when resection is feasible.

# Functional tumours of the pancreas

These rare tumours arise from the pancreatic islets, usually as single or multiple adenomas and come to attention because symptoms result from the increased amounts of hormone(s) being produced. The commonest example is insulinoma (page 492), and gastrinoma (Zollinger–Ellison syndrome) described on page 356. Rarer tumours include those producing glucagon and vasoactive intestinal polypeptide (VIP). The glucagonoma syndrome includes a characteristic rash and mild diabetes mellitus. VIPomas produce severe chronic diarrhoea.

# Cystic fibrosis (fibrocystic disease of the pancreas; mucoviscidosis)

See page 295.

## THE LIVER

# Viral hepatitis

The most important causes of acute and chronic viral hepatitis are the hepatotropic viruses A, B, C, D and E.

## HEPATITIS A

Hepatitis A virus (HAV) is a 27 nm enveloped picornavirus transmitted via the faecal–oral route. The genome has been cloned and sequenced. There is only one serotype worldwide. In developing countries most preschool children are infected and become immune without jaundice. In countries in which hygiene has improved, infection takes place later in life, with a corresponding increase in clinically apparent cases, but a lower overall rate of infection.

Typical vectors in the developed world are uncooked shellfish and foods washed in water contaminated with sewage. The disease also spreads readily in such institutions as boarding schools, army camps and prisons. The incubation period is 3 to 5 weeks.

## HEPATITIS B

This DNA virus consists of a 40 nm spherical particle (Dane particle) with an envelope (hepatitis B surface antigen – $HB_sAg$). The nucleic acid is surrounded by a core protein ($HB_cAg$) of which a subunit ($HB_eAg$) is a useful serum marker of infectivity (Table 15.8). During replication the DNA is produced from RNA by a reverse transcriptase (DNA polymerase). The viral DNA can be integrated into hepatocyte DNA.

Hepatitis B virus is present in blood, saliva and semen of infected individuals. Transmission of hepatitis B virus (HBV) is via percutaneous or transmucosal routes, including sexual transmission and by transfusion of blood or blood product. The mean incubation period is 11 weeks.

**Table 15.8** Serological tests for viral hepatitis A, B and C.

| Hepatitis | Test | Diagnosis |
|---|---|---|
| A | HAV IgM | Acute infection |
| | HAV IgG | Past infection |
| B | $Hb_sAg$ | Acute or chronic infection |
| | $Hb_eAg$ | High infectivity – viral replication |
| | $Hb_sAb$ | Past infection or vaccination |
| | $Hb_eAb$ | 'Seroconversion' after past infection |
| | $Hb_cAb$ IgG | Sometimes sole serum marker of past infection or low infectivity carriage |
| | $Hb_cAb$ IgM | Acute infection or reactivation |
| C | $NS_{1-5}$ | Various phases of acute and chronic infection |

NS = non-structural part of genome.

Hepatitis B occurs sporadically in Western Europe, North America and other developed countries. The risk factors associated with $HB_sAg$ infection in these countries are given in Table 15.9.

In endemic areas children acquire infection either at parturition – 'vertical transmission' – or from preschool siblings or playmates. During this period, infection is usually anicteric and the chronic carrier state, especially in males, is the usual sequel due to relative immune tolerance to HBV.

**Table 15.9** Main risks of hepatitis B virus (HBV) infection in developed countries.

Intravenous drug abuse
Male homosexuality
Residence in prisons or institutions for mental handicap
Persons having tattoos with inadequate precautions
Heterosexual promiscuity
Ethnic group
Low socioeconomic status
Blood or blood product recipients
Employment in health professions
Family members of HBV carriers

## HEPATITIS C

It was known for many years that transfusion-associated hepatitis occurred in the absence of HBV. Many of these cases can now be ascribed to hepatitis C virus (HCV). The genome of the virus has now been cloned and sequenced. It appears to be related to the flaviviruses, has a diameter of 30–60 nm and an RNA genome of almost 10 kB. Most patients suffer a rather mild hepatitic illness. There is a very high chronic carrier rate in certain parts of the world, such as the Far East and Africa. It is rarely transmitted perinatally or sexually. At risk groups are shown in Table 15.10.

## HEPATITIS D

The D (delta) agent is an incomplete RNA virusoid which requires the presence of HBV for transmission. It can either coinfect with that virus or cause a worsening of liver disease in chronic HBV carriers. The incubation period is about 5 weeks. It is rare in Britain, occurring principally in South America, Sub-Saharan Africa, the Mediterranean, Middle East and Asiatic parts of the former USSR.

## HEPATITIS E

Epidemic, enterically transmitted hepatitis due to this 27–34 nm RNA virus was first reported from India but has since occurred in South America, North Africa and South-East Asia or in people returning from those areas.

Other viruses which can cause acute hepatitis include the cytomegalovirus (CMV), Epstein–Barr virus (EBV) or infectious mononucleosis,

**Table 15.10** Main risk groups for hepatitis C virus (HCV) infection.

Intravenous drug abusers
Multiple transfusion recipients
    Haemophiliacs
    Haemodialysis patients
    Thalassaemics
    Hypogammaglobulinaemics
Alcoholics
Organ transplant recipients
Those from high incidence areas
Health care workers

yellow fever and herpes simplex. There are many others with occasional hepatitic manifestations and other 'non-A, non-B, non-C' viruses probably exist.

# Acute hepatitis

## CLINICAL FEATURES

All the viruses produce a similar illness with only minor features distinguishing one from another. Virological diagnosis depends on specific laboratory testing.

The onset usually occurs after a week or two of a non-specific illness with malaise, loss of appetite, characteristically a distaste for cigarettes, backache, fever and sometimes right upper quadrant pain. Serum sickness-like symptoms, with fever, urticaria and joint pains, are more common with hepatitis B, and headache and mild meningism with hepatitis A. A particular predilection for, and high mortality in, pregnant women is a feature of hepatitis E only. Jaundice soon follows, and can last from 2 to 3 days to many weeks; characteristically the duration is 2 to 3 weeks. There can be a cholestatic phase with deepening jaundice and itching, especially with hepatitis A.

## PATHOLOGY

The viruses all produce a similar abnormality with enlargement of the liver, diffuse lobular necrosis and acute inflammation predominantly near the central veins. In severe cases there is massive destruction of the lobules with shrinking of the liver ('acute yellow atrophy') but, if the patient survives, the liver can recover completely. However, there may be irreversible damage to the liver architecture even during an apparently mild attack. This will heal by nodular regeneration, fibrosis and cirrhosis (postnecrotic scarring or posthepatitic cirrhosis). Sometimes a more chronic, active inflammatory and necrotic process ensues and leads to the clinical and histopathological entity of chronic active hepatitis (page 399).

These longer term complications of hepatitis are most likely to follow hepatitis B or especially C infection, which may be mild clinically or asymptomatic. It seems to be exceptionally rare for HAV, EBV or CMV to produce chronic liver disease.

Physical signs are usually restricted to jaundice and modest, tender enlargement of the liver. Liver function tests will show marked elevation of the transaminases with rather more modest increase in the alkaline phosphatase. Serum albumin is usually well maintained, but blood coagulation tests are abnormal in all but the mildest cases. Marked prolongation of prothrombin time is an indicator of severe disease. In EBV infection there are usually other signs of infectious mononucleosis (glandular fever, page 731). In herpes simplex infection there may be obvious signs of the virus around the mouth or evidence of infection elsewhere (e.g. encephalitis, page 694).

## DIAGNOSIS

This is confirmed by appropriate serological tests on the plasma (Table 15.8). As with all infections, only IgM antibodies indicate that the infection is current or recent.

In patients with evidence of hepatitis B (i.e. positive B surface antigen), it is advisable to determine whether another marker of this virus – the e antigen – is present in the serum. Its presence indicates continuing viral replication in the liver cells, high infectivity of the blood and a continuing risk of progressive liver disease. The development of antibodies to this antigen heralds an improved prognosis. It is too early to be confident about the relevance of the antibodies for hepatitis C.

## COMPLICATIONS

The major acute complications are bleeding as a result of impaired coagulation and the development (over days) of encephalopathy, hypoglycaemia and oliguric renal failure (fulminant hepatic failure). The remote complications of hepatitis B and C include chronic active hepatitis, cirrhosis and hepatocellular carcinoma (page 408). Rare complications include aplastic anaemia, myocarditis, vasculitis and cryoglobulinaemia.

## TREATMENT

This is supportive in the expectation that resolution will occur over several weeks. There is much current interest in the use of antiviral drugs and interferon in the management of hepatitis B and C, but this is still at the stage of clinical research and is not being generally applied in acute hepatitis. Acyclovir is usually given to patients with severe local and systemic herpes simplex infections. There is no evidence that corticosteroids are helpful and they are best avoided – their use in hastening the resolution of severe cholestasis is controversial.

In most cases, supportive therapy merely means a light, palatable diet and bed rest if the patient feels weak. Enforced bed rest is of no benefit.

Alcohol should be avoided completely at least until liver function tests have returned to normal. All unnecessary drugs should be withheld, especially those that are known to be potentially hepatotoxic. In more severe cases, intravenous hydration may be required and blood glucose levels must be maintained with adequate intravenous administration. Sedatives should be avoided for fear of masking encephalopathy. Prothrombin time prolongation should be treated with parenteral vitamin K only if bleeding occurs when transfusion of fresh frozen plasma or blood will be required. In severe acute liver failure, intensive care is required with monitoring of central venous pressure, arterial pressure, blood gases and renal function. Anaesthesia and artificial ventilation with hyperventilation may be helpful. Cerebral oedema may develop and monitoring and treatment of raised intracranial pressure are crucial. Late infective complications may prove fatal. Liver transplantation is now being used successfully in those who are otherwise unlikely to survive.

## PROGNOSIS

This is usually excellent in hepatitis A and in infections with EBV and CMV, although there may be a prolonged period of morbidity. Generalized herpes simplex virus (HSV) infection has a high mortality rate. The risk of developing late complications of hepatitis B and C is uncertain.

Fulminant hepatic failure is very rare and carries a poor prognosis which depends on the virus responsible and on the criteria used to define the condition. If the patient is drowsy and confused, the chances of survival are less than 30 per cent. Poor prognostic factors include age over 50, hepatitis C, slow onset, prothrombin time over 120 s, bilirubin over 300 µmol/l.

## PREVENTIVE CARE

Care must be taken with venepuncture and the handling of blood and other body fluids in the laboratory. Faeces must be treated with antiseptic fluid and disposed of carefully. In general, a safe technique should be used for all patients as not all carriers will be necessarily tested for viruses causing hepatitis. Strict barrier nursing is not essential if these precautions are taken. Attendants must sterilize their own hands before handling food. Ideally patients should be treated out of hospital or in separate sidewards or cubicles if admission is necessary.

If contamination occurs, passive immunization with immunoglobulin (for hepatitis A) or hyperimmune immunoglobulin (for hepatitis B) should be undertaken as soon as possible. This is particularly important for contacts of hepatitis B cases if the patient has e antigen in the serum.

Active immunization against hepatitis B is now available, using a genetically engineered, yeast-derived vaccine. It is given to dental, medical and nursing personnel on a selective basis and is effective in preventing the spread of infection among high-risk homosexuals. It is also highly effective against vertical spread in endemic areas where its major drawback is cost. Revaccination may need to be performed after about 5 years, depending on initial antibody response. This vaccine naturally also protects against hepatitis D. A live, attenuated vaccine for hepatitis A is now available to replace the gamma globulin previously used for travellers to endemic areas. Vaccine for hepatitis C is not yet available.

# Chemicals, drugs and the liver

## AETIOLOGY

Many drugs and chemicals can damage the liver (ethyl alcohol will be considered in the next section). The precise mechanism of action is often uncertain. Some reactions are dose-related and predictable, suggesting a direct toxic effect on the liver (e.g. carbon tetrachloride, chloroform, paracetamol). Most drug reactions are idiosyncratic, unpredictable and can be produced by very low doses. A classification of the major drugs responsible for liver disease is shown in Table 15.11.

In the case of acute paracetamol (acetaminophen) poisoning the mechanism of action and protection has been established. Glutathione within the hepatocyte plays a protective role and is consumed by the products of paracetamol metabolism. These toxic products denature intracellular proteins and destroy the liver cells. This understanding has led to rational treatment (page 819).

## PATHOLOGY

Some drugs produce hepatocellular necrosis and the lesions resemble those of viral hepatitis (hepatitis-like reactions). Others produce predominant bile stasis with damage to the excretory membrane of the hepatocyte and accumulation of bile plugs in distended canaliculi (cholestatic reactions). There may be various combinations of both reactions. There are sometimes features of an acute allergic response with eosinophil leukocyte infiltration into the portal tracts in addition to other acute inflammatory features.

**Table 15.11** Drugs responsible for liver disease.

| Pattern of liver damage | Examples of drugs |
| --- | --- |
| Liver cell necrosis | Paracetamol |
| Acute hepatitis | Halothane |
| | Rifampicin |
| | Diclofenac |
| Chronic hepatitis | Oxyphenisatin |
| | Methyl dopa |
| | Isoniazid |
| Cholestasis | Oral contraceptives |
| | Phenothiazines |
| | Flucloxacillin |
| Portal tract fibrosis | Methotrexate |
| Hepatic vein thrombosis (Budd–Chiari syndrome) | Oral contraceptives |

Exceptionally chronic liver disease may ensue and a lesion resembling chronic active hepatitis has been described following the use of oxyphenisatin (a laxative now withdrawn), methyl dopa and other drugs. Some drugs can produce chronic portal tract fibrosis without any initial inflammatory reaction, for example, methotrexate. These chronic drug-related lesions will often improve slowly following withdrawal of the drugs.

## CLINICAL FEATURES

There is usually either an acute hepatitis-like illness or a cholestatic syndrome with any or all the clinical features which have already been described. Occasionally there is evidence of generalized allergy with skin rashes and bronchospasm.

Jaundice after an operation may result from infection, drugs including the anaesthetic agent halothane. The risk is greatest in patients who have several general anaesthetics using halothane within short intervals (<6 months). The clinical picture is of an acute hepatitis-like illness with fever, which can rarely progress to fulminant hepatic failure and death. A suitable, reasonably cheap alternative to halothane has not yet found wide acceptance.

**Paracetamol** (acetaminophen) poisoning has a well-defined clinical pattern with clinical and laboratory abnormalities evolving over 48 hours after ingestion. Elevation of the transaminases and prolongation of the prothrombin time precede the onset of encephalopathy and bleeding by several days. Timely intervention with agents such as methionine or N-acetylcysteine (page 819) during the first 24 hours is crucial if severe liver disease is to be prevented. There is recent evidence that late administration of N-acetylcysteine is beneficial. Prior enzyme induction by alcohol or anticonvulsants appears to worsen the prognosis.

## DIAGNOSIS

This is based almost entirely on the drug history and the exclusion of other causes of jaundice. There may be other features to suggest an allergic illness (e.g. rashes, bronchospasm). Liver biopsy may show features very suggestive of drug damage but is often not necessary if the drugs can be withdrawn and if the patient recovers quite rapidly. Rechallenge with the drug following recovery is sometimes justifiable, but potentially dangerous, and is the only way to establish the relationship with certainty.

## DIFFERENTIAL DIAGNOSIS

This is from all other causes of jaundice. It is especially important to exclude virus infection and extrahepatic obstruction if there are cholestatic features (page 378).

## COMPLICATIONS

Acute hepatitis-like lesions can progress to acute liver failure and death. Prolonged cholestasis may lead to steatorrhoea and deficiency of fat-soluble vitamins.

## TREATMENT

All potentially culpable drugs must be withdrawn. In some cases (e.g. rifampicin in the treatment of tuberculosis), it may be justifiable to ignore mild disturbances of liver function because they can resolve even if treatment is continued. In the cholestatic syndrome associated with the contraceptive pill, the condition will resolve if very low oestrogen or progestogen-only preparations are substituted.

Otherwise the patient is treated in the same supportive way as for viral hepatitis and full liver intensive care may be required. Prolonged cholestatic jaundice usually requires the parenteral use of fat-soluble vitamins and oral cholestyramine for itching.

## PROGNOSIS

This is usually excellent provided the drug is withdrawn completely. Full recovery of liver structure and function can be predicted in the vast majority of cases. Prognosis regarding the outcome of acute damage by paracetamol can be predicted with some accuracy by blood levels of the drug over the first 12 hours after its ingestion.

# *Ethyl alcohol and the liver*

## AETIOLOGY

Alcohol is the most familiar liver toxin and its first metabolite, acetaldehyde, is probably the compound which damages the liver cell directly. Acute alcohol poisoning produces a predictable and rapidly reversible acute liver injury, which is usually inapparent clinically if the liver was initially healthy. The continued ingestion of large amounts of alcohol over many years is associated with a number of different clinical syndromes. There is considerable variation in individual susceptibility and this is probably determined genetically.

The continued drinking of 80 g alcohol (8 units) or more daily in males and 40 g or more in females over many years is likely to damage the liver and many other organs. However, the risk of chronic liver disease increases in males with any consumption over 30 g (3 units) per day and in females the level is as low as 20 g (2 units) per day.

It is helpful to remember that a standard drink, or 'unit' (half pint of beer, single unit of spirits or a glass of wine or sherry), contains about 10 g alcohol. It cannot be assumed that a lower consumption is totally safe and some organs, especially the brain, may suffer subtle damage in the absence of any evidence of disease of the liver or other organs.

## PATHOLOGY

There are several types of liver injury depending on the amount of alcohol consumed and the chronicity of the habit. In **fatty liver** (steatosis) the hepatocytes are swollen by collections of intracellular fat which form large globules displacing the nucleus. This is usually a subacute process with little or no inflammation and is completely reversible if the patient stops drinking. **Acute alcoholic hepatitis** is a severe inflammatory and necrotic process affecting the lobules diffusely with relatively little fatty change. This is again fully reversible, but if the patient has repeated bouts of hepatitis, the liver architecture is damaged permanently and cirrhosis will result.

**Alcoholic cirrhosis** usually develops insidiously without overt episodes of acute hepatitis. There is variable inflammation, necrosis and fat accumulation and a frequent feature is Mallory's hyaline, an eosinophilic material which accumulates in damaged hepatocytes. All three features can be present in a single liver biopsy, but none is specific to alcoholic liver disease.

## CLINICAL FEATURES

Simple steatosis is often asymptomatic and may present with hepatomegaly or abnormal liver function tests as chance findings.

Acute alcoholic hepatitis is a severe illness with fever, nausea and vomiting, jaundice and tender hepatomegaly. The condition can progress to liver failure with bleeding and encephalopathy. The liver function tests show elevations of alkaline phosphatase and of transaminases, although rarely to levels as high as those seen in viral hepatitis. There are often other features of alcohol abuse such as poor nutrition and withdrawal symptoms, especially convulsions and delirium tremens. Parotid swelling is a characteristic feature. Histological hepatitis may be present without the clinical syndrome.

Chronic alcoholic cirrhosis presents insidiously with non-specific symptoms and the gradual development of the characteristic signs of chronic liver disease (Table 15.2). Feminization with gynaecomastia and impotence is common in the male. The course is eventually that of slow deterioration if drinking continues, with the later development of complications. These patients are prone to acute and chronic infections in the lungs, ascitic fluid and elsewhere. Malnutrition is common with loss of muscle bulk, weakness and the development of specific deficiencies, especially of folic acid and thiamine (vitamin $B_1$).

## DIAGNOSIS

This depends on the finding of clinical or laboratory evidence of acute or chronic liver disease in a known or suspected heavy drinker. The taking of an alcohol history requires experience and most patients underestimate and some deny consumption. Interviewing friends, relatives and partners is often revealing. Liver biopsy is required to determine the type and severity of the liver disease and to indicate the likely reversibility if the patient stops drinking.

The combination of macrocytosis and a raised gamma glutamyl transpeptidase suggests heavy alcohol consumption and the measurement of blood alcohol will confirm the suspicion if the sample is taken at an appropriate time. In a cooperative patient a period of abstinence will often clarify the nature of the biochemical abnormalities of liver function.

## DIFFERENTIAL DIAGNOSIS

A fatty liver can be produced by obesity, diabetes mellitus and severe malnutrition. Acute alcoholic hepatitis must be distinguished from viral and drug-induced hepatitis. There is typically a heavy neutrophil infiltrate into the lobules in alcoholic disease, but liver biopsy may not be feasible if the patient is ill with disturbed coagulation tests.

Alcoholic cirrhosis must be distinguished from the other identifiable forms of chronic liver disease, especially those related to hepatitis B and autoimmune phenomena. There may be confusion with haemochromatosis because alcoholics tend to accumulate iron in the liver (page 401). The coexistence of hepatitis B or C viruses tends to accelerate alcoholic liver damage.

## COMPLICATIONS

Acute alcoholic hepatitis or an acute exacerbation of chronic alcoholic liver disease can lead to acute liver failure and a fatal outcome. Superadded infections, including tuberculosis, are common and may be lethal if not treated vigorously.

The major complications of chronic liver disease will be discussed separately on page 403.

## TREATMENT

Alcohol withdrawal is the essence of treatment, irrespective of the stage of the disease or the severity of its complications. In the acutely ill patient, it is important to recognize and treat hypoglycaemia, thiamine deficiency and infections, especially of the chest and of any ascitic fluid. Full supportive therapy for acute liver failure may be required as discussed on page 392. The treatment of ascites, encephalopathy and variceal bleeding are described on page 403–8.

A severely agitated patient will require careful sedation with chlormethiazole or chlordiazepoxide which should then be tailed off over 6 to 7 days. The use of these drugs in an outpatient setting is hazardous due to possible overdose or to the risk of dual drug and alcohol dependence developing.

How much alcohol should a patient be 'allowed' to drink after recovery from an acute episode of hepatic dysfunction? The ideal answer is none at all, especially if there is evidence of chronic liver damage. Patients whose livers have recovered could presumably tolerate small amounts of alcohol with impunity (e.g. 20 g daily in men, <10 g daily in women). However, the major risk is that this level of consumption will not be maintained with the passage of time and the resumption of full social and business activities. Attention should be directed to changing lifestyle. If job or social activities are built entirely around alcohol the outlook is poor.

## PROGNOSIS

This depends entirely on the ability of the patient to abstain. Fatty liver and acute hepatitis carry very good prognosis if the patient survives the acute illness and abstains. The course of chronic disease can be modified by abstinence although cirrhosis itself is by definition irreversible. However, the progress of the disease can be halted and it is always worth trying very hard to achieve abstinence. In patients presenting with major complications, the prognosis is poor and the chance of survival to 5 years is 10 per cent or less if drinking continues, but 50 per cent if they abstain. In those who genuinely abstain, but continue to deteriorate, liver transplantation is sometimes performed.

# *Cholestasis of pregnancy*

## AETIOLOGY

This is a hypersensitivity phenomenon which occurs in the last 3 months of pregnancy and ceases after delivery. It is related to a rise in circulating oestrogens and can be reproduced in sensitive women by oestrogen-containing contraceptives. The prevalence of the sensitivity shows marked geographic variation and it is notably common in Scandinavia and Chile.

## CLINICAL FEATURES

There is itching and mild jaundice with elevation of the serum alkaline phosphatase. There are no histopathological features of note. The condition is usually quite mild, although the itching can be intense. The condition will probably recur in future pregnancies. There is an increased risk of fetal death and also a twice normal incidence of gall stones.

## TREATMENT

Severe itching should be treated with cholestyramine otherwise it is necessary to await spontaneous delivery. Rarely this may be an indication for an early induction of labour.

The prognosis is good and chronic liver disease does not ensue. Future contraception should be achieved using low oestrogen or progestogen only pills or other methods.

# *Fatty liver of pregnancy*

## AETIOLOGY

This poorly understood and rare entity develops late during the last 3 months of pregnancy, usually in primiparous women. The histopathological features are distinctive – a microvesicular distribution of globules of fatty acid within the hepatocyte, a feature shared with Reye's syndrome and sodium valproate hepatotoxicity.

## CLINICAL FEATURES

The onset is insidious with malaise, anorexia, vomiting followed by progressive deterioration of liver function. Jaundice is often delayed and mild. Coagulopathy and encephalopathy may ensue rapidly after a week or more of prolonged severe vomiting. There is a high mortality rate from acute liver failure. Death may be averted by prompt recognition of the syndrome and induction of labour or operative delivery.

## TREATMENT

Full supportive therapy, as described on page 392, and prompt delivery of the fetus is required. The prognosis is bad, but if the patient survives the acute illness the long-term prognosis is excellent. In the few cases where second pregnancies have occurred, there has been no recurrence.

# Budd–Chiari syndrome

## AETIOLOGY

This is produced by occlusion of the hepatic veins by thrombosis, by tumour or occasionally by webs in the upper inferior vena cava. Venous thrombosis may be caused by the contraceptive pill and by hypercoagulable states such as polycythaemia vera (page 618), the lupus anticoagulant syndrome (page 647) or paroxysmal nocturnal haemoglobinuria (page 613). Tumours may compress from without or obstruct from within by intraluminal spread. A rare cause is drinking herbal infusions (e.g. bush tea which is consumed by AfroCaribbeans).

## PATHOLOGY

The liver enlarges and there is haemorrhagic necrosis of the central parts of the liver lobules. Venous collaterals develop, but in spite of this portal pressure rises and, in survivors, cirrhosis may ensue as complete resolution of the lesion is unlikely.

## CLINICAL FEATURES

In classical cases, there is hepatic enlargement with pain and rapidly developing ascites over a period of days or weeks. The time course is, however, variable and in some patients only part of the hepatic venous system is occluded giving a more chronic and less dramatic clinical picture.

The liver is enlarged or tender with variable ascites and later splenomegaly will be apparent. The ascitic fluid has no distinctive features and a variable protein content.

An isotopic (technetium-99 m sulphur colloid) liver scan shows a relatively normal or large caudate lobe with grossly impaired uptake elsewhere. Ultrasound will reveal characteristic venous collaterals and occluded hepatic veins. The liver histology is very distinctive and clear proof can be provided by hepatic venography.

## TREATMENT

The underlying disease should be corrected where possible. Anticoagulants or thrombolytic therapy have not met with much success. Surgery or angioplasty may be helpful in patients with caval webs. Most patients are treated with the various supportive measures outlined elsewhere for complicated liver disease.

## PROGNOSIS

This is usually poor with about 50 per cent of the patients dying within a year from liver failure or bleeding varices. However, long-term survival is possible and depends, in part, on the nature of the underlying cause, if any. Liver transplantation may be appropriate if liver failure ensues.

# Chronic active hepatitis

## AETIOLOGY

This is most commonly produced by viruses (especially hepatitis B and C) and by autoimmune phenomena which often affect other organs or systems. A similar clinical syndrome can be produced by Wilson's disease (page 402). Some drugs have been implicated, including the now withdrawn laxative oxyphenisatin and methyl dopa.

## PATHOLOGY

There is diffuse lobular inflammation and necrosis of hepatocytes. A distinctive feature is the breakdown of the boundary zone between the lobules and the portal tracts (limiting plate) as inflammatory cells infiltrate the lobules and surround small islands of hepatocytes. The activity of the necrosis and inflammation can be greatly modified by treatment, but if it is unchecked, permanent damage to the liver architecture will result with the usual risks of nodular regeneration and bands of fibrosis, i.e. cirrhosis (page 396).

## CLINICAL FEATURES

During an active episode there is malaise, muscle aching, jaundice, hepatomegaly and biochemical evidence of acute hepatocellular necrosis, i.e. marked elevation of the transaminases. Acute liver failure may, rarely, ensue with coagulopathy and encephalopathy. In most cases the symptoms are milder and persist for months or years with variable jaundice and disturbances of biochemical tests.

The autoimmune type of disease affects mainly middle-aged women and there is often evidence of inflammatory disease of other organs, for example, the thyroid and joints.

## DIAGNOSIS

This is based on clinical and biochemical evidence of chronic remitting and relapsing liver disease in a person who has evidence of past viral infection or autoimmune phenomena. Past viral B infection is indicated by the carriage of hepatitis B surface antigen (Hb$_s$Ag) or by antibodies to the surface or core antigens. Hepatitis C viral antibodies or RNA can also be shown.

The commonest autoimmune markers are a positive anti-nuclear or smooth muscle antibodies. Two types of auto antibody profile are found in chronic active hepatitis (Table 15.12). Liver biopsy is required to establish a firm diagnosis and to indicate the severity of the disease and its potential reversibility. There is a rather poor correlation between symptoms, the elevation of transaminases and the histological abnormality.

## DIFFERENTIAL DIAGNOSIS

In a young person (<30 years), Wilson's disease must be excluded (page 402). Chronic persistent hepatitis is the name given to a similar but very much milder illness. It is often asymptomatic, the biochemical disturbances are mild and histologically the inflammation is confined to the portal tract. This may progress to more florid active hepatitis and it is probably part of the same illness, although formerly regarded as always having an excellent prognosis.

## COMPLICATIONS

The main risks are the development of an acute episode of severe liver failure and, after a very variable and often prolonged period of time (5–10 years), the complications of end-stage disease (page 403).

## TREATMENT

For hepatitis B-associated chronic hepatitis the antiviral agent interferon is now the treatment of choice although response is variable. The best

**Table 15.12** Autoantibodies in immune liver disease.

| | Anti-nuclear antibody | Smooth muscle antibody | Liver–kidney microsomal antibody | Anti-mitochondrial antibody |
|---|---|---|---|---|
| Autoimmune chronic active hepatitis | | | | |
| Type I | ++ | ++ | – | ± |
| Type II | + | – | ++ | – |
| Primary biliary cirrhosis | ± | ± | – | +++ |

predictor of response is a low hepatitis B viral DNA level in the blood. Hepatitis C-associated disease can also be treated with interferon and trials with other antiviral agents are in progress for both viruses. Corticosteroids are best avoided as they may allow increased viral replication.

With hepatitis B the aim is to convert from the active viral replicative phase, characterized by $HB_eAg$ positivity to $HB_eAb$ with a concomitant reduction in activity of liver disease and infectivity. Patients with high viral DNA and low transaminase levels in the blood are unlikely to respond. With hepatitis C the aim is to reduce the level of alanine aminotransferase in the blood, which goes along with an improvement in liver histology and well-being. Chronic viral hepatitis can run a relatively silent clinical course until complications develop.

Autoimmune chronic active hepatitis produces more clinical and biochemical disturbances, which usually respond very well and quickly to corticosteroids. There can be remarkable histological resolutions, but steroid withdrawal is often followed by relapses which may be more difficult to treat. It is exceptional for permanent resolution to follow short courses of steroids and long-term treatment is usually advised. In view of the risks incurred by this, the immunosuppressive drug azathioprine is often added for its 'steroid sparing' effect in order to keep the dose of prednisolone below 10 mg daily. The course of the disease is monitored by biochemical tests and ideally by liver biopsy.

## PROGNOSIS

This used to be considered grave with progression to death over a 5 to 7 year period. However, this applied to untreated florid autoimmune disease and the use of anti-inflammatory drugs has improved the outlook considerably. Milder cases are now being treated and long survival can be predicted.

The prognosis of prolonged liver disease after hepatitis B and C is less certain and may improve with the use of antiviral drugs in the future. Chronic hepatitis B and C are the main causes of cirrhosis worldwide which means that they are the primary causes of hepatocellular carcinoma, one of the commonest causes of fatal cancer in the world.

# *Primary biliary cirrhosis*

## AETIOLOGY

This relatively rare disease has an autoimmune basis but the initiating trigger factor is not known. Environmental factors including drugs have been implicated and the disease's great predilection for women suggests a role for female sex hormones.

## PATHOLOGY

The histopathological features in typical cases include chronic inflammation around the small bile ducts in the portal tracts, small granulomas and a marked accumulation of copper within the hepatocytes. The duct epithelium is ultimately destroyed, but lobular architecture is preserved for long periods with relatively little damage to the hepatocytes. In the later stages of the disease, the hepatocytes are damaged and the lobular architecture is eventually destroyed leading to cirrhosis (the name of the disease is misleading because cirrhosis is a late feature).

## CLINICAL FEATURES

The most distinctive features are chronic itching and jaundice in middle-aged women. The disease is often diagnosed in asymptomatic patients in whom the laboratory abnormalities are discovered by chance.

In severe long-standing disease, there are deep jaundice, marked pigmentation and all the stigmata of chronic liver disease. Splenomegaly is particularly common. Hypercholesterolaemia is frequent and may be shown clinically by xanthelasmata or xanthomata. Well-recognized clinical associations include the sicca syndrome of dry eyes and dry mouth, caused by immunological damage to the lacrimal and salivary glands, and renal tubular abnormalities (page 467).

Steatorrhoea is common but seldom severe, but fat-soluble vitamin deficiency may arise and lead to bleeding, osteomalacia and, rarely, night blindness. Bone pains and vertebral collapse are caused by vitamin D deficiency and accelerated osteoporosis, the reason for the latter being uncertain.

## DIAGNOSIS

This is suggested by the finding of greatly raised alkaline phosphatase, hypercholesterolaemia, raised IgM and a positive anti-mitochondrial antibody in the serum (Table 15.12). The latter is positive in 95 per cent of cases. Liver biopsy is needed to confirm the diagnosis.

## DIFFERENTIAL DIAGNOSIS

If the history is short and jaundice prominent, other causes of obstructive jaundice must be excluded (page 377). After more prolonged illness the differential diagnosis is narrower and includes sclerosing cholangitis (pager 379) and cholangiocarcinoma (page 383). In atypical cases, especially if the anti-mitochondrial antibody is negative, ERCP should be undertaken to exclude biliary tract pathology.

## COMPLICATIONS

These include fat-soluble vitamin deficiencies, portal hypertension and ultimately liver failure. Malignant transformation occurs rarely.

## TREATMENT

There is no known effective therapy. Corticosteroids are ineffective and contraindicated in view of the frequency of osteoporosis. Azathioprine has a small beneficial effect. Although pencillamine will reduce the amount of copper in the liver it is ineffective as treatment. Cyclosporin is currently under trial. Methotrexate, colchicine and the bile acid ursodeoxycholic acid have all shown promise in clinical trials and work continues with all three agents.

Treatment is therefore supportive and includes the use of cholestyramine for itching, a low fat diet for steatorrhoea and fat-soluble vitamin replacement. The vitamins are most conveniently given in large intramuscular doses every 2 months, but 1-$\alpha$-hydroxyvitamin $D_3$ is effective orally. Oestrogen therapy can be used to prevent osteoporosis and rarely causes cholestasis, especially if it is administered by a patch to avoid 'first pass' metabolism.

# Primary sclerosing cholangitis

In addition to presenting like gallstones (page 379) primary sclerosing cholangitis may have clinical and laboratory features in common with primary biliary cirrhosis.

# Haemochromatosis

## AETIOLOGY

This term applies to a rare familial disorder in which the intestine absorbs iron excessively because the normal regulatory mechanism is ineffective. It is inherited as an autosomal recessive trait and there is an association with histocompatibility antigens HLA-A3 and -B14.

## PATHOLOGY

There is a slow accumulation of iron in the liver, pancreas, heart, testes and joints. Pigmentation of the skin is caused by the accumulation of melanin rather than of the iron itself.

In the liver, iron accumulates in hepatocytes and in reticuloendothelial cells within the portal tracts. Eventually the hepatocytes are damaged and undergo necrosis, with little active inflammation. Finally lobular architecture is destroyed with resultant cirrhosis, but this can take many years even after clinical features have become apparent. Similar damage with fibrosis of the pancreas is evident in most cases.

## CLINICAL FEATURES

The disease presents in males in middle age (30–50 years) and in females considerably later because of the menstrual losses of iron during the reproductive years. There are usually mild non-specific symptoms with slow liver enlargement. The skin becomes progressively pigmented and insulin-dependent diabetes develops eventually ('**bronze diabetes**'). Joint symptoms may be troublesome and the knees are commonly affected. Loss of libido and feminization occur frequently. In severe untreated disease, there may be clinically overt heart disease with arrythmias and congestive cardiac failure. The liver function tests are variably abnormal without any distinctive features.

## DIAGNOSIS

Serum iron is raised with a normal iron binding capacity so that iron saturation is high and the serum ferritin level is very high. A liver biopsy stained for iron is required to make a firm diagnosis, to assess the extent of iron accumulation and liver cell damage and to assess reversibility and prognosis. Determination of liver iron stores chemically gives the most precise diagnosis.

## DIFFERENTIAL DIAGNOSIS

The main differential diagnosis is from other causes of iron overload. Excess hepatic iron is commonly seen in alcoholic liver disease owing to increased iron intake (e.g. from certain wines) and inappropriately high absorption rates. However, the total accumulation of iron in the body is far less than that seen in haemochromatosis.

Iron accumulates to excess in chronic haemolytic anaemia, after years of inappropriate iron therapy and in patients who require repeated blood transfusions.

## COMPLICATIONS

To the usual complications of chronic liver disease are added diabetes mellitus and cardiac failure. Joint disease and testicular failure are common. There seems to be a particularly high risk of hepatocellular carcinoma.

## TREATMENT

The only effective treatment is to remove iron by venesection and to keep body iron stores near normal by repeated venesection over the years. Iron chelating agents are much less effective in quantitative terms and require systemic administration. Subcutaneous infusions of desferrioxamine are given to patients with chronic haematological disorders requiring frequent transfusions to prevent iron accumulation.

One unit of blood (500 ml) contains approximately 250 mg of elemental iron. Haemochromatosis may cause a total accumulation of 20–40 g of iron compared with the normal stores of about 4 g. Therefore venesections at the rate of one unit every 2 weeks will be required for 1–2 years to rid the body of its excess iron. Treatment is monitored by measurement of haemoglobin (to avoid anaemia) and serum ferritin. Life-long observation is required.

## PROGNOSIS

This is good with a chance of long survival if the condition is detected early enough and treated adequately. The risk of hepatocellular carcinoma may not, however, be averted by venesection.

## FAMILY CONSIDERATIONS

It is important to persuade other family members, especially males, to have tests of liver function, serum iron and ferritin and HLA status. If indicated by these tests, a liver biopsy should be performed and venesection started in the hope of preventing disease later.

# Wilson's disease (hepatolenticular degeneration)

## AETIOLOGY

In this rare disease, copper accumulates to excess in the liver and in certain parts of the brain and other organs. The primary abnormality is unknown but there is usually a low level of the plasma protein caeruloplasmin, which is responsible for the transport of copper in the blood. There is also impaired excretion of copper in bile. The condition is inherited as an autosomal recessive trait.

## CLINICAL FEATURES

The main features are hepatic and cerebral. The hepatic manifestations are variable and include progression to cirrhosis with all the usual long-term complications, a more symptomatic disease resembling chronic active hepatitis clinically and histologically and an acute fulminating illness presenting as acute hepatic failure. The onset of overt liver disease is usually before the age of 15 years.

The neurological features include extrapyramidal tract signs and slowly developing dementia. These tend to occur in late adolescence. The main diagnostic features are the distinctive deposition of copper around the periphery of the cornea (**Kayser–Fleischer rings**), which are best seen by slit-lamp examination, depressed level of serum caeruloplasmin, variable serum copper and increased urinary copper excretion, especially after a dose of penicillamine. Orcein staining of liver biopsy material shows considerable accumulation of copper binding protein in the hepatocytes. Chemical determination of liver copper content or radiocopper scanning are sometimes helpful.

## MANAGEMENT

Penicillamine is the drug of choice. It chelates copper and increases its urinary excretion. Treatment is life long but may be complicated by side effects, which are usually dose related and reversible. These include rashes and heavy proteinuria. Trientine is an alternative to penicillamine. If neither drug is suitable, zinc, dimercaprol and a low copper diet may have a limited beneficial effect.

Young relatives should be examined clinically and biochemically for evidence of liver and neurological disease at a presymptomatic stage so that early treatment can be started. Successful pregnancy has been reported in women taking penicillamine continuously.

The prognosis has improved considerably since the introduction of penicillamine and survival for many years is now possible.

# Complications of chronic liver disease

## ASCITES

### Aetiology

The combination of hypoalbuminaemia and portal hypertension allows the retention of sodium and water in the extravascular space and especially in the peritoneal cavity where the portal capillary pressure is raised. This, coupled with vasodilatation of the splanchnic vasculature leads to an apparent reduction in circulating volume. The latter encourages a number of reflexes to increase salt and water retention including renin release by the kidney which stimulates aldosterone production, an increase in antidiuretic hormone and ACTH levels, and a reduction in atrial natriuretic peptide. The resulting intense renal conservation of sodium does not, however, restore the apparent circulating plasma volume and oliguric renal failure may ensue.

### Clinical features

Ascites is often very gross indeed, 10–20 litres may accumulate with relatively little dependent oedema in the legs or over the sacrum. In severe cases, especially if there has been vigorous diuretic therapy, the patient may be hypovolaemic with a low blood pressure, and depressed venous pressure in the neck and oliguria. Despite this, the cardiac output and plasma volume are characteristically increased. The umbilicus may be everted and there are often venous collaterals over the distended abdomen indicating portal hypertension.

### Differential diagnosis

The many other causes of ascites (Table 15.13) are usually excluded on clinical grounds and by suitable examination of the ascitic fluid obtained at an initial small volume paracentesis (50 ml). In hepatic cases the ultimate diagnosis usually requires liver biopsy, which is generally not advisable until the ascites has cleared. However, laparoscopically or ultrasonically guided biopsies may be obtained with greater safety

**Table 15.13** Causes of ascites.

Primary liver disease, including Budd–Chiari syndrome
Abdominal malignancy
Infection especially tuberculosis
Pancreatic ascites
Chylous ascites due to lymphatic block

(page 378). In uncorrectable cases with prolonged coagulation transjugular liver biopsy may be used; any haemorrhage then occurs into the patient's venous system.

Malignancy and peritoneal infection can complicate long-standing liver disease, so initial cytological and bacteriological examination of ascitic fluid is required even when a firm diagnosis of chronic liver disease is already well established. Pancreatic ascites occasionally develops in heavy drinkers and is indicated by a high amylase concentration in the fluid.

Ascites is rare in acute or subacute liver disease. Its rapid development suggests the possibility of hepatic venous thrombosis (Budd–Chiari Syndrome, see page 398). In chronic liver disease, the sudden onset of ascites might suggest portal vein occlusion especially if infection and malignancy are excluded.

Ascites is frequently infected (so-called spontaneous bacterial peritonitis), usually by Gram-negative organisms or by *Streptococcus pneumoniae*. An ascitic fluid neutrophil count of more than 300 per mm³ should be regarded as diagnostic and intravenous antibiotics must be commenced. The normal symptoms and signs of peritonitis are usually absent.

### Treatment

The mainstays of treatment are the restriction of sodium and water intake and the careful use of diuretics. Forty-eight hours of bed-rest and observation will establish a baseline weight, allow time to exclude problems requiring specific treatment, especially infection, and permit measurement of urinary flow and sodium losses. Salt should not be added to the ward diet, salty foods must be avoided (40–50 mmol Na⁺ daily) and fluid intake should be restricted to 1000 ml daily if the serum sodium concentration is <130 mmol/l (this usually indicates impaired

excretion of 'free water'). The need for greater restriction of salt (22 mmol daily) and water (1 litre daily) intake will be determined by the measured urinary losses and by a falling level of serum sodium.

Spironolactone is the diuretic of choice and should be introduced on the second day at a dose of 50 mg daily, doubling every 2 days to 200 mg daily and by 100 mg increments thereafter according to response as measured by careful daily weighing and urinary outputs (including sodium concentration). A dose above 400 mg/day is rarely helpful. The ideal rate of weight loss is 0.5 kg/day in the absence of and 1 kg/day in the presence of peripheral oedema, and a greater rate should be avoided for fear of producing hypovolaemia and impaired renal function. Urinary sodium concentrations <30 mmol/l indicate intense salt conservation and the need to increase the dose of spironolactone. If the urinary concentration is higher, additional salt and water losses will only be achieved by a more proximally acting diuretic such as frusemide or a thiazide.

Serum potassium concentrations must be closely monitored and values between 4 and 5 mmol/l should be maintained by oral supplementation. Tissue K⁺ depletion is common in these patients and will be aggravated by the use of proximally acting diuretics (especially if spironolactone is not being used simultaneously).

Most patients will respond to this treatment, but additional measures may be required. If the ascites is very tense, a slow paracentesis of 4–5 litres will relieve distress without harm. Repeated paracentesis should be avoided unless some of the protein lost is replaced by infusions of salt poor albumin, for example, 40 g daily intravenously. Albumin infusion is also appropriate if the patient becomes hypotensive and oliguric because this will re-expand the circulating volume and should improve renal function. The infused albumin has a relatively short half-life (7–8 days) so the benefits will be short-lived and, moreover, it is very expensive. In recent years the use of large volume paracenteses with appropriate colloid replacement has regained fashion. The risks are no greater than with diuretic therapy if the diuretics are stopped at least 48 hours earlier, the flow rate is slow and carefully monitored, and sufficient attention is paid to cardiovascular status and colloid replacement. In addition there is a great reduction of hospital stay. A central venous pressure monitor is a useful safety measure.

In very resistant cases, it is possible to insert shunts between the peritoneal cavity and the great veins of the neck, for example, the LeVeen shunt. This can be dramatically effective in promoting diuresis but carries many hazards including cardiac failure and intravascular coagulation. Truly resistant ascites is fortunately rare if the patient complies with the regime and if complicating factors have been excluded. A high albumin concentration in the ascitic fluid (>30 g/l) would indicate the need to search again for malignancy, infection, pancreatitis and myxoedema.

## Prognosis

This is usually good if the patient complies with treatment and if the progression of the underlying liver disease can be halted, for example, by abstaining from alcohol or by the use of corticosteroids in patients with chronic active hepatitis. Poor response to the above measures and the development of other complications will, however, indicate a poor overall prognosis with little chance of surviving for more than a few months. Overall, once ascites appears, mortality is approximately 50 per cent in 2 years.

## HEPATIC ENCEPHALOPATHY (PORTAL–SYSTEMIC ENCEPHALOPATHY)

### Aetiology

This reversible cerebral syndrome is caused by the accumulation in the blood of a number of nitrogenous compounds which are produced by bacterial action on proteins in the large bowel, and would normally be detoxified and excreted by the healthy liver. It is especially likely to occur if there is major shunting of portal venous blood directly into the systemic circulation. Surgical shunts are created much less commonly than in the past, but numerous small shunts can develop spontaneously during the development of cirrhosis.

No single chemical has been linked unequivocally with hepatic encephalopathy. Ammonia has been the most widely studied putative neurotoxin and plasma levels of ammonia are high in these patients. However, there is a poor correlation between the level of ammonia and the severity of the encephalopathy. Other candidates include more complex amines with false neurotransmitter properties (e.g. octopamine) which can interfere with the action of true neurotransmitters such as noradrenaline and dopamine.

### Clinical features

Minor changes include somnolence, sleep reversal, i.e. awake at night, sleepy in the daytime, impaired memory for recent events and a characteristic difficulty with spatial orientation as shown by an impaired ability to draw shapes such as five-pointed stars, clock faces etc. (constructional apraxia).

In more severe cases somnolence can progress to stupor or even coma. The physical signs include a distinctive oral fetor, flapping tremor of the outstretched hands (asterixis) and symmetrical hyperreflexia with variable plantar responses.

There may be clinical or laboratory evidence of a precipitating cause, such as constipation, inappropriate use of sedatives, a recent gastrointestinal haemorrhage, hypokalaemia or an infection in the lungs, urinary tract or ascitic fluid.

### Differential diagnosis

There is nothing absolutely pathognomonic and similar encephalopathic features can be observed in other metabolic disorders, for example, renal and respiratory failure. Signs of chronic liver disease and high blood ammonia concentration would strongly suggest the diagnosis. Severity can fluctuate markedly depending on the nature of the precipitating cause, if any, and on the treatment given.

There are characteristic EEG abnormalities, especially increased slow frequency activity, but this cannot be regarded as diagnostic.

In the neglected alcoholic patient, there are many possible sources of confusion including withdrawal symptoms, hypoglycaemia, cerebral abscess, subdural haematoma and vitamin $B_1$ deficiency.

## Treatment

The first essential is to try to identify a precipitating cause which can be corrected. Sedatives and opiates must be withdrawn and severe constipation corrected with a phosphate enema and oral lactulose. Gastrointestinal bleeding must be identified and residual blood in the gut expelled by purgation to reduce the protein load. Hypokalaemia and other metabolic disturbances should be sought and corrected. Infections must be treated with the appropriate antibiotics.

Otherwise, the mainstays of treatment are a low protein (40–60 mg), high energy diet accompanied by gentle daily purgation with lactulose (40–60 ml daily as required). Two soft stools daily is a reasonable goal. It may be necessary to feed the patient through a nasogastric tube or even intravenously initially and an intake of approximately 2000 non-protein calories should be encouraged.

Antibiotics, especially neomycin, have been much used in an attempt to suppress bacterial production of toxic nitrogenous compounds in the gut. Neomycin, 2–4 g, daily can be very effective but, if used for long periods, it can damage the kidneys and the inner ear. Vancomycin has been claimed to be safer but this remains unproven and it is much more costly.

## Prognosis

As with ascites, this depends on the nature of the underlying liver disease, on the patient's compliance with dietary and drug regimes, and on whether a correctable precipitating cause can be identified. Many patients survived for long periods (years) after portocaval shunt operations but had chronic encephalopathy which greatly reduced the quality of their lives. This is the main reason for the recent disenchantment with this type of surgery (page 408).

## PORTAL HYPERTENSION

A high pressure in the portal venous system can open up previously unused vessels, producing unusual features such as the caput Medusae. Portal hypertension leads to enlargement of the spleen and formation of oesophageal varices.

## BLEEDING FROM OESOPHAGEAL VARICES

### Aetiology

The pathological processes of hepatic fibrosis and cirrhosis produce profound effects on the hepatic circulation leading to portal hypertension and collateral vessels between the portal and systemic venous systems. Collaterals develop most notably along the submucosa of the oesophagus (varices) and deep to the anorectal mucosal junction as haemorrhoids.

Other causes of varices include hepatic venous obstruction (Budd–Chiari syndrome) and portal vein obstruction. The Budd–Chiari syndrome is a relatively acute illness (page 398) with predominant ascites, and varices only develop later if survival is prolonged. Portal vein thrombosis may complicate cirrhosis or can occur as an isolated entity especially in the neonatal period as a result of sepsis spreading along the umbilical vein.

Fibrosis of the portal tracts without cirrhosis is characteristic of hepatic schistosomiasis and is the commonest cause of varices in parts of the world where this disease is prevalent, such as in Egypt, parts of South America and the Far East.

### Clinical features

The bleeding is usually sudden and severe, without any obvious precipitating cause. Gastro-oesophageal reflux and oesophagitis are often invoked as aggravating factors and, if present, should be treated appropriately. A minor upper respiratory tract infection is a common preceding event. There is almost always marked enlargement of the spleen and usually other features of chronic liver disease depending on the cause of the portal hypertension.

### Differential diagnosis

This is from other causes of severe upper gastrointestinal bleeding and depends on gastroscopy, which should be undertaken as soon as possible after initial resuscitation. Varices often coexist with ulcers and diffuse gastric erosions, and gastroscopy is necessary even when varices are known to be present in order to exclude other sources of blood loss.

## Treatment

The first priority is to restore and maintain the circulating blood volume, with CVP monitoring. Oral lactulose and phosphate enemas should be given if bleeding produces encephalopathy.

At the time of the initial gastroscopy, if a suitably skilled endoscopist is available, or within 6 hours at any rate, the varices should be injected with sclerosant (2–3 ml ethanolamine oleate into each varix under direct vision). This usually prevents further bleeding and the procedure is repeated every 1 to 2 weeks until the varices are thrombosed. Endoscopy is repeated at intervals of 3 to 6 months – and recurrences are re-injected in the hope of preventing further bleeding. An alternative procedure which is gaining acceptance is the 'banding' technique, when small elastic bands are placed over the varices in a similar manner to treating haemorrhoids. Sclerotherapy or banding may be impractical during active bleeding when pharmacological treatment or balloon tamponade may be used.

Vasopressin can be given either as a bolus (20 units in 200 ml 5 per cent glucose infused over 20 minutes) or as a continuous infusion (0.4 units/min) into a peripheral vein over about 2 hours. This constricts the splanchnic arterioles and reduces portal pressure but produces significant side effects, including gut colic and hypertension. It can be dangerous in patients with ischaemic heart disease and slow continuous infusion is probably the safer method of administration.

Safety, and probably efficiency are improved by coinfusion of nitroglycerin. An alternative drug is the long-acting analogue of somatostatin, octreotide, given by subcutaneous bolus or intravenous infusion. The use of vasopressin or octreotide allows time to perform sclerotherapy or to prepare the Sengstaken–Blakemore tube, which should be passed with minimal sedation into the stomach through the mouth (Fig. 15.9). Meticulous attention to detail is required and there are many hazards in its use. Successful balloon tamponade will usually control bleeding and after about 24 hours the balloons should be deflated and the tube withdrawn later. If the Sengstaken tube and sclerotherapy are ineffective, a surgical approach is usually required. The current favoured procedure is to ligate the submucosal veins at the gastrooesophageal junction with an automatic stapling device inserted from below through a gastrotomy incision. This should control bleeding for a few months but varices tend to recur and will require sclerotherapy at subsequent gastroscopy.

Portocaval shunts were widely performed until recently, but fell into disrepute because of the high risk of disabling chronic encephalopathy.

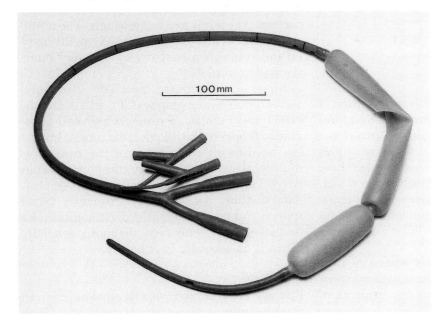

**Figure 15.9** A Sengstaken–Blakemore tube, the distal balloon is inflated with contrast material in the stomach and the proximal tube with air in the oesophagus. The proximal port is continuously aspirated to prevent inhalation of saliva. The distal port is used for gastric aspiration and for the administration of drugs.

The recent development of the transjugular intrahepatic portosystemic stent shunt (TIPSS) looks set to tip the balance back towards reducing portal pressure by shunting. Initial results are very promising, but long-term studies are awaited.

## Prognosis

The outlook is good if bleeding can be controlled and if the underlying functional reserve of the liver is adequate. All too often, bleeding precipitates encephalopathy through the protein load in the GI tract and an acute deterioration of liver function as shown by impaired coagulation, jaundice and ascites. In such patients, even if the bleeding can be controlled, the prognosis is very poor. If bleeding is due to non-cirrhotic portal hypertension, prognosis is excellent.

## Prophylaxis

The place of sclerotherapy or banding in the prevention of bleeding remains controversial but they may be effective when large varices are present in patients with otherwise well compensated liver disease. β-Blockade by propranolol is an alternative approach which has proven beneficial in appropriately selected groups.

# Malignant disease of the liver

## PRIMARY HEPATOCELLULAR CARCINOMA

### Aetiology

This tumour is common globally, and in parts of the developing world it is the commonest form of cancer (Table 15.14). It almost always develops in an abnormal liver, usually with pre-existing cirrhosis, although this may not have been apparent clinically. In much of the world, there is a close relationship between the prevalence of hepatitis B and C in the community and the incidence of hepatocellular carcinoma (HCC).

Other chronic liver diseases especially alcoholic cirrhosis and haemochromatosis predispose to primary carcinoma without any evidence of previous viral infection. The disease is seven to

**Table 15.14** Incidence rates of primary liver cancer.

| Area | Rate per 100 000 males/year |
|---|---|
| Mozambique | 98 |
| China | 17 |
| South Africa | 14 |
| UK | |
| USA | 2–3 |
| Central America | |

ten times more common in males. The role of male hormones is an area of intense study.

### Clinical features

Enlargement of the liver, accompanied by continuous pain caused by stretch of the liver capsule, suggests the presence of a liver tumour if the patient is known to have chronic liver disease or to be from an area of high incidence.

There is commonly a low-grade fever and tenderness, and a vascular bruit may be heard over a palpable mass. There are a number of associated endocrinological syndromes, especially, hypercalcaemia, hypoglycaemia and polycythaemia. The most helpful laboratory test is the serum α-fetoprotein (AFP), but this is not specific for HCC and is not invariably associated with it. However, using sensitive radioimmunoassay, 70–90 per cent of patients with HCC will have detectable AFP and in most patients, the levels will be very high. The serum des-γ-carboxyprothrombin assay is equally helpful and has only a partial overlap with AFP but is not widely available.

Imaging techniques, especially ultrasound and computed tomography (CT), will define the extent and number of tumours and will allow guided biopsy for histological diagnosis. Images can be difficult to interpret if the tumour is multifocal and arises in a very non-homogeneous liver. Hepatic angiography is often helpful. Ascitic fluid, if present, is frequently blood stained and must be examined cytologically for neoplastic cells. However, diagnosis generally depends on adequate liver biopsy.

### Treatment

Primary HCC is often slowly growing and can remain confined to one lobe of the liver for long periods (months) so that surgical excision must be considered if the patient is relatively young and otherwise fit. It is unlikely that the rest of the liver will be absolutely normal histologically and, provided that there is good overall liver function, cirrhosis is not an absolute contraindication to surgery. Careful preoperative assessment will include CT scanning and hepatic arteriography to determine the limits of the tumour. In well selected cases, 20–50 per cent 5-year survivals can be expected in those who survive the immediate postoperative period. This outlook can be improved if sufferers are detected at an early and even asymptomatic stage. Screening programmes based on AFP or ultrasound scanning have been introduced in parts of the world where HCC is common and the medical services are available (e.g. Hong Kong). However, the markers of HCC are usually present only when the disease is at an advanced, irresectable stage.

Medical treatment for HCC is not well established but tumours sometimes respond to chemotherapy, which usually consists of doxorubicin. Clinical trials continue and firm guidelines cannot yet be given. The value of direct portal infusions of cytotoxic agents with or without gel foam remains unproven.

## *Prognosis*

This is very poor if the tumour is not resectable and survival beyond a few months cannot be expected. Resection does however offer a real hope of cure in a small number of cases, and liver transplantation may eventually become more widely available for patients in whom resection is not possible. However, recurrence after transplantation is very common.

## METASTATIC TUMOURS

In general, metastatic tumours are treated by chemotherapy or hormonal therapy if appropriate and prolonged survival can be achieved, for example, in breast cancer and in lymphoma. For many patients with the common carcinomas arising from the gut, pancreas or lungs, no treatment other than simple palliation is available. Surgical excision of a solitary metastasis or metastases confined to one lobe of the liver is undertaken occasionally, for example, for colonic adenocarcinoma or renal carcinoma.

## CARCINOID TUMOURS AND THE CARCINOID SYNDROME

### *Aetiology*

These tumours arise from enterochromaffin cells situated in the gut, bronchial mucosa and elsewhere. The commonest site is the appendix, where they are found incidentally during appendicectomy and usually have no sinister long-term significance unless they are large.

### *Clinical features*

Localized tumours in the ileum (the second commonest site) can obstruct the lumen or bleed if the mucosa is ulcerated. Spread to the liver is frequent (30–60 per cent) and the metastases are large and multiple. The carcinoid syndrome is almost always associated with large hepatic metastases. The natural history is of slow progression over many years.

Functional tumours produce 5-hydroxytryptamine, bradykinin and other vasoactive compounds. The symptoms are facial flushing, abdominal cramps and diarrhoea and, less commonly, asthma and right-sided heart failure secondary to fibrotic valvular changes. The symptoms are often intermittent but can persist with permanent changes in facial colour.

### *Diagnosis*

The diagnosis is based on the finding of a big liver with ultrasonic evidence of multiple tumour deposits. The urinary excretion of 5-hydroxyindole acetic acid (5HIAA), a metabolite of 5-hydroxytryptamine, is greatly increased. Ultrasonically guided liver biopsy will enable a firm histological diagnosis to be made. Not all carcinoid tumours are functional (those arising from stomach and rectum are usually not) and, in such cases, histology is required to differentiate the lesions from the much more common metastatic carcinoma.

### *Treatment*

Pharmacological treatment using antagonists of 5-hydroxytryptamine (e.g. cyproheptadine) or inhibitors of its synthesis (e.g. parachlorophenylalanine) or release (Octreotide) can be helpful, but in severe cases, treatment designed to reduce tumour bulk is usually more satisfactory if feasible. Ultrasound, CT scanning and hepatic angiography indicate whether limited hepatic resection is feasible and this is probably the treatment of choice.

An alternative approach is embolotherapy with boluses of gel foam or wire coils injected at arteriography in the hope of reducing by necrosis the size of some of the larger deposits. There is a risk of abscess formation or of producing a massive release of vasoactive compounds and pharmacological blockade must be achieved before the procedure is undertaken.

Radiotherapy and cytotoxic drugs (streptozotocin) are relatively ineffective and seldom used.

### Prognosis

This is relatively good, compared with carcinoma, but the carcinoid syndrome can be distressing and very difficult to treat. Survival is very variable, but in one large series, the median survival was 8 years (range 1–20 years).

# Nutrition

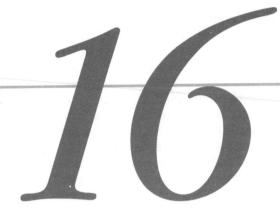

# *I*NTRODUCTION

Nutrition plays an important role in many diseases. Deficiencies or excesses in the diet can lead to clinical problems. An appropriate diet is important for the maintenance of health and recovery from debilitating illness. The aspects relevant to various renal, hepatic, cardiovascular and gastrointestinal disorders are dealt with in their appropriate chapters. This chapter will deal with nutritional assessment, obesity and starvation, specific dietary deficiencies, vitamins and supplemental feeding.

Food intake varies a great deal between cultures and within communities. The necessary elements of the diet are calories, water, the essential amino acids, the essential fatty acids, some carbohydrate, various vitamins and elements. Generally these essential nutrients are provided in adequate quantities by any varied diet of sufficient quantity. However, when intake is strictly controlled, as with parenteral feeding, attention must be paid to specific supplementations. When taken in excess many constituents of the diet such as calories, fat and various vitamins produce their own health problems.

The physical characteristics and preparation of the food are of importance. Cereals and other substances may be deprived of some of their nutrient value by inappropriate preparation. Fibre in the diet may not have nutritive value of its own but will affect the absorption of other substances and alter the behaviour of the bowel. It has been suggested that these effects are important in the prevention of a number of conditions prevalent in Western society including appendicitis, diverticular disease, carcinoma of the colon and haemorrhoids.

Recommended dietary intakes for adults in sedentary employment are 2500 kcal/day for men and 2000 kcal/day for women, but 300 kcal/day less over 75 years of age.

# *T*HE ASSESSMENT OF NUTRITION

One of the simplest methods of assessment is by weighing the person. The scales must be accurate, and beam or lever balances are best for this purpose. Fluctuations of up to 1 kg occur in normal subjects even if care is taken to ensure the same quantity of clothing each time the individual is weighed. Calorimetry suggests that, relating energy to weight change, 1 kg represents around 6000 kcal.

A brief dietary history should be part of the initial assessment of most patients. When dietary factors are felt to be important then a more detailed history is necessary. This is best done by asking:

1. What do you eat on a typical day?
*or*
2. What have you had to eat and drink over the last 24 hours?

*or*
3. Write down everything you eat and drink over the next 7 days.

These methods depend on the honesty of the patient and the experience and knowledge of the interviewer. With practice and attention to detail they can provide reasonably accurate information. The contents of various foods can be obtained from standard food tables to produce a detailed analysis of the diet. A good idea of the general adequacy of the diet can be obtained just from a careful description of a typical day. Recommended dietary amounts of some important nutrients are shown in Table 16.1.

Other methods of assessment of nutrition are measurement of mid upper arm circumference, skinfold thickness, serum albumin.

**Table 16.1** Recommended daily intakes of essential nutrients.

| Nutrient | Recommended daily intake for young adult males | Nutrient | Recommended daily intake for young adult males |
|----------|-----------------------------------------------|----------|-----------------------------------------------|
| Energy | 2500 kcal | Vitamin E | 10 mg |
| Protein | 63 g | Folate | 200 µg |
| Thiamine | 1.0 mg | Sodium | 40–100 mmol |
| Riboflavin | 1.6 mg | Potassium | 50–140 mmol |
| Nicotinic acid equivalents | 18 mg | Calcium | 600 mg |
| Vitamin C | 30 mg | Iron | 12 mg |
| Vitamin A | 750 retinol equivalents µg | Zinc | 15 mg |
| Vitamin $B_6$ | 2.2 mg | Iodine | 150 µg |
| Vitamin $B_{12}$ | 3.0 µg | | |

# Clinical problems

## UNDERNUTRITION

Most malnutrition worldwide is related to economic problems of food supply. In developing world countries this is a considerable problem and has its most devastating effects on children. In higher income countries problems of malnutrition still occur, particularly in the elderly and the socially deprived, in association with alcohol abuse or food avoidance as in anorexia nervosa (page 886). There is some risk also when diets are restricted to certain categories of food. For example, vegans who avoid all animal products are at considerable risk of vitamin $B_{12}$ deficiency and may have inadequate intake of calcium, iron and zinc.

Many chronic diseases lead to inadequate nutrition. Disorders of the gastrointestinal tract may reduce appetite, cause discomfort on eating or interfere with absorption of food. Malignant diseases and some chronic diseases are associated with anorexia and weight loss.

## Malnutrition in the developing world

The majority of the world's population lives in economically poor countries. These countries tend to have a relatively young population and an increasing population because of high birth rates. The problems related to an inadequate food supply are compounded by poor medical and public health resources with increased risks of infection without facilities to cope with these. Malnutrition is a constant problem in such areas with around 100 million children suffering moderate to severe starvation at any time. Major local disasters on top of this background problem are often related to drought or war. Grades of starvation related to height and weight are shown in Table 16.2.

**Table 16.2** Criteria and management for starvation.

| Degree of starvation | Body mass index | Management |
|---|---|---|
| Mild | 20–18 | Feed |
| Moderate | 18–16 | Rehydrate orally + feed + supplements |
| Severe | 16 | Resuscitate in hospital |

**Wellcome classification**

| *Weight/weight of a normal child of same age* | *Oedema present* | *No oedema* |
|---|---|---|
| 60–80% | Kwashiorkor | Undernutrition |
| 60% | Marasmus/ kwashiorkor | Marasmus |

## CLINICAL FEATURES

Severe malnutrition in children is sometimes separated into marasmus and kwashiorkor although the two overlap. **Marasmus** is equivalent to childhood starvation leading to severe weight loss with muscle wasting. In **kwashiorkor** the diet is particularly inadequate in protein compared to carbohydrate. Muscles tend to be spared but the liver is affected with fatty change and later hypoalbuminaemia and oedema (Table 16.2). The skin may show areas of depigmentation and hair loss.

Early features of malnutrition are weight loss in adults and a failure of normal growth in children. Thirst and hunger develop together with weakness and apathy. Nocturia may occur and there is intolerance to cold. The risk of infection is increased and compounds the problem.

As weight loss occurs the muscles become weak and wasted, hair becomes thin and straight and may change colour, the skin becomes dry, pale and inelastic. There may be bradycardia, hypotension and hypothermia. The abdomen becomes distended and diarrhoea occurs. The associated apathy, weakness and depression increase the difficulties in obtaining and eating food.

All organs and tissues other than the brain are reduced in size.

## INVESTIGATIONS

There may be anaemia, leucopenia and thrombocytopenia. Albumin levels are often maintained but blood sugar falls and ketones rise. The electrocardiogram shows a slow rate and small complexes. Measurements of basal metabolic rate indicate that this slows with a consequent reduction in oxygen consumption.

## TREATMENT

The management depends upon the severity of the malnutrition (Table 16.2). The first essential in severe malnutrition is resuscitation with replacement of fluids, electrolytes and glucose. At the same time any associated infections must be dealt with. This phase should be followed by a gradual increase in the intake of calories and protein together with vitamin supplements.

Initial supplementation must be followed by plans for future care and prevention. This involves questions of economics, public health and planning including education on family planning, breast feeding, oral rehydration and growth monitoring.

# Vitamins

Vitamins are organic substances or groups of substances which are required in the diet in very small quantities. They act as cofactors for metabolic processes. The necessary vitamins are shown in Table 16.3.

# Vitamin A

Vitamin A (retinol) is available preformed in some animal foods particularly liver, fish liver

**Table 16.3** The essential vitamins.

| Vitamin | Alternative name |
| --- | --- |
| Vitamin A | Retinol |
| Thiamine | Vitamin $B_1$ |
| Riboflavin | Vitamin $B_2$ |
| Niacin | Nicotinic acid, nicotinamide |
| Vitamin $B_6$ | Pyridoxine |
| Folate | – |
| Pantothenic acid | – |
| Biotin | – |
| Vitamin $B_{12}$ | Cobalamin |
| Vitamin C | Ascorbic acid |
| Vitamin D | Calciferol |
| Vitamin E | Tocoferols |
| Vitamin K | – |

oils and dairy products. Polar bear and seal liver have been a source of vitamin A toxicity in Arctic explorers. Carotenes are yellow or orange pigments found in vegetables and fruits and β-carotene produces two molecules of vitamin A. This is then stored in the liver where most adults hold 1 to 2 years' stores of vitamin A. Deficiency occurs with an inadequate intake or malabsorption.

## CLINICAL FEATURES

Vitamin A is important in maintaining mucus-secreting epithelia, particularly the cornea and conjunctiva. Xerophthalmia and keratomalacia resulting from vitamin A deficiency are important causes of blindness in developing countries, particularly in Asia. There may be an association also with skin tumours. Mild deficiency causes night blindness which responds rapidly to therapy, but more severe, destructive lesions are irreversible.

The toxic effects of excess vitamin A are desquamation of the skin and raised intracranial pressure in acute toxicity, and weakness, dry skin, liver damage and exostoses in chronic toxicity. Large intakes of carotene-containing vegetables produce carotenaemia in which the skin and plasma are coloured yellow, but this is otherwise harmless. Carotenaemia also occurs in myxoedema, diabetes mellitus and anorexia nervosa. Treatment of vitamin A deficiency consists of retinol acetate, 66 mg (200 000 units) orally or retinol palmitate intramuscularly. A retinoic acid derivative, etretinate, is used in the treatment of skin conditions such as psoriasis and acne.

# Thiamine

Thiamine (vitamin $B_1$) is found in cereals and some meats. It is important in carbohydrate and amino acid metabolism and deficiency occurs in the presence of poor nutrition with a diet mainly of polished rice and, particularly in Western countries, in alcoholics. The Wernicke–Korsakoff syndrome occurs in thiamine deficiency especially in alcoholism. Body stores are minimal and problems can arise in starvation for around a month.

## CLINICAL FEATURES

**Wernicke's encephalopathy** consists of ataxia, external ophthalmoplegia, nystagmus and suppression of consciousness while **Korsakoff's psychosis** involves mainly memory problems, often with confabulation.

Peripheral neuropathy (dry beri-beri) occurs with marked muscle tenderness. Cardiovascular beri-beri (wet beri-beri) involves high output cardiac failure and is seen in areas of severe deficiency and when prolonged parenteral nutrition is given without supplementation.

## DIAGNOSIS

Diagnosis is based on the clinical picture and the red cell transketolase level.

## TREATMENT

Treatment is with thiamine replacement. Cardiac failure and Wernicke–Korsakoff syndrome are treated with parenteral thiamine hydrochloride, 50 mg, daily. Peripheral neuropathy responds to oral therapy, 30–50 mg, daily. Other nutritional deficiencies will need to be dealt with at the same time. Underlying causes such as alcohol consumption need to be dealt with to avoid future problems.

# Riboflavin

Riboflavin (vitamin $B_2$) comes from dairy products, liver, kidney and cereals and is an essential coenzyme in cellular oxidation.

## CLINICAL FEATURES

Deficiency of riboflavin causes anaemia, angular cheilitis, a sore, atrophic oral mucosa and tongue, corneal vascularization and seborrhoeic dermatitis. The diagnosis can be confirmed by measuring the 24-hour urinary output of riboflavin. There are no effective body stores.

## TREATMENT

Treatment is by oral replacement, 10 to 30 mg, daily and ensuring a suitable change in the diet.

# Niacin

Niacin (nicotinic acid) acts as a coenzyme in a number of metabolic processes. It occurs in meat, fish and some cereals. Niacin can be formed from tryptophan. Deficiencies of niacin occur in alcoholics, Hartnup disease, where tryptophan absorption is impaired, and carcinoid tumours where tryptophan is converted to 5-hydroxytryptamine rather than niacin. In Africa those on a predominantly maize diet are at particular risk.

## CLINICAL FEATURES

The classic picture of niacin deficiency is pellagra consisting of dermatitis of exposed skin, dementia, diarrhoea, and a raw, red and painful tongue.

## DIAGNOSIS

Diagnosis can be confirmed by the low urinary excretion of N-methyl nicotinamide and metabolites.

## TREATMENT

Nicotinic acid, 50 mg, is used orally in mild deficiency, and up to 500 mg daily for severe cases.

# Pyridoxine

Pyridoxine (vitamin $B_6$) is found in meat, fish, cereals and some fruits and nuts. Deficiencies occur in malabsorption and with certain drugs which antagonize pyridoxine, particularly isoniazid, hydralazine, penicillamine and possibly, oestrogens.

## CLINICAL FEATURES

Anaemia may develop in children deprived of pyridoxine. In adults cheilosis, glossitis, seborrhoeic dermatitis and peripheral neuropathy may occur.

## DIAGNOSIS

Plasma and urinary pyridoxine levels are low.

## TREATMENT

Treatment consists of pyridoxine replacement, 10–50 mg daily, and attention to the underlying cause. Pyridoxine should be given prophylactically to patients on isoniazid therapy when high doses are used or when nutrition is poor. Excess pyridoxine can itself produce a peripheral neuropathy.

# Biotin

Biotin deficiency is rare; it produces a rash and painful tongue.

# Folate

Folate is found in many vegetables and fruits and in bread and flour products. Deficiency occurs with poor dietary intake, malabsorption, pregnancy, increased cell turnover in haematological malignancies and with antagonism by drugs such as methotrexate and alcohol. Body stores are small and folate deficiency can develop quickly.

## CLINICAL FEATURES

Folate deficiency results in a megaloblastic anaemia similar to vitamin $B_{12}$ deficiency. This is discussed further on page 604.

# Vitamin $B_{12}$

Vitamin $B_{12}$ is available preformed in animal foods, particularly from liver, but also from fish and milk. After combination with intrinsic factor in the stomach it is absorbed in the ileum. Considerable stores exist in the liver. Deficiency of vitamin $B_{12}$ from dietary deficiency, lack of intrinsic factor or small bowel disease can result in megaloblastic anaemia (page 605), subacute combined degeneration of the cord (page 713), peripheral neuropathy, optic atrophy and dementia.

# Vitamin C

Most vitamin C (as ascorbic acid) in the diet comes from fruit, green vegetables and potatoes. It is easily destroyed by heat and alkalis and dissolves in water so cooking methods for vegetables should take account of this. The body has stores to last 2 to 3 months. The recommended intake of vitamin C is 30 mg/day in the UK. Ill patients require a larger intake as needs increase with stress, surgery and various drugs. Lack of vitamin C affects collagen formation, capillary and platelet function.

## CLINICAL FEATURES

In infants the features are anaemia, bone pains from subperiosteal bleeding and enlarged painful costochondral junctions (scorbutic rosary). Amongst adults the elderly are at greatest risk of vitamin C deficiency (scurvy). Bones, joints and muscles become painful and two characteristic features develop. The first is keratosis and haemorrhage at the hair follicles and the second is swelling, infection and bleeding in the gums. The latter changes only occur in the presence of teeth or underlying roots and not in edentulous patients. Large spontaneous haemorrhages appear together with anaemia and delayed wound healing.

## DIAGNOSIS

Vitamin C can be measured in the plasma but is only unequivocally low in advanced disease. Better assessments come from measurement of vitamin C in the blood buffy coat (white cells) or urinary excretion after a loading dose.

## TREATMENT

In adult scurvy, vitamin C, 1 g, should be given daily in divided doses. Larger doses have been recommended for prophylaxis of viral infections, particularly colds, and tumours with very little supporting evidence. Large doses can produce diarrhoea and oxalate or urate stones in the urinary tract.

# Vitamin D

Vitamin $D_3$ (cholecalciferol) comes from fish oils and fortified margarine and from the action of ultraviolet light on dehydrocholesterol in the skin. Deficiency of vitamin D results in rickets in children and osteomalacia in adults, the clinical features and treatment of which are described on page 503.

# Vitamin E

Vitamin E comes from vegetable oils, wholegrain cereals, eggs and butter.

## CLINICAL FEATURES

The vitamin prevents the oxidation of polyunsaturated fatty acids in cell membranes and deficiency results in red cell fragility. A mild haemolytic anaemia occurs and prolonged severe deficiency can produce ataxia, areflexia and retinal pigmentation.

## TREATMENT

Treatment is with oral supplementation or by the intramuscular route in the presence of malabsorption. There is no evidence to support the popular belief that vitamin E supplements increase athletic or sexual performance.

# Vitamin K

Vitamin K is needed for synthesis of prothrombin (factor II) and other clotting factors (VII, IX and X). Dietary sources of vitamin K are mainly vegetables containing vitamin $K_1$ (phytomenadione). Bacteria produce vitamin $K_2$ (menaquinones) but this is not an important dietary source.

## CLINICAL FEATURES

Vitamin K deficiency occurs in newborn infants and in adults in the presence of obstructive jaundice and malabsorption. Common oral anticoagulants act by antagonism of the formation of vitamin K-dependent coagulation factors in the liver. Clinical features of vitamin K deficiency are hypoprothrombinaemia and haemorrhage. Vitamin K-dependent factors, including prothrombin, will be low.

## TREATMENT

Vitamin $K_1$, up to 10 mg intramuscularly or, in emergency, slowly intravenously replaces the deficiency. In severe liver disease the lack of clotting factors is not helped by vitamin K.

# Trace Elements

Fifteen trace elements (by definition less than 0.005 per cent body weight) are accepted as essential. Iron (page 600) and iodine (page 520) are considered separately.

## COPPER

Children with malnutrition may develop anaemia, neutropenia and bone changes from copper deficiency. In adults copper toxicity occurs in Wilson's disease (page 402).

## FLUORINE

Dental caries is more common where the level in drinking water is below 1 ppm, and fluoridation of the supply or topical use reduces such caries.

Where the supply of fluoride is excessive fluorosis develops with white patches on the teeth, pitting and discolouration of the enamel, and bone exostoses.

## ZINC

Zinc deficiency in children leads to impaired growth. An inherited disease, acrodermatitis enteropathica is related to zinc malabsorption and produces diarrhoea, dermatitis and delayed growth. Zinc deficiency in adults occcurs in liver disease and malabsorption and may produce night blindness and interfere with wound healing. Acute zinc deficiency during parenteral feeding can result in diarrhoea and dermatitis.

# ADVERSE EFFECTS OF FOOD

## Obesity

The body mass index or Quetelet index of weight/height squared (kg/m²) is a suitable index of relative weight independent of height. Around 13 per cent of men and fifteen per cent of women in the UK have a body mass index of >30, the threshold for obesity. Gross obesity occurs when the index exceeds 40. Mortality increases with body mass index over the desirable range of 20 to 25 but also at low weights perhaps because of associated diseases causing the weight loss.

Obesity usually results primarily from taking in more calories than are consumed. Only rarely is it secondary to thyroid or hypothalamic disorders although these must be considered.

There are many complications of obesity particularly glucose intolerance, hypertension and cardiovascular disease, respiratory insufficiency and psychiatric problems.

The treatment of obesity is dealt with on page 507. Most patients require intensive support and encouragement to be successful.

## Food intolerance

This may occur with a specific intolerance such as the gluten sensitivity of coeliac disease (page 358) or enzyme deficiencies such as lactase (page 342) or with various less well defined responses. Allergy to food has received a great deal of media attention although many problems are an intolerance rather than a true allergic response.

### CLINICAL FEATURES

The clinical features of food intolerance vary. Early symptoms such as swelling of the lips and urticaria are easiest to pin down because of their close temporal relationship to the food. It is much more difficult to be certain about responses such as eczema or arthralgia. Most symptoms have been related to food intolerance at some time, but perhaps the best documentation is for urticaria, asthma, eczema, migraine and irritable bowel syndrome.

### DIAGNOSIS

When the patient is not certain about a relationship to food then a food diary of everything eaten or drunk may help. The next step is to try eliminating foods: either those suspected of giving trouble or a general elimination of all but a few basic foods with a gradual reintroduction and assessment of individual items. Skin tests are often negative even in the face of documented food sensitivity, particularly if this is not immediate. Skin tests and the radioallergosorbant test (RAST) look for specific IgE but false positives and negatives are quite common.

The best way of diagnosing food sensitivity is by double blind challenge. Usually this should be performed in hospital to deal with any late reactions.

Reactions to food vary. They include IgG and IgE antibodies, but may also occur with a direct response to chemicals in the food such as histamine.

### TREATMENT

Treatment consists of identifying the particular food causing the problem or problems and then avoiding it. Patients often develop their own complicated diets and it is then important to check that they are nutritionally adequate. Introduction of a relevant allergen after a period of avoidance may result in an augmented reaction.

# THERAPEUTIC DIETS

## Arterial disease

Premature atherosclerosis is related to lipid abnormalities which result in increased low density lipoprotein (LDL) and cholesterol in the blood. This may be an inherited metabolic defect or be related to diet. There seems little doubt that subjects with substantially abnormal levels of these substances should be encouraged to bring these down and the earlier in life this treatment starts, the better. Although coronary artery disease is correlated with a population's median cholesterol there is less convincing evidence that changing the eating patterns of a nation can be successful and worthwhile. However, it seems likely to be helpful and should be encouraged whilst greatest help is concentrated on those known to have very high levels. Foods which need to be avoided or reduced are shown in Table 16.3 along with those suitable for use instead.

## Hypertension

Much attention has been devoted to sodium and potassium levels in hypertension. Each day the body requires approximately 20 mmol sodium

**Table 16.3** Reducing saturated fat and cholesterol in the diet.

| Avoid or reduce | Use |
| --- | --- |
| Butter, lard | Polyunsaturated margarine |
| Cream | Skimmed or semi-skimmed milk |
| Meat, sausages | Poultry, fish |
| Cheese | Cottage cheese |
| Cakes | Vegetables, fruit |
| Pastries, biscuits | Cereals |

although the average intake is much more than this. Reduction in sodium intake will produce a small drop in blood pressure but the restriction needs to be quite severe at around 50 to 60 mmol/day and some patients are not able to tolerate the diet. Substituting potassium and magnesium may help the palatability of the diet and possibly further reduce blood pressure.

## Other conditions

Dietary manipulation in diabetes, renal disease and coeliac disease is described in the appropriate chapters. Various dietary factors such as spices, vitamins and fat have been associated with malignancies of the oesophagus, stomach and large bowel but not to a degree convincing enough to modify routine diets.

# ENTERAL AND PARENTERAL FEEDING

Many patients who come into hospital for medical or surgical conditions suffer from poor nutrition related primarily to their underlying disease or to a secondary diminution in appetite. Substantial nutritional deficits interfere with the recovery from operations and medical conditions. Guides to the diagnosis of malnutrition in the UK are shown in Table 16.4. Intensive care unit patients may have had poor nutrition before admission and are often more catabolic because of sepsis. Usually they are not able to take food for themselves and it is important to start supplemental nutrition early in their stay in the intensive care unit using the enteral route if possible.

The options for supplementing nutrition are to encourage suitable high calorie, high protein feeds; to introduce feeds into the gastrointestinal

**Table 16.4** Criteria for malnutrition in the UK.

10% recent weight loss
Bodyweight <80% ideal
Albumin <30 g/l
Lymphocyte count <1.2 × 10⁹/l

tract by way of a tube (enteral feeding) or to feed intravenously (parenteral feeding). They should be regarded in this same order of desirability.

# Enteral feeding

Enteral feeding is used in patients who cannot or will not swallow appropriate nutrition readily but in whom gastrointestinal absorption is adequate (Table 16.5). It is much safer and cheaper than parenteral feeding. Enteral feeding tubes are of fine bore and are able to take commercially designed feeds but not liquidized food. Enteral feeds can be given by way of a gastrostomy tube inserted percutaneously into the stomach at endoscopy or by a radiologist under fluoroscopic screening. This technique avoids the discomfort of a nasogastric tube and is often preferable if feeding is likely to be necessary for more than 2 weeks. It does not interfere with the patient's own swallowing as recovery begins.

Various commercial feeds are available for enteral feeding providing approximately 2000 kcal in 2 litres of fluid with around 60 to 70 g protein. Fat provides around one-third of the energy requirements. A higher calorie input is needed in the presence of severe sepsis or burns. Trace elements and vitamins need to be added when feeding is necessary for more than 4 weeks. A low sodium feed may be necessary in patients with cardiac failure or renal failure. Elemental

**Table 16.5** Indications for enteral feeding.

Inadequate airway protection (depressed level of
  consciousness, neurological deficit)
Severe catabolic states (burns)
Chemotherapy for malignancy
Short bowel syndrome*
Inflammatory bowel disease*
Intestinal fistulae*
Obstructive lesion in the pharynx or oesophagus (if a
  tube can be passed under radiological control)

*Parenteral feeding may be needed for short periods.

feeds in which the protein is predigested to amino acids and oligopeptides may be necessary in the presence of severe intestinal or pancreatic disease.

The complications of enteral feeding include aspiration, vomiting, diarrhoea, hyperglycaemia, oesophageal erosions and misplaced tubes.

# Parenteral feeding

This is necessary when the gastrointestinal tract cannot cope with oral or enteral feeding. This may occur in the short term after surgery or in the longer term with inadequate absorptive surface of the bowel. In the latter situation it can be used for long-term outpatient care. Access to the circulation is best into a large vein such as the superior vena cava. The cannula should be inserted by a strictly aseptic procedure and tunnelled under the skin to reduce further the risk of infection.

The constituents of the nutrition are nitrogen as amino acids, carbohydrate (glucose) and fat for calories together with electrolytes, vitamins and trace elements. Various commercial preparations are available. The most suitable arrangement is to have the hospital pharmacy produce, under sterile conditions, a 2.5–3 litre bag containing each day's supply. This will provide around 2500 kcal (30 per cent as lipid) and 12 g nitrogen. The details of feeds needed in particular situations are best decided by a designated parenteral feeding team in the hospital. The team should include a specialised nurse dedicated to the care of the insertion sites and the aseptic changing of bags and giving sets.

The complications of parenteral nutrition are shown in Table 16.6.

**Table 16.6** Complications of parenteral nutrition.

Pneumothorax
Air embolus
Catheter fracture
Catheter infection
Venous thrombosis
Fluid overload
Lack of essential nutrient (in long-term feeding >1
  month)
Increased $CO_2$ production (relative excess of
  carbohydrates)
Hyperglycaemia

# **D**isorders of the Kidney

# SYMPTOMS AND SIGNS

The kidneys are inconvenient organs in that many diseases can be silent as far as symptoms are concerned and unlike, for example, the heart, the lungs or the nervous system, they do not lend themselves easily to physical examination. On the other hand, unless function is grossly disturbed so that the patient is anuric, examination of the urine provides a swift and simple means of gaining information in many diseases. In numerous patients renal disease is discovered by chance on routine examine, or when they present with a systemic illness such as diabetes mellitus, which is then found to be involving the kidneys. Symptoms arising from the lower urinary tract, i.e. ureters, bladder and urethra, are often marked and result in early consultation.

# Symptoms

## PAIN

Loin pain, usually accurately located by the patient, is most often caused by infection, stones or obstruction. Ureteric or renal colic is a very severe variety of loin pain usually caused by passage of a stone, but also sometimes by a necrotic papilla or blood clot. The pain is incapacitating, radiates to the iliac fossa, groin and genitalia, and is accompanied by nausea, vomiting and sweating.

Renal tumours can also cause loin pain.

## HAEMATURIA

The patient will usually recognize that blood is causing the change in colour of the urine because it is bright red. Sometimes, however, particularly in glomerulonephritis, the urine may be a very dark brown colour, like tea. Haematuria always merits full investigation.

## DYSURIA

This is urethral and sometimes there is suprapubic pain during and after micturition. The commonest cause is infection, but trauma and chemical injury to the epithelium of the bladder or urethra can cause similar symptoms.

## FREQUENCY

This is often associated with dysuria and refers to the frequent passage of small volumes of urine. When this occurs at night it is known as nocturia. The commonest causes are infection and prostatism. It may also occur when the capacity of the bladder is diminished, as in chronic infection, for example, tuberculosis or malignancy.

## URGENCY

Urgency of micturition, a painful desire to micturate which cannot be controlled, usually accompanies frequency.

## STRANGURY

This is the passage of blood with dysuria, and is associated with infections and tumours.

## ENURESIS

Enuresis or bed-wetting is normal in children until they are trained. When pathological it is due to infections or neurological disease affecting the bladder (neurogenic bladder).

## RETENTION

This may be acute or chronic. Chronic retention is usually caused by obstruction, usually due to prostatism, and is often not noted until the bladder becomes so large that overflow incontinence occurs. Chronic retention also occurs in a neurogenic bladder.

Acute retention is painful, unless there is a neurological cause which also results in loss of sensation.

## SYSTEMIC SYMPTOMS

There are two types of systemic symptoms. First, patients may have systemic symptoms due to acute or chronic renal failure, whatever the cause of the disease, and these are described on pages 428 and 433. Secondly, patients with renal disease may have symptoms which are entirely due to a systemic disease involving organs other than the kidneys, but in whom the renal disease, although asymptomatic, may be the major determining prognostic factor. For example, a patient with systemic lupus erythematosus may present with a rash and joint pains, but the underlying nephritis and renal failure are the most important aspects of the disease.

## SYMPTOMLESS

Symptomless renal disease is commonly uncovered at routine medical examination, for example, for insurance or employment purposes, during pregnancy or when patients consult their doctors because of an unrelated illness. Hypertension, which commonly complicates renal disease, may be found on examination; urinalysis may reveal proteinuria and/or haematuria; and the multichannel analysis of blood samples, now routine, may reveal a raised plasma concentration of urea or creatinine.

## *Signs*

During the complete examination, particular attention should be paid to the possibility of hypertension and fluid retention, as well as to the abdominal examination.

### HYPERTENSION

As high blood pressure often accompanies renal disease, the blood pressure must be noted, and if elevated, evidence sought for end organ damage due to hypertension, i.e. retinal changes and evidence of heart disease.

### FLUID RETENTION

Failing kidneys cannot excrete a salt and water load so if these are present in excess then peripheral oedema, ascites, pleural effusions and pulmonary oedema will develop.

### ABDOMINAL EXAMINATION

Enlarged kidneys and/or an enlarged bladder should be excluded. If present, then in males the external genitalia should be inspected to exclude a local cause of obstruction, such as stricture or phimosis. In addition rectal examination in both sexes and pelvic examination in women should be done to exclude tumours, which can cause obstruction.

## *I*NVESTIGATIONS

Investigations have two aims. First, to assess renal function in the patient and, second, to define the structure, macroscopic or microscopic, of the kidneys and urinary tract.

any response to treatment. Knowledge of renal function is also important for the proper prescription of drugs which are excreted by the kidney.

## *Assessing renal function*

This is necessary to measure the severity of the disease's effects on the kidney, to follow the progress of the disease, and particularly to assess

## *Glomerular filtration rate*

Glomerular filtration rate (GFR) is the most widely used test of renal function. The commonest method is to measure the plasma urea and creatinine from which an indirect assessment of GFR can be made. Plasma creatinine and urea do not have a linear relationship with GFR (Fig. 17.1) so that they rise very slowly as the first 50 per cent of GFR is lost, and then progressively more rapidly when the second 50 per cent of GFR is lost. **Creatinine** is an endogenous product of muscle metabolism and is therefore relatively constant, although it will fall when there is muscle wasting. Plasma urea is, by contrast, rapidly altered by protein intake and catabolism. Common causes of a raised plasma urea not due to renal disease are a large protein meal, haemorrhage into the gastrointestinal tract (which is the equivalent of a protein meal), muscle injury, burns and corticosteroid therapy.

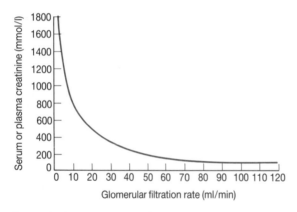

**Figure 17.1** Relationship of plasma creatinine to glomerular filtration rate (GFR). Note the increasingly and eventually large changes in plasma creatinine for equal reductions in GFR once the latter has fallen below 50%.

Various formulae are available to calculate the GFR from measurements of the plasma urea and creatinine alone. A more formal estimate may be made by measuring **creatinine clearance** (urea clearance is rarely used). This requires collection of a timed sample of urine, usually for 24 hours, and measurement of the plasma creatinine during that period. Despite its apparent simplicity this test is often valueless due to errors in timing of the urine collection or its incompleteness.

The most accurate and widely available method of measuring GFR is to use a nuclide such as chromium-51 ethylenediamine tetra-acetic acid (EDTA). This is cleared virtually completely by the kidneys and allows estimation of the GFR by measuring its disappearance curve from the blood following intravenous injection, i.e. urine collection is not required.

The classic method of measuring GFR by inulin clearance is now only used as a research procedure as it requires bladder catheterization.

## INTERPRETATION OF PLASMA CREATININE/UREA/GLOMERULAR FILTRATION RATE

There are three common pitfalls. First, the lack of a linear relationship between plasma creatinine/urea and GFR has been referred to above: the mistake made is to miss impaired renal function before 50 per cent of the GFR is lost because the plasma urea and creatinine have not risen sufficiently to alert the clinician. If impaired renal function is suspected, then the GFR must be measured directly. The second and third pitfalls are interrelated. The GFR falls with age (Fig. 17.2), but the plasma creatinine does not rise because, as the individual ages the muscle mass falls. The error made is to assume that a raised plasma creatinine in an elderly patient is due to 'old age'. The reduced GFR of elderly patients, despite their normal creatinine, must be remembered when prescribing drugs, and also makes them more susceptible to acute renal failure because they have less reserve of renal function.

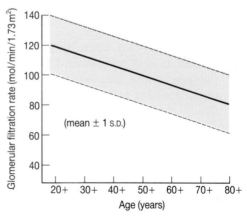

**Figure 17.2** Change of glomerular filtration rate with age (corrected to standard surface area).

# Tubular function

Tubular function tests are performed much less frequently as tubular disorders provide only a small portion of nephrological practice.

## URINARY CONCENTRATION

This is now most usually assessed by osmolality. An early morning sample of greater than 550 mosmol/kg indicates normal concentrating ability. If the osmolality is less than 550 mosmol/kg a concentration test is performed by giving desmopressin (a synthetic analogue of vasopressin), usually in the morning, and urine collected 6 or 8 hours later. In younger subjects an osmolality of 750 mosmol/kg, or greater, should be achieved, but in older individuals, due to progressive reduction in concentrating ability, 550–600 mosmol/kg should be attained.

## URINARY ACIDIFICATION

The pH of an early morning urine sample should be 5.4 or less. If greater, an acidification test should be performed using ammonium chloride, 100 mg/kg of body weight, given in the morning, and urine pH measured over the succeeding 8 hours. Blood is taken to measure plasma bicarbonate at the beginning and end of the period to demonstrate sufficient acidification, i.e. a fall in plasma bicarbonate. The normal response is a urine pH of 5.3 or less.

## OTHER TUBULAR FUNCTION TESTS

Clearance of phosphate, urate and amino acids may be performed to study proximal tubular damage and for assessing transport defects.

# Urine analysis

Urine testing is simple and provides important and immediate information. The specimen should be a mid-stream specimen, i.e. collected after the passage of urine has begun to avoid contamination, particularly in women. Occasionally a suprapubic aspiration of the bladder will be necessary to avoid contamination. Conventional bladder catherization, although providing easy access to urine samples, is often complicated by a contaminated specimen.

## DIPSTICK TESTING

This is a very sensitive method for detecting microscopic haematuria and proteinuria. The test for proteinuria will detect normal amounts of protein in the urine, i.e. up to 250 mg protein excreted per 24 hours, usually equated with concentrations as low as 50 mg/l.

## URINE MICROSCOPY

This is aimed at detecting cells and casts. Both are found in normal urine, and increase after exercise. Normal casts are formed from Tamm Horsfall protein. Diseased casts are more numerous and in infection will contain leukocytes and bacteria, and in glomerular disease will contain leukocytes and erythrocytes. Casts containing cellular elements are often described as granular casts. The presence of leukocytes indicates infection. Red cells are found in disorders associated with haematuria.

# *Clinical problems*

## $A$CUTE RENAL FAILURE

Acute renal failure (ARF) is a sudden fall in GFR which causes uraemia. It is a serious condition because the overall mortality rate is 50 per cent. The onset of ARF may be on a background of completely normal renal function, or on preceding chronic renal failure in which the kidneys are much more susceptible to the insults which cause ARF. Although ARF is often accompanied by oliguria, or anuria, the definition of ARF does not include the passage of a small volume of urine, or no urine, as occasionally it can occur with normal or large volumes of urine.

## *Causes*

It is very useful in the diagnosis and management of ARF to divide its causes into prerenal, renal and postrenal. Table 17.1 shows the common causes of acute renal failure, and the wide range of diseases which can cause this condition.

## *Presenting features*

Patients may present with symptoms and signs due to kidney failure itself, or to the underlying cause of ARF, or a combination of both.

### ABNORMAL KIDNEY FUNCTION

The patient may note anuria or oliguria or, if the patient is already in hospital then the change in urine output may be noted by nursing or medical staff. The accumulation of fluid may cause breathlessness due to pulmonary oedema or swelling of the feet and legs. The patient may also complain of the symptoms caused by uraemia (page 425).

### THE UNDERLYING DISEASE

As Table 17.1 shows, the list of possible causes is very extensive: there are some general guidelines.

### *Prerenal causes*

These occur in patients who have had surgery, burns, haemorrhage or excessive diarrhoea and/or vomiting. All these events lead to a reduction in intravascular volume and hypoperfusion of the kidneys. Patients may have postural hypotension, a low jugular venous pressure, cool extremeties and tachycardia. A particularly severe form of ARF occurs in patients with concomitant liver failure: the 'hepatorenal syndrome'. Acute tubular necrosis, which is a histological description, will result when hypotension, hypovolaemia and renal hypoperfusion are severe, or allowed to persist. It can also be caused by drugs, for example, the antibiotic gentamicin, by haemoglobinaemia as in haemolytic anaemia, and by myoglobinaemia following severe damage to muscles, known as rhabdomyolysis, for example, following heat stroke.

**Acute tubular necrosis** causes 50 per cent of cases of ARF. Its pathogenesis is not clearly understood, but hypoperfusion of the tubules causing ischaemia, with damaged tubular cells forming debris which obstructs the tubular lumen, and leakage of glomerular filtrate across the damaged tubule into the peritubular capillaries are thought to be likely factors. Fortunately the tubules regenerate in the great majority of cases.

**Table 17.1** Main causes of acute renal failure.

**Prerenal**

| | |
|---|---|
| Extracellular volume loss | Gastrointestinal |
| | Urinary |
| | Burns |
| Intravascular volume loss | Sepsis |
| | Haemorrhage |
| | Hypoalbuminaemia |
| Decreased cardiac output | Heart failure |
| | Cardiac tamponade |
| Other causes | Hypercalcaemia |
| | Hepatorenal syndrome |

**Renal**

| | |
|---|---|
| Nephrotoxic agents | Analgesics |
| | Antibiotics |
| | Contrast media |
| | Heavy metals |
| | Solvents |
| Glomerulonephritis | |
| Acute interstitial nephritis | Antibiotics |
| | Analgesics |
| | Leptospirosis |
| | Viral infections |
| | Myeloma |
| Intratubular obstruction | Urate |
| Coagulopathies | Haemolytic uraemic syndrome |
| | Thrombotic thrombocytopenic purpura |
| | *Post-partum* renal failure |

**Postrenal**

| | |
|---|---|
| Renal tract obstruction | Stones |
| | Tumour (prostate, bladder, uterus, other) |
| | Retroperitoneal fibrosis |
| | Bladder dysfunction |

**Vascular**

| | |
|---|---|
| Major vessel occlusion | Renal artery thrombosis |
| | Renal artery embolism |
| | Renal artery stenosis |
| | Renal vein thrombosis |

## Renal causes

### Glomerulonephritis

A previous history of proteinuria, oedema or a nephrotic syndrome suggests the possibility of glomerulonephritis. Painful joints or a vasculitic rash, suggests the nephritis may be complicating systemic diseases, such as systemic lupus erythematosus or vasculitis. Patients with vasculitis and antiglomerular basement membrane nephritis may cough up blood (haemoptysis).

### Acute interstitial nephritis

This usually occurs secondary to antibiotics, diuretics or non-steroidal anti-inflammatory drugs and may be accompanied by fever and a rash.

## Vascular causes

Patients with renal arterial disease may present with acute renal failure. The usual setting is of a middle-aged or elderly person with a history of smoking and previous coronary or cerebral vascular disease who has already lost all or most of the function of one kidney, often silently, due to vascular disease. When the remaining kidney develops arterial thrombosis or, less frequently, an embolus complicating a myocardial infarct, ARF develops. The diagnosis is usually suspected by small but unequal-sized kidneys on ultrasound examination, and is confirmed by radionuclide scanning or arteriography to show the impaired perfusion.

Renal vein thrombosis, usually as a complication of the nephrotic syndrome (page 444), can cause ARF.

## Postrenal causes

Obstruction of the urinary tract is suggested by anuria or oliguria, occasionally alternating with polyuria. A history of a poor urinary stream suggests prostatic disease, causing obstruction in elderly men, or urethral valve obstruction in young boys. Altered bowel habit, rectal bleeding, haematuria and, in women, vaginal bleeding, suggest malignancy of the lower bowel, bladder or uterus, which has spread locally to obstruct the ureters. A story of ureteric colic suggests obstruction due to stones or renal papillae. Renal failure will only occur if the obstruction is bilateral or has developed in a solitary kidney, the other being either congenitally absent or lost through previous disease. A rare, but preventable type of ARF is due to uric acid crystallization in the renal tubules in patients with tumours, usually a leukaemia or a lymphoma. Treatment with cytotoxic drugs causes destruction of tumour cells with formation of uric acid from nucleic acids (tumour lysis syndrome (page 464).

## DIAGNOSIS

There are two requirements for a diagnosis to be made. First, the presence of ARF must be established and, second, the cause of ARF must be defined. Diagnosing ARF is not difficult – the main problem is to recognize it as a potential diagnosis. An oliguric or anuric patient with a raised plasma creatinine, with or without evidence of fluid overload in the peripheral or pulmonary circulations, has ARF until proved otherwise. The main differential diagnosis is of oliguria and a moderate rise in plasma creatinine (e.g. up to 200 μmol/l) in patients with renal hypoperfusion, usually due to hypovolaemia. In this phase, which precedes the development of acute tubular necrosis, the ratio of urea concentration in urine to plasma is raised, being at least 10:1, and urine sodium is low. In ARF, due to acute tubular necrosis, the ratio is low, being 1:1 to 4:1, and the urine sodium is not low as the renal tubules have lost their ability to conserve this ion. If the patient has been treated with diuretics to try and increase the urine flow, the measurement of urine sodium is invalidated.

Diagnosing the cause of ARF ranges from very easy, for example, in a patient with burns and sepsis with consequent hypotension and hypovolaemia, to very difficult, as in some forms of drug-induced renal failure. It is essential that obstruction, because it is so easily reversible, is excluded or proven, and therefore ultrasound examination, now widely available, should be performed. Ultrasound examination will define whether one or two kidneys are present, their size, whether obstruction is present and, if so, may demonstrate the cause, for example, stones or prostatic enlargement. If ultrasound is not available, then an intravenous urogram using a high dose of contrast medium can demonstrate the number and size of the kidneys. With the aid

of tomography (page 114) the ureters and pelvic calyceal system can be outlined to demonstrate obstruction and the level at which it is occurring.

## PLASMA CHEMISTRY

As well as assessing the degree of renal failure by measuring creatinine and urea concentrations, the plasma potassium, which is often raised in ARF and may cause sudden fatal cardiac arrhythmias, sodium and bicarbonate should be measured to assess the degree of acidaemia. The pH and concentration of oxygen and carbon dioxide in the blood should also be measured to provide further information on the acid–base status of the patient.

## URINALYSIS AND MICROSCOPY

Haematuria, proteinuria and red cell casts strongly suggest glomerulonephritis as the cause, but these abnormalities can also occur in acute tubular necrosis. White cell (granular) casts suggest infection, and eosinophils in the urine suggest interstitial nephritis caused by drugs.

## BLOOD COUNT

Acute renal failure is accompanied by anaemia which is normocytic and normochromic. Anaemia more profound than expected and accompanied by fragmented red cells indicates that disseminated intravascular coagulation (page 645) or the haemolytic uraemic syndrome (page 464) are causing the renal failure.

## BACTERIOLOGY

Acute renal failure is frequently caused by infections, especially when septicaemia complicates the underlying infection. Therefore, culture of blood, urine if available, sputum and any other substance such as diarrhoea or pus, should be performed.

## RENAL BIOPSY

This is not always required in patients with ARF, for example, when there is good historical, clinical and biochemical evidence of acute tubular necrosis. However, a renal biopsy will be necessary in patients in whom a diagnosis of glomerulonephritis or interstitial nephritis is suspected, or who have unexplained ARF.

## OTHER INVESTIGATIONS

These will be indicated by the history and examination, and will form part of the search for any underlying disorders causing the ARF. For example, if myeloma (page 636) is suspected, then electrophoresis of serum and urine, if available, for paraprotein, and bone marrow examination for histology should be done.

Two general principles in the search for a diagnosis of ARF are important. The first is that more than one cause may be producing ARF and therefore one does not stop searching for causes after one has been found. For example, an elderly patient may develop a gastrointestinal infection which causes diarrhoea with consequent hypovolaemia and hypotension, a myocardial infarction follows due to the hypotension and, finally, the patient is treated with inappropriate antibiotics which are nephrotoxic. Second, if ARF is suspected, then a small number of investigations which are swift and simple to perform can make the diagnosis, i.e. plasma and urine biochemistry and urine microscopy, the results of these being available in 1–2 hours at the most. In addition, ultrasound can be performed quickly and easily, again often within the space of an hour or two.

# Management

## INITIAL ASSESSMENT

After taking the history and examining the patient, the following investigations should be done for the reasons described above:

1. Plasma creatinine, urea, sodium, potassium and bicarbonate
2. Urine urea and sodium
3. Culture blood and urine
4. Microscopy of urine

5. Insert a bladder catheter to exclude lower urinary tract obstruction and measure urine output
6. Chest X-ray to assess pulmonary oedema
7. Insert central venous pressure line to assess hypo/hypervolaemia
8. Ultrasound of the urinary tract

With the completion of these investigations it should be clear whether the patient has prerenal failure, correction of which may prevent the establishment of ARF due to acute tubular necrosis, and whether urgent dialysis is required because of hyperkalaemia or pulmonary oedema. A plan for further investigation to establish the cause of the renal failure should be made. Obstruction will have been demonstrated or excluded. From this point on the management of the patient depends on whether the ARF is established or reversible.

## REVERSIBLE ACUTE RENAL FAILURE

If hypovolaemia is present, as shown by a low blood pressure with a postural drop and a low central venous pressure measurement, then swift correction may allow the renal function to improve. Hypovolaemia should be corrected using the appropriate fluid to compensate for that which has been lost, for example, plasma for burns, blood for haemorrhage, salt and water for diarrhoea and vomiting. The amount of replacement is assessed by central venous pressure measurement and blood pressure. This treatment must be very carefully supervised as, if the patient is not going to respond because ARF is established, too much fluid will cause pulmonary oedema. Various drugs are also used at this stage to try and improve renal perfusion. Diuretics are often used, although the evidence that they prevent the development of acute tubular necrosis is not conclusive. They should only be given when hypovolaemia has been corrected. A common method is to give intravenous frusemide to a total of 500 mg at a rate not more than 4 mg/min: high concentrations of frusemide can cause deafness. Dopamine acts as a renal vasodilator at low rates of infusion (1–5 μg/kg/min). Intravenous mannitol (10–20 g) has been used for its osmotic diuretic effect.

If the patient has heart failure as a cause of the renal hypoperfusion then measurements of the left atrial pressure, either direct or with a wedged pulmonary artery catheter, facilitate management.

If these manoeuvres are successful, then urine volume will increase and the plasma urea and creatinine will begin to fall.

## Obstructive uropathy

If obstruction is diagnosed, then rapid relief of the obstruction may prevent progression to ARF. If the obstruction is at the bladder outlet, or below, then bladder catheterization, either *per urethram* or suprapubically, will suffice. However, although the ultrasound examination defines obstruction, the level and cause of obstruction are quite commonly not evident. Percutaneous nephrostomy, which allows urine to drain from the kidneys and antegrade ureteropyelography (page 447) which will define the site of obstruction, and possibly its pathology, is the next step.

If correction of hypovolaemia or obstruction results in urine output, then great care must be taken to maintain the patient in proper water and electrolyte balance, replacing the losses in the urine and making good any pre-existing deficits.

## ESTABLISHED ACUTE RENAL FAILURE

Whatever the cause, the following factors are important in the management of established renal failure.

## Dialysis

The indications for dialysis are:
- Plasma urea concentration greater than 30 mmol/l
- Plasma potassium concentration greater than 7.0 mmol/l
- Pulmonary oedema
- Acidosis – with a pH of 7.2 or less
- A poor or deteriorating clinical state, even if none of the above requirements is met

The above are to be interpreted with common sense, for example, if it is clear that a patient has

established ARF, is septic and has a plasma potassium of 6.8 mmol/l, there is no point waiting until it reaches 7.0 mmol/l to begin dialysis.

The main modes of dialysis are:

1. Peritoneal dialysis can be used for patients with mild degrees of renal failure, i.e. not hypercatabolic.
2. Haemodialysis, which will require an arteriovenous shunt, or insertion of a central venous catheter (neckline) for access to the circulation is required for hypercatabolic patients and can only be done by suitably trained staff.
3. Haemofiltration, performed continuously, will allow removal by ultrafiltration of water, urea, creatinine and ions from plasma. It is an attractive alternative to intermittent dialysis as it does not require highly trained staff and is more easily tolerated by patients with poor cardiac function and hypotension.

## Hyperkalaemia

This is a lethal complication of ARF because it can cause cardiac arrest. The plasma potassium concentration can rise extremely quickly, particularly in patients who are hypercatabolic due to infection and trauma. Measures to reduce the hyperkalaemia will often be required before dialysis can commence. Hyperkalaemia should be treated by:

1. Infusion of dextrose and insulin: this causes potassium to move into cells and therefore total body potassium is not affected.
2. Calcium gluconate intravenously reduces the effect of high potassium concentration on cardiac muscle, but does not alter potassium concentration.
3. Cation exchange resins, given either orally or per rectum, will exchange calcium in the resin for potassium in the circulation. This is a slow procedure and will not be effective in reducing a potentially lethal hyperkalaemia.

## Fluid and electrolyte balance

The patient must be regularly assessed for the state of hydration by accurate measurement of fluid intake, output, weight, blood pressure and central venous pressure. Fluid intake is restricted to 500 ml daily, plus extra loss via the urinary and gastrointestinal tracts. The intakes of sodium and potassium are restricted according to losses and dialysis.

## Acidaemia

If the patient is acidotic then dialysis is indicated; hypertonic sodium bicarbonate may cause pulmonary oedema if used as the sole treatment because of the sodium and water overload.

## Drugs

Daily review of the drug chart is an important part of management. Many drugs are excreted by the kidneys and will therefore accumulate in renal failure with possible toxic effects. Dialysis and haemofiltration variably affect the clearance of drugs; it must not be assumed that all drugs will be cleared from the circulation by these treatments.

## Gastrointestinal bleeding

There is a high risk of gastrointestinal bleeding in ARF, and prophylaxis with histamine type 2 receptor ($H_2$) antagonists (e.g. cimetidine/ranitidine), antacids and sucralfate is advisable. Magnesium-containing antacids can cause hypermagnesemia and should be avoided.

## Nutrition

Although urea is derived from protein, restricting protein can lead to a negative nitrogen balance which, in the medium and long term, is deleterious for the patient. A large amount of muscle mass can be lost and the immune response will be depressed, making infection more likely. A diet of 1 g of protein per kg of body weight and 14 000 kJ/day is the aim. As the patients are often unwell, or have nausea and anorexia due to uraemia, enteral or parenteral feeding may be required. These procedures require large volumes of fluid to deliver these amounts of protein and calories, and so daily dialysis or continuous haemofiltration will be necessary.

# Prognosis

The prognosis of ARF overall is poor, the mortality rate being 50 per cent. Any disease which develops ARF as a complication increases its mortality rate eightfold. Within these figures lies a range of survival. Thus, a young previously fit person with only ARF and without complications has an almost 100 per cent chance of survival, whereas an elderly patient with ARF complicated by septicaemia, respiratory failure and bleeding will only have a 10 per cent chance of survival.

The prognosis for return of renal function depends on the disease causing the ARF. Most patients with acute tubular necrosis have a full return of renal function, which may take as long as 8 weeks. During the recovery period the patient must be assessed for hypovolaemia, hyponatraemia and hypokalaemia due to the impaired function of the recovering tubules. A very small number of patients with acute tubular necrosis may have sustained such severe ischaemic damage that they develop necrosis of the renal cortex and chronic renal failure.

# CHRONIC RENAL FAILURE

Chronic renal failure (CRF) is a permanent reduction in glomerular filtration rate (GFR) caused by a loss of nephrons. A raised plasma urea or creatinine concentration does not define CRF as these biochemical abnormalities can occur in acute renal failure, and in the early stages of reduction of GFR the plasma urea and creatinine will not be raised (Fig. 17.1).

# Epidemiology

In the UK and similar countries all ages are affected, but the incidence rises with age, especially in those over 60 years. Treatment is not necessarily indicated in all patients, for example, if a malignancy with a poor prognosis is causing CRF. The incidence of patients requiring treatment is therefore calculated at 50–80/ million per annum.

# Aetiology

The main causes of CRF are shown in Table 17.2 in approximate order of frequency. Diabetes mellitus, both insulin and non-insulin dependent is increasing, whereas glomerulonephritis is decreasing in incidence, albeit gradually.

**Table 17.2** Causes of chronic and end-stage renal failure.

| Cause | % (approx.) |
| --- | --- |
| Glomerulonephritis | 25 |
| Diabetes mellitus* | 20 |
| Hypertension | 10 |
| Pyelonephritis/reflux nephropathy | 10 |
| Polycystic kidneys | 10 |
| Interstitial nephritis | 5 |
| Obstruction | 3 |
| Miscellaneous | 5 |
| Unknown† | 12 |

*The incidence of chronic renal failure due to diabetes mellitus is increasing, and in some countries, e.g. USA, it is now the commonest cause.
†'Unknown' usually means the patient has two very small kidneys – too small to biopsy – and there is no past history to suggest a diagnosis.

# Pathophysiology and effects

The metabolism of the body is very disordered in CRF. The reasons are complicated and still not completely understood. The main abnormalities are due to the disordered physiology of the diseased kidney, the effects of uraemia on the tissues and organs of the body, and the impaired endocrine function of the kidney.

## DISORDERED PHYSIOLOGY

As the number of nephrons reduces, whatever the cause, certain physiological effects inevitably occur. The GFR falls, and so urea and creatinine plasma concentrations rise. The remaining nephrons have to deal with an increased solute load and eventually they become unable to concentrate urine. This causes polyuria and thirst, and a failure to compensate for salt and water loss, for example, if the patient is vomiting or has diarrhoea. In the early stages of CRF there may be a 'salt-losing nephropathy' due to excessive sodium loss in the urine. As more nephrons are lost, sodium retention occurs after the maximum filtration fraction of sodium is passed. Fluid retention in the lungs and peripheries, and systemic hypertension result. Failure to excrete potassium, hydrogen, phosphate and urate also follow from the lack of nephrons, with consequent hyperkalaemia, acidaemia and phosphate retention leading to osteodystrophy (see below) and gout from urate retention.

Urea and creatinine themselves have slight or no toxicity; the effects of uraemia are due to the retention of molecules which are still not clearly defined but are normally excreted by the kidney. The term 'uraemia' is a handy label and measurements of plasma urea and creatinine are biochemical signs of renal failure.

## EFFECTS OF URAEMIA ON TISSUE AND ORGANS

The accumulating toxic metabolites in uraemia affect many parts of the body. Most symptoms occur late in the course of CRF when the GFR is 10–15 ml/min.

### Gastrointestinal tract

Anorexia, nausea and vomiting are common symptoms: with the attendant weight loss a mistaken diagnosis of carcinoma of the stomach is sometimes made. The incidence of peptic ulceration is increased, owing to raised gastrin levels; any peptic ulcers which develop have an increased tendency to bleed (see below).

## Skin

Itching is a common and distressing symptom in uraemia. The cause is not completely understood, but is thought to be related to retained phosphate, increased parathormone secretion and increased histamine concentrations. The combination of anaemia (see below) and retained urochromes, which are breakdown products of haemoglobin giving urine its normal yellow brown colour, give the skin a characteristic unhealthy pale, sallow, browny tinge. When urea concentrations are extremely high urea may crystallize in the sweat and give an appearance on the skin known as uraemic frost. This is very rare.

## Blood and bone marrow

Uraemia depresses bone marrow function and, combined with erythroprotein deficiency (see below) causes a normocytic, normochromic anaemia. Red cell survival is decreased in uraemia. There is also an increased bleeding tendency due to platelet dysfunction and fragility of the capillary walls.

## Nervous system

Tiredness and impaired mental ability, often noted by the patient, and frequently accompanied by depression and irritability, are common symptoms. If not treated, then, as CRF progresses, drowsiness, fits and coma will ensue. In the elderly these symptoms of uraemia may be put down to 'old age' or 'dementia'. Peripheral neuropathy may occur in the late stages of CRF.

## Cardiovascular system

Hypertension, due to kidney disease (page 220) and fluid retention combine to cause heart failure with pulmonary and peripheral oedema. Patients with CRF have an increased incidence of coronary artery disease due to atheroma, which is related to hypercholesterolaemia, hypertriglyceridaemia, increased low density lipids and reduced high density lipids, all of which are caused in an unknown way by CRF.

## Bones

Renal osteodystrophy is a complex mixture of increased bone resorption due to secondary hyperparathyroidism and inadequate vitamin D production and therefore osteomalacia (page 503). Chronically diseased kidneys are less able to hydroxylate vitamin D from its 25-OH form to the 1-25-OH form, thus causing vitamin D deficiency. The secondary hyperparathyroidism is due to a sequence of phosphate retention, due to diminished GFR which, in turn, causes hypocalcaemia which stimulates the parathyroid glands to increase parathormone secretion. Eventually the increased parathormone secretion may become autonomous and cause hypercalcaemia with all its complications (page 500). In its early stages renal osteodystrophy may be asymptomatic, but if unchecked it will cause bone pain and, in particular, the proximal myopathy of osteomalacia.

## DIMINISHED ENDOCRINE FUNCTION

The kidneys are the body's main source of erythroprotein and lack of this hormone in CRF contributes to the characteristic anaemia. Hyperreninaemia develops in some patients and contributes to the development of hypertension but hyperreninaemia is not present in every patient with CRF. Vitamin D deficiency also occurs (see above).

# Presenting features

Because CRF can disturb so many parts of the body and its functions it may present in many different ways and thus, in hospital practice, to many different medical and surgical specialties. In practice, the presenting features of CRF can be grouped as follows.

## TYPICAL SYMPTOMS

Typically a patient exhibits malaise, tiredness, drowsiness, anorexia and vomiting with weight loss, itching and fluid retention.

## EFFECTS AND COMPLICATIONS OF CHRONIC RENAL FAILURE

These have been described above and may occur in various combinations with or without the typical symptoms. In children an important effect of CRF is failure to grow and, in babies, failure to thrive.

## ACUTE RENAL FAILURE

The first clue that the patient has CRF may be presentation with acute renal failure superimposed on the chronic disease. The more severe the CRF the less the severity of the insult required to cause acute renal failure because of the diminished reserve of GFR. Relatively benign events in normal healthy people, such as a chest infection or elective surgery, may be sufficient to cause this presentation.

## SYMPTOMLESS CHRONIC RENAL FAILURE

A routine medical examination may reveal hypertension, proteinuria or haematuria, all of which indicate measurement of plasma urea or creatinine. Alternatively, the patient may present with features due to an underlying disease which is causing symptomless chronic renal failure, for example, a patient with stones and CRF may present with loin pain, ureteric colic, urinary infection or macroscopic haematuria; another patient may present with the nephrotic syndrome.

# Diagnosis

As with acute renal failure, diagnosis consists of two stages. First the functional impairment needs to be defined, either by measuring the GFR if the plasma urea or creatinine are not significantly elevated or, in the later stages, the abnormal plasma biochemistry will suffice. To prove that the loss of function is at least partly permanent, evidence of structural damage to the kidney is required. Imaging techniques, such as ultrasound, intravenous urography or radionuclide scanning will show gross structural changes and reduction in normal kidney tissue, such as polycystic kidneys, bilaterally small kidneys or obstruction causing hydronephrosis. If imaging shows apparently normal kidneys, then renal biopsy will be indicated to search for structural damage at a microscopic level, for example, glomerulonephritis.

Second, the cause of CRF must be defined as it may require treatment in its own right, which may also prevent possible progression of the CRF. Examples of these important conditions are stone formation, treatable forms of glomerulonephritis, such as vasculitis, hypertension and renovascular disease (Fig. 17.3). If the patient will eventually require transplantation for end-stage renal failure, the cause may be relevant because of the possibility of recurrent disease.

# Management

Management has two aims: to prevent decline in renal function and thereby, if possible, to avoid end-stage renal failure, and to prevent complications.

## PREVENTING DECLINE

Patients with CRF often have reversible factors which, if not treated, would certainly promote decline in renal function. These reversible factors are:

1. Hypertension
2. Obstruction
3. Infection
4. Electrolyte and fluid retention
5. Dietary factors

There may also be **exacerbation of a primary cause** such as a flare-up in an inflammatory condition, for example, vasculitis or systemic lupus, or reformation of stones which can worsen function. These are, in their different ways, preventable.

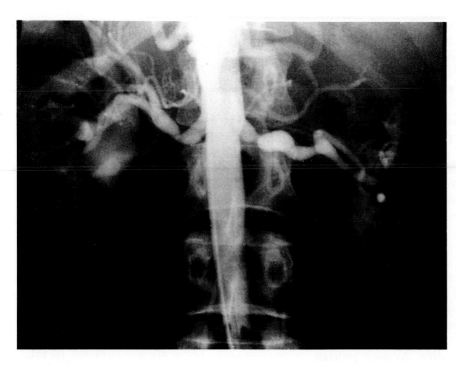

**Figure 17.3** Renal arteriogram in a 20-year-old woman showing fibromuscular hyperplasia causing renal stenosis of both renal arteries. Note the smooth, beaded appearance with stenosis and dilations. The patient presented with hypertension and a moderate degree of renal failure, both of which were cured by percutaneous angioplasty. In this patient the arteriogram was obtained by injecting the aorta through a catheter inserted into a femoral artery; the catheter can be seen ascending the right side of the aorta.

## Hypertension

Unless the patient has a salt-wasting nephropathy, hypertension is almost universal in CRF, either secondary to the renal disease or as the primary disorder causing it. Meticulous control of blood pressure in CRF reduces the rate of its progression. Conventional treatment such as β-blockers (e.g. propranolol), vasodilators (e.g. prazosin) and calcium antagonists (e.g. nifedipine) are effective. Atenolol, a β-blocker with a long half-life, and which is renally excreted, should be used with extreme care when the GFR is below 50 ml/min. Loop diuretics (e.g. frusemide) can be used for their hypotensive effect, but at low values of GFR they become ineffectual, and diuretics such as bendrofluazide used to treat mild hypertension with normal or slightly impaired renal function, are inadequate. More recently angiotensin-converting enzyme (ACE) inhibitors (e.g. captopril) have been effectively used, but if renal artery stenosis is present they may cause deterioration in renal function (page 220).

## Obstruction

Any cause of obstruction (page 446) must be relieved. A surprising degree of long-standing recovery of renal function can result.

## Infection

Infection in the urinary tract must be eradicated; nephrotoxic antibiotics should be avoided.

## Electrolyte and fluid depletion

Gross lack of salt and water is easily detected, but patients with CRF may have a surprising amount of negative salt and water balance which has developed slowly. Postural hypotension and a low jugular venous pressure point to this condition.

## Drugs

Nephrotoxic drugs must be removed from the patient's medication and proscribed rather than prescribed.

## Dietary factors

Much attention has been paid to dietary means of preventing deterioration in CRF in recent years.

### Protein restriction

Observations in experimental animals and humans have shown that an increased protein intake in CRF causes glomerular hyperfiltration and glomerular hypertension. These dynamic glomerular changes cause structural damage and reduction in protein intake reverses the physiological and structural changes and results in prolonged survival in animals. These observations remain controversial, particularly in their application to humans, and the case for protein restriction remains unproven and is the subject of current large-scale trials. Nonetheless, some physicians advise a low protein diet of approximately 0.6 g of protein per kg of body weight; it is important to avoid a negative nitrogen balance, which will simply make the patient ill. If a low protein diet is used it is not yet clear at what stage of renal failure it should be introduced.

### Phosphate restriction

A similar case has been made for reducing dietary phosphate intake. This, however, is a difficult aim as it usually entails decreased calcium intake which can worsen renal osteodystrophy. Phosphate binders can be given by mouth to reduce phosphate availability. As with protein restriction the indications for phosphate restriction are not available.

## PREVENTING OR TREATING COMPLICATIONS

### Renal osteodystrophy

The mainstays of treatment are to maintain plasma calcium and phosphate concentrations in the normal range. The plasma calcium is low in chronic renal failure and should be elevated into the normal range by treatment with vitamin D analogues such as 1-hydroxycholecalciferol, or 1,25-dihydroxycholecalciferol. Hypercalcaemia should be avoided as it can cause further impairment of renal function, pruritis, vomiting and metastatic calcification. The plasma phosphate is elevated in CRF and should be reduced by dietary restriction and use of phosphate binders, the most appropriate of which is calcium carbonate. This can cause hypercalcaemia, but aluminium hydroxide can be used as an alternative. However, excessive use of aluminium phosphate binders can cause severe side effects, such as dementia and a bone disease similar to renal osteodystrophy. If aluminium phosphate binders are used then plasma aluminium concentration should be monitored.

### Hypertension

Chronic renal disease is likely to cause hypertension and it should therefore be treated as described above.

### Acidaemia

Symptoms are not usually profound, but when the plasma bicarbonate concentration is 15 mmol/l or less, sodium bicarbonate can be used to treat acidaemia. However, the extra sodium load may prove a problem by contributing to hypertension and fluid retention.

### Anaemia

The availability in the last few years of human erythropoietin produced by genetic engineering has transformed the treatment of anaemia. Hitherto this depended on blood transfusion which, although practicable, has two major disadvantages. These are sensitization to HLA antigens which reduces the chances of finding a compatible kidney for transplantation, and the development of iron overload. Erythropoietin, although a normal human substance, is not free of side effects when used as a drug; it can cause hypertension, hyperkalaemia and cerebrovascular accidents. The aim is to achieve a haemoglobin of 10–11 g/per dl of plasma. Many symptoms improve, such as tiredness and poor exercise tolerance.

### Peripheral neuropathy

Little can be done for peripheral neuropathy apart from dialysis or transplantation, and excluding other factors which may contribute, such as drugs.

### Hyperlipidaemia

This causes atheroma and therefore an increased incidence of coronary artery and cerebrovascular disease in CRF. With hypertension and anaemia it contributes to the heart failure which can develop in anaemia.

### Sexual dysfunction

Patients suffer both a loss of libido and infertility. The latter is curable only by a successful renal transplant.

# *Prognosis*

Chronic renal failure, by definition, is permanent, but not all patients inevitably progress to end-stage renal failure requiring dialysis and transplantation. Whether progression occurs depends on two important factors, which are the amount of remaining and salvageable renal tissue at the time of diagnosis of CRF, and the underlying cause, which may range from being completely reversible to untreatable. Thus, for example, a patient with a plasma creatinine level of 200 µmol/l due to renal stones which have caused obstruction and infection may have no more deterioration if the stones are removed, obstruction relieved and infection swiftly treated, and then further infections prevented. On the other hand, a patient with glomerulonephritis, such as focal sclerosing glomerulosclerosis (page 459) who, at presentation, also has a plasma creatinine of 200 µmol/l will, with only rare exceptions, progress to end-stage renal failure in 5–10 years.

Part of the management of chronic renal failure includes the preparation, both physical and mental, of patients who will develop end-stage renal failure for appropriate treatment.

# *E*ND-STAGE RENAL FAILURE

End-stage renal failure (ESRF), or terminal renal failure, occurs when kidney function is so poor that the patient requires treatment by dialysis or transplantation in order to survive. The causes and presentation are similar to those of chronic renal failure, as described above, and are shown in Table 17.2. The patient may be treated by haemodialysis, chronic peritoneal dialysis or transplantation. These forms of treatment are interchangeable and over months or years an individual patient may employ each in various sequences, depending upon circumstances.

# *Haemodialysis*

Blood from the patient is passed through an extracorporeal circulation system and exposed to dialysis fluid, from which the blood is separated by an artificial semipermeable membrane. Solutes at high concentration in the blood will pass to low concentration in the dialysis fluid across the semipermeable membrane, sometimes known as the artificial kidney. Haemodialysis equipment is based on a complex machine which generates the dialysis fluid from a concentrate, has pumps to circulate the blood through the extracorporeal circulation, and has many inbuilt safety checks and alarms. Modern machines have electronic controls which can adjust the machine's function during dialysis according to the patient's individual requirements. The artificial kidney itself is small and disposable, and is constructed of either hollow fibres or layered plates with a total surface area of approximately 1 m². To provide access to the haemodialysis machine the patient has an arteriovenous fistula fashioned in the forearm by joining a major artery and vein, usually the radial vessels (Fig. 17.4). A successful fistula should supply blood at approximately 200 ml/ min to the machine.

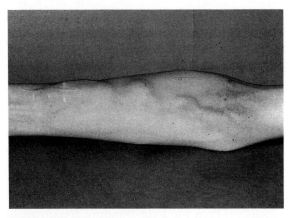

**Figure 17.4** Arteriovenous fistula in the forearm of a patient on haemodialysis. Note the tortuous and dilated vein and the surgical scar over the radial artery where this vessel was joined to the accompanying vein to form the fistula.

These days patients require 8–12 hours of haemodialysis each week in two or three sessions. Patients can be trained to dialyse themselves at home, ideally with the help of a relative, and thus gain independence from the hospital.

Patients must restrict their intake of potassium to 60 mmol/day, and their sodium and fluid intake according to their urine output. Many patients with ESRF continue to pass some urine. Failure to follow these restrictions will result in hyperkalaemia, hypertension and peripheral and pulmonary oedema.

## COMPLICATIONS OF HAEMODIALYSIS

### Hypotension and cramps

These are usually due to excess or too rapid removal of salt and water and usually respond to adjustments in sodium concentration in the dialysis fluid, or altering the rate of removal. Cramps can be a persistent problem, however, and curiously often respond to quinine, better known for its antimalarial effect.

### Hypertension

As patients have largely lost their renal function their blood pressure is very dependent on their salt and water balance. If this is properly controlled, then usually antihypertensive drugs can be stopped. A minority of patients continue to require them, and amongst these are a few patients who have severe hypertension due to hyperreninaemia. Extreme thirst and weight loss are typical in these patients who may need bilateral nephrectomy.

### Anaemia

Anaemia occurs because of erythropoietin deficiency, as described above in the section on chronic renal failure. Erythropoietin, given intravenously, or subcutaneously, will cure the anaemia. If erythropoietin is unavailable, or, for financial reasons, cannot be supplied (it is very expensive) then the long-standing treatment of intermittent blood transfusions may be used. This has two potential disadvantages: sensitization to HLA antigens, making cross-matching a kidney for transplantation difficult, and iron

overload which may cause haemochromatosis (page 401).

### Renal osteodystrophy

This problem continues in dialysis patients, but is treated as described under chronic renal failure.

### Dialysis arthropathy

In recent years it has become clear that patients who have been on haemodialysis for 10 years or so develop an unusual type of amyloid which affects the bones and joints. The amyloid deposits consist of $\beta_2$-microglobulin, a normal serum protein with raised plasma levels in chronic and end-stage renal failure. Particular sites affected are the shoulder joints and wrists, where carpal tunnel syndrome (page 689) may develop. At present there is no treatment to reverse or prevent the amyloid deposition other than transplantation. Carpal tunnel syndrome will require surgical treatment.

### Hyperlipidaemia

Type II hyperlipidaemia, i.e. elevated concentrations of triglyceride and very low density lipoproteins, is common and contributes to the high rate of cardiovascular complications.

### Cardiovascular disease

There is an increased incidence of atheroma, particularly affecting the coronary arteries, with an increased mortality and morbidity due to myocardial and cerebral infarction.

### Cystic renal disease

Whatever the original renal disease causing ESRF, patients on long-term dialysis may develop cysts in the kidney which, in turn, may cause haematuria or develop into benign or malignant tumours.

### Aluminium toxicity

Aluminium hydroxide was the favoured method of preventing phosphate retention in the long-term to control renal osteodystrophy. The water used for dialysis may also contain a high concentration of aluminium, depending on the local water authority. Aluminium is retained in ESRF and may cause an osteodystrophy and an encephalopathy, which is often fatal, during the course of which the patient becomes distressingly demented (dialysis dementia). Treatment relies on prevention by using other phosphate binders, such as calcium carbonate, reducing the aluminium level in the dialysate and, if the patient has high aluminium plasma levels, then removal by desferrioxamine, a chelating agent, is indicated.

# Chronic peritoneal dialysis

The basis of this is extremely simple, relying on a permanent dialysis catheter in the abdomen, through which dialysis fluid is inserted and then drained out, using the peritoneal membrane as the dialysis membrane. Most patients employ continuous ambulatory peritoneal dialysis (CAPD) which, as the term implies, allows the patient to be mobile while dialysis is performed, in contrast to haemodialysis. On average a patient performs four exchanges of fluid every day, at approximately 6-hourly intervals. A variation is intermittent peritoneal dialysis which may be performed only at night by using a machine which automatically inserts and drains fluid from the peritoneal cavity and relieves the patient of these chores during the day.

## COMPLICATIONS OF PERITONEAL DIALYSIS

### Infection
The exit site of the catheter and the track along which the catheter runs are prone to infections because they are exposed to the open air. They require treatment with appropriate antibiotics and if this is not successful the catheter may have to be removed and resited. Peritonitis is, unfortunately, a common complication, but not so common as to exclude this mode of treatment. The commonest organisms are *Escherichia coli* and Enterobacter species.

### Catheter displacement or obstruction
The ideal position of the catheter is deep in the pelvis. It may wander from there and poor drainage may result, or the omentum may block the catheter tip. In both of these instances the catheter will need repositioning.

### Loss of ultrafiltration
Because of infection or adhesions the peritoneal membrane may become inefficient as a dialysing membrane, and then this mode of treatment will have to be abandoned. A rare complication is sclerosing peritonitis in which the peritoneum becomes fibrotic and may cause intestinal obstruction.

# Other consequences of dialysis

It is important to realize that any form of dialysis does not cure uraemia, unlike transplantation. The patient remains in chronic renal failure and remains prone to its effects and complications. The burden of having to live with long-term treatment can cause psychological stress, with social consequences, not only for the patient but also for the family. Dialysis patients have an increased rate of divorce and suicide.

# Renal transplantation

Ideally, all patients should be assessed for transplantation as it provides the only cure for chronic renal failure. There are two forms of transplantation: cadaveric and live donor transplantation.

## CADAVERIC TRANSPLANTATION

This is the main source of kidneys in the UK and similar countries. Most donors come from intensive care units where they have been declared brain dead following the strict application of rigorous tests (page 263). As the cardiovascular system is still intact, i.e. the donor's heart is beating at the time of donor nephrectomy, the kidneys have not been ischaemic. Most donors will have died from accidents, cerebrovascular accidents or suicide. Occasionally donors who have died without being on a ventilator but with a functioning cardiovascular system are used, but the donor kidneys must be taken quickly before ischaemia causes permanent damage.

## LIVE DONOR TRANSPLANTATION

In most instances the donor is a first degree blood relative, i.e. a parent, child or sibling. Blood group compatibility is required. Occasionally second degree relatives i.e. aunts, uncles, nephews, nieces or first cousins are used. Unrelated living donors are used in the UK in only very exceptional circumstances, but are a common source of kidneys in developing countries where cadaveric donation is either unacceptable for religious or cultural reasons, or not practicable for administrative and medical reasons.

Living donor nephrectomy does not affect renal function in the long term, although there is some evidence that some donors may develop very mild hypertension.

## PROCEDURE

Transplanted kidneys are placed in an iliac fossa with anastomosis of the donor vessels to the recipient's iliac vessels and of the donor ureter to the recipient's bladder. If the graft does not function immediately dialysis will be required. Apart from urine output and plasma creatinine and urea measurement, assessment of the graft relies on radionuclide scanning techniques which measure renal perfusion and excretion, and percutaneous biopsy to exclude rejection. The patient requires immunosuppression and the following drugs are used in various combinations:

1. Prednisolone, which reduces the numbers of circulating B- and T-cells and inter-leukin-2 (IL-2) production
2. Azathioprine, which prevents a primary antibody response
3. Cyclosporin A, which prevents activation of T-cells by preventing IL-2 production
4. Antilymphocyte sera, polyclonal or monoclonal, to remove lymphocytes

These drugs are used for three purposes: to initiate immunosuppression at the time of trans-

plantation, to treat rejection which affects most patients, and for long-term maintenance of immunosuppression. There are no agreed best protocols for any of these three indications, consequently there is considerable variation between transplant units and the details of the drug regimes.

## COMPLICATIONS

Early infections (particularly viral, fungal and parasitic) are common and may be fatal. Cytomegalovirus infection, usually acquired from the donor of the kidney, causes a swinging fever which may be accompanied by leukopenia, hepatitis and impairment of graft function. Lung infection due to cytomegalovirus, tuberculosis, or aspergillosis may occur, but pneumonia due to *Pneumocystis carinii* is the most serious problem because of its high fatality rate. Treatment with high dose cotrimoxazole or pentamidine is life-saving. Brain infections with Nocardia, Herpes simplex and Cryptococcus occur and are difficult to diagnose and eradicate. Other early complications include those related to corticosteroids, azathioprine, wound infections and renal artery stenosis. Most cases of acute rejection which can cause graft failure occur during the first 3 months.

The most important late complication is malignancy. There is a two or three times greater chance of developing cancer, but some specific tumours such as microglioma of the brain, skin cancer (both basal cell and squamous) and lymphoma are very much more common. Other late complications include graft failure due to chronic rejection or recurrent or *de novo* glomerulonephritis. Avascular necrosis of bone is common with high-dose steroid regimens. There is an increased rate of cardiovascular disease.

## PROGNOSIS

Graft survival is 80–85 per cent at 1 year, and 50–60 per cent at 5 years. Patient survival depends on age and underlying fitness, for example, patients with diabetes mellitus causing ESRF have a worse prognosis than non-diabetics. Transplant patients have a lower life expectancy than normal due to cardiovascular disease and malignancy.

# PROTEINURIA

Proteinuria is the presence of protein in the urine which can range from low but normal values to large amounts which cause serious disease.

Many patients are found to have proteinuria during a routine medical examination. Patients with slight proteinuria, i.e. 'trace' or '1+' on stick testing should have repeated urinalysis to confirm its presence. Occasional positive tests in this range are usually of no importance, especially if unaccompanied by haematuria. If, however, a consistent slight proteinuria is confirmed, or if it is immediately clear that there is moderate or heavy proteinuria, it should be quantified by a 24-hour urine collection. The normal range of proteinuria varies between laboratories and is usually quoted as 200–400 mg/24 hours. It is more accurate at these low levels to express the proteinuria as $mg/m^2$ of body surface for 24 hours; more than 200 $mg/m^2$ is abnormal.

In the nephrotic syndrome the proteinuria is usually greater than 3 g/24 hours. Many text books and papers now quote a 'nephrotic' proteinuria and variously define it between 3 and 5 g/24 hours (page 444).

## PATHOGENESIS

Proteinuria is caused by damage to either the glomeruli or the tubules. Glomerular proteinuria is much more common. It is a result of increased permeability of the glomerulus. Normally blood in the glomerular capillaries is separated from the glomerular filtrate in the urinary space by:

- The fenestrated capillary endothelium
- The glomerular basement membrane which consists of glycoproteins and collagen
- The glomerular epithelium which covers the surface of the glomerulus exposed to the urinary space

These structures, together, form the barrier to the loss of large molecules such as albumen by providing a physical barrier and also a charge barrier. These three structures, and particularly the glomerular basement membrane, are negatively charged, and therefore repel negatively charged molecules such as albumen and other proteins. Glomerular permeability is increased either by structural damage or by chemical alterations, causing loss of negative charge.

## PRESENTING FEATURES

Proteinuria may present with no symptoms, the proteinuria having been found on routine examination. Alternatively it may be discovered when a patient complains of macroscopic haematuria, for example, in glomerulonephritis, or presents with a nephrotic syndrome (see below), an acute nephritic syndrome (see below) or with the features of a systemic disease which has glomerular involvement such as diabetes mellitus. Asymptomatic proteinuria and the nephrotic syndrome are considered at this point while the remaining topics are dealt with elsewhere.

## MANAGEMENT OF ASYMPTOMATIC PROTEINURIA

It is first necessary to show that the proteinuria is significant by demonstrating that it is persistent and that it is above the normal 24-hour excretion value. Thus repeated urine testing followed by a 24-hour urine collection and analysis will either exclude or indicate further investigation. If the proteinuria is significant the patient has renal disease and requires further investigation. The history may elicit points indicating systemic disease, for example, diabetes mellitus or systemic lupus. Family history is important as some types of nephritis and other conditions such as polycystic kidneys are inherited. Important points in the physical examination are blood pressure since if the patient is hypertensive then it indicates that the renal disease is serious.

Microscopic examination of the urine can prove the presence of glomerular disease if red cell or granular casts are found. Glomerular filtration rate should be measured to assess whether kidney function is reduced. Patients with significant proteinuria who also have hypertension, diminished GFR and/or suspected systemic disease, should have a renal biopsy. This investigation is not so clearly indicated if the only abnormality is proteinuria between 0.5 and 1 g/24 hours because, with a normal GFR and with no ill effects from this proteinuria, there will be no improvement from any treatment of the renal disease. Patients themselves often wish to have a renal biopsy to establish the prognosis, or to clarify their suitability for employment.

The treatment of a patient with proteinuria depends on the underlying cause (Table 17.3).

## PROGNOSIS

This is very dependent upon the underlying disease. Patients with persistent small amounts of proteinuria have no long-term increased morbidity or mortality.

**Table 17.3** Common causes of proteinuria.

**Excretion of excess plasma proteins**
Myeloma

**Glomerulonephritis**

**Tubular disease**
Interstitial nephritis
Acute tubular necrosis
Specific tubular defects

**Vascular disease**
Hypertension
Renal vein thrombosis

**Bladder/prostate**
Infections
Tumours

# NEPHROTIC SYNDROME

The nephrotic syndrome is the combination of proteinuria, hypoalbuminaemia and oedema. The definition does not include any degree of renal failure; the nephrotic syndrome can occur in patients with a normal GFR. Although the nephrotic syndrome is sometimes defined as proteinuria greater than 3–5 g/24 hours ('nephrotic proteinuria'), this is incorrect unless hypoalbuminaemia and oedema have developed. It is important to realize that not all patients with this amount of proteinuria will develop a nephrotic syndrome. The biochemical consequences of heavy proteinuria often depend upon the age of the patient. In young patients who have good hepatic function the liver can compensate by increased protein synthesis for the proteinuria (and hypoalbuminaemia), whereas in elderly people the liver has a much reduced capacity for increasing protein synthesis and such patients become nephrotic at lower values of proteinuria.

## CAUSES

Many diseases can cause a nephrotic syndrome. They are best thought of as primary, in which the kidney alone is diseased, or secondary, in which the kidney is involved as part of a systemic disease. Table 17.4 shows the commonest causes of nephrotic syndrome.

## PRESENTING FEATURES

The patient complains of oedema of the feet and legs, and may note swelling of the hands and face, particularly in the mornings, after having redistributed the excess body fluid when asleep during the night. Heavy proteinuria causes frothy urine and some patients will spontaneously describe this. Other patients may present with a complication of the nephrotic syndrome (see below) or with the symptoms and signs of underlying disease in secondary nephrotic syndrome.

## MANAGEMENT

This is aimed at treating the underlying cause of the nephrotic syndrome, or lessening the effects of the heavy proteinuria. The former will depend on the underlying disorder (Tables 17.3 and 17.4). The main target in the second aim is to reduce the oedema, which is achieved with varying degrees of success by diuretics. Large doses of powerful diuretics are frequently required, for example, frusemide, 500 mg bd or metolazone, 2.5 mg bd. The additional diuretic

**Table 17.4** Causes of nephrotic syndrome.

**Primary forms of glomerulonephritis**
Membranous nephropathy
Minimal change nephropathy
Focal glomerulosclerosis
Mesangiocapillary glomerulonephritis

**Systemic diseases**
Diabetes mellitus
Amyloidosis
Vasculitis
Systemic lupus erythematosus
Henoch–Schönlein purpura
Cryoglobulinaemia

**Infections**
Streptococcal and staphylococcal infections
Malaria
Schistosomiasis
Hepatitis B
Syphilis

**Drugs**
Gold
Penicillamine
'Street' heroin

**Tumours**
Carcinoma
Sarcoma
Leukaemia and lymphoma

**Familial disorders**
Congenital nephrotic syndrome

**Miscellaneous conditions**
Renal vein thrombosis
Allergic reaction to insect bites, pollen and vaccines

effects of amiloride which acts on the distal tube, and of spironolactone, which inhibits the action of aldosterone, are often helpful. Care must be taken not to produce too rapid a diuresis as this can cause hypovolaemia, hypotension and acute renal failure; elderly people and children are particularly susceptible to this iatrogenic effect of diuretics, which can be fatal. Some patients are so nephrotic that they require admission for intravenous protein in the form of plasma or albumen to raise the plasma concentration of protein. Although frequently practised, it is not completely evident that this is appropriate treatment, as increasing the plasma concentration of protein often simply causes increased proteinuria. In very resistant cases salt and water restriction are necessary, but they should not be employed routinely as they are not pleasant forms of treatment and are not usually necessary with the diuretics now available.

## COMPLICATIONS

### Thrombosis

Loss of antithrombin III in the urine and increased plasma concentrations of factor VIII and fibrinogen cause hypercoagulability. Patients are often immobile and have a high haematocrit because of loss of intravascular fluid. Any vessel, artery or vein, may thrombose, but the commonest are the deep veins of the legs and pelvis, with consequent pulmonary embolism as a further complication, or the renal veins themselves, which can cause even heavier proteinuria, or acute renal failure.

### Acute renal failure

This may complicate the nephrotic syndrome as a consequence of renal vein thrombosis or because of profound hypovolaemia, due to the nephrotic syndrome itself, diuretic treatment, or both.

### Infection

Children are particularly prone to infection, especially pneumococcal peritonitis. This may be related to loss of IgG in the urine.

# OBSTRUCTIVE UROPATHY

Obstruction occurs when urine flow is prevented anywhere from the tubules to the point at which urine is voided from the body.

## EFFECTS OF OBSTRUCTION

The increase in pressure in the obstructed urinary tract diminishes glomerular filtration, although urine formation may continue, even when obstruction is complete. In the latter case, however, eventually glomerular filtration ceases after a period. Obstruction causes dilation of the renal pelvis and swelling of the kidney. When persistent the kidney tissue atrophies so that eventually a very large kidney, but with only a thin rim of cortex, may result. The enlarged obstructed kidney with a dilated collecting system is known as **hydronephrosis**.

In chronic partial obstruction impairment of concentrating mechanisms may paradoxically cause polyuria and sodium loss.

## AETIOLOGY

Table 17.5 shows the common causes of obstructive nephropathy. In an individual the likely cause will depend upon the age and sex of the patient.

## CLINICAL FEATURES

A dramatic symptom, often timed precisely in its onset by the patient, is complete anuria. Any patient with anuria must have a diagnosis of complete bilateral obstruction or complete obstruction of a single functioning kidney excluded. Some patients with retroperitoneal fibrosis (page 472) or stones have an unusual but striking picture of intermittent anuria and polyuria, the latter occurring as a diuretic phase after the anuric phase.

Obstruction of the upper urinary tract may cause no symptoms, or mild loin pain which may be caused or exacerbated by a large fluid intake or diuretics (which include alcohol). The increased urinary volume causes painful distension of the collecting system.

**Table 17.5** Causes of obstructive nephropathy.

**Intraluminal**
Calculi
Bladder or ureteric tumours
Necrotic papillae
Blood clot

**Mural**
*Congenital*
Pelvi-ureteric junction obstruction
Bladder neck obstruction
Urethral valves
Phimosis

*Acquired*
Neurogenic bladder
Urethral stricture
Ureteric stricture

**Extramural**
Prostatic obstruction
Pelvic tumours
Trauma including surgery
Retroperitoneal fibrosis

Most cases of obstruction are caused by a lesion preventing outflow from the bladder and the symptoms differ according to the speed of onset. In acute obstruction, most commonly due to prostatism, there is painful retention of urine, the patient being agitated and complaining of suprapubic and perineal pain. However, when chronic, symptoms may be very slight and the patient may make very little of them as they have come to be accepted as normal. A diminished stream with hesitancy, terminal dribbling of urine, and a sensation of incomplete bladder emptying are typical. When there is retention with overflow there is frequent passage of small volumes of urine. All the above may occur on a background of symptoms caused by infection, chronic renal failure and a past history indicating the cause of the presenting episode of obstruction, for example, a previous illness caused by stones or previous unsuccessful prostatic surgery.

Examination may reveal palpable, enlarged

kidneys, which may be tender if infected. If the obstruction is below the bladder then it may be enlarged, sometimes to a very large size. The external genitalia, particularly in males, may reveal a phimosis (a congenital narrowing of the prepuce) or strictures which may be palpable in the penile urethra. The pelvic organs must be examined to exclude responsible lesions, especially carcinoma.

## DIAGNOSIS AND TREATMENT

It is extremely important not to miss the diagnosis of urinary obstruction as in most cases the obstruction can be reduced if not removed entirely, the exceptions mainly being due to malignant disease. In addition, the swift treatment of obstruction will reduce the likelihood of permanent damage to the kidneys. It is a tragedy for patients to end up requiring dialysis or transplantation for a benign obstructing lesion which has been missed. Clinical suspicion must therefore be high and a good rule of thumb to adopt is that patients with anuria or oliguria, or with acute or chronic renal failure have obstruction until proved otherwise. The proof is easily obtained by ultrasound, which has replaced the intravenous urogram (IVU) in most centres as the initial imaging technique. Ultrasound will exclude obstruction, i.e. by not showing a dilated system, although it must be remembered that in early acute obstruction dilation may be slight at first. The ultrasound may not only show dilation of the system, but may also show the cause of the obstruction, for example, stones or a bladder tumour.

If an IVU is performed, then typically there will be a delayed appearance of the nephrogram which develops to show a negative pyelogram due to the failure of contrast medium to go into the renal pelvis, which therefore appears as a dark (negative) shadow against the nephrogram demonstrated by the contrast medium. When dye eventually enters the pelvis of the kidney and the ureters dilation will be shown down to the site of the obstruction. If this is below the bladder then a distended bladder which empties poorly after micturition can be seen.

Having made the diagnosis of obstruction on either of these initial investigations, then two important questions remain: at what level is the obstruction and what is its cause? If these have not already been answered, then computed tomography (CT) can give very precise information, especially when the procedure is performed with the intravenous contrast medium. It is particularly useful when obstruction is due to pelvic or retroperitoneal masses. Computed tomography has now largely replaced retrograde pyelography in which contrast medium was introduced via catheters placed at cystoscopy into the ureters. This required general anaesthesia and had a high risk of infection.

The technique of antegrade pyelography is most useful. The procedure may be performed

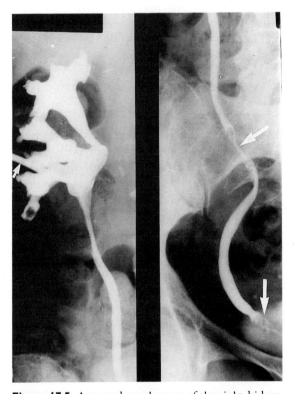

**Figure 17.5** Antegrade pyelogram of the right kidney and ureter. The lower part of the left picture joins the upper part of the right picture, showing the right renal tract throughout its length. As the ureter enters the bladder there is a marked lessening in the amount of contrast medium due to a stricture (large arrow) eventually shown to be due to carcinoma of the bladder. There is also a stricture further up the ureter (large arrow) due to metastases in lymph nodes compressing the ureter. A similar picture was seen on the left side. The patient had presented with anuria and acute renal failure, caused by the bilateral obstruction. This had been relieved by a nephrostomy tube in each kidney (small arrow) which relieved the obstruction and renal failure, and allowed injection of contrast medium.

under local anaesthesia and relies upon the distended pelvis of the kidney to facilitate the manoeuvre. A catheter is passed percutaneously through the loin into the dilated renal pelvis. The catheter *in situ* has two important uses: it will allow drainage of the urine, thus relieving the obstruction and improving renal function, and contrast medium can be injected into the catheter into the dilated system to define the level and possibly the nature of the obstruction (Fig. 17.5). The catheters, also known as nephrostomy tubes, can be left in for several days with only a relatively slight risk of infection. In dubious cases of obstruction they can also be used to measure the pressure in the collecting system.

When the bladder or urethra are considered likely sites of obstruction, then cystoscopy, urethroscopy, cystography, urethrography and urodynamics may all provide diagnostic information.

If the obstruction is relieved and renal function returns, the patient will not need dialysis. Some patients, as renal function returns, develop a huge diuresis, and will need careful replacement of salt and water. The outcome for renal function depends on how much renal tissue has been destroyed during the obstructive phase and ranges from normal to end-stage renal failure. The overall outcome depends on the cause of the obstruction.

# *U*RINARY TRACT INFECTION

This is a common illness, especially in women. It causes much misery and morbidity, even when there are no serious underlying abnormalities causing the infection and, at its worst, can cause chronic and end-stage renal failure. The appropriate use of prophylactic antibiotics has much improved the outcome of urinary tract infections.

## AETIOLOGY AND PATHOGENESIS

Any structural abnormality of the kidney or the urinary tract can predispose to infection:

- **Kidneys**: stones, obstruction causing hydronephrosis, scars from previous infections or infarctions and papillary necrosis (see below)
- **Ureters**: congenital duplex formation (Fig. 17.6), vesicoureteral reflux, normal physiological dilation during pregnancy
- **Bladder**: neurogenic bladder, tumours, diverticula, stones, catheter, obstruction
- **Urethra**: any form of stricture, enlarged prostate

Organisms can be introduced during sexual intercourse, by instrumentation such as catheterization or the insertion of nephrostomy tubes, or

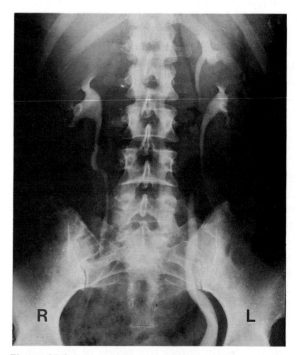

**Figure 17.6** Intravenous urogram in a young woman with recurrent acute pyelonephritis showing a left-sided duplex collecting system.

by formation of fistulae between the urinary tract, usually the bladder, and the intestine.

Nonetheless, many infections occur in apparently completely normal organs. The normal female lower urinary tract predisposes to infection because of its relative shortness compared to the male, and its nearness to the perianal area with easy access for faecal flora. In addition, some bacteria are more prone to cause urinary tract infection because they produce mucinase, can adhere to mucosal surfaces, and are relatively resistant to phagocytosis. The commonest bacteria causing infections are *E. coli*, *Streptococcus faecalis* and *Proteus mirabilis*.

# Acute Pyelonephritis

This can be a very serious illness causing septicaemia and shock, and when severe and bilateral, or affecting a single functioning kidney, acute renal failure may develop.

## CLINICAL FEATURES

The patient typically complains of loin pain and fever, usually with rigors, frequency of micturition and dysuria, and sometimes notes foul-smelling urine and macroscopic haematuria. There may be a history of a predisposing problem, as noted above.

The physical findings are loin tenderness in a feverish and ill-looking patient.

## DIAGNOSIS

The immediate diagnosis is made clinically from the above features, and confirmed by microscopy of the urine, which will usually show easily seen organisms without any need for staining. Urine and blood cultures should be taken but as the results will not be known for 24–48 hours then expectant antibiotic treatment must be given, intravenously if the patient is seriously ill.

## TREATMENT

Amoxycillin, ampicillin or trimethoprim are appropriate drugs pending the reports of cultures and sensitivities to antibiotics. Management is not complete unless the patient is investigated to exclude lesions predisposing to infection, the most common of which are obstruction or stones (or both) which can be excluded by ultrasound. Prophylactic antibiotics should be used if infections are recurrent.

# Chronic pyelonephritis

## AETIOLOGY

This is chronic interstitial inflammation of the kidney caused by prolonged or recurrent bacterial infection. It accounts for 15–20 per cent of patients in end-stage renal failure. The commonest causes are vesicoureteric reflux (see below), obstruction or stones.

## CLINICAL FEATURES

Patients present with chronic or end-stage renal failure, and not always with a previous history of overt infections, recurrent infection, hypertension or stone formation secondary to the infection. The physical findings may vary from none to those caused by high blood pressure, acute infection at the time of presentation or chronic renal failure.

## DIAGNOSIS

The diagnosis is made from the history and demonstrating, by ultrasound, IVU or radionuclide scan, the presence of scars in the kidneys, which themselves may be significantly and unequally smaller than normal.

## TREATMENT

Treatment (page 450) is aimed at preventing further infection, treating acute attacks swiftly and effectively, and correcting any underlying causes, e.g. stones.

# Reflux nephropathy

## AETIOLOGY

This disease is caused by **vesicoureteric reflux** (VUR) which is due to an incompetent vesicoureteric junction. Vesicoureteric reflux is graded as follows from the findings on a micturating cystogram:

Grade 1    There is incomplete filling of the urinary tract by contrast medium, which does not reach the kidney, with a normal ureteric orifice

Grade 2    The contrast medium completely fills the urinary tract, but with little or no dilation of the calyces

Grade 3    Complete filling of the urinary tract with dilation of the calyces by contrast medium

Most cases are due to a congenital abnormality whereby the ureter remains patent at the vesicoureteric junction during bladder contraction. This allows the reflux of urine during micturition. Reflux is accompanied by increased pressure within the kidney which causes damage and scarring, which in turn becomes subject to infection.

The damage caused by VUR occurs in the early years, usually before the age of 4–5 years. If the kidneys have been scarred, then further scarring is likely, but if they have remained grossly normal, then they will probably not become scarred in the future. The reflux itself frequently disappears, so that it is not demonstrable when the patient presents in later life. The diagnosis of reflux nephropathy is then made on grounds of probability and in the absence of any other obvious cause.

## CLINICAL FEATURES AND DIAGNOSIS

There are no findings on examination which lead to the diagnosis of reflux nephropathy itself. The patient may have hypertension, infection or chronic renal failure.

## TREATMENT

If VUR is demonstrable at diagnosis, surgical correction, although apparently logical has little to offer unless infection is not controlled by antibiotics. Prophylaxis with a broad-spectrum antibiotic is the mainstay of treatment.

# Cystitis

## AETIOLOGY

Although inflammation of the bladder can be caused by drugs, toxins and radiation, the term 'cystitis' is commonly used to mean bacterial cystitis. It is common in females and rare in males. In most adult women no structural abnormality is found, but in children abnormalities predisposing to urinary tract infection are more frequent.

## CLINICAL FEATURES

The typical symptoms are frequency, which can be extreme, nocturia, dysuria, malodorous urine and sometimes macroscopic haematuria. In contrast to acute pyelonephritis, fever is uncommon, and the patient does not have the systemic symptoms of infection, i.e. malaise, muscle aching and tenderness. Suprapubic pain or discomfort is common; if there is loin pain or tenderness of renal origin then the patient does not have simple cystitis but pyelonephritis as well.

## TREATMENT

Management consists of treatment of the acute attacks and prophylaxis. The acute attack can be treated immediately with an antibiotic, to which the commonest organism causing the infection, *E. coli*, will be expected to be sensitive. Thus trimethoprim or ampicillin can be given until the result of the urine culture is known. If the patient has frequent infections long-term prophylatic antibiotics, for example, trimethoprim, 100 mg each night, can significantly reduce the incidence of infections. Other prophylactic measures are to keep the anal and vulval areas clean, particularly before sexual intercourse, and to empty the bladder following intercourse.

Investigation in adult women usually shows no abnormality and is only worth doing if infections are recurrent. In these cases, and in men and children, an ultrasound examination of the urinary tract is usually sufficient to exclude any serious abnormality.

## PROGNOSIS

Cystitis in the presence of a structurally normal urinary tract does not cause renal damage, and therefore renal function will remain normal. From this point of view the prognosis is good, although recurrent infections, which are not always responsive to treatment, undoubtedly cause much misery.

# Asymptomatic bacteriuria

This is the growth of significant amounts of bacteria from women who have no symptoms to suggest urinary tract infection. In practice it is detected when pregnant women or healthy women in population studies have their urine cultured. This finding in the absence of structural abnormalities does not indicate that any serious consequences will follow. In follow-up studies, overt urinary tract infections occur in a proportion, but in 50 per cent of the women the urine will be sterile. On the other hand, in those women who have sterile urine in the first examination, 25–50 per cent will have asymptomatic bacteriuria on follow-up. Thus, the finding of positive urine cultures in asymptomatic, healthy women appears to be a normal phenomenon. No treatment is required unless the woman is pregnant, when asymptomatic bacteriuria carries a risk of pyelonephritis and the organism should therefore be eradicated.

# Prostatitis

Infection arising in the prostate gland can cause recurrent urinary tract infection. It occurs characteristically in middle-aged or elderly men who present with pain in the perineum and dysuria. Diagnosis is proven by culture of the urine after prostatic massage, performed by the examiner via the rectum. The patient provides a mid-stream urine (MSU) specimen both before and after the massage which will allow comparison of the bacterial growths. Treatment is with appropriate antibiotics. Some men develop chronic prostatitis which requires a 3 month course of appropriate antibiotic. There is no particular association of prostatitis with benign prostatic hypertrophy or carcinoma of the prostate.

# Tuberculosis

This is still a common problem in developing countries, and is still seen, but uncommonly, elsewhere. Infection commences in the kidney and then spreads to the ureters, bladder and, in males, to the seminal vesicles, epydidimes and vasa deferentia. The usual symptoms are dysuria, frequency, haematuria and loin pain. The clue to the diagnosis is the demonstration of multiple strictures in the urinary tract, demonstrated by ultrasound or IVU, but the diagnosis is proven by the culture of mycobacteria from the urine. The patient should provide three early morning urine (EMU) specimens, as it is in these that the concentration of bacteria is at its highest. Six to twelve months' treatment with at least two appropriate drugs is recommended and, because the formation of ureteric strictures which can eventually cause obstruction and renal failure is one of the most important ways in which tuberculosis causes morbidity, the use of corticosteroids to prevent scarring is also recommended.

# CALCULI

Renal calculi are common in the UK and similar countries, but bladder calculi have become very uncommon over the last 200–300 years. Renal calculi can occur at any age, but are most common in 30–60 year-olds with a 3:1 preponderance in males.

# Types of stones

In practice there are four main types of stones:

1. Calcium oxalate stones which cause 80 per cent of all renal stones. Calcium oxalate also occurs as a mixture with calcium phosphate in its hydroxyapatite form.
2. Calcium phosphate (triple phosphate) stones which cause approximately 10 per cent of renal calculi. They comprise magnesium ammonium phosphate, also known as struvite, and calcium phosphate.
3. Uric acid stones which cause 5–10 per cent of renal stones and occur in association with gout.
4. Cystine stones which account for 1 per cent of renal calculi develop in cystinuria. The amino acids cystine, arginine, lysine and amithine are malabsorbed in the intestine and renal tubules by a recessively inherited mechanism. The only important factor is the cystinuria which, because of cystine's relative insolubility, causes stones.

Stones form when the urine is supersaturated with the stone-forming crystals. Urine normally contains substances which prevent cystallization such as glycosaminoglycans. Supersaturation may arise from a combination of:

1. Increased urinary concentration of the cystalloid due to increased urinary excretion or reduced urinary volume
2. Alterations in pH of the urine, with accompanying changes in crystal solubility
3. Deficiency of the substances which prevent crystallization

# Presenting features

The characteristic symptom is **ureteric colic**, also known, but erroneously, as renal colic. This is an extremely severe pain due to the passage of a stone(s) down the ureter. The pain extends from the loin and the groin, and may radiate to the testes in men, and to the labia majora in women. Its character is usually described as 'like a knife'. The severity of the pain is so well recognized that it is often mimicked by drug addicts seeking an injection of pethidine, or by patients with the Munchausen syndrome (page 885).

Not all patients with stones develop ureteric colic. Others may present with loin pain, symptoms of urinary tract infection, macroscopic haematuria with or without ureteric colic, chronic renal failure and acute renal failure. This is particularly likely to occur when the function of one kidney has been lost due to the calculi (which can occur silently), and the remaining kidney, the function of which in itself may not be normal, develops acute obstruction or pyelonephritis.

By no means do all patients with stones give a history of passing stones. This may be for two reasons: they may indeed never have passed stones, or it is not uncommon, particularly in women, for stones to be passed without the knowledge of the patient. Some patients describe the passage of grit, or particulate matter which they do not recognize themselves as stones. The findings on examination will vary according to the presentation outlined above. In ureteric colic the patient is clearly in great distress. There may be marked loin tenderness, with swelling if there is obstruction. The signs of chronic or acute renal failure (see above) may be present, and if infection is severe, then the patient may have septicaemia.

## DIAGNOSIS AND INVESTIGATIONS

The diagnosis of calculi is usually evident from the history of the presenting complaints and confirmation is usually easily provided by imaging. Ultrasound can demonstrate stones, as they cast an 'acoustic shadow' if obstruction is present, and the size of the kidneys, in particular the amount of renal parenchyma. A plain X-ray of the abdomen will show the number, size and site of radio-opaque stones. Eighty per cent of calculi are radio-opaque; urate stones account for the majority of non-radio-opaque stones. An IVU can be used if ultrasound is not available or is not informative enough (Fig. 17.7). The IVU will

which have a typical hexagonal shape, do not occur in normal urine and thus their presence diagnoses cystinuria.

Biochemical investigations required are analysis of any available stone and measurement of urine excretion of calcium, oxalate, urate and cystine. Hypercalcaemia, hyperuricaemia and renal failure should be excluded by the appropriate blood tests. If any metabolic abnormality is uncovered then this must be further investigated.

## COMPLICATIONS

Calculi are a potent cause of much illness, and a significant cause of end-stage renal failure.

## TREATMENT

The aims of treatment are to remove stones which are causing symptoms or complications, to deal with the complications themselves, and to prevent recurrence of stones.

### Removal of stones

Recent years have seen the development of a number of methods of stone removal which have largely replaced the direct operative removal of stones from the urinary tract. They share a common advantage over surgical removal by being less invasive, causing less pain and requiring fewer days as a hospital in-patient and a shorter period of convalescence.

#### Percutaneous stone removal

A needle is inserted percutaneously through the loin into the kidney under X-ray control. The track made by the needle can be enlarged by dilators and various instruments then introduced through the track to remove the calculi. Ultrasonic and laser probes have been used to shatter the stone. The pieces are then passed in the urine. Larger pieces or a whole stone, if it is less than 7 mm in diameter, can be removed *in toto* by retrieval baskets.

#### Retrograde stone removal

This is not a new technique but it has developed recently due to the introduction of ultrasound and laser probes. These can be introduced via the urethra and bladder into the relevant ureter(s) and the stone disintegrated and retrieved or passed normally.

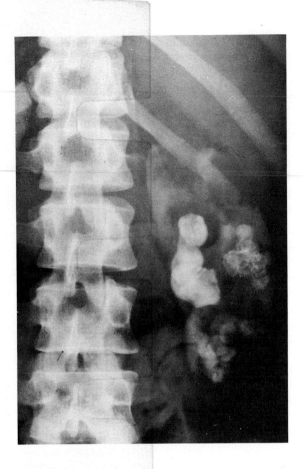

**Figure 17.7** Calcium phosphate stones in the left kidney. Note how the densest stones have the same density as the vertebral column. This film was taken in the very early phase of an intravenous urogram and therefore the early nephrogram shows the outline of the kidney.

show precisely the relationship to the urinary tract of the stones and the site of obstruction and will also show non-opaque renal calculi because they cause negative shadows within the contrast. In obstructed patients antegrade pyelography or, now less often, retrograde pyelography can be used to show the level of obstruction, more particularly when a kidney is not functioning because of infection or severity of obstruction, or to outline non-radio-opaque calculi.

Urine culture is necessary to exclude infection. Microscopy of the urine may define the types of stones which are present. Although normal urine can contain crystals of calcium and uric acid, these are more numerous, larger and often aggregated in patients who have stones composed of these substances. Cystine crystals,

### Extracorporeal shockwave lithotripsy

This method uses ultrasound shockwaves which are focussed on the calculus which is then fragmented. There is no invasion of the patient and the ultrasound waves do not cause damage to surrounding tissues. The new models allow the procedure to be performed on an unanaesthetized, conscious patient.

In many instances, when the stone is 5 mm in diameter or less and is lodged in the ureter, it will pass spontaneously. This waiting game does require checking by ultrasound to ensure that the stone has been passed and that, if still present, obstruction is not developing.

## Prevention of recurrent stones

If an underlying cause such as hyperparathyroidism, gout or obstruction has been found then successful treatment will prevent recurrence. Most calculi, however, have no known cause, but several different manoeuvres, such as control of fluid intake and diet or treatment with drugs are available to try and prevent recurrence depending on the type of stone.

### Fluid intake

This simple measure is one of the most effective. The urine volume should be kept at 2.5–3.5 l/24 hours and, at its most effective, the patient should drink before retiring and during the night to prevent nocturnal concentration.

### Dietary control

Many patients with idiopathic calcium stones are put on a low calcium diet and calcium absorption from the gut prevented with oral phosphate. However, these regimes are not very effective and, indeed, dietary calcium restriction produces an increased absorption of oxalate from the bowel, which causes hyperoxaluria and itself, therefore, predisposes to stone formation. A low oxalate diet is not effective except in the rare instance of intestinal oxalosis in which there is hyperabsorption of oxalate from the intestine. A diet free or low in purines in patients with gout is difficult for the patient to follow as so many foods must be restricted, and compliance is difficult. The use of allopurinol to prevent urate formation has much reduced the emphasis on low purine diets.

### Thiazide treatment

The thiazides, usually used as diuretics or antihypertensives, increase tubular calcium reabsorption and therefore reduce hypercalcuria.

### Potassium citrate

Many cases of calcium oxalate stones are associated with hyperuricosuria, but in the absence of classical gout. The urine can be made alkaline by potassium citrate, which increases the solubility of the uric acid, which is less likely to crystallize and form the nidus on which the calcium oxalate crystallizes.

### Cystine stones

The solubility of cystine increases markedly in alkaline urine, above pH 8.0. A high fluid intake must be tailored to the size of the patient and their working environment (many patients work in central heating which increases insensible loss), so that a 70 kg man in a normal environment should drink 5 litres of fluid per day with sodium bicarbonate taken orally to alkalinase the urine. The increased fluid intake must be spread over the 24 hours so that the dilute alkaline urine is formed at night as well as during the day. Patients must therefore get up during the night to drink. When this approach is insufficient then penicillamine reduces cystine stone formation by altering the cystine to cysteine, which is much more soluble and prevents recurrence. The other amino acids at greater concentration in the urine do not form stones as they are easily soluble whatever the circumstances.

# Nephritis

The term nephritis covers two main types of inflammatory disease of the kidney other than inflammation due to direct infection of renal tissue. The commoner type is glomerulonephritis in which the inflammation is primarily in the glomeruli, and the second type is interstitial nephritis (pages 455 and 472) in which the interstitial tissue and tubules are affected. Sometimes both types occur together (when the disease is usually just called glomerulonephritis). Glomerulonephritis accounts for 25–30 per cent of patients with end-stage renal failure. Interstitial nephritis is, however, increasing in frequency and importance, mainly due to the drugs which cause it (page 472).

# Glomerulonephritis

This is often perceived as a confusing topic. Some general statements should help to explain, if not lessen, the confusion. First there is no satisfactory system of classification. Whichever system is adopted will include considerable overlap between types and therefore imprecision. In practice, because of the ease of performing percutaneous renal biopsy, and therefore obtaining a histological description, a morphological classification is usually used. However, identical histological pictures can occur in different diseases, for example, membranous nephropathy may be found as an idiopathic form, in systemic lupus erythematosus, or as a result of treatment with pencillamine. In many instances, therefore, a histological description of glomerulonephritis leads to a search for associated diseases or causes, and is not a diagnosis in itself (just as iron deficiency anaemia requires an explanation for the iron deficiency).

Second, the aetiology of nephritis is usually unknown, and therefore this cannot serve as a basis for classification (unlike, for example, the pneumonias).

Third, the effects of glomerulonephritis on renal function are relatively few, and although there are clusters of a typical histological picture accompanying a particular group of clinical features, very few of these are circumscribed enough to allow this as a system of classification. To take membranous nephropathy as an example again, patients with identical histological appearances can have slight proteinuria, heavy proteinuria causing a nephrotic syndrome, normal renal function or renal failure and, in resolved cases, there may be normal renal function, no proteinuria, but persistence of the histological changes.

In summary, glomerulonephritis is best described in an individual patient in three terms:

1. The histological picture, obtained by biopsy
2. Its description as idiopathic, or associated with or caused by another disease
3. The clinical effect of the glomerulonephritis.

Thus, we have, for example, a patient with membranous nephropathy due to gold toxicity causing a nephrotic syndrome and renal failure.

## AETIOLOGY AND PATHOGENESIS

By analogy with experimental work, most cases of nephritis are thought to be mediated by immune mechanisms. The commonest is formation of antigen–antibody complexes (immune complexes) which initiate inflammation in the kidney. The immune complexes may be deposited in the kidney, as such, from the circulation, or may form in the kidney, where the antigen and antibody arrive separately but combine in the organ to form the immune complex. In a small number of cases antibody is formed against normal structural components of the kidney as, for example, the glomerular basement membrane and tubular basement membrane. Because monocytes have been found in the glomeruli and interstitium it is thought that cell-mediated immunity also causes tissue damage in nephritis.

As antigen–antibody complexes are thought to be responsible for most cases, an obvious question is the nature of the responsible antigens. In only a relatively small number of cases in humans has the pathogenic antigen been identified either in the kidney or in the circulation. Most of these are infectious organisms and the most commonly occurring examples are shown in Table 17.6. Other antigens, for example, drugs, tumours and endogenous antigens such as nuclear antigens in systemic lupus erythematosus have also been defined.

Susceptibility to some types of nephritis is associated with particular HLA types, hinting that the patient's immune system is a factor which increases the likelihood of developing the disease.

**Table 17.6** Infectious organisms associated with human nephritis.

**Bacteria**
Streptococcus (Group A haemolytic and viridans)
Staphylococcus aureus and Staph. albus
Streptococcus pneumoniae
Meningococcus
Salmonella typhi
Klebsiella pneumoniae
Mycobacterium tuberculosis
Mycobacterium leprae
Treponema pallidum
Brucella spp
Yersinia enterocolitica
Leptospira

**Viruses**
Hepatitis B
Epstein–Barr
HIV
Oncornavirus
Mumps
Measles
Rubella
Cytomegalovirus
Coxsackie
Variola
Varicella
Vaccinia
Guillain–Barré agent

**Rickettsiae**
Coxiella burnetti

**Mycoplasma**
Mycoplasma pneumoniae

**Fungi**
Candida albicans

**Parasites**
Plasmodium malariae and P. falciparum
Schistosoma mansonii and S. Haematobium
Toxoplasma
Filaria spp

In clinical practice nephritis is conveniently regarded as 'primary' in cases in which the kidney alone is affected, or 'secondary' when the kidney is involved as part of a systemic disease. This is a useful way of approaching nephritis as the management of the patient will differ in these two categories.

## CLINICAL FEATURES

Glomerulonephritis may present in a number of different ways, and in an individual patient the features can change over time – a patient may present with asymptomatic proteinuria which increases so that a nephrotic syndrome ensues, with a final phase of chronic and then end-stage renal failure.

### Proteinuria with or without microscopic haematuria

When the proteinuria is not suffcient to cause a nephrotic syndrome (see below), this presentation is usually incidental when a patient's urine is examined for health screening, insurance purposes, during pregnancy etc.

### Macroscopic haematuria

In nephritis this usually gives a brown, rather than red colour to the urine, which is often compared to tea or coca cola.

### The nephrotic syndrome

Nephrotic syndrome (page 444) will develop when hypoproteinaemia results from the urinary protein loss, with the consequent formation of oedema.

### The nephritic syndrome

This comprises hypertension, the retention of salt and water, expansion of the intravascular volume (often causing bradycardia), all resulting from reduction in glomerular filtration. When the nephritic syndrome is at its most severe acute renal failure occurs.

### Chronic renal failure

This is the end result of several types of nephritis.

### Acute renal failure

As noted above, this may occur as part of the nephritic syndrome or when severe types of proliferative nephritis develop so quickly that the patient presents with acute renal failure.

### Loin pain

This symptom is often overlooked by clinicians; it rarely occurs alone, however.

# PRIMARY GLOMERULONEPHRITIS

## Membranous nephropathy

This usually affects adults who generally present with a nephrotic syndrome, but in other cases with symptomless proteinuria. In the majority of cases the disease is idiopathic, but in a minority associated aetiological factors such as drugs (e.g. gold or penicillamine) or a carcinoma, occurring in the usual common sites, are found.

The renal biopsy (Fig. 17.8) shows a thickened glomerular basement membrane (hence 'membranous') with deposits of immunoglobulin and complement; there is usually only a minor degree of inflammation.

Approximately one-third of patients undergo spontaneous remission, one-third continue to have proteinuria, with or without nephrotic syndrome, and in the remainder there is a slow progression over many years to chronic and end-stage renal failure.

Although improvement has been reported with steroids and immunosuppressive drugs, this treatment is not widely accepted. It is particularly difficult in membranous nephropathy to assess the effects of treatment because of the relatively high spontaneous rate of remission. Many centres reserve a trial of treatment for patients with severe nephrotic syndrome, or with a more than usually rapid progress towards renal failure.

## IgA nephropathy

This has gained prominence over the last 10 years or so through its recognition as the most common form of nephritis in developed countries. Children and young adults usually present with macroscopic haematuria, often occurring with, or shortly after, upper respiratory tract infections. Older patients usually present with hypertension with or without renal impairment. In countries with a high alcohol consumption such as France, an association with alcoholic liver disease has been noted.

The renal biopsy (Fig. 17.9) characteristically shows the deposition of IgA in the mesangium of the glomeruli, with proliferative changes. The pathogenesis of this curious finding is not understood, but may reflect either an increased production of IgA or some abnormality in the mucosae (where most of the body's IgA is produced) which allows IgA-containing antigen–antibody complexes into the circulation and to deposit in the kidneys.

Although originally thought to be benign, it is now recognized that 10–20 per cent of patients can eventually develop chronic or end-stage renal failure. No treatment has been shown to be effective.

## Acute exudative proliferative nephritis

This usually follows infections and was a common disease, particularly amongst children after

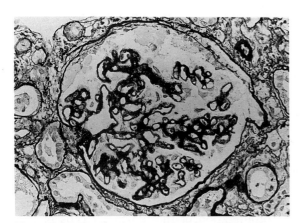

**Figure 17.8** Membranous nephropathy. Glomerular cellularity is normal, but the capillary walls are thickened and spikes of basement membrane material can be seen on the subepithelial (outer) aspect (arrowed).

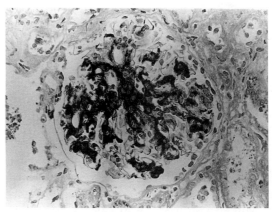

**Figure 17.9** IgA nephropathy. Immunoperoxidase stain performed on fresh frozen tissue, using anti-human IgA antibody. The dark granular reaction product is mainly localized in the mesangial areas. Nuclei are revealed with a haematoxylin counterstain.

streptococcal infection, in developed countries until 20–30 years ago. The decreased incidence has been explained by a healthier and more hygienic population, the more widespread use of antibiotics to treat upper respiratory tract infections, which was the usual antecedent type of infection, and possibly a change in the antigenic structure of the Streptococci themselves. Poststreptococcal nephritis is still common in developing countries, where it often follows streptococcal skin infection complicating scabies. Other bacteria such as Pneumococci, Staphylococci and Meningococci, can cause a similar clinical picture.

The typical presentation is with the acute nephritic syndrome (see above). If this is recognized in association with a typical antecedent infection then renal biopsy is not necessary for management. If performed, histology (Fig. 17.10) shows proliferation of glomerular cells, infiltration of the glomeruli with polymorphonuclear leukocytes and deposition of immunoglobulins and complement in the glomeruli. These deposits of immune material are often so large that they can be seen on light microscopy as 'humps'.

Most patients recover completely, although small amounts of haematuria and proteinuria may continue for many months without ill effect. A minority may develop chronic renal failure later in life.

The management consists of treatment of any infection and maintenance of appropriate fluid and electrolyte balance, with dialysis for acute renal failure if this occurs.

## Rapidly progressive or crescentic glomerulonephritis

This histological descriptive name arises from the proliferation of cells around the glomerulus which surround it like a cap, so that when the biopsy is cut to make the histological specimens, the section of the cap appears like a crescent. The condition usually presents as oliguric renal failure developing over days (hence rapidly progressive) or weeks. Macroscopic haematuria and loin pain are common. Most cases of crescentic nephritis occur as part of a systemic disease, the most common being vasculitis and systemic lupus erythematosus; other cases appear to be idiopathic.

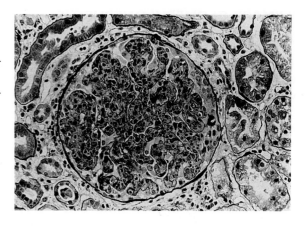

**Figure 17.10** Postinfectious nephritis. There is an enormous increase of cells, mainly within the capillary loops (endocapillary). Large numbers of these can be seen to be polymorphs. A small cellular crescent can be seen between 2 and 4 o'clock inside Bowman's capsule (extracapillary).

However, if treated early enough with immunosuppressive drugs and steroids, and in some severe cases plasma exchange, a marked improvement in renal function can be obtained. Patients who were dialysis-dependent can return to normal renal function or an acceptable degree of mild to moderate chronic renal failure. For treatment to be effective, the diagnosis must be made early in the course of the disease. It can only be made with certainty by renal biopsy.

## Mesangiocapillary glomerulonephritis

In developed countries mesangiocapillary glomerulonephritis (also known as membranoproliferative glomerulonephritis) has become less common over the last 20 years, whereas by contrast it remains common in developing countries. It aetiology is unknown, but with this rapid change in incidence an environmental cause such as infection is obviously a possibility. It is typically a disease of older children and young adults who present with proteinuria, haematuria which may be macroscopic, nephrotic syndrome, and sometimes with acute or chronic renal failure.

The histological, descriptive name indicates the proliferation of the mesangial cells of the glomeruli with a thickening of the basement membrane. A striking association of this condition is with prolonged hypocomplementaemia due to a low plasma C3 concentration.

The disease has a poor prognosis as progression to end-stage renal failure occurs in 50–70 per cent of patients. No effective treatment has been described.

## Focal glomerulosclerosis

This is a serious condition of unknown aetiology. Patients usually present with the nephrotic syndrome or, less commonly, with lesser degrees of proteinuria. The nephrotic syndrome can be particularly profound and the majority of patients develop end-stage renal failure over 5–10 years.

The aetiology is unknown. Histology shows a sclerosing lesion affecting some glomeruli. A small proportion of cases have a partial, occasionally complete, response to steroids and immunosuppressive drugs, with diminution or cure of the nephrotic syndrome and arrest of the progression to renal failure.

## Minimal change nephropathy

This is mainly a disease of children, in whom it causes 80–90 per cent of cases of the nephrotic syndrome, but has a lower incidence in adults. Although the typical presentation is with nephrotic syndrome, a minority can present with proteinuria.

It is a curious condition in that there is no abnormality on light microscopy (Fig. 17.11). It is therefore something of a misnomer to label this as 'a nephritis', although this is conventionally done, hence the term 'minimal change'. In most patients the nephrotic syndrome responds completely to steroids with complete loss of proteinuria. This is difficult to explain in the absence of any inflammatory changes.

The pathogenesis is unknown but there is some evidence to suggest that the proteinuria is due to increased permeability of the glomerular basement membrane, caused by a cytokine secreted by lymphocytes.

Treatment relies on steroids. Many patients require only one course of this drug over 4–8 weeks. However, in some patients the condition relapses, requiring further courses of steroids, and in others proteinuria is continuous, requiring long-standing treatment with steroids to reduce the proteinuria to acceptable levels. In some patients who are resistant to steroids an

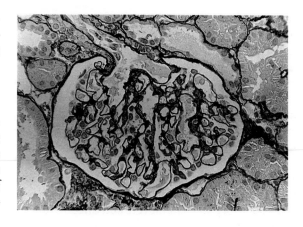

**Figure 17.11** Minimal change nephropathy. A normal glomerulus. Glomerular capillary and tubular basement membranes revealed with deposition of silver. Nuclear and cytoplasmic detail revealed with haematoxylin and eosin counterstain.

8-week course of cyclophosphamide can produce partial or complete remission.

The prognosis is good, apart from possible complications of the nephrotic syndrome or its treatment; a particular point is the risk of gonadal damage and sterility in adult life if excessive amounts of antimitotic drugs are used. Chronic renal failure does not develop.

## Antiglomerular basement membrane nephritis

Although rare, accounting for approximately 2 per cent of cases of nephritis, antiglomerular basement membrane (anti-GBM) nephritis is of considerable interest. The typical clinical picture is of a rapidly progressive nephritis which, in some patients, is accompanied by pulmonary haemorrhage, presenting variously as haemoptysis, respiratory failure, 'unexplained' lung shadowing on chest X-ray or a normocytic, normochromic anaemia greater than would be expected from the patient's degree of renal failure. When the nephritis and pulmonary haemorrhage occur together the condition is known as **Goodpasture's syndrome**.

The disease is caused by circulating antibody to the glomerular basement membrane. Histologically there is a crescentic proliferative nephritis with deposition of anti-GBM antibody on the glomerular basement membrane in a typical linear fashion. The aetiology is unknown, although in some cases there seems to be a connection between a preceding respiratory infection or exposure to hydrocarbons, in which case the disease may primarily arise because antibody is formed to damaged alveolar basement membrane, and these antibodies then cross-react with the glomerular basement membrane.

Treatment with steroids, immunosuppressive drugs and plasma exchange can effect marked improvements in both renal and pulmonary damage by removing and diminishing the production of antibody. In some cases the pulmonary haemorrhage is so severe and uncontrollable that death occurs. The prognosis for renal function depends on how soon in the course of the disease treatment is begun; if too late then end-stage renal failure may rapidly ensue.

## SECONDARY GLOMERULONEPHRITIS

Secondary forms of nephritis occur in systemic disease. In such patients the involvement of many organs may be evident when the patient presents, while in others only one system, for example, the kidney, may produce the only presenting signs and symptoms. The diagnosis and management of these patients is more complex as investigation and management of the other aspects of their disease is necessary as well. The secondary forms of glomerulonephritis can be divided into those which are thought to be immune mediated, as in primary glomerulonephritis, or not.

### Systemic lupus erythematosus

For a general account of systemic lupus erythematosus (SLE) see page 571. Only the renal aspects will be dealt with here.

#### Presenting features

The whole range of presentation of glomerular disease is seen, i.e. rapidly progressive glomerulonephritis, nephrotic syndrome, proteinuria and/or haematuria, all of which may occur with varying degrees of renal failure, either acute or chronic. Most patients present with other features of the disease, most commonly arthritis and rash.

#### Pathology

Any histological type of nephritis may occur in SLE. There is therefore no particular light or electron microscopic picture, nor immunohistological pattern, which is typical of this condition.

#### Diagnosis

From the above it should be clear that the diagnosis of SLE may be suspected but not proven from the nephrologist's point of view. Diagnosis relies on demonstrating a raised anti-DNA antibody level in the blood, with or without hypocomplementaemia.

#### Management

The mainstays of treatment are steroids and immunosuppressive drugs, either azathioprine or cyclophosphamide; chlorambucil is used occasionally. In severe renal disease, i.e. rapidly progressive glomerulonephritis with acute renal failure, the patient requires high doses of steroids, for example, intravenous pulse steroid or high-dose oral therapy, with azathioprine or cyclophosphamide. Plasma exchange to remove anti-DNA antibodies is used as an adjunct, but with no strict evidence that it is helpful. A nephrotic syndrome would also require steroids and immunosuppressive drugs, but proteinuria alone with normal renal function is usually managed with steroids only. Once the initial problem, if acute, has been dealt with, then the dose of steroids can be reduced and the patient is then continued on maintenance therapy, which is low-dose steroids, with or without immunosuppressive drugs.

Extrarenal manifestations of SLE may be more severe than the renal involvement and may determine the treatment.

Patients with end-stage renal failure can be managed with dialysis or transplantation. There is very little risk of recurrent disease in the transplanted kidney. Overall the prognosis for SLE with renal involvement, although it remains a very serious condition, has improved markedly over the last 15 to 20 years, so that end-stage renal failure or chronic renal failure can be averted in many cases, and the nephrotic syndrome successfully treated.

### Vasculitis

For a general description of vasculitis see page 574. Vasculitis of the kidney can occur very swiftly, either as an isolated manifestation of the disease or with the other clinical features. There is increasing evidence that vasculitis is becoming more common. In the UK it now represents the commonest disease causing acute renal failure due to glomerulonephritis.

### Clinical features

The nephritis usually presents with acute or subacute renal failure, i.e. developing over days or weeks. The patient may present with other symptoms affecting other parts of the body, and the renal involvement is then noted during investigation. Vasculitis very rarely causes a nephrotic syndrome.

Wegener's granulomatosis is often used as a synonym for vasculitis when there is evidence of pulmonary involvement. The accurate definition of Wegener's granulomatosis requires histological definition of the granulomata, the distinguishing feature of this variant. However, when there is evidence of pulmonary involvement, such as haemoptysis, intrapulmonary haemorrhage, or multiple shadows on chest X-ray, many clinicians assume a diagnosis of Wegener's granulomatosis without the histological proof.

### Pathology

The inflammation of the vessel is intermittent along the course of the vessel, and therefore histology may show no abnormality. It is therefore important to realize that normal vessels, in any organ, do not exclude a diagnosis of vasculitis. The size of the vessel affected may be medium or large (polyarteritis nodosa) so that infarction of organs or tissues often results. In most cases the affected vessels are small and, when this occurs in the kidney, there is a crescentic glomerulonephritis and ischaemia of the glomeruli.

### Diagnosis

A circulating antibody – anti-neutrophil cytoplasmic antibody (ANCA) – is associated with vasculitis and is now in common use as an aid to diagnosis, and evidence is accumulating to suggest that an increase in antibody titre can predict relapse. It is not yet known whether the antibody plays a part in causing the disease or is simply a secondary event.

The diagnosis of vasculitis rests heavily on initial clinical suspicion. It must be made swiftly so that the effective treatment for this condition can be given before serious morbidity or death ensues. Thus the diagnosis can very well be made on clinical grounds alone. Supporting evidence comes from measuring ANCA and histology.

### Management

The mainstay of treatment for acute vasculitis affecting the kidneys is high-dose steroids, which may be given orally, for example, 60–80 mg prednisolone per day, or intravenously, for example, 1 g methlyprednisolone daily for 3 days, with either cyclophosphamide or azathioprine. In addition, plasma exchange, antiplatelet drugs, anticoagulants and, more recently, pooled gammaglobulin (page 641) are added in various combinations in some centres. From the renal point of view treatment of vasculitis must be given as soon as possible as the disease is eminently reversible, but this chance will be lost if the patient is allowed to progress to anuria. After control of the acute illness maintanence treatment with steroids and immunosuppression is usually required, the patient being monitored for clinical and serological evidence of the current disease which will require an increase of the maintenance treatment.

The survival rate of patients with renal vasculitis is now 80 per cent at 5 years, which again emphasizes how worth while it is to diagnose and treat these patients at an early stage.

## Variants of vasculitis

### Churg–Strauss syndrome

The patient's predominant problem is asthma, accompanied by eosinophilia, due to pulmonary vasculitis.

### Henoch–Schönlein purpura

This is rare in adults, occurring mainly in children. The typical features are a non-thrombocytopaenic purpura, characteristically affecting the extensor surfaces of the limbs and buttocks, accompanied by arthritis, gastrointestinal bleeding and nephritis. Acute renal failure may be the main presenting feature.

Although vasculitis is seen histologically, the appearances differ from those of microscopic polyarteritis and polyarteritis nodosa as they are accompanied by the deposition of IgA in skin and the mesangium of the kidney. The glomeruli show a variety of appearances ranging from mesangial proliferation to crescentic nephritis. The cause of the disease is unknown, as also is the reason for the deposition of IgA. Episodes are often preceded by infections or drugs, but no particular organisms or chemicals are associated.

The diagnosis of Henoch–Schönlein purpura is clinically easy and if confirmation is required this is provided by the finding of IgA in the histological lesions. In most cases no treatment is necessary as recovery is complete; a small number of patients have a severe crescentic nephritis with acute renal failure and treatment similar to that of vasculitis appears effective.

### Systemic sclerosis

In systemic sclerosis (page 577) the arterial walls become grossly thickened with narrowing or occlusion of the lumen. Involvement of the kidneys produces hypertension, often severe, and renal failure which may be of acute or chronic onset. Steroids and immunosuppressants have little effect. The angiotensin-converting enzyme inhibitors, for example, captopril, may improve renal function in some patients, probably by altering intrarenal arterial blood flow, with an improvement in glomerular perfusion.

### Rheumatoid arthritis

Curiously, in view of the systemic nature of this disease and its mediation by the immune system, there is no recognized nephritis associated with the disease itself. Nephritis, due to the drugs used to treat rheumatoid arthritis, such as membranous nephropathy caused by penicillamine or gold, are quite common.

## Infections

We are all exposed to viruses, bacteria and fungi, all of which are potential antigens, so it is not surprising that many infections can cause nephritis, usually of an immune complex type (Table 17.6). Some of the infections causing nephritis are discussed briefly.

### Post-streptococcal glomerulonephritis

This has now become uncommon in the UK and similar countries, but remains a frequent cause of nephritis in developing countries. In the latter, the preceding streptococcal infection is usually of the skin, often secondary to scabies (page 801), whereas streptococcal throat infection is the usual antecedent in the developed countries. The normal presentation is of an acute nephritic syndrome, with or without a nephrotic syndrome, occurring 10 to 20 days following the original infection. The Streptococcus is of the Lancefield group A β-haemolytic type. Histologically there is an exudative proliferative glomerulonephritis, with or without crescents. There is no specific treatment apart from eradicating any remaining streptococcal infection. The nephritic and/or nephrotic syndrome should be managed appropriately. The prognosis is excellent, assuming that any acute renal failure is treated, and both recurrence and long-term chronic renal failure are very uncommon.

Similar illnesses may follow acute infections with Staphyloccoci, Pneumococci and Meningococci.

### Infective endocarditis

Many patients with endocarditis have proteinuria and haematuria and, in a smaller number, renal failure occurs due to the nephritis. Histologically this is usually a focal proliferative nephritis, sometimes occurring with crescents. Any organism causing endocarditis is associated with glomerulonephritis. Treating the nephritis requires eradication of the endocarditis by antibiotics or surgery, or both.

### Shunt nephritis

This is similar to infective endocarditis in that the aetiology is due to chronic infection. This occurs on a shunt of synthetic material used for draining hydrocephalus. The organism most frequently found is *Staphylococcus albus* and histologically the nephritis is usually of the mesangiocapillary type. The presenting features range from haematuria and proteinuria to a nephrotic syndrome and renal failure. The basic treatment of the nephritis is to cure the infection, which usually requires removal of the shunt.

## Parasitic diseases

Chronic nephritis complicating malaria, schistosomiasis and filariasis are common in countries where those diseases are endemic.

# SYSTEMIC DISEASES WHICH ARE NOT IMMUNE MEDIATED

## Diabetes mellitus

This is an increasingly important cause of chronic and end-stage renal failure. In the UK it accounts for 20–30 per cent of patients requiring dialysis or transplantation. Both insulin-dependent and non-insulin-dependent diabetes lead to diabetic nephropathy.

### CLINICAL FEATURES

The presenting features are the development of proteinuria, succeeded successively by a nephrotic syndrome and renal failure in patients with known diabetes. Patients with nephropathy frequently have other complications of diabetes, thus affecting their management, in particular diabetic retinopathy almost always accompanies diabetic nephropathy. A particular complication of diabetes mellitus is **acute papillary necrosis**, when a papilla becomes ischaemic due to the impaired intrarenal blood supply. Sometimes a papilla becomes detached and causes obstruction of that kidney.

### PATHOLOGY

Histology shows thickening of the basement membranes of the glomeruli and the tubules, and arterial disease. The Kimmelstiel–Wilson lesion is characteristic and consists of an area of sclerosis in the glomerular mesangium. As with the other complications of diabetes such as retinopathy and neuropathy, the underlying aetiology is not understood.

### DIAGNOSIS

The diagnosis is usually straightforward, and biopsy is often considered unnecessary when proteinuria etc. develops in a setting of diabetes mellitus.

### MANAGEMENT

The management is that of renal hypertension which frequently accompanies diabetic nephropathy, and the nephrotic syndrome, chronic renal failure and end-stage renal failure as they develop. Control of high blood pressure in diabetics is extremely important as good control decelerates the complications, including nephropathy.

Diabetic nephropathy cannot be reversed. The most important factor in delaying progression is good control of hypertension. There is new evidence that very strict control, if possible, of the diabetes improves outcome. Currently there is much interest in the possibility of improvement produced by angiotensin-converting enzyme inhibitors, for example, captopril. This drug reduces proteinuria in the early stages of diabetic nephropathy and trials are under way to establish whether it results in, or is associated with, an improvement in the long-term outcome. When end-stage renal failure develops, both dialysis and transplantation are effective and appropriate if other severe complications, such as peripheral or coronary vascular disease, do not contraindicate these measures. Pancreatic transplantation as a treatment for diabetes is practicable, but is still undergoing assessment; it is not widely practised yet.

## Hyperuricaemia

Nephropathy due to hyperuricaemia occurs in two settings: gouty nephropathy and acute hyperuricaemic nephropathy.

Gout may affect the kidney by causing uric acid stones (page 580), or by a chronic interstitial nephritis with deposition of sodium urate crystals in the kidney substance. Hypertension is very commonly associated.

The renal presentation is usually that of chronic renal failure, often found by chance in patients whose gout and hypertension are being supervised. The management is that of the hypertension and gout itself, i.e. prescribing allopurinol, which reduces the formation of uric acid. The dose of allopurinol must be carefully measured against the patient's renal function, as this drug is renally excreted and accumulation causes bone marrow toxicity.

Acute hyperuricaemic nephropathy occurs in patients with lymphoproliferative and myelo-proliferative disorders who are receiving chemo-therapy. The massive cell destruction causes hyperuricaemia and hyperuricosuria, in consequence the precipitation of uric acid crystals in the tubules causes intratubular obstruction and acute renal failure (tumour lysis syndrome). Acute oliguria in this setting is the usual presenting feature. The condition is preventable by prophylactic prescription of allopurinol with, or preferably before, the chemotherapy. If, however, the condition develops in addition to allopurinol, the solubility of uric acid in the urine should be increased by giving sodium bicarbonate to raise the urine pH above 7.

# Haemolytic uraemic syndromes

A number of syndromes are characterized by acute intravascular haemolysis and acute renal failure. The commonest is the haemolytic uraemic syndrome of childhood. A similar disorder occurs in adults, and also haemolytic uraemic syndrome in the puerperium, or related to oral contraceptives, and thrombotic thrombocytopenic purpura (Moschowitz's syndrome).

## CLINICAL FEATURES

These are mainly an acute haemolytic anaemia, bleeding due to thrombocytopenia and acute renal failure. In children there is often a preceding infection of the gastrointestinal or respiratory tract. In adults the only recognizable antecedent factors are parturition and oestrogens (usually the contraceptive pill). Other systems may be involved, especially the brain: indeed involvement of the brain is a central feature of thrombotic thrombocytopaenic purpura. Hypertension, which may be severe, often develops.

## PATHOLOGY AND PATHOGENESIS

The arterioles are occluded by fibrin and have fibrinoid necrosis in their walls. The glomeruli are ischaemic. The aetiology is unknown, but is thought to be due to a sequence of endothelial damage, coagulation with consumption of platelets and clotting factors, and haemolysis due to mechanical damage to red cells by the abnormal vessel wall and fibrin strands. This damage causes the fragmented and distorted erythrocytes characteristic of this condition, and has given rise to the term microangiopathic haemolytic anaemia (page 618). It has been suggested that in some patients there is a deficiency of plasma factor(s) necessary for the production of prostacyclin which prevents platelet aggregation.

## DIAGNOSIS

The combination of microangiopathic haemolytic anaemia, thrombocytopenia, bleeding and renal failure, with or without the involvement of other organs, is unmistakable. Renal biopsy is not easy because of the thrombocytopenia and indeed is not strictly necessary.

## MANAGEMENT AND PROGNOSIS

There is a spontaneous remission rate, particularly in children. However, other patients rapidly develop terminal renal failure, emphasizing the need for effective treatment. There is no convincing evidence that steroids, immunosuppressive drugs or anticoagulants are useful. Plasma infusion or plasma exchange may produce improvement, presumably by correcting a deficiency of plasma factor(s). However, not all cases respond to this treatment.

# Amyloidosis

The kidney may be affected by primary and secondary amyloid (page 494); the commonest cause of the latter now is rheumatoid arthritis, although occasionally cases of renal amyloid are seen with tuberculosis, bronchiectasis and osteo-myelitis.

The renal presenting feature is proteinuria, which in many patients causes a nephrotic syndrome.

The diagnosis is confirmed by renal biopsy, but powerful histological support for the diagnosis is provided by biopsy of easily available tissue from the gum, rectum, involved skin or abdominal wall fat. If amyloid is not found in these extrarenal sites renal involvement is not excluded.

Secondary amyloid may regress if the underlying cause can be treated, but treatment of primary amyloid, with the possible exception of colchicine for familial Mediterranean fever, is ineffectual. The outcome for the patient with renal involvement mainly depends on the involvement of other organs and the underlying cause. If end-stage renal failure develops then both dialysis and transplantation are suitable if other circumstances allow.

# *Neoplasms*

## MYELOMA

Patients presenting with typical features of myeloma are often found incidentally to have impaired renal function. Other patients may present with acute renal failure or proteinuria. The renal damage is caused by the light chains themselves, hypercalcaemia, intratubular obstruction due to precipitation of proteins, amyloidosis and hyperuricaemia due to treatment (page 464) if proper prophylaxis is not employed.

The diagnosis is made on the usual bone marrow and biochemical findings, when renal biopsy is not usually necessary. If the latter is performed it can provide the diagnosis by the presence of typical myeloma cases in the tubules – these are large, homogenous and eosinophilic.

The treatment is the same as that for myeloma, with dialysis for end-stage renal failure if appropriate. The prognosis of myeloma with renal failure is that of the myeloma itself; the renal failure confers a worse prognosis only if it is left untreated.

## CARCINOMA

There is an association between membranous nephropathy and the common carcinomas, for example, bronchus. The renal disease itself is undistinguishable from the idiopathic form. There is suggestive, but inconclusive evidence that complexes of tumour antigen and antibody cause the nephritis.

## LYMPHOMA

Minimal change nephropathy is associated rarely with lymphomas. The explanation is not clear, but may be due to abnormal lymphocyte function (page 633). Treatment of the underlying neoplasia alone can cause remission of the proteinuria, indicating its causal role.

# *F*AMILIAL RENAL DISEASE AND TUBULAR DISORDERS

There are many familial disorders with a renal component; involvement of other organs or tissues such as the eyes or ears, may predominate in the presentation.

# *Hereditary glomerular disease*

## ALPORT'S SYNDROME

Inheritance is autosomal dominant with a varying degree of penetrance. Twenty per cent of cases are the result of new mutations. The disease is due to a defect in the synthesis of basement membranes, giving a typical appearance on electron microscopy. The commonest features are persistent or recurring macroscopic haematuria, which may be preceded by an upper respiratory infection, and proteinuria, which very rarely causes a nephrotic syndrome. The renal disease leads to chronic renal failure, usually in adult life. Women are usually less severely affected than men, few of whom survive beyond the age of 40 years without dialysis or transplantation. Nerve deafness is commonly associated and about 15 per cent of patients have abnormalities in the lens, such as lenticonus – a cone-shaped lens. The eye and ear defects may be asymptomatic. There is no single explanation for the variability of the disease presentation, or for the considerable variation between sexes. Antenatal diagnosis is not yet possible.

## FAMILIAL RECURRENT HAEMATURIA

Familial recurrent haematuria is dominantly inherited. It is a benign disease without deafness. Although the characteristic ultrastructural lesion of Alport's syndrome is absent, the glomerular basement is abnormally thin.

## CYSTIC DISEASE

### *Adult polycystic disease*

The inheritance is autosomal dominant. The gene responsible has not yet been identified, but marker genes have been identified, allowing prenatal diagnosis with some certainty. The presentation is in middle age, but the disease may occur in childhood. It is a common cause of renal failure in adults. The cause is unknown. The cysts are distributed so that renal enlargement is usually unequal. The cysts vary in size, are present in cortex and medulla, and affect all parts of the nephron, including the glomerulus. The liver contains cysts in 50 per cent of patients and about 10 per cent of patients have aneurysms of the cerebral arteries.

Presenting features include renal pain, stones, haematuria, infection or chronic renal failure. The kidney masses are usually palpable. Proteinuria is common, but rarely clinically significant.

Diagnosis is confirmed by ultrasonography or urography (Fig. 17.12).

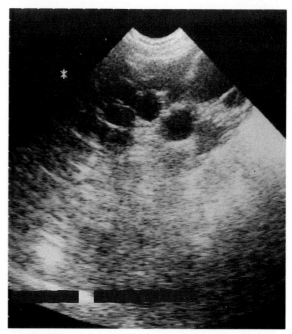

**Figure 17.12** Ultrasound of a polycystic kidney. Note the multiple cysts in the parenchyma.

The progression is variable, some patients have a normal lifespan, but more commonly, terminal renal failure occurs within 10 years of diagnosis. Liver disease very rarely develops in the adult form. Many patients are diagnosed because they refer themselves for investigation when the disease is found in a relative.

Treatment is that of chronic renal failure. Some patients require supplements for salt loss.

### Infantile polycystic disease

The cause in unknown; inheritance is recessive. Cases range from the newborn baby with huge renal masses to the older child presenting with cystic kidney and liver disease. Liver disease is a serious component of the illness, with hepatic failure, portal hypertension and cirrhosis as severe complications. Infantile polcystic disease may be diagnosed prenatally using ultrasound. The baby often looks abnormal with Potter facies (low set ears, a broad flat nose and micrognathos). The large kidneys may obstruct labour. Moderate kidney enlargement and hepatomegaly are found in older children. The progression of hypertension and renal insufficiency is variable. As there is no specific treatment, the management is that of progressive renal failure and of the liver disease, which may require liver transplantation.

### Medullary cystic disease (nephronophthisis)

These conditions can be regarded as synonymous. In children the disease may progress insidiously and the child presents with chronic renal failure and dwarfism. Hepatic, ophthalmic, neurological and bony abnormalities also occur. Thirst and polyuria are common, but hypertension is rare because of renal wasting of potassium and sodium. Proteinuria is absent. The cause is unknown. Inheritance is recessive although dominant forms usually occur, particularly in young adults. There is no specific treatment; there is no contraindication to dialysis or transplantation.

### Medullary sponge kidneys

Although medullary sponge kidneys are mostly sporadic, there are reports of familial cases. The papillary medulla contains cavities and cysts connected to tubules so that the cut surfaces of the kidney resemble a sponge. Patients present with haematuria, infection or stone formation. Management depends upon the last two complications and, when it occurs, on chronic renal failure.

# Renal tubular disorders

These may be inborn metabolic errors which alter transport systems across the tubular epithelium, or acquired from toxic, immunological or inflammatory causes. The consequences may be excretion of substances absent in normal urine, excessive excretion of a component of normal urine or failure to reabsorb. Most tubular disorders are rare, and only the commonest of them are described.

## RENAL TUBULAR ACIDOSIS

Abnormalities of renal tubular acidification may be quantitative when the number of functioning nephrons is too few to cope with the metabolic acid load, for example, in chronic renal failure. In such cases individual tubular function is normal. Qualitative abnormalities occur in the proximal and distal types of renal tubular acidosis (RTA).

### Proximal renal tubular acidosis

The defect is a bicarbonate leak with excessive bicarbonate appearing in the urine at serum bicarbonate levels lower than expected. The primary form presents in infancy with growth failure, vomiting, hypercholoraemic acidosis and alkaline or slightly acid urine. The disorder may also occur at other ages accompanying generalized tubular diseases such as Fanconi syndrome and cystinosis, and following renal transplantation. These patients excrete normal quantities of acid and can form an acid urine in the presence of severe acidosis. There are no bone changes, nor is there nephrocalcinosis. Treatment is with large amounts of alkali, 10 mmol/kg. Thiazide diuretics may decrease these requirements by reducing the extracellular fluid volume and increasing bicarbonate reabsorption. Potassium supplements are required. The prognosis of primary proximal RTA is good and treatment may be reduced or discontinued in later life.

### Primary distal renal tubular acidosis

Abnormal distal tubular cell metabolism results in failure of $H^+$ secretion into tubular fluid in the presence of systemic acidosis. It may occur in early life with failure to thrive, polyuria, dehydration and constipation. Some cases are not diagnosed until growth retardation is noted in adolescence. Renal stones, rickets and osteomalacia are common and nephrocalcinosis invariable (Fig. 17.13). Weakness due to potassium deficiency occurs occasionally. Diagnosis depends on demonstrating a urine pH above 6 with either spontaneous or ammonium chloride-induced acidaemia. Titratable acid and ammonium excretion concentrations are low.

Treatment is with small amounts of alkali, 1–3 mmol/kg/day (1–3 mEq/kg/day) equivalent to daily endogenous production of $H^+$, and potassium. The dose should be adjusted to keep the urine calcium below 0.05 mmol/kg/day (2 mg/kg/day). If nephrocalcinosis has not developed, the prognosis can be good.

Secondary forms of distal RTA occur in vitamin D poisoning, idiopathic hypercalcaemia, amphotericin nephrotoxicity and chronic active hepatitis.

## THE FANCONI SYNDROMES

A number of multiple tubular disorders are characterized by glycosuria, phosphaturia, aminoaciduria and tubular acidosis. They are best considered as: Lignac–Fanconi syndrome (cystinosis), idiopathic 'adult' Fanconi syndrome (non-cystinotic Fanconi syndrome) and secondary Fanconi syndrome.

### Cystinosis

Cystinosis is an autosomal recessive condition. Its pathogenesis is unknown but is thought to be a lysosomal storage disease with impairment of the transport mechanisms responsible for removing cystine from the lysosome. Cystine crystals are widely deposited in the soft tissues. The proximal tubule is shortened and thickened (swan-neck deformity) but this is not specific. This disease occurs in about 1 in 40 000 live births. It is usually diagnosed in the first year. Prenatal diagnosis is possible by analysis of the amniotic fluid cells for cystine.

Failure to thrive in infancy, rickets, polydipsia and polyuria, recurrent vomiting and dehydration are typical symptoms in childhood. Ocular involvement causes photophobia and later, especially in transplanted patients, hypothyroidism occurs. On investigation a metabolic acidosis with low plasma levels of potassium and phosphate is found. The urine contains glucose, phosphate and amino acids, and there is a concentrating defect. A diagnosis is easily made by demonstrating cystine crystals in the cornea, the bone marrow or skin, or by measuring the cystine content of leukocytes.

Recently treatment with phosphocysteamine has been introduced. It reduces plasma concentration of cystine, but any long-term benefit awaits proof. The usual course is progression to end-stage renal failure by puberty. Symptomatic biochemical abnormalities should be corrected. Dialysis and transplantation have been performed – cystine reaccumulates in the grafted kidney but has not yet been shown to cause renal failure. Recently a small number of cases of dementia, presumably due to cystine deposition, have occurred, with eventual death.

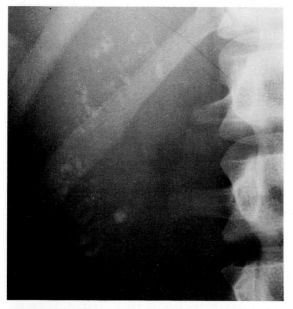

**Figure 17.13** Plain X-ray (i.e. without contrast medium) showing multiple deposits of calcium within the renal substance of the right kidney (nephrocalcinosis) in a patient with renal tubular acidosis.

## Idiopathic 'adult' Fanconi syndrome

Recessive and dominant forms occur and usually present in early adulthood. There is no cystinosis but intestinal transport defects are found. The presentation is usually with bone pain and muscle weakness due to osteomalacia.

## Secondary Fanconi syndromes

These arise from a number of causes such as myeloma, intoxication with heavy metals and drugs, inborn errors of metabolism such as Wilson's disease (page 402) or glycogen storage diseases.

## PRIMARY TUBULAR CONCENTRATING DEFECTS

Nephrogenic diabetes insipidus (page 552) is caused by a block in the antidiuretic hormone—cyclic AMP pathway affecting water permeability of the distal tubular cell. Inheritance is X-linked and carrier females have a partial defect in concentration.

## SECONDARY TUBULAR CONCENTRATING DEFECTS

Hypercalcaemia and hypokalaemia impair cyclic adenosine monophosphate (AMP) production in the distal tubular cell and water reabsorption. The effects are reversible in the short term but not if structural damage has resulted. Drugs, for example, lithium carbonate and methoxy-flurane, may cause a similar concentrating defect.

## AMINOACIDURIAS

These are primary, with impaired tubular reabsorption but normal blood amino acid levels (e.g. cystinuria, Hartnup disease), or secondary to hyperaminoacidaemias, for example, phenylketonuria in which tubular reabsorption is insufficient to deal with the load presented.

## BARTTER'S SYNDROME

Bartter's syndrome is a recessively inherited condition which usually presents with failure to thrive, a normal blood pressure and polyuria and polydipsia due to failure to conserve salt and water. Hypokalaemia, metabolic acidosis, hyperreninaemia and aldosteronism and a vasopressin-resistant concentrating defect are biochemical features, and histologically there is hyperplasia of the juxtaglomerular apparatus. The pathogenesis of this heterogeneous condition is unknown: defective tubular sodium handling, angiotensin resistance and excessive prostaglandin synthesis have all been suggested. Symptomatic improvement may occur by correcting the electrolyte abnormalities by diet, potassium supplements or spironolactone. Propranalol has been used to suppress renin and prostaglandin synthetase inhibitors, for example, indomethacin or ketoprofen, have also been reported as being successful.

# ANATOMICAL ABNORMALITIES

# Vesico-ureteric reflux

Vesicoureteric reflux (page 449) occurs in one-third of children with urinary tract infection and surveys of relatives have demonstrated that it is familial. Inheritance is multifactorial with a 10 per cent chance of a first-degree relative being affected.

## URETERIC DUPLICATION

Ureteric duplication is one of the more common forms of urogenital abnormality with an incidence of 1 in 200. Renal damage may occur from obstructed ectopic ureters or vesicoureteric reflux. An autosomal dominant form of inheritance is thought to be responsible.

# DRUGS AND THE KIDNEY

Many drugs can cause renal damage because the kidney is the final common pathway for excreting drugs and their metabolites. If renal failure from any cause is present, those drugs excreted renally will accumulate unless dosage is modified.

# Renal disease caused by drugs

The main effects of drugs on the kidney are direct nephrotoxicity – acute tubular or interstitial damage and renal papillary necrosis – prerenal effects, obstructive uropathy, allergic or immunological damage, for example, vasculitis or nephritis.

Up to 20 per cent of cases of acute renal failure are caused by drugs and chemicals, but minor degrees of damage may pass undetected. Chronic damage usually occurs insidiously and the role of drugs may be unrecognized. The clinical features of drug-induced renal diseases are no different to those of spontaneous renal disease apart from the obvious history of exposure to drugs. An accurate drug history must be obtained from any patient with renal disease.

## TUBULAR AND INTERSTITIAL DAMAGE

Drugs and their metabolites are selectively taken up and concentrated by the renal tubular cells before excretion. As high intracellular concentrations occur particularly in the renal medulla, direct toxic damage tends to affect the renal tubular cells and renal papillae and is usually dose dependent.

Acute tubular necrosis is the lesion usually found due to drug-induced renal failure and antibiotics, especially the aminoglycosides, are the commonest cause. Aminoglycosides are excreted unchanged by the kidney. Renal damage is dose dependent and occurs typically in de-

hydrated patients and in those presenting with renal failure. Nomograms should be used for calculating the initial dose according to the age, weight and serum creatinine levels of the patient, and subsequent doses should be adjusted according to plasma levels. Potentiation can occur with other nephrotoxic agents. Other antibiotics causing acute tubular necrosis are cephalosporins, colistin and polymyxin B. Frusemide may potentiate the nephrotoxicity of aminoglycosides, cephalosporins and polymyxins. Amphotericin is an antifungal agent which causes acute proximal and distal tubular damage, causing renal tubular acidosis, hypokalaemia and nephrocalcinosis. Gold and mercurial compounds produce proximal tubular damage. Both paracetamol and aspirin, in overdosage, may cause renal tubular necrosis.

Acute renal failure may follow contrast radiography, especially in patients with diabetes, jaundice, myeloma, dehydration or pre-existing renal disease. Liver disease prolongs excretion of contrast medium through the kidneys, resulting in tubular damage. Modern urographic media, for example, diatrizoate and iothalamate, are relatively safe, even in renal failure where high doses may be required, but dehydration must be avoided. It is essential that dehydration is avoided in all ill or uraemic patients undergoing contrast radiography, including computed tomography.

Fluorinated anaesthetic agents such as methoxyflurane cause acute distal tubular damage, resulting in polyuria and hypernatraemia. This effect is less common with enflurane and halothane. Lithium salts can cause nephrogenic diabetes insipidus, unresponsive to vasopressin and aldosterone. Polyuria and dehydration result in renal damage and increasing plasma lithium levels. Both acute and chronic renal failure may occur, with scarring of the interstitium. Lithum salts cause tubular acidosis, hypocalciuria and membranous nephropathy. Lithium therapy must be monitored by plasma levels and regular tests of renal function.

Demethylchlortetracycline also causes diabetes insipidus. It is used to treat inappropriate antidiuretic hormone secretion, but care must be taken to avoid dehydration and the development of acute renal failure.

## ANALGESIC NEPHROPATHY

This is the commonest form of chronic drug-induced renal damage. It is an important cause of renal failure, accounting for 5–30 per cent of patients with end-stage renal failure in different countries. Analgesic nephropathy is preventable, and discontinuation of analgesics often produces stabilization or improvement in renal function.

### Aetiology and pathogenesis

No analgesic drug can be considered completely safe. In practice, virtually all patients with this condition have taken several drugs over the years, often as mixtures, and it is impossible to single out any one as the causative agent, although phenacetin has been described as the main cause. Papillary necrosis can occur following the consumption of 1–2 kg of analgesics, equivalent to six tablets a day for 3–5 years, but many patients have taken more than this amount by the time the diagnosis is made.

### Presenting features

Analgesic nephropathy may arise secondary to a chronic disease accompanied by much pain, for example, rheumatoid arthritis. The incidence is higher in women than in men. Apart from features of chronic renal failure, the patients with the idiopathic type are characterized by depression or other psychiatric disorders, the abuse of purgatives or alcohol, dyspepsia, ischaemic heart disease, recurrent urinary tract infections, and an appearance of premature aging. Patients may also present with complications (see below). There is an 'idiopathic' group in which the long-term reason for taking analgesics is often headaches or back pain the cause of which is hard to elucidate.

### Diagnosis

This requires a high index of suspicion and an accurate drug history. All patients with renal problems should be asked about their intake of analgesics, especially patent remedies for headaches, migraine, backache or rheumatism. A sample of urine, sent for estimation of salicylates and paracetamol, will measure analgesic intake within the previous 48 hours.

Ultrasound or urography shows scarred kidneys with absent papillae in many patients due to papillary necrosis.

### Complications

Ureteric obstruction may result from the passage of a necrotic papilla or ureteric fibrosis. Transitional cell tumours of the renal pelvis and ureter occur in about 10 per cent of patients.

### Treatment

The treatment is to reduce the intake of analgesic, which is often not achieved, either because of the underlying painful condition, or because of the very nature of the abuse.

## ALLERGIC OR IMMUNOLOGICAL DAMAGE

### Glomerulonephritis

Many drugs cause glomerular damage associated with the deposition of immunoglobulins and complement, i.e. evidence of inflammation and/or immunological damage. It is thought that the drug acts as a hapten or in some other way alters a protein to form an allergen, resulting in the formation of circulating immune complexes. Two important forms of drug-induced glomerular disease are discussed in more detail.

#### Membranous nephropathy

Gold therapy for rheumatoid arthritis may cause membranous nephropathy which may progress to renal failure. Gold treatment must be accompanied by regular urine tests for protein and treatment must be discontinued if proteinuria develops. Penicillamine produces proteinuria in 10–20 per cent of patients, which remits on withdrawal of the drug. Membranous nephropathy has also been described with lithium therapy.

*Drug-induced systemic lupus erythematosus
syndrome*

The reported incidence with hydralazine varies between 10 and 20 per cent of patients treated, but renal involvement is rare. The liability to develop hydralazine-associated systemic lupus erythematosus (SLE) is genetically linked to the human leukocyte antigen DR4. Procainamide may cause the SLE syndrome in up to 30 per cent of patients on long-term therapy. It occurs both in fast and slow acetylators. Renal involvement is uncommon. Complement levels are generally normal in drug-induced SLE, and antibodies to double-stranded DNA are rare.

## Vasculitis

Vasculitis is a rare form of drug-induced renal damage. It may follow thiazide diuretics or penicillamine, and occur as part of drug-induced SLE. 'Street' heroin contains impurities which can cause vasculitis.

## Interstitial nephritis

Acute interstitial nephritis is quite common, and may be accompanied by fever and rash. Eosinophilia may be noted in the blood. In most cases, renal function improves when the drugs are withdrawn. Interstitial nephritis is seen most commonly with the penicillins, diuretics and non-steroidal anti-inflammatory drugs. It also occurs with rifampicin, sulphonamides, cotrimoxazole, cephalosporins, phenytoin, phenindione and phenazone.

## PRERENAL DAMAGE CAUSED BY DRUGS

Water and electrolyte loss occurs with excessive use of diuretics or laxatives. Lithium carbonate has similar effects, which will be exacerbated if diuretics are coprescribed. Non-steroidal anti-inflammatory drugs are an increasingly common cause of acute renal failure. The action of these drugs is to inhibit the production of prostaglandin synthetase and therefore the production of prostacyclin. If there is impairment of renal perfusion the kidneys normally respond by increasing prostacyclin, which is a vasodilator. Non-steroidal anti-inflammatory drugs prevent this protective effect, with consequent glomerular hypoperfusion and ischaemia.

## OBSTRUCTIVE UROPATHY

### Retroperitoneal fibrosis

Retroperitoneal fibrosis has been attributed to several drugs, including methysergide and methyldopa.

### Ureteric fibrosis

Ureteric fibrosis and obstruction due to a sloughed papilla are complications of analgesic nephropathy (see above).

### Tubular blockage

*Crystalluria*

Uric acid may be deposited in the renal tubules during the treatment of myeloproliferative disorders with cytotoxic agents. Allopurinol and a high fluid intake prevent urate deposition. The early sulphonamides were relatively insoluble and crystallized in acid urine. Modern sulphonamides rarely cause problems, but a high fluid intake must be maintained. Acetazolamide, which is structurally related to sulphonamides, may precipitate in the urine.

## INCREASED CATABOLISM

Glucocorticoids raise the blood urea by increasing catabolism. Tetracyclines inhibit the incorporation of amino acids into protein, causing a rise in blood urea. In renal failure, tetracycline excretion is delayed, tetracyclines should therefore be avoided in patients with renal impairment, except for doxycycline which has minimal anti-anabolic effects and even in renal failure is eliminated rapidly.

## VASCULAR OCCLUSION

Arteriolar and/or venous occlusion may occur with oestrogen therapy. It is usually reversible but occasionally causes acute renal failure.

## HAEMORRHAGE

Anticoagulants or fibrinolytic agents may cause ureteric obstruction by a blood clot within the urinary tract, or by retroperitoneal haemorrhage.

## CALCIUM NEPHROPATHY AND RENAL CALCULI

Vitamin D preparations can cause hypercalcaemia and calcium deposition in the kidney. 1-α-Hydroxycholecalciferol is safer than earlier preparations, since its effects are briefer and reversible, but serum calcium levels must be carefully monitored. Renal calculi have been described following excessive consumption of vitamin D and antacids containing calcium (milk-alkali syndrome). Rarely xanthine nephropathy occurs with allopurinol therapy.

# Prescribing in renal failure

Renal failure has several different effects. It can diminish renal excretion, alter drug metabolism by diminishing protein binding with consequent greater bioavailability of the drug, change the volume of distribution, and reduce gastrointestinal absorption.

Prescribing for patients with renal failure therefore requires a knowledge of the metabolism and activity of the drug, its duration of action and method of excretion. General principles to be followed are to choose the drug with minimal nephrotoxic effects, to use plasma levels to prescribe the dose, to avoid prolonged courses of toxic drugs and to avoid nephrotoxic combinations of drugs. Therapeutic drug levels may be maintained either by reducing doses or by increasing the intervals between doses.

# Renal disease in pregnancy

# Hypertension and eclampsia

In a normal pregnancy the diastolic blood pressure falls by approximately 15 mm Hg, thus the diastolic blood pressure should be below 75 mm Hg. A raised blood pressure is a common complication of renal disease in any patient, and is evident from an early stage in pregnancy. Hypertensive disorders of pregnancy can be divided into two categories: idiopathic hypertension (pre-eclampsia) and hypertension due to underlying renal disease. Pre-eclampsia seldom recurs after the first pregnancy. When hypertension in pregnancy is a manifestation of latent essential hypertension, or occurs as a complication of renal disease, it usually recurs in all subsequent pregnancies.

# Glomerulonephritis and pregnancy

It is important to exclude glomerulonephritis as a cause of proteinuria, hypertension or impaired renal function because patients with this condition constitute a high-risk group during pregnancy. Urine microscopy is the most sensitive method for detecting glomerulonephritis as the presence of increased numbers of glomerular erythrocytes in the urine is a specific indicator of glomerulonephritis. While it is not definite that pregnancy affects the natural history of glomerulonephritis, some patients with lesions which are normally benign, such as membranous glumerulonephritis, may deteriorate sharply during pregnancy.

# Urinary tract infection

Bacteriuria (i.e. $10^5$ organism/ml) accompanies pregnancy in 5–10 per cent of women; approximately 30 per cent of untreated patients with bacteriuria will develop acute pyelonephritis. Treatment of bacteriuria with antibacterial agents prevents acute pyelonephritis and it is therefore important to treat bacteriuria promptly. A high proportion of pregnant women with bacteriuria will have underlying renal disease if investigated during the *post-partum* period.

# Reflux nephropathy

This is a common condition, and a large proportion of these patients are at risk of urinary tract infections. If renal failure is already present then they may undergo an accelerated deterioration to end-stage renal failure. Prophylactic antibiotics are indicated during the pregnancy.

# Acute renal failure

Acute tubular necrosis may develop during pregnancy due to either sepsis or haemorrhage. The most common context in which acute tubular necrosis accompanies septicaemia is in septic abortions performed in early pregnancy. The incidence of this condition has fallen to negligible levels in countries where abortion has been legalized. Acute tubular necrosis may accompany haemorrhage in late pregnancy, when the much more serious complication of acute cortical necrosis may occur. Patients with acute cortical necrosis may recover gradually over 3–6 months to a level at which their own kidneys can sustain adequate function, but for most patients the prognosis is very poor, most requiring maintenance dialysis or transplantation.

# Renal calculi

Renal calculi are common and there may be a particular propensity to form stones during pregnancy, most likely due to infection. Stones can grow rapidly during pregnancy.

# Pregnancy and chronic renal failure

Patients with plasma creatinine greater than 200 μmol/l are at considerable risk of accelerating to end-stage renal failure if they become pregnant and are generally advised not to do so. In addition, those women with active glomerular disease, for example, mesangiocapillary glomerulonephritis or lupus glomerulonephritis should avoid pregnancy.

# **D**isorders of Metabolism

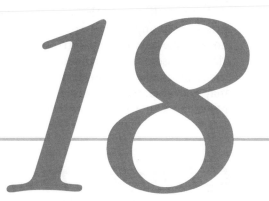

18

# INTRODUCTION

Metabolic disorders are a diverse group of diseases ranging from the common, such as diabetes mellitus, to the very rare. They comprise a very important part of medical practice, not only because of their intrinsic problems, but also because of their influence on the management of unrelated disorders which the patient may develop, for example, management of pneumonia in a patient with diabetes mellitus requires more than antibiotics and simple continuation of the routine treatment of the underlying metabolic disease.

Increased understanding of cell biology and genetics have begun to define the precise abnormalities in several of these disorders, with the prospect of new treatments such as gene therapy bringing about the cure of hitherto lifelong diseases.

# Clinical problems

# DIABETES MELLITUS

## INTRODUCTION

Diabetes mellitus is the name given to an heterologous group of conditions characterized by hyperglycaemia (high blood glucose concentration) and other metabolic derangements secondary to insufficient insulin action. Thus, the clinical picture can be created by absolute insulin deficiency, as in **type I** or **insulin-dependent diabetes mellitus (IDDM)** or by insulin resistance and failure of compensatory additional insulin secretion as in **type II** or **non-insulin-dependent diabetes mellitus (NIDDM)**.

## EPIDEMIOLOGY

Diabetes mellitus is common: the prevalence in the UK is quoted as 1.2 per cent (1988 figures) and is probably rising. It is estimated that, of the calculated one million people in the UK with diabetes, about 250 000 are not known. Ascertainment may increase as a result of some of the recent reforms in primary health care in the UK. Non-insulin-dependent diabetes mellitus is much more common than IDDM (about 90%). It is in part a disease of ageing (4 per cent in the over 60s). Its increasing prevalence may relate to the increasing mean age of the British population. Non-insulin-dependent diabetes mellitus is also a condition that relates to lifestyle and particularly affects immigrant populations in Britain. Amongst British Asians, prevalence in the over 60s is over 16 per cent. The incidence and prevalence of IDDM is also rising, for reasons that are not yet clear. The incidence rate of diabetes mellitus in the under 20s (which will be almost exclusively IDDM) is over 20 per 100 000 population per year. It has doubled since 1968 and there are 18 000 young people with diabetes in the UK today.

## PATHOPHYSIOLOGY

Insulin is a polypeptide hormone secreted by the $\beta$ cells of the islets of Langerhans in the pancreas directly into the portal vein. This endogenous insulin goes directly to the liver. The liver denatures approximately 70 per cent of the insulin presented to it, so that in health peripheral blood levels of insulin are always considerably lower than portal levels. The principal actions of insulin are listed in Table 18.1. It

**Table 18.1** The metabolic actions of insulin.

### 1. Hypoglycaemic
Suppression of hepatic glucose production
  (glycogenolysis and gluconeogenesis)
Stimulation of glucose uptake and oxidation by muscle
  and fat

### 2. On fat metabolism
Suppression of lipolysis – reduction of circulating non-
  esterified fatty acids (NEFA)
Stimulation of fat synthesis
Inhibition of ketogenesis
Stimulation of ketone utilization

### 3. On protein metabolism
Inhibition of protein breakdown
Stimulation of protein synthesis

should be noted that higher plasma levels of insulin are required to stimulate peripheral glucose uptake than to reduce hepatic glucose production.

In the absence of adequate insulin action, hepatic glucose production proceeds unchecked, peripheral tissues, such as muscle and adipose tissue, are unable to take up or oxidize glucose and hyperglycaemia results. Lipolysis proceeds unchecked with elevated circulating free fatty acid levels encouraging ketogenesis (ketone body formation) and increasing hepatic glucose production by providing further substrate for gluconeogenesis (synthesis of 'new' glucose from non-carbohydrate substances). Proteolysis (protein breakdown) provides further gluconeogenic fuel in the form of free amino acid. The underlying biochemical derangements explain the clinical manifestations of uncontrolled diabetes mellitus.

## AETIOLOGY

The clinical syndromes of diabetes mellitus can be divided on clinical and aetiological grounds into categories. Table 18.2 lists the main features of the two major categories of diabetes.

There is a strong link to human leukocyte antigen (HLA) haplotypes DR3 and DR4 in IDDM. In NIDDM the familial link is strong but there is no link to particular HLA types. Pancreatic islet cell antibodies are often found in the serum in IDDM and there is lymphocytic infiltration of the pancreas. The pancreatic damage gives rise to the deficiency in insulin. In NIDDM there is no evidence for an immune role in the aetiology. Insulin levels may be high but not high enough to deal with the glucose levels and there may be a degree of insulin resistance.

The World Health Organization also recognizes a third category, namely, diabetes associated with malnutrition, a ketosis-resistant diabetes seen in countries where nutritional deprivation is common. This category could strictly be considered a secondary form of the disease. Fibrocalcification of the pancreas occurs in association with protein deprivation and cyanide toxins from the consumption of cassava in one form. Protein deficiency can also produce diabetes without fibrocalcinosis, in which case the exocrine pancreatic function is preserved. Ketoacidosis does not occur. Other malnutrition related disorders coexist.

In addition to the three primary types of

**Table 18.2** Characteristics of insulin and non-insulin-dependent diabetes mellitus.

|  | IDDM | NIDDM |
| --- | --- | --- |
| Insulin deficiency | Absolute | Relative |
| Insulin resistance | Secondary | May be primary |
| Age of onset | Young | Generally over 40 years |
| Duration of prodrome | Days to weeks | Months to years |
| Ketosis | Prone | No |
| Genetics | Associated with certain HLA types | Multigenetic inheritance |
| Aetiology | Autoimmune | Variable |
| Treatment | Insulin essential | Insulin may be used |

IDDM = insulin-dependent diabetes mellitus.
NIDDM = non-insulin-dependent diabetes mellitus.

diabetes mellitus, we also recognize secondary and gestational diabetes.

## Secondary diabetes mellitus

The clinical picture of diabetes mellitus occurs secondary either to pancreatic disease or to insulin resistance in the presence of some degree of pancreatic insufficiency. In diabetes mellitus secondary to pancreatic disease, there are usually associated defects of the exocrine pancreas. Such secondary diabetes may occur late in advanced chronic pancreatitis, or in haemochromatosis, where iron deposition interferes with the function of the pancreas, liver and other endocrine organs, for example, testes, and colours the skin (bronze diabetes).

Insulin is the major hypoglycaemic hormone of the body. Avoidance of hypoglycaemia is very important for survival (the brain is, in normal circumstances, almost exclusively dependent upon a steady supply of glucose from the blood) and the body has several hormones which counteract the blood glucose lowering effect of insulin (Table 18.3). These hormones are released during hypoglycaemic stress but also in response to non-hypoglycaemic stress. Excessive production of these hormones may result in hyperglycaemia and frank diabetes mellitus if the pancreas is not able to compensate with sufficient insulin output. Thus, diabetes mellitus in a susceptible individual will manifest at times of stress (e.g. intercurrent infection); at times when insulin antagonist hormone levels are elevated, either physiologically as with growth hormone during puberty or oestrogens during pregnancy or pathologically as with growth hormone in acromegaly or adrenocorticosteroids in Cushing's syndrome; or iatrogenically as during steroid therapy. Drugs such

as thiazide diuretics can provoke diabetes, particularly in older patients by increasing insulin resistance.

## Gestational diabetes

This is diabetes mellitus occurring during, but regressing after, pregnancy. It is important for two reasons. Firstly, because the hyperglycaemia of the mother stimulates hyperinsulinaemia in the fetus, with subsequent risk of macrosomia (insulin being a very important growth factor) and neonatal hypoglycaemia *postpartum*. Secondly, because gestational diabetes is a very strong prognostic factor of NIDDM in the mother as she ages. However, affected women are very often obese and loss of the obesity with chronic maintenance of ideal body weight greatly reduces the risk of subsequent diabetes.

## CLINICAL FEATURES

Hyperglycaemia causes glycosuria, as blood levels exceed the renal tubular threshold and glucose is excreted in the urine. The high glucose concentration of the urine produces an osmotic diuresis, causing polyuria. The fluid loss of the polyuria leads to dehydration and stimulates thirst, giving rise to polydipsia. Clinically, these symptoms are often best detected and quantified as nocturia and nocturnal drinking. Fluid loss and, if the disease progresses untreated for any time, protein and fat breakdown, result in weight loss and muscle wasting. In severely insulin-deficient states, ketogenesis produces ketonuria, contributing to the osmotic diuresis and dehydration, and ketosis, which may produce nausea and a metabolic acidosis.

The physical signs of poorly controlled or untreated diabetes mellitus follow logically. Dehydration causes tachycardia, postural hypotension and reduced skin turgor (often difficult to assess) and may lead to acute renal failure; acidosis causes hyperventilation as the respiratory centre attempts to compensate for the metabolic acidosis; the breath may smell of ketones (but only 50 per cent of the population are able to smell the ketones). High plasma osmolality is associated with confusion and impaired conscious level.

The time course of the presenting illness in a

**Table 18.3** Insulin antagonists.

| Counterregulatory hormones | Drugs |
| --- | --- |
| Adrenaline | Steroids |
| Noradrenaline (reflecting activation of sympathetic nervous system) | Thiazides |
| | Diazoxide |
| Glucagon | |
| Growth hormone | |
| Cortisol | |

newly diagnosed patient varies greatly: the patient may present in an advanced stage of hyperglycaemia with ketoacidosis and impaired consciousness, severely dehydrated and ill with a short history of polydipsia, polyuria and weight loss lasting only a few days. More commonly, the history is insidious and older people with NIDDM may have had their disease for years before presenting clinically. Chronic complications of diabetes (page 481) may thus be present at diagnosis. Often an acute stress will precipitate the presentation, and infection (particularly of the genitourinary tract, skin or chest) or other acute illness such as myocardial infarction must be sought in newly presenting diabetes or in established disease during a loss of metabolic control.

## Diagnosis

Diabetes mellitus can be diagnosed by:

1. The presence of unequivocal hyperglycaemia (greater than 11.1 mmol/l glucose in venous plasma) in association with symptoms.
2. A fasting (6 hours without calories) blood glucose of greater than 7.8 mmol/l.

Only in cases of doubt is the **oral glucose tolerance test** required. In this test, 75 g glucose (exactly 389 ml chilled Lucozade for convenience) is given orally after an overnight fast. Diabetes is diagnosed if the venous plasma glucose exceeds 7.8 mmol/l fasting or 11.1 mmol/l at 2 hours after the glucose load. Values differ if capillary sampling or blood rather than plasma is tested (Table 18.4). Subjects with normal fasting levels but 2 hour levels between fasting levels and levels required for diagnosis of diabetes are classified as having impaired glucose tolerance (IGT). Four per cent

per year of these individuals develop diabetes, one-third regress to complete normality, the rest continue to show IGT.

## THE SOCIOECONOMIC COSTS OF DIABETES MELLITUS

Diabetes mellitus is a diagnosis for life. Young people with diabetes are most commonly insulin-dependent and are committed to a treatment regimen that will significantly interfere with lifestyle, dietary and exercise habits, and career opportunities, requiring daily injection therapy with no possibility of 'days off' treatment. In personal terms the costs are large. The economic costs to the community are also substantial. Twenty thousand people die prematurely because of diabetes per year. The risks of premature death (especially from ischaemic heart disease, which, together with renal disease, is the major cause of diabetes-related death in the under 50s) are particularly exaggerated in women. Women with diabetes stand 2.7 times the risk of death from a myocardial infarction (relative risk for diabetic men 1.9), or 11.5 times the risk if under 45 years of age. Death from renal failure was 40 times more common in the under 50s in the presence of diabetes. These figures from 1981 may have been substantially improved upon by the recent increased availability of renal support and replacement therapy to people with diabetes. In terms of morbidity, diabetes is the most common cause of blindness in people aged 46 to 65 years in the UK and it increases the risk of limb loss after foot ulceration manyfold. Modern management may be able to alter many of these gloomy statistics and it is not easy now to give a true prognosis to the newly diagnosed patient: the problems that beset the last generation may be reduced, if not avoided.

**Table 18.4** Oral glucose tolerance test (glucose values for the diagnosis of diabetes mellitus in mmol/l).

| | Venous | | Capillary | |
| --- | --- | --- | --- | --- |
| | **Blood** | **Plasma** | **Blood** | **Plasma** |
| Fasting | ≥6.7 | ≥7.8 | ≥6.7 | ≥7.8 |
| At 2 hours to diagnose diabetes | >10.0 | >11.1 | >11.1 | >12.2 |
| At 2 hours to diagnose IGT | 6.7–10.0 | 7.8–11.1 | 7.8–11.1 | 8.9–12.2 |

IGT = impaired glucose tolerance.

## ACUTE COMPLICATIONS

### *Hyperglycaemic coma*

#### *Diabetic ketoacidosis*

Diabetic ketoacidosis (DKA) is characteristic of IDDM and an absolute indication of the need for insulin therapy. In fact less than 50 per cent of patients with IDDM actually present in DKA, but it may occur at any time during the course of the disease, either because of withdrawal of adequate insulin therapy or because of an intercurrent stress.

#### *Clinical features*

The patient presents as dehydrated, ketoacidotic (i.e. with ketones in the plasma and urine and acidotic with a low arterial pH and reduced venous bicarbonate) and a reduced conscious level. The condition may be complicated by gastroparesis, renal failure, hypothermia and an underlying event which has precipitated the ketoacidosis, such as pneumonia. Until renal perfusion is diminished by dehydration, patients may be able to control the hyperglycaemia by renal glucose loss and high fluid intake, so the blood glucose level does not necessarily reflect the severity of the patient's state.

#### *Management*

Immediate treatment consists of urgent rehydration, together with insulin therapy optimally given as a low-dose intravenous infusion (Table 18.5) with careful monitoring of potassium replacement. Often plasma potassium levels are high at presentation but total body potassium is diminished and levels fall quickly as therapy commences. Electrocardiographic monitoring is useful to assess potassium needs. Arterial pH, blood glucose, plasma potassium, conscious level, blood pressure, respiratory rate and fluid output must be closely monitored and intravenous insulin therapy continued until ketones have been cleared from the urine for 24 hours. Intravenous insulin must not be stopped until a subcutaneous dose has been administered.

Rapid correction of blood glucose levels can produce fluid shifts which predispose to cerebral oedema, especially in children. Glucose fall should not exceed 5 mmol/h. It is rarely necessary to give bicarbonate to correct pH and can be dangerous as intracerebral pH takes longer to equilibrate. As blood glucose levels reach 13 mmol/l, insulin infusion should continue but intravenous dextrose used as the fluid replacement to avoid blood glucose falling below 10 mmol/l. A suggested regimen for initial therapy in DKA is given in Table 18.5. The principle of good management is close monitoring.

Any underlying cause (e.g. myocardial infarction, infection) must be sought and treated.

The most common errors in the management of diabetic ketoacidosis are late diagnosis, in-

**Table 18.5** Initial treatment of diabetic ketoacidosis: suggested regimen.

| Time | Investigation | Fluid | Insulin | Additives | Observations |
|---|---|---|---|---|---|
| 0–30 min | Plasma glucose, $K^+$, pH, $HCO_3^-$, ECG monitor | Normal saline 1000 ml i.v. | — | — | Pulse, blood pressure, temperature, respiration every 15 min |
| 30–90 min | Glucose hourly from this point | Normal saline 1000 ml i.v. | 6 U/hour i.v. (0.1 U/kg/hour) | 20 mmol $K^+$ i.v. | Every 30 min |
| 90–120 min | Plasma glucose, $K^+$, pH, $HCO_3^-$ | Normal saline 500 ml i.v. | 6 U/hour i.v. | 20 mmol $K^+$ i.v. | Every hour |

Further replacement depends upon clinical state. It is suggested that fluid replacement continue with N/saline until blood glucose reaches 15 mmol/l, after which 5 per cent glucose is used. Insulin should be kept at 6 U/hour until blood glucose is ≤11 mmol/l, when it may be reduced to 3 U/hour if necessary to maintain blood glucose. Plasma glucose should be reduced by approximately 5 mmol/l/hour. Potassium should be measured 2 hours after starting therapy and at least 4-hourly thereafter.

adequate monitoring, inadequate fluid replacement, too rapid a reduction in insulin infusion, and omitting to start subcutaneous insulin therapy before discontinuing intravenous infusion.

## Hyperosmolar non-ketotic coma

### Clinical features

This is most commonly seen in older people, often as their presentation, and seems particularly common in older black patients. Often thirst quenching with sugary drinks (Lucozade, Colas, orange juice) during the prodrome contributes to the degree of hyperglycaemia. Blood glucose is very high but ketosis is absent and, although insulin is necessary initially, later maintenance therapy may not include insulin.

### Management

Treatment is by rehydration and intravenous insulin therapy. There is discussion about the most appropriate fluid to use for rehydration – half-normal saline may be used but the first litre of fluid should probably be normal saline as in DKA, given that even this will be hypotonic to the hyperosmolar patient. Later, half-normal saline, dextrose saline and dextrose are used as appropriate. Insulin is also necessary, often at lower doses than in DKA, although the low dose regimen advised currently for DKA can be used (Table 18.5) Cerebral oedema and renal failure may develop.

## Lactic acidosis

This complication (page 512) of diabetes mellitus is rarely seen in the UK today since the withdrawal of phenformin as a treatment for diabetes and more careful use of the related compound metformin. It carries a 50 per cent mortality and requires careful correction of the acidosis by using small amounts of bicarbonate as well as fluid replacement and insulin.

## Hypoglycaemia

The brain, in normal circumstances, is dependent upon glucose as a metabolic fuel, and because it can neither synthesize nor store glucose, it depends upon a well-maintained supply from the blood. If blood glucose falls too low, cerebral dysfunction ensues, starting with confusion and ending in coma. Usually as blood glucose falls, a series of protective responses occur (including the release of adrenaline and stimulation of the sympathetic nervous system) which act both to restore blood glucose and to create a symptom complex (e.g. sweating, palpitations, tremor, hunger) which alerts the patient to eat. In many patients with diabetes, especially of long duration or with frequent hypoglycaemia in the past, these protective responses are impaired. Such patients are prone to severe hypoglycaemia without warning.

### Clinical features

Diabetic hypoglycaemia is typically of rapid onset, from a few minutes to an hour or so. A period of confusion may be the first feature. This, or the ensuing coma if not averted, can be very dangerous if the patient lives alone or is doing something which requires full concentration such as driving or operating machinery. Sometimes, hypoglycaemia results in abnormal behaviour such as uncharacteristic violence. Treatment is by giving glucose, ideally by mouth, but, if the patient has become unconscious, the oral route is dangerous and either intravenous glucose (25–50 ml 50 per cent) or intramuscular glucagon (0.5–1 mg) should be administered, followed by a meal or some long-lasting carbohydrate to maintain recovery.

Hypoglycaemia is not just a complication of insulin therapy but also occurs in patients on sulphonylureas, especially the elderly (e.g. the old lady with poor appetite and low income living on the occasional jam sandwich) and especially with longer acting drugs. The shorter acting sulphonylureas such as tolbutamide, glipizide and gliclazide are to be preferred. Sulphonylurea-induced hypoglycaemia may be very prolonged and needs admission to hospital.

## CHRONIC COMPLICATIONS

### Microvascular complications

#### The eye

The eye can be affected at all levels in diabetes (Table 18.6). Of particular note are the effects of diabetes on the lens and retina.

#### Cataracts

Specific snowflake diabetic cataracts occur rarely now and may respond to improved glycaemic control. Most common is premature development of the so-called senile cataract.

**Table 18.6** Eye complications in diabetes mellitus.

Cataract – diabetic or 'senile'
Retinopathy
Maculopathy
Ischaemic optic neuropathy
External ocular muscle palsy
   (cranial neuropathy)
Blepharitis
Conjunctivitis
Iritis
Rubreosis iridis
Glaucoma
Vitreous haemorrhage

*Retinopathy*

Retinopathy probably results from damage to microvessels in the retina with subsequent ischaemia of the retina itself. Capillary closure is an early change. Background retinopathy comprises small microaneurysms (seen as dot haemorrhages) in the walls of small retinal blood vessels, small numbers of fluffy white soft exudates which mark the presence of areas of retinal infarction. Venous beading and formation of interretinal microvascular abnormalities (IRMA) occur later. Hard exudates are shiny yellow-white deposits of lipid in the retina, probably subsequent upon leakage from small blood vessels, and may mark the onset of pre-proliferative retinopathy. The dead tissue stimulates the growth of new blood vessels, which are tortuous and fragile, and leak and bleed. This **proliferative retinopathy** is sight-threatening and needs urgent treatment with laser ablation of the vessels themselves or of the ischaemic retina stimulating their formation. Bleeding into the retina or the vitreous impairs sight and healing may cause scars and fibrosis with further loss of vision and risk of retinal detachment. Recurrent bleeding may darken the vitreous and vitrectomy may then help. Macular oedema is difficult to detect by direct inspection and is picked up by diminishing visual acuity, especially if performance deteriorates when tested with a pin-hole which corrects for refractile errors. Urgent laser therapy, good glycaemic control and control of hypertension may help this. The sudden introduction of strict glycaemic control can however provoke deterioration in preproliferative or proliferative retinopathy, which should be treated with laser therapy first. There may be an apparent worsening of background retinopathy with the institution of intensified insulin therapy but this seems to be a temporary increase in soft exudates and does not persist.

With the use of laser therapy to destroy leaking blood vessels and areas of ischaemia likely to stimulate new vessel growth, 70 per cent of blindness due to diabetes is preventable if detected early enough. People with diabetes must have visual acuities measured and the retinae inspected through dilated pupils at least once a year, once past puberty.

**The kidneys**

Forty per cent of insulin-dependent diabetic patients die of renal failure. Greater availability of renal support and replacement therapy is reducing mortality and prevention of diabetic renal disease is beginning to be a real possibility. The natural history of diabetic kidney disease progresses through a phase of hyperfiltration (increased glomerular filtration rate), then a selective leakage of small amounts of small proteins (microalbuminuria is defined as a loss of more than 30 mg but less than 200 mg albumin per 24 hours), leading to significant proteinuria (greater than 500 mg per day) with progressive loss of filtration rate and rising levels of plasma urea and creatinine thereafter. Once beyond the stage of microalbuminuria, the progress is inexorable; before this, rigorous maintenance of normal blood pressure (i.e. 120/80 or less), rigorous optimization of glucose control and possibly reduction in dietary protein intake may avert progression. Patients with diabetic nephropathy may therefore present with symptomless proteinuria, a nephrotic syndrome, or with the symptoms of chronic renal failure.

Diabetic renal disease almost invariably is associated with retinopathy; in the absence of the latter, renal dysfunction in a diabetic may have a different explanation. Investigation of renal dysfunction in diabetes should in any event allow exclusion of obstructive nephropathy, renal artery stenosis (more common in hypertensive diabetic as opposed to non-diabetic patients) and infection which should be vigorously sought and treated. Apparent diabetic nephropathy with normal eyes should lead one to consider renal biopsy to establish the diagnosis of the renal disease.

## Diabetic neuropathies

The neuropathies of diabetes are conveniently classified as microvascular, although their pathogenesis is complex and unlikely to be purely vascular. There are several classifications, but one of the most clinically relevant is to divide the clinical syndromes into:

1. Acute painful neuropathies
2. Chronic symmetrical somatic polyneuropathy
3. Nerve compression syndromes

### Clinical features

**Acute painful neuropathies** are in general self-limiting and are unrelated to disease duration. They last from weeks to, occasionally, years and are unrelated to disease duration. The typical symptoms are symmetrical, often exquisite, burning pain, in the feet and lower limbs, worse at night and exacerbated by warmth and pressure. Numbness is often felt but there may be little in the way of physical signs. It sometimes follows the start of insulin therapy. There may be associated severe weight loss ('diabetic cachexia') and poor nutrition has been implicated.

**Diabetic amyotrophy** is a painful wasting of the proximal, usually lower, limb muscles (and very rarely of the trunk), associated with loss of knee reflexes. It sometimes occurs at presentation in older, male NIDDM patients and may improve more rapidly with insulin treatment. Amytrophy may start unilaterally but may spread to the other limb within the first few weeks or may present bilaterally.

Truncal nerve roots may be involved in **radiculopathy** (compression must be carefully excluded) which sometimes masquerades as abdominal pathology.

**Isolated cranial neuropathies** most commonly affect the IVth or VIth nerves, but not exclusively. The aetiology is uncertain. Spontaneous recovery is the rule.

The chronic neuropathies include **symmetrical peripheral polyneuropathy**. The dying back of the longest axons first leads to alteration and loss of sensation in the feet, then the hands and arms. Loss of sensation and reflexes can be demonstrated objectively, small fibres (pain, temperature) being lost first. The foot becomes susceptible to unperceived injury and later loss of proprioception leads to deformation and disorganization of the articular surface (**Charcot's joints**) which is occasionally acute. The neuropathy is a progressive, unremitting condition, untied to duration of the diabetes. **Mixed neuropathy** with motor loss or **pure motor neuropathy** also occurs.

**Autonomic neuropathy** can affect all systems of the body (Table 18.7). It is frequently associated with peripheral neuropathy, and likewise is unrelated to the duration of the diabetes. The prognosis of diabetic autonomic neuropathy is poor once patients have symptomatic postural hypotension with 50 per cent mortality at 3 years. Although there are suspicions that cardiac arrhythmias may occur, this has never been

**Table 18.7** System and effect of autonomic nerve dysfunction.

| System | Effect |
| --- | --- |
| Gut | Diarrhoea, especially alternating with constipation, or nocturnal; gastroparesis with early satiety and bloating |
| Sweating | Loss of sweating to the lower limbs increases the risks of ulceration at the feet; excessive sweating of the trunk at night and after eating |
| Cardiovascular system: | Resting tachycardia; postural hypotension; increased risk of arrhythmia and sudden death; increased and disorganized flow through the microcirculation |
| Genitourinary | Impotence in men (may be manageable with intracavernosal vasodilators, vacuum devices to create an erection or, as a last resort, surgical implants; bladder dysfunction with incomplete emptying |

proven. Death has usually been due to concomitant nephropathy, but this may be reduced with increasing rates of treatment for diabetic end-stage renal failure.

**Nerve compression syndromes** are most often seen in the median nerve (carpal tunnel syndrome), lateral popliteal nerve or lateral cutaneous nerve of the thigh (meralgia paraesthetica).

*Management*

Treatment of neuropathy is unsatisfactory. Intensified insulin therapy can speed remission of painful types and may improve electrophysiological parameters. Healing has been attempted with aldose reductase inhibitors (to reduce sorbitol and increase myoinositol), myoinositol gangliosides, gamma-linoleic acid and others. Improvement in nerve function has been documented with these agents but long-lasting significant benefit remains to be proven. Symptomatic treatment for the peripheral neuropathy is simple analgesia, anticonvulsants and tricyclics for pain and percutaneous nerve stimulation. The extremely unpleasant symptoms of autonomic neuropathy require several different approaches.

## Macrovascular complications

Premature atherosclerosis occurs in diabetes, so that there is a greatly increased risk of ischaemic heart disease. Angina is common and asymptomatic ischaemic heart disease can be found if sought. Diabetes increases the risk of death from myocardial infarction more so in women than in men (page 479). Stroke and transient ischaemic accidents (TIA) (page 703) are more common also. Peripheral vascular disease with increased incidence of claudication and ischaemic limb loss is also more common in diabetes.

It is probable that the metabolic derangements of diabetes underlie the increased risk of vascular disease. Hyperinsulinaemia has long been (though not without controversy) implicated in the aetiology. Diabetic patients tend to be hyperinsulinaemic either as a result of insulin resistance or as a result of therapy with exogenous insulin which is delivered peripherally and so bypasses the normal route direct to the liver. The hyperinsulinaemia has been thought to encourage premature atheroma. More recently, an association has been described between obesity, hyperlipidaemia, hypertension and glucose intolerance, perhaps with hyperinsulinaemia as the link. Otherwise healthy people with impaired glucose tolerance tend to show insulin resistance and hyperinsulinaemia and they too have an increased risk of ischaemic heart disease.

Hypercholesterolaemia is probably no more common in diabetic populations than in non-diabetic ones although high levels may be seen in individuals if control is poor. Hypertriglyceridaemia is common in non-insulin-dependent diabetics and increasingly believed to be important in the pathogenesis of ischaemic heart disease.

## PATHOGENESIS OF CHRONIC COMPLICATIONS

There is an increased prevalence of microvascular complications in diabetic patients with very poor glycaemic control and it has been suggested that chronic hyperglycaemia may underline such complications. Glucose reacts with amine groups on protein molecules and undergoes an irreversible binding. This glycosylation of structural proteins may contribute to microvascular pathology. Another theory of the pathogenesis of chronic complications of diabetes implicates the increased formation of sorbitol and loss of myoinositol in the tissues, again a result of increased glucose levels.

However, hyperglycaemia is unlikely to be the sole cause of diabetic complications. There is increasing evidence to suggest that an individual patient's risk is a combination of genetic predisposition and environmental factors of which hyperglycaemia is likely to be one. At least as important in the aetiology of microvascular disease are even minor degrees of hypertension. Smoking increases the risk for macrovascular disease but the link with microvascular disease is not known. Hypercholesterolaemia increases macrovascular risk and, in NIDDM, hypertriglyceridaemia is also common.

The diabetic foot is cause for particular interest. Ulceration is encouraged by loss of sensation which allows minor trauma to go unnoticed; the opening of shunts between small arteries and veins, bypassing the capillary circulation (thought to relate to autonomic neuropathy); loss of sweating, due to autonomic neuropathy which encourages cracking and subsequent infection of the skin and maldistribution of weight on small areas. Poor perfusion secondary to large vessel disease also contributes. Many diabetic foot ulcers thus have a mixed aetiology with vascular and neurological elements, although neurological defects are more common.

## MANAGEMENT

Correct management of a patient with diabetes should include screening of and if necessary treatment for minor hypertension (although care must be used in the selection of drug therapy for treating fertile females), hyperlipidaemia and smoking habits, as well as optimizing glucose control.

Good foot hygiene encouraged by professional chiropody, avoidance of constricting footwear, early intervention to remove bunions, adaption of footwear to avoid ulceration of pressure points and early detection of minor damage with rapid responses in terms of antibiotic therapy and rest may reduce the necessity for amputation by half. Vascular surgery may enable rescue of even an infected foot. Palpable pedal pulses should imply a good prognosis. Underlying bone infection, requiring more intensive antibiotic therapy and perhaps limited surgical excision of infected bone, is not uncommon in diabetes and should be sought in all but the most minor of lesions.

## TREATMENT

Treatment of diabetes mellitus includes acute management to control blood glucose, regular screening for early treatable complications, and the detection and possible elimination of risk factors for such complications. Glucose control comprises three main principles – diet, exercise and the use of hypoglycaemic agents.

### Diet

All patients with diabetes require dietary advice. Regular spacing of meals is particularly important once hypoglycaemic medication is introduced but is also beneficial even as part of a dietary modification to limit the demands made upon a failing pancreas. The principles of dietary advice for diabetic patients are similar for NIDDM and IDDM. Rapidly absorbed 'pure' simple carbohydrates likely to cause sudden surges in blood glucose should be avoided. They are replaced with complex carbohydrates which, being slowly absorbed, provide a gradual increase in blood glucose which does not stress the failing pancreas or the absorption profile from subcutaneous insulin injections. Soluble fibre (in contrast to bran) is especially useful and guar gum has been used as a (not very palatable) medication to help slow absorption of other foods from the gut. Total caloric intake depends upon the patient's weight, activity level and disease but should be divided approximately into 50–60 per cent complex carbohydrates, 10–15 per cent protein and not more than 30 per cent fat, especially monounsaturated (olive oil) and polyunsaturated fat. Obesity is related to insulin resistance and reduction of obesity may relieve the diabetic condition in a substantial number of NIDDM patients. However desirable, it is important not to concentrate on weight reduction as the sole aim of diet – failure becomes very discouraging for patients and adherence to the principles of sensible diet can produce remarkable improvement in diabetic control even without weight loss.

'Diabetic foods' are hardly ever useful and can be dangerous as they may lull the patient into a sense of false security. Low sugar beers are very high in alcohol (and vice versa); the patient is better off consuming ordinary beer! Small amounts of sugar can be used in cooking where its absorption will be modified by the ingredients, but sugar substitutes such as aspartame are useful to sweeten drinks and cereals for those with a very sweet tooth.

Suggestions that protein restriction or the use of vegetable protein may be beneficial in early nephropathy are under investigation.

### Exercise

Care must be taken not to suggest jogging to patients with neuropathies or squash, or similar violent exercise, to patients who might have asymptomatic ischaemic heart disease. In the latter an exercise electrocardiogram (ECG) will be useful first. Otherwise exercise is to be recommended both for weight control and to improve insulin sensitivity. In well-controlled diabetic patients on insulin, vigorous exercise reduces blood glucose acutely (i.e. during and immediately after the game), and subacutely (during the ensuing night). If an exercise programme is pursued the patient needs a reduction in insulin usage or increased carbohydrate intake. Straining exercises should be avoided, especially in patients with microvascular complications. In pregnancy, exercises unlikely to stimulate uterine contractions (arm exercises especially) may be permitted.

## Hypoglycaemic agents

### Oral agents

Sulphonylureas stimulate insulin secretion. Later, improved glycaemic control also results in improved insulin sensitivity. The main risk of these agents is hypoglycaemia, especially with long-acting agents such as chlorpropamide and glibenclamide which are probably better avoided. Chlorpropamide, one of the earliest, is rarely used today. There are newer shorter acting sulphonylureas, such as gliclazide, which is excreted via the liver and glipizide which is excreted via liver and kidneys and must be used with caution in renal failure. Patients with more than minor degrees of renal dysfunction should be managed on insulin. There is probably not much to choose between the new sulphonylureas, and there is never an indication to use two sulphonylureas together. Nor is it likely that one will be more effective than another. The only one of this group to be a little different is the old tolbutamide, which is a rather weaker agent with a short action that is safer in renal failure and in the elderly. Allergic responses to this class of drugs may occur and very rarely agranulocytosis.

Because they stimulate insulin secretion, sulphonylureas tend to encourage weight gain. **Biguanides**, on the other hand, act by increasing insulin sensitivity and slowing glucose absorption from the gut. The main side effect of metformin, the only biguanide in use, is gastrointestinal upset which may limit its use. Metformin must be avoided in renal failure and low cardiac output because it is cleared by the kidneys and accumulation of the drug encourages lactic acidosis. Lactate can also accumulate in hepatic impairment. Liver function can be upset by metformin and should be monitored.

### Insulin therapy

Exogenous insulin was originally extracted from animal pancreas and contaminated by many non-insulin pancreatic products. Furthermore, beef insulin differs from human insulin by three and porcine insulin by one amino acid – the relevance of these differences is not clear. Chromatography allowed the purification of insulin alone from pancreas extracts. The resulting single peak or monocomponent insulins were purer and therefore faster acting with a slightly shorter duration of action than their old counterparts – a difference in pharmacokinetics which is enhanced by the reduced antigenicity of the newer insulins and the loss of anti-insulin antibodies from the circulation of patients using them. The loss of anti-insulin antibodies is probably beneficial in reducing the risks of hypoglycaemia and in pregnancy, where insulin-binding antibodies can carry insulin across the placenta. They slow the onset of the action and prolong the duration of any given insulin preparation. Most recently porcine insulin has been chemically altered to mimic human insulin and finally insulin molecules have been synthesized by micro-organisms carrying the human insulin gene to provide a pure therapy for human patients. The very pure human insulin has a rapid onset of action in its soluble form and the intermediate acting forms probably do not last as long as their animal counterparts. Adjustments may need to be made in therapeutic regimens if converting a patient from one form of insulin to another. Unexpectedly, there do not appear to be any real benefits of human insulin compared with the highly purified porcine preparations, except in rare cases of insulin allergy. It has been suggested that the use of human insulin is associated with reduced awareness of the warning symptoms of hypoglycaemia. This is an area of controversy but patients uncomfortable using human insulins could be allowed to return to animal preparations.

Ketosis-prone diabetes requires insulin therapy, as do other forms of diabetes if satisfactory control cannot be achieved by other means. Other indications for insulin therapy of diabetes

**Table 18.8** Indications for insulin therapy.

**Absolute indications**

Diabetic ketoacidosis and ketosis-prone diabetes
   mellitus

Pregnancy

**Relative indications**

Inadequate glucose control by other means*

Weight loss due to poor diabetic control

Intercurrent events: Surgery
                     Illness
                     Myocardial infarction

Diabetic amyotrophy
Painful neuropathy

---

*Inadequate glucose control must be defined for each patient. Acceptable control is not the same for an adolescent or a pregnant woman as for a patient in his 80s.

**Table 18.9** Examples of commonly used insulins and their characteristics.

**Short-acting (soluble)**

Onset of action    15–30 min
Peak action        1–2 hours
Duration of action  6–10 hours

Actrapid* (pork)
Velosulin* (pork)
Human Actrapid† (human)
Humulin S† (human)

**Intermediate acting**

Onset of action    1–2 hours
Peak action        4–8 hours
Duration of action 14–18 hours

*Protamine*
Isophane (beef)
Insulatard* (pork)
Human Insulatard† (human)
Protaphane† (human)
Humulin I† (human)

*Zinc*
Lente (beef and pork)
Monotard* (pork)
Human Monotard† (human)

**Long-acting**

Peak action        8–12 hours
Duration of action 30–40 hours

Humulin Zn

**Mixed**

Mixtard

---

Note that purified insulins (*) are faster acting and shorter acting than their older counterparts and human insulins (†) are probably the fastest and shortest acting of all.

are listed in Table 18.8. Exogenous insulin is given by the subcutaneous route; it is only after absorption into the blood stream that it is active. Various insulin preparations are formulated to be absorbed at different rates. They therefore have different times on onset and duration of action (Table 18.9). Thus soluble insulin starts to act within 20 to 30 minutes of subcutaneous injection, has peak effects from 1 to 2 hours and is dissipated within 8 hours. Insulin complexed with protamine or zinc is absorbed much more gradually (onset 1 to 2 hours, peak action 4 to 8 hours, duration 18 hours). There are a few insulins designed for slow constant absorption from the subcutis into the blood stream, so that they provide a background insulin against which preprandial soluble insulin can be administered. On the whole these ultra-long-acting insulins are difficult to use, their absorption is less gradual than one would wish and their long half-life makes them inflexible.

The aim of exogenous insulin therapy should be to reproduce the pattern of normal pancreatic insulin secretion (Fig. 18.1). A small background insulin effect is always necessary even after an overnight fast to limit hepatic glucose output. Ideally, a narrow peak of hyperinsulinaemia would then accompany every food intake but this cannot be fully accommodated by presently available insulins and techniques of administration. A simple regimen is to give a mixture of short- and intermediate-acting in-

sulins before breakfast to cover breakfast and lunch, and before the evening meal to cover that meal and the night, but overlap of the insulins' action profiles means that intermediate food ingestion (snacking) is usually essential. Greater flexibility can be achieved by administering short-acting insulins immediately before every meal, with a bedtime intermediate-acting insulin to cover the night. However, this necessitates multiple injections. Such therapy has been greatly facilitated by the introduction of injection devices that hold a reservoir of soluble insulin from which doses can be administered without the necessity of drawing up the drug

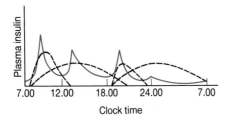

**Figure 18.1** Twenty-four hour profile of blood insulin levels. Peripheral insulin levels from a non-diabetic pancreas are shown by the solid line, with a constant background secretion and peaks at mealtimes. Least insulin is required to control endogenous glucose release at 3 a.m. The dotted lines show hypothetical blood insulin levels from a regimen of two injections of mixed insulins, superimposed. Hyperinsulinaemia is virtually inevitable postprandially and in the night. Reproduced with kind permission from *Hypoglycaemia*, the editor B. M. Frier and publisher Edward Arnold.

into a conventional syringe (an example of such a pen device is shown in Fig. 18.2). Originally introduced for soluble insulin only, these devices are convenient to use and have now been made available with intermediate-acting insulins and premixed (ready-made mixtures of soluble and intermediate-acting insulins in various proportions in a single solution) preparations. These 'pen' devices are convenient and popular with patients. Less popular in the UK, though useful for the occasional patient, is the technique of continuous subcutaneous insulin infusion (CSII). Soluble insulin is kept in a small reservoir and delivered by a pump continuously through a fine cannula to a needle implanted under the skin. The pump is activated by the patient to deliver larger boluses as needed, for example, preprandially. With CSII, the infusion site needs to be changed regularly and small interruptions in insulin delivery (e.g. air in the cannula, temporary disconnection) can have serious effects as the patient has no insulin reserve and is at risk of developing hyperglycaemia and ketoacidosis.

All conventional insulin therapy is given subcutaneously and will cause peripheral hyperinsulinaemia if portal insulin levels are to be maintained to control hepatic glucose production. Intraperitoneal insulin has been used to deliver insulin to the portal system first but the practicalities have not been fully worked out. In renal failure treated by continuous ambulatory

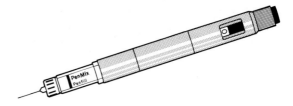

**Figure 18.2** Diagrammatic representation of a pen injection device for insulin administration.

peritoneal dialysis (CAPD) insulin is added to the dialysis bags and provides satisfactory control.

Attempts have been made to eliminate the need for injection of insulin but this is difficult because insulin, a polypeptide, is digested in the gut. Recent attempts to find an oral insulin that was active foundered, but the use of the nasal mucosa as an absorption site continues to attract attention and nasal preparations of insulin are under investigation.

### Side effects of insulin therapy

Insulin is a normal body product and, apart from hypoglycaemia, side effects are rare. Problems at the injection site can occur with inadvertent intradermal injection causing skin necrosis and constant injection into the same site causing local lipohypertrophy, which is unsightly and can impair subsequent insulin absorption. It is probably a local tissue response to the growth promoting actions of insulin and will resolve if the site is abandoned for a time. Lipoatrophy, atrophy of the subcutaneous tissue at the site of injection, is probably the result of immune complex deposition. It was seen particularly with the older more immunogenic insulins and can be relieved by injection of highly purified insulin into the site. Fluid retention can be a problem when starting insulin therapy. There are also concerns about the possible effects of hyperinsulinaemia on lipid deposition in arterial walls. A very few patients are allergic to insulin, or more probably to the preservative in a particular preparation.

A truly insulin-dependent diabetic patient can never stop taking insulin. Hyperglycaemia and ketosis will result. It is important to realize that when unwell, stress responses may increase rather than decrease insulin needs even if the patient is unable to eat. This problem can be managed at home if patients can test their own blood glucose levels by using small doses of soluble insulin and using sugary fluids to provide glucose. Once ketosis or vomiting occurs, hospitalization for parenteral fluid and insulin glucose is necessary.

### Monitoring diabetes therapy

Clinical monitoring (is the patient well, avoiding hypoglycaemia and symptomatic hyperglycaemia?) is important but not adequate for any except the very elderly. In younger patients, blood glucose should be kept as near to normal as possible to diminish risks of chronic hyper- or hypoglycaemia. There are a variety of testing strips in which enzymes and reagents needed to react with glucose and produce a colour change proportional to the amount of the sugar are immobilized on a plastic strip for convenience. Patients can assess their control themselves by measuring the plasma glucose content of blood samples obtained by pricking the finger. By testing regularly at different times of day (never within 2 hours of eating unless feeling unwell) they can build up a picture of their usual insulin requirements. The technique used and especially the timing of such tests is critical.

In patients striving for really 'good' glycaemic control, frequent home blood testing may be necessary, both to help design treatment regimens and to guard against hypoglycaemia that may otherwise go unnoticed. Less frequent measurement is usually acceptable, with patients trying to build up a picture of the usual blood glucose levels at any given time of day with readings made at different times on several occasions scattered over several weeks. Home glucose testing is particularly useful for management of 'sick days' and identification of episodes of asymptomatic hypoglycaemia, especially at night.

Measurement of the level of fructosamine or glycosylated haemoglobins gives an indication of the average blood glucose level over the previous week or 3 months, respectively, but does not alert the patient to possible swings in glucose levels. Such measurements are, however, an invaluable check on chronic control, to ensure that aims of therapy are being achieved and risks of chronic poor control are avoided. Changes in regimen usually require home blood testing to identify which part of an insulin regimen requires attention. The fasting blood glucose is a useful indication of control in NIDDM, where the glucose profile is often similar and hyperglycaemia dependent upon the starting glucose of the day.

Urine glucose testing is easy to do and useful to check glucose control where tight control is not required – the urine should really always be glucose-free so no indication of hypoglycaemia can be obtained – but if the patient is clinically well and the other indices of control are acceptable, it still has a place. Urine testing is invaluable to check for ketones and of course for the identification of people with or at risk of diabetic nephropathy.

# Special cases

## DIABETES AND PREGNANCY

Maternal whole-body insulin sensitivity diminishes throughout pregnancy, secondary to all the hormonal changes, although an initial fall in insulin needs may occur. Insulin requirements rise towards the end of the second trimester in diabetic women, and women who are not already diabetic but who have limited pancreatic reserve may develop impaired glucose tolerance or frank diabetes in pregnancy. Maternal mortality is higher in diabetic women (0.1 versus 0.009 per cent, USA 1965–85), but this number continues to fall with improved management.

If either parent has IDDM, the genetic susceptibility to development of the disease may be inherited, leaving the child with a fivefold increase in risk. Surprisingly, the risk may be greater if the father has diabetes.

The risks of congenital abnormalities can be reduced almost to that of the background non-diabetic risk if maternal metabolic control is normal at conception. Babies of diabetic mothers had a greatly increased incidence of congenital abnormalities (7–13 versus 1–2 per cent in the non-diabetic population) and of spontaneous abortion (17–30 versus 9 per cent). Good glycaemic control immediately before pregnancy is essential and gives normal babies in up to 90 per cent of deliveries. These risks do not apply to women with gestational diabetes whose hyperglycaemia develops only as pregnancy progresses.

Babies of mothers with diabetes in poor control after the first 12 to 16 weeks of pregnancy risk macrosomia – the baby is not diabetic and responds to maternal hyperglycaemia with hyperinsulinaemia. This encourages excessive and pathological growth. This risk, unlike that of congenital malformation, is shared by babies of mothers with gestational diabetes. Macrosomia increases maternal as well as perinatal mortality. Mothers with microvascular complications of diabetes, especially if hypertensive, have a contrasting risk of small babies, presumably because of poor placental function. Perinatal mortality rises with mean blood glucose levels in the third trimester, reaching almost 100 per cent if DKA occurs. Good glycaemic control throughout pregnancy is thus essential. Finally, if the mother is hyperglycaemic in labour, the baby will likewise be hyperinsulinaemic at birth and is at especial risk for neonatal hyperglycaemia, so good glycaemic control throughout labour is also essential.

Fertile women with diabetes should be counselled about planning their family and supported from the time they first decide to start a family. The presence of advanced complications or macrovascular disease should discourage pregnancy but there is no firm evidence to suggest that pregnancy *per se* worsens microvascular complications. Control should be stabilized before pregnancy. Sudden tightening of control during pregnancy can lead to deterioration of advanced retinopathy as at any other time. Pre-eclampsia and toxaemia are more common in diabetes, especially if complicated, and hypertension worsens the prognosis for mother and child. Glucose control should aim for preprandial levels of 4.0–6.5 mmol/l and 2 hour postprandial levels of 7.0 mmol/l (some authorities recommending 1 hour postmeal), which is very strict indeed. Hypoglycaemia (often without much warning) is a risk of such control but fortunately does not seem to harm the fetus. Most women (and their carers) accept the risk for the duration of the pregnancy although obviously steps should be taken to minimize hypoglycaemia without jeopardizing overall control.

Oral hypoglycaemic agents should not be used in pregnancy; sulphonylureas cross the placenta to cause fetal hyperinsulinaemia.

Gestational diabetes should be sought by glucose screening and if suspected its presence confirmed by formal glucose testing. In Europe, the WHO criteria for the diagnosis of diabetes or IGT in the non-pregnant state are traditionally used in pregnancy, although there are indications that glucose tolerance deteriorates a little during late normal pregnancy and the criteria for diagnosing IGT may need to be relaxed in the future. Once diagnosed, it seems reasonable to have the same goals for glycaemic control in these women as in true diabetes. Diet may be very effective in IGT especially, but insulin should be started soon if necessary.

During labour, diabetes is managed with intravenous glucose and insulin. Insulin requirements fall to prepregnant levels as soon as delivery is complete.

## DIABETES IN ADOLESCENTS

Diabetes in the young must be managed carefully. Severe growth retardation, with hepatomegaly, is now fortunately rare but children with diabetes do not achieve their full growth potential if poorly controlled and good control accelerates linear growth. However, prepubertal diabetes does not appear greatly to influence the development of microvascular complications.

Puberty is a difficult time for all individuals and their families but it is especially tough for the young patient with diabetes. The hormonal changes of puberty, perhaps especially the growth hormone, result in a degree of insulin resistance which, coupled with the brisk neurohumoral responses which young people have during even quite moderate hypoglycaemia, offers a physiological explanation for the diabetic instability of adolescents. It is especially important not to alienate young diabetic patients at this time. The evidence would suggest that it is after puberty that risks for microvascular complications of diabetes begin to accumulate.

For diabetic girls the issue of contraception must be discussed. While it would be preferable not to give oestrogens to diabetic patients, the risks of unwanted pregnancy during a time of poor control are probably greater and oral contraceptives (preferably with lower oestrogen doses) may be used.

Weight gain may be a serious issue for young diabetic girls especially. Recent research suggests that true eating disorders are no more common in diabetic than in non-diabetic youths, but they are common and skipping insulin as a means of weight reduction is not rare! Obesity and high androgen syndromes may occur (polycystic ovaries, page 537).

## DIABETES AND SURGERY

Surgery is a stress which might be expected to elevate glucose levels. A more important problem is the difficulty of maintaining good metabolic control while a patient takes nil by mouth. The simplest and most effective management is to give intravenous glucose and insulin, ideally separately so one can be adjusted without the other (Table 18.10). If nursing facilities for strict supervision are not available, it may be safer to put one-quarter of the patient's total

**Table 18.10** Suggested regimen for management of diabetic patient who is taking nil by mouth.

| Glucose |
| :-: |
| Intravenous infusion |
| 5% glucose 500 ml + 20 mmol K+ 6 hourly |

| Insulin | | |
| :-: | :-: | :-: |
| Intravenous sliding scale | | |
| Blood glucose (hourly) | Insulin (50 units soluble in 50 ml saline) | |
| mmol/l | U/hour | ml/hour |
| <4 | 0 | 0 | but check in 30 min |
| 4–7 | × 12 | × 12 |
| 7–11 | × | × |
| 11–17 | × + 1 | × + 1 |
| >17 | × + 3 | × + 3 |

*Notes:* Progress should be checked after 1 or 2 hours and if necessary the sliding scale adjusted up if the blood glucose is rising or down if the blood glucose is falling outside desired ranges.

Sliding scales should only EVER be used with intravenous insulin regimens, when alteration in dose is immediately effective.

× = total daily dose of insulin ÷ 24.

daily insulin dose (12 to 20 units if the patient is not already on insulin) into 500 ml of 5 per cent glucose, add 20 mmol potassium and infuse the mixture over 6 hours. The disadvantage of this is that the whole infusion will need to be replaced if blood glucose control is not ideal. But at least insulin cannot be given without glucose or vice versa. These infusions should be regarded as additional to the patient's other requirements except in terms of volume. Whichever regimen is used, blood glucose should be carefully monitored, at least hourly until control is stable.

Hyperglycaemia creates a dehydrated, haemoconcentrated patient who may be more susceptible to infection. Neutrophil function is impaired once blood glucose exceeds 15 mmol/l. Ideally, normoglycaemia should be maintained throughout surgery and recovery. Regular bedside glucose monitoring allows the treatment regimen to be adjusted to avoid hypoglycaemia.

# *The future*

## PREVENTION

Because IDDM results from immune destruction of β cells, investigations to find the triggering antigen continue. Immune modulation therapy has been tried in early diabetes to attempt to delay progression – and with some success. The drugs used (e.g. cylcosporin, azathioprine, prednisolone) are however too toxic. New trials with nicotinamide are beginning but probably newer more specific strategies will be needed. For NIDDM, reduction in obesity is important. Because of the role of genetic factors in NIDDM and the high rate of NIDDM in women with a history of gestational diabetes, education and help with weight reduction are particularly important for women with a relevant family or personal history.

## CURE

Over 3000 pancreatic transplants have been performed with some success in reducing or eliminating insulin requirements. However, the immunosuppressive therapy required to prevent rejection (and recrudescence of the diabetic process) has mainly restricted this to patients receiving renal transplant. The transplantation of isolated cells is under continued investigation. Here problems of rejection could be diminished in theory by processing the islets *in vitro* or wrapping them up to isolate them from large molecules. Supply is a problem, and at least two donors are required for success. There are five patients worldwide who have come off insulin after islet transplantation and one has rejected the graft, but the other four were functioning at more than 3 months.

# NON-DRUG-INDUCED HYPOGLYCAEMIA

Diagnosis of hypoglycaemia depends upon documenting a low blood glucose (less than 2.8 mmol/l by convention) in the presence of symptoms which are rapidly relieved by the administration of glucose. Clinical symptoms of autonomic activation and catecholamine release (sweating, tremor, palpitations, feeling hot, feeling anxious) are associated with stimulation of hepatic glucose production and a tendency for recovery and cerebral dysfunction due to glucose lack generally occurs at lower blood glucose levels, although this relationship is often altered in disease states.

Hypoglycaemia rarely occurs in individuals not on exogenous blood glucose lowering agents. Rare diseases in children can produce hypoglycaemia. In nesidioblastosis, diffuse growth of β cells throughout the pancreas creates hyperinsulinaemia and intractable hypoglycaemia in neonates. Premature and small-for-date babies are prone to hypoglycaemia because of inadequate glycogen stores or enzymes for gluconeogenesis. In glycogen storage diseases I (and III) enzymes required for glycogenolysis are deficient. Glucose cannot be released from liver stores and hypoglycaemia ensues. Enzyme defects in glycogen synthesis or gluconeogenesis probably underlie ketotic hypoglycaemia, a condition seen in young children where hypoglycaemia causes low insulin levels and ketosis.

Hypoglycaemia may also occur as a result of increased insulin sensitivity when hormones which act as insulin antagonists are absent as in hypopituitarism, hypoadrenalism or growth hormone deficiency. Severe liver disease may result in hypoglycaemia as a result of failure of hepatic glucose stores, as can ethanol which suppresses hepatic glucose production.

In adults, hypoglycaemia occurs as a result of rare pancreatic insulin-secreting tumours. Such **insulinomas** can be very small. Clinical presentation includes episodes of neuroglycopenia much more commonly than episodes of acute autonomic symptoms – episodic (especially morning) confusion or even seizures lead to psychiatric or neurological referrals. Diagnosis is made by finding inappropriately high insulin and c-peptide levels during frank hypoglycaemia (less than 2 mmol/l) which can be induced (or excluded) by supervised 3-day fasting. Inability to suppress endogenous insulin (reflected by c-peptide levels) with exogenous insulin is sometimes used for diagnosis but is not necessary if hyperinsulinaemia is demonstrated during hypoglycaemia and surreptitious sulphonylurea taking can be ruled out. Much of the secretion may be proinsulin. The tumour can sometimes be localized by computed tomography or superior mesenteric or coeliac axis arteriography. Transhepatic selective venous sampling to find the source of insulin secretion is sometimes used in specialist centres but a new technique using calcium gluconate to stimulate insulin secretion from the tumour is gaining favour. Intraoperative ultrasonography, using a specially adapted probe placed directly onto the pancreas has been very successful. There is no place for blind partial pancreatectomy now. Insulinomas are rarely malignant or multiple and occasionally secrete other neuropeptides. Rare tumours secreting insulin-like growth factors (IGFs) and large sarcomas can occasionally produce hypoglycaemia, possibly through excess utilization of glucose, but probably through IGF secretion also.

**Reactive hypoglycaemia** is said to occur as a result of excessive insulin responses to food intake. It might occur in healthy people but then it does not cause severe neuroglycopenia. It can happen if meal absorption is excessively fast, as may occur after gastric surgery (page 354). The diagnosis can be made by teaching patients how to collect small capillary tube blood samples at home during an episode which can then be measured for glucose content in a laboratory. Autonomic responses can be triggered by quite minor degrees of hypoglycaemia, giving rise to symptoms.

# STORAGE DISEASES

A number of conditions, mostly hereditary, result in the overproduction of a normal product of metabolism which builds up in tissues. The storage of an abnormal amount of the substance interferes with the normal function of the storage organ or tissue. Glycogen storage diseases caused by errors in carbohydrate metabolism make up one group. Others are some of the hyperlipidaemias, the porphyrias and defects in amino acid metabolism such as cystinosis (page 468). Abnormalities in lysosomal enzymes result in the lysosomal storage diseases.

## Glycogen storage diseases

Defects in enzymes involved in the breakdown of glycogen result in abnormal storage of glycogen especially in the liver (e.g. von Gierke disease with a defect in glucose 6-phosphatase) or the muscle (e.g. muscle phosphorylase deficiency in McArdle disease. In von Gierke disease glucose cannot be produced from stored glycogen; a remarkable improvement occurs with continuous intragastric feeding with glucose through a nasogastric or gastrostomy tube.

## Disorders of fructose metabolism

The commonest type of hereditary fructose intolerance is inherited as an autosomal recessive and results in vomiting, sweating and even convulsions after ingestion of fructose.

## Lysosomal storage diseases

The two most important groups of lysosomal storage diseases are the sphingolipidoses and the mucopolysaccharidoses.

### SPHINGOLIPIDOSES

#### Neimann–Pick disease

Inheritance is autosomal recessive. Sphingomyelin builds up in reticuloendothelial cells. Most cases have hepatosplenomegaly and neurological involvement with death in childhood. Milder types without neurological problems may present in adulthood.

#### Gaucher disease

The adult form of Gaucher disease is an autosomal recessive condition with storage of glucocerebroside. It is particularly common in Ashkenazi Jews and leads to hepatosplenomegaly and bone marrow failure.

#### Fabry disease

Inherited as an X-linked recessive, female carriers are mildly affected or not at all. A glycosphingolipid builds up in blood vessel walls and reticuloendothelial cells. Affected males die in middle age from renal failure, cerebro- or cardiovascular disease. There is a typical rash with raised or flat telangiectasia, angiokeratoma corporis diffusum.

### MUCOPOLYSACCHARIDOSES

There are seven types of mucopolysaccharidoses, Hurler (Type IH) and Hunter (Type II) are best known. Others are Scheie (Type IS), Sanfilippo (Type III), Morquio (Type IV) and Maroteaux-Lamy (Type VI).

## IH Hurler

Inherited as an autosomal recessive the thickened facial appearance led to the use of the term Gargoylism for Hurler and Hunter diseases. Skeletal and central nervous system involvement are prominent and survival beyond 10 years is unusual.

## II Hunter

This has a sex-linked recessive inheritance, features are similar to Hurler disease except that corneal clouding is rare. A mild form is compatible with normal intelligence and survival into the 20s or 30s.

# AMYLOIDOSIS

Amyloidosis is a general term describing various disorders of protein metabolism in which insoluble protein, in the form of fibrils, is deposited in many different parts of the body. Amyloid is defined histologically; on light microscopy it is amorphous and homogeneous, staining red with congo red stain, which fluoresces a green colour in polarized light. Immunohistology, using monoclonal antibodies, can also define the amyloid, and electron microscopy will show the typical fibrillar pattern of the proteins.

## PATHOGENESIS

The excess proteins deposited as amyloid have many different sources.

### Protein A

This is a precursor of a normally occurring serum protein, serum amyloid A, which is an acute phase protein. Overproduction of serum amyloid A and its precursor, amyloid A, occurs in chronic infections such as tuberculosis, osteomyelitis; in chronic inflammation such as rheumatoid arthritis; in malignancy such as Hodgkin's disease and carcinoma; and in familial Mediterranean fever (FMF, page 589). It is laid down as AA amyloid.

### Amyloid light chains (AL)

These are produced by B-cell malignancies, for example, myeloma, Waldenström's macroglobulinaemia, and non-Hodgkin's lymphoma.

### Pre-albumin

This is found in a rare hereditary form of amyloidosis, most commonly seen in Portugal.

### $\beta_2$ Microglobulin

Deposition of this protein occurs for unknown reasons in patients on long-term dialysis for end-stage renal failure.

### A4 amyloid

There has been considerable interest in this because it is found in the brains of patients with Alzheimer's disease, and also Down's syndrome.

## CLINICAL FEATURES

The amyloid found in long-standing infections and inflammations (secondary amyloid, reactive systemic amyloidosis, AA amyloid) usually is deposited in the liver, spleen, kidneys and adrenal glands. Hypofunction and failure of these organs may occur, with the addition, when the kidneys are involved, of proteinuria which may produce a nephrotic syndrome. The underlying disease will form part of the picture in many patients, for example, bronchiectasis, or rheumatoid arthritis, although in other patients these chronic infections and inflammations may become quiescent or, as in the case of tuberculosis, may never have been diagnosed. The presentation with amyloid may be many years after the infection or inflammation. The commonest associated cause now is rheumatoid, the chronic infections being much less common than previously. On examination the affected organs may be enlarged, sometimes to a great degree.

In the other forms of amyloid, the clinical findings are more variable. The heart may be involved, with heart failure. There may be a neuropathy, for example, carpal tunnel syndrome, or peripheral neuropathy (which is typical of the Portuguese type) and deposition in the tongue, causing macroglossia. Involvement of the kidneys, liver and spleen appears less frequently than in secondary amyloid.

## DIAGNOSIS

Biopsy of an affected organ will allow the diagnosis to be made histologically. Amyloid in small amounts is frequently deposited in the gum, the fat of the abdominal wall and the rectal mucosa and, in the absence of clinical involvement, these tissues can be biopsied instead of major organs, avoiding the added risk.

In some laboratories measurement of the elevated serum protein, or their precursor is available, and radionuclide scans, using monoclonal antibodies to amyloid proteins, can also demonstrate amyloid deposits.

## TREATMENT

In secondary amyloid, treatment of the underlying infection or inflammation may halt, or rarely in some cases even reverse the disorder. In the other forms of amyloid, particularly those related to malignancy of the B or T cells, chemo-therapy has been tried, without uniform success, but with a small minority improving. In familial Mediterranean fever colchicine produces some improvement in the amyloid, but this effect is not seen in other types of amyloid. In the amyloid due to $\beta_2$-microglobulin in renal failure, the only sure way of improving the patient is to provide a renal transplant.

The diminished function of any affected organs should be treated appropriately, for example, hypoadrenalism.

## PROGNOSIS

This is variable, depending upon the type of amyloid, and the organ affected. Sometimes the disease can progress very rapidly, with, for example, death due to heart failure. Other patients have a very slowly progressive or unchanging course. The nature of the underlying disorder also governs the outcome.

# HYPERLIPIDAEMIA

## PATHOPHYSIOLOGY

Fat is carried in the plasma in complex molecules called lipoproteins. Density or the electrophoretic mobility of the particles are used to separate the lipoproteins. The proportions of cholesterol and triglyceride in each type of particle determine its size and its density. Hyperlipidaemia occurs when either circulating cholesterol or triglycerides or both are high, caused by increased production or diminished clearance.

Lipids enter the circulation either from the gut after meals (carried in very large low-density lipoprotein structures called chylomicrons in the exogenous pathway) or from endogenous synthesis of cholesterol and triglyceride in the liver, when they are exported into the blood stream in large particles – very low density lipoproteins (VLDL). Gradually these are metabolized by removal of triglyceride by lipoprotein lipase in the endothelium to form intermediate density and then low density lipoproteins (LDL), which are increasingly concentrated in cholesterol. Apoproteins expressed on the surface of the lipo-proteins assist in lipid clearance by activating lipoprotein lipase (apo cII) and by allowing receptor-mediated uptake of the lipoprotein for subsequent intracellular oxidation or metabolism of the lipid (e.g. apos E and B). High density lipoprotein (HDL) carries esterified cholesterol and is involved in its clearance from vessel walls and the circulation (reverse transport pathway). Thus high HDL cholesterol is beneficial and it is a high LDL:HDL ratio which is of particularly ominous prognostic significance for atherosclerosis.

## CLASSIFICATION AND AETIOLOGY OF HYPERLIPIDAEMIA

About 20 per cent of hyperlipidaemias are secondary to other pathology, as listed in Table 18.11. The remaining primary hyperlipid-aemias are often genetically inherited, usually as autosomal dominants, with heterozygotes often showing intermediate degrees of hyperlipid-aemia and risk of associated disease. Genetic

**Table 18.11** Causes of secondary hyperlipidaemias.

| Primary condition | Main lipid component |
|---|---|
| Diabetes mellitus | Triglyceride |
| Hypothyroidism | Cholesterol |
| Alcohol excess | Triglyceride |
| Cholestasis | Cholesterol |
| Renal failure | Triglyceride |
| Nephrotic syndrome | Mixed |
| Myeloma and paraproteinaemia | Mixed |
| Drugs: Thiazides | Triglyceride |
| Chlorthalidone | Cholesterol |
| Corticosteroids | Mixed |
| Contraceptive pill and oestrogens (premenopausal) | Triglyceride |

considerations give a useful alternative method of classification.

Table 18.12 shows the Frederickson classification of the hyperlipidaemias, together with the causes that may underlie each one and the main clinical features and potential complications. Increasingly, laboratories are introducing measurements of the apoprotein content of lipids to give a more detailed diagnosis.

## CLINICAL FEATURES

The clinical features of hyperlipidaemia depend upon which stage of metabolism is at fault.

Hypercholesterolaemia is associated with increased risk of premature atherosclerosis and ischaemic heart disease. Xanthomata (lipid deposits) are seen especially around the eyes and in a thickened Achilles tendon. Raised triglycerides are associated with eruptive xanthomata, especially in the skin and around joints, retinal lipaemia (lipid visible in the small blood vessels of the retina on ophthalmoscopy), pancreatitis (although beware that the hyperlipidaemia may interfere with the laboratory measurement of amylase), impaired glucose tolerance and hepatosplenomegaly.

**Familial hypercholesterolaemia** is an autosomal dominant condition of impaired receptor-mediated clearance of LDL. Homozygotes have hyperlipidaemia IIa and present with ischaemic heart disease, including myocardial infarction, in their 20s and 30s, with a high risk of premature death. A positive family history for such premature cardiac death is important diagnostic information. Others may show type IIb. All patients show the typical clinical syndrome of high cholesterol: xanthoma, xanthelasma and ischaemic heart disease.

**Familial combined hyperlipidaemia**, in which both triglycerides and cholesterol are raised, may be inherited in an autosomal dominant manner and results from overproduction of VLDL and LDL (phenotypically presenting as types IIa, IIB, IV). Apo B levels are high. Patients may have arcus, xanthelasma and increased risk of ischaemic heart disease.

**Table 18.12** Frederickson's classification of hyperlipidaemia.

| Type | Lipoprotein | Lipid in excess | Causes – primary (secondary) |
|---|---|---|---|
| I | Chylomicron | CHOLESTEROL, triglyceride | Lipoprotein lipase deficiency Apo C II deficiency |
| IIa | LDL | CHOLESTEROL | Familial hypercholesterolaemia (hypothyroidism) |
| IIb | LDL + VLDL | CHOLESTEROL, triglyceride | Familial combined hyperlipidaemia (nephrotic syndrome, diabetes, anorexia) |
| III | IDL VLDL | Triglyceride, CHOLESTEROL | Familial (hypothyroidism, diabetes, obesity) |
| IV | VLDL | Triglyceride | Familial combined hyperlipidaemia Familial hypertriglyceridaemia (diabetes, chronic renal failure) |
| V | Chylomicron VLDL | Triglyceride, CHOLESTEROL | Familial hypertriglyceridaemia Apo C II deficiency |

LDL = low density lipoprotein. VLDL = very low density lipoprotein. IDL = intermediate density lipoprotein.

**Familial hypertriglyceridaemia** is inherited as an autosomal dominant and may have the phenotypes of IV or V. There is increased synthesis and decreased clearance of VLDL without affecting LDL levels. Patients may present with eruptive xanthomata, pancreatitis and neuropathy. Retinal lipaemia and hepatosplenomegaly can be seen on examination. Impaired glucose tolerance may be associated. A similar clinical picture may be seen with disorders of lipoprotein lipase activity, inherited as an autosomal recessive condition, where chylomicrons (type I) and/or (type V) VLDL accumulate.

**Mixed hyperlipidaemia type III** is a broad β disease or dys-β-lipoproteinaemia which results from decreased catabolism of IDL and VLDL due to defective or absent apo EIII. The hyperlipidaemia is mixed. Low density lipoprotein cholesterol is low and the B-VLDL probably causes the atherosclerosis. The broad β band on electrophoresis of the plasma is unique and diagnostic. The clinical picture tends to present after puberty in boys or the menopause in women, with corneal arcus, palmar xanthomata (unique to this condition), pancreatitis, arteriopathy (peripheral vascular and ischaemic heart disease), abnormalities of glucose tolerance including frank diabetes mellitus and hyperuricaemia.

**Common hypercholesterolaemia** is a polygenic condition, phenotypically type IIa, and presenting later in life than the familial form. Tendon xanthoma are seen and premature ischaemic heart disease.

## INVESTIGATIONS AND DIAGNOSIS

To investigate a hyperlipidaemia, the precise nature of the lipid abnormality should be determined because the treatments are different. Electrophoresis is particularly useful to identify dys-β-lipoproteinaemia and it is important to quantify LDL cholesterol in high cholesterol states in order to assess the risk of ischaemic heart disease. (The Friedman equation can be used to estimate LDL cholesterol if triglyceride levels are less than 5 mmol/l: LDL cholesterol then = total cholesterol minus HDL cholesterol minus triglyceride/2.2.) Less than 4.1 mmol/l is regarded as ideal in the USA. The European Atherosclerosis Society currently suggest that a total cholesterol over 5.2 mmol/l is excessive. Analysis of the apoproteins helps precise diagnosis. Low density lipoprotein B may be measured instead of LDL cholesterol which is usually calculated from other measurements. Apo B may indeed be a better predictor of risk for ischaemic heart disease, even in the absence of hypercholesterolaemia. Lipoprotein (a) [Lp(a)] is considered an independent risk factor because of its homology with elements of the clotting system.

Secondary causes of hyperlipidaemia, such as thiazide drug use, hypothyroidism and diabetes mellitus must be ruled out. First degree relatives should be checked, especially if familial hypercholesterolaemia (type II) is diagnosed in a proband.

There has been controversy about the place of screening for high cholesterol levels and their treatment. When a high level is found the general lipoprotein profile should be measured and treated as appropriate at the same time as other risk factors.

## TREATMENT

The principal reason for reducing lipid levels is to diminish the risk of ischaemic heart disease. Initial treatment is dietary — avoidance not so much of dietary cholesterol, which has little influence on plasma cholesterol levels, as weight reduction and avoidance of saturated fat (dairy products, animal fat, red meat) and excess alcohol. Hyperlipidaemia secondary to disorders of lipoprotein lipase activity is especially sensitive to fat-free dieting which is used as a simple diagnostic test, but familial hypertriglyceridaemia is very insensitive. Attention should be directed towards other factors which increase risk of ischaemic heart disease. Hypertension doubles the risk of any given cholesterol level. Treatment of hypertension reduces the risk of cerebrovascular disease, but results in coronary artery disease are less impressive, perhaps because of adverse metabolic effects of some of the hypotensive agents used. Smoking increases fibrinogen levels and reduces HDL cholesterol, both increasing the risk of vascular disease. Aerobic exercise can raise HDL cholesterol and lower triglycerides but must be used with caution in patients at increased risk of ischaemic heart disease.

If dietary measures fail, hypercholesterolaemia may be helped by interruption of the enterobiliary circulation, reducing resorption of bile salts of high cholesterol content, by means of bile acid binding resins (e.g. cholestyramine). Apart from interference with absorption of other lipid-soluble drugs (e.g. digoxin and warfarin) and vitamins (e.g. folate), these are safe and simple drugs, but bulky and not very palatable, with a risk of causing gastrointestinal upset, including severe constipation. They are used as first-line drug therapy for type IIa or b phenotypes, but tend to result in a rise in triglyercide. Inhibition of cholesterol synthesis by inhibition of β-hydroxy-β-methylglutaryl coenzyme A (HMG CoA) reductase is a later treatment of hypercholesterolaemia which seems effective and safe, although these drugs (e.g. simvastatin) have not been in use for long. They can be effective in type IIa or b or III but will not work in homozygous familial hypercholesterolaemia where the problem is caused by lack of LDL receptors and diminished LDL clearance.

Hyperlipidaemia which is primarily hypertriglyceridaemia may respond to fibrates which stimulate lipoprotein lipase. Fibrates produce a useful reduction in VLDL triglyceride and increase HDL cholesterol in type III, IV and V hyperlipidaemia. In type IV, increased conversion of VLDL into LDL may occur. The most useful drug in this class is bezafibrate, or the more expensive gemfibrozil. Neither of these drugs seems to increase the risk of cholelithiasis, a problem with the original drug in this class because of increased biliary cholesterol. Side effects of the fibrates include gastrointestinal upset and reversible myopathy. Dosage must be reduced in impaired renal function.

Nicotinic acid derivatives decrease lipolysis, non-esterified fatty acid levels, VLDL synthesis and HDL clearance. Side effects of nicotinic acid itself, especially flushing, and a tendency to raise plasma glucose and urate levels seem less troublesome with later derivatives such as acipimox, which may even improve glucose tolerance. Liver function tests should be monitored and the drugs should not be used in patients with peptic ulcer.

If monotherapy fails, combinations of resins with fibrates or nicotinic acid derivatives may be useful in type IIb. Resins and HMG CoA reductase inhibitors have been effective in lowering cholesterol in heterozygotes with familial hypercholesterolaemia. β-Hydroxy-β-methyl glutaryl CoA reductase inhibitors can cause rhabdomyolysis in patients on cyclosporin A. Combining a statin and a nicotinic acid derivative may be safer.

There are some other agents which have been used for hyperlipidaemia. Neomycin precipitates cholesterol in the intestinal lumen and may be effective in familial hypercholesterolaemia and it lowers Lp(a) but it may be toxic and its safety for long-term use has not been accepted. Probucol, which may reduce LDL cholesterol by about 15 per cent also tends to reduce HDL cholesterol, but its antioxidant action is being explored for possible benefit in prevention of atheroma. Fish oils reduce triglyceride levels and are also under investigation. There are concerns about their effect on glucose metabolism.

In very severe cases of hypercholesterolaemia plasma exchange or selective extracorporeal removal of LDL may be used to remove cholesterol, and surgical interruption of the enterobiliary circulation has also been used, but will probably be less useful with the introduction of the HMG CoA reductase inhibitors. Even liver transplant has been considered for intractable homozygotes with familial hypercholesterolaemia.

# *H*EPATIC AND CUTANEOUS PORPHYRIAS

Rare disorders of the synthetic pathways of haemoglobin result in accumulation of haem precursors, including the porphyrins. Individual porphyrias occur when there are defects of specific enzymes in the synthetic pathway (Fig. 18.3). Diagnosis is established by demonstra-

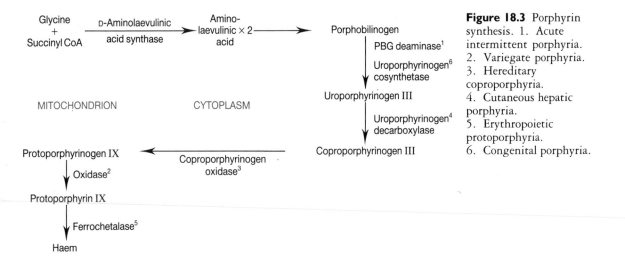

**Figure 18.3** Porphyrin synthesis. 1. Acute intermittent porphyria. 2. Variegate porphyria. 3. Hereditary coproporphyria. 4. Cutaneous hepatic porphyria. 5. Erythropoietic protoporphyria. 6. Congenital porphyria.

tion of elevated precursors (up to the affected reaction) in red cells, urine and faeces. Activity of the initial enzyme in the synthetic pathway, amino-laevulinic acid (ALA) synthase, activity is enhanced so ALA and, in acute porphyrias, porphobilinogen, are elevated.

## Acute porphyrias

The acute porphyrias are inherited as autosomal dominant conditions. **Acute intermittent porphyria** presents most commonly in young women with abdominal pain, neuropsychiatric symptoms, neuropathy and sometimes seizures, hypertension and tachycardia. **Variegate porphyria** includes photosensitive bullous skin lesions (which may be the only evidence of the disease), with a preponderance of skin manifestations in young men, and neuropsychiatric and abdominal symptoms in young women. **Hereditary coproporphyria** is rare but has similar clinical features, occurring with equal sex incidence from childhood to old age.

Attacks of all the acute porphyrias are precipitated by drugs which induce hepatic enzymes. Sulphonamides, barbiturates, anticonvulsants and oral contraceptives are absolutely contraindicated. All drugs should be checked against full lists for complicity in precipitating attacks before prescriptions are given to porphyria sufferers.

## Non-acute porphyrias

The non-acute porphyrias are characterized by photosensitive skin pathology but neurologic involvement does not occur, perhaps because elevated porphobilinogen deaminase limits the accumulation of ALA.

In **cutaneous hepatic porphyria** a photosensitive, bullous eruption occurs on exposed skin with pruritis, hyperpigmentation and hirsutism. There are associated abnormalities of liver function, exacerbated by the alcohol excess that is causally related in most patients. Increasing liver dysfunction diminishes the biliary excretion of the porphyrins, with diversion into plasma, skin and urine. Venesection to remove circulating porphyrins, avoidance of alcohol and increasing urinary excretion of uroporphyrin are useful treatments. Twenty-five per cent of patients have diabetes mellitus.

**Erythropoietic protoporphyria** is an autosomal dominant condition manifesting as a painful, pruritic and burning photosensitive urticarial or erythematous rash. The protoporphyrins may cause liver damage and cholelithiasis. β-Carotene may reduce the photosensitivity, and bile salt binding resins reduce the protoporphyrin levels.

**Congenital porphyria** is fortunately very rare but manifests as very severe photosensitive bullous eruptions, pigmentation and hypertrichosis. Scarring can lead to blindness and nail and hand deformity. Porphyrin deposition in the teeth stains them pink, and anaemia and splenomegaly occur.

Circulating porphyrins may also be elevated in lead poisoning, iron deficiency and in alcoholic and other liver disease.

# CALCIUM METABOLISM

## PHYSIOLOGY

Most of the body's calcium is in the skeleton. Apart from its role in maintaining skeletal integrity, calcium is important in tissue excitability, including neuromuscular conduction, in muscle cell contractility and in mediating the action of most, if not all hormones. Blood calcium levels are determined by input from two sources – the diet and skeleton – and the rate of calcium excretion through the kidney. Calcium homeostasis is controlled principally by parathyroid hormone (PTH) and vitamin D. Calcitonin, from the clear cells of the thyroid, antagonizes PTH and lowers calcium by inhibiting calcium resorption from bone and decreasing renal tubular absorption of calcium and phosphate. Its role in day-to-day calcium balance is uncertain.

Parathyroid hormone secretion by the parathyroid glands is stimulated by hypocalcaemia. It stimulates renal tubular calcium resorption and has a phosphaturic effect, mediated by cyclic adenine monophosphate (cAMP) – the loss of phosphate in the urine lowers the product calcium $\times$ phosphate in the blood, encouraging removal of calcium from the skeleton to the circulation. Parathyroid hormone stimulates calcium absorption from the gut via activation of vitamin D and inhibits tubular resorption of bicarbonate. The resulting mild hyperchloraemic acidosis further encourages bone calcium release. There may be a direct stimulation of bone turnover.

Vitamin $D_3$ (calciferol) is drawn from the diet and is also synthesized from cholesterol derivatives in the skin under the influence of sunlight. 25-Hydroxycalciferol is formed in the liver, then further hydroxylated in the kidney to the very active 1,25-dihydroxycalciferol and 24,25-hydroxycalciferol. These pathways of activation are stimulated by PTH but may be impaired in renal disease. Vitamin D and its derivatives are metabolized in the liver and kidney. They act by increasing absorption of calcium and phosphate from the gastrointestinal tract and increase bone resorption, leading to hypercalcaemia and hyperphosphataemia. Ergocalciferol (vitamin $D_2$) has the same metabolic fate and actions as calciferol and is available therapeutically.

# Hypercalcaemia

Causes of hypercalcaemia are listed in Table 18.13.

**Table 18.13** Causes of hypercalcaemia.

| |
| --- |
| Hyperparathyroidism |
| Malignancy: Myeloma |
|         Squamous carcinoma of the lung |
|         Bony metastases |
| Immobilization |
| Vitamin D intoxication |
| Sarcoidosis |
| Milk-alkali syndrome |
| Thiazide diuretics |
| Hyperthyroidism |
| Benign familial hypercalcaemia |

## INVESTIGATION

Preliminary investigation must include measurement of plasma fasting uncuffed calcium, albumin, phosphate, erythrocyte sedimentation rate (ESR), protein electrophoresis, PTH, thyroid function and urine analysis for Bence Jones proteins, measurement of 24 hour urine calcium excretion, glomerular filtration rate and chest X-ray.

Only free calcium ions are relevant to metabolism. About 50 per cent of calcium in the circulation is protein bound, mostly to albumin, so measured levels will be higher if protein levels are high. Indeed, to obtain a clearer idea of clinically relevant calcium levels, the measured result should be corrected according to the plasma albumin level:

Total calcium + 0.02 × (Mean normal albumin − Measured albumin)

Free (ionized) calcium can be measured directly but this is not an easy or readily available assay. Finally, albumin binding is pH dependent and will increase (with the possibility of hypocalcaemic symptoms and signs) in alkalosis (e.g. hyperventilation).

Measurement of renal tubular reabsorption of phosphate, urine hydroxyproline and cAMP may be useful in the differential diagnosis.

## HYPERPARATHYROIDISM

Primary hyperparathyroidism is now commonly diagnosed as a chance finding of hypercalcaemia. It is most common in the elderly, where it is twice as common in women (younger patients show no sex difference). Over 80 per cent of cases are due to a single parathyroid adenoma, 4 per cent are multiple, and most of the rest have diffuse hyperplasis of all four glands (approximately 11 per cent). They are sometimes associated with tumours of other endocrine tissues in the syndromes of multiple endocrine neoplasia (page 553): MEN 1 (hyperparathyroidism, pancreatic islet cell tumour, pituitary adenoma) and MENIIa (hyperparathyroidism, medullary carcinoma of the thyroid and phaeochromocytoma). Carcinoma is rare (less than 2 per cent).

### Clinical features

Asymptomatic hypercalcaemia may be detected as part of a blood chemistry screen or may be associated with the following symptoms. Polyuria causes dehydration and polydipsia. Hypercalciuria may result in renal calculi and renal colic (a common presentation) and nephrocalcinosis. Chronic renal failure occurs in 5 to 10 per cent. Depression is common.

Chronic hyperparathyroidism can lead to significant demineralization of bone with characteristic X-ray appearances of subperiosteal erosion occurs in about 2 per cent of patients. Loss of the distal tufts of the phalanges is a typical appearance on X-ray, and, rarely, cystic

areas through which fracture can occur. Diffuse changes are also seen. Patients with involvement of large bones may complain of bone pain and tenderness, even without fractures.

The reasons for treating asymptomatic hyperparathyroidism are to prevent skeletal and renal damage.

### Diagnosis and management

Diagnosis is established by demonstrating hypercalcaemia in an uncuffed fasted blood sample, hypophosphataemia and hypercalciuria in the presence of inappropriately high PTH levels. Failure to suppress the hypercalcaemia by high-dose steroids, an old test for hyperparathyroidism, is no longer necessary since the advent of easily available PTH assays. Measurement of renal tubular phosphate resorption is sometimes used: it will be decreased. 1, 25-OH-vitamin D will be elevated. Parathyroid hormone stimulates bone turnover so both alkaline phosphatase (from osteoblasts) and urinary hydroxyproline (evidence of osteoclast activity) are raised and urine cAMP rises.

Ultrasound or thallium pertechnetate scanning are used to visualize the parathyroids and identify a tumour. Exploration of the neck is usually indicated even if the scans are negative. Some surgeons inject methylene blue intravenously to help identify the parathyroids, which take up the dye, during surgery. Occasionally parathyroid tissue is found in the mediastinum rather than in the neck. Selective venous sampling of the neck veins can confirm the source of the PTH if the source of excess hormone is uncertain. If a single adenoma is the cause the other glands will be atrophic but should recover. If diffuse hyperplasia is found, attempts are sometimes made to leave a remnant or to remove all glands and implant a remnant in an accessible subcutaneous site to avoid subsequent hypoparathyroidism but make recurrence easy to treat.

## SECONDARY AND TERTIARY HYPERPARATHYROIDISM

Secondary hyperparathyroidism occurs owing to phosphate levels rising as a response to calcium loss. Tertiary hyperparathyroidism occurs when the parathyroid glands, stimulated by calcium depletion, become autonomous and hyper-secrete, leading to frank hypercalcaemia. These conditions occur in renal failure, where calcium loss occurs in part because of failure of hydroxylation of 25-hydroxycalciferol by the kidneys (page 435).

## MALIGNANT HYPERCALCAEMIA

Hypercalcaemia, secondary to malignant disease, may relate to the presence of extensive bone metastases but is not usually directly due to bone destruction. Humoral hypercalcaemia factor of malignancy is, as its name suggests, a circulating factor secreted by tumour cells and was sequenced a few years ago. Squamous carcinoma of the lung can also secrete PTH. Hypercalcaemia of malignant disease may respond to steroid suppression but treatment of the primary disease is indicated. In myeloma and other haematological malignancies, hypercalcaemia may be due to the release of osteoclast-activating factors from leukocytes. This is often very sensitive to steroids.

## OTHER CAUSES OF HYPERCALCAEMIA

Hypercalcaemia may also accompany sarcoidosis where it is clinically indistinguishable from excessive action of vitamin D and probably due to hydroxylation to active 1,25-dihydroxycalciferol by granulomas. Parathyroid hormone levels may be quite low. It is steroid sensitive. The clinical picture may be similar to hypervitaminosis D (which usually results from excessive consumption of vitamin supplements) in which hypercalcaemia and hyperphosphataemia are seen due to increased bone resorption. If undetected, bone loss can be significant but it is the renal effects that do most damage. Standard vitamin D supplements have very long half-lives, so resolution may be slow. Hyperthyroidism, excess intake of milk and antacids, and use of thiazide diuretics are other uncommon causes.

Benign familial hypercalcaemia is an autosomal dominant condition, usually asymptomatic, which may be indistinguishable from primary hyperparathyroidism but it does not have the same pathogenesis. It is due to decreased renal excretion of calcium so 24-hour urinary calcium is low. It is not helped by parathyroidectomy.

## HYPERCALCIURIA

Hypercalciuria occurs in hypercalcaemia due to hyperparathyroidism, sarcoidosis and malignancy, but may also occur in the presence of a normal blood calcium in familial normocalcaemic hypercalciuria. Nephrolithiasis and/or nephrocalcinosis may result in chronic renal failure. Treatment is by low calcium diet and thiazide diuretics. Such therapy may unmask undiagnosed hyperparathyroidism so hypercalcaemia must be excluded after initiating therapy.

## MANAGEMENT OF HYPERCALCAEMIA

Emergency treatment may be necessary to prevent renal damage and death. Initial management consists of vigorous fluid replacement. Frusemide, which has a calciuric action, can be useful once dehydration is fully corrected. Although oral phosphate therapy lowers calcium, and may still be used orally in well-hydrated, hypophosphataemic patients with normal renal function, the risks of deposition of calcium salts in the tissues and especially in the kidney with intravenous phosphates are too great. Dietary restriction and oral calcium-binding resins may have a small role in hypervitaminosis D and sarcoidosis. Steroids may be effective in reducing the hypercalcaemia of hypervitaminosis D, sarcoidosis and myeloma. Calcium may be lowered very effectively by biphosphate infusion (e.g. etidronate) which raises the solubility product of calcium and phosphate, inhibiting bone resorption. Mithramycin, a chemotherapeutic agent, has calcium-lowering activity and has been used in the hypercalcaemia of malignancy. Calcitonin, from salmon, is an expensive but safe agent for calcium control, but its efficacy is not always sustained. In the long term the primary condition must be treated. The treatment of primary hyperparathyroidism is surgical (page 501).

# Hypoparathyroidism

In hypoparathyroidism failure of PTH secretion leads to hypocalcaemia. This may present clinically with weakness and muscle cramp and, if severe, carpopedal spasm and seizure. It is detected at the bedside by demonstrating positive Chvostek and Trousseau's tests. In the former, muscle hyperreactivity is demonstrated by a facial twitch on tapping the patient's facial nerve in front of the tragus. In the latter, the hand can be forced into spasm by using a blood pressure cuff to occlude arterial supply for up to 3 min.

Hypocalcaemia and hyperphosphataemia are the rule. Hypocalcaemia may occur acutely after parathyroid or thyroid surgery, and the plasma calcium should be measured every 6–12 hours for 2–3 days postoperatively. Hypocalcaemia will need urgent treatment but does not always imply permanent loss of parathyroid tissue or function. Urgent treatment is by intravenous calcium and then by oral replacement. If long-term treatment is necessary it is now usually by 1-α-cholecalciferol rather than calcium salts.

**Pseudohypoparathyroidism** is a congenital abnormality of tissue resistance to the actions of PTH. Levels of PTH are normal or high, despite the clinical picture of hypoparathyroidism. Associated structural abnormalities of short stature, round face, and shortened 4th metacarpals lead to diagnosis. Similar physical features occur in the absence of any abnormality of calcium metabolism in pseudohypoparathyroidism.

# Rickets and osteomalacia

Bone diseases are importantly linked with calcium metabolism. Rickets is a condition of failure of skeletal hardening seen in young people – lack of calcium prevents adequate mineralization. It presents as stunted growth or severely painful joint lesions. Dietary deficiency of vitamin D is usually responsible. Children of Asian immigrants to the UK are especially susceptible through lack of adequate calcium and vitamin D intake, consumption of foods that inhibit absorption and inadequate exposure to sunlight. The condition responds to vitamin D supplementation, but if diagnosis is delayed permanent structural deficits remain. Rickets is a disease of growing bone and does not occur in adults in whom osteomalacia (demineralization of bone) is seen instead.

Osteomalacia occurs when bone mineralization cannot proceed normally.

## AETIOLOGY

Lack of vitamin D results in calcium deficiency and may be due to a number of factors including dietary deficiency (the elderly and vegans are particularly prone); lack of exposure to sunlight; malabsorption (especially where the enterohepatic recirculation of vitamin D is interrupted as in steatorrhoea, gluten sensitivity and biliary fistula); failure of hydroxylation of vitamin $D_3$, as in hypoparathyroidism, chronic renal failure, genetic enzyme defects; and defective tissue sensitivity to 1,25-dihydroxycalciferol. Osteomalacia may also result from hypophosphataemia which may occur in vegans; in malabsorption due to intake of aluminium hydroxide antacids; in association with certain haemangiomas and fibromas; in diseases of excessive renal loss as in renal tubular acidosis; and in X-linked familial hypophosphataemia. Systemic acidosis, such as in renal tubular acidosis, also precipitates bone demineralization. Finally, some anticonvulsant drugs may cause osteomalacia.

## CLINICAL FEATURES

Clinically, osteomalacia may present as nonspecific bone pain and muscle weakness with preserved, or even brisk, reflexes. The weakness particularly affects the proximal muscles.

## DIAGNOSIS

Loss of bone density with symmetrical pseudofractures (Looser's zones) may be seen on X-ray. In cases of doubt, pseudofractures also show up on radionuclide bone scanning. Plasma calcium, phosphate and 25-hydroxycalciferol will be variably low, with high PTH levels according to the severity of the disease. Plasma alkaline phosphatase tends to be high and low urinary excretion of calcium is characteristic. If in doubt, bone biopsy after two timed administrations of oral tetracycline to label the mineralization front of the bone will provide the diagnosis. Underlying conditions such as steatorrhoea or the inability to acidify urine must be excluded.

## TREATMENT

Treatment of rickets or osteomalacia is by vitamin D therapy with calcium supplements to prevent hypocalcaemia as bone remineralization begins. Ergocalciferol is effective in low doses in cases of dietary or sunlight exposure lack. In malabsorption much larger doses are needed, but the primary cause should be treated too. Renal disease requires calcitriol (1, 25-$(OH)D_2$), and hypophosphataemia requires the rather unpalatable phosphate therapy and calcitriol to prevent secondary hyperparathyroidism. When long-term maintenance therapy is needed, care must be taken to avoid hypercalcaemia with regular monitoring. Renal tubular acidosis requires bicarbonate therapy.

# Osteoporosis

This is a condition where bone is lost quantitatively. The 'thinner' bones are prone to fracture, especially the vertebrae, the wrist and the femoral neck which may break after minimal trauma, causing loss of height and severe morbidity.

## PATHOGENESIS AND AETIOLOGY

The sex hormones have an antagonist effect against PTH action on bone and osteoporosis occurs most commonly in post menopausal females. An individual woman's risk of trouble is related to her bone mass at the time she enters her menopause. Forty per cent of women over 65 experience fractures and they are a major cause of morbidity and mortality. Men begin to lose bone mass progressively from their 60s onwards, but the loss is less pronounced than in women. Calcium deficiency exacerbates the problem by stimulating PTH release. Alcohol excess, smoking, immobilization and inertia contribute. Corticosteroid excess as in Cushing's syndrome (page 530) and in treatment regimens have a direct inhibitory effect on osteoblast collagen synthesis, enhance tissue sensitivity to PTH and inhibit intestinal and renal calcium transport mechanisms, causing decreased intestinal absorption and increased renal loss of calcium with subsequent hyperparathyroidism. Rapid bone loss ensues. Osteoporosis also occurs in vitamin C deficiency (the vitamin being a cofactor of hydroxyproline synthesis), in haemochromatosis, in immobilization, hyperthyroidism and anticonvulsant therapy. Juvenile osteoporosis is rare and may be self-limiting, but a form occurs in young adults which is severe and rapidly progressive. Apparent osteoporosis can occur in localized areas where it is painful and may progress to fibrous replacement of bone. Osteogenesis imperfecta is a disease of impaired collagen synthesis that results in osteoporosis of varying degree.

## DIAGNOSIS

Bone mass can now be measured in several ways. X-ray changes are unlikely to be perceptible until 30 per cent of bone has been lost, and it is rarely possible to scan the whole skeleton. However, changes in the vertebrae are particularly characteristic. Thinned bone is eroded by the intervertebral discs (codfish spine) and unsuspected wedge fractures occur. Trabecular patterns are lost from the femoral head and neck. Dual photon absorptiometry or dual energy radiography, as well as computed tomography (CT) techniques are used for quantitative measurements and can detect loss of 20 per cent or more of the bone mass.

## TREATMENT

Treatment should ideally be preventative, with replacement of low-dose oestrogens for women at risk. Women who still have a uterus will need this treatment to be cycled with intermittent progesterone to allow endometrial shedding and diminish the risks of uterine cancer. A history (and probably a family history) of breast cancer or thromboembolic disease are contraindications. Dietary calcium supplementation with exercise programmes may be beneficial in retarding bone loss. Calcitonin, PTH and vitamin D, fluoride and diphosphonates are under investigation as therapeutic options.

In the established individual case, osteoporosis cannot be reversed. The above means should be used to prevent further deterioration, and any reversible primary causes should be treated.

# *Paget's disease*

Paget's disease of bone occurs in the elderly. It is not a metabolic condition but will be mentioned for completeness. It is a focal disease of abnormal bone modelling, where structured bone is replaced by disorganized woven and trabecular bone.

## CLINICAL FEATURES

The usual bones affected are the long bones of the legs, and the skull. It can be painful and the affected bone is fragile. Increased blood flow to the area and its overlying skin causes local redness. The increased cardiac output may be so great as to precipitate heart failure. There is an increased risk of osteosarcoma developing in the diseased bone.

## DIAGNOSIS

Alkaline phosphatase levels are very high and urinary hydroxyproline levels are high. Typical X-ray appearances of enlarged bones with expanded cortex are diagnostic.

## TREATMENT

Treatment is not ideal. If anti-inflammatory drugs do not control symptoms, other treatment options include calcitonin (to decrease bone resorption) or 3–6 month courses of diphosphonates.

# *D*EFECTS OF NUTRITIONAL STATUS

# *Obesity*

A body weight significantly in excess of ideal, if maintained over years, is associated with increased morbidity and mortality. Definitions of obesity are indeed derived from mortality data garnered from statistics from life insurance companies anxious to weight their premiums appropriately. Clinically, obesity can be defined from several measurements, as set out in Table 18.14.

Obese people have an increased lean body weight (i.e. body tissue excluding adipose tissue), but the major component of the excess weight is fat. Healthy men should have less than 20 per cent fat, and women less than 25 per cent fat. Fat content falls during childhood until puberty and subsequently rises.

Fat distributed intra-abdominally rather than subcutaneously has particularly poor prognostic implications, hence the value of the waist:hip ratio in determining risk to health. The fat

**Table 18.14** Definitions of excessive weight.

| | Method | Acceptable | Overweight | Obesity |
|---|---|---|---|---|
| Adults | Weight for height (% of 'normal' derived from life insurance tables) | <110% | 110–120% | >120% |
| | Skinfold thickness | <40 mm | 40–80 mm | >80 mm |
| | Weight/height$^2$ | 20–25 kg/m$^2$ | 26–29 kg/m$^2$ | >30 kg/m$^2$ |
| | Waist : hip ratio | | | >0.8 |
| Children | Weight for height from 'normal' | <110% | 110–120% | >120% |
| Adolescents | Skinfold thickness | <20 mm | 20–40 mm | >40 mm |

content of an individual can be assessed by the low density of fat in radiological studies and by the low proportion of body water to total body mass measured by isotope techniques.

## DISEASE ASSOCIATIONS OF CHRONIC OBESITY

### Ischaemic heart disease

High LDL cholesterol, low HDL cholesterol and high triglycerides are found in obese subjects. These improve with weight loss and may contribute to the 1.6–1.8 mortality ratios from ischaemic heart disease for those 25 per cent over their ideal body weight. Decreased activity contributes both by diminishing energy expenditure and encouraging further weight gain and by loss of the lipid lowering effects of exercise.

### Hypertension

The basis for the association between hypertension and obesity is unclear. A standard size blood pressure cuff tends to overestimate blood pressure on a very fat arm, and a thigh cuff gives a closer approximation to true blood pressure in the obese, but even with accurate recording there is a significant association between obesity and hypertension. Activation of the sympathetic nervous system by carbohydrate ingestion may be a causative assocation. Hypertension contributes to the excess mortality and morbidity from heart disease and from stroke in the obese.

### Diabetes mellitus

The association between non-insulin-dependent diabetes mellitus (NIDDM) and obesity is strong. There is a major (probably multifactorial) genetic component to NIDDM, but the risk of diabetes in first degree relatives of patients with NIDDM is much increased if they become obese. Particularly striking is the link between gestational diabetes, obesity and later development of NIDDM. If women with a history of gestational diabetes can achieve and maintain ideal body weight, their risk of NIDDM may be halved. The link between obesity and diabetes may relate to the relative insulin resistance of obese people. Most obese people have normal glucose tolerance, but only

at the cost of high insulin levels. If there is a genetic predisposition to pancreatic β cell failure, the increased demands for insulin by the obese body will precipitate glucose intolerance and frank diabetes as the pancreas fails to keep up with the increased demand for insulin. Syndrome X comprises obesity, hyperlipidaemia, hypertension and glucose intolerance and it has been postulated that insulin resistance is the underlying pathological mechanism.

### Osteoarthritis

The transmission of excessive body weight through the relatively small weight-bearing surfaces of the skeleton, especially the knees, predisposes to osteoarthritis. Back pain is probably a result of strain on the ligaments supporting the paunch. Arthritis limiting mobility exacerbates the problem in a vicious circle.

### Cholelithiasis

Obesity is associated with increased hepatic cholesterol synthesis. This is probably a response to accelerated cholesterol metabolism but results in a lithogenic bile and increased risk of gallstones. An associated stimulation of cholesterol synthesis by oestrogens makes this complication particularly common in obese females.

### Menstrual irregularities and subfertility

Obesity is a common feature of the polycystic ovarian syndrome and, in some women, may contribute to its clinical features (hirsutism and menstrual irregularities) because adipose tissue metabolizes oestrogen into active androgen. Progesterone stimulates appetite and the contraceptive pill, by inhibition of ovulation preventing the increase in metabolic rate associated with the second phase of the menstrual cycle, may contribute to obesity.

### Respiratory disease

Dyspnoea is a common complaint of the obese and respiratory disease will be exacerbated by the splinting of the diaphragms seen in obesity, although true hypoventilation is rare.

### Other associations of obesity

Obesity also predisposes to varicose veins, ankle oedema, endometrial and breast cancers, poor wound healing and increased anaesthetic risk, although the last has become less of a problem with current techniques.

## PATHOGENESIS

Excess weight is due to an energy intake in excess of requirements. People with obesity do have some metabolic abnormalities that contribute to their difficulties in losing weight. Basal metabolic rate (BMR) (energy expended in protein synthesis, carbohydrate and fat metabolism, maintenance of intracellular electrolyte status etc.) is lower than normal in obese patients if expressed per unit lean body mass and in the non-obese children of obese parents, facilitating weight gain and delaying its loss. In obesity BMR may actually be high because, although significant amounts of the weight are adipose tissue, there is also an increase in lean body mass. Thermogenesis from fat is diminished with only about 3 per cent of the caloric content of ingested fat being converted to heat. Simple fat overfeeding of the non-obese does not cause substantial weight gain as most of the excess energy is expended in heat.

Although obesity is unquestionably familial, the role of genetic factors is unclear. Twin studies suggest a role for genes, but this is not the whole story. Intrauterine nutrition is important. Fat mothers tend to have large placentae and big babies who develop into fat children, but if other factors result in a small placenta, a small baby results. There is little factual evidence to support the commonly held theory that fat cell number is determined by early nutrition, but over 30 per cent of fat infants will be obese adults compared with 14 per cent of non-obese infants.

There are rare genetically inherited syndromes which include obesity, usually also including hypogonadism, mental retardation and retinal degeneration, and sometimes polydactyly. The most common one (1/20 000) is the Prader–Willi syndrome consisting of hypotonia, mental retardation, obesity, short stature, hypogenitalism, hyperphagia (page 63). These genetic syndromes contrast with the much more common simple obesity in children which is usually associated with increased height for age.

Underlying endocrine abnormalities in obesity are also very rare. Hypothyroidism is found in about 1 per cent of attendees at specialist obesity clinics, and Cushing's syndrome even less commonly. Increased urinary 17-hydroxy-corticosteroids and impaired suppression of endogenous cortisol with dexamethasone may be found in simple obesity but diurnal rhythms, urinary-free cortisol and plasma-free cortisol are normal.

## TREATMENT

The mainstay of treatment for obesity is exercise and restriction of caloric intake. That over 30 per cent of British adults are dieting at any time suggests that current therapies are not successful in the long term. It is not easy to lose weight – a loss of 1 kg fat represents a deficit of over 7000 kcal. Exercise is beneficial, it helps improve unfavourable lipid profiles and contributes to a negative caloric balance. Small imbalances in energy consumption and expenditure will contribute to maintenance of obesity and loss of muscle bulk with inactivity will lower BMR. Basal metabolic rate is over 1000 kcal/day (4.2 kJ) in most adults; it is increased by 3 per cent by light physical activity, and up to 100 per cent by hard physical work, such as lumberjacking!

There is some feedback control of appetite from energy expenditure and some obese people do not eat more than their non-obese peers but need to eat less. Strenuous exercise leads to increased food intake and experimental dilution of the calorie content of food leads to increased appetite. Gastric distension plays a role in satiety however, and high energy foods do not produce satiety as quickly as low energy foods which need to be taken in greater volume to achieve the same energy intake. New tastes will also stimulate appetite in the satisfied person – thus western diets with great variety and high energy content carbohydrate foods particularly encourage weight gain. Weight-reducing diets should be based on long-term restriction of sugars and fat. Although protein and carbohydrate restriction produce rapid results, this is because of large water loss associated with glycogen and protein loss and is not a true loss of adiposity. Thus initial weight loss may be rapid (the basis of the success of 'one week wonder diets'), but then slows. Even a small increase in carbohydrate intake thereafter leads to rapid glycogen synthesis with water retention and apparent weight gain. The constipating and cholelithogenic effects of low fibre diets must also be guarded against. Starvation regimens are not recommended because they are associated with decreased energy expenditure. Very low calorie diets, marketed as protecting against protein loss, can be effective initially, but early systems were associated with cardiovascular deaths, thought to relate to electrolyte and mineral deficiencies and should be used with great care. In any event, initially good results (with any diet) are seldom maintained. The use of behaviour modification techniques and re-training eating habits are thought to encourage longer term success. Self-help groups and slimming clubs work for some patients, especially if they encourage exercise and motivation, but may suffer from single diets being applied universally. Other patients benefit from close supervision (e.g. every 2 weeks) by trained dietitians. Food diaries may help both in the assessment of intake and retraining of eating habits. Measurement of 24-hour potassium and urea excretion can be used if in real doubt of a patient's own impressions of caloric intake. Daily weighing should be strongly discouraged.

Drugs to suppress appetite should be used only with close supervision and only as an adjunct to diet. Amphetamines stimulate catecholamine receptors and thermogenesis, and produce anorexia, but also may produce agitation, insomnia and addiction. Structurally related compounds such as diethylpropion and mazindol are not addictive but cause significant cerebral stimulation. Fenfluramine is metabolized to norfenfluramine and acts through the serotoninergic neurons to cause anorexia. The newly formulated pure D-isomer of fenfluramine, dexfenfluramine, is an exciting new concept in drug synthesis – it is believed that using only the isomer with the required action will reduce side effects. The drug is licenced for short courses of therapy and seems effective and safe, although there have been a few reports of pulmonary hypertension in people on it.

Smoking tends to keep body weight down because of its anorexic effects and the stimulation of metabolic rate. However, the health hazards of smoking greatly outweigh the potential effects of the moderate weight gain that tends to occur with giving up. Part of the weight gain may be avoided by providing some less fattening occupation for the hands and mouth.

Surgical treatment of obesity is a last resort. Jaw wiring is not recommended by most practitioners now. The teeth can suffer from the ingestion of high carbohydrate fluids. Energy intake can easily be maintained with fluids and recurrent obesity later is the rule. Intestinal bypass produces significant side effects, including diarrhoea and malabsorption. Stapling the stomach to induce early satiety is probably technically the safest option and can be beneficial.

# Endocrine and metabolic aspects of anorexia nervosa

Anorexia (literally loss of appetite) accompanies many stresses. Anorexia nervosa is a specific condition (page 886), believed to have a strong psychological basis, in which voluntary restriction of carbohydrate intake leads to weight loss and loss of reproductive function. It is classically a disease of young women (male:female 1:10–20), with one in every 250 schoolgirls over 18 experiencing the condition. Over 6 per cent of ballerinas have anorexia nervosa.

Diagnosis is based on severe weight loss, expression of a fear of becoming fat and amenorrhoea. The disease usually starts soon after puberty and is attributed to a fear of developing into a mature adult. The patient is thin, with marked loss of subcutaneous fat, often bradycardic and hypotensive, with decreased core temperature and a development of fine lanugo hair over the face. Body image is abnormal. There is often an excessive devotion to exercise and paradoxically, a keen interest in cooking, with abuse of laxatives or diuretics. Proximal myopathy and vitamin deficiency related peripheral neuropathies may occur. Prolonged malnutrition and amenorrhoea increase the risk of osteoporosis. Psychiatric conditions such as depression or obsessive behaviour are common.

Amenorrhoea or absent libido and erectile dysfunction have an endocrine basis. Gonadotrophins and circulating oestrogen (or testosterone in males) are low, but the follicular-stimulating hormone (FSH) response in luteinizing hormone releasing hormone (LHRH) is normal, and the luteinizing hormone (LH) responses only slightly diminished, suggesting a defect in the hypothalamus rather than the pituitary. The LH response to the oestrogen receptor blocker clomiphene is diminished and oestrogen does not rise in response to elevations in LH. Thyroxine levels may be reduced, with increased conversion to reverse T3 rather than to tri-iodothyronine (T3, the most metabolically active thyroid hormone), and the thyroid-stimulating hormone (TSH) response to thyrotropin-releasing hormone (TRH) may be delayed. Cortisol and growth hormone may be elevated, possibly as a response to glucose lack and starvation stress. Cholesterol rises. Hypokalaemia is exacerbated by diuretic or laxative abuse, and vitamin deficiency, especially thiamine, is common. In the rare prepubertal case, linear growth is impaired.

Large amounts of calories are required to make up the deficit but rapid refeeding can precipitate gastric dilation, clinical evidence of the thiamine deficiency (beri-beri) and oedema. Psychological therapy, often involving the whole family, is necessary for success. Indeed, family dynamics are often abnormal for patients with anorexia. Often patients need to overshoot their ideal body weight to resume menstruation, although clomiphene may help once weight gain is achieved. Inpatient therapy is usually indicated initially, and about 66 per cent of patients eventually adjust to a more normal body image and food intake. The remainder have a poor prognosis, with continuing morbidity, and the overall death rate is 20 per cent.

Bulimia nervosum is characterized by bouts of excessive carbohydrate intake, followed by self-induced vomiting to avoid weight gain. This may follow a period of anorexia nervosum, but often patients are frankly obese. Depression is common and the advocated treatment is cognitive behaviour therapy.

# $A$CID–BASE AND ELECTROLYTE DISTURBANCES

The pH of the blood is normally kept within a narrow range of 7.36–7.42. Values outside the range can seriously affect the function of vital organs because intracellular pH will be altered too. Severe changes in pH can be lethal, particularly in acidosis. These effects reflect the importance of the $H^\times$ ion in metabolic pathways and membrane transport.

Certain terms need defining:

## Acidaemia/alkalaemia
pH below/above the normal range

## Acidosis/alkalosis
These terms are used in two ways:
(a) equivalent to acidaemia and alkalaemia
(b) to describe a potential acidaemia/alkalaemia, but which is compensated so that the pH is actually normal

## Base deficit
The number of mmol of alkali necessary to restore 1 litre of blood to normal (pH 7.40 at an arterial $PCO_2$ of 5.33 kPa)

## Base excess
The number of mmol of alkali to be removed from 1 litre of blood to achieve normal pH (as above)

## Standard bicarbonate
Correction of the actual bicarbonate value to its value calculated for blood with a normal arterial $PCO_2$ (5.33 kPa)

## Anion gap
The difference between the sum of the main cations ($Na^+$ and $K^+$) and anions ($Cl^-$ and $HCO_3^-$) in the blood. This is normally 10–18 mmol/l, the sum of anions being the lesser; the gap is closed by $PO_4^-$, $SO_4^-$ and proteins. The gap is increased pathologically when other anions (e.g. lactate or ketones) are present, as they will not be included in the calculation.

# Production of H⁺

The body is a net producer of $H^+$ ions, which must be eliminated to maintain homeostasis. There are three main sources of production which require different methods of elimination and which are not interchangeable.

1. $CO_2$ production by tissues generates $H^+$ through its formation of carbonic acid which, in turn, is eliminated by expiration of $CO_2$, leaving water. As this daily production of $H^+$ measures 15 mol, the lungs must be regarded as the main organs of $H^+$ elimination, the daily production of $H^+$ from the other two sources being much less.
2. Synthesis of organic acids. These mainly comprise hydroxybutyric, lactic and free fatty acids produced in the liver, muscles and fat. These are eliminated by metabolism, the liver itself playing the major part. Daily production is 2.5–3.0 mol.
3. Phosphoric and sulphuric acids. These derive from the diet, the former from metabolism of organic phosphate compounds, the latter from dietary proteins containing sulphur. Daily production is only 0.1 mol, but this apparently small amount belies the importance of this source of $H^+$ ions which can only be eliminated by renal excretion. Renal failure therefore inevitably results in acidosis.

# Excretion of H⁺

Excretion of $H^+$ ions is via the lungs and the kidneys. The former provide the most important route of excretion, eliminating the 15 mol produced daily by the process of respiration as explained above. An increased respiratory rate can increase elimination of $H^+$ ions by this route. The kidneys excrete sulphuric and phosphoric acids unchanged, but also control acid–base balance by the following means:

1. Ammonia production. Ammonia ($NH_3$) is produced in the tubular epithelium by metabolizing glutamine. The $NH_3$ combines with $H^+$ ions and is excreted as ammonium ($NH_4^+$).
2. Bicarbonate reabsorption. The proximal and distal tubular epithelia reabsorb bicarbonate from the glomerular filtrate. This combines with the $H^+$ ions in the cell to form $H_2CO_3$. Carbonic anhydrase then catalyses the dissociation of the carbonic acid to form $H_2O + CO_2$; the $CO_2$ recombines with $H_2O$ within the cell, which then dissociates to $H^+$ and $HCO_3^-$. The $H^+$ exchanges with sodium in the lumen of the tubule so that sodium bicarbonate is retained and $H^+$ is excreted.
3. Sodium phosphate in the glomerular filtrate will act as a buffer by binding to $H^+$ ions in the lumen. This accounts for a very small amount of acid excretion.

# Buffers

The most important buffer, because of its large amount and easy availability, is bicarbonate. Other buffers are phosphate and proteins. The large capacity of the bicarbonate buffer system is related to the large excretory load undertaken by the lungs through its elimination of $H^+$ ions as carbonic acid.

# Measurement of acid–base status

In most instances the data used to diagnose and guide the management of acid–base disturbances come from measuring the plasma concentration of bicarbonate and analysis of arterial blood samples.

## PLASMA BICARBONATE

This is often provided routinely on multichannel analysers and low concentrations (metabolic acidosis, respiratory alkalosis) or high concentrations (respiratory acidosis, metabolic alkalosis) may occasionally be the first signal that the patient has an important biochemical disturbance. Abnormal concentrations of chloride and/or potassium may also indicate acid–base disturbance.

## BLOOD GASES

Arterial samples, usually obtained from the brachial or radial artery, provide values for oxygen ($PO_2$), carbon dioxide ($PCO_2$), the pH, bicarbonate concentration and the base excess/standard bicarbonate. The pH, which is the reciprocal of the $\log_{10}$ of the hydrogen ion concentration, indicates whether there is acidosis (pH <7.35) or alkalosis (pH >7.42). The standard bicarbonate or calculated bicarbonate excess (shown as a negative value for the excess if there is, in fact, a deficit) is an artificial value and does not allow for buffering of $H^+$ ions in the blood by interstitial and intracellular fluid. Other measurements which may be made are:

*The anion gap*
See above. Cases with metabolic acidosis are helpfully divided into those with a normal or an increased anion gap (see below).

*Serum lactate*
Accumulation of lactate contributes to certain types of metabolic acidosis (lactic acidosis); measurement of serum lactate not only defines and quantifies the acidosis, but could then be used as an indicator of effective treatment.

*Interpretation of data*
The values for serum bicarbonate and arterial pH etc. are easily obtained in most hospitals, but they must be interpreted very carefully in the context of the patient's illness. This may be simple, for example, chronic respiratory failure with retention of $CO_2$ (respiratory acidosis), or complex, for example, diabetic ketoacidosis (metabolic acidosis) with vomiting (metabolic alkalosis) and acute renal failure (metabolic acidosis). In the early stages the metabolic and respiratory systems may balance each other, for

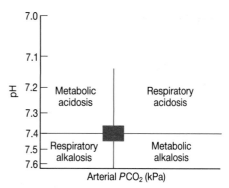

**Figure 18.4** The common disorders of acid–base metabolism.

example, hyperventilation (respiratory alkalosis) compensating a metabolic acidosis. A useful aid is to plot the measurements of arterial pH and $PCO_2$ on a graph (Fig. 18.4) and use the area in which the value falls to indicate the type of acid–base disturbance. If a metabolic acidosis is diagnosed then the serum lactate may be relevant.

# Types and causes of acid–base disturbance

These are conveniently divided into four categories: metabolic and respiratory acidosis and alkalosis. The two forms of acidosis are the more important because of their greater frequency and potentially more lethal effects. Many of the causes are dealt with in detail elsewhere in this book.

## METABOLIC ACIDOSIS

This may arise through loss of alkali or retention or overproduction of acid. It is the commonest acid–base disturbance in clinical practice and several medical emergencies are among its causes (Table 18.15). Measuring the anion gap helps to define the cause and to assess the effect of treatment in metabolic acidosis with a high anion gap.

## Metabolic acidosis with a high anion gap

This is caused by retention or generation of acids which are buffered by $HCO_3^-$, so producing a

**Table 18.15** Causes of metabolic acidosis.

| High anion gap | Normal anion gap |
|---|---|
| Uraemia (page 426) | Gastrointestinal loss of |
| Diabetic ketosis | $HCO_3^-$ |
| (page 480) | Diarrhoea (page 333) |
| | Pancreatic fistula |
| | Renal tubular acidosis |
| Drugs/poisons | (page 467) |
| Salicylates (aspirin) | Artificial feeding |
| (page 818) | (page 420) |
| Ethylene glycol | |
| (page 823) | |
| Methanol | |
| Lactic acidosis | |

fall in this anion's concentration and therefore an increase in the anion gap. The main causes are:

1. **Ketoacidosis.** This is most frequently seen in diabetic ketoacidosis (page 480), but it also occurs in starvation and acute alcohol toxicity. Excess amounts of keto-acids and lactic acid are produced.
2. **Renal failure.** Acute and chronic renal failure cause a relatively slow accumulation of phosphoric and sulphuric acids, which can be excreted only via the kidneys (page 426).
3. **Salicylate poisoning** (page 818).
4. **Methanol and ethylene glycol poisoning** (page 823).
5. **Lactic acidosis.** Many conditions can cause lactic acidosis, which is usually defined as a blood lactate concentration >5 mmol/l (normal range 0.6–1.2 mmol/l). Two types are recognized:

   *Type A:* This is caused by severe hypoxia or hypoperfusion when anaerobic metabolism produces excess lactate. A physiological form occurs in strenuous exercise which may elevate lactate levels to 2–3 mmol/l. The pathological causes are any type of shock (page 249) and any cause of hypoxia.
   *Type B:* This is caused by drugs, toxins, uncommon inherited metabolic defects, liver failure and anaerobic metabolism by large masses of malignant cells such as lymphoma and leukaemia. The drug which

most frequently caused lactic acidosis was phenformin, a biguanide used for non-insulin dependent diabetes. Phenformin has been withdrawn for this reason; a similar compound, metformin, has a much lower risk and when used carefully has not been associated with this complication to date.

## Metabolic acidosis with a normal anion gap

This results from loss of bicarbonate or, very uncommonly, the ingestion of hydrochloric acid or a substance metabolized to it such as ammonium chloride. The anion gap remains unchanged because bicarbonate loss results in renal retention of chloride and hyperchloraemia, and intake of hydrochloric acid, although lowering bicarbonate, provides chloride ions. Bicarbonate loss occurs from the gastrointestinal tract, by diarrhoea or pancreatic fistula, or from the kidneys by renal tubular acidosis (page 467).

## RESPIRATORY ACIDOSIS

Any cause of respiratory failure (page 290) will result in $CO_2$ retention and the formation of carbonic acid:

$$CO_2 + H_2O \rightarrow H_2CO_3 \rightarrow H^+ + HCO_3^-$$

## METABOLIC ALKALOSIS

The commonest cause of metabolic alkalosis is vomiting in which hydrogen and chloride are depleted, causing a hypochloraemic alkalosis. There is an associated hypokalaemia, due to loss of potassium in the urine. The urine exhibits a characteristic triad of findings – no, or very low chloride, excess potassium, and an acid urine despite the systemic alkalosis.

Other causes are diuretic therapy which also causes hypochloraemic alkalosis with hypokalaemia. The blocking of the tubular reabsorption of chloride is the underlying mechanism.

In hyperaldosteronism there is increased renal bicarbonate reabsorption with hypokalaemia.

Ingestion of excess amounts of alkali, usually taken for indigestion or peptic ulcer, can cause metabolic alkalosis. As the alkali is often taken with milk, used to reduce the indigestion, this alkalosis is known as the 'milk-alkali syndrome'.

Hypercalcaemia is another important metabolic derangement in this syndrome (page 500).

## RESPIRATORY ALKALOSIS

Hyperventilation causes loss of $H^+$ leading to respiratory alkalosis. Common causes are over-breathing in anxiety states, and stimulation of the respiratory centre as in, for example, salicylate poisoning.

## EFFECTS AND CLINICAL FEATURES

### Acidosis

Metabolic acidosis stimulates the respiratory centre and eventually produces deep 'sighing' respirations (described by Kussmaul and named after him – Kussmaul breathing). The hyperventilation tends to compensate the metabolic acidosis by eliminating excess $H^+$ ions through the lungs.

Acidosis has a negative inotropic effect on the heart, which is particularly important in the acutely ill patient. Peripheral arteries dilate, which may contribute to hypotension, but peripheral veins contract. This transfers blood volume to the central portion of the circulation, putting the patient at risk of pulmonary oedema. The haemoglobin oxygen dissociation curve is shifted to the right (page 271), which results in improved oxygen uptake by the tissues.

Confusion, drowsiness and eventually coma can develop.

Acidosis produces two important metabolic effects. Intracellular potassium is displaced by $H^+$ ions, causing hyperkalaemia. If renal function is moderate or normal, potassium may be excreted, resulting in a net loss of body potassium, despite the raised concentration in the blood. Second, bone acts as a buffer, and acidosis will result in loss of calcium carbonate, in exchange for hydrogen–phosphate molecules. In chronic acidosis, for example, in chronic renal failure, the negative calcium balance contributes to the accompanying bone disease.

### Alkalosis

The effects of alkalosis are less severe and fewer than those of acidosis. There is a small amount of positive cardiac inotropism, and the cerebral arterioles constrict. The haemoglobin–oxygen dissociation curve is shifted to the left, i.e. making oxygen less available. Coupled with the change in cerebral vessels this may account for the slight confusion sometimes seen in alkalosis.

Tetany (page 502) is a feature of respiratory alkalosis; the explanation is not clear but there may be increased binding of calcium ions to proteins.

The kidneys lose potassium because $H^+$ ions are no longer excreted by the renal tubules and the normal exchange of potassium (retained) for hydrogen (excreted) no longer occurs. In the most common cause of alkalosis, vomiting, there is loss of chloride and a similar mechanism, i.e. renal retention of chloride and lack of its exchange for potassium, compounds the potassium loss. Hypokalaemia and total body potassium depletion eventually result, with symptoms of fatigue and weakness due to impaired muscle function. The cause of the alkalosis itself, for example, diarrhoea, may also directly contribute to the hypokalaemia.

## DIAGNOSIS AND TREATMENT

It is important to remember the conditions which can cause acid–base disturbance as the diagnosis may be overlooked until considerable deterioration, which is preventable, has occurred. Clues may be seen in routine plasma biochemical measurements, for example, hyper-hypokalaemia, hyper-hypochloraemia, changes in plasma bicarbonate concentration. For a complete diagnosis, in addition to measuring plasma $Na^+$, $K^+$, $Cl^-$ and $HCO_3^-$, an arterial blood sample should be taken for measurement of the arterial blood pH and $PCO_2$; these will help define the severity and type of acid–base disturbance. It is helpful to place these two values on the graph of arterial pH versus arterial $PCO_2$ (Fig. 18.4) for guidance towards the type of disturbance. Urine concentrations of potassium and chloride will confirm metabolic alkalosis.

The treatment of an acid–base disturbance will obviously differ according to its type. Each shares, however, some general principles. First, the cause of the disturbance should be removed or reversed, for example, insulin for diabetic ketoacidosis, dialysis for acute renal failure, treatment of circulatory failure in cardiogenic shock, ventilation for neuromuscular diseases causing respiratory failure. Second, if the first measure is accompanied by appropriate repletion of any lost fluid and electrolytes, the body's own compensatory mechanisms will usually suffice to return the acid–base balance to normal. This will not be so if there is severe damage and failure of the organ(s) required for elimination of acid, i.e. lungs, kidneys and liver. Particular measures for the type of disturbance are as follows:

### Acute metabolic acidosis

While it may seem logical to reverse the acidosis with alkali, there may be disadvantages. The haemoglobin–oxygen dissociation curve may be shifted to the left, i.e. making oxygen less available with serious effects if there are circulatory failure and hypoperfusion of tissues and organs. If sodium bicarbonate is used the $PCO_2$ may rise because of reaction of the bicarbonate with the excess $H^+$ ions and subsequent dissociation into $H_2O$ and $CO_2$, and because reducing the acidosis in turn reduces the compensatory hyperventilation. The latter effect will not pose a problem if the patient is being ventilated. The rise in $PCO_2$ may be disadvantageous because it can reduce intracellular pH still further. This apparent paradox in the face of giving bicarbonate in acidosis is explained by the greater solubility of $CO_2$ compared to $HCO_3^-$ across cell membranes, including the blood–brain barrier. Alternative alkalinizing agents can present their own problems, for example, sodium lactate must be metabolized in order to alkalinize.

In practice, sodium bicarbonate is used in severe cases of acute metabolic acidosis, but care must be taken to monitor any deterioration it may be causing. Small quantities, repeated only after rechecking arterial blood pH, are given using an isotonic continuous intravenous infusion. Hypertonic bicarbonate can render the blood hyperosmotic: it is best reserved for the treatment of cardiac arrest.

Lactic acidosis type A requires, in addition, treatment with oxygen for the hypoxia and appropriate expanders of circulatory volume to improve cardiac output and tissue perfusion.

### Respiratory acidosis

This requires appropriate treatment of the respiratory failure, which in many cases may require ventilation (page 256).

### Metabolic alkalosis

Most cases are corrected easily by appropriate fluid and electrolyte replacement, with particular attention to replacing potassium and chloride, depletion of which are usually inherent in the acid-losing types of metabolic alkalosis. Only very rarely is acid replacement needed, the indication being severe tetany or circulatory disturbances affecting the brain. Either ammonium chloride or arginine hydrochloride can be given intravenously.

### Respiratory alkalosis

This is best managed by removing the cause; if this is not possible, and in the unlikely event that intervention is needed, artificial ventilation to slow the rate of respiration may be used.

## PITFALLS IN TREATMENT

In the complex and sometimes rapidly changing circumstances contributing to acid–base disturbances, it is all too easy to make errors which can profoundly worsen the outcome. The following are traps for the unwary:

1. Misinterpreting venous blood $PCO_2$ as arterial. In the hypoxic and peripherally vasoconstricted patient it can be difficult to puncture the brachial or radial artery to take the blood sample, and so a venous sample is obtained instead. Since venous blood has a lower $PO_2$ and pH, and higher $PCO_2$ than normal arterial blood, and as values of this nature may be expected in the ill patient, the error may not be spotted when the results become available.
2. Omitting potassium replacement in metabolic acidosis. The patient may already have total body potassium depletion, particularly if the acidosis has been present for days or weeks, despite hyperkalaemia. Alkalinization causes hypokalaemia as potassium enters cells, and in the potassium-depleted patient this can

develop rapidly and profoundly, with the possibility of an ensuing cardiac arrest, unless potassium is given intravenously.

3. Failing to replace fluid loss adequately. In diabetic ketoacidosis (page 480), for example, giving insulin before rehydration will encourage circulatory collapse as water follows glucose into the cells.

4. Causing fits and tetany in uraemia. In moderate to severe uraemia there is a metabolic acidosis with a low serum/plasma bicarbonate and hypocalcaemia. Succumbing to the temptation to correct the acidosis by rapid alkalinization with sodium bicarbonate will cause tetany and fits. Patients with chronic renal failure will very likely have renal osteodystrophy (page 435) and the weakened bones can fracture during the intense muscle contractions of a fit or tetany.

## OUTCOME

This is very dependent on the type of acid–base disturbance. The most serious is metabolic acidosis; patients with shock and lactic acidosis type A have the worst outlook, with a mortality rate of 80 per cent.

# Electrolyte disturbance

## SODIUM

Sodium is the main extracellular cation. The kidneys regulate body sodium in response to the renin–angiotensin–aldosterone system and natriuretic peptide.

### Hyponatraemia

In practice this is most commonly due to excess water, but without a deficit of sodium. The commonest causes of excess body water are inappropriate intravenous fluid replacement or impaired renal function; inappropriate secretion of ADH is rare (page 548). Treatment is by reducing the fluid replacement or, in renal failure, dialysis.

Hyponatraemia due to sodium loss occurs from the gastrointestinal tract, caused by vomiting, diarrhoea, gastrointestinal fistulae, and from the kidneys in chronic renal failure, after relief of urinary obstruction and during recovery from acute tubular necrosis. Inappropriate diuretic treatment also causes hyponatraemia. Patients with sodium depletion have hypotension and peripheral vasoconstriction due to reduced circulating and extracellular fluid volume and should be treated with appropriate sodium replacement by intravenous saline or oral salt intake.

### Hypernatraemia

The commonest cause of hypernatraemia is water depletion, usually seen in excessive sweating, fever, gastrointestinal loss in which the water loss exceeds the sodium loss, diabetes insipidus and diabetes mellitus. The extra- and intracellular fluid compartments are reduced, and hyperosmolarity develops. The patient is thirsty, and may become confused and comatose. Treatment requires isotonic or hypertonic intravenous fluids which should be administered slowly, otherwise a rate form of brain damage (pontine myelinolysis) can occur.

True sodium excess is uncommon, arising through inappropriate intravenous sodium infusions or, more rarely, saline enemas or emetics. The symptoms are the same, but treatment is to remove the cause and replete with water orally or dextrose intravenously.

## POTASSIUM

Only 2–3 per cent of body potassium is extracellular, so major changes in total body potassium are not necessarily reflected in plasma potassium levels.

### Hypokalaemia

This usually arises from excess loss of potassium from the kidneys or gastrointestinal tract (Table 18.16). The symptoms are muscle weakness, paralytic ileus, cardiac failure and arrhythmias. Chronic hypokalaemia can cause renal failure. Management requires oral or intravenous potassium chloride, with careful monitoring of plasma potassium concentration, particularly if the patient has renal disease.

## *Hyperkalaemia*

See page 432.

## MAGNESIUM

Hypomagnesaemia is caused by malabsorption, urinary loss due to diuretics or renal tubular acidosis, gastrointestinal loss due to vomiting or diarrhoea and diminished intake, usually seen in parenteral feeding. Muscle weakness, tetany, drowsiness, fits and cardiac arrhythmias may occur. As well as treating the cause, magnesium should be replaced intravenously or orally.

Hypermagnesaemia is seen in patients with chronic renal failure who ingest magnesium as antacids or laxatives. Cardiac arrhythmias or drowsiness may result. The treatment is to remove the cause and, if necessary, to dialyse the patient. Intravenous calcium gluconate will correct arrhythmia.

**Table 18.16** Causes of hypokalaemia.

**Renal**
Diuretics
Solute diuresis (glucose, urea, saline)
Aldosteronism (primary and secondary)
Cushing's syndrome
Bartter's syndrome
Renal tubular acidosis

**Gastrointestinal**
Prolonged vomiting
Ileostomy
Fistulae
Purgative abuse
Villous adenoma of the rectum

**Intracellular shifts**
Alkalosis
Peiodic paralysis

# **E**ndocrine Disorders

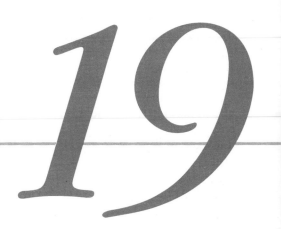

19

# INTRODUCTION

Endocrine secretions, acting in one sense as another nervous system, coordinate and control a wide variety of functions. As in the nervous system, positive and negative feedback are crucial, and this feedback is exerted either by hormones themselves or by the metabolic effects of hormones. Top-level control, in the hypothalamus, integrates these forms of feedback and the signals related to the subject's environment, such as dark or light, sleep or wakening, stress and excitement. The network of endocrine control is also held together by influences between the different hormone 'channels', both at hypothalamic–pituitary level and at the periphery where hormones act. Table 19.1 outlines the principal control mechanisms of the pituitary gland and Fig. 19.1 illustrates in more detail some of the interactions between the pituitary gland and the gonads.

The variety of levels at which modulation or feedback can occur deserves emphasis. Some hypothalamic factors act on tissues other than the pituitary; for example, gonadotrophin-releasing hormone (GnRH) influences the mood (a cerebral effect) and the uterus, and somatostatin occurs in high concentration in the islet cells of the pancreas and the wall of the gut. Pituitary hormones may act directly on tissue

**Table 19.1** Anterior pituitary and hypothalamic hormones.

| Anterior pituitary hormones | | Hypothalamic hormones |
|---|---|---|
| Adrenocorticotrophic hormone (ACTH) and melanocyte-stimulating hormone | *released by* | Corticotrophin-releasing hormone (CRH); the negative feedback is through cortisol |
| Follicle-stimulating hormone (FSH) which in the male stimulates spermatogenesis | *released by* | GnRH Gonadotrophin-releasing hormone (GnRH, previously LRH or LHRH), a decapeptide; positive and negative feedback through gonadal hormones including oestradiol, progesterone and inhibin and other peptides (Fig. 15.1) |
| Luteinizing hormone (LH) which in the male stimulates interstitial Leydig cells to produce testosterone | *released by* | |
| Growth hormone (GH) which stimulates production of insulin-like growth factor (IGF, somatomedin) | *released by* | Growth hormone-releasing hormone (GHRH), the dominant control |
| | *inhibited by* | Growth hormone release inhibitory hormone (GHRIH), somatostatin which also inhibits TSH release and several pancreatic hormones |
| Thyroid-stimulating hormone (TSH, thyrotrophin) | *released by* | Thyrotrophin-releasing hormone (TRH), a tripeptide, the dominant control |
| | *inhibited by* | Thyroid hormones and GHRIH |
| Prolactin | *inhibited by* | Dopamine. This is the dominant control, so there is an increase in prolactin secretion if control is 'impaired' in any way |
| | *released by* | TRH; but only significant at supraphysiological levels |

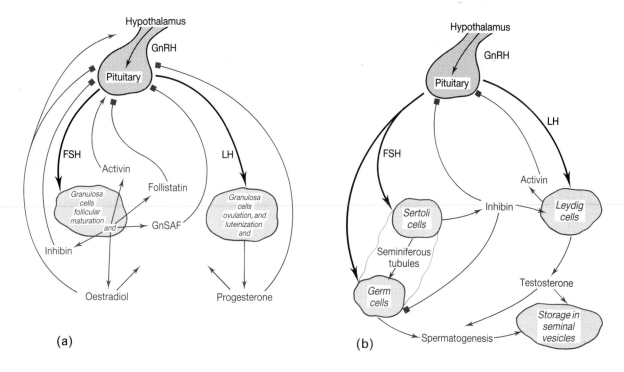

(a)

(b)

**Figure 19.1** Interactions between hormones of the hypothalamus, pituitary and gonads. (a) Hypothalamus–pituitary–ovaries. (b) Hypothalamus–pituitary–testes. GnRH = gonadotrophin-releasing hormone. FSH = follicle-stimulating hormone. LH = luteinizing hormone. GnSAF = gonadotrophin surge-activating factor. ➤ = stimulation. ─■ = inhibition. Reproduced with permission from *Clinical Endocrinology* 1991; 35: 403.

receptors (e.g. prolactin on milk-producing cells), on 'non-endocrine' tissues to release secondary 'hormones' (e.g. growth hormone, GH, on the liver to release somatomedin), or on other endocrine glands (e.g. thyroid-stimulating hormone, TSH, on the thyroid). The hormones secreted by target glands in their turn activate receptors which usually elicit the cellular response through a mechanism involving a second messenger, in many cases cyclic adenosine monophosphate (cAMP).

The 'adrenergic' effects of thyroid hormones are a result of interaction at this sort of level, and it is likely that local factors such as prostaglandins also act here. Within the pancreatic islet the various cell types and their products, including insulin, glucagon and somatostatin, operate and interact as a functional metabolic unit.

The nervous and endocrine systems share evolutionary origins in primitive chemical mediators, and even in humans the borderline between the two systems is often blurred. The 'posterior pituitary' hormones oxytocin and vasopressin (antidiuretic hormone, ADH, page 551) are synthesized in the hypothalamus and secreted down axons of the nerve fibres, to be released in the posterior lobe. Adrenaline at the nerve endings is a neurotransmitter; adrenaline released from the adrenal medulla is a hormone. Hormones of the gut and pancreas, responsive particularly to stimuli from the gut and to levels of various substrates in the blood, are strongly influenced by autonomic nervous signals and themselves influence the gastrointestinal response to the vagus nerve.

# Clinical problems

## THYROID DISORDERS

## Goitre

A goitre is an enlarged thyroid gland. If it occurs in the absence of thyrotoxicosis it is a **non-toxic goitre**. The term **simple goitre** is used for the diffuse non-toxic goitre that is not uncommon in adolescent girls; it usually resolves spontaneously. In the context of thyroid disease the word toxic means thyrotoxic, in other words a thyroid condition accompanied by the disorder of function known as thyrotoxicosis. This is defined and discussed in more detail below.

Iodine deficiency is a potent cause of non-toxic goitre, and goitre is or was endemic in certain areas where the levels of iodine in the drinking water are low or the iodine is diverted from the thyroid gland by pollutants, fluorine or other factors. Endemic goitre has been eliminated in many areas by iodination of table salt. For reasons unknown, endemic goitre is much more frequent in women than men. The incorporation of iodine into thyroid hormone may also be blocked by antithyroid drugs, phenylbutazone, sulphonylureas (which are therefore goitrogens), or by congenital deficiencies of the enzymes involved in thyroid hormone synthesis resulting in so-called goitrous cretinism; this presents in childhood and may lead to permanent intellectual and neurological damage.

## Thyrotoxicosis

This is the clinical state associated with raised circulating levels of free tri-iodothyronine (FT3) and usually thyroxine (FT4). The metabolic rate is increased, and the patient's resting state may mirror that of an athlete after a run – hot, flushed, sweaty, with a fast pulse. In adults it is due to one of two disorders: either Graves' disease, which would classically be accompanied by a diffuse toxic goitre; or toxic nodular goitre (Table 19.2 and Fig. 19.2).

## CLINICAL FEATURES OF THYROTOXIC STATES

A staring appearance results as eyelid retraction widens the palpebral fissure. When the patient looks up and then down a rim of white sclera appears between the iris and upper lid during the downward movement (so-called 'lid-lag').

In terms of behaviour there is nervousness and irritability, an inability to relax or stay still and visible hyperkinesia, with shaking and fine tremor. Rarely a psychotic state may develop. Conversely, in some older persons, there is apathy and depression.

There is hypermetabolism with weight loss but increased appetite, warm, moist skin (with or without fever) and diminished tolerance of warm temperatures.

There is general weakness and fatigue of the muscles with weakness and sometimes myopathy, especially of proximal muscles. Dyspnoea on exertion is partly related to respiratory muscle weakness.

Diarrhoea (increased frequency and/or looseness) is common, but nausea and vomiting occur rarely.

There are palpitations, tachycardia persisting during sleep or occurring in paroxysms, atrial fibrillation, angina and high-output state with flow murmurs, bounding pulse, and sometimes heart failure.

Increased rates of bone turnover may result in

**Table 19.2** Features of thyrotoxicosis.

| Features specific to Graves' disease | Common features, related directly to high thyroine and T3 levels | Features specific to autonomous nodules |
|---|---|---|
| Goitre *diffuse* classically (but see text) | Stare and lid-lag<br>Nervousness, or apathy | Goitre *nodular* classically (but see text) |
| Graves' eye signs: exophthalmos may be severe, with external ophthalmoplegia, diplopia, stretch of optic nerve with loss of visual acuity, pain, i.e. malignant exophthalmos | Hyperkinesia<br>Fine tremor<br>Psychosis (rare)<br>Weight loss, or<br>Weight gain (rare)<br>Appetite increase<br>Heat intolerance<br>Fatigue and weakness | Relatively more common in the elderly |
| Rarely: thyroid acropachy and pretibial myxoedema | Proximal myopathy<br>Dyspnoea on exertion<br>Diarrhoea | |
| Autoimmune associations with: insulin-dependent diabetes mellitus, myasthenia gravis, etc. | Tachycardia at rest<br>Palpitations<br>Atrial fibrillation<br>High cardiac output<br>Angina if prone<br>Heart failure<br>Osteoporosis<br>Periodic paralysis | |

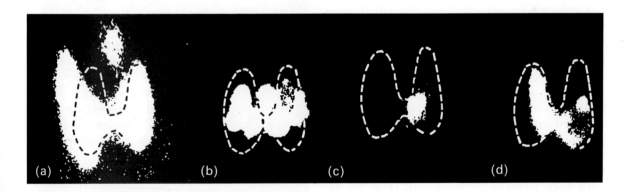

(a)          (b)          (c)          (d)

**Figure 19.2** Typical thyroid isotope scans. The dashed line indicates the outline of a 'normal' thyroid gland, which is of course variable. (a) Graves' disease, diffuse toxic goitre with obviously active left pyramidal lobe. (b) Multi-nodular toxic goitre, with several adenomata (nodules). (c) Autonomous toxic nodule in left lobe, suppressing the remainder of the gland (d) 'Cold nodule' – the white area of low uptake within the left lobe. As 10 per cent are malignant lesions, surgery is indicated unless an ultrasound scan suggests that it is cystic and/or needle aspiration cytology confirms its benign nature.

net resorption of bone, so osteoporosis or hypercalcaemia can occur.

## GRAVES' DISEASE

In this condition the **goitre is usually diffuse** and there are changes outside the thyroid gland which are *not* a direct consequence of elevated levels of T3 and T4, as if some unknown factor was acting both on the thyroid and on those other tissues. Many years ago it was shown that pituitary TSH was not the factor, and indeed the concentrations of TSH are suppressed to low or undetectable levels in all forms of thyrotoxicosis. The factor is an IgG immunoglobulin, or a group of such immunoglobulins. The plasma of most patients with Graves' disease contains immunoglobulins which bind specifically to thyroid membranes, can be displaced by TSH, and activate adenylate cyclase in thyroid preparations (human thyroid stimulator, HTS; thyroid-stimulating immunoglobulin, TSI). The gland is often infiltrated by activated lymphocytes. There is an association with autoimmune conditions such as myasthenia gravis and pernicious anaemia.

The disorder particularly affects women aged between 20 and 40, but the age range is wide and men are sometimes affected. In one-third of patients it remits spontaneously within 1 or 2 years.

The thyroid is diffusely enlarged (Fig. 19.2), but if the condition occurs in a previously lumpy gland (with previous non-toxic nodules) then one may find what is clinically a **toxic nodular goitre**. It is important to distinguish this descriptive term, literally 'a clinically nodular goitre in a thyrotoxic patient', from the aetiologically distinct disorder described below.

A systolic bruit is sometimes audible over the gland.

**Exophthalmos** (protrusion of the eyeball) may aggravate the staring appearance associated with both forms of thyrotoxicosis (Fig. 19.3). There is inflammation of the tissue in the orbit with a lymphocytic infiltrate. An antibody directed against retro-orbital tissue is thought to be responsible. Infiltration of the extraocular muscles may occur, with consequent diplopia and/or paralysis of upward gaze. In severe cases, conjunctival irritation, chemosis (inflammation of the eyelids) and even corneal ulceration may occur. Malignant exophthalmos is the progression of these changes to a condition of raised intraocular pressure, with pain, fall in visual acuity and a risk of permanent damage to the optic nerve. Guanethidine eye drops and systemic steroids at high doses may reduce the intraocular pressure; but if sight is seriously threatened then surgical decompression may be necessary.

In ophthalmic Graves' disease the eye changes occur in the absence of thyrotoxicosis, levels of FT4 and FT3 being normal. About half of these patients progress eventually to thyrotoxicosis.

**Pretibial myxoedema** (mucopolysaccharide infiltration under the skin of the shin) and **thyroid acropachy** (a form of finger clubbing which is secondary to periosteal new bone formation and soft tissue thickening) are rare but pathognomonic signs of Graves' disease (Fig. 19.4).

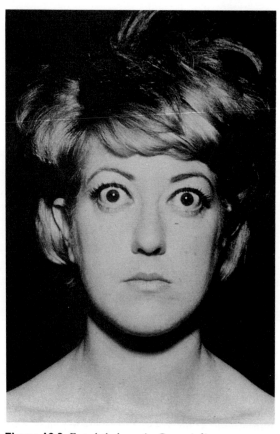

**Figure 19.3** Exophthalmos in Graves' disease.

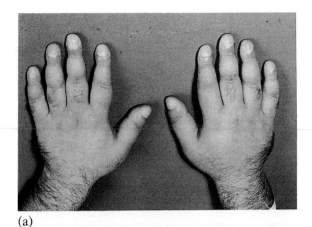

(a)

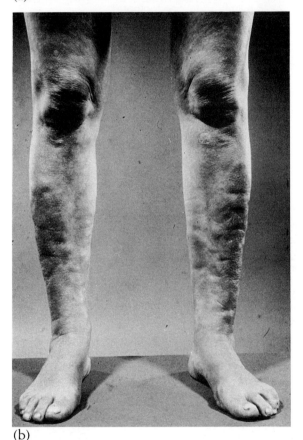

(b)

**Figure 19.4** Graves' disease. (a) Thyroid acropachy. (b) Pretibial 'myxoedema'.

be normal but not influenced by changes in circulating TSH. The patient usually presents when FT4 and FT3 are elevated, with features of thyrotoxicosis, and by this time the TSH levels are suppressed by the high thyroid hormone concentrations, with a consequent 'suppression' of the normal thyroid tissue around the adenoma (see Fig. 19.2). On palpation, such a thyroid gland may feel lumpy, one or more nodules enlarging part or parts of the gland. The nodule may be immersed in the gland and then a goitre may seem clinically 'diffuse'.

Because this form of thyrotoxicosis affects an older age group than Graves' disease, and the eye signs are less noticeable, its presentation is often more subtle. Thus many older patients present with cardiac or bowel symptoms, unexplained weight loss, or myopathy, and they may be lethargic or depressed rather than overactive and anxious (apathetic thyrotoxicosis). This form of thyrotoxicosis is often misdiagnosed as depression, idiopathic heart failure in elderly people, or malignancy.

## INVESTIGATION AND DIAGNOSIS OF THYROTOXICOSIS

Tests of thyroid function are summarized in Table 19.3. The serum FT3 (tri-iodothyronine, not the resin uptake) is a more reliable index than FT4 in diagnosing thyrotoxicosis because the FT4 is normal in some patients with thyrotoxicosis. Suppression of TSH to below its physiological level is the most sensitive indicator of excessive or autonomous thyroid activity. The structure and tissue diagnosis can be further explored by technetium and ultrasound scanning and (rarely in toxic patients) needle aspiration biopsy. A thyroid scan will show a single 'hot' nodule with the rest of the gland suppressed in a toxic nodule. In Graves' disease the whole gland will be enlarged and active (Fig. 19.2).

## TOXIC NODULAR GOITRE

A disorder which is essentially 'local' in origin, the toxic nodule is an actively secreting thyroid adenoma which has become autonomous, i.e. independent of control by the pituitary. Early in its development the levels of FT4 and FT3 will

## TREATMENT OF THYROTOXICOSIS

Graves' disease may remit spontaneously, and since surgical or radio-iodine therapy which restores normal thyroid function is accompanied by the later emergence of hypothyroidism in 2–3 per cent of patients per year of follow-up, a

**Table 19.3** Thyroid function tests.*

| Abbreviation | What does it measure? | Typical normal range (varies with laboratory) | Comment |
|---|---|---|---|
| FT4 | Free unbound T4 | 10–25 pmol/l | Low in hypothyroidism (FT3 occasionally normal) |
| FT3 | Free unbound T3 | 3–9 pmol/l | High in thyrotoxicosis (FT4 occasionally normal) |
| T4 or TT4 | Total T4 including bound T4 | 70–170 nmol/l | Increased by increased TBG† |
| T3 or TT3 | Total triiodothyronine | 1.2–3.0 nmol/l | Increased by increased TBG† |
| TBG | Thyroid-binding globulin | 12–28 μg/ml | See footnote† |
| TSH | Hypothalamic–pituitary function, or the degree of suppression by T4 and T3 secreted autonomously | 0.15–5.0 mU/l | Low in pituitary failure; high in primary hypothyroidism; response to TRH 200 μg increased in primary hypothyroidism, suppressed in thyrotoxicosis, diminished in hypopituitarism |
| Scan ($^{99}Tc^m$ or $^{131}I$) | Degree and localization of trapping of Iodine | See Fig. 19.2 | The pattern of uptake may indicate the likely nature of a thyrotoxic state, Graves' disease or adenomata. Viral or inflammatory thyroiditis may block uptake completely. Retrosternal extension of the gland may be seen |

*Tests appropriate only in very special circumstances or now superseded by improved methods are omitted from this list.
†*Binding of thyroid hormones to plasma proteins:* Both thyroxine (T4) and tri-iodothyronine (T3) are largely in bound form in the plasma, the main carrier proteins being albumen and the specific thyroid-binding globulin (TBG). The concentrations of T4 and T3 are therefore increased when the TBG level is increased (as during pregnancy and treatment with oestrogens), and decreased when TBG is decreased. The physiologically important levels are those of the *free* unbound hormones (FT4, FT3).

*Drug interference with test results:* By displacement of T4 and T3 from TBG, salicylates and other non-steroidal anti-inflammatory drugs may lower total T4 and T3 while free levels – and the thyroid-stimulating hormone (TSH) – remain normal. Phenytoin may also have this effect, but additionally shares with phenobarbitone a hepatic enzyme induction which increases the rate of clearance of T4; the TSH may rise slightly and those with limited thyroid reserve may be made hypothyroid. Amiodarone and lithium may cause hypothyroidism through other mechanisms.
TRH = thyrotrophin-releasing hormone.

trial of drug therapy is indicated. In contrast, the toxic 'hot nodule' will not remit spontaneously and so merits definitive treatment as soon as convenient. Having temporarily suppressed any iodine uptake by the normal thyroid tissue, a hot nodule will take up virtually the whole of a dose of therapeutic radio-iodine, leaving the normal thyroid to resume normal function. But these comments and the following are in the nature of general guidance, the actual choice of treatment being tailored to the clinical state, age and circumstances of each patient.

## Surgery (thyroidectomy)

This is appropriate in the following situations:

- Significant possibility of carcinoma
- Very large goitres

- Pressure symptoms whatever the apparent size of the goitre (e.g. deviation or compression of the trachea, or dysphagia). This is particularly likely when the goitre extends down behind the trachea (**retrosternal goitre**)
- Alternative methods of treatment refused, impossible (e.g. allergies to antithyroid drugs, or radio-iodine contraindicated) or failed

Patients must be rendered euthyroid by carbimazole and iodine aqueous solution (Lugol's iodine) before operation, and the use of propranolol considered.

## Radio-iodine

This is the standard method of definitive therapy, either at the time of diagnosis or after an appropriate trial of antithyroid drugs. The full effect of the radiation will not be seen for several months, during which time antithyroid drugs should be prescribed. It is contraindicated only in patients who are, or may be, pregnant or breast feeding. There are some who argue against the use of radio-iodine in fertile subjects, but the radiation dose to the gonads is less than that associated with a barium enema or intravenous urogram, and follow-up studies have shown no increase in congenital abnormalities in the offspring of those so treated.

## Antithyroid drugs

The drugs in common use are carbimazole (40 mg daily, reducing to 5–15 mg daily) and propylthiouracil (100 mg four times a day, reducing to 50 mg daily). Carbimazole is the less toxic but even so causes rashes in 3 per cent, neutropenia in 1–2 per cent and agranulocytosis in about 0.5 per cent of cases. Patients should be asked to report at once any sore throats, malaise or abnormal lymphadenopathy. Several weeks will elapse before the clinical improvement is complete. At the end of 1 or 2 years of treatment of Graves' thyrotoxicosis the drug may be discontinued and the TSH measured. If this is normal then remission has probably occurred and no further treatment is necessary, but prolonged annual follow-up is advisable.

## Propranolol

This acts peripherally through its β-sympathetic antagonism to relieve those toxic symptoms due to sympathetic overactivity. Although the levels of T3 are slightly diminished, the blocking effect is largely independent of thyroid hormone concentrations. It may be of special value in three situations:

1. For rapid control of cardiac effects of T4 and T3
2. For symptomatic relief while investigations proceed
3. For rapid preparation of the thyrotoxic patient and the thyrotoxic gland for thyroidectomy, as a fast-acting supplement to iodine aqueous solution and carbimazole.

## Thyroxine

At a dose of 0.1–0.2 mg daily this is sometimes prescribed during or after antithyroid treatments to protect the patient from iatrogenic hypothyroidism. It will always be required where an ablative dose of radio-iodine is employed as standard therapy for Graves' disease.

## THYROTOXICOSIS IN PREGNANCY

Treatment of thyrotoxicosis in pregnancy is best managed with carbimazole, using the minimum dose which will keep FT4 and FT3 just inside the normal range (Table 19.3). The baby may be born with maternal thyroid stimulator (a thyroid-stimulating immunoglobulin) in the circulation, causing neonatal thyrotoxicosis. This needs immediate and careful control by those with special experience, so delivery should be arranged in an appropriate centre. As carbimazole is excreted in breast milk, the baby must not be breast fed.

## THYROID CRISIS

Also known as thyroid 'storm', this consists of an acute exacerbation of thyrotoxicity, with especially marked hyperpyrexia and tachycardia. It can occur after thyroid surgery (or occasionally radio-iodine therapy) but is rare since patients have been rendered scrupulously euthyroid before surgery. Treatment may include physical cooling (*not* aspirin which may unbind even more T3 and T4), iodine aqueous solution, carbimazole, propranolol and hydrocortisone.

# Thyroiditis

## AUTOIMMUNE THYROIDITIS (HASHIMOTO'S DISEASE)

A diffuse firm goitre develops, usually insidiously but sometimes in a subacute manner with pain and tenderness, characteristically in a middle-aged woman. Lymphocytic infiltration of the gland and auto-antibodies to thyroglobulin and thyroid microsomes are to be expected. Early in the disease mild thyrotoxicosis may occur transiently, but 20 per cent present with, and many more progress to, overt hypothyroidism. Other autoimmune disorders may be associated with this disease and with those cases of Graves' disease and 'primary' myxoedema who exhibit thyroid auto-antibodies.

## SUBACUTE THYROIDITIS (DE QUERVAIN'S DISEASE)

Although mild cases occur, the thyroid generally becomes acutely enlarged, firm, tender and painful, in a patient who is unwell and feverish. Transient hypothyroidism may be noted. There is often a history of recent respiratory infection, and the aetiology is thought to be viral. If the symptoms are not relieved by simple anti-inflammatory analgesics, prednisolone or low-dose radiotherapy may be necessary. Rarely thyroid abscess can mimic this disorder.

## WOODY THYROIDITIS (RIEDEL'S DISEASE)

The thyroid gland becomes hard as a result of intensive and locally invasive fibrosis (analogous to retroperitoneal fibrosis). It is rare, non-metastatic and can only be treated by resection. Thyroid function may be normal or, in the advanced case, slightly diminished.

# Hypothyroidism

In the infant, thyroid deficiency produces **cretinism**, evident by slowing of growth, mental and physical retardation, a characteristic appearance and a hoarse cry. The adult form of the disease was first described by Sir William Gull in 1874; its name, **myxoedema**, derives from the mucoprotein thickening of subcutaneous tissue which is found in severe cases (Table 19.4 and Fig. 19.5).

**Table 19.4** Features of hypothyroidism.

Myxoedema (puffy features)
Skin dry, coarse, cool
Pale and/or lemon tint
Hair dry, coarse, thin
Eyebrows: loss laterally
Slowness of thought and action
Reflexes: delayed relaxation
Bradycardia
Constipation
Memory loss or dementia
Depression
Psychosis* (rare)
Weight gain (usually modest)
Appetite poor
Cold intolerance
Hoarseness of voice
Angina: part metabolic, part vascular
Menorrhagia
Hypothermia, possibly to coma
Hypertension (variable, mild)
Intermittent claudication (similarly)
Effusions: pericardial and pleural

*'Myxoedema madness'.

## CLINICAL FEATURES

There is myxoedema, a boggy non-pitting oedema, which may be diffuse but is especially noticeable around the eyes and on the hands and feet.

The skin is cool, dry and coarse in texture, pale or faintly yellow in colour (aggravated by the anaemia which is often present). The hair is also dry, coarse and thin, with particular loss of the outer third of eyebrows.

There is slowness of thought, of action, of

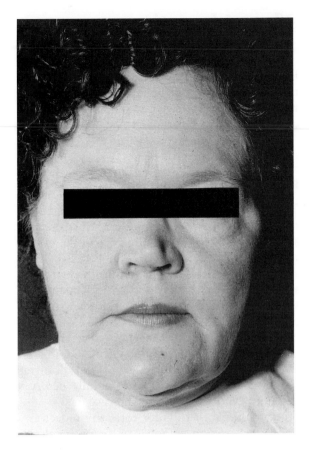

**Figure 19.5** Hypothyroidism. Note the puffy, pasty appearance and thinning of the eyebrows laterally.

speech and of relaxation of the muscle after a reflex has been elicited (particularly at the ankle). The pulse is slow and constipation may be a feature. The mental state may exhibit memory loss, dementia, depression or psychosis (so-called 'myxoedema madness').

There is hypometabolism with poor appetite yet mild weight gain and diminished tolerance of the cold. Hypothermia may occur, even to the point of coma in a severe case.

The voice may become hoarse as the vocal cords thicken.

One-third of patients show systolic hypertension until treated. Some have angina and/or palpitations, which are not always relieved by treatment of the hypothyroidism. Some are dyspnoeic on exertion and intermittent claudication has been reported. Pericardial and pleural effusions occur.

Menorrhagia is a common complaint.

## INVESTIGATION AND DIAGNOSIS

Tests of thyroid function are summarized in Table 19.3. The key finding is an elevated level of TSH. (Fortunately, TSH-secreting tumours are exceedingly rare.) Auto-antibodies to thyroid microsomal antigen and thyroglobulin occur commonly, often at high titre. Non-specific findings may include a normochromic normocytic or macrocytic anaemia, a raised plasma cholesterol, low-voltage waves on the electrocardiogram (ECG), flattening of the glucose tolerance curve and elevation of muscle enzymes.

### Primary failure of the thyroid gland

Even in those without a convincing history of Hashimoto's disease there is a high frequency of thyroid auto-antibodies, suggesting an auto-immune aetiology. Congenital defects in thyroidal enzymes, and thus thyroid hormone synthesis, do occur but they are rare and are usually discovered in early childhood in the form of goitrous cretinism. The latter accompanied by congenital deafness constitutes Pendred's syndrome.

### External factors affecting the thyroid

Previous treatment for thyrotoxicosis is the commonest such cause of hypothyroidism. Severe iodine deficiency within the thyroid, associated with trapping or blocking of iodine, is a rare cause, usually presenting with goitre.

The anti-arrhythmic drug amiodarone lowers FT3 and FT4 levels by interference in thyroid hormone metabolism; rebound thyrotoxicosis may occur if the drug is stopped abruptly. Lithium and phenobarbitone may also cause hypothyroidism, while other drugs alter binding to thyroid-binding globulin (TBG) (Table 19.3).

### Secondary failure, due to low TSH levels

This usually occurs as part of a panhypopituitary state, which is discussed on page 549. Thyrotrophin-releasing hormone (TRH) is a very potent stimulus to TSH secretion and a TSH response to TRH may persist even in the presence of a pituitary lesion; the hypothyroidism in such cases is presumed to reflect a low average level of pituitary drive.

## TREATMENT

Whatever the cause of the hypothyroidism, most patients need to be treated by gradual restoration of normal thyroid hormone levels using oral thyroxine commencing with 50 μg daily increasing over 6–12 weeks to 150 μg. After several further weeks the TSH will indicate whether the dose of thyroxine is appropriate. Excessive, or even normal, levels of hormone activity may precipitate angina or left ventricular failure, especially in the old. There may then be an advantage in substituting liothyronine (T3) tablets: these are quicker to act and are more rapidly cleared than thyroxine, and hence more flexible in use. The patient must clearly understand the lifetime nature of the medication.

In external and secondary types of myxoedema the primary cause must be remedied where possible.

## MYXOEDEMA COMA

Especially in the cold of winter, the hypothyroid condition of an elderly patient may progress to such a degree that bradycardia, shallow breathing, hypoxia, carbon dioxide retention, hypoglycaemia, hyponatraemia and hypothermia all contribute to a lapse into coma (see hypothermia, page 834). The patient is cold to the touch, with depression of central and peripheral body temperatures, *often below the range of the standard clinical thermometer*, so that the severity of the problem is not recognized. Mortality is high and care must be intensive but not hasty – vigorous rewarming must be avoided, the gentle action of warm blankets being safer. Rapid-acting rapidly metabolized liothyronine (20 μg 8-hourly) and hydrocortisone (100 mg 8-hourly) should be administered intravenously, and the ECG and body functions, including the central venous pressure (CVP) closely monitored. As for any patient in coma and in shock, or on the brink of it, the airway, oxygenation and circulation must be maintained by appropriate means.

# Thyroid carcinomas

Papillary, follicular and anaplastic tumours arise in the follicular epithelium of the thyroid, whereas the medullary carcinoma has a quite distinct origin in the parafollicular or C-cells (Table 19.5).

## PAPILLARY CARCINOMA

This tumour is the most common thyroid malignancy, occurring in the second and third decades and in later life. The solitary nodule in the thyroid gland may be unobtrusive and asymptomatic, and the first clinical sign may be an enlargement of the local nymph nodes, by which time more extensive metastasis may have occurred. These tumours usually take up iodine but much less avidly than normal thyroid, so they appear as a 'cold' nodule on a thyroid scan (see Fig. 19.2) and solid or semisolid on ultrasound examination. Any such nodule deserves excision: evidence of recent increase in size or of frank malignancy calls for total thyroidectomy and total excision of nodes or tissue involved. Some weeks later, if malignancy is confirmed, a large ablative dose of radio-iodine is administered, and a whole-body iodine scan is carried out. Tumour tissue (in the absence of the thyroid gland) now takes up the radio-iodine, both displaying the extent of any local or distant metastases and receiving treatment by irradiation. Because the tumours are TSH-responsive in their rate of growth, thyroxine is administered from this point onwards so as to suppress TSH secretion completely. At intervals of 3–6 months, the ablative and diagnostic radio-iodine scan is repeated after a brief pause in the thyroxine suppression to allow TSH levels to rise and stimulate iodine uptake by any surviving thyroid tissue. Apart from these pauses, thyroxine should be continued for life.

## FOLLICULAR CARCINOMA

Histologically and functionally this tumour is closest to normal thyroid tissue. It tends to metastasize through the bloodstream earlier than the papillary form, so it may be first

**Table 19.5** Characteristics of thyroid cancers.

| Type | Relative incidence (%) | ♀:♂ | Typical origin | Typical spread | Typical uptake | Typical series survival (%) at | |
|------|----|----|----|----|----|----|----|
| | | | | | | 5 years | 20 years |
| Papillary | 60 | 2:1 | Multifocal | Lymph nodes (bone, lung) | $^{131}I ++$ | 95 | 85 |
| Follicular | 30 | 3:1 | Solitary lesion | Venous | | 80 | 70 |
| Well differentiated | (15) | | | (Unusual) | $(^{131}I +++)$ | (90) | (80) |
| Poorly differentiated | (15) | | | (Bone, lung) | $(^{131}I +)$ | (70) | (60) |
| Anaplastic | 5 | 1:1 | Unifocal but very invasive | Locally invasive and lung | — | 10 | 2 |
| Medullary | 5 | 1:1 | Diffuse (±MENIIb) | Local (and bone) | DMSA, MIBG (secretes calcitonin) | 80 | 50 |

Note: Lymphomas also occur, accounting for less than 5% of primary thyroid neoplasms.
MEN = multiple endocrine neoplasia. DMSA = dimercaptosuccinic acid.
MIBG = metaiodobenzyl guanidine.

identified through its distant metastases or by the finding of a stony hard nodule, which becomes subsequently locally invasive. The uptake of iodine may be similar to that of the thyroid gland, or even excessive, with the production of thyrotoxicosis. Management is along the lines of that for papillary carcinoma.

## ANAPLASTIC CARCINOMA

The rapid painful enlargement of a 'cold' nodule may indicate the presence of this highly malignant form, which is fortunately less common than the related papillary and follicular carcinomas. Anaplastic tumours rarely concentrate radio-iodine so, following surgery, consideration should be given to external radiotherapy. If there should be a recurrence, cytotoxic therapy may be useful.

## MEDULLARY CARCINOMA

This C-cell tumour, which accounts for between 5 and 10 per cent of all thyroid carcinomas, secretes calcitonin. Even so, it usually presents clinically as a malignant tumour of the thyroid, often with regional lymph node involvement, sometimes with early extensive blood-borne metastases. The tumour carries a worse prognosis than papillary or follicular carcinomas, even if local thyroidectomy, neck dissection and radiotherapy are instituted promptly. High calcitonin levels, basal or stimulated by alcohol, are useful as a 'marker' for the tumour. Furthermore, like many tissues thought to be of neural crest origin, these tumours may demonstrate avid uptake of metaiodobenzylguanidine (MIBG), the basis of an isotope scan.

Medullary carcinoma may occur sporadically but it tends to be familial, with an autosomal dominant pattern. In the familial cases there is a particular association with **multiple endocrine adenomatosis (MEA) syndromes** (page 553), both MEA type II-A (with phaeochromocytoma and hyperparathyroidism) and MEA type II-B (with phaeochromocytoma and mucosal neuromas). Relatives of an affected patient should therefore be screened for raised calcitonin levels; if such an elevation is found and confirmed, total thyroidectomy is appropriate before the cancer becomes clinically overt.

# ADRENAL DISORDERS

# Cushing's syndrome

The term refers to the clinical state induced by prolonged elevation of cortisol levels, whatever its aetiology. The *disease* that Harvey Cushing described was that in which pituitary adenomas, usually small and basophilic, induced and driven by excessive hypothalamic corticotrophin-releasing hormone (CRH), overproduce the adrenocorticotropic hormone (ACTH) (Table 19.6).

**Table 19.6** Causes of Cushing's syndrome (excluding iatrogenic causes).

| | |
|---|---|
| 80% | ACTH-dependent,* of which 80% are pituitary in origin 20% are ectopic (or uncertain) |
| 20% | ACTH-independent of which 80% are adrenal adenomas 20% are adrenal carcinomas |

*Inducing bilateral adrenal hyperplasia.
ACTH = adrenocorticotropic hormone.

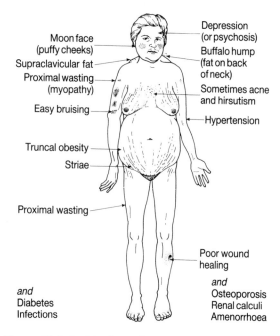

**Figure 19.6** Cushing's syndrome.

## CLINICAL FEATURES OF CUSHING'S SYNDROME

### Those related to the effects of cortisol

Many of the clinical features reflect impaired protein synthesis or redistribution of fat. The face is typically plethoric and mooned as the skin gets thinner and adipose tissue rounds out the chin and cheeks. The supraclavicular notch may be filled, and posteriorly fat in the upper thoracic/lower cervical area produces the 'buffalo hump'. Obesity especially affects the trunk (Fig. 19.6).

As muscle wasting occurs the thin legs and arms contribute to the 'lemon-on-sticks' shape, and the patient suffers from fatigue and weakness, sometimes severe (steroid myopathy). These signs, and the pathological bruising, are those with the most discriminatory power in the differential diagnosis.

Purpura or easy bruising is common and

important. The blood pressure may be moderately raised. Polycythaemia may be a feature.

Depression or psychoses related to the condition are relieved as steroid levels return to normal.

Osteoporosis leads to compression fractures of the vertebrae and thus spinal curvature, and pathological fractures of the ribs. Renal stones commonly occur.

Glucose tolerance is often impaired. The mineralocorticoid effects of cortisol and related compounds may result in a low serum potassium with alkalosis, but this is prominent only when very high levels of cortisol are circulating, and so more common in cases of ectopic ACTH production.

### Androgenic effects (especially if an adrenal tumour is present)

In men there may be impotence, increasing baldness, and acne; in women, hirsutism (increased body and beard hair), recession of hair at the temples, menstrual irregularities or amenorrhoea, enlarged clitoris, and an increase in musculature.

## Other effects

Most often the pituitary tumour is a rather small basophil adenoma, which will produce no local signs.

Signs related to an adrenal tumour are unusual but an adenocarcinoma may metastasize. Eighty per cent of tumours are benign adenomas, 20 per cent are carcinomas.

Some 20 per cent of cases of adrenal hyperplasia are caused by secretion of ACTH by a tumour outside the pituitary (ectopic tumour). Typically the ACTH level and therefore the adrenal output of cortisol is very high in such cases, the result being a severe Cushing's syndrome with hypokalaemic alkalosis and pigmentation. Oat-cell carcinoma of the bronchus, carcinoid, thymic and pancreatic islet cell tumours are especially associated with this picture. Anaemia rather than polycythaemia may then occur. However, some are virtually undistinguishable from pituitary cases.

## INVESTIGATION AND DIAGNOSIS

Non-specific findings may include polycythaemia, a neutrophilia between 10 000 and 20 000, depressed lymphocyte and eosinophil counts, mild glucose intolerance with or without a raised fasting blood glucose, and hypokalaemic alkalosis.

This is one of several endocrine disorders in which the diagnostic process divides into two quite separate phases: first, 'Is the hormonal function normal (physiological) or abnormal (autonomous)?' – a *biochemical* question; second, 'Once an abnormality of function is proven, what is the source of abnormality?' – a *pathological* and *anatomical* question. A basic scheme for the investigation of Cushing's syndrome is shown in Fig. 19.7, the normal ranges for function tests are listed in Table 19.7 and specific tests are discussed below.

## Plasma cortisol

This is often the most convenient measurement, and a low or low normal level virtually excludes

**Table 19.7** Adrenal function tests (normal ranges vary slightly between laboratories).

| Test | Healthy, non-stressed | Cushing's syndrome | Addison's disease |
|---|---|---|---|
| **Plasma cortisol (nmol/l)** | | | |
| Diurnal levels: 09.00 h | 150–700 | >400 | <150 |
| 24.00 h | 80–220 | >400 | n/a |
| Dexamethasone-suppressed (see text for details) | <50 | >150 | n/a |
| Tetracosactrin-stimulated: 0 min | 150–700 | >400 | <150 |
| 30 min | 700–1050 | 800–2000 | <400 |
| 60 min | 700–1050 | 800–2000 | <400 |
| CRH-stimulated (see text) | Rise | See text | n/a |
| **Plasma ACTH (ng/l)** | | | |
| Diurnal levels: 09.00 h | 10–80 | High or low | >100 |
| 24.00 h | <10 | | n/a |

| **Urinary corticosteroid excretion in 24 hours (adults)** | Normal male | Normal female |
|---|---|---|
| Urinary free cortisol (nmol) | 130–160 | 130–160 |
| *Dexamethasone-suppressed* | <100 | <100 |
| Urinary pregnanetriol (μmol) | 1–3 | 1–3 |
| 17-Hydroxy corticoids (μmol)* | 11–45 | 11–30 |
| 17-Oxogenic corticoid (μmol)* | 15–60 | 11–48 |
| 17-Oxosteroids (μmol)* | 18–64 | 11–51 |

*Now rarely measured in UK.
CRH = corticotrophin-releasing hormone. ACTH = adrenocorticotrophic hormone. n/a = not appropriate.

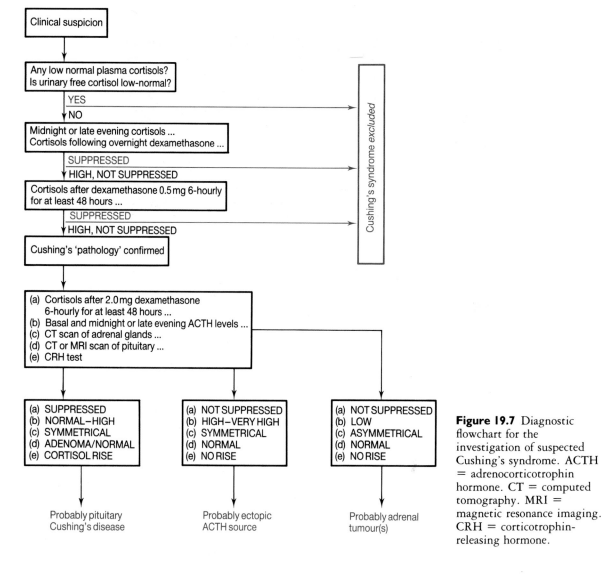

**Figure 19.7** Diagnostic flowchart for the investigation of suspected Cushing's syndrome. ACTH = adrenocorticotrophin hormone. CT = computed tomography. MRI = magnetic resonance imaging. CRH = corticotrophin-releasing hormone.

Cushing's syndrome. The levels may be misleadingly high in the anxious or obese subject, or in patients with high levels of the carrier protein transcortin in the blood such as those who are on 'the pill' or pregnant. A useful screening test for outpatients requires blood samples at 9.00 a.m. and 6.00 p.m. on the first day followed by dexamethasone (2 mg) taken by mouth at 11.00 p.m. on the first day. The cortisol level is repeated at 9 a.m. on the second day. In Cushing's syndrome and in some stressed patients the normal diurnal variation is lost and the second 9.00 a.m. cortisol is *not* suppressed to less than 50 mmol/l as it should be in a normal subject. If the result of this study is not completely normal then further investigation is required.

### Urinary free cortisol

This is unaffected by transcortin concentrations and reflects the secretion rate of cortisol, provided the urine collection is accurately timed. It may be mildly elevated by illness or continued stress.

### Dexamethasone suppression tests

Cortisol production (and excretion) is suppressed in most normal or obese subjects by dexamethasone (0.5 mg 6-hourly) and in most patients with adrenal hyperplasia due to pitui-

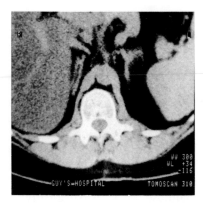
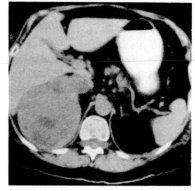
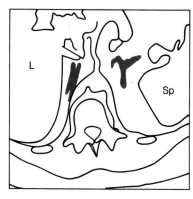
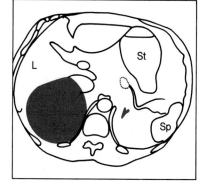

**Figure 19.8** Computed tomography of normal adrenal glands (left) and a large adrenal tumour causing Cushing's syndrome (right). On the line diagrams below each scan the adrenal tissue is shown in colour. L = liver. Sp = spleen. St = stomach.

tary ACTH by dexamethasone (2 mg 6-hourly) (but *not* by 0.5 mg 6-hourly). In most patients with adrenal tumours or an ectopic source of ACTH-like substance it cannot be suppressed even by the higher dose. However, the localization suggested by this test can be unreliable, and it is most useful in confirming the pathological nature of borderline hypercortisolism.

## Plasma ACTH levels

These are depressed in the presence of adrenal carcinoma or adenoma, and modestly elevated in Cushing's syndrome of pituitary or hypothalamic origin. Most ACTH assay systems give very high readings in most but not all cases of *ectopic* peptide production (Fig. 19.7). An injection of corticotrophin-releasing factor (CRH) will usually provoke a significant rise in ACTH

levels in disease of pituitary origin, but will rarely do so in cases of ectopic origin.

## Anatomical localization

Computed tomography (CT) of the suprarenal area will usually define the adrenal glands and/or an adrenal tumour (Fig. 19.8), while an isotope uptake adrenal scan employing radio-labelled cholesterol will show the level of activity of one or both glands and/or tumour(s). The investigation of the adrenals may occasionally be taken further by arteriography or venography. Bilateral enlargement and active function favour hyperplasia secondary to an excess of ACTH, whereas unilateral 'suppression' as reflected by atrophy and loss of function of one adrenal with marked enlargement and/or activity on the other side, suggests a primary adrenal tumour.

The search for a source of excess ACTH will require X-rays and CT scans of the pituitary gland and the chest, the latter because so many of the ectopic sources are bronchial or thymic tumours. Selective venous sampling by an experienced radiologist may suggest the source of the ACTH by the finding of an especially high concentration of ACTH in a particular vein. If the vein is draining from an area which includes a pituitary adenoma, for example, an inferior petrosal sinus, then a preceding injection of CRH will markedly enhance the difference in ACTH concentrations compared with a simultaneous sample from control veins on the other side and elsewhere in the body.

**TREATMENT**

An adrenal tumour must be removed with the whole of the affected gland and the other gland must be carefully inspected. In the case of inoperable adrenal carcinoma, the excessive steroid synthesis may be controlled by the drug $o'p'$-DDD (mitotane), which is generally too toxic to use in other situations. A non-pituitary tumour secreting ACTH is resected.

When adrenal hyperplasia is secondary to pituitary overproduction of ACTH, transphenoidal adenectomy or hypophysectomy is usually effective. Bilateral adrenalectomy followed by pituitary irradiation offers an alternative with the putative advantages of an immediate reduction in cortisol levels, the temporary maintenance of pituitary function and the positive exclusion of an adrenal tumour. Maintenance therapy with corticosteroids and other hormones will be necessary following treatment. The disadvantage is the risk of developing **Nelson's syndrome** (in which an ACTH-secreting tumour of the pituitary produces generalized pigmentation and local signs of expansion) during the period before the pituitary gland is irradiated.

If eradication of the tumour producing ACTH is not possible, or the source of the ACTH cannot be identified, drugs such as metyrapone or ketoconazole may be valuable in diminishing cortisol synthesis. This will usually relieve symptoms but androgen levels will rise, a particular problem in female patients. The long-term objective is removal of the ACTH source.

# Aldosteronism (Conn's syndrome)

In its primary form this is related to an adenoma or hyperplasia of the adrenal cortical zona glomerulosa, producing a raised level of aldosterone in plasma and urine and (to a variable degree) hypertension, metabolic alkalosis and a low serum potassium which may lead to polyuria, periodic paralysis and paraesthesias. It is a rare cause of hypertension, but is important to diagnose as it is surgically correctable. The condition is diagnosed by the finding of persisting high levels of aldosterone which cannot be suppressed by loading the patient with sodium, and *low* levels of renin which cannot be raised by sodium depletion. These tumours can be imaged by uptake of labelled cholesterol, but are often too small for a positive CT scan. Selective venous catheterization with measurements of aldosterone may be helpful. Correction of hypertension and hypokalaemia may be initiated with spironolactone, but surgical excision of tumours is advised.

Aldosterone excess secondary to *high* renin and angiotensin levels is well documented in accelerated hypertension (page 225), heart failure, cirrhosis of the liver, nephrotic syndrome, salt depletion and conditions of low blood volume.

# Adrenal insufficiency

Atrophy of the glands occurs with prolonged administration of corticosteroids in pharmacological doses. Apart from this, the presence of auto-antibodies to adrenal tissue is the most common cause of deficient corticosteroid production. Tuberculous infiltration was once common, and even now this aetiology may be betrayed by adrenal calcification and an appropriate history. Rare causes include carcinoma, various infiltrations, and haemorrhage in the gland in the course of meningococcal septicaemia (Waterhouse–Friderichsen syndrome, page 745). A new problem is the frequent occurrence of adrenalitis – viral, bacterial or candida – in acquired immune deficiency syndrome (AIDS). The circulating levels of ACTH are high in these conditions, which constitute true 'Addison's disease', but secondary adrenal insufficiency may occur with low ACTH levels in hypopituitary states (page 549). In patients with diminished adrenal reserve, rifampicin may cause insufficiency by induction of liver enzymes which increase the rate of metabolism of circulating cortisol and thus shorten its half-life.

## CLINICAL FEATURES

### Chronic insufficiency (Addison's disease)

The principal features are listed in Table 19.8. The pigmentation reflects the sustained high level of compensatory ACTH, so will not occur in insufficiency secondary to pituitary disorders. It is characteristically prominent over elbows and knuckles, in flexures and skin creases, in scar tissue, and on the gums and buccal mucosa.

The specific craving for salt is caused by an alteration in the taste threshold for salt.

### Acute insufficiency (Addisonian crisis)

This often occurs on a background of chronic deficiency, and it may therefore include any of the features listed in Table 19.8, particularly severe hypotension, fever, profound weakness, nausea, vomiting and diarrhoea, progressing if

**Table 19.8** Features of Addison's disease.

Pigmentation
Weakness, fatigue, lassitude
Decreased muscle mass
Weight loss
Anorexia
Nausea, vomiting, diarrhoea
Dehydration, hypovolaemia
Hypotension, especially postural
Dizziness and faintness, especially postural
Hypoglycaemia
Salt-craving
Abdominal aches and cramps
Hypothermia
Hair loss
Vitiligo

untreated to coma. The coma may be complicated by hypoglycaemia or hypothermia. The precipitation of the crisis in a patient with chronic insufficiency may be provoked by some major stress (e.g. an infection, an accident, an operation), or by increased salt loss (e.g. in sweat), or by raising the level of thyroid hormones without covering the inevitable rise in the rate of metabolism of cortisol.

Acute adrenal insufficiency without preceding chronic deficiency occurs in sepsis, such as the Waterhouse–Friderichsen syndrome in meningococcal septicaemia.

## INVESTIGATION AND DIAGNOSIS

During the acute illness the patient is in danger of fatal collapse, so treatment should not be delayed. In the stress of any severe acute illness *other* than adrenal insufficiency the plasma corticosteroids will be elevated (certainly >300 nmol/l) so plasma cortisols in samples of blood taken on admission will later confirm or refute the diagnosis of Addisonian crisis. The plasma ACTH, if available, indicates directly whether the condition is that of hypothalamic–pituitary failure (low ACTH) or that of primary adrenal failure (raised ACTH). The clinical clue to the level of ACTH is the degree of pigmentation, the pallor of chronic pituitary insufficiency contrasting with the 'tan' of chronic adrenal failure. It should be borne in mind, however, that increased pigmentation may also occur in chronic renal failure, hepatic cirrhosis, malabsorption, haemochromatosis, collagen disorders, folate or vitamin $B_{12}$ deficiency, acromegaly and chronic skin infestation.

If the situation is not acute, or if a loss of adrenal reserve rather than manifest insufficiency is suspected, the diagnostic tests fall into three groups.

### Baseline measurement

Plasma control or urinary free cortisol are persistently depressed in adrenal insufficiency (Table 19.7).

### Response to ACTH

This is a test of adrenal function which is independent of the hypothalamic–pituitary axis. For safety and convenience ACTH is given in the form of the synthetic analogue tetracosactrin, Synacthen. A normal response in the 'Synacthen test' indicates adequate function of adrenal cortical tissue (Table 19.7). A poor response indicates *either* adrenal gland destruction *or* a state of disuse atrophy because ACTH secretion has been chronically low (e.g. hypopituitarism, or use of oral corticosteroid drugs). If the response is poor, a 3-day course of intramuscular Synacthen-depot (2 mg daily) is followed by a second 60-min Synacthen test. A marked improvement over the result of the first test suggests that disuse atrophy was the cause of the poor response; a persistently poor response points to primary adrenal disease.

## Total response

If the adrenal gland is not primarily at fault, the response of the entire system, hypothalamus–(CRH)–pituitary–(ACTH)–adrenal–cortisol, can then be tested by inducing hypoglycaemia with soluble insulin (0.15 units/kg body weight intravenously). Hypoglycaemia should cause sharp rises in ACTH and plasma and urinary levels of cortisol. The 'Metopirone (metyrapone) test' may precipitate acute adrenal crisis as it lowers cortisol levels even lower than they already are, and this method of testing the system should be *avoided* in cortisol-deficient patients.

Aldosterone secretion is usually reduced, as well as cortisol, and a considerable loss of sodium and water with shifts across cell membranes produces a low plasma sodium and chloride, a raised blood urea and often a high potassium, in a hypovolaemic patient. Antidiuretic hormone secretion may be increased and aggravate the lowering of the plasma sodium. The blood sugar may be low.

Diagnostic procedures will include, where appropriate, a search for infective and neoplastic conditions which can destroy the adrenals. Only the autoimmune type of adrenal atrophy leaves adrenal medullary secretion intact, but it is not usually necessary to measure catecholamines.

## TREATMENT

The acute Addisonian crisis requires immediate and generous infusion of normal saline and dextrose to restore circulating volume and correct hypoglycaemia. Hydrocortisone sodium succinate (100 mg intravenously) is administered immediately and 6-hourly or as required. Infections must be vigorously treated. The patient's blood pressure and salt–fluid status must be carefully followed.

The long-term treatment should be based on oral hydrocortisone (20–40 mg daily) and fludrocortisone (0.1–0.2 mg daily) to supplement the mineralocorticoid effect. In establishing the proper maintenance dose, these factors should apply: the patient's subjective response, the supine and erect blood pressure, the absence of oedema, the plasma cortisol levels, and possibly the ACTH level. These patients are absolutely dependent on their steroid medication, which should be trebled in dose in the event of transient illness or stress and then gradually restored to normal levels. They must understand their condition and carry a card stating their situation, maintenance dose and procedure in the event of accident, and ideally wear a Medic-Alert bracelet or necklace.

# Virilization

This is the clinical state associated with excessive androgenic effect in the female. While commonly of adrenal or ovarian origin, an abnormal end-organ sensitivity to androgens may also be important in many patients. Hirsutism (increased body and facial hair) is marked, pubic hair becomes masculine in distribution, and recession of the hairline at the temples occurs. The voice becomes deep, muscles increase in size and the clitoris enlarges. In postpubertal women there is amenorrhoea, reduced fertility and shrinkage of the breasts. This picture may be associated with:

1. Adrenal tumours with or without Cushingoid clinical features
2. Congenital adrenal hyperplasia (see below)
3. Arrhenoblastoma of the ovary or hilus cell tumours (high plasma testosterone with normal urinary 17-oxosteroids) (Table 19.11)

Hirsutism with no major virilization, but often with menstrual irregularities and acne, is more common. Major causes include those of virilization and:

4. Polycystic ovaries
5. Mild androgen excess (compensated partial enzyme defects along the pathways of synthesis of cortisol or oestrogens in the adrenal gland or ovary)
6. Simple familial hirsutism (diagnosed by family history) or 'constitutional' hirsutism with no obvious cause. Certain races, families and individuals are naturally more hirsute than others, and the problem is often as much a cultural or social problem as it is hormonal.

## INVESTIGATION AND DIAGNOSIS

This is especially directed at the identification of patients with tumours. Both ACTH and the gonadotrophins stimulate the adrenal glands *and* the ovary to produce androgens, and in the absence of an obvious mass on examination (which will include a full gynaecological examination), localization of the source of the androgen can be difficult. Free testosterone is the most relevant hormone in this condition, but other specific androgens (such as androstenediol) are said to correlate highly with hirsutism, and sex hormone binding globulin (SHBG) levels are consistently low. 17-Oxosteroids tend to be especially high in adrenal disorders. Ultrasound

examination of the ovaries is usually required (Fig. 19.9) and laparoscopy will be appropriate in doubtful cases.

## TREATMENT

This is a condition in which it is particularly important to treat the patient and not just the disease. Apart from those patients in whom a tumour can be identified and removed, the long-term response to treatment is generally disappointing. Tumours should be resected. Corticosteroids (e.g. prednisolone, 5 mg, at night) and cyclical oestrogen therapy – separately or together – may be effective in reducing plasma testosterone levels. Cyproterone acetate, which blocks the effect of androgens on the androgen receptor, is used cyclically with low-dose oestrogens. Spironolactone has a similar action and may be effective when used with a combined oral contraceptive.

# Congenital adrenal hyperplasia

In these disorders (adrenogenital syndromes) there are enzyme defects along the pathway of cortisol synthesis. In the absence of a feedback system the cortisol levels would fall markedly, but plasma cortisol is protected by a very effi-

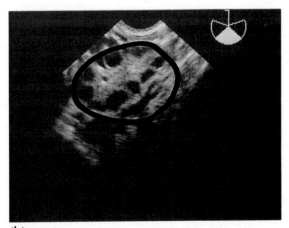

(a) (b)

**Figure 19.9** Ultrasound scans. (a) A normal ovary. (b) A polycystic ovary. (Each has been ringed in black to aid interpretation.)

cient homeostatic mechanism, and indeed this hormone is the only major restraint on the secretion of CRH and hence ACTH. The result of the enzyme deficiency is therefore an increased ACTH drive, which has the effect of increasing the concentration of cortisol precursors 'proximal' to the 'block', so restoring towards normal the concentrations of substances 'distal' to the block (including cortisol itself). Some of the common levels of 'block' are illustrated in Fig. 19.10. In every case the accumulating precursor steroids have an androgenic effect overall, and in some syndromes potent mineralocorticoids are also formed in excess. While a common feature, valuable diagnostically, is the increased concentration of 17-OH-progesterone and hence urinary pregnanetriol, the presentation depends not only on the level of the 'block' but also on severity and age at presentation.

## CLINICAL FEATURES

Typical clinical presentations include:

1. Perinatal and infantile: In the male there is phallic enlargement and the 'infant Hercules' appearance (musculature overdeveloped). In the female there is pseudohermaphroditism with genital abnormalities. In both sexes there is early fusion of epiphyses; adrenal insufficiency depends on severity of block.
2. Delayed female puberty, primary amenorrhoea.
3. C-21 hydroxylase partial block: High levels of 17-OH-progesterone etc. produce virilization and high levels of ACTH-producing pigmentation.
4. C-11 hydroxylase partial block: Features are the same as for C-21 with the addition of hypertension produced by high levels of 11-desoxycorticosterone (a potent mineralocorticoid).

## TREATMENT

Corticosteroids will abolish the excessive ACTH drive in these patients and restore normal androgen levels. If adrenal insufficiency is present this is treated as would a case of Addison's disease (page 536).

# *Phaeochromocytoma*

This very rare tumour of the adrenal medulla is important as a curable cause of hypertension, and as a 'mimic' of anxiety neurosis, thyrotox-

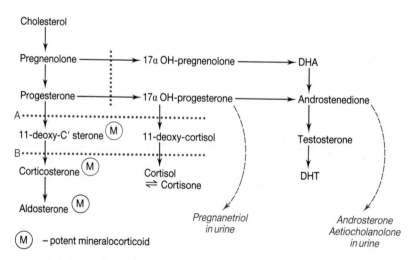

**Figure 19.10** Outline of adrenal steroid synthesis. The dotted lines indicate levels at which enzyme deficiencies may occur, acting as a block to synthesis and so causing accumulation of precursors 'above' the block. The upper horizontal dotted line (A) indicates C-21 hydroxylase level; the lower one (B) indicates C-11 hydroxylase level. The dashed lines indicate metabolites excreted in urine. DHT = dihydrotestosterone.

icosis and diabetes mellitus. About 10 per cent of the tumours are malignant and 10 per cent bilateral, and about the same proportion are associated with parathyroid adenomas or medullary carcinoma of the thyroid. The clinical features are related to the effects of excess adrenaline and/or noradrenaline. Phaeochromocytomas arise in cells of neuroectodermal origin and can be found wherever there is sympathetic tissue from the neck to the pelvis.

## CLINICAL FEATURES

Most patients are hypertensive and many complain of headaches. The hypertension is usually constant but there sometimes occurs a characteristic picture of paroxysmal hypertension, with concurrent headaches, nose bleeds or pulmonary oedema. Palpitations with or without tachycardia are common. Increased perspiration is a frequent complaint. Tremor, weakness, weight loss, feeling of warmth, even psychosis, with an increased metabolic rate, may at first suggest thyrotoxicosis. Anorexia and constipation are not uncommon. Although few patients complain of postural symptoms, the blood pressure may drop sharply on standing.

## INVESTIGATION AND DIAGNOSIS

Tests currently in use include:

1. As a screening test: vanillyl-mandelic acid (VMA, metabolite of adrenaline and noradrenaline) in urine. It is normally less than 25 μmol in 24 hours (2.4 mmol/mol creatinine excreted); it is slightly higher in patients with hypertension, renal artery stenosis, or thyrotoxicosis, or those on tricyclic or related antidepressant drugs; it is usually over 50 μmol in 24 hours (4.8 mmol/mol creatinine) in cases of phaeochromocytoma.
2. As definitive tests: adrenaline and noradrenaline in plasma and/or urine.
3. For localization (especially of second or secondary tumours): CT scans and isotope scans employing metaiodobenzylguanidine (MIBG).

Suppression and provocation tests, such as those employing phentolamine or glucagon, are potentially dangerous and rarely indicated. Levels of blood glucose, free fatty acids and the haematocrit may be elevated. Calcium and calcitonin levels should be checked to exclude parathyroid adenomas and medullary carcinoma of the thyroid.

## TREATMENT

Radiological investigations and surgery should be preceded and covered by combined adrenergic blockade, anti-α (phenoxybenzamine by mouth or phentolamine intravenously) and anti-β (propranolol to protect against a sudden surge in catecholamines). During surgery both adrenal glands must be inspected. Following resection, precipitous falls in blood pressure may occur and rapid volume repletion and vasoconstrictor therapy may be necessary to anticipate and prevent this.

# *R*EPRODUCTIVE HORMONE DISORDERS

# *Menopause (female climacteric)*

This can be regarded as physiological ovarian failure, leading to cessation of menstruation (menopause), sometimes preceded by menstrual irregularity. Episodes of 'hot flushes', with sweating and warmth, and symptoms of anxiety or depression may be prominent. Luteinizing hormone (LH) and follicle-stimulating hormone (FSH) levels are high. If symptoms are severe then a combined or sequential low-dose preparation of oestrogen and progesterone should be prescribed. Changes consequent upon the drop in oestrogen production include osteoporosis, which may become severe (page 504), a rise in the risk of cardiovascular disease, a reduction in vaginal secretions (which may lead to vaginitis and dyspareunia), and some involution of the uterus and breasts. There is a good case for long-term hormone replacement therapy (HRT) in any postmenopausal woman who exhibits significant problems of this nature.

# Delayed puberty in the female

Regular menstruation normally commences between the ages of 10 and 16, with a mean of 13 years, the so-called menarche. The other major changes of puberty include breast development and nipple pigmentation, growth of pubic hair of increasingly coarse dark curled type, axillary hair growth, thickening of the vaginal epithelium and growth of the genitalia; the pelvis gradually becomes gynaecoid in shape and the subcutaneous fat assumes the typical female distribution. Delayed puberty may be physiological and/or familial, especially in the presence of obesity. In primary ovarian failure the delay in fusion of the epiphyses eventually leads to overgrowth of the long bones, such that span exceeds height, and 'bone age' on X-ray may for a time be less than actual age.

## INVESTIGATION AND DIAGNOSIS

Any major disease, particularly thyroid disorders, diabetes, renal failure or chronic infection, may be contributary to such a delay. As discussed on page 537, the barrage of androgens secreted in congenital adrenal hyperplasia may impair female development. Beyond these possibilities, the main question is whether a primary ovarian defect or a failure of gonadotrophin secretion exists. If plasma and urinary FSH levels are low, the possible causes of hypopituitarism (page 549) are pursued. Isolated gonadotrophin deficiency may be found, usually

responsive to GnRH, suggesting that the basic problem may be GnRH failure; the line between such patients and 'late developers' is often indistinct and the initial treatment should be conservative. High levels of FSH are consistent with:

- The first hint of puberty
- Absence of ovaries, as in Turner's syndrome or testicular feminization
- Damage to the ovaries by cysts, tumours, trauma, surgery or irradiation

# Turner's syndrome (gonadal dysgenesis)

The patients are phenotypically women, but they have an XO or XO-mosaic karyotype and consequent dysgenesis of the gonads. Having neither ovaries nor testes they develop into phenotypic females (as do all mammals lacking testosterone *in utero*, whatever their genetic sex). Secondary sexual characteristics and the normal menstrual cycle do not appear spontaneously.

They usually present as short women or girls, under 5 feet tall, who have failed to undergo sexual maturation (Fig. 19.11). Numerous other clinical features occur but are variable in their expression, as might be expected from the variety of karyotypes found in the syndrome. The features may include webbing of the neck, a short neck, increased carrying angle at the elbow (cubitus valgus), widely separated nipples, shield-like chest, coarctation of the aorta (20 per cent), abnormalities of the urinary tract (on investigation, 60 per cent), recurrent otitis media and sometimes deafness, lymphoedema (especially of the feet), hypoplastic nails and numerous pigmented naevi. Mild mental handicap with well-preserved verbal ability is not uncommon.

Ethinyloestradiol (0.02 mg daily) given cyclically with norethisterone (5 mg daily) on the last 10 days of the cycle will induce menses and sexual characteristics without overrapid fusion of the epiphyses. Higher doses of oestrogen will improve the rate of sexual development but may reduce the patient's final height.

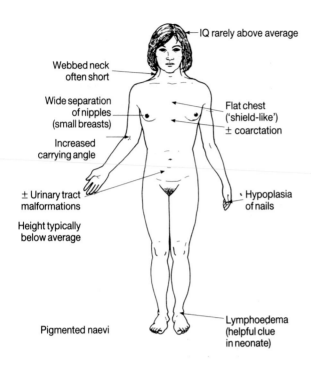

IQ rarely above average

Webbed neck
often short

Wide separation
of nipples
(small breasts)

Increased
carrying angle

± Urinary tract
malformations

Height typically
below average

Pigmented naevi

Flat chest
('shield-like')
± coarctation

Hypoplasia
of nails

Lymphoedema
(helpful clue
in neonate)

**Figure 19.11** Turner's syndrome (typically XO).

# Androgen resistance syndromes (testicular feminization)

Several syndromes exist but in the classical form most patients present as females, seeking medical advice because of primary amenorrhoea or infertility. They are genetic males with an XY karyotype whose testes may be located in the abdomen, inguinal canal or 'labia'. Breasts and external genitalia are female in development with occasional slight enlargement of the clitoris, and only on investigation does it become apparent that the vagina ends blindly and there is no uterus. Testosterone production is normal in these patients, and the condition represents a diminished response to testosterone. There is diminished conversion of testosterone to the more active dihydrotestosterone and/or a deficiency of the appropriate receptors.

# Amenorrhoea

The failure to initiate menstruation is termed by convention primary amenorrhoea and it is usually accompanied by the other deficiencies in sexual development discussed above ('delayed puberty in the female'). Mechanical factors obstructing menstrual flow may also require exclusion, and a gynaecological assessment is essential.

Secondary amenorrhoea implies the *cessation* of menstruation; the condition represents the end of a spectrum that runs from regular ovulatory menstruation, through regular menses that are often anovulatory, through irregular and/or infrequent cycles (oligomenorrhoea) that are all anovulatory, to amenorrhoea. Conditions that give rise to amenorrhoea may cause the lesser disorders in their early stages or milder forms. These various conditions are classified in Table 19.9.

# Subfertility

The availability of new modes of investigation and successful treatment, both hormonal and surgical, has transformed this subject in recent years. Nevertheless, the enthusiasm of patients and doctors should be restrained because a large proportion of couples who have failed to achieve conception after 6 months 'trying' will be sucessful without treatment within the following year or so. It is also important to confirm that 'trying' includes normal coitus of reasonable frequency, especially at the time of suspected ovulation, an assumption that proves to be untrue in a surprising number of cases.

In genuinely subfertile couples a reproductive problem of some sort will be found in 65–85 per cent of the women and about a third of the men, while in some a partial deficit is identified in both partners. The partners should be interviewed and examined independently in every instance. A cost-effective approach is then to:

1. Follow any leads given by the history or physical signs

**Table 19.9** Scheme for main causes of secondary amenorrhoea.

| | Hormone lack | Hormone block |
|---|---|---|
| | **Diminished or disordered function of hypothalamus and/or pituitary** | **Hyperprolactinaemia** (see page 548) |
| **Central** | *Specific conditions* Functional (any major physical or psychological stress) Anorexia nervosa Isolated LH, FSH deficiency Panhypopituitarism, idiopathic or secondary to: Pituitary tumour, trauma or infarct Pituitary irradiation or surgery | *Specific conditions* Tumours, including prolactinomas Drugs Hypothyroidism Renal/hepatic failure etc. |
| | *Major hormonal findings* LH, FSH (basal, and/or after GnRH): low | *Major hormonal findings* Prolactin, high LH, FSH: normal or slightly low |
| **Peripheral** | **Diminished function of ovaries** | **Excess of androgens or thyroid hormones** (see page 536) |
| | *Specific conditions* Mild forms of ovarian dysgenesis or testicular feminization (see text) Premature menopause (autoimmune?) Mumps oophoritis Ovarian irradiation or surgery | *Specific conditions* Adrenal tumours Congenital adrenal hyperplasia Arrhenoblastoma of ovary Polycystic ovaries Thyrotoxicosis |
| | *Major hormonal findings* Oestrogens: low LH, FSH: high | |

LH = luteinizing hormone. FSH = follicle-stimulating hormone. GnRH = gonadotrophin-releasing hormone.

2. Check the sperm count on semen analysis
3. Establish the presence or absence or ovulation

If a normal sperm count is confirmed and regular ovulation is occurring, further investigation should take place to look for tubal blockage by hysterosalpingography, pelvic disease by laparoscopy, ovarian status by biopsy and mucus hostility to the sperm by study of postcoital cervical mucus.

## FEMALE SUBFERTILITY

The occurrence of ovulation may be suggested by a history of transient mid-cycle ovarian pain, by a modest elevation of the basal body temperature during the luteal phase, by characteristic changes in the vaginal lining (hence 'serial smears') and the cervical mucus, or by more direct evidence of the hormonal changes illustrated in Fig. 19.12, such as a mid-luteal plasma progesterone exceeding 30 nmol/l. The absence of ovulation, or amenorrhoea, may be secondary to any of a large number of conditions which have been listed under the heading of secondary amenorrhoea (Table 19.9). Prolactin is particularly important in subfertility, because even moderate elevation of prolactin may prevent ovulation or proper luteinization of the follicle.

Hyperprolactinaemia is corrected by removal of the cause, or use of bromocriptine, as discussed on page 548. Specific treatments of the other conditions listed are discussed in the relevant parts of the text. Ovulation may be provoked

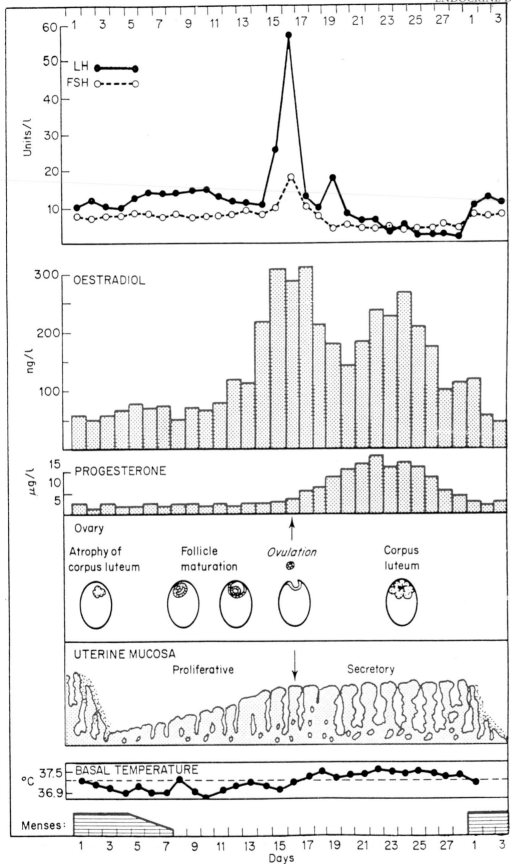

**Figure 19.12** Hormonal patterns during a normal menstrual cycle.

in some cases by the use of clomiphene, which blocks the oestrogen receptors of the hypothalamus, and induced in most cases by the programmed administration of gonadotrophins or synthetic GnRH.

Causes of female subfertility in the presence of ovulation include genital tract abnormalities such as blockage of the Fallopian tubes secondary to past or present infection, disease of the endometrium preventing implantation, and abnormalities of the cervical mucus or the sperm which impair penetration. Some of these are now treatable by specialist techniques which bypass the problem, for example, *in vitro* fertilization (IVF) or gamete intra-Fallopian transfer (GIFT).

## MALE SUBFERTILITY

Although sperm counts as low as 10 million/ml have been associated with fertility, the normal range for fresh semen lies between 50 and 150 million/ml in at least 2 ml, of which at least 60 per cent of sperm are motile and normal in morphology. A low count (oligospermia) or total absence of motile sperm (azoospermia) may rarely be accompanied by impotence and signs of feminization, such as gynaecomastia and small soft testes, suggesting androgen deficiency or oestrogen excess. Usually the problem is confined to the germinal cells of the testis, and levels of testosterone and the oestrogens are within normal limits: a raised level of FSH is then a useful indicator of germinal cell failure or aplasia. Sometimes the process of spermatogenesis is normal but the delivery of sperm is obstructed by a lesion of the vas deferens, and this possibility needs consideration if the FSH level proves to be normal despite the occurence of azoospermia. The more common specific causes to be considered are:

1. With gynaecomastia: Klinefelter's syndrome (Fig. 19.13, described on page 545); testes damaged by trauma, surgery or irradiation or drugs; chronic liver disease (page 403), androgen resistance syndromes (page 541).
2. With germinal cell failure or aplasia: idiopathic ('Sertoli cell only syndrome'); cryptorchidism (undescended testes); maturation arrest; mumps orchitis; cytotoxic

drugs; varicocele; any chronic endocrine or debilitating disease.
3. With hypothalamic/pituitary deficiency: hypogonadotrophic hypogonadism, either selectively (such as in Kallmann's syndrome, see below) or as one feature of panhypopituitarism.

Unless a particular hormonal deficiency can be identified and corrected, or a disorder such as obstruction of the vas or a varicocele corrected surgically, treatment has little to offer. Traditional advice includes maintenance of a cool scrotal environment, hence loose underwear and cold douches, and intermittent androgen therapy (such as mesterolone). Recent work supports the use of clomiphene for patients with the less severe degrees of oligospermia. The fertile effectiveness of a semen in which the sperm count is borderline can be enhanced by the use of artificial insemination (AI), a fresh sample of the husband's semen being applied direct to or through the os of the uterine cervix (AIH). More effective, but more complex, is the use of *in vitro* fertilization techniques with direct transfer of the fertilized ovum.

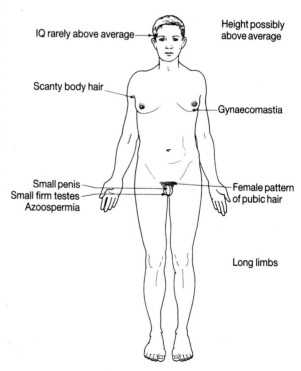

**Figure 19.13** Klinefelter's syndrome (typically XXY).

# Delayed puberty in the male

In normal boys the earliest changes include enlargement of the testes and growth of coarse hairs in the pubic region. The scrotum develops rugal folds and darkens, the penis enlarges, axillary and then facial hair appears and the voice deepens. A mild degree of gynaecomastia is not uncommon. When the patient or his parents complain of 'delay' a family history of late puberty may be reassuring. In true gonadal failure the 'bone age' by X-ray falls behind actual age and, in the absence of the epiphyseal fusion, the eunuchoid physique emerges with span exceeding height and ground to pubis exceeding pubis to crown.

## INVESTIGATION AND DIAGNOSIS

Any endocrine disorder or debilitating illness may delay puberty. When those are excluded, the diagnosis lies between a primary gonadal disease, with high levels of FSH and LH, and a hypothalamic–pituitary disorder, with low levels of gonadotrophins and bilaterally small soft testes (see hypopituitarism, page 549). An isolated deficiency of the hypothalamic factor GnRH occurs in **Kallmann's syndrome**. Anosmia may be an associated feature.

The only cause of primary testicular failure commonly to affect puberty is **Klinefelter's syndrome**, in which very small firm testes are associated with variable degrees of eunuchoidism, gynaecomastia, impairment of intelligence, azoospermia, sterility and typically an XXY karyotype (Fig. 19.13). Very rare versions of Turner's syndrome also occur in the phenotypic male.

# Tumours of the testis or ovary

Tumours of the testes are rare (Table 19.10) but occur particularly in the 20–35 age group. If the tumour is functional gonadotrophin secretion is suppressed and the other testis may be atrophied.

Most cysts and neoplasms of the ovary are non-secretory, but the tumours listed in Table 19.11 usually secrete hormones.

**Table 19.10** Tumours of the testis.

| Type | Five-year mortality | Special features |
| --- | --- | --- |
| Seminoma | 10% | FSH frequently raised |
| Teratoma | 30% | Spread by blood not lymph |
| Choriocarcinoma | 100% | Raised HCG; gynaecomastia |
| Leydig cell tumours | ± benign | Oestrogens or androgens |

FSH = follicle-stimulating hormone. HCG = chorionic gonadotropin.

**Table 19.11** Secretory tumours of the ovary.

| Androgens secreted | Oestrogens secreted |
| --- | --- |
| Arrhenoblastoma | Granulosa cell tumour |
| Hilus cell tumour | Theca cell tumour |
| | Luteoma (and → progesterone) |
| | Teratoma, chorionepithelioma (and → HCG) |

HCG = chorionic gonadotropin.

# $P$ITUITARY HYPERSECRETION

For discussions of hypersecretion of ACTH, ADH and prolactin refer to pages 530, 548 and 548, respectively.

Tumours secreting TSH or gonadotrophins are exceedingly rare.

# Growth hormone excess

The syndromes of growth hormone (GH) excess are usually related to an eosinophil adenoma of the pituitary, characteristically slow in growth and insidious in clinical presentation. Only in retrospect may it be realized that the disease has been active for 20 or more years before the patient presents.

## GIGANTISM

This results from excessive GH effect before the epiphyses are fused, producing the features of acromegaly but in addition long limbs and abnormal height. The all-time record for height was held by Robert Wadlow of Illinois, who died in 1940 at an authenticated height of 8 feet 11 inches; the better known case of Goliath is not so well documented!

## ACROMEGALY

There are many clinical features of this disorder (Fig. 19.14):

- Headache; sometimes visual field defects, especially temporal; excessive tiredness.
- Muscular aching; proximal muscle weakness.
- Excessive sweating; skin thick, sebaceous, wrinkled.
- Tingling in the fingers; carpal tunnel syndrome.
- Progressive enlargement of hands and feet and head (perhaps noticed by change in size of gloves, shoes or hat); spade-like hands; soft and mushy grip; big feet; lips thick; nose bulbous; supraorbital ridges enlarged.
- Dentures stop fitting; bite overrides; teeth become separated as the mandible enlarges.

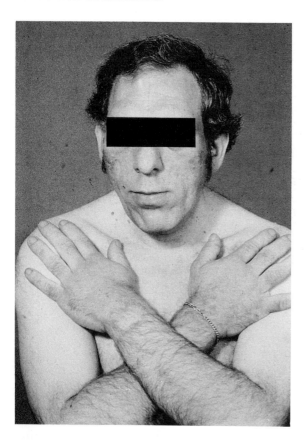 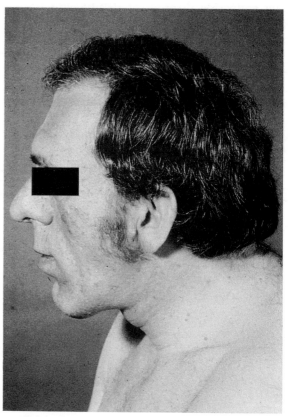

**Figure 19.14** Acromegaly. Note the coarsened features, large hands, and prominent supraorbital ridges and mandible.

- Arthritis and backache; kyphosis; enlarged vertebrae.
- Loss of secondary sexual characteristics. In women, menstrual irregularities and/or amenorrhoea. In men, loss of libido and/or impotence.
- Hoarseness of voice; larynx enlarges; vocal cords thicken.
- A few patients have galactorrhoea, or uncinate fits (hallucinations of taste or smell), or rhinorrhoea.
- Soft tissue enlargement may include thyroid (goitre), liver and spleen.
- Excessive pigmentation is frequently present.

## Investigation

X-rays of the hands show increased soft-tissue thickness, tufting of the tips of the distal phalanges, increased width of phalanges and exostoses. Skull X-rays show an enlarged mandible, prominence of all the sinuses but notably the supraorbital, and in most cases enlargement of the sella. Computed tomographic or magnetic resonance imaging scans of the pituitary usually demonstrate the tumour (Fig. 19.15). The calcaneal skin pad may exceed 30 mm in thickness. Over 10 per cent of patients are frankly diabetic, and most have an impaired tolerance of glucose. Levels of GH in plasma are elevated even at rest and are not suppressed during an oral glucose tolerance test, the ultimate diagnostic test for this condition.

## TREATMENT

Transphenoidal hypophysectomy, yttrium implantation and proton beam irradiation are effective treatments. Bromocriptine, ergotamine derivatives with dopaminergic properties, and

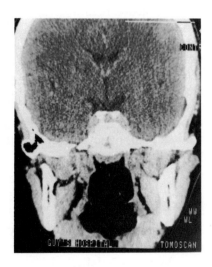
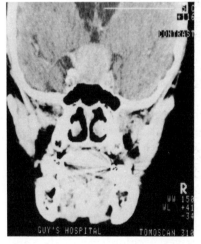
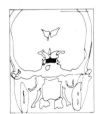
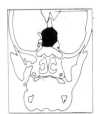

**Figure 19.15** Computed tomography of normal pituitary gland (left) and large non-functioning pituitary tumour (right). On the line diagrams below each scan the pituitary tissue is shown by the solid black.

analogues of somatostatin (growth hormone release inhibitory hormone, GHRIH, Table 19.1) will usually suppress high levels of GH, and are especially valuable for the occasional patient in whom pituitary 'ablation' fails to control the GH hypersecretion.

# Hyperprolactinaemia

The effects of hyperprolactinaemia recognized as clinically important are the stimulation of lactation, the inhibition of ovulation (with or without amenorrhoea), and the inhibition of spermatogenesis (with or without impotence). Prolonged hyperprolactinaemia is known to diminish bone density, probably through an anti-oestrogenic effect. An elevated prolactin level may also assume greater significance as a sign of some other pathology or disorder previously unsuspected such as:

- Secretion of prolactin by a pituitary adenoma or microadenoma (e.g. a 'pure' prolactinoma, or an eosinophilic tumour also producing GH).
- Interference by a tumour, trauma or inflammatory disease in the normal transmission of dopamine, the prolactin inhibitory hormone, between the hypothalamus and the pituitary, so 'releasing' the prolactin-secreting cells.
- Pharmacological interference in the synthesis, release or activity of dopamine, with effects analogous to above by phenothiazines, methyldopa, reserpine, tricyclic antidepressents, opiates, oral contraceptives, chlordiazepoxide and perhaps diazepam.
- Secretory response to increased levels of thyrotrophin-releasing hormone (TRH) such as occurs in the presence of hypothyroidism.
- Prolactin levels raised by chronic renal failure, hyperparathyroidism or hepatic cirrhosis.

If the cause of the hyperprolactinaemia cannot be removed, corrected or identified, dopaminergic agents such as bromocriptine usually suppress prolactin levels to within the normal range.

# Syndrome of inappropriate antidiuretic hormone secretion (SIADH)

Excessive levels of ADH may be of pituitary origin, through hypothalamic pathways, and yet be truly pathological as in many cases of cerebral irritation or trauma, or *appropriately* compensatory to real or false 'volume signals' in various chest disorders, or in patients on ventilators. Malignant tumours, especially small cell undifferentiated carcinomas of the bronchus, may secrete such quantities of ADH as to produce an acute neurological disturbance, from confusion and nausea to fits, focal signs and coma. This reversible state is mainly caused by severe hyponatraemia, a dilutional effect seen also in the low blood urea concentration. Oedema is unusual. (The dilutional changes distinguish this hyponatraemia from that seen in severe sodium depletion, when there will be a tendency to hypovolaemia, hypotension, low CVP and tachycardia.)

## DIAGNOSIS

The urine osmolality in SIADH is inappropriately 'normal' (i.e. it is high *relative* to the *low* plasma osmolality): in a normal subject a fairly modest fall of plasma osmolality below the individual normal range will stimulate a marked diuresis and *very* low urine osmolalities.

## TREATMENT

In management, removal of an ectopic source (or the bulk of it), water restriction, and the use of demeclocycline to block ADH effect on the renal tubules, may be helpful.

# $H$YPOPITUITARY STATES

For the purposes of discussion these can be classified as:

1. Isolated hormone deficiencies, for example, of TSH, ACTH or FSH. Pure growth hormone deficiency impairs growth in an otherwise normal child.
2. Pituitary chromophobe adenoma producing varying degrees of hypopituitarism and hypothalamic disorder.
3. Panhypopituitarism in the juvenile and adult.

## *Pituitary chromophobe adenoma*

Tumours of chromophobe histology often secrete prolactin and occasionally secrete ACTH (especially following adrenalectomy) or GH, but typically act as 'non-functioning' space-occupying lesions within the sella and then the brain.

### CLINICAL FEATURES

The pressure within the sella may cause a classical 'bursting' bitemporal headache and radiologically visible expansion of the sella with erosion of the clinoid processes. The pressure on the optic chiasma causes loss of visual acuity, bitemporal hemianopia and optic atrophy. Olfactory nerves may be involved with consequent anosmia. Signs of raised intracranial pressure may appear.

Local effects on the pituitary include progressive failure of most of the hormones of the anterior and posterior lobes, and the clinical picture may gradually move towards adult panhypopituitarism (see below).

Pressure on the hypothalamus may aggravate the pituitary failure, and also provoke characteristic hypothalamic features of weight gain, somnolence and polydipsia.

### INVESTIGATION AND DIAGNOSIS

For these and other tumours in the region of the sella turcica special investigations should include:

- A combined pituitary test (Table 19.12)
- Full visual testing including perimetry for visual fields (page 658)
- Computed tomography of the pituitary area (Fig. 19.15) and/or magnetic resonance imaging (Fig. 19.16)
- Arteriography if an aneurysm must be excluded
- Plain X-rays of the skull if other diagnoses are under consideration

### TREATMENT

Surgery and/or radiotherapy should be advised depending on the position and extent of the adenoma.

## *Panhypopituitarism*

This condition may be congenital causing pituitary dwarfism with adult body proportions and combined failure of thyroid, adrenal and gonad function; this is rare and it is discussed fully in specialist and paediatric texts.

In the adult, panhypopituitarism (**Simmonds' disease**) may be caused by infiltration of the pituitary by neoplasms or granulomas, by trauma or by infarction. The latter is the major cause, being especially associated with major haemorrhage at the time of parturition (**Sheehan's syndrome**). Hypopituitarism may follow surgery or irradiation of the pituitary gland or hypothalamus.

### CLINICAL FEATURES

There may be a history of *ante-* or *post-partum* haemorrhage. After delivery there is a failure of lactation and failure to resume menstruation

**Table 19.12** The combined anterior pituitary function test.*

The following are injected intravenously at about 09.00 h:

1. *Soluble insulin:* 0.1 units/kg body weight in suspected hypopituitarism, 0.3 units/kg in conditions of insulin resistance, 0.15 units/kg otherwise. (The blood glucose must fall to 2.5 mmol/l or below for the test to be valid. It is necessary for a doctor to be present or immediately available throughout in case severe hypoglycaemia occurs and administration of glucose becomes necessary.)
2. *TRH:* 200 μg (caution! TRH is risky in the presence of ischaemic heart disease)
3. *GnRH:* 100 μg

**Normal adult blood levels and responses (typical ranges)**

| Sample | GH (μ/l) | Cortisol (nmol/l) | TSH (mu/l) | Prolactin (mu/l) | LH (male) (u/l) | FSH (male) (u/l) | LH (female) (u/l) | FSH (female) (u/l) |
|---|---|---|---|---|---|---|---|---|
| Basal | 1–10 | 150–170 | 1–3 | <500 | 3–10 | 1–8 | 3–10† | 3–8† |
| 30′ | Peak exceeds 12 | Peak exceeds 800 | 5–20 | 300–3000 | 8–35 | 15–11 | 8–25 | 4–11 |
| 60′ | | | 4–18 | 200–3000 | 6–35 | 1–11 | 6–20 | 6–12 |
| 90′ | | | | | | | | |
| 120′ | | | | | | | | |

*This is a combination of the insulin hypoglycaemia, TRH and GnRH tests. In its complete form the test measures the capacity of the anterior pituitary to secrete all the anterior pituitary hormones. In some patients a more selective test may be adequate. The hypothalamic factors corticotrophin-releasing hormone (CRH) and growth hormone-releasing hormone (GHRH) are sometimes employed in the detailed analysis of deficiencies. In children exhibiting poor growth velocity the more relevant observation may be the nocturnal levels and patterns of growth hormone (GH) secretion.
†Figures obtained in the follicular phase of the cycle. Levels are generally lower than this during the luteal phase, having risen to a peak at mid-cycle (see Fig. 19.12).
TRH = thyrotrophin-releasing hormone. GnRH = gonadotrophin-releasing hormone. GH = growth hormone. TSH = thyroid-stimulating hormone. LH = luteinizing hormone. FSH = follicle-stimulating hormone.

(FSH, LH deficiency). The uterus and vagina shrink and vaginal secretions are reduced. There is secondary infertility. Patients often notice loss of libido, reduced pubic and axillary hair and impotence (FSH, LH and ACTH deficiency). Mild adrenal deficiency may occur with depigmentation and pallor (ACTH deficiency). Thyroid-stimulating hormone deficiency produces secondary myxoedema. The skin is characteristically soft, fine and wrinkled. Hypoglycaemic episodes may occur through ACTH and GH deficiency but mineralocorticoid function is well maintained by the renin–angiotensin system.

## INVESTIGATION AND DIAGNOSIS

The several gland deficiencies should be quantified by appropriate tests. Basal levels of anterior pituitary hormones may be low, but deficiencies will be more obvious under the conditions of a combined pituitary test (Table 19.12).

## TREATMENT

Substitution by hydrocortisone (20–40 mg daily), regular androgens, and cyclical oestrogens are advisable. Thyroxine may be added gradually when the adrenal insufficiency has been abolished. As the best treatment for the pituitary remnant is another pregnancy, a trial of gonadotrophins may be in order. Patients should take the same precautions as those with Addison's disease (page 536). Some adults may benefit from GH replacement therapy.

## *Hypopituitary coma*

This rare event, which should be prevented by good management, is dangerous in that it may involve the conjunction of hypoglycaemia, hypoadrenalism, hypothyroidism and hypothermia. The patient is treated specifically for these conditions and generally for shock.

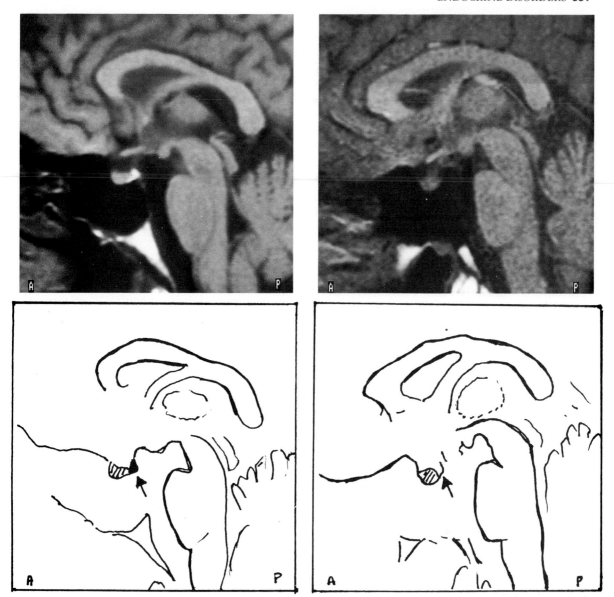

**Figure 19.16** Magnetic resonance images of normal hypothalamus and pituitary (left). A patient with diabetes insipidus (right). On the scans, the posterior lobe of the pituitary appears white. On the line diagrams below each scan the posterior pituitary tissue is shown in solid black. Note the *absence* of such tissue in the patient with diabetes insipidus.

## POSTERIOR PITUITARY DEFICIENCIES

## *Diabetes insipidus*

This is a rare disease, characterized by the excretion of a large (10–20 litres in 24 hours) urinary volume and consequent great thirst. It is caused by either a deficiency of antidiuretic hormone from the posterior pituitary gland (Fig. 19.16), or an inability of the distal renal tubule to respond to its action (nephrogenic diabetes insipidus). Failure of secretion may occur when disease processes affect the region of the pituitary, for example, tumour (50 per cent), inflammatory disease (25 per cent), vascular changes (10 per cent), trauma (10 per cent) and Hand–Schüller–Christian disease and histiocytosis X (2–3 per cent).

## CLINICAL FEATURES

The effect of the diuresis is to cause intense thirst. The condition should be suspected in all patients passing over 4 litres of urine per 24 hours and drinking more than 5 litres per 24 hours. It must be differentiated from diabetes mellitus (glycosuria), chronic renal failure (proteinuria, uraemia) and compulsive overdrinking. Only the last is difficult to separate. The most useful confirmatory test is to deprive the patient of water for 8 hours. Normal subjects will achieve a urine concentration of at least 600 mOsmol/kg, whereas those with diabetes insipidus will achieve only a small rise in urine osmolality. This test requires care as it is possible to dehydrate the patient seriously: it should not be performed if the plasma osmolality is above 300 mOsmol/kg, and it must be terminated if the patient passes so much urine that the body weight falls by more than 2 kg.

## TREATMENT

The ADH analogue desmopressin is given in a dose of 10–20 μg intranasally once or twice daily, or 2 μg intramuscularly daily. Some patients are helped by thiazide diuretics and chlorpropamide which sensitize the tubules to endogenous vasopressin. Cure can only be achieved by treating the cause.

# Nephrogenic diabetes insipidus

This is almost always congenital, very rarely the result of destruction of the distal renal tubule in pyelonephritis. The congenital form is easily recognized by the family history, its early onset, male predominance, and failure to respond to desmopressin.

Prognosis is poor, but some sensitization to low levels of ADH may be achieved by use of thiazide diuretics, or chlorthalidone, or chlorpropamide (but not other sulphonylureas), or carbamazepine.

# HYPOTHALAMIC DEFICIENCIES

Some typical pathological lesions leading to hypothalamic deficiencies are shown in Table 19.13.

## CLINICAL FEATURES

Visual defects tend to occur early. In a small minority, hyperphagia, weight changes, temperature disturbance and drowsiness occur.

Hyperprolactinaemia, with or without galactorrhoea, may arise, and diabetes insipidus may occur in association with the anterior lobe hormone deficiencies (page 549).

Magnetic resonance imaging is especially valuable in identifying hypothalamic and posterior pituitary lesions (Fig. 19.16).

**Table 19.13** Causes of hypothalamic deficiencies.

*Tumours*
Craniopharyngioma (calcification visible on skull X-ray; common in children)
Chromophobe adenomas (early visual changes usually occur)

*Trauma*

*Granulomas*
Sarcoidosis (look for disease elsewhere)
Tuberculosis (look for disease elsewhere)
Hand–Schüller–Christian disease (histiocytosis X)

# PLURIGLANDULAR DISORDERS

These are disease states in which two or more endocrine glands are involved in the same patient.

## COMBINED GLAND FAILURES

- Hypopituitary states (page 549)
- Autoimmune group (associated with HLA-DW3 and DW4):
  Hashimoto's disease, Graves' disease, myxoedema
  Pernicious anaemia
  Addison's disease
  Insulin-dependent diabetes mellitus
  Hypoparathyroidism
  Hypogonadism

## COMBINED GLAND HYPERSECRETION

Multiple endocrine adenomatosis (MEA) or neoplasia (MEN) may occur sporadically or as a familial disorder. It is classified into three types:

| | |
|---|---|
| Type I | Especially pituitary, parathyroid and pancreatic adenomas |
| Type IIA | Parathyroid adenomas, phaeochromocytomas and medullary carcinoma of thyroid |
| Type IIB | Phaeochromocytomas, medullary carcinoma of the thyroid and mucosal neuromas |

# ENDOCRINE FUNCTIONS OF 'NON-ENDOCRINE ORGANS'

## THE KIDNEY

The kidney is responsible for the secretion of at least three substances that are hormonal in character:

- Erythropoietin controlling red cell production
- Renin, controlling angiotensin production (page 162)
- 1,25-dihydroxycholecalciferol (1-25-OH-vitamin $D_3$) (page 5)

## THE GASTROINTESTINAL TRACT

The gut wall secretes a number of identified peptides, such as pancreozymincholecystokinin, gastrin, secretin, gastric inhibitory polypeptide, vasoactive inhibitory polypeptide (VIP), enteroglucagon, pancreatic polypeptide, secretin, motilin, neurotensin, enkephalin, substance P, bombesin, somatostatin and probably many others. Occasionally overproduction of such peptides by tumours in the pancreas can produce clinical problems, for example gastrinomas producing recurrent duodenal ulceration (Zollinger–Ellison syndrome) and VIPomas producing watery diarrhoea.

# ECTOPIC SECRETION OF HORMONES

Many tumours arising in apparently non-endocrine tissues are found to contain or secrete peptide hormones or biochemically similar peptides. A wide variety of tumours and peptides have been associated, but the more common and important syndromes are described here.

## ECTOPIC CUSHING'S SYNDROME

Very high levels of ACTH typically produce marked hypokalaemia and weakness. Sources include small cell carcinoma of the bronchus, thymomas, carcinoids, and carcinomas of the stomach, colon, gallbladder and ovary.

**Table 19.14** Hypercalcaemia in malignant disorders.

| Malignant disorder (and see text) | Usual main pathophysiology | | | | | Known and probable tumour-derived factors |
|---|---|---|---|---|---|---|
| | Bone resorption | Bone formation | Renal calcium resorption | Renal GFR | Gut calcium absorption | |
| Squamous cell carcinoma of the bronchus | ↑ | ↓ | ↑ | — | — | Parathyroid hormone-related proteins(s) (PTHrP) Prostaglandins |
| Carcinoma of the breast | ↑ | ↑ | ↑ | — | — | Transforming growth factors? (TGFα and perhaps β) |
| Myeloma | ↑ | — | — | ↓ | — | |
| Some lymphomas (e.g. T-cell) | (↑) | ? | ? | — | ↑ | 1, 25-OH-vitamin D |

GFR = glomerular filtration rate.

## INAPPROPRIATE ADH SECRETION

See page 548.

## HYPERCALCAEMIA

This is a well-recognized complication of carcinoma of the breast, squamous cell carcinoma of the bronchus, head and neck, carcinomas of kidney, ovary and pancreas, of myeloma and of some lymphomas. Some of the known and postulated mechanisms are shown in Table 19.14. Dehydration and/or confinement to bed will aggravate any tendency to hypercalcaemia. The keystones of management are rehydration, mobilization of the patient if possible, and the judicious use of biphosphonates or calcitonin when necessary.

## POLYCYTHAEMIA

This occurs secondary to erythropoietin secretion. Sources include hypernephroma, fibromyoma of the uterus and stomach cancer.

# Disorders of Joints and Connective Tissues

# 20

# INTRODUCTION

Rheumatic diseases constitute a heterogeneous group of conditions affecting joints, muscles and ligaments and causing much suffering in the community through pain, stiffness and loss of mobility. A very significant part of the work of a general practitioner involves rheumatic disorders. Although acute episodes and life-threatening complications may be seen in certain of the conditions under consideration, the bulk of the problems encountered are less spectacular in their presentation and give rise to prolonged discomfort and disability without seriously impairing the general health of the patient. A wide spectrum of disease is seen in this group, including hereditary, inflammatory (both acute and chronic; infective and non-infective), metabolic, traumatic, degenerative, neoplastic, neuropathic and psychogenic disorders. The aetiology and pathogenesis is in many cases unknown or poorly understood but advances in immunology, genetics and molecular biology are beginning to shed light on some of the causes and mechanisms of disease.

Treatment is aimed at suppressing inflammation, reducing the disease activity and preserving and restoring the function of the locomotor system by physical therapy or surgical intervention or by adapting the environment to suit the patient's limited capabilities. Few of the diseases are amenable to eradication by medical means, but fortunately there is, in many cases, a strong tendency towards spontaneous recovery or remission.

The terms rheumatism, fibrositis and lumbago have imprecise meanings and are best avoided (Table 20.1).

**Table 20.1** Definitions.

| | |
|---|---|
| Ankylosis | Complete loss of joint movement |
| Arthralgia | Pain in a joint |
| Arthritis | Inflammation in a joint |
| Arthropathy | Any lesion affecting a joint |
| Bursitis | Inflammation in a bursa |
| Capsulitis | Inflammation in a joint capsule |
| Chondritis | Inflammation in cartilage |
| Crepitus | Cracking sound or grating feeling |
| Cruralgia | Pain in the distribution of the femoral nerve |
| Effusion | Presence of fluid in a synovial cavity |
| Enthesopathy | Inflammatory lesion at the point of insertion of a tendon or a ligament in bone |
| Fasciitis | Inflammation of deep fascia |
| Monoarthritis | Inflammation in a single joint |
| Myalgia | Pain in a muscle |
| Myositis | Inflammation in a muscle |
| Oligoarthritis | Inflammation in two, three or four joints |
| Osteitis | Inflammation in a bone |
| Osteoarthritis | Degeneration in a peripheral joint |
| Polyarthritis | Inflammation in five or more joints |
| Sciatica | Pain in the distribution of the sciatic nerve |
| Spondarthritis | Inflammation in the spine and peripheral joints |
| Spondylitis | Inflammation in the spinal joints |
| Spondylosis | Degeneration in the spinal joints |
| Subluxation | Partial dislocation of a joint, some contact is preserved between joint surfaces |
| Synovitis | Inflammation of synovial membrane |
| Tendonitis | Inflammation of a tendon |
| Tenosynovitis | Inflammation in a tendon sheath |

# ASSESSMENT OF THE ARTHRITIC PATIENT

The clinical history provides important clues to the diagnosis of rheumatic diseases, and so the time devoted to a careful history taking is well spent. Aspects such as mode of onset, duration, aggravating and relieving factors, response to treatment, effects on ability to function normally in the home and at work, are all essential for a complete understanding of the patient's condition. Important and relevant information can be gleaned by enquiry of the patient's past medical, family and occupational histories. Of particular importance from the diagnostic point of view, in both the acute and chronic rheumatic diseases, is the pattern of progression of the ailment, whether it follows a self-limiting, recurrent, acute or chronic course.

# Symptoms

The principal symptoms of arthritis are pain, stiffness, swelling and limitation of movement (Table 20.2).

**Table 20.2** Symptoms and signs of arthritis.

| Symptoms | Signs |
| --- | --- |
| Pain | Heat |
| Stiffness | Redness |
| Swelling | Swelling |
| Limitation of movement | Limited/excessive movement |
| | Mechanical dysfunction |

## PAIN

Pain is the most frequent symptom of musculo-skeletal disease. It is a complex symptom, difficult to define and difficult to measure. Being a subjective phenomenon its perception is strongly influenced by a patient's emotional state.

The site of the pain (whether it is felt in joint, muscle, bone or ligament) is often indicative of the anatomical site of the lesion. The exception to this is so-called referred pain (e.g. hip joint pain referred to the knee region, shoulder joint pain referred to the insertion of deltoid, and sciatica and cruralgia seen in intervertebral disc prolapse). The nature of the pain and the effect of movement may be helpful. Aching around and within a joint suggests an arthropathy, whereas a burning or lancinating nature suggests a pain of nerve origin. Pain due to inflammatory joint disease is usually present both at rest and with movement, whereas pain of degenerative or mechanical origin is often present only on movement.

## STIFFNESS

True stiffness implies the need to apply additional effort to overcome resistance to movement. Prolonged stiffness after a period of immobility (usually early-morning stiffness on waking or less commonly evening stiffness) is the hallmark of inflammatory joint disease, its duration (e.g. from half an hour to all day) being directly proportional to the severity of the inflammatory process. By contrast, in osteo-arthritis stiffness (known as articular gelling) lasts only a few moments.

## SWELLING

Although strictly speaking joint swelling is a physical sign (see below), it may also be a presenting symptom and cause the patient to seek medical advice.

## LIMITATION OF MOVEMENT

Diminution of range of movement is a cardinal feature of joint disease and may render the patient incapable of performing normally because of reduced flexibility. Patients with hip disease complain of difficulty with putting on socks or mounting on to a bus platform; patients with spinal disease notice difficulty in getting in and out of the car and in reversing; loss of knee extension leads to difficulties in walking.

# Signs

Physical signs in joint disease can be broadly categorised into those determined by inflammation within joints and those features, largely mechanical in nature, which result from damage to the joints. Since joint damage may result from the effects of inflammation, the two sets of features are by no means mutually exclusive.

## SIGNS OF INFLAMMATION

Because the synovial joints (with the notable exception of the hips and spinal joints) are so accessible to inspection and palpation, the cardinal signs of inflammation can readily be recognized. Redness of the overlying skin and swelling can be observed, while tenderness and heat are detected by manual palpation. Loss of function is translated to limitation of active and passive movement and inhibition of strength of movement by pain. An important sign of inflammation is the detection of an effusion (synovial fluid exudate) within the joint cavity by means of careful palpation for fluctuation.

## SIGNS OF MECHANICAL DYSFUNCTION

These include crepitus, loss of range of movement, deformity and instability.

### Crepitus

A fine crepitus on passive movement is the clinical hallmark of the osteoarthritic joint, being caused by movement between roughened surfaces. A coarser form of crepitus is seen in any condition where the articular cartilage has been damaged by disease (e.g. in rheumatoid arthritis). Loud clicks emanating from a joint are usually of no pathological significance and, provided they are painless, may be ignored.

### Loss of range of movement

This can arise when a joint is distended by thickened synovium and by an effusion, the sheer bulk impeding movement by its very presence. When articular cartilage is eroded by disease, the extremes of ranges of movement are initially lost. As the condition progresses, so the range decreases progressively until ankylosis occurs. The sudden complete loss of movement is known as 'locking'. This occurs when a 'loose body', for example, a detached fragment of cartilage or torn meniscus, becomes impacted in the joint.

### Deformity

This refers to any malalignment of articulating bones which is liable to occur when joint surfaces are severely damaged, or sometimes where supporting structures (e.g. ligaments, tendons or muscles) are weakened or ruptured. The presence of deformities greatly reduces the efficiency and effectiveness of movement, whether it be in the upper limb where hand and wrist involvement drastically reduce hand function or in the lower limbs where locomotion may be severely impaired. Specific deformities are discussed under the sections relating to individual diseases.

### Instability

Loss of the normal joint stability may also arise from damage to joint surfaces or supporting structures. It too can have a disastrous effect on function; for example, a strong hand grip depends on normal wrist joint stability and standing relies on stability of the knee joint. Inflammatory joint diseases such as rheumatoid arthritis can cause irreversible damage, not only to joints but also to articular ligaments whose prime function is to maintain stability. Joint laxity and instability may arise from an inherent weakness of collagen, as in the hypermobility syndrome.

The vertebral column poses particular problems because it is a composite structure of 25 interarticulating vertebral segments which also articulate with the skull (via the atlanto-occipital joints), the thoracic cage (via the costo-vertebral joints) and the pelvis (via the sacroiliac joints). Because of the inaccessibility of the spinal articular structures, the examination is limited to (a) elicitation of tenderness by deep palpation over individual intervertebral joints; (b) observation of spinal posture – exaggeration or diminution of the normal curvature in the anteroposterior plane or the presence of abnormal curves e.g. scoliosis, curvature laterally, and (c) observation of restriction (painful or otherwise) of normal movements pertaining to the region in question. Thus for the cervical spine the movements tested are rotation to the left and right, flexion, extension and lateral flexion to the left and right; for the dorsal spine, rotation of the trunk to the left and to the right; and for the lumbar region flexion and extension and lateral flexion to the left and right. An integral part of the examination of the spine involves a complete neurological examination of the upper and lower limbs, since the spinal cord and the nerve roots which constitute the brachial, lumbar and sacral plexuses are very vulnerable to pressure from degenerative changes in the intervertebral discs especially disc prolapse and osteophyte formation. Evidence for tension of L2/3/4 roots and the L5/S1 roots may be obtained by performing the femoral nerve stretch tests and the straight leg raise combined with the sciatic nerve stretch test, respectively.

No consideration of the locomotor system can be complete without full examination of the other systems and an assessment of the patient as a whole. Features such as the presence of rheumatoid nodules or tophi are helpful in confirming rheumatoid arthritis and gout, respectively. Other features such as psoriasis, uveitis, genitourinary or inflammatory bowel diseases should be sought. Many rheumatic diseases have characteristic clinical features so that clinical diagnosis is often not difficult.

## DIAGNOSTIC AIDS IN RHEUMATOLOGY

The following diagnostic tests are helpful in difficult cases and as confirmation of the clinical diagnosis.

The erythrocyte sedimentation rate (ESR) distinguishes inflammatory from degenerative and mechanical joint disease. The tests for rheumatoid factor, a serum antibody directed against the person's own denatured gammaglobulin, (latex fixation test and sheep cell agglutination test) and are positive in two-thirds of patients with rheumatoid arthritis but also in a substantial number of patients with systemic lupus erythematosus (SLE) and in 5 per cent of the normal population. **Antinuclear factor** (a set of serum antibodies directed against the components of cell nuclei) is positive in most patients with SLE and in substantial numbers of patients with rheumatoid arthritis and scleroderma. The pattern of immunofluorescent staining varies from disease to disease. Whilst the homogenous pattern may be seen in all the connective tissue diseases as well as the drug-induced lupus erythematosus, the speckled pattern is particularly seen in the sera of patients with SLE, rheumatoid arthritis, systemic sclerosis and Sjögren's syndrome. The DNA-binding test which demonstrates serum anti-DNA antibody is more specific for SLE. Plasma urate is raised in primary and secondary gout.

X-rays can provide diagnostic pointers to rheumatoid arthritis (periarticular osteoporosis, joint space narrowing and erosion of cortical surface of articulating bone, Fig. 20.1), osteo-

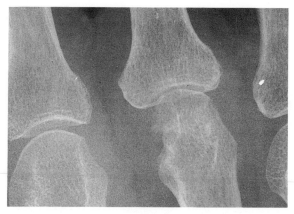

**Figure 20.1** The second right metacarpophalangeal (MCP) joint (shown in the centre) shows typical erosion of the head of MCP laterally with associated juxta-articular osteoporosis and joint space narrowing.

arthritis (periarticular osteosclerosis, joint space narrowing with osteophyte formation), ankylosing spondylitis (with sacroiliitis, syndesmophyte, i.e. ossification of spinal ligaments, formation leading to bony ankylosis, gout (presence of bony tophi) and pseudogout (chondrocalcinosis articularis, page 582). Contrast radiology is used as arthrography (in the diagnosis of ruptured Baker's cyst and ruptured rotator cuff lesions) and in radiculography or myelography in the investigation of disc prolapse and other spinal lesions. The use of these techniques is currently surplanted by newer imaging methods such as computed tomography and magnetic resonance imaging (page 119).

Synovial fluid analysis should be undertaken whenever the diagnosis is uncertain and a joint effusion is detected. Bacteriological examination by Gram stain and culture are of paramount importance in patients suspected of having infective arthritis, and gout and pseudogout are diagnosed by recognizing crystals of sodium urate (page 581) and calcium pyrophosphate respectively by polarizing microscopy. Arthroscopy allows (as yet only routinely in the knee joint) inspection of the inside of the joint whilst synovial biopsy undertaken during arthroscopy or by closed needle biopsy can provide useful histological information on the underlying pathology.

No assessment of the chronic arthritic patient

is complete without a consideration of the capacity to undertake the basic tasks of daily living and return to work, preferably undertaken by an occupational therapist.

# Clinical problems

## RHEUMATOID ARTHRITIS (RHEUMATOID DISEASE)

Rheumatoid arthritis is the most common form of chronic inflammatory disease affecting synovial joints. It is a multisystem disease of connective tissue which produces systemic manifestations in viscera as well as the locomotor system.

### AETIOLOGY AND PATHOLOGY

The precise aetiology is still unknown. There is a distinct familial tendency, and an important recent discovery is a significant association (70 per cent rheumatoid arthritis patients, 28 per cent controls) between occurrence of the disease in Europeans and an inherited major histocompatibility complex (MHC) antigen DR4 (page 84). In certain other racial groups the association is with DR1. The presence of an autoantibody, rheumatoid factor (page 559) in approximately 70 per cent of sufferers and the occasional finding of circulating immune complexes has led to the theory that the disease has an 'autoimmune' pathogenesis. The current prevailing view is that these features of autoimmunity have some pathogenetic significance, but are triggered by a virus or other infective agent yet to be identified. The resultant synovial inflammatory response is characterized by hyperplasia, increased vascularity and a dense infiltration of lymphocytes and plasma cells, sometimes aggregated into follicles. The granulation tissue, commonly known as pannus, releases enzymes including collagenase, a neutral protease and lysosomal cathepsin D capable of destroying cartilage, ligament and bone. The process may result in destruction of the joint with subluxation and instability, ultimately leading to fibrous and, occasionally, bony ankylosis. A characteristic feature is the formation of the **rheumatoid nodule** over the ulnar aspect of the forearm (Fig. 20.2) and other points of pressure. Histologically, these are examples of a 'pallisading granuloma' with a central zone of connective tissue necrosis surrounded by radiating histiocytes and a peripheral zone with small round-cell infiltration.

The non-articular manifestations of the disease (Table 20.3) are explained on the basis of an arteritis occasioned by the deposition of immune complexes. This usually takes the form of a mild endarteritis, but occasionally a more serious necrotizing arteritis is seen. Secondary amyloid deposition may also occur in a small percentage (5–20 per cent) of patients with rheumatoid arthritis which, owing to the falling prevalence of chronic sepsis, now constitutes the major cause of secondary amyloid.

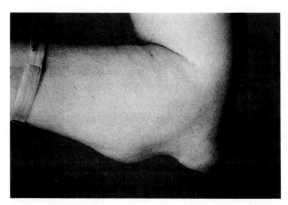

**Figure 20.2** A rheumatoid nodule over the olecranon.

**Table 20.3** Extra-articular manifestations of rheumatoid arthritis.

| Lesion | Site | Clinical features | Complications |
|---|---|---|---|
| Rheumatoid nodule | Subcutaneous Tendon | Palpable swelling | — |
| | Pleura Lung | Effusion Asymptomatic | Bronchopleural fistula |
| | Pericardium | Effusion | Tamponade, constriction |
| | Myocardium | Myocarditis | Cardiac failure |
| | Endocardium | Valvulitis | Cardiac failure |
| | Sclera | Scleritis | Scleromalacia perforans |
| Endarteritis | Digital arteries (small calibre 15 μm diameter) (Fig. 20.3) | Raynaud's phenomenon Sensory neuropathy | Digital 'nail-fold' infarcts (Fig. 20.4) |
| | Eye | Episcleritis | — |
| Necrotizing arteritis | Large arteries | Necrotic skin ulcers Sensorimotor neuropathy | Rupture/occlusion of mesenteric or other visceral arteries (life threatening) |
| Amyloid deposition | Bowel, liver, kidney, spleen | Proteinuria Nephrotic syndrome | Renal failure |
| 'Rheumatoid lung' | Lung parenchyma | Fibrosing alveolitis Caplan's syndrome (in coal miners) (page 313) | Respiratory failure |
| Sjögren's syndrome | Lacrimal and salivary glands | Dry eyes (keratoconjunctivitis sicca), dry mouth (xerostomia) | Keratitis, corneal ulcer, lymphoma |
| Felty's syndrome | Haematopoietic system, spleen | Splenomegaly Neutropenia Thrombocytopenia 1/3 | Infections |

## EPIDEMIOLOGY

Rheumatoid arthritis may affect all ethnic and geographical groups but it is certainly more common and more severe in temperate than in tropical climates. In the UK the prevalence of adult rheumatoid disease is of the order of 1 per cent with an annual incidence of new cases of approximately 0.02 per cent. The comparable figures for chronic juvenile arthritis are 0.06 and 0.006 per cent a year, respectively. The adult disease is seen in between 3 and 8 per cent of first-degree relatives of patients. There is evidence to suggest that life expectancy is reduced, particularly in those patients in whom the disease starts before the age of 45 years and those with more severe disease at the time of first diagnosis. Women are affected three times more often than men.

## CLINICAL FEATURES

The disease usually commences with articular symptoms, namely pain, swelling and stiffness

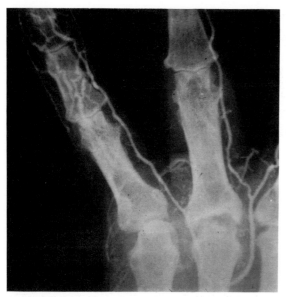

**Figure 20.3** Arteriogram showing occlusion of the radial digital arteries of the 4th and 5th digits due to rheumatoid digital vasculitis. Note the severe erosive changes at the metacarpophalangeal and proximal interphalangeal joints.

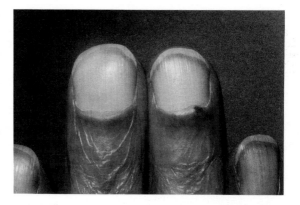

**Figure 20.4** Close up view of a nail-fold lesion seen in the ring finger. This 'microinfarct' is the result of digital arterial occlusion due to arteritis.

in one or more synovial joints. The onset is usually insidious but may be acute, particularly in the aged. Classically, the joints favoured are the proximal interphalangeal joints, and metacarpophalangeal joints of the hands (the distal interphalangeal joints are usually not affected), the wrists, elbows, shoulders, hips, knees, ankles, tarsal joints and metatarsophalangeal joints. In the spine the cervical region is the only area commonly involved. Occasionally one encounters arthritis of the temporomandibular joints, the sternoclavicular joints, and even the cricoarytenoid joint may be affected.

A typical feature of all inflammatory arthritides is the early-morning stiffness experienced by the patient on rising. The affected joints are tender, swollen and often warm and an effusion may be detected. In the hands the soft tissue swelling produces a spindling of the fingers with increased sweating of the skin and visible muscle atrophy. Involvement of weight-bearing joints causes difficulty in standing, walking and climbing stairs. Occasionally, the disease commences in one solitary joint or two or three simultaneously, from which it may spread to become a widespread polyarthritis.

As the disease progresses unchecked, defor-

mities commonly develop. These are seen as the characteristic ulnar deviation and eventually subluxation (Fig. 20.5) of the metacarpophalangeal joints, the 'swan-neck' or 'boutonniere' deformities of the fingers, fixed flexion deformities of the wrists, hip, knee and ankle, valgus deformity of the knee, hind foot and big toe and subluxation of the metatarsophalangeal joints. Subluxation of the cervical spine may occur in approximately 25 per cent of rheumatoid arthritis patients, either at the atlantoaxial joint (C1/C2) (Fig. 20.6) or lower. This may cause compression of the cervical cord, but fortunately tetraparesis from this is surprisingly uncommon. Cricoarytenoid involvement when present may give rise to hoarseness, laryngeal discomfort and even stridor.

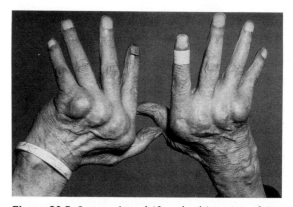

**Figure 20.5** Severe ulnar drift and subluxation of the metacarpophalangeal joints in rheumatoid arthritis. Note the nail-fold lesions on both ring and left index fingers.

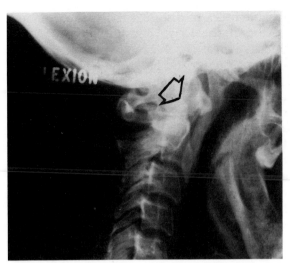

**Figure 20.6** Atlantoaxial subluxation in rheumatoid arthritis. Note the posterior movement of the odontoid peg in relation to the anterior arch of the axis in this lateral cervical spine X-ray taken in flexion (arrow).

A common feature of knee involvement is the development of a **Baker's cyst**. This arises when synovial fluid under pressure is forced from the knee joint into a communicating bursa which enlarges to produce a palpable and often painful swelling in the popliteal fossa or upper calf. While often asymptomatic, a Baker's cyst may rupture its contents into the tissues of the calf to produce pain and oedema mimicking a deep-vein thrombosis (Fig. 20.7). Rheumatoid synovitis also commonly affects tendon sheaths and bursae, producing soft tissue swelling over the dorsum of the hand, the flexor aspect of the fingers (Fig. 20.8), the olecranon, the deltoid region and the malleoli. Synovial swelling may give rise to compression of peripheral nerves (in particular, the median nerve at the wrist), causing carpal tunnel syndrome (page 689). Rheumatoid arthritis may be complicated by pyogenic joint infection, either blood-borne or introduced at the time of an intra-articular injection through faulty technique. Suspicion of this is aroused when a single joint appears to be more actively inflamed than the remainder.

## Extra-articular manifestations (Table 20.3)

Weight loss, lethargy, anorexia, pyrexia and symptoms of anaemia may be seen in varying degrees of severity and exemplify the systemic nature of rheumatoid arthritis. Fever is common

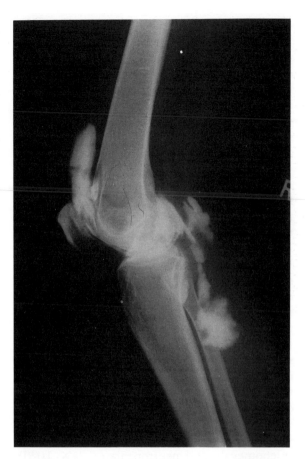

**Figure 20.7** Contrast arthrogram showing a popliteal cyst (Baker's cyst) that has ruptured its contents into the calf.

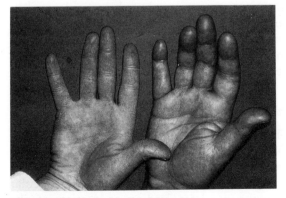

**Figure 20.8** Swelling of the fingers due to flexor tenosynovitis in rheumatoid arthritis on the right. Normal hand on the left for comparison.

during acute exacerbations of the disease and tends to settle with anti-inflammatory drugs. A mild anaemia occurs and is usually nor-mochromic, normocytic or, less often, hypochromic, microcytic (page 603). There is usually 'anaemia of chronic disease' associated with low serum iron, low iron binding capacity and normal serum ferritin level (page 597). However, iron deficiency anaemia may occur from blood loss associated with the use of non-steroidal anti-inflammatory drugs. Reactive depression not infrequently results from the pain, disability and frustration that ensues.

Subcutaneous rheumatoid nodules, most commonly seen over the ulnar border of the forearm and olecranon (Fig. 20.2) over the sacrum, the fingers and in large tendons, notably the Achilles, occur in one-third of patients. Although unsightly and occasionally liable to infection, these are painless and cause little trouble. Their presence is of diagnostic significance in that it helps to confirm the diagnosis of rheumatoid disease and implies a liability to more destructive joint disease and vasculitis. Patients with nodules are invariably seropositive with a high titre of rheumatoid factor. Various forms of visceral involvement may occur (as a result of arteritis, nodule formation, or amyloid deposition (Table 20.3).

The term **Felty's syndrome** is used to describe the triad of rheumatoid arthritis, splenomegaly and neutropenia ($<2 \times 10^9/l$). Although it may occur early in the course of rheumatoid arthritis, the common presentation is in severe destructive disease of long duration. Infections are common but their incidence does not correlate with the degree of neutropenia. Other features include skin pigmentation, chronic leg ulceration and occasionally nodular degenerative hepatic hyperplasia.

## DIAGNOSIS

The diagnosis is made by the clinical features of the joint disease, and confirmed radiologically and serologically.

The X-ray appearances include juxta-articular osteoporosis, later leading to erosion of the articular surface and loss of joint space. Finally, total destruction of a joint may be seen with or without bony ankylosis.

The erythrocyte sedimentation rate is raised whilst the disease remains active. Recently it has been suggested that measurement of acute-phase proteins (e.g. C-reactive protein) may be a more reliable index of disease activity. Anaemia is a feature of the active disease. The degree and progression of the X-ray appearances can also indicate activity and progression of the disease.

Rheumatoid factor is present in approximately 60 per cent of patients with established rheumatoid disease. It is an auto-antibody against immunoglobulin G and may be IgG, IgM or IgA. The tests commonly in use include the Rose–Waaler test in which sheep red cells are coated with gammaglobulin agglutinate in the presence of a patient's serum, or the latex fixation test in which similarly coated polystyrene particles are used. The latter is more sensitive but less specific, being positive in a variety of other conditions, including bacterial endocarditis, tuberculosis and cirrhosis. A high titre is associated with an increased development of nodules and arteritic manifestations. Rheumatoid factor is by definition negative in the so-called seronegative arthropathies (see below), but may be positive in systemic lupus erythematosus (SLE), scleroderma and Sjögren's syndrome. A positive antinuclear factor test may be seen in the serum of up to 20 per cent of patients with rheumatoid arthritis, and this occasionally causes diagnostic confusion. Such patients, however, follow the pattern of rheumatoid disease rather than SLE. Plasma electrophoresis frequently reveals an increase in the $\alpha_2$ and gammaglobulin fraction during the active phase of the disease.

Synovial fluid analysis generally reveals a loss of the normal viscosity, and a cellular exudate (predominantly polymorphonuclear leukocytes) containing between 5 and 60 billion ($10^9$) per litre. Synovial biopsy, performed when the diagnosis is in doubt, may reveal the characteristic synovial pathology.

## TREATMENT

Since the aetiological agent is unknown, it is not yet possible to eradicate the disease. Much however, can be done to mitigate the effects of the disease. The principal aims of treatment are:

1. To control the synovitis thereby relieving symptoms and reducing the likelihood of erosion. This is achieved by rest, anti-inflammatory drugs, disease-modifying

drugs and, when single joints are involved, by intra-articular steroid injections, and where these fail by surgical or radioisotope synovectomy.

2. To prevent deformities by splinting inflamed joints such as the hand, wrist, knee or ankle, which would otherwise develop serious flexion contractures.

3. Where irreversible damage has occurred to a joint, to improve joint and muscle function by physiotherapy, exercises, appropriate surgical appliances (splints, collar, calliper, corset etc.) and surgical means where necessary (prosthetic joint replacement).

Acute exacerbations respond to a short period of joint immobilization by splinting in the case of a single joint, or by a short period (one week) of bedrest in the presence of a polyarthritis. The latter must be carefully supervised since bedrest carries certain risks (bed sores, deep-vein thrombosis, contractures, muscle atrophy and pneumonia) especially in the elderly or debilitated. Light resting splints are essential when joints of the hand, wrist, knee or ankle are involved if serious deformity is to be avoided. A cervical collar is helpful if the cervical spine is affected. Isometric exercises at this stage help to prevent muscle atrophy. The most actively inflamed joints may be aspirated and injected with corticosteroid (e.g. hydrocortisone acetate, 25–50 mg, methylprednisolone acetate, 20–40 mg, or triamcinolone hexacetonide, 5–20 mg), the dose depending on the size of the joint. The effect of these injections is often dramatic. The duration of benefit varies and is often prolonged, particularly with the longer acting preparations.

## Non-steroidal anti-inflammatory drugs

These drugs are also administered at this stage and will continue to be required for as long as the synovitis remains active, in most cases over a period of several years or even decades. It is essential, therefore, to choose the best drug for each individual patient, which is a process of trial and error. Many non-steroidal anti-inflammatory drugs (NSAIDs) are currently available.

### Aspirin

Potent and still widely used, this drug is liable to cause tinnitus, deafness, and overt or occult gastrointestinal bleeding in therapeutic doses. These side effects and the large numbers of tablets required reduces its acceptability and thereby patient compliance. Alternative formulations including enteric-coated and micro-encapsulated forms, for example, benorylate (an ester of aspirin with paracetamol) have proved more acceptable than soluble aspirin.

### Indomethacin

This, too, is potent and liable to cause headache and dizziness in many patients. Long-term use may give rise to prepyloric gastric ulceration. The dose is 25–50 mg three times daily. A sustained-release oral preparation, 75 mg, and a suppository, 100 mg, is available for night use and helps to control morning stiffness. Sulindac, 200 mg b.d., is a chemically related preparation which has fewer side effects.

### Phenylbutazone

This is pyrazole which may cause fluid retention, gastric ulceration and bone marrow depression, particularly with long-term use. It is, therefore, suitable only for short-term use for acute exacerbations. In the UK this drug is only available for hospital-treated patients with ankylosing spondylitis. The chemically related preparation azapropazone, 600 mg b.d., is less toxic.

### Propionic acid derivatives

These are ibuprofen, 400–600 mg t.d.s, naproxen, 250 mg in the morning, 500 mg at night, ketoprofen, 50 mg t.d.s., fenoprofen, 300–600 mg t.d.s., flurbiprofen, 150 mg q.d.s., and fenbufen, 600–900 mg daily.

### Aryl-acetic acid derivatives

These are diclofenac, 25–50 mg t.d.s., and tiaprofenic acid, 200 mg t.d.s.

### Miscellaneous

These are tolmetin, 200–400 mg t.d.s., a pyrole derivative, piroxicam, 20 mg once daily, an oxicam derivative, etodolac, 200–300 mg b.d., and nabumetone, 1g at night.

By and large, all the drugs listed in the last three groups above have been shown in clinical trials to be comparable in terms of efficacy with the older drugs. They are undoubtedly better tolerated, although rashes occur. Gastric intolerance is common and occasionally gastric haemorrhage may be seen. They should be used with extreme caution in the elderly, patients suffering from known peptic ulceration and those on anticoagulants, and they should all be avoided in pregnancy. Non-steroidal anti-inflammatory drugs should be avoided in the presence of borderline or impaired renal function as they can precipitate serious renal failure. All the newer preparations are more expensive than the earlier ones. With few exceptions their mode of action is believed to be inhibition of prostaglandin synthetase. Their use is applicable in other forms of inflammatory joint disease, including acute gout. They may also be helpful in degenerative joint disease and soft tissue lesions when symptoms merit their use.

## Disease-modifying agents in rheumatoid disease

These drugs are introduced as second-line drugs where NSAIDs have failed to control joint inflammation and/or where erosions have developed on X-rays. They include gold salts, D-penicillamine, sulphasalazine, chloroquine, immunosuppressive and immunopotentiating drugs, and corticosteroids.

### Gold

Injections of sodium aurothiomalate are given by weekly intramuscular injections of 50 mg (after a test dose of 10 mg) until a total of 1 g has been given. If by the end of that time a favourable response is seen, treatment is continued indefinitely on a monthly basis, provided that side effects do not develop. Skin reactions are common and may be severe. Temporary suspension of the injections is recommended. Many patients, however, are subsequently able to resume the course. Gold nephropathy is a rare complication which may lead to nephrotic syndrome. Proteinuria should be looked for at each attendance and gold is withdrawn if it is present. It may take a year before the kidney recovers. Of greatest importance is the liability to bone marrow depression which may lead to serious (even fatal) aplastic anaemia. Fortunately this is rare but thrombocytopenia alone is more common. These haematological complications can only be

prevented by careful and regular monitoring of blood and platelet counts, preferably before each injection. With these precautions gold salts have proved themselves over a half century to be a useful and effective means of suppressing rheumatoid synovitis, although the mode of action is uncertain. Gold-induced remissions are accompanied by an improvement in systemic features. An oral gold preparation 'Auranofin' is also available. It is less effective than i.m. gold and is liable to cause diarrhoea.

### D-Penicillamine

This drug has been introduced for the treatment of rheumatoid arthritis in the past three decades and has been shown in trials to be equivalent to gold in its efficacy, though similar and serious side-effects do occur. These include rashes, proteinuria which may progress to nephrotic syndrome, loss of taste (which is transient), nausea, anorexia and thrombocytopenia (rarely aplastic anaemia). Like gold its effect does not become apparent until 3–6 months after starting treatment. It has the advantage of being administered orally.

### Sulphasalazine

This drug, widely used in the treatment of inflammatory bowel disease, was originally introduced 50 years ago for the treatment of rheumatoid arthritis. However, it fell from favour and only recently with the successful conclusion of controlled comparative studies has it been used again. It is given orally in a dose of 0.5 g per day rising by monthly increments of 0.5 g to a maintenance dose of between 2 and 3 g per day. Although generally well tolerated, it can cause rashes, methaemoglobinaemia and occasionally bone marrow depression. It is degraded in the intestine to its two components, 5-aminosalicyclic acid and sulphapyridine. Whereas the former is not absorbed and is the active ingredient for treatment of ulcerative colitis, it has been shown that it is either the sulphapyridine which is absorbed or the intact molecule itself that is responsible for the improvement in rheumatoid arthritis. It is also responsible for most of the adverse affects.

### Chloroquine and hydroxychloroquine

These antimalarial drugs were introduced in the 1950s for rheumatoid arthritis. They have somewhat fallen out of favour owing to their propensity for causing retinal damage and should only be used if facilities are available for an ophthalmological examination at 6-monthly intervals.

### Methotrexate

Low dose methotrexate, 7.5–15 mg/week, has recently become very widely used having been originally successfully introduced for the treatment of psoriatic arthritis. Safety monitoring should include monthly blood counts and liver function tests. Patients on the drug should avoid alcohol.

### Immunosuppressive drugs

These include azathioprine, chlorambucil and cyclophosphamide. They are reserved for the treatment of serious arteritic complications because of their tendency to serious side effects, including bone marrow depression (page 607).

### Corticosteroids

Oral corticosteroids are now rarely used in the long-term treatment of rheumatoid arthritis owing to the cumulative side effects of osteoporosis, skin atrophy, peptic ulceration, steroid myopathy, steroid cataracts and suppression of the hypophyseal–pituitary–adrenal axis. If they are to be used at all, it should be at a low dose (e.g. 5–7.5 mg prednisolone daily). Alternative-day therapy is less harmful, particularly in children in whom suppression of growth is an additional hazard. Pulse steroid as 1 g prednisolone i.v. is advocated for the treatment of severe rheumatoid arthritis with arteritis. A single 100 mg i.m. dose of depot methyl prednisolone is helpful in tiding a patient over the induction period of disease-modifying drugs or over a flare in the disease.

### Synovectomy

Persistent refractory inflammation in a single joint may be treated by synovectomy – removal of the synovial membrane – by either medical or surgical means. In either case, relief of pain and stiffness and restoration of movement is achieved, although relapse may occur subsequently. Medical synovectomy is obtained by the intra-articular injection of a radioisotope (e.g. yttrium-90) in colloidal form. The isotope is taken up by the synovial cells and the membrane is thereby ablated by the ionizing radiation (β particles). This form of treatment is reserved for patients over the age of 45 because of the (largely theoretical) risk of oncogenesis.

Surgical synovectomy is the surgical excision of the synovial membrane as far as this is possible, and it is most widely used in the knee and small finger joints. Postoperative stiffness of the joint is a hazard, which usually responds to manipulation under anaesthetic and vigorous physiotherapy.

### Other surgical measures

Total joint destruction may be treated either by arthrodesis (still widely practised in the wrist, big toe and thumb joints), or total joint replacement in those joints where a satisfactory prosthesis is available. This is most successful in the hip joint where the Charnley type of low-friction arthroplasty (metal on plastic) is the most widely used. Many total knee protheses are now available and prostheses are available for the shoulder, elbow, ankle and the metacarpophalangeal and proximal interphalangeal joints of the hands. In other joints attempts at joint replacement have been less successful. The main problems of joint replacement are the complications of infection and/or loosening of the prosthesis which may require it to be removed. Subluxation of the cervical spine which causes cord compression requires cervical fusion.

## REHABILITATION

Total management of the patient with rheumatoid arthritis requires a team approach in which specialist medical and nursing skills are supplemented by those of the trained physiotherapist, occupational therapist, chiropodist/podiatrist and medical social worker. Careful assessment of the patient's ability to cope with daily living, together with monitoring of progress, enables realistic goals to be set for the patient to return to as full and as active a life as possible. Skills lost as a result of the ravages of the disease may be restored partly by retraining and partly by adapting the environment to the needs of the handicapped patient. Many devices and adaptations are available to assist in everyday tasks and to maintain independence. Both home and work environments need to be considered, and it is essential that the patient, his or her family and employer be put into the picture in order to achieve an optimal result (Table 20.4).

**Table 20.4** 'The team'.

| | |
|---|---|
| The patient | Nurse |
| General practitioner | Physiotherapist |
| Rheumatologist | Occupational therapist |
| Orthopaedic surgeon | Podiatrist/chiropodist |
| | Social worker |

# THE SERONEGATIVE SPONDARTHRITIDES

This group of chronic arthritic conditions is characterised by the absence of rheumatoid factor in the serum, the absence of nodules, a largely asymmetrical distribution of peripheral joint involvement, and a tendency towards bilateral sacroiliitis progressing, in some cases, to a picture of ankylosing spondylitis. The presence of spinal disease is commonly associated with the MHC antigen HLA B27 (page 84). Despite this important hereditary factor, the precise aetiological agent responsible for these diseases is as yet unknown.

## *Ankylosing spondylitis*

### AETIOLOGY AND PATHOLOGY

This disease predominantly affects young men and has a prevalence of approximately 1 per 1000 of the population. Recent epidemiological studies suggest that it may be considerably more common than this. This condition has a predilection for synovial joints of the vertebral column commencing in the sacroiliac joints and spreading cranially. Larger peripheral joints may also be affected. The MHC antigen HLA B27 is present in 90–95 per cent of cases compared with 5–10 per cent in the normal population. Recent evidence suggests that *Klebsiella pneumoniae* may be an important pathogen in this disease, but this is as yet unconfirmed. Although the synovial histopathological reaction is similar to that seen in rheumatoid arthritis, the tendency is for bony ankylosis to occur. Syndesmophytes or bony bridges form between ad-

jacent vertebrae and ultimately the facet joints, intervertebral discs and ligaments ossify, giving rise to the classical radiological appearance of the 'bamboo spine' (see below).

### CLINICAL FEATURES

Persistent low back pain with morning stiffness in the young adult male is the classical presentation. Imperceptible progressive loss of spinal movement occurs, with flattening of the lumbar spine, dorsal kyphosis and a compensatory cervical hyperlordosis (Fig. 20.9). Loss of chest expansion results from costovertebral joint involvement. As the spinal deformity develops the patient tends to adopt a hyperextension of the hips in order to maintain his centre of gravity. Symptoms may be so mild that the condition remains undiagnosed until advanced or it may be ascribed in error to intervertebral disc disease or psychogenic backache. On occasion the pain may be severe, particularly at night, waking the patient in the early hours. Pain and limitation of movement in the hip joints and shoulder and/or effusions in the knees indicate peripheral joint involvement which adds to the disability imposed by an increasingly rigid spine. Enthesopathies (tender lesions at the site of tendinous insertions, for example, plantar fasciitis) are common, and alternating sciatic pain may occur as well as discomfort around the thoracic cage.

A tendency to recurrent, acute iritis occurs in 20 per cent of cases. A normochromic, normocytic anaemia is common during active phases of the disease, which may be aggravated by gastrointestinal blood loss caused by NSAIDs.

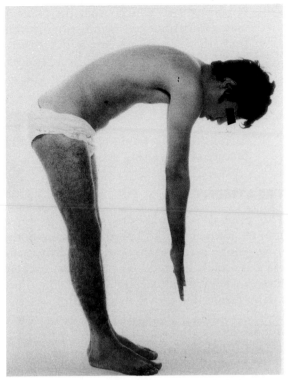

**Figure 20.9** Loss of spinal mobility in ankylosing spondylitis.

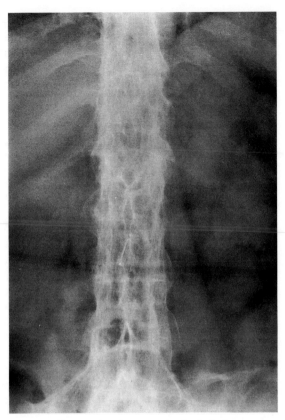

**Figure 20.10** The 'bamboo spine' of ankylosing spondylitis.

Amyloid deposition (see above) is said to occur in 6 per cent of patients coming to necropsy. Rare complications are cardiac involvement with conduction defects (e.g. complete heart block) and/or aortic regurgitation due to aortitis and bilateral upper lobe fibrosis of the lungs.

## DIAGNOSIS

The diagnosis is based on the clinical history and examination and is confirmed by the radiological appearance of the spine, notably the sacroiliac joints (blurring of the joint margins, sclerosis, erosion and ultimately ankylosis) and the vertebral bodies (formation of syndesmophytes, squaring of the vertebrae and ultimately the appearance of the 'bamboo spine', (Fig. 20.10). The erythrocyte sedimentation rate and serum C-reactive protein is raised while the disease remains active.

A quantitative radionuclide scintiscan is sometimes helpful in detecting sacroiliitis before the radiological changes have become established.

Ankylosing spondylitis can occur in subjects who do not have HLA B27, so that this test is of no value in establishing the diagnosis.

## TREATMENT

The aim is to relieve pain and stiffness by the application of non-steroidal anti-inflammatory drugs which permit the patient to take part in vigorous physiotherapy necessary to restore and maintain the spinal mobility and to prevent flexion deformity of the spine. The patient is encouraged to lie prone as much as possible and to practise mobilizing exercises daily for the rest of his life.

Evidence to date suggests that the disease-modifying drugs such as gold and penicillamine are ineffective. Corticosteroids are contraindicated owing to the risk of osteoporosis, and deep X-ray therapy (formerly used widely to relieve pain and stiffness) is no longer used owing to the increased risk of leukaemia. Total hip replacement is indicated in the presence of advanced hip joint destruction, and spinal osteotomy is occasionally used in the presence of severe spinal deformity. Acute iritis is treated along conventional lines by local corticosteroid drops and mydriatics.

# Psoriatic arthritis

## AETIOLOGY

Arthritis occurs some six to ten times more frequently in psoriatic patients than in controls. Psoriasis and psoriatic arthritis occur in 2 and 0.1 per cent of the population, respectively. It is slightly more common in males than in females. There is a strong genetic component with a raised frequency of B27, Cw6 and DR7.

## CLINICAL FEATURES

Arthritis associated with psoriasis may take one of the following forms:

1.  A widespread polyarthritis typically involving the distal interphalangeal joint (Fig. 20.11), the interphalangeal joint of the thumb and great toe as well as larger joints.
2.  A severe mutilating arthritis affecting the hands, causing widespread osteolysis as well as total destruction of the small finger joints.

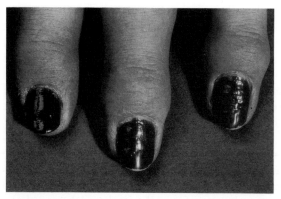

**Figure 20.11** Distal interphalangeal joint involvement in psoriatic arthropathy. Note the characteristic pitting of the nails.

3.  A polyarthritis which, from the point of view of distribution, is indistinguishable from that seen in rheumatoid arthritis. This is the most common variety. It does, however, pursue a more benign course, though erosions do occur. Rheumatoid nodules and rheumatoid factor are, of course, absent.
4.  Sacroiliitis progressing in many cases to a picture of ankylosing spondylitis.

## TREATMENT

The general principles are similar to those adopted for rheumatoid arthritis. Because of the more benign nature of the condition, drug treatment is usually limited to the NSAIDs. In more severe cases gold injections and low dose methotrexate (see above) may be effective, but D-penicillamine is ineffective and oral corticosteroids are rarely indicated.

# Reactive arthritis

## AETIOLOGY

This term denotes the development of arthritis in a patient suffering from an infective process elsewhere in the body (usually in the gastrointestinal or genital tracts), but without evidence of infection in the joint itself. It occurs almost exclusively in patients showing the MHC antigen HLA B27 who develop enteric infection with *Salmonella*, *Shigella*, *Yersinia* or *Campylobacter* organisms. It may also occur as sexually acquired reactive arthritis (SARA), and there is evidence to suggest that the offending organism here may be *Chlamydia trachomatis*. In most cases the symptoms settle spontaneously within 2 to 3 weeks.

# Reiter's syndrome

This was originally described as a triad of urethritis, conjuctivitis and arthritis, but it often presents additional features including balanitis circinata or sicca on the penis, keratoderma blenorrhagica (a pustular rash starting on the palms and soles), uveitis, aortitis, sacroiliitis and ankylosing spondylitis. It has long been known that Reiter's syndrome may complicate dysentery or sexually acquired non-specific urethritis, but living micro-organisms have never been isolated from the affected joints. For this reason Reiter's syndrome is now classified as a form of reactive arthritis.

Acute rheumatic fever can be considered as a form of reactive arthritis and is considered on page 189.

imately one-half of whom proceed to the full picture of ankylosing spondylitis. In these circumstances the activity and progression of the spinal disease appear to bear no temporal relationship to the activity of the underlying bowel condition.

Arthritis is also a feature in about 15 per cent of patients suffering from the multisystem disease that follows intestinal bypass surgery used as a treatment for obesity. The cause of the arthritis is believed to be due to immune complex deposition. Bacterial antigens of intestinal origin have been implicated.

# Arthritides associated with bowel disease

An inflammatory polyarthritis may occur in patients suffering from ulcerative colitis (page 365), Crohn's disease (page 362) and Whipple's disease (page 360). This tends to be a recurrent, acute or persistent affection of large, predominantly lower, limb joints. By and large, the activity of the arthritis mirrors that of the underlying intestinal disease. In addition some 18 per cent of patients suffering from inflammatory bowel disease will develop sacroiliitis, approx-

# Behçet's syndrome

A subacute or chronic, usually non-destructive, arthritis with a predilection for knee joint involvement, but with occasional involvement of the axial skeleton, is seen in association with buccal and genital ulceration, erythema nodosum, meningoencephalitis and uveitis in Behçet's syndrome. It is rare in the UK (1 in 200 000 prevalence) but commoner in Japan and the countries surrounding the Mediterranean. Skin, mucosal and joint symptoms respond to high-dose corticosteroids, uveitis to chlorambucil.

# *I*NFLAMMATORY DISORDERS OF CONNECTIVE TISSUE

The group of diseases included under this heading (formerly referred to as the collagen diseases) include systemic lupus erythematosus (SLE), vasculitis, dermatomyositis and polymyositis, and scleroderma (systemic sclerosis). The members of this group have a number of features in common, namely, abnormal immunological reactivity, multisystem involvement, a (variable) therapeutic response to corticosteroids, and a usually unremittant course. Syndromes which overlap the standard diagnostic categories also occur.

# Systemic lupus erythematosus

(See also page 460).

## AETIOLOGY

Systemic lupus erythematosus (SLE) is a multisystem disease with protean manifestations. It is nine times more common in women than in men, with an onset during the child-bearing years, though occasional onset during childhood or advanced age occurs. It appears to be much more common in Chinese and Blacks than Caucasians and a familial tendency is seen.

## AETIOLOGY AND PATHOGENESIS

The aetiology is unknown. Autoantibodies and high gammaglobulin levels suggest increased activity of B-lymphocytes. Immune complexes are found in the serum and deposit in the glomeruli and the junction of dermis and epidermis in the skin.

A wide variety of humoral antibodies is encountered in the serum. These include antinuclear antibodies directed against a variety of nuclear constituents, native double- and single-stranded DNA, DNA–histone, double-stranded nuclear ribonucleoprotein (RNP), two other RNP antigens, SS-A (previously called Ro) and SS-B (previously called La) and Sm antigen. In addition, both IgG and IgM rheumatoid factors and a biological false positive test for syphilis (BFP) are found in approximately one-third of patients. Serum complement levels (C3, C4 and total haemolytic complement) are lowered, particularly in the presence of renal involvement, and cryoglobulins and antibodies directed against erythrocytes (detected by the antiglobulin test), leukocytes, lymphocytes and platelets are widely seen. Antibodies against phospholipid (including anti-cardiolipin antibodies) result in circulating lupus anticoagulants. These cause a false positive serological test for syphilis (Venereal Disease Research Laboratory, VDRL) (page 760) in 10 per cent of patients and a tendency to thrombosis (page 647). In addition, there is also evidence of impaired cellular immunity in SLE resulting from an impairment of suppressor T-lymphocyte activity. A possible viral aetiology responsible for the immunological abnormalities is likely, but as yet no viral agent has been identified. An SLE-like illness occurs in some patients treated with drugs such as hydralazine, penicillamine, procainamide, practolol, insoniazid and anticonvulsants. In patients so afflicted renal involvement is rare and complete recovery is seen on withdrawal of the offending drug.

## CLINICAL FEATURES

See Table 20.5.

**Table 20.5** Clinical and laboratory findings in systemic lupus erythematosus (based on four large series totalling 365 patients).

| | % |
|---|---|
| Facial erythema (butterfly rash) | 40–65 |
| Discoid lupus | 20–30 |
| Raynaud's phenomenon | 20–44 |
| Alopecia | 40–70 |
| Photosensitivity | 17–41 |
| Oral or nasopharyngeal ulceration | 15–36 |
| Arthritis without deformity | 86–100 |
| Biological false positive test for syphilis | 8–26 |
| Proteinura >3.5 g/day | 16–25 |
| Cellular casts in urine | 16–48 |
| Pleurisy and/or pericarditis | 30–60 |
| Psychosis and/or convulsions | 16–20 |
| Haemolytic anaemia | 14–16 |
| Leukopenia <4.0 × $10^9$/dl | 40–54 |
| Thrombocytopenia <100 × $10^9$/dl | 11–14 |
| Venous or arterial thrombosis | 5–10 |

### General

Systemic lupus erythematosus is a chronic fluctuating disease which affects a large number of systems. Fever, malaise, anorexia and weight loss are common.

### Skin

The classical rash of SLE is the erythema seen typically in the butterfly region of the cheeks and bridge of the nose but also in areas exposed to ultraviolet light to which the skin in this condition is particularly sensitive. Other skin lesions include discoid lupus, urticaria, periungual erythema and cutaneous vasculitis. Alopecia is a frequent feature limited to SLE within this group of conditions.

### Joints

A symmetrical peripheral polyarthritis affecting predominantly small finger joints and reminiscent of rheumatoid arthritis is a common finding. Symptoms are often more severe than clinical findings. Ulnar deviation of the fingers may occur, but erosions are characteristically absent. Subcutaneous nodules are uncommon.

### Tenosynovitis

This may occur in the hands and is a common symptom.

## Aseptic necrosis

Aseptic necrosis of the femoral head (osteonecrosis) is a common finding even in the absence of corticosteroid treatment.

## Respiratory system

Pleurisy with effusion is common, and parenchymal pulmonary involvement (pneumonitis) may be seen. Diffuse pulmonary fibrosis is less common. Diaphragm weakness through myopathy may cause loss of lung volume.

## Cardiovascular system

Raynaud's phenonemon may be a presenting symptom. Pericarditis with effusion, myocarditis and verrucose (Libman–Sacks) endocarditis, cardiac failure, arrhythmias and conduction defects may all occur.

## Kidney (page 460)

Renal involvement occurs in most patients, although in only a half is it clinically significant. Four pathological types of lupus nephritis have been defined: focal proliferative (mild), diffuse proliferative (severe), membranous and mesangial (minimal). Presentation is with proteinuria which may be heavy and lead to nephrotic syndrome and be associated with hypertension and renal failure. Clues to the prognosis may be gleaned from renal biopsy, examined by immunohistology, light and electron microscopy.

## Haematopoietic and reticuloendothelial systems

Anaemia (usually normocytic but in 10 per cent of patients haemolytic), neutropenia and thrombocytopenia are common events and may be severe. Hepatosplenomegaly and lymphadenopathy are commonly seen. Thrombotic complications occur in association with the presence of anti-cardiolipin antibodies.

## Gastrointestinal tract

Sjögren's syndrome (dry eyes and dry mouth in association with rheumatoid arthritis or SLE) may be present, and abdominal pain and diarrhoea occasionally occur owing to intestinal arteritis, pancreatitis or peritonism. Mild elevations of liver enzyme occur but significant involvement of the liver does not occur. The formerly styled 'lupoid hepatitis', thought to be a feature of SLE, is now termed 'chronic active hepatitis' and considered to be a separate entity.

## Central nervous system

Brain involvement is now known to be one of the most common features, presenting as a neuropsychiatric disorder (e.g. depressive state), convulsions, hemiplegia, cranial and peripheral nerve lesions, cerebellar disorder or aseptic meningitis. Transverse myelitis may also occur. Conventional neurological investigations (angiography, brain and computed tomography, CT) are generally unhelpful. Electroencephalography may show a non-specific diffuse abnormality. By contrast, magnetic resonance imaging appears to be promising.

## Eyes

Retinal haemorrhages and exudates are common but major ocular disturbances are rare.

## Pregnancy

*Post-partum* exacerbations and spontaneous abortions, related to anti-phospholipid antibodies, are common in SLE. Congenital heart block is seen in infants born of mothers with SLE, especially those carrying serum anti-Ro (SS-A) antibodies.

## DIAGNOSIS

This is based on the clinical features discussed above. The anti-nuclear antibody (ANA) immunofluorescent test is positive in virtually all cases, although it is not specific for the disease (see above). The DNA binding test for double-stranded (native) DNA is a more specific indicator of SLE, although it may be negative during inactive phases of the disease. It may therefore be used as an index of disease activity, and in this context is a more reliable pointer than the erythrocyte sedimentation rate which is often markedly elevated in this condition.

## PROGNOSIS

There has been a remarkable improvement in the prognosis of this disease in recent years, due in part to the wider (and earlier) recognition of this condition, and in part to the greater restraint in the use of corticosteroids for treatment. The 5-year survival has virtually doubled in the last 25 years and is now over 90 per cent. Severe renal and neurological complications carry the poorest prognosis.

## TREATMENT

Non-steroidal anti-inflammatory drugs are valuable in treatment of articular complaints, while antimalarial drugs are also capable of suppressing the disease, particularly in those patients with skin and joint involvement. Severe manifestations are treated by oral corticosteroid, usually with immunosuppressive drugs (e.g. azathioprine or cyclophosphamide). The side effects of these drugs carry a morbidity and mortality, and they should be used with caution. In very ill patients, in whom a rapid response to treatment is sought, the steroids may be given intravenously in large doses (e.g. 0.5–1.0 g daily for 3 days) – known as pulse steroids – and plasma exchange can be used to remove the antibodies. Both these forms of treatment still require full evaluation.

# Vasculitis

Polyarteritis nodosa (PAN) is characterized by a necrotizing arteritis of small and medium-sized vessels. The aetiology is not yet understood. Hepatitis B antigen has been found in the serum and in the arteritic lesions, which suggests that serum hepatitis virus may be participating in the pathogenesis. The arteritic lesions are widely disseminated throughout the body and may lead to aneurysm formation, rupture and haemorrhage, thrombosis and ultimately recanalization. Variants are Wegener's granulomatosis (WG), a locally destructive arteritic lesion affecting the nasal passages and upper and lower respiratory tract and PAN which affects large arteries causing palpable swellings. Vasculitis is frequently associated with glomerulonephritis.

## CLINICAL FEATURES

Males predominate with an incidence rising with age. Features include fever, weight loss, hypertension, tachycardia, gangrene of the extremities, pneumonitis, an acute abdomen (due to mesenteric arteritis), proteinuria and renal failure, arthralgia and myalgia, cutaneous vasculitis and peripheral neuropathy of the mononeuritis multiplex type. In addition, focal brain and spinal cord involvement and ocular vascular accidents complete the truly protean nature of the disease. As any artery in the body can be affected, there are many other rare manifestations due to ischaemic infarction of other parts of the body.

## DIAGNOSIS

High titres of anti-neutrophil cytoplasmic antibodies (ANCA) may be found in the serum. Other serological tests such as the anti-nuclear antibody (ANA) and rheumatoid factor are usually negative. Confirmation is usually obtained histologically by skin, kidney or nerve biopsy. The lesions consist of lymphocytes within and surrounding the vessel wall with fibrinoid necrosis. They are not present along the entire length of the vessel so a normal portion of vessel may be seen. The absence of inflammatory change does not exclude the diagnosis. Hepatic or renal arteriography may reveal multiple small aneurysms which are said to be diagnostic of this condition (Fig. 20.12).

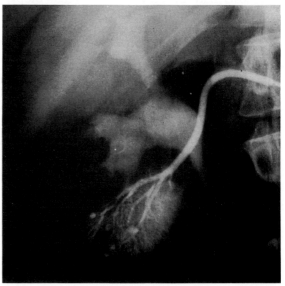

**Figure 20.12** Renal arteriogram in a patient suffering from vasculitis, showing the presence of multiple aneurysms.

## PROGNOSIS

This depends on the distribution of organ involvement. The survival rate is 80 per cent with treatment, compared with less than 15 per cent in untreated cases.

## TREATMENT

High-dose corticosteroids (prednisolone, 40–50 mg daily) are generally recommended initially with a view to slowly reducing and eventually withdrawing the drug in the light of the subsequent progress. Immunosuppressive drugs, for example, cyclophosphamide or azathioprine 2 mg/kg/day are also used. Severely ill patients may be treated with pulse steroids, intravenous cyclophosphamide and plasma exchange.

As organ damage can progress very rapidly, for example, to end-stage renal failure in a matter of days, it is important to initiate treatment swiftly. It may be appropriate to treat on clinical grounds alone, before diagnostic tests are completed.

# Giant cell (temporal) arteritis

## PATHOLOGY AND AETIOLOGY

This is a granulomatous form of arteritis affecting predominantly the branches of the external carotid artery, notably the temporal and facial arteries, and certain branches, notably the ophthalmic, of the internal carotid artery. Only occasionally are arteries emanating from the aorta (e.g. coronary arteries) involved. A possible immunological mechanism has been suggested by the finding of increased cellular immune responses by lymphocytes from patients with the condition to constituents of the arterial wall. The condition is predominantly seen in middle and old age. No consistent relationship has been observed with HLA-A, B- or C- antigens, although an association with DR4 has been recorded.

## CLINICAL FEATURES

The common presentation is with pain in the head and face due to ischaemia, and intermittent claudication of the muscles of mastication has been reported. The temporal arteries are characteristically thickened, tender and pulseless, and the overlying scalp may be reddened and occasionally frankly gangrenous. Other modes of presentation include sudden visual failure owing to ophthalmic artery thrombosis, polymyalgia rheumatica (page 586), pyrexia of unknown origin, anaemia or high ESR for no obvious reason.

## DIAGNOSIS

The erythrocyte sedimentation rate is invariably elevated, often markedly so. Since the arteritis may be distributed patchily, the temporal arteries may be normal on palpation, and where doubt exists it is prudent to perform a temporal artery biopsy. The characteristic features are thickening of the media with infiltration by inflammatory cells, including giant cells, and intimal proliferation leading to gross narrowing of the lumen. The condition should be suspected in particular in elderly patients suffering from (often vague) headaches or rheumatic symptoms in the presence of a raised ESR.

## TREATMENT

Oral corticosteroid treatment is indicated as soon as the diagnosis is made in order to prevent blindness, since this is irreversible. Prednisolone, 40–60 mg a day, may be required to bring the condition under control, the dose being tapered in response to the fall in the erythrocyte sedimentation rate. Steroids taken for 1–3 days do not effect the biopsy appearances. Long-term surveillance is essential if relapse is to be avoided. The condition may remain active for months or years.

# Other forms of necrotizing arteritis

## RHEUMATOID VASCULITIS

Manifestations of necrotizing arteritis indistinguishable from those seen in vasculitis are encountered in rheumatoid disease which enters a 'polyarteritic' or 'malignant' phase.

## HYPERSENSITIVITY ANGIITIS

In this group of conditions, small blood vessels are infiltrated with polymorphonuclear leukocytes with destruction of the vessel wall. Such changes are seen in Henoch–Schönlein purpura, cryoglobulinaemia, serum sickness, as well as vasculitis seen in association with Sjögren's syndrome, hypergammaglobulinaemic purpura, chronic active hepatitis, ulcerative colitis and primary biliary cirrhosis.

## CHURG–STRAUSS VASCULITIS (ALLERGIC GRANULOMATOSIS)

The association of vasculitis with asthma, eosinophilia and extravascular granulomas is known as Churg–Strauss vasculitis. It is a rare syndrome, more common in males. The cause is unknown. Small granulomas with eosinophilic centres are seen in the small arteries and veins. Vasculitis and granulomas are seen similarly through the viscera including liver, spleen, kidney and lymph nodes. Cardiac involvement is common and the treatment of choice is high-dose corticosteroids.

## LYMPHOMATOID GRANULOMATOSIS

This is a rare disease of unknown aetiology. There is widespread evidence of vasculitic infiltration about the major viscera, and a high proportion progress to malignant lymphoma.

## TAKAYASU'S DISEASE

In this condition (otherwise known as 'pulseless disease') which affects mainly children and young women, the aorta, its branches and other main vessels are involved in an arteritic process which leads to thickening of the arterial wall and progresses to occlusion. The media is infiltrated with lymphocytes and plasma cells and the intima is proliferated. Its highest incidence is in the Indian subcontinent and in Japanese subjects who show an association with HLA BW 52 implying an important hereditary component. Clinical features depend on the pattern of arteritic narrowing or occlusion. In its early stages the disease may be reversed by treatment with corticosteroids.

## KAWASAKI'S DISEASE (MUCOCUTANEOUS LYMPH-NODE SYNDROME)

This is mainly seen in infants and consists of fever, conjunctivitis, erythema in the mouth and on the palms and soles, and lymphoedema. Ischaemic heart disease may occur also.

## ERYTHEMA NODOSUM

This term is given to the presence of raised, red, tender lumps on the surfaces of the lower legs which are thought to represent a hypersensitivity reaction to a variety of agents, including infection (e.g. tuberculosis, *Streptococcus*, *Yersinia*, leptospirosis, psittacosis, certain mycotic infections), drugs (e.g. halides, oral contraceptives and sulphonamides) and other conditions (e.g. sarcoidosis, ulcerative colitis and Crohn's disease). There is a self-limiting symmetrical arthritis notably affecting the knees and ankles. Treatment is with NSAIDs. Occasional courses of corticosteroids may be required. Essentially the management is that of the underlying condition.

## SUBACUTE NON-MIGRATORY PANNICULITIS

This is a variant of erythema nodosum and occurs primarily in Caucasian females between the ages of 50 and 60. Individual lesions spread to considerable size and show central clearing. The aetiology is unknown and the prognosis is excellent. Treatment is symptomatic.

# Scleroderma (systemic sclerosis)

This uncommon condition is characterized by an excessive deposit of collagen in the dermis and viscera (notably the gastrointestinal tract), together with a small-vessel arteritis involving, in particular, the extremities.

## AETIOLOGY

The cause is unknown. The finding of auto-antibodies such as anti-nuclear antibodies which include a very specific antibody to a nuclear protein SCl 70, and altered cellular immunity all suggest a possible immunopathogenetic mechanism.

## CLINICAL FEATURES

Scleroderma is three times more common in women than in men. The onset, usually at 30–50 years of age, is often insidious and Raynaud's phenomenon may antedate other symptoms by several years. Pain and stiffness in the small joints and tendon sheaths are common early symptoms. Gradually the skin of the distal extremities becomes thickened, tethered and rigid, inhibiting movement. This process gradually extends proximally and may envelop the whole body. Puckering of the mouth leads to a characteristic appearance. Calcinotic nodules appear over the fingertips and pressure areas. Telangiectasia are seen on the skin of the extremities, face and on the tongue (Fig. 20.13). Joint and tendon-sheath involvement causes pain and additional stiffness and flexion deformities of the fingers. A palpable crepitus is a feature of tenosynovitis of the wrist. Tapering of the fingers is due to osteolysis occasioned by ischaemia. Muscle involvement also commonly occurs although this may be mild.

Gastrointestinal involvement occurs in 70 per cent of patients. The most common manifestation is in the oesophagus, where there is loss of peristalsis, acid reflux and stricture formation, resulting in dysphagia, which may be severe.

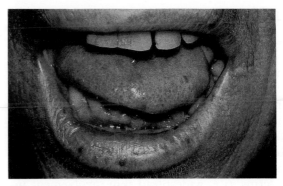

**Figure 20.13** Puckering of the mouth in a patient suffering from systemic sclerosis. Note the presence of telangiectasia on the tongue and lips.

Recurrent aspiration may occur. Small bowel involvement gives rise to malabsorption, which may be aggravated by bacterial overgrowth. A rare complication is the presence of collections of gas in the intestinal wall (pneumatosis intestinalis). Coexistent primary biliary cirrhosis or chronic active hepatitis may be seen. Colonic involvement is common but usually asymptomatic. Occasionally distension or perforation may occur.

Pulmonary fibrosis is common, although it may be asymptomatic in the initial stages. Pulmonary vascular disease and pulmonary hypertension also occur. In the heart, pericarditis and myocardial fibrosis may be present. A variety of ECG changes is seen, including arrhythmias and heart block. Frank renal involvement tends to lead to a rapidly progressive spiral of hypertension and renal failure. Central nervous system involvement does not occur but trigeminal neuropathy has been described. Sjögren's syndrome may occur in association with scleroderma.

## DIAGNOSIS

Characteristic changes in the skin biopsy include increased dermal collagen, a thinning of the epidermis and a loss of the normal appendages. Anti-nuclear antibody is present in over 50 per cent, and anti-Scl 70 in 25 per cent of patients. The ESR is raised in two-thirds of patients, while one-third give a positive test for rheumatoid factor.

## PROGNOSIS

In the absence of major organ involvement, scleroderma may pursue a relatively benign, though usually progressive course. Over 70 per cent of patients survive for 5 years. In the presence of lung, but no heart or kidney involvement, or heart but no kidney involvement, the corresponding figures are 50 and 30 per cent. Renal involvement indicates a survival of less than 1 year without dialysis. 'Diffuse scleroderma' (i.e. widespread skin involvement including the trunk) is usually associated with major organ involvement and a poorer prognosis, whereas the **CREST** syndrome (Calcinosis, Raynaud's phenomenon, Oesophageal involvement, Sclerodactyly and Telangiectasia) carries a more favourable outlook. It has recently been shown that anti-centromere antibodies are common in this subgroup.

## TREATMENT

There is no really effective treatment for this disorder. D-Penicillamine has been used and may be helpful with regard to the skin condition if instituted early. Corticosteroids are of little benefit except in relieving the rheumatic symptoms, which are probably better treated by NSAIDs. Raynaud's phenomenon and digital ischaemia have been treated by intra-arterial reserpine and a variety of other vasoactive drugs (e.g. nifedipine) but with limited success. The use of infusions of commercially available prostacyclin is currently under investigation. Cervical sympathectomy, plasmapheresis and hyperbaric oxygen give only limited and transient relief. Cardiac, pulmonary, renal and gastrointestinal symptoms are treated on their own merits along conventional lines. Hands and feet should be carefully protected in cold weather.

## VARIANTS OF SCLERODERMA

### Eosinophilic fasciitis

In this condition, which affects mainly young males, thickening of the skin occurs in the extremities in the absence of Raynaud's phenomenon. Visceral abnormality does not occur, but eosinophilia (up to 50 per cent of granulocytes) is seen with hypergammaglobulinaemia and elevated immunoglobulin levels. Biopsy of the skin shows a mononuclear infiltration, often with eosinophils, which affects the deep fascia producing dense fibrosis.

### Scleredema

This is a rare self-limiting condition which follows bacterial infection. It, too, is not associated with Raynaud's phenomenon or visceral involvement and carries a good prognosis.

### Toxic-oil syndrome

Scleroderma-like skin changes were seen in the chronic phase of the epidemic of poisoning which occurred in Spain in 1981 resulting from the adulteration of rapeseed oil. Severe respiratory symptoms and muscle weakness, fatal in many cases, were also seen. A noteworthy feature was the increased frequency of the haplotype HLA DR3–4 in these patients.

### Morphoea

This is a localized form of scleroderma of the skin which only rarely progresses to systemic sclerosis.

# Dermatomyositis and polymyositis

## CLINICAL FEATURES

These are inflammatory disorders of striated muscle of unknown aetiology, which present with weakness of the limbs and trunk, respiratory difficulties, dysphagia and diplopia. The term dermatomyositis denotes muscle and skin involvement, notably the heliotrope discolouration around the eyelids, periungual erythema, and an inflammatory oedema of the skin causing induration and later atrophy, collodion patches (atrophic lesions over the knuckles also known as Gottron's papules) and subcutaneous calcinosis (Fig. 20.14). Other features include Raynaud's phenomenon, arthralgia and arthritis, cardiac failure, and occasionally pulmonary fibrosis. An association between malignancy and both dermatomyositis and polymyositis is generally

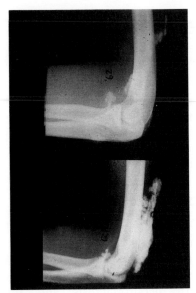

**Figure 20.14** Subcutaneous calcinosis in a patient suffering from dermatomyositis. Note the partial disappearance of the subcutaneous calcinotic deposits which has occurred spontaneously over a 3-year period.

accepted (incidence 15–20 per cent in dermatomyositis, 2–3 per cent in polymyositis). Carcinoma of the lung, prostate, uterus, ovary, breast and large bowel are the most common tumours. There is a juvenile form which presents at 5–14 years and is not associated with malignancy.

## DIAGNOSIS

This is confirmed by typical electromyographic (EMG) changes and on muscle biopsy by histological evidence of degeneration of muscle fibres, regeneration and chronic inflammatory infiltration. The serum creatine phosphokinase is elevated. The ESR may be mildly elevated or normal in the presence of active disease, and serological tests may reveal the presence of Jo-1 antibody (directed against histidyl-tRNA synthetase).

## TREATMENT

Oral corticosteroids (prednisolone, 40–60 mg, daily initially) are used to suppress the disease and are usually effective. The addition of methotrexate, azathioprine or cyclophosphamide may be helpful in resistant cases. During acute phases the patient is treated with bedrest with appropriate splinting to avoid contractures and deformities. Even in the absence of an associated malignancy the prognosis may be poor, particularly in older subjects with heart or lung complications. Overall the 5-year survival rate is 70 per cent.

# Overlap syndrome

Not infrequently, clinical features of two or more of the inflammatory disorders of connective tissue are seen in the same patient, causing diagnostic difficulty. A particular subset, called 'mixed connective tissue disease' (MCTD) has been identified by the presence in the serum of antibodies to extractable nuclear antigen (ribonucleoprotein (RNP) component). Testing for anti-nuclear antibody shows a speckled pattern. There may be features of SLE, polymyositis, scleroderma and rheumatoid arthritis. The commonest symptoms are joint pains, Raynaud's phenomenon, swollen hands, myositis, oesophageal problems and lymphadenopathy. Pulmonary, cardiac and neurological complications occur. Treatment relies on non-steroidal anti-inflammatory drugs, with corticosteroids and immunosuppressive drugs used in severe cases. Some patients have full remission, others remain clinically affected requiring long-term treatment. Mixed connective tissue disease is generally not responsive to steroids and claims that it carried a better prognosis have not been borne out.

# METABOLIC ARTHRITIS, GOUT, PSEUDOGOUT AND OCHRONOSIS

Acute synovitis may be provoked by the liberation into the joint cavity of microcrystals — monosodium urate monohydrate in the case of gout and calcium pyrophosphate dihydrate in pseudogout.

# Gout

The peak age of onset of gout is in the fifth decade and 90 per cent of sufferers are male. When females develop gout it is usually postmenopausal. Gout is associated with hyperuricaemia, but only occurs in one-third of those with a raised uric acid level. There is an association with obesity, hypertension, high alcohol consumption, hyperlipidaemia, coronary artery disease and a family history of gout. Other conditions in which hyperuricaemia is seen include lead poisoning, toxaemia of pregnancy, starvation, hyperparathyroidism and hypothyroidism.

## AETIOLOGY

The concentration of urate in plasma and body fluids represents a fine balance between production and excretion. Owing to the limited solubility of urate, its accumulation leads to precipitation of crystals, particularly in joints, subcutaneous tissues and in the renal collecting system. This may arise as a result of increased *de novo* purine synthesis from excessive intake of high purine foods, or from excessive catabolism of nucleoproteins as occurs in the myeloproliferative disorders, leukaemia, myeloma and polycythemia rubra vera (secondary hyperuricaemia) particularly when these conditions are treated by cytotoxic agents (tumour lysis syndrome). Failure of the kidney to excrete urate, as in renal failure, or tubular retention of urate, as occurs with certain drugs (e.g. oral diuretics and pyrazinamide), also results in accumulation.

Only in very rare instances can the increased *de novo* synthesis be ascribed to an hereditary enzyme deficiency (hypoxanthine-guanine-phosphoribosyl transferase, HGPRTase) in the case of the Lesch–Nyhan syndrome).

## PATHOLOGY

Urate deposits are seen as tophi in and around joints and bursae, in cartilage such as the pinnae, over bony prominences and (rarely) in the kidney. Renal changes are those of hypertension with nephrosclerosis and interstitial nephritis. Urate calculi may be seen in 8 per cent of patients.

## CLINICAL FEATURES

An intense self-limiting attack of acute arthritis favouring the first metatarsophalangeal joints is the classical presentation of gout. The joint is hot, swollen and tender with reddened overlying skin. Other joints such as the knee, ankle and hand joints may also be affected. The attacks may be associated with pyrexia, leukocytosis and an elevated erythrocyte sedimentation rate. Spontaneous remission (if the attack has not been aborted by medical treatment) occurs within a week in most patients, though a migratory polyarthritis is sometimes seen. The natural history is for recurrent acute attacks to occur with increasing frequency, and eventually a chronic deforming arthropathy may result from tophus formation. Tophi may discharge releasing a chalky material, composed of urate crystals, which are readily identified as such by microscopic examination or chemical analysis. Hypertension and renal impairment due to gout can cause renal failure.

## DIAGNOSIS

Clinical diagnosis is confirmed by the finding of hyperuricaemia and the identification of urate crystals, seen on polarizing microscopy as negatively birefringent needles within synovial fluid

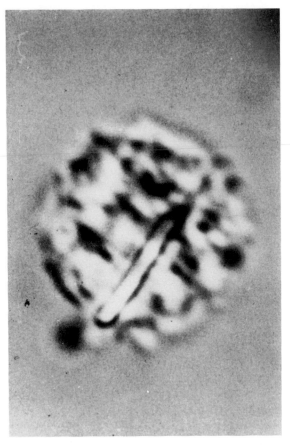

**Figure 20.15** Intraleukocytic polymorph containing a needle-shaped urate crystal diagnostic of classical (urate) gout as seen on polarizing microscopy.

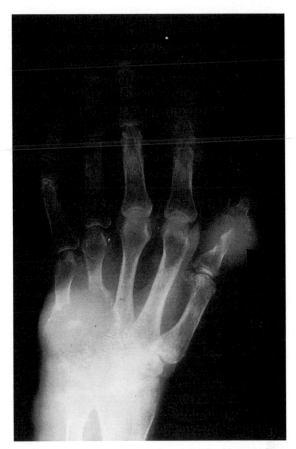

**Figure 20.16** Severe tophaceous gout. Note the destructive changes affecting the interphalangeal joint of the thumb, the distal interphalangeal joint and distal phalanx of the fingers and the bases of the 4th and 5th metacarpal bones and adjacent carpals. These changes are due to the deposition of urate crystals (tophi).

polymorphs (Fig. 20.15). X-rays are normal in the early stages, but eventually punched-out areas caused by the tophi are seen in relation to the chronically affected joints (Fig. 20.16).

## TREATMENT

Acute gouty episodes respond to oral colchicine (0.5 mg 4 hourly until relief or diarrhoea ensues) or full doses of indomethacin. The newer NSAIDs (e.g. naproxen, fenoprofen, ibuprofen or piroxicam) constitute a promising and better-tolerated alternative. An intra-articular steroid injection often aborts an attack. Systemic steroids are reserved only for the most intractable cases. In the face of recurrent acute attacks it is justified to institute hypouricaemic drugs, probenecid or sulphinpyrazone, which are uricosuric agents promoting the excretion of urate, or allopurinol which is a xanthine–oxidase inhibitor which curtails urate synthesis by blocking the last stage of the pathway. All these drugs require to be taken indefinitely and compliance may be a problem. Their institution may result in a temporary exacerbation of acute attacks during the first few months and it is wise, therefore, to cover this period by the concurrent administration of an anti-inflammatory drug. Allopurinol is the drug of choice in the presence of renal failure, renal stone or overproduction of uric acid, particularly when cytotoxic drugs are used to treat malignant disease. The usual daily dose is 300 mg but is adjusted in response to serum urate level.

Smaller doses are required in patients with renal failure because allopurinol is renally excreted and accumulation causes bone marrow suppression. Asymptomatic hyperuricaemia in chronic renal failure does not require treatment.

# Pseudogout (pyrophosphate arthropathy)

## AETIOLOGY

This disorder is principally seen in elderly subjects and is rarely encountered in early life. It occurs as a result of calcium pyrophosphate dihydrate ($CaP_2O_7 + 2H_2O$) crystal deposition in cartilage (**chondrocalcinosis**) which in most patients appears to be a feature of ageing of cartilage. In a few patients it is a manifestation of a metabolic disorder (e.g. hyperparathyroidism or haemochromatosis). A familial variety has been recorded.

## CLINICAL FEATURES

Recurrent acute episodes of arthritis occur predominantly in the larger joints (knee, wrist etc.) resembling urate gout, and following a similarly self-limiting course. The average duration of attack is 9 days. Precipitating factors include trauma, surgical operations or other acute illnesses. Occasionally polyarticular involvement occurs and a destructive arthropathy resembling either rheumatoid or osteoarthritis may be seen.

## DIAGNOSIS

The erythrocyte sedimentation rate may be elevated during an attack but other blood investigations are normal (except when there is an associated metabolic disorder). Plain radiographs will reveal fine stippling of chondrocalcinosis seen in the fibrocartilaginous menisci of the knee or wrist joints, or as a fine line within the articular cartilage of involved joints. Chondrocalcinosis is a common finding in elderly subjects, only a small percentage of whom suffer from pseudogout. It should not be assumed therefore, that the presence of chondrocalcinosis is pathognomonic of pseudogout. Confirmation of this diagnosis can only be made satisfactorily by identifying the intraleukocyte crystals of calcium pyrophosphate on polarizing microscopic examination of synovial fluid aspirated from an affected joint. These crystals (unlike those of gout) are oblong in shape and are weakly positively birefringent.

## TREATMENT

Acute attacks are treated by resting the affected joint and by the administration of NSAIDs. An intra-articular steroid injection is helpful in aborting an attack. There is no known means whereby the deposited articular calcification can be removed or recurrence prevented. Even treatment of an associated metabolic disorder (e.g. removing a parathyroid adenoma in hyperparathyroidism or venesection in haemochromatosis) fails to halt the (albeit slow) progression of the chondrocalcinosis.

# Hydroxyapatite arthropathy

Another crystal capable of inciting an inflammatory reaction in and around joints is hydroxyapatite. Examples of this phenomenon include calcific tendinitis of the shoulder (see below), and a particularly destructive form of arthropathy known as the 'Milwaukee shoulder' associated with the presence of large quantities of collagenase and neutral proteinase within the synovial fluid. The role of hydroxyapatite crystals in the pathogenesis of inflammation in osteoarthritis generally remains controversial.

# Ochronosis (alkaptonuria)

The inborn error of metabolism allows accumulation of homogentisic acid in cartilage. The resultant premature degeneration of cartilage results in destructive changes in the inter-vertebral discs and larger peripheral joints. The disc spaces become extremely narrowed, with sclerosis of vertebral plates. The result is a severe loss of spinal movement. In the peripheral joints the features are those of severe osteoarthritis. Urine turns black on standing or addition of alkali and the diagnosis is confirmed by the detection of homogentisic acid in the urine. Treatment is of the resulting osteoarthritis.

# *I*NFECTIVE ARTHRITIS

Invasion of a synovial joint by pathogenic micro-organisms occurs in a wide variety of infections caused by bacteria, viruses and fungi. For practical purposes, the most important infections are those due to pyogenic bacteria, including *Staphylococcus, Streptococcus, Gonococcus, Meningococcus, Pneumococcus, Escherichia coli, Salmonella, Haemophilus, Brucella* and *Mycobacterium tuberculosis*.

Spread to the joint is usually via the blood stream, although direct invasion may occur from adjacent osteomyelitis, or when organisms are inadvertently introduced into the joint during an aspiration procedure or a surgical operation. Predisposing factors include the presence of debilitating illness (diabetes, alcoholism, uraemia, malignant disease) or treatment with steroid or immunosuppressive agents.

# Bacterial arthritis

Involvement of one or more joints may arise in the presence of bacteraemia in the course of an infection from a wide variety of bacteria (see above). A focus of infection elsewhere in the body would be an important clue to this diagnosis. However, any patient with an acute monoarthritis should be suspected of suffering from bacterial arthritis, particularly in the presence of unexplained fever until proved otherwise. Bacterial endocarditis may present with this manifestation. Rheumatoid arthritis sufferers are particularly prone to secondary bacterial joint infection.

The only way to confirm (or exclude) this diagnosis with certainty is to obtain a sample of synovial fluid by aspiration of the affected joint and submit it to full bacteriological examination, including Gram staining of the smear and culture. This procedure has the added advantage of permitting antibiotic sensitivity testing to be undertaken and correct therapy to be instituted. Undiagnosed (and therefore untreated) bacterial arthritis may rapidly lead to total destruction of the joint – a tragedy in a condition so readily amenable to treatment.

In gonococcal arthritis a febrile illness is seen, particularly in female subjects presenting with fever and oligoarthritis, or migratory poly-arthritis, and tenosynovitis in association with a widespread skin eruption composed of macules, petechiae, vesicles or pustules.

Though arthralgia is a common event in brucellosis, a true arthritis, usually monoarticular, and favouring the hip or knee joint is seen. Spondylitis may also occur.

Tuberculous infection frequently occurs in bone, notably the spine, where it may give rise to serious destructive changes and compression of the spinal cord (Pott's disease). Peripheral joint involvement may also occur, particularly in the knee or hip with pain and gradual loss of mobility. Severe destructive changes are seen on X-ray. Other manifestations include tenosynovitis, particularly involving the flexor tendon sheaths at the wrist, and tuberculous dactylitis which presents as a painless swelling in relation to a metatarsal or metacarpal bone.

Arthritis is a prominent feature of Lyme disease (page 751), caused by the spirochaete *Bor-*

relia burgdorferi and transmitted by a tick *Ixodes ricinus* which lives mainly on deer. Suggestive clues to this diagnosis would be a recent tick bite, visiting an endemic area such as the New Forest in the UK or the eastern USA or the presence of erythema chronica migrans. Anti-Borrelia antibodies are helpful in diagnosis.

# Viral infections

A symmetrical self-limiting polyarthritis occurs in rubella at about the time that the rash develops, and it is particularly common in young, adult female subjects suffering from this condition. A similar complication is seen after rubella immunization with live attenuated virus. Acute polyarthritis may occur in human parvovirus infection, accompanied by fever, rash and lymphadenopathy. Arthritis is occasionally seen in other viral infections such as mumps, chicken-pox, smallpox, infectious mononucleosis and infective hepatitis. In some of these conditions the arthritis is due to the presence of live virus within the joint, while in others it appears to be due to the deposition of immune complexes.

## TREATMENT OF INFECTIVE ARTHRITIS

Treatment will depend on identifying the pre-cise aetiological agent involved, and no amount of effort should be spared to this end. It is important that specimens for bacteriological culture should be sent immediately on suspicion of the diagnosis and before antibiotic treatment is instituted, otherwise negative cultures will result, confusing the issue. Bacterial arthritis is a medical emergency and needs to be handled as such. Antibiotic therapy with broad-spectrum drugs (e.g. erythromycin and fucidin given intravenously) is instituted as soon as synovial fluid and blood have been sent to the laboratory for culture pending the result of antibiotic sensitivity testing. The joint should be treated by splinting and anti-inflammatory analgesic drugs prescribed as appropriate. Full parenteral antibiotic therapy obviates the need for intra-articular installation of antibiotics, though daily aspiration of the joint should be performed to remove accumulated purulent exudate. As the bacterial inflammation subsides the joint may be gently mobilized, although antibiotic therapy should be continued for 6–12 weeks depending on the severity of the condition. Surgical drainage is performed for bacterial arthritis only when medical treatment fails. Tuberculous infection in bone and joint (which can only be confirmed by histological and bacteriological examination of biopsy material) is treated by antituberculous drugs (page 302). Lyme disease usually responds well to antibiotic therapy with either penicillin or ceftriaxone.

# DEGENERATIVE JOINT DISEASES (OSTEOARTHRITIS, SPONDYLOSIS)

## AETIOLOGY

These common conditions result from degeneration of cartilage, both articular cartilage in synovial joints and fibrocartilage in the intervertebral discs. The prevalence increases sharply with advancing age, but other factors, notably previous fracture in relation to a joint, recurrent dislocation, occupational overuse, previous joint or spinal diseases whether congenital or acquired, are important. Hereditary factors may also play an important aetiological role. Epi-demic forms due to unidentified environmental agents also occur (e.g. Kashin–Beck disease in Siberia and China, and Mseleni disease in South Africa).

Where five or more joints are involved the term 'generalized osteoarthritis' is used. One particular variety, in which Heberden's nodes (Fig. 20.17) are a common feature, shows a strong hereditary tendency, tending to present chiefly in females at around the time of the menopause.

## PATHOLOGY

The primary event in osteoarthritis is believed to be a break-up in the articular cartilage. There is increased proteoglycan synthesis, but this is believed to be a compensatory response to the degradation of cartilage by enzymatic breakdown of proteoglycans by neutral proteinases and collagenase.

## CLINICAL FEATURES

Osteoarthritis is suspected in any middle-aged or elderly patient who presents with pain, stiffness and deformity of one or more joints in the absence of symptoms and signs of inflammation. Commonly involved joints are the distal interphalangeal and proximal interphalangeal joint of the hands (with bony deformities known as the **Heberden** and **Bouchard** nodes, respectively; Fig. 20.17), the first carpometacarpal joint at the base of the thumb, ankle and metatarsophalangeal joint of the great toe. Hip involvement causes a limp and difficulty in climbing stairs, and examination reveals limitation of passive movement, notably rotation. Knee involvement gives rise to pain on walking and difficulty with stairs and may be recognized by crepitus on passive movement, deformity (genu varum) and loss of joint range, both flexion and extension. Quadriceps wasting is usually evident and an effusion may be present, although this is usually small. A Baker's cyst may be present (page 563). Cervical spondylosis may cause local pain and restriction of movement of the neck; pain, paraesthesiae and weakness in the upper limb due to cervical nerve root compression by osteophytes, (rarely) cord compression known as cervical myelopathy; or brain stem ischaemia due to vertebral artery compression. Dorsal spine involvement is usually asymptomatic but may give rise to local pain or referred pain radiating around the side of the chest. The lumbar spine is particularly vulnerable to acute and chronic trauma occasioned by lifting, bending etc. Prolapse of a lumbar intervertebral disc is a common disorder affecting adults of both sexes. Herniation of the nucleus pulposus through a rent in the annulus fibrosis may compress one or more of the nerve roots constituting the cauda equina. The clinical

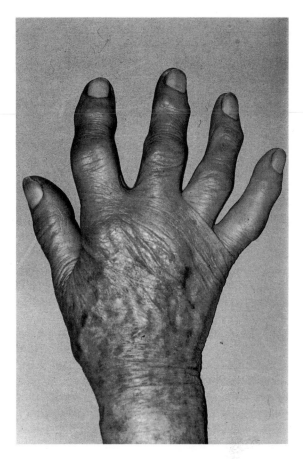

**Figure 20.17** Polyarticular (generalized) osteoarthritis with bony swelling and deformity affecting the distal (Heberden node) and proximal (Bouchard nodes) interphalangeal joints of the hand. Because of its polyarticular pattern, this condition is commonly misdiagnosed as rheumatoid arthritis.

picture is one of acute lumbar pain after strenuous activity, inability to move the spine followed by pain down the leg in the distribution of either the femoral or sciatic nerve on tension (femoral nerve stretch test and reduced straight leg raising test, respectively). An associated neurological deficit may be present, and cauda equina compression may occur. Causes of acute lumbar pain in the absence of evidence of nerve root compression include a central disc prolapse, facet joint dysfunction, muscle and ligamentous injury, vertebral fracture due to trauma or secondary to infective, metabolic or neoplastic disease of the bones, spondylolysis or spondylolisthesis, as well as visceral causes. Chronic low back pain is a serious problem both in human and economic terms. Any of the above mentioned causes may participate and there may be a strong pyschogenic element. The syndrome of 'intermittent claudication of the cauda equina' in which symptoms of lumbar nerve root compression are brought on by exercise is due to further reduction in the capacity of the vertebral canal, for example, disc protrusion in those with a congenitally small canal (spinal stenosis).

## DIAGNOSIS

This is usually made on clinical grounds. Evidence of systemic disease is absent and blood tests are usually normal. Radiological appearances are characteristic and include narrowing of the joint space. Subchondral sclerosis and loss of the normal joint contour and the presence of osteophytes. Such changes may, however, be present in asymptomatic individuals and undue importance should not be placed on their finding in the absence of appropriate clinical features. In spondylosis confirmatory evidence of cord and/or nerve root compression may be found using contrast radiculography, myelography, computed tomography (CT) or magnetic resonance imaging (MRI).

## TREATMENT

There is no known way of halting the progress of this condition. Painful episodes may be treated by short courses of NSAIDs or analgesics coupled with physiotherapy in the form of heat and exercises, hydrotherapy or gentle manipulation. Intra-articular injections of corticosteroids are generally not indicated except in the presence of a joint effusion. Compression of nerve roots should be treated by immobilization, with a collar in the case of cervical spine or with bedrest in an acute lumbar intervertebral disc prolapse.

Most episodes of acute low back pain (including that associated with acute disc prolapse) respond to a short period of complete bedrest lasting from a few days to a week. Patients should be on a firm mattress or should use a board under a poorly supported mattress. Some patients prefer to lie directly on the floor! The patient is allowed up to use the toilet but should remain flat at other times. With this regime, the majority of the lesions will remit. However, patients with persistent referred pain with or without neurological signs may benefit from epidural corticosteroid injections or, failing that, discectomy. Preoperative investigations include the performance of either a radiculogram using a water-soluble contrast medium, CT or MRI of the lower lumbar region. Worsening neurological signs, in particular, evidence of an acute cauda equina compression with difficulty in micturition and defaecation, need urgent neurosurgical consultation and possible decompression.

Advanced osteoarthritis affecting the hip or knee joint may be satisfactorily treated by total joint replacement.

# NON-ARTICULAR RHEUMATIC DISORDERS

## *Polymyalgia rheumatica*

This condition of elderly patients presents with muscle pain and stiffness predominantly affecting the muscles of the shoulder and the pelvic girdle and the proximal limb muscles. Muscle weakness and tenderness are not seen, though occasionally synovitis of central joints (e.g. the sternoclavicular joint) may be present. Some patients also experience malaise, weight loss and anaemia and a proportion show features of temporal (cranial) arteritis (page 575). Tests for rheumatoid and antinuclear factor are usually absent, although an increase in the serum gamma globulins may be present and the immunoglobulin levels may be raised. Striking elevation of the ESR is a hallmark of the condition. Another characteristic feature is the dramatic response to oral corticosteroid medication, response being evident within hours of starting. The usual dose is between 10 and 20 mg prednisolone daily until such time as the ESR falls to within normal limits, whereupon the dose may be tapered accordingly. Although the aim is to withdraw steroids completely as soon as possible, the condition may remain active for several years which precludes this. Because of the close relationship between polymyalgia rheumatica and temporal arteritis (with the attendant risk of retinal artery occlusion) it is important that this condition is recognized and adequately treated without delay and careful follow-up is instituted. Because of the rather non-specific nature of the symptoms, alternative diagnoses – including myeloma, carcinomatosis and polymyositis – should be borne in mind. A temporal artery biopsy, protein electrophoresis, a creatinine phosphokinase estimation and an EMG are helpful in this regard.

# Soft tissue lesions

Under this heading is included a group of common, benign, though troublesome, conditions which may mimic arthritis and cause diagnostic difficulties for the unwary. For convenience they may be divided into five main categories.

### 1. Enthesopathies
These may be either acute traumatic episodes or chronic overuse injuries affecting sites of attachment of ligaments, tendons or fascial bands. Common examples include lateral epicondylitis ('tennis elbow'), medial epicondylitis ('golfer's elbow') and plantar fasciitis.

### 2. Periarthritis (including capsulitis and periarticular tendonitis)
These lesions affect predominantly the shoulder joint which, being a shallow ball and socket, depends to a considerable extent for its stability on the complex of muscles, tendons and joint capsule known collectively as the rotator cuff. Four syndromes are commonly described within this entity; tendonitis of supraspinatus, infraspinatus, subscapularis or the long head of biceps – identified by a painful arc of movement when the affected muscle is moved; subacromial bursitis with tenderness over the site of the bursa; acute calcific tendonitis associated with a brisk inflammatory reaction due to crystals of hydroxyapatite reminiscent in its ferocity of acute gout and distinguished by the presence of calcific material seen on X-ray; and adhesive capsulitis ('frozen shoulder') in which gross restriction of movement in the shoulder joint is apparent in all directions, though pain is variable. Adhesive capsulitis is commonly seen after pleurisy, myocardial infarction, hemiplegia and certain operations in the region, notably mastectomy. An extension of this condition is known as the shoulder/hand syndrome in which the hand becomes diffusely swollen and tender followed by progressive atrophy of the muscle, bone and skin with severe contractures and deformities. It is believed to be due to a reflex neurovascular dystrophy (algodystrophy).

### 3. Entrapment neuropathy
The carpal tunnel syndrome (page 689) is the most commonly seen variety. Tarsal tunnel syndrome and meralgia paraesthetica are other examples.

### 4. Bursitis
Excessive friction between bone and overlying moving soft tissues may give rise to bursitis. Commonly affected sites include olecranon bursitis, prepatellar bursitis and pre-achilles bursitis.

### 5. Tenosynovitis
Inflammation of synovium of the tendon sheaths occurs in a wide variety of conditions of overuse, particularly involving the long flexor tendons of the fingers or the extensor and abductor tendons of the thumb. Blocking of the movement of the tendon within the sheath may result in 'triggering'. This condition is known as stenosing tenosynovitis or de Quervain's disease.

For a more detailed description of the conditions mentioned in this section the reader is referred to standard rheumatological and orthopaedic texts. The majority of the conditions listed are amenable to treatment, which may be on the basis of local corticosteroid injections, physiotherapeutic techniques or minor surgical procedures. Oral drug treatment has little part to play in the management of these conditions, although the recently introduced transdermal preparations of NSAIDs may be helpful.

# Psychogenic rheumatism

This term is used to denote a condition whereby rheumatic-type symptoms manifest an underlying psychological disorder such as depression, anxiety or compensation neurosis. Arthralgia and low back pain in the absence of clinical signs of organic disease are characteristic features of this condition.

# Tietze's syndrome (costal chondritis)

In this obscure condition pain and tenderness are observed in the costochrondral junctions. It is usually self-limiting, but local infiltrations of corticosteroids may be helpful and are required occasionally.

# Heritable disorders of connective tissue

These are multisystem disorders resulting from the inheritance of abnormalities in either the fibrous proteins (collagen, fibrillin and elastin) or the ground substance (glycosaminoglycans).

The disorders of fibrous proteins share a common feature, namely, generalized laxity of ligaments, resulting in hypermobility of joints which may give rise to articular symptoms. They include:

1. The **Marfan syndrome** (long, slender extremities, arachnodactyly, high arched palate, dislocation of the lens and aneurysm of the ascending aorta).
2. **Homocystinuria** (due to a deficiency of the enzyme cystathionine synthetase and similar to Marfan syndrome with the addi-

tional features of thrombosis in medium-sized arteries, and osteoporosis).
3. The **Ehlers–Danlos syndrome** characterized by hyperextensible and fragile skin, a tendency to bruising and rupture of arteries (Fig. 20.18).
4. **Osteogenesis imperfecta** (fragilitas ossium) or 'brittle bone disease' in which a marked tendency to fractures of bone and a blue appearance of the sclera of the eye are the most characteristic features.

With the exception of homocystinuria which is inherited as a recessive gene, all these conditions are inherited as a dominant gene. The term 'hypermobility syndrome' denotes generalized laxity of ligaments in otherwise healthy subjects. It, too, is a benign hereditary disorder, albeit mild, of connective tissue. Hypermobility, irrespective of the cause, may result in synovitis of the joints, recurrent dislocation and, possibly, premature osteoarthritis.

The disorders of ground substance comprise the **mucopolysaccharidoses**, a group of eleven diseases with differing manifestations (including the Hurler, Hunter, Scheie, Sanfilippo, Morquio and Maroteaux–Lamy syndromes). Patients manifest a variety of features including dwarfism, stiff joints, clouding of the cornea, aortic regurgitation, hepatosplenomegaly and learning difficulties. Excessive quantities of mucopolysaccharides are found in the urine. In a number of these conditions the underlying enzyme defect has been identified.

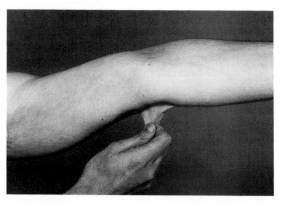

**Figure 20.18** Hyperextensible skin seen in a patient suffering from the Ehlers–Danlos syndrome. Note that the elbow joint shows hyperextension (hypermobility).

# MISCELLANEOUS RHEUMATIC CONDITIONS

## SARCOIDOSIS

In early sarcoid (page 314) the arthopathy associated with erythema nodosum may be seen. Later in the disease sarcoid granulomata may appear in the synovial membrane or bone, causing synovitis and destructive arthropathy, respectively.

## FAMILIAL MEDITERRANEAN FEVER

Episodic arthritis of short duration with spontaneous remission is common and a chronic destructive arthritis has also been reported. The episodes of arthritis respond to colchicine which is also capable of preventing amyloidosis (page 494) – a recognized complication.

## HYPERLIPOPROTINAEMIAS (page 495)

A migratory polyarthritis is seen in type II, whilst in type IV an episodic arthropathy is reported.

## HYPOGAMMAGLOBULINAEMIA

An arthropathy similar to rheumatoid arthritis is seen, although destructive changes are rare.

## HAEMOPHILIA AND CHRISTMAS DISEASE

In these bleeding diatheses (page 639) recurrent haemarthroses give rise to acute episodes of joint pain and swelling and eventually to severe destructive changes, deformity and fibrous ankylosis.

## LEUKAEMIA

Arthralgia, arthritis and bone pain are frequent symptoms in acute leukaemia, whilst in chronic leukaemia asymmetrical arthritis of larger joints results from infiltration of articular structures. Secondary gout may also occur in these conditions.

## SICKLE CELL DISEASE

In this condition bone infarction, arthralgia or synovitis may occur during crises.

## PIGMENTED VILLONODULAR SYNOVITIS

This granulomatous condition of synovium may affect joint, tendon sheath or bursa. It presents as a painless swelling of a single joint, usually of the knee, leading to erosion and cyst formation. Treatment is by synovectomy.

## HYPERTROPHIC (PULMONARY) OSTEOARTHROPATHY

This is a combination of finger clubbing with painful, tender swelling of ankles and wrists with characteristic periosteal new bone formation seen radiologically. Joint effusions may occur. It is most often associated with lung carcinomas but may occur with other neoplastic or infective intrathoracic or intra-abdominal pathology.

## AVASCULAR NECROSIS OF BONE (OSTEONECROSIS)

The femoral head is the most commonly affected site, although the humeral head and femoral condyles may be affected. It is seen in trauma, sickle cell disease, caisson disease (decompression problems in divers), high-dose corticosteroid therapy, SLE and alcoholism.

## NEUROPATHIC (CHARCOT'S) JOINTS

This is a severe form of destructive arthropathy seen in certain neurological diseases with loss of pain sensation. Common causes are diabetes mellitus with peripheral neuropathy and paraplegia; rare causes are tabes dorsalis, syringomyelia, and congenital indifference to pain.

## POLYCHONDRITIS

Polychondritis is an inflammatory condition that gives rise to destructive changes in hyaline and fibrocartilagenous structures.

# JUVENILE CHRONIC ARTHRITIS

Many patients carry their chronic rheumatic disease from childhood into adult life. It is for this reason that a note on juvenile chronic arthritis is not out of place in a volume devoted to adult medicine. It is now known that several clinical and pathological entities fall within this broad title and the use of the term 'Still's disease' to cover them all is no longer tenable. Rheumatic fever is not included and is dealt with separately (page 189). The following entities have been delineated.

## SEROPOSITIVE (ADULT-LIKE) JUVENILE RHEUMATOID ARTHRITIS

This variety is very similar to the adult one with IgM rheumatoid factor, nodules and erosive disease.

## JUVENILE ANKYLOSING SPONDYLITIS

This presents in childhood (mainly in boys) as a peripheral arthropathy, and only in the late teens do the classical features of ankylosing spondylitis develop with spinal involvement. These patients are almost exclusively HLA B27 positive and have a tendency to recurrent acute iritis.

## JUVENILE CHRONIC ARTHRITIS

This comprises three entities:

1. There is a systemic onset, with fever, lymphadenopathy, splenomegaly and pericarditis, which may all precede the polyarthritis and cause diagnostic confusion.
2. Pauciarticular disease, as its name implies, commences in a small number of joints (1–4). Although the articular disease may not be very severe there is a real danger of severe eye problems following chronic iritis, which may be insidious in its onset and pass undetected. The antinuclear factor is commonly positive.
3. Polyarticular disease develops in five or more joints, particularly in the knees and wrists. Small finger joints may also be involved, including the distal interphalangeal joints. The cervical spine may also be involved.

## OTHER

The following are uncommon childhood ailments and their clinical presentation follows the general pattern of adult disease (see above):

- Juvenile scleroderma
- Juvenile dermatomyositis
- Juvenile systemic lupus erythematosus
- Juvenile psoriatic arthritis
- Polyarthritis associated with ulcerative colitis and regional enteritis

# Disorders of the Blood

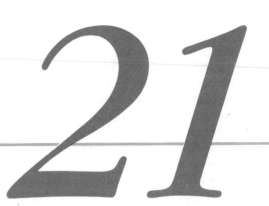

# INTRODUCTION

In the UK, among the Caucasian population, intrinsic disease of blood cells is rare, but changes in their number, shape, size and function can be detected in many illnesses. Among the Black, Asian and Oriental populations congenital disorders of blood cells are much commoner. The advances in prenatal diagnosis of diseases such as thalassaemia and sickle cell disease have made a huge impact on the management of these disorders by providing genetic counselling and the opportunity for termination of pregnancy.

Worldwide, anaemia is a major cause of morbidity and mortality, mainly due to infection and malnutrition in the developing countries. Correction of this continues to pose an apparently insurmountable challenge, but for economic and social reasons rather than lack of medical knowledge.

Advances in the chemotherapy of the lymphomas and the leukaemias, and improvement in the techniques of bone marrow transplants and postoperative immunosuppression have resulted in improved survival, and even cure for some malignant and aplastic diseases, although several of these disorders still have a distressingly high mortality rate. The increase in understanding of the genetic aspects of leukaemias and lymphomas, and the continuing advances in chemotherapy hold the promise of further improvements in survival for these patients.

# THE BLOOD CELLS

All blood cells are derived from a common, pluripotential stem cell which, by division and differentiation, forms distinct types of blood cells. In the fetus this takes place in liver and spleen, but from the fifth month of fetal life the medullary cavity of the bones becomes increasingly responsible. In adults, the haematopoietic bone marrow is mainly confined to the flat bones of the axial skeleton. Haematopoiesis is shown diagrammatically in Fig. 21.1.

All stem cells look like small lymphocytes. The pluripotential stem cell is self-perpetuating but also gives rise to a series of progenitor cells which are committed to a particular type of differentiation. This process corresponds to changes in demand and is under humoral control.

# Haematopoietic growth factors

Control of haematopoiesis is through the interaction of a complex mixture of growth factors or cytokines which are derived from lymphocytes, macrophages and bone marrow stromal cells. Because of the way that they were discovered or are assayed, they are generally known as either interleukins (IL) or colony-stimulating factors (CSFs). Although most have a number of activities, they are listed in Table 21.1 according to the one most relevant to haematopoiesis.

Some cytokines have been produced in recombinant form in pharmacological quantities by molecular techniques and are used, for example,

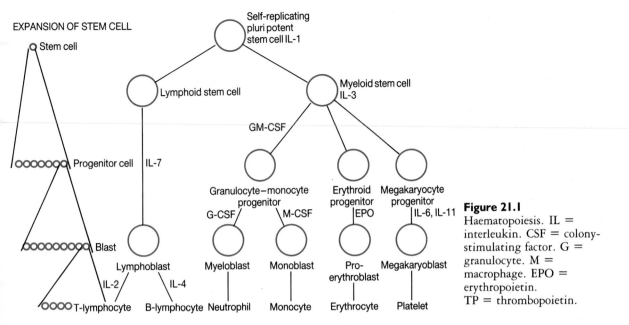

**Figure 21.1**
Haematopoiesis. IL =
interleukin. CSF = colony-
stimulating factor. G =
granulocyte. M =
macrophage. EPO =
erythropoietin.
TP = thrombopoietin.

**Table 21.1** Activities of cytokines.

| Cytokine | Haematopoietic activity |
| --- | --- |
| IL-1 | Stimulates multipotent stem cells |
| IL-2 | T-cell growth factor |
| IL-3 | Stimulates myeloid stem cells |
| IL-4 | B-cell growth factor |
| IL-5 | Eosinophil differentiation factor |
| IL-6 | Stimulates plasma cells and megakaryocytes |
| IL-7 | Stimulates lymphoid stem cell |
| IL-11 | Stimulates megakaryocytes |
| GM-CSF | Stimulates granulocyte/macrophage progenitors |
| G-CSF | Causes neutrophil differentiation |
| M-CSF | Causes monocytic differentiation |
| Erythropoietin | Causes red cell differentiation |
| Thrombopoietin | Causes megakaryocytic differentiation |

IL = interleukin. CSF = colony-stimulating factors. G = granulocyte. M = macrophage.

to speed recovery from neutropenia following large doses of cytotoxic drugs (granulocyte colony-stimulating factor, G-CSF; granulocyte macrophage colony-stimulating factor, GM-CSF) or to correct the anaemia of renal failure (erythropoietin).

# Red blood cells (erythrocytes)

The earliest cell recognizably committed to red cell differentiation is the proerythroblast. This large cell will divide three to four times at roughly 24-hour intervals, becoming progressively smaller and acquiring increasing quantities of haemoglobin in the cytoplasm, while its nucleus condenses and is finally extruded. The newly formed erythrocyte, when released from the bone marrow contains RNA and a reticular formation of condensed ribosomes. Such cells are therefore known as reticulocytes.

The mature red cell, a biconcave disc 7 μm in diameter, is extremely pliable and able to pass through spaces one-third of its size. It is a very simple cell comprising a membrane, haemoglobin, and a non-renewable enzyme system to maintain the integrity of the membrane and the respiratory pigment. The function of the cell is to transport oxygen from lungs to tissue by means of haemoglobin. This molecule consists of a protein (globin) which is made up of four folded polypeptide chains. In each chain, in a pocket between the folds, sits the red pigment, haem, which consists of four porphyrin rings surrounding a molecule of ferrous iron. Red cell production depends on the availability of iron salts, needed for haemoglobin; vitamin $B_{12}$ and folic acid, required for DNA metabolism; and erythropoietin, a hormone produced by the kidney in response to hypoxia, which provides the erythroid 'drive' for the marrow.

Red cells survive in the circulation for about 120 days during which time their enzyme systems gradually decay. Effete cells are destroyed by macrophages in the bone marrow, liver and spleen. The iron from the haemoglobin is re-utilized by the marrow, the porphyrin structures are broken down to bilirubin which is excreted by the liver, and the protein is recycled.

# White blood cells (leukocytes)

Whereas red cells spend their entire life-span within the circulation, the white cells spend relatively short periods there en route to the tissues. There are three types of white cell: lymphocytes, monocytes and granulocytes.

## LYMPHOCYTES

The committed lymphoid progenitor cell is believed to arise from the pluripotent stem cell earlier than other committed cells. T-lymphocytes migrate to the thymus where they are processed before circulating to the peripheral lymphoid organs. They are responsible for cellular immune responses and control of the immune system. B-lymphocytes mature in the bone marrow before migrating to lymph nodes, spleen and other lymphoid tissue. They are programmed to produce specific antibody in response to antigenic stimuli, by differentiating into plasma cells. A third population, natural killer (NK) cells, is responsible for non-specific killing of virus-infected cells, some cancer cells and antibody-coated cells. They may also down-regulate haematopoiesis. They have abundant cytoplasm and azurophil granules and are sometimes known as large granular lympho-

cytes. Lymphocytes are discussed more fully in Chapter 8.

## MONOCYTES

Monocytes are large cells with irregular oval or horseshoe-shaped nuclei and abundant cytoplasm with small numbers of granules. They derive from the same committed progenitor cell as granuloytes, and recognizable intermediate cells are monoblasts and promonocytes. Maturation takes 2–5 days within the bone marrow. Monocytes circulate in the blood for 3 days, before passing to the tissues where they become long-lived macrophages with a variety of names depending on the particular tissue: for example, alveolar macrophages in the lung, Langerhans cells in the skin, microglial cells in the brain, Kupffer cells in the liver, littoral cells in the spleen, osteoclasts in the bone, and histiocytes in many tissues.

## GRANULOCYTES

Between the committed progenitor cell and the myeloblast, the earliest recognizable granulocyte precursor, at least five doubling divisions occur. Maturation of the myeloblast involves between four and six divisions over 5 or 6 days. The nucleus become eccentric, kidney-shaped and then lobulated. The cytoplasm becomes increasingly granular with the granules containing peroxidase, acid hydrolases, lysozyme and other enzymes hostile to bacteria.

Neutrophil polymorphonuclear phagocytes (often called neutrophils or 'polys') are held in the bone marrow as a 'reserve' pool for 5–10 days, but they eventually migrate into the blood where they circulate for 6 or 7 hours before passing towards the margins of the blood vessels (the 'marginated' pool) and thence into the tissues, either to die, or when attracted by chemotactic factors, such as complement breakdown products, to act as effector cells in an immune response.

The number of circulating neutrophils increases in response to 'stress' factors such as exercise, emotion or infection, and this increase comes from the mobilization of the reserve and marginated pools. Infection leads to the early release of neutrophils before nuclear lobulation has occurred (a shift to the left).

Eosinophil granulocytes have bilobed nuclei and large red granules in Romanowsky-stained films. They have IgE–receptors and are thus involved in allergic reactions, and can phagocytose.

Basophil granulocytes are the blood phase of mast cells. They are involved in immediate hypersensitivity reactions. The Fc portion of IgE is bound to the basophil surface. Reaction of the IgE molecule with specific antigen causes the release of histamine and heparin from the basophilic granules.

# *Platelets*

Platelets are small granular bodies 2–4 μm in diameter derived from cytoplasmic budding of megakaryocytes in the marrow. The megakaryocyte is a very large cell with a multilobulated nucleus and abundant cytoplasm.

If they are not consumed in thrombosis, platelets survive in the circulation for 10 days. Their function is to adhere to any break in the blood vessel wall, to aggregate to one another and to release factors which enhance the formation of the haemostatic plug.

# $S$YMPTOMS

Although symptoms of blood diseases may be referred to almost any system of the body, a surprising number of disorders are asymptomatic.

## ANAEMIA

Anaemia is frequently symptom-free, especially when it is of slow onset. Even when it does draw attention to itself many of its symptoms are non-specific (tiredness, lassitude, malaise and headache), while others are more clearly related to cardiac decompensation (angina, dyspnoea, orthopnoea and ankle oedema).

## INFECTION

Infections are common in blood diseases because of lymphopenia, neutropenia and hypogammaglobulinaemia. Fever may be the only symptom of infection in such patients, although there may be features which localize the infection to the mouth, infusion sites or lung. Fever may also be caused by allergic reactions to drugs or blood products and sometimes as a direct consequence of the disease itself. Night sweats are often a symptom of low-grade fever and may occur in lymphoma and leukaemia.

## EXTERNAL BLEEDING

External bleeding and bruising are features of platelet disorders, whereas clotting factor deficiencies are more likely to cause spontaneous bleeding into muscles and joints.

## PAIN

Pain in the left hypochondrium or left shoulder tip is a feature of splenic infarction, but patients otherwise seldom notice an enlarged spleen. On the other hand enlarged lymph nodes are often discovered by patients, although many such nodes have no serious pathological significance.

# $S$IGNS

## PALLOR

This is notoriously easy to misdiagnose since the colour of skin is the product of the pigment contained within it and the blood flowing through it. Facial colour is particularly difficult to assess since it varies with emotion, exposure to sunlight, race and covering with cosmetics. The mucous membranes give a better guide, although the conjunctivae and gums may be red because of inflammation and the tongue pale because of a coating. Nail beds and palmar creases have the advantage of being comparable with the examiner's own hands. Palmar creases remain pink in a fully opened hand unless the haemoglobin level is less than 70 g/l.

## PURPURA

The term refers to a haemorrhagic rash which may be due to platelet deficiency or damage to the vascular endothelium (e.g. vasculitis). It may consist of *petechiae*, small (1–3 mm) round, red or brown lesions or *ecchymoses*, which are larger confluent areas of skin haemorrhage ranging from red or purple to blue or green in colour.

## LYMPHADENOPATHY

Lymph nodes are distributed widely throughout the body but are normally palpable only in the groins of adults, whereas in children they may also be felt in the cervical region. In the lymphomas and other blood disorders they may be enlarged and readily palpable in cervical, axillary, epitrochlear, inguinal and femoral regions. Very large para-aortic glands may sometimes be detected by deep palpation of the abdomen.

## SPLENOMEGALY

The normal adult spleen, which weighs about 150 g, is not palpable on physical examination. As it enlarges in disease states it appears from under the left costal margin advancing towards the right iliac fossa. It is dull to percussion and moves on respiration. The examining hand cannot get above it. The splenic notch may be felt along the medial border. Masses in stomach, colon, kidney or pancreas, and the left lobe of the liver, are often mistaken for splenic enlargement.

## HEPATOMEGALY

The normal liver may be palpable as much as 5 cm below the costal margin in certain normal individuals but is seldom normally palpable in the epigastrium. Hepatic enlargement below the costal margin should be measured in the mid-clavicular line. Hepatic size is best measured by determining both the upper and lower borders by percussion. The normal vertical span is up to about 11 cm.

# $S$PECIAL INVESTIGATIONS

## FULL BLOOD COUNT

This is normally performed on a blood sample anticoagulated with sodium ethylenediamine tetra acetic acid (EDTA). Nowadays, most laboratories are equipped with electronic blood cell counters which rapidly and reproducibly provide precise measurements of haemoglobin concentration, red cell, white cell and platelet number and mean red cell volume. They also calculate from these measurements a number of red cell indices (Table 21.2). More sophisticated machines are able to determine white cell differential counts. Normal ranges are given in the Appendix.

## BLOOD FILM

An examination of a blood film stained with one of the Romanowsky stains is the essence of diagnostic haematology. The sizes and shapes of red cells are noted and a differential white count performed. Abnormal cellular inclusions and the presence of certain parasites may be recognized. Terms used to describe abnormalities seen in the blood film are given in Table 21.3. Supravital staining with brilliant cresyl blue allows the detection of reticulocytes, Heinz bodies (denatured haemoglobin seen in certain haemolytic anaemias), and haemoglobin H inclusions (the golf-ball appearance seen in $\alpha$-thalassaemia).

## BONE MARROW EXAMINATION

Examination of the bone marrow yields far more diagnostic information than the blood film.

Bone marrow aspirates may be obtained, using a hollow steel Salah needle, from sternum or iliac crest. The aspirated bone marrow is spread, like blood, on glass slides. Cytochemical and immunochemical staining are useful to

**Table 21.2** Red cell indices.

| | |
|---|---|
| Haemoglobin (Hb) | Measured by conversion to cyanmethaemoglobin and calculating absorbance at 540 nm<br>Expressed in either g/l or g/dl |
| Red blood count (RBC) | Measured directly by light scattering or changes in potential difference<br>Expressed as number $\times 10^{12}$/l |
| Packed cell volume (PCV) | May be measured by centrifuging blood in a capillary tube in a microhaematocrit or by calculation<br>PCV (in %) = MCV × RBC |
| Mean cell volume (MCV) | Measured directly by electronic counters or derived from PCV and RBC<br>Expressed in femtolitres (fl) = $10^{-15}$l |
| Mean corpuscular haemoglobin (MCH) | Calculated from Hb ÷ RBC<br>Expressed in pg |
| Mean corpuscular haemoglobin concentration (MCHC) | Calculated from Hb ÷ PCV<br>Expressed in g/dl |
| Red cell distribution width (RDW) | Electronically derived estimate of degree of anisocytosis |

identify particular cells. Dispersed bone marrow cells may be examined by immunofluorescence to detect surface markers. They may also be examined cytogenetically to detect abnormal karyotypes (Chapter 7).

Bone marrow trephine biopsies are usually obtained with the Jamshidi needle, a wide-bore hollow needle with a tapered tip which obtains a core of bone marrow from anterior or posterior iliac crest. The specimen is examined histologically. Trephine biopsies are performed when aplastic anaemia, lymphoma, secondary cancer and myeloproliferative diseases are suspected or when aspiration has yielded a 'dry tap'.

## ERYTHROCYTE SEDIMENTATION RATE

The erythrocyte sedimentation rate (ESR) is a measure of the rate (mm/hour) of settling of red cells in the patient's own plasma. The test must be performed in a standardized way. The rate is mainly determined by the fibrinogen level, but very high immunoglobulin levels will also accelerate settling. In patients over 60 the upper limit of normal increases and in pregnancy the test has no value. The test is mainly used as an index of inflammation and as a screening test for myeloma. In some laboratories plasma viscosity is measured as an alternative to the ESR.

## PAUL BUNNEL TEST

Eighty to ninety per cent of patients with infectious mononucleosis develop an antibody which cross-reacts with sheep red blood cells. Detection of this by agglutination is the Paul Bunnel test. Many laboratories substitute the Monospot or similar test which relies on the agglutination of formalin-treated horse red cells.

## TESTS OF IRON METABOLISM

Serum iron is measured by a variety of colorimetric methods. Iron-containing medicines should be avoided for 72 hours before estimation. There is a diurnal variation with lower levels in the evening. Total iron-binding capacity (TIBC) is an indirect measurement of the serum transferrin content and is raised in iron deficiency. Iron is stored as haemosiderin and ferritin. Haemosiderin may be visualized in bone marrow macrophages with Perl's stain and is the best indication of the presence of storage iron. A small fraction of the water-soluble iron–protein complex, ferritin, is present in the serum. Serum ferritin may be measured by a radioimmunoassay; in health it correlates with total body iron stores, but it also operates as an acute inflammatory protein and may be raised in connective tissue disorders and cancer.

## TESTS OF MEGALOBLASTIC ANAEMIA

In some laboratories vitamin $B_{12}$ and folic acid are still measured by microbiological assays in which the vitamin in the patient's serum provides a critical growth factor for a particular micro-organism. However, these assays have largely been supplanted by methods making use of radioisotope dilution. For a full assessment of

**Table 21.3** Terms used when reporting blood films.

| Term | Meaning | Significance |
| --- | --- | --- |
| Hypochromasia<br>Microcytosis | Pale staining cells<br>Small red cells | Iron deficiency; thalassaemia trait;<br>anaemia of chronic disorders |
| Macrocytosis<br>Anisocytosis | Large red cells<br>Variation in red cell size | See Table 21.10<br>Non-specific, but marked anisocytosis<br>is seen in megaloblastic anaemia |
| Poikilocytosis | Variation in red cell shape | Seen in megaloblastic anaemia, severe<br>iron deficiency, myelofibrosis etc. |
| Spherocytes | Red cells are spherical instead of<br>biconcave discs | Hereditary spherocytosis or<br>autoimmune haemolytic anaemia |
| Elliptocytes | Red cells are elliptical | Hereditary elliptocytosis or<br>myelofibrosis |
| Polychromasia | Some red cells appear bluish | Increased numbers of young red cells;<br>haemolysis, haemorrhage or<br>myelofibrosis |
| Target cells | Thin cells with dark central areas | Liver disease; thalassaemia; post-<br>splenectomy; HbC disease |
| Tear drop cells | Red cells shaped like teardrops | Myelofibrosis |
| Anisochromasia | Two populations of palely and<br>normally staining cells | Iron deficiency with treatment or<br>sideroblastic anaemia |
| Leucoerythroblastic picture | Nucleated red cells and myeloid<br>precursors seen | Marrow infiltration |
| Acanthocytosis | Irregularly shaped cells | Uraemia, microangiopathy, liver<br>disease |
| Rouleaux | Red cells appear stacked like piles of<br>coins | Raised fibrinogen or immunoglobulin,<br>especially seen in myeloma |
| Basophilic stippling | Fine blue staining inclusions | Lead poisoning; thalassaemia |
| Howell–Jolly bodies | Dark blue regular inclusions; remnants<br>of nuclei | Splenectomy or splenic atrophy |

Hb = haemoglobin.

megaloblastic anaemia it is necessary to assay serum $B_{12}$ and both serum and red cell folate (Table 21.4).

The **Schilling test** is a measure of the absorption of vitamin $B_{12}$. Radioactively labelled $B_{12}$ is given orally and this is followed by an intramuscular injection of the unlabelled vitamin to saturate tissue stores so that the test is not just a measure of $B_{12}$ deficiency. If the labelled $B_{12}$ is absorbed it will be rapidly excreted in the urine

**Table 21.4** Interpretation of vitamin $B_{12}$ and folate measurements.

| Serum $B_{12}$ | Serum folate | Red cell folate | Interpretation |
| --- | --- | --- | --- |
| Low | High or<br>normal | Low | Vitamin $B_{12}$ deficiency |
| Normal | Low | Low | Folic acid deficiency |
| Normal | Low | Normal | Poor diet recently |

(normals excrete more than 12 per cent in 24 hours). Those who malabsorb the $B_{12}$ should be tested again with the addition of oral hog intrinsic factor. If this corrects the malabsorption it suggests that the absence of intrinsic factor is the problem and the diagnosis of pernicious anaemia is likely. Vitamin $B_{12}$ absorption can also be measured by whole body counting, measuring faecal excretion or plasma concentration of the radioisotope.

## TESTS OF HAEMOLYSIS

Tests of haemolysis are directed first to establish that haemolysis is occurring, and then to find out why. Evidence for haemolysis is gained from the following.

### Increased red cell production

This is accompanied by reticulocytosis and bone marrow erythroid hyperplasia.

### Increased red cell breakdown

Signs of this are raised serum bilirubin, increased urinary urobilinogen, undetectable serum haptoglobins (the haemoglobin-binding proteins of serum) and decreased red cell survival. In the measurement of red cell survival, the patient's own red cells are labelled by incubating them with radioactive chromium (chromium-51) and then reinjecting them into the patient. The radioactivity of blood samples taken on successive days measures the rate of decay. The normal half time of these cells is around 30 days: in significant haemolysis it is usually less than 15 days.

Variations on this test will yield further information. Surface counting of the radioactivity over the liver, spleen and sacrum indicates where red cell destruction is taking place.

The measurement of radioactivity 30 minutes after reinfusion of the chromium-15-labelled red cells gives an indication of the total red cell content of the body (known as the red cell mass), and this usefully distinguishes between true and relative polycythaemia in which the red cell mass is elevated and normal, respectively. The total body plasma volume may be estimated in a similar way using albumin labelled with radioactive iodine.

## TESTS FOR THE CAUSE OF HAEMOLYSIS

Clues to the causes of haemolysis may be found on the blood film, otherwise the following tests may be helpful.

### Osmotic fragility

This tests for lysis of red cells in a series of salt solutions of decreasing concentration. Spherical cells (spherocytosis, page 613) are less able to swell under osmotic stress than are biconcave discs, and therefore lyse at a higher concentration of salt.

### Coombs' test

The direct Coombs' test is used to detect antibody or complement on the surface of cells. IgG antibodies are too small to bridge the gap between adjacent red cells and are unable to cause agglutination in the way that IgM antibodies do (Fig. 21.2). Washed red cells coated with

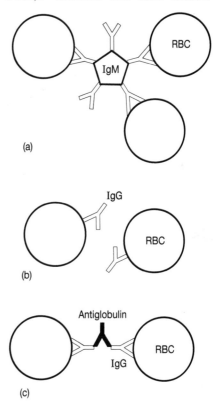

**Figure 21.2** The direct Coombs' test. (a) IgM is large enough to agglutinate adjacent red cells. (b) Surface charge keeps red cells so far apart that the IgG molecule cannot react with adjacent cells. (c) Antiglobulin reagent bridges the gap. RBC = red blood cell.

immunoglobulin or complement may be agglutinated by a second layer of antibody directed against the bound immunoglobulin or complement.

An indirect Coombs' test is employed in cross-matching blood to detect a putative anti-red cell antibody in the recipient's serum.

## TESTS OF COAGULATION AND BLEEDING

### Bleeding time

This test is best performed in a standard way. The modified Ivy test uses a template to make a standard incision on the volar surface of the forearm while a sphygmomanometer cuff is pumped to a constant 40 mm Hg. The blood is absorbed every 30 seconds on to a piece of blotting paper which is not allowed to touch the incision. The result is mainly influenced by platelet number and platelet function.

### Prothrombin time

The time taken for citrated plasma to clot after the addition of tissue thromboplastin (extracted from rabbit brain) and calcium is usually expressed as a ratio to a normal control, corrected by a reference value (the International Normalized Ratio, INR). It is prolonged by deficiencies of factors II, V, VII and X, and fibrinogen.

### The kaolin cephalin clotting time

The kaolin cephalin clotting time (KCCT) measures the activity of the intrinsic clotting system (page 639). The variable steps in this pathway are the activation of contact factors and the release of phospholipid (platelet factor 3) from platelets. The test avoids these variables by fully activating contact factors with kaolin and providing a platelet substitute (cephalin). The test is sensitive to deficiencies of factors II, V, X, VIII, IX, XI and XII, and fibrinogen.

# Clinical problems

# THE ANAEMIAS

Anaemia is defined as a level of haemoglobin (Hb) lower than expected for the age and sex of the patient. Since the concept of a normal range is a statistical one the figures chosen are to a degree arbitrary. The newborn baby has an Hb as high as 200 g/l because the fetus has lived in a relatively hypoxic condition. By 3 months of age the Hb falls to just over 100 g/l. Because of the stimulating effect of androgens, after puberty males have Hbs on average 20 g/l higher than females. The anaemias are classified in Table 21.5, although this should be regarded as a tentative classification. Most anaemias are multifactorial. Even iron deficiency has a haemolytic element when it is severe.

# Iron deficiency anaemia

## AETIOLOGY

Iron deficiency is the commonest cause of anaemia in every country in the world but myths about it abound (Table 21.6). Although iron is one of the most plentiful elements on earth its absorption is carefully regulated according to what is needed (Table 21.7). This careful balance is disturbed in thalassaemia and haemochromatosis, and in these conditions excessive iron is absorbed and laid down in tissues.

Table 21.8 summarizes the main causes of iron deficiency. A normal diet which includes

**Table 21.5** Classification of anaemia.

**Decreased production of red cells**

Disturbed Hb synthesis
  Iron deficiency
  Anaemia of chronic disorders
  Thalassaemias

Disturbed DNA synthesis
  Vitamin $B_{12}$ deficiency
  Folic acid deficiency

Disturbed proliferation of stem cells
  Aplastic anaemia
  Dyserythropoietic anaemias

Insufficient humoral stimulus
  Chronic renal failure
  Thyroid deficiency

Bone marrow infiltration
  Malignancy
  Myelofibrosis

**Increased loss or destruction of red cells**

Red cell loss
  Acute bleeds

Intrinsic disorders of red cells
  Membrane (hereditary spherocytosis)
  Enzymes (glucose 6-phosphate deficiency)
  Haemoglobin (sickle cell disease)

Extrinsic disorders affecting red cells
  Antibodies
  Physical (heart valves)
  Chemical (drugs)
  Infections (malaria)
  Hypersplenism

**Relative/apparent anaemia due to expanded plasma volume**
Pregnancy
Splenomegaly
Macroglobulinaemia

**Table 21.6** Eight myths about iron.

| Myth | Truth |
|---|---|
| 1. The MCHC is the best index of iron deficiency | A low MCHC was a methodological artefact; the MCV is the most useful index |
| 2. Iron deficiency is a diagnosis | It is only an indication of underlying abnormality |
| 3. Poor diet is a common cause of iron deficiency | It is very rare in the UK; blood loss is the commonest cause |
| 4. Spinach is a good source of iron | A nineteenth century chemist misplaced the decimal point; it is no better than lettuce leaves |
| 5. Hiatus hernia is sufficient diagnosis for cause of blood loss | Significant numbers also have large bowel pathology |
| 6. Malabsorption is an important cause of iron deficiency | Even in coeliac disease increased iron loss is more important |
| 7. Sideroblastic anaemia is an important differential diagnosis of a low MCV | Most cases of sideroblastic anaemia are macrocytic |
| 8. Parenteral iron raises the Hb faster than oral iron | Oral iron is just as quick and far safer |

MCHC = mean corpuscular haemoglobin concentration. Hb = haemoglobin.

**Table 21.7** Daily iron requirements.

| | Loss in faeces sweat and urine (mg) | Menstrual loss (mg) | Growth (mg) | Growth of fetus and uterus (mg) | Total (mg) |
|---|---|---|---|---|---|
| Men and postmenopausal women | 0.5 | | | | 0.5 |
| Menstruating women | 0.5 | 0.5–1.0 | | | 1.0–1.5 |
| Children | 0.5 | | 0.5 | | 1.0 |
| Adolescent girls | 0.5 | 0–1.0 | 0.5 | | 1.5–2.0 |
| Pregnant women | 0.5 | | | 1.0–2.0 | 1.5–2.5 |

**Table 21.8** Causes of iron deficiency.

**Inadequate**

| | |
|---|---|
| Poor diet | Seldom the sole factor in the UK but may contribute when there is increased demand |
| Malabsorption | Contributes to anaemia of atrophic gastritis; postgastrectomy syndrome; coeliac disease |

**Increased demand**

| | |
|---|---|
| Growth | Growth spurts of childhood and puberty |
| Pregnancy | For uterus, fetus and increased blood volume |
| Blood loss | |
| Uterine | Fibroids; carcinoma; 10% normals |
| Gastrointestinal | Hiatus hernia; oesophageal varices; aspirin; hereditary telangiectasia; peptic ulcer; carcinoma of stomach; Meckel's diverticulum; angiodysplasia of colon; carcinoma of colon and rectum; hookworm; colitis; piles |
| Urological | Haematuria |
| Increased iron loss | |
| Gastrointestinal | Coeliac disease 3.5 mg/day; postgastrectomy syndrome 2 mg/day |
| Renal | Intravascular haemolysis leads to haemoglobinuria or haemosiderinuria |

meat or fish every day provides most people with their requirements, and in the UK poor diet is seldom a cause of iron deficiency. Fresh vegetables are not a good source of iron (not even spinach). Most iron deficiency is caused by chronic blood loss and the commonest source is the uterus. More than 80 ml loss per month usually leads to anaemia, but most women find it difficult to know whether or not their periods are heavy. Passing clots or having to use both sanitary towels and tampons together are signs that they are. Heavy periods do not necessarily

mean disease. Ten per cent of women without gynaecological pathology lose more than 80 ml of blood per month.

Gastrointestinal blood loss is the next most important cause of iron deficiency. Aspirin and other non-steroidal anti-inflammatory drugs are a major cause of occult bleeding from the stomach. In the elderly, colonic cancer is common, clinically silent and often operable. Worldwide, hookworm is very common and the main cause of iron deficiency.

The iron deficiency associated with coeliac disease and the postgastrectomy syndrome is mainly caused by the greatly increased iron loss from desquamating intestinal cells: 3.5 mg/day in coeliac disease and 2 mg/day in postgastrectomy syndrome.

## PATHOPHYSIOLOGY

Iron absorption occurs mainly through the duodenum and is favoured by acid and reducing agents (like vitamin C). Phytates and phosphates (present in bread and rice) inhibit absorption. The iron content of the gut mucosal cells controls the amount of iron absorbed, which is therefore greater in iron deficiency. Iron passes from gut to bone marrow bound to transferrin. It is stored mainly in macrophages, first as ferritin, from which it is readily exchangeable, and then in its condensed form, haemosiderin. Most iron is delivered to developing erythroblasts for the manufacture of haemoglobin. In the absence of iron, erythroblasts are small with ragged cytoplasm and the red cells they produce are small, thin and irregularly shaped. In severe cases their survival is shortened. Iron is also required by other tissues, particularly for myoglobin and cytochrome C.

## CLINICAL FEATURES

Mild cases are often asymptomatic, but as the Hb falls the symptoms of anaemia (see above) appear. In severe cases glossitis (smooth, sore, red tongue) and koilonychia (ridged, brittle, spoon-shaped nails) appear. Dysphagia due to postcricoid webs (Paterson–Brown–Kelly syndrome or Plummer–Vinson syndrome) is rare, as is pica (craving to eat unusual substances). Mild splenomegaly is sometimes present. Itching may be a feature even in the absence of anaemia.

## DIAGNOSIS

The blood count shows a low Hb, mean cell volume (MCV) and mean corpuscular Hb (MCH) (Table 21.2). The value of the mean corpuscular Hb concentration (MCHC) depends on how it is measured. When calculated from the Hb and spun packed cell volume (PCV), or measured by the new generation of Technicon electronic counters, it falls in iron deficiency; when measured by Coulter technology it does not. The blood film shows hypochromia, microcytosis with pencil-shaped poikilocytosis and some target cells. The main differential diagnoses are the anaemia of chronic disorders and thalassaemia traits. These can be distinguished by measurement of serum iron and TIBC which are respectively low and raised in iron deficiency. Serum ferritin, decreased in iron deficiency, may be helpful in sorting out difficult cases, but sometimes it is necessary to stain a bone marrow with Perl's stain in order to estimate iron stores (Table 21.9). The diagnosis of iron deficiency is not complete until the cause of the iron loss is determined. This may involve a complete investigation of the gastrointestinal tract.

## TREATMENT

Treatment should be directed at the underlying condition. Heavy periods, in the absence of gynaecological pathology, may be reduced by the contraceptive pill or treatment with an antifibrinolytic agent such as tranexamic acid, 500 mg t.d.s., on the days of the period.

For replenishment of iron, oral ferrous sulphate, 200 mg three times daily, is usually satisfactory. Its main side effects are dyspepsia, constipation or diarrhoea. These are similar for all oral iron preparations. Those with less severe side effects contain less iron (ferrous sulphate 200 mg = 62.5 mg elemental iron; ferrous gluconate 300 mg = 35 mg elemental iron). Slow-release tablets are often not absorbed at all. Parenteral iron has no real advantages except that the physician can be sure that it has been taken. (There is a small group of patients so intolerant of oral iron that they refuse it.) The haemoglobin rises no more quickly than with oral iron. Intravenous iron may cause anaphylactic reactions. Intramuscular iron stains the skin and a small number of fibrosarcomas at injection sites has been reported.

# Anaemias of chronic disorders

Chronic inflammatory diseases (particularly rheumatoid arthritis) and neoplastic diseases produce a blood picture that mimics iron defi-

**Table 21.9** Differential diagnosis of hypochromic anaemia.

|  | Iron deficiency | Anaemia of chronic disorders | Thalassaemia trait | Sideroblastic anaemia |
|---|---|---|---|---|
| Mean cell volume | Reduced | Reduced | Reduced | Usually raised, reduced in rare congenital type |
| Serum iron | Reduced | Reduced | Normal | Raised |
| Total iron-binding capacity | Raised | Reduced | Normal | Normal |
| Serum ferritin | Reduced | Normal or raised | Normal or raised | Raised |
| **Bone marrow** |  |  |  |  |
| Macrophage iron | Absent | Present | Present | Present |
| Erythroblast iron | Absent | Absent | Present | Ring forms |

ciency anaemia, although the MCV seldom falls as low as it may in iron deficiency. The syndrome is produced by macrophage iron being unavailable for haemoglobin production. Measurement of serum iron and TIBC usually distinguishes between the two (Table 21.9), but in complicated cases (such as rheumatoid arthritis with chronic blood loss due to consumption of anti-inflammatory drugs) bone marrow iron stores should be estimated.

Not all anaemia in chronic disease is of this type. In uraemia, the anaemia is a product of shortened red cell survival and lack of erythroid drive from low erythropoietin production. The anaemia of myxoedema is often macrocytic and its origin complex. Thyroxine increases bone marrow activity. Frequently there is an associated iron deficiency due to menorrhagia or megaloblastic anaemia due to the coexistence of pernicious anaemia.

## TREATMENT

This is of the underlying condition. Parenteral iron is inappropriate and may provoke a severe reaction with arthralgia, myalgia and fever.

# Sideroblastic anaemia

The condition is characterized by the presence of rings of iron within mitrochondria around the nucleus of developing erythroblasts in the bone marrow. Such rings may be seen in a minority of cells in some patients with haemolytic anaemia, lead poisoning, or rheumatoid arthritis or those on isoniazid treatment, but the commonest form of sideroblastic anaemia occurs in the elderly and is associated with a raised MCV. It is one of the myelodysplastic syndromes (see below). It is only the rare X-linked congenital type of sideroblastic anaemia that has microcytic red blood cells.

## TREATMENT

Some of the congenital sideroblastic anaemias and some of those secondary to other conditions respond to treatment with pyridoxine, 100–

200 mg/day. Others may require regular blood transfusion but there is a danger of iron overload.

# Megaloblastic anaemias

The megaloblastic anaemias are a group of disorders which display a characteristic abnormality in the erythroblasts of the bone marrow, the maturation of the nucleus being retarded compared with that of the cytoplasm. The underlying abnormality is a defect in DNA synthesis. In practice this is almost always due to a shortage of vitamin $B_{12}$ or folic acid, although there are rare enzyme deficiencies and some cytotoxic drugs which produce the same effect. By far the commonest cause of megaloblastic anaemia in the UK is pernicious anaemia (PA), which was described first by Thomas Addison of Guy's Hospital in 1855 and has an incidence of 1:10 000. It occurs predominantly in women over the age of 50 with a male:female ratio of 1:1.5. It is associated with blood group A and purportedly in those whose hair turns grey at an early age. There is frequently a family history of PA, and both patients and relatives have a high incidence of autoimmune thyroid disease and vitiligo.

## PATHOLOGY

Vitamin $B_{12}$ consists of a group of cobalt-containing compounds that are produced by micro-organisms. The main source is food of animal origin, especially liver; strict vegans are at risk of developing $B_{12}$ deficiency. Vitamin $B_{12}$ is released from food in the stomach where it binds to **intrinsic factor** (IF), a glycoprotein secreted by parietal cells. This $B_{12}$/IF complex binds to receptors in the terminal ileum from where the $B_{12}$ is absorbed into portal blood. It is carried in the blood bound to transcobalamin II and thence transferred to the bone marrow. Storage of $B_{12}$ is mainly in the liver but also in the blood bound to transcobalamin I which is produced mainly by granulocytes. Normally, enough $B_{12}$ is stored in the body to sustain haematopoiesis for 5 years.

Folic acid (pteroylglutamic acid) is the parent compound of a large group of folates present in leafy vegetables and yeast products. Folates occur in food as polyglutamates and are absorbed as monoglutamates. They appear in the plasma as methyl tetrahydrofolate (methyl THF). In order to be taken-up from the plasma methyl THF must be converted to 5, 10-methylene THF. This reaction requires vitamin $B_{12}$ as a co-enzyme. Once inside the cell 5, 10-methylene THF catalyses the conversion of deoxyuridine to thymidine, a step that is essential for DNA synthesis (Fig. 21.3).

# Pernicious anaemia

**Pernicious anaemia** is caused by a failure to secrete IF due to an immunological attack on the gastric parietal cells by autoantibodies and reactive lymphocytes. The gastric mucosa becomes atrophic and acid secretion is also reduced. Other mechanisms of $B_{12}$ and folate deficiency together with a full list of causes are given in Table 21.10.

## CLINICAL FEATURES

The onset of anaemia is usually insidious. Sometimes glossitis is present together with mild jaundice (a lemon-yellow tint) due to haemolysis. Purpura may be a presenting feature, and this is particularly likely in intensive care units where patients may become acutely and unexpectedly short of folate. Mild splenomegaly is sometimes present and the fea-

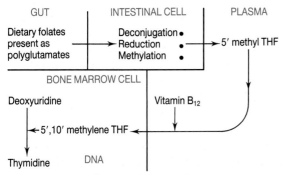

**Figure 21.3** Metabolism of folic acid. THF = tetrahydrofolate.

Rees/Williams  Fig 21.3  67% (second colour)

**Table 21.10** Causes of megaloblastic anaemias.

| | |
|---|---|
| **Vitamin $B_{12}$ deficiency** | |
| Decreased intake | Only in vegans |
| Gastric causes | Pernicious anaemia |
| | Gastrectomy (total and partial) |
| | Congenital deficiency of intrinsic factor |
| Intestinal causes | Consumption of vitamin $B_{12}$ by bacteria in stagnant intestinal loops or by the fish tapeworm *Diphyllobothrium latum* |
| | Malabsorption due to coeliac disease or tropical sprue |
| | Disorders of the terminal ileum: resection, Crohn's disease, congenital malabsorption |
| **Folate deficiency** | |
| Decreased intake | Old age, poverty, alcoholics, patients in intensive care units |
| Malabsorption | Coeliac disease, tropical sprue, bowel resection |
| Excessive utilization | Pregnancy, lactation |
| | Blood diseases: haemolytic anaemia, myelofibrosis |
| | Neoplasms: lymphoma, cancer |
| | Inflammation: rheumatoid arthritis, exfoliating skin disease, patients in intensive care units |
| Drugs | Anticonvulsants: phenytoin |
| | Antifolates: methotrexate |
| **Unresponsive to vitamin $B_{12}$ or folic acid** | |
| Rare congenital diseases | Orotic aciduria, Lesch–Nyhan syndrome (page 580) |
| Metabolic inhibitors | 6-Mercaptopurine, 6-thioguanine, 5-fluorouracil, hydroxyurea, cytosine arabinoside |

tures of any underlying disease may be apparent. In vitamin $B_{12}$ deficiency a neurological syndrome may dominate (see below).

## DIAGNOSIS

A macrocytic anaemia is usually apparent, although cases with a normal MCV undoubtedly occur. The blood film shows oval macrocytes, marked anisocytosis and poikilocytosis. Circulating megaloblasts may be seen. There is usually neutropenia and thrombocytopenia and occasionally this is severe. Hypersegmented neutrophils are usually seen.

The differential diagnosis involves the other causes of macrocytosis (Table 21.11) and to establish the diagnosis of megaloblastic anaemia a bone marrow aspirate is necessary. This usually shows erythroid hyperplasia with the characteristic megaloblastic picture, the red cell precursors being large with lacey nuclear chromatin but normal haemoglobinization and the white cell series showing giant metamyelocytes. Both vitamin $B_{12}$ and folate deficiency give the same blood and bone marrow picture and to distinguish them serum $B_{12}$ and folate and red cell folate measurements are necessary (Table 21.4). It is futile and a waste of money to ask for $B_{12}$ and folate measurements on patients being treated with $B_{12}$ or folate. A Schilling test will distinguish between malabsorption of vitamin $B_{12}$ and lack of intrinsic factor. Antibodies to gastric parietal cells are present in the serum of

**Table 21.11** Causes of macrocytosis.

---

Megaloblastic anaemias

Reticulocytosis
   Haemorrhage
   Haemolysis
   Response to treatment for anaemia

Increased surface membrane
   Liver disease
   Myxoedema
   Postsplenectomy

Dyshaematopoiesis
   Myelodysplastic syndromes
   Aplastic anaemia
   Alcohol
   Cytotoxic drugs (especially hydroxyurea)

---

95 per cent of patients with pernicious anaemia (but are also present in large numbers of patients with thyroid disease, iron deficiency and Addison's disease and in 20 per cent of women over 40). Intrinsic factor antibodies are present in 50 per cent of patients with PA and are virtually confined to this condition.

## COMPLICATIONS

Vitamin $B_{12}$ deficiency is associated with a number of neurological complications:

1. Subacute combined degeneration of the cord (page 713)
2. Glove and stocking peripheral neuropathy
3. Dementia
4. Optic atrophy (very rare)

Carcinoma of the stomach is commoner in PA than in the general population. There is an association with other organ-specific autoimmune conditions for example, hyper- and hypothyroidism and Addison's disease.

## TREATMENT

In vitamin $B_{12}$ deficiency, hydroxocobalamin (1 mg i.m. $\times$ 6) over 2 weeks should be given to replenish the stores. Thereafter 1 mg should be given every 3 months for life. In folate deficiency 5 mg of oral folic acid daily should be given at least for as long as the underlying condition persists. In either condition response is signified by a rise in the reticulocyte count, peaking at 7 days, although there is often subjective improvement within 48 hours. Vitamin $B_{12}$ deficiency will also respond initially to folic acid treatment, but this is hazardous since neurological complications are likely to be precipitated because the increased red cell population consumes the already low stores of vitamin $B_{12}$, directing them from the nerves and spinal cord. If an urgent response is necessary before the full diagnosis is made, vitamin $B_{12}$ and folic acid should be given together. In the elderly, potassium supplements may be necessary during the first 10 days of treatment since hypokalaemia, due to uptake of the new erythrocytes, is common and may be fatal. Blood transfusion should be avoided unless absolutely essential, but if given, packed cells should be transfused slowly. Prophylactic folic acid is often given during pregnancy, but physiological doses (0.5 mg/day) are all that are required.

# Aplastic anaemia

This is a very rare but extremely serious disorder of bone marrow stem cells in which there is failure of production of erythrocytes, granulocytes and platelets. Each cell line may be affected individually, producing pure red cell aplasia, agranulocytosis, thrombocytopenia or any combination. The causes are given in Table 21.12.

**Table 21.12** Causes of aplastic anaemia.

| |
|---|
| Radiation or cytotoxic drugs |
| Idiosyncratic reaction to drugs<br>   Phenylbutazone and oxyphenbutazone<br>   Chloramphenicol<br>   Gold salts<br>   Troxidone<br>   Sulphonamides and derivatives including thiazides<br>     and sulphonylureas |
| Postinfection<br>   Hepatitis, human parvovirus |
| Rare congenital conditions<br>   Fanconi syndrome |

## PATHOLOGY

There is a destruction of stem cells and/or an inhibition of those remaining to divide and repopulate the bone marrow. In some cases this is immunologically mediated through antibodies or T suppressor cells.

## CLINICAL FEATURES

The features are of anaemia, neutropenia and thrombocytopenia. The onset is insidious. Infections in the mouth with necrotic ulcers and thrush are very troublesome, and life-threatening haemorrhage, particularly intracranially is a constant risk.

## DIAGNOSIS

Severe pancytopenia is characteristic (Table 21.13). There is usually a normochromic, normocytic anaemia, although the MCV may be moderately raised. Reticulocytes are reduced. Granulocytes are fewer than $1.5 \times 10^9$ per litre and platelets reduced in severe cases to fewer than $10 \times 10^9$ per litre. A bone marrow trephine biopsy is essential to make the diagnosis. It shows patchy cellular areas on a fatty, hypocellular background.

Some cases are associated with paroxysmal nocturnal haemoglobinuria, and in these a positive Ham's test is found (page 614).

**Table 21.13** Differential diagnosis of pancytopenia.

| |
|---|
| Aplastic anaemia |
| Megaloblastic anaemia |
| Myelodysplastic syndrome |
| Acute leukaemia |
| Bone marrow infiltration<br>   Lymphoma<br>   Carcinoma<br>   Myeloma<br>   Myelofibrosis<br>   Gaucher disease (rare)<br>   Osteopetrosis (very rare) |
| Hypersplenism |
| Infection<br>   Disseminated tuberculosis<br>   Overwhelming sepsis<br>Systemic lupus erythematosus |
| Immune pancytopenia (rare) |

## TREATMENT

Good supportive care as described for the treatment of acute leukaemia (page 627) is the cornerstone of management. The milder cases sometimes respond to treatment with anabolic steroids in high doses (e.g. oxymethalone, up to 250 mg/day). Treatment for up to 6 months may be necessary before there is a response, and the side effects are troublesome. All such drugs are androgenic to a degree and may cause cholestasis and fluid retention. Approximately 50 per cent of patients will improve on treatment with anti-T-cell antibodies (usually horse polyclonal antibodies, although mouse monoclonal antibodies are under evaluation). The best results are achieved by the centres that have the best supportive care.

Bone marrow transplantation (page 629) should be considered in cases of severe aplasia (reticulocytes $<20 \times 10^9/l$, granulocytes $<0.5 \times 10^9/l$, platelets $<20 \times 10^9/l$). The procedure differs from that used in acute leukaemia in that the recipient does not receive total body irradiation (TBI), since there is no leukaemic clone to obliterate, but only cyclophosphamide, 50 mg/kg, for 4 days for immunosuppression. Since the degree of immunosuppression obtained is less, rejection is more likely. However, this degree of immunosuppression may be sufficient to switch off the autoimmune process if this is the cause of the disease, and some patients regrow their own marrow rather than that of the donor.

## PROGNOSIS

More than 50 per cent of patients die in the first year. It the patient can be kept alive by good supportive care for more than a year, then improvement is likely. Bone marrow transplantation in the young is effective, with 50 to 70 per cent survival over 5 years.

# Pure red cell aplasia

The mode of inheritance of the rare congenital form Diamond–Blackfan syndrome, is unknown. It sometimes responds to treatment with corticosteroids. The acquired form often seems to have an immunological basis, and may be associated with a (usually benign) thymoma and/or myasthenia gravis. Removal of the thymoma is often beneficial, and other cases respond to immunosuppressive treatment. Some cases are associated with the myelodysplastic syndrome. Human parvovirus is an important cause of transient pure red cell aplasia, especially in congenital haemolytic anaemias. In patients with immunodeficiency syndromes chronic human parvovirus infection may cause persistent pure red cell aplasia which can be aleviated by infusions of normal human IgG.

# Haemolytic anaemias

Haemolytic anaemias are those anaemias caused primarily by increased red cell destruction. They may be caused by intrinsic disorders of the red cell or by external agents acting upon them. Many anaemias have a haemolytic element, but those with another major cause are not usually included within the classification (Table 21.14).

## CLINICAL FEATURES

Pallor, mild jaundice and splenomegaly are the usual findings in haemolytic anaemia. Leg ulcers (particularly over the lateral malleolus) are a feature of chronic congenital haemolytic anaemias. Acute intravascular haemolysis is often associated with back pain and dark urine.

## PATHOLOGY

After a life-span of some 120 days red cells are destroyed mainly in the bone marrow and spleen. Increased destruction leads to a compensatory production in the marrow which can increase up to eight times before anaemia results.

When blood cells are destroyed within the circulation (intravascular haemolysis) the haemoglobin released is bound to haptoglobin and the complex cleared by the macrophages so that serum haptoglobin is reduced or undetectable. Excess haemoglobin is filtered by the kidney. Some will be processed by renal tubular cells and appear in the urine as haemosiderin; the remainder is excreted as haemoglobinuria which causes red urine, but is differentiated from haematuria by the absence of red cells. Some of the plasma haemoglobin is processed to methaemalbumin which circulates in the blood and may be detected spectroscopically. Unconjugated bilirubin is raised from breakdown of haemoglobin. Extravascular haemolysis takes place mainly in the spleen, which is an environment especially hostile to damaged red cells.

## DIAGNOSIS

A scheme for the diagnosis of haemolytic anaemia is shown in Fig. 21.4.

**Table 21.14** Types of haemolytic anaemia.

**Intrinsic red cell defects**

| | |
|---|---|
| Disorders of haemoglobin | Sickle cell syndromes<br>HbC disease<br>Rare amino acid substitutions (thalassaemias) |
| Disorders of red cell membrane | Hereditary spherocytosis<br>Hereditary elliptocytosis<br>Paroxysmal nocturnal haemoglobinuria |
| Disorders of red cell enzymes | Glucose 6-phosphate deficiency<br>PK deficiency |

**Extrinsic disorders**

| | | |
|---|---|---|
| *Immune* | | |
| Autoimmune | | Warm antibodies<br>Cold agglutinins<br>Paroxysmal cold haemoglobinuria |
| Isoimmune | | Rhesus haemolytic disease of the newborn<br>Incompatible transfusion |
| *Non-immune* | | |
| Physical | | March haemoglobinuria (due to walking or running on a hard surface)<br>Heart valve damage<br>Microangiopathic haemolytic anaemia (TTP, haemolytic uraemic syndrome, carcinomatosis, haemangiomas) |
| Chemical | | Drugs<br>Toxins |
| Infections | | Malaria<br>*Clostridium welchii* |
| Hyperactivity of monocyte/ macrophage system | | Hypersplenism |

PK = pyruvate kinase. TTP = thrombotic thrombocytopaenic purpura.

# Disorders of haemoglobin

These may be acquired or inherited, the latter being among the commonest single gene disorders.

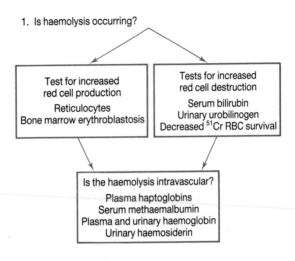

1. Is haemolysis occurring?

| Test for increased red cell production | Tests for increased red cell destruction |
|---|---|
| Reticulocytes<br>Bone marrow erythroblastosis | Serum bilirubin<br>Urinary urobilinogen<br>Decreased $^{51}Cr$ RBC survival |

Is the haemolysis intravascular?
Plasma haptoglobins
Serum methaemalbumin
Plasma and urinary haemoglobin
Urinary haemosiderin

2. What is the cause of the haemolysis?

Blood film
Special tests

**Figure 21.4** Investigation of haemolytic anaemia. RBC = red blood cell.

## THE THALASSAEMIAS

The thalassaemias are common in a broad band stretching from the Mediterranean to South-East Asia. Generally speaking, α-thalassaemia is commoner in the east and β-thalassaemia in the west. They are caused by inherited defects of globin chain synthesis. The heterozygous conditions (*thalassaemia minor*) manifest as abnormalities of the blood count which mimic iron deficiency, although anaemia is seldom present. The homozygous form (*thalassaemia major*) produces a severe anaemia which may be incompatible with life. *Thalassaemia intermedia* is a clinical term used to describe the condition of a number of patients with the blood features of thalassaemia minor who have a moderate to severe anaemia. It may be caused by the interaction of several congenital abnormalities of haemoglobin synthesis.

### Pathology

Each molecule of haemoglobin A consists of two α chains and two non-α chains, β, γ or δ. The major haemoglobin in the fetus is HbF ($\alpha_2, \gamma_2$) which has a relatively high oxygen affinity. After 3 months of age, although small amounts of HbF continue to be made, the major haemoglobin is HbA ($\alpha_2$, $\beta_2$). HbA$_2$ ($\alpha_2$, $\delta_2$) is also produced in small amounts. β-Thalassaemia trait is caused by the inheritance of an abnormal β-chain gene from one parent which results in a reduced synthesis of β-chains, but their lack is compensated for to a degree by increased synthesis of γ- and δ-chains. Homozygous β-thalassaemia is a much more severe condition characterized by the production of small dysplastic red cells with a short life-span.

Almost all cases of β-thalassaemia are the result of single nucleotide substitutions in the DNA which lead to defects in transcription, RNA splicing or translation through frame shifts or nonsense codons, or else to production of a highly unstable β-globin which cannot be used. Because of the wide variety of genetic lesions there is a degree of variability in the clinical picture and uncertainty about prenatal diagnosis unless the familial lesion is known.

Production of α-chains is controlled by four α-chain genes, two from each parent. Therefore, it is possible to have deficiencies of one, two, three or four α-chains in α-thalassaemia. The commonest genetic abnormality is the complete deletion of one or more genes. Four-gene deletion leads to death *in utero* from hydrops fetalis with the formation of Hb Barts ($\gamma_4$), and three-gene deletion produces HbH disease ($\beta_4$). One- and two-gene deletion produce α-thalassaemia minor.

## Clinical features

Thalassaemia minor is a clinically silent condition with gives rise to an abnormal blood count, although the Hb remains near normal. β-Thalassaemia major is not clinically apparent until the production of HbF decays at about 3 months of age. The clinical features of the untreated disease are those of severe anaemia, hypersplenism, iron overload and marrow expansion (Fig. 21.5). The characteristic facial appearance is of bossing of the skull, prominent frontal and parietal bones and enlarged maxillae.

HbH disease is a chronic haemolytic anaemia with Hb levels between 80 and 100 g/l, and splenomegaly.

Interaction between different types of thalassaemia and the haemoglobinopathies is common so that the phenotypic expression of any particular genotype is difficult to predict.

## Diagnosis

The disease may be suspected from the blood count and film appearance which shows microcytosis, hypochromia, target cells, basophilic stippling and normoblasts. In β-thalassaemia both HbA$_2$ and HbF levels are raised, and in α-thalassaemia HbH inclusions may be seen by supravital staining with cresyl blue. In thalassaemia major, X-rays show expansion of bones, with the skull showing a typical 'hair-on-end' appearance. Precise genetic diagnoses are now possible with the use of cDNA probes, and these may be used on chorionic villus samples taken at the tenth week of pregnancy allowing the parents the option of termination of pregnancy.

## Treatment

Thalassaemia minor requires genetic counselling, especially in countries where the disease is common.

β-Thalassaemia major should be treated with regular blood transfusions. The aim is to keep the Hb near normal so that the marrow may be sufficiently suppressed to prevent the bony changes. This policy leads to iron overload syndrome with diabetes, delayed puberty, liver damage and congestive cardiac failure, but the increased iron absorption found in the inadequately treated patient has a similar consequence. To prevent this iron chelation therapy is given: 2 g of a chelating agent, desferrioxamine, which binds to the iron, in each unit of blood transfused, together with pump-driven subcutaneous infusion of desferrioxamine, up to 4 g over 12 hours. Vitamin C, 200 mg/day, enhances the urinary iron excretion produced by desferrioxamine. Folic acid supplements are also necessary. Splenectomy may be necessary for hypersplenism.

Transfusion and chelation therapy is far from ideal. Many teenagers resent being coupled to a pump for prolonged periods and default on the treatment. Furthermore, desferrioxamine has side effects which include cataracts. Several oral iron chelaters are undergoing clinical trial; bone marrow transplantation is being used and gene therapy may eventually be applicable.

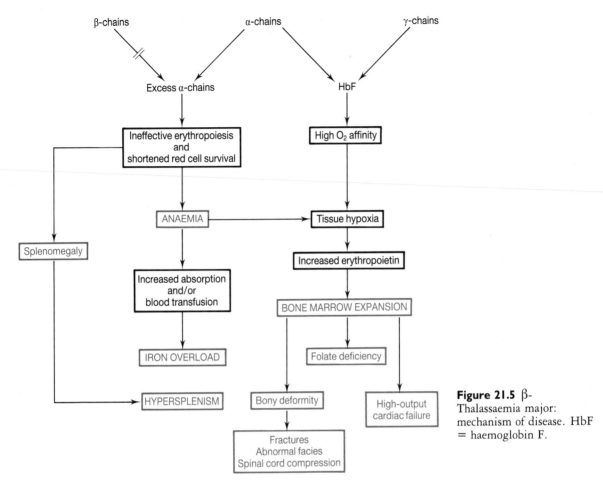

**Figure 21.5** β-Thalassaemia major: mechanism of disease. HbF = haemoglobin F.

## Prognosis

Thalassaemia minor and HbH disease are compatible with a normal life-span. Untreated thalassaemia major is fatal in childhood or adolescence owing to infection and the anaemia itself. Transfusion and chelation therapy are expensive and beyond the reach of many of the countries where the disease is commonest, but they hold out hope for a prolongation of life to near normal.

# Disorders of haemoglobin structure

## AETIOLOGY

Point mutations of the genes coding for the α- and β- chains of globin lead to amino acid substitutions which may alter the structure and function of haemoglobin. Some of these have had a survival advantage (particularly in the heterozygous state) in malarious areas. The haemoglobinopathies are relatively common in patients whose origins are in Africa or Asia (Fig. 21.6). In the third world they are a major health problem.

## SICKLE CELL SYNDROMES

These diseases are caused by an amino acid substitution at position 6 of the β-chain (valine for glutamic acid). This gives rise to a haemoglobin molecule HbS that is insoluble in the reduced state and which when exposed to low oxygen tension forms crystals; the red cells adopt a sickle shape which prevents their normal circulation through small blood vessels and leads to microinfarcts in various organs.

Homozygous HbS disease is generally a severe

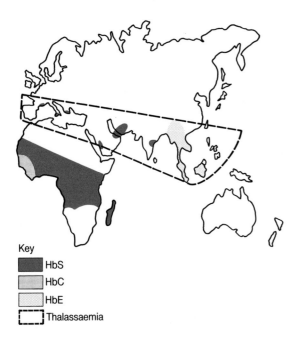

**Key**

- ■ HbS
- ▦ HbC
- ▢ HbE
- ⌐⌐ Thalassaemia

**Figure 21.6** Distribution of thalassaemias and haemoglobinopathies. Hb = haemoglobin.

disease, although it may be modified by conditions which increase the amount of HbF in the cell. The heterozygous condition, sickle cell trait, is a benign condition except in extreme anoxia. It affords some protection against *Plasmodium falciparum* malaria which probably accounts for the high gene frequency in certain geographical areas. Combination of HbS with HbC or thalassaemia produces syndromes of varying severity.

## Clinical features

There is a moderate haemolytic anaemia with an Hb of between 80 and 100 g/l in homozygous HbS disease. This steady state is punctuated by crises. Infarctive crises, which are characteristically severely painful, may occur in any organ. In children the bones of the hands and feet are most frequently affected causing dactylitis. Recurrent splenic infarcts result in hyposplenism in most adults. The combination of infection and infarction can produce a rapidly progressive intra-alveolar consolidation with the risk of respiratory failure. Painful occlusive crises may occur in the limbs, back, abdomen or trunk. Infarctive crises are precipitated by hypoxia, dehydration and infection. Aplastic crises

occur either in association with human parvovirus infections or because of folate deficiency.

Leg ulcers are a feature of many haemolytic anaemias but are particularly common in adults with sickle cell disease. Occlusions in the retinal vessels can lead to vitreous haemorrhage and retinal detachments, especially in HbS/C disease. Aseptic necrosis of the femoral heads is not uncommon. Cerebral infarction may lead to hemiplegia and epilepsy.

## Diagnosis

The diagnosis may be suspected on the blood film, but this shows characteristic sickled red cells only in the homozygous condition. A solubility test rapidly screens for sickle cell disease and sickle cell trait, and this is valuable preoperatively. The definitive test is haemoglobin electropheresis.

## Complications

Pregnancy is hazardous in sickle cell disease but careful antenatal care has brought maternal mortality down from about 1 in 3 to 1 per cent.

Infections are common, and osteomyelitis caused by *Salmonella* is a particular risk. As with all chronic haemolytic anaemias, pigment gallstones are common. Painful priapism which usually results in impotence is one of the most unpleasant of the results of occlusion in the microvasculature.

## Treatment

There is no specific treatment. Avoidance of the factors that precipitate crises is important together with the cultivation of a good standard of health and hygiene. Raising living standards in the developing world helps to prevent complications. Infections should be treated promptly and acidosis and dehydration avoided or rapidly remedied. Pregnancy and anaesthesia carry special risks and for these prophylactic transfusions are often helpful; the aim should be to reduce the HbS level to less than 20 per cent. Patients should receive oral folic acid at a dose of 5 mg/ day. Immunization against pneumococci and long-term prophylactic oral penicillin reduce the sequelae of splenic infarction. Painful crises are treated with rest and adequate analgesia (opiates if necessary) together with treatment of the precipitating cause. Genetic counselling may be necessary for patients with sickle cell trait. Antenatal diagnosis is possible with the option of termination of pregnancy.

## Prognosis

In areas with a high standard of living sickle cell disease is compatible with an average survival of 50 years, but in the poor, and especially in developing countries it is often a cause of early death and much disability.

## OTHER HAEMOGLOBINOPATHIES

Other amino acid substitutions lead to HbC, HbE and HbD. They are quite common in Africa and Asia but produce only mild haemolytic anaemias. There are over 100 different types of haemoglobinopathy that occur sporadically, most of which produce no clinical effect, although a minority cause a chronic haemolytic anaemia. The commonest of the latter is Hb Köln.

# Red cell membrane abnormalities

## HEREDITARY SPHEROCYTOSIS

This is the commonest hereditary haemolytic anaemia in Europe and is due to an abnormality of the structural protein, spectrin, in the red cell membrane. As a consequence the red cell loses its typical biconcave shape and becomes spherical. It is consequently less able to pass through small apertures and prone to destruction in the spleen. It is inherited as an autosomal dominant characteristic.

## Clinical features

Hereditary spherocytosis may present at any age. The typical features of haemolytic anaemia are present and a family history is usual. The anaemia is sometimes revealed following a virus infection such as infectious mononucleosis or parvovirus. The severity varies from family to family. Moderate splenomegaly is almost always present. Pigment gallstones are common.

## Diagnosis

The diagnosis is made by the finding of spherocytes in the blood film and confirmed if this finding is seen in the film of family members. The other common cause of spherocytosis is autoimmune haemolytic anaemia, and therefore in hereditary spherocytosis the direct Coombs' test (page 599) should be negative. The presence of spherocytes causes a positive osmotic fragility test (page 599).

## Treatment

Splenectomy results in complete resolution of the anaemia and all other symptoms. It should certainly be offered to all patients who have suffered from the effects of anaemia or haemolysis, including those with pigment gallstones. Since splenectomy leads to an increased susceptibility to some infections (particularly those due to pneumococci and meningococci), it should be avoided in those with asymptomatic abnormalities and delayed in young children. Prophylaxis against such infection is indicated in young people by immunization with pneumococcal vaccine before splenectomy and long-term oral penicillin following it. Folic acid supplements are usually required.

## HEREDITARY ELLIPTOCYTOSIS

Elliptical red cells are normal in camels but a rare finding in humans. These are of unknown cause and are inherited as an autosomal dominant trait but they seldom cause anaemia. Occasionally haemolysis is severe; when it is, splenectomy is indicated.

## PAROXYSMAL NOCTURNAL HAEMOGLOBINURIA

This exceptionally rare acquired defect of the red cell membrane leads to episodes of acute intravascular haemolysis characteristically, but by no means exclusively, at night. An abnormal clone of cells with an exquisite sensitivity to the alternative complement pathway is produced. Chronic intravascular haemolysis leads to iron loss in the urine and thus iron deficiency. Recurrent thromboses are common, most seriously involving the hepatic vein or cerebral sinuses. Transformation to aplastic anaemia or even acute leukaemia may occur. Diagnosis is by demonstrating haemolysis at a pH of 6.4 (Ham's test); the low pH activates the alternative complement pathway, so demonstrating the sensitivity of the erythrocytes to lysis. Treatment is based on transfusion with washed red cells to avoid activating complement.

# Disorders of red cell enzymes

The functions of the red cell enzyme systems are (a) the generation of hydrogen ions to prevent oxidation of the membrane and the haemoglobin molecule, and (b) the production of ATP to fuel the metabolic processes of the cell (Fig. 21.7).

Although congenital deficiency of many enzymes may occur, only two are likely to be encountered.

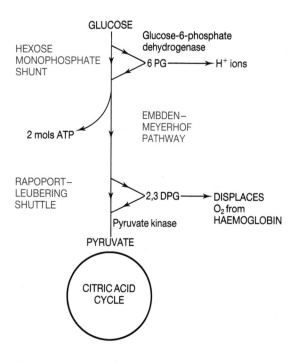

**Figure 21.7** Important red cell enzyme pathways in haemolytic anaemia. PG = phosphoglycerate. DPG = diphosphoglycerate.

## GLUCOSE 6-PHOSPHATE DEHYDROGENASE DEFICIENCY

Glucose 6-phosphate dehydrogenase (G6PD) deficiency is present in over 100 million people in the world. It is inherited as an X-linked recessive characteristic and there are three common abnormalities, the Afro-Caribbean, Mediterranean and Chinese variants, but there are over 160 sporadically occurring ones.

### Pathology

Failure to generate hydrogen ions makes the red cell susceptible to oxidative stress causing denaturation of haemoglobin which precipitates to form Heinz bodies in the red cells. Cells containing Heinz bodies cannot traverse the splenic pulp. In severe cases intravascular haemolysis occurs.

### Clinical features

Three clinical syndromes are recognizable.

*1. Chronic haemolytic anaemia*
This is mainly seen in the sporadic variants.

*2. Episodes of acute intravascular haemolysis*
These are mainly in response to exposure to oxidative drugs or fava beans. The Mediterranean type is more susceptible than the Afro-Caribbean type to such stress. Most of the drugs quoted in large textbooks produce haemolysis that is only detectable in the test-tube. Those still in the British National Formulary that produce clinical haemolysis are given in Table 21.15.

Favism is confined to the Mediterranean type. The mechanism is unknown but is presumed to be in part allergic. Ingestion of beans or even inhalation of pollen leads to the most severe

**Table 21.15** Drugs inducing haemolysis in glucose 6-phosphate dehydrogenase deficiency.

| |
| --- |
| Primaquine |
| Quinine* |
| Sulphamethoxazole |
| Nitrofurantoin |
| Nalidixic acid |
| Chloramphenicol* |
| Dapsone |

*In Mediterranean type only.

attack of intravascular haemolysis. Fava beans (*Vicia fava*) are the common broad beans.

### 3. Haemolytic disease of the newborn

This occurs particularly in the Chinese variant.

## Diagnosis

During haemolytic episodes small clumps of denatured haemoglobin attach to the red cell membrane (Heinz bodies) and may be demonstrated by supravital staining with brilliant cresyl blue, which will also reveal a reticulocytosis. Heinz bodies are removed by the spleen and the resulting cells appear to have been nibbled at the periphery (bite cells). A screening test for the integrity of the hexose monophosphate shunt may be performed and the level of the red cell G6PD may be estimated.

## Treatment

Removal of the toxic agent is required together with blood transfusion as indicated.

## PYRUVATE KINASE DEFICIENCY

This is the second commonest red cell enzyme defect; 250 cases have been described. It is inherited as an abnormal autosomal recessive characteristic and its chief unusual feature is the mildness of the symptoms for the degree of anaemia. This is because the block in the Embden Meyerhof pathway causes a build-up of 2, 3-diphosphoglycerate. This displaces oxygen from the haem pocket making it more available to tissues. Diagnosis is by measurement of the specific enzyme. The blood film shows a characteristic poikilocytosis. Splenomegaly is common.

# Autoimmune haemolytic anaemia (AIHA)

## WARM-REACTING ANTIBODIES

### Pathology

Self-tolerance to red cell antigens may be by-passed in a variety of ways (Table 21.16), but in 50 per cent of cases the cause in unknown. Some

**Table 21.16** Causes of autoimmune haemolytic anaemias.

**Warm antibodies**
50% of cases are idiopathic

Secondary to drugs
  Methyldopa type
  Hapten type
  Immune complex type

Secondary to autoimmune disease
  Systemic lupus erythromatosus
  Rheumatoid arthritis

Secondary to lymphoid malignancy
  Chronic lymphocytic leukaemia
  Non-Hodgkin's lymphoma

**Cold antibodies**
Idiopathic (cold haemagglutination syndrome)
Secondary to infection
  *Mycoplasma pneumoniae*
  Infectious mononucleosis

Secondary to lymphoid malignancy
  Non-Hodgkin's lymphoma

**Paroxysmal cold haemoglobinuria**
Secondary to
  Syphilis
  Measles
  Varicella

drugs such as methyldopa induce autoantibodies directed against the red cell membrane. About 20 per cent of patients taking methyldopa develop red cell autoantibodies although overt haemolysis is seen in fewer than 1 per cent.

Warm antibodies are most active at 37°C and are usually IgG in type. They are usually directed against rhesus antigens and a minority of them fix complement, although intravascular haemolysis is rare. Antibody-coated cells attach to macrophages in the spleen, whereas those coated with complement can also be destroyed by macrophages elsewhere.

### Clinical features

The features are those of a haemolytic anaemia of variable severity with splenomegaly.

### Diagnosis

The blood film shows spherocytes and the direct Coombs' test is positive. Features of any underlying disease should be sought.

## Treatment

Most cases respond to treatment with oral prednisolone 60 mg/day. The dose is subsequently reduced to the lowest compatible with a normal Hb. If an acceptably low dose cannot be reached, then splenectomy may be indicated depending on results of the $^{51}$Cr-labelled red cell splenic-uptake test. In some patients there is a place for immunosuppressive treatment with cyclophosphamide or azathioprine.

## COLD-REACTING ANTIBODIES

### Aetiology

Cold antibodies are most active at 4°C and are IgM in type. They may appear as part of the immune response to infections with Epstein–Barr (EB) virus or *Mycoplasma pneumoniae*, in which case they are polyclonal; or they may be a version of benign monoclonal gammopathy (page 638) in which the antibody specificity of the monoclonal immunoglobulin happens to be directed against autologous red cells. Occasionally a monoclonal cold agglutinin is produced by malignant lymphoma. The specificity of the antibody is usually within the Ii blood group system. Antibody attaches to red cells in the cold (e.g. when passing through skin blood vessels) and fixes the C3 component of complement. At body core temperatures the IgM antibody disassociates from the cell but the C3 remains. C3-coated cells may be cleared from the circulation by macrophages. Low-titre cold agglutinins are frequently present in normal people and complicate blood cross-matching done at room temperature. The only clinically significant antibodies are those of high titres which are active at temperatures greater than 30°C.

### Clinical features

In most patients the haemolysis is minor, although after chilling severe intravascular haemolysis sometimes occurs. In many patients the major symptoms relate to sludging of red cells within the peripheral circulation, leading to acrocyanosis and Raynaud's phenomenon (page 232).

## Diagnosis

The first clue to the presence of cold agglutinins is often a very high MCV caused by the electronic cell counter erroneously counting two cells for one. Red cell agglutination may be seen on the blood film. The direct Coombs' test shows the presence of complement (C3) on the red cells.

## Treatment

The patient should keep warm. Electrically heated gloves and socks may be a help. Corticosteroids, immunosuppressives, splenectomy and plasmapheresis all have their advocates for the chronic syndrome, but the treatment is generally unsatisfactory. Cases associated with acute infection resolve spontaneously within a few weeks.

## PAROXYSMAL COLD HAEMOGLOBINURIA

This rare condition used to be seen in association with congenital syphilis but is now more frequently a transient complication of childhood virus infections especially human parvovirus infections. It is caused by the Donath–Landsteiner antibody (IgG with anti-P (a blood group) specificity) which reacts with red cells in the cold and fixes complement. When the temperature is raised, intravascular haemolysis occurs.

# Isoimmune haemolytic anaemia

## HAEMOLYTIC DISEASE OF THE NEWBORN (HDN)

Although only 20 years ago this was a major cause of infant mortality and morbidity, the widespread use of anti-D immunoglobulin has greatly reduced the prevalence, so that fewer than 70 infants per year die of this condition in the UK.

### Aetiology

Sensitization of the mother to the baby's red cells usually occurs at the delivery of the first child, but fetomaternal leaks may occur during pregnancy, especially during obstetric intervention (such as amniocentesis) or threatened miscarriage. Although Rh(D) has been by far the most important antigenic system, immunoprophylaxis has rendered it rare, so that other Rh groups, and the Kell, Duffy and Kidd blood groups have assumed more prominence. ABO incompatibility is a special case since naturally occurring IgG anti-A antibodies may occur in the sera of group O mothers, and no prior sensitization is needed.

Only IgG antibodies are able to cross the placenta, but those that do so induce a warm antibody immune haemolytic anaemia in the fetus.

## Clinical features

These vary from mild anaemia to severe hydrops fetalis, a condition in which profound anaemia causes cardiac failure, oedema, hepatosplenomegaly and ascites, leading to intra-uterine death in the worst cases. In utero, unconjugated bilirubin is cleared via the placenta, but after birth the immature liver cannot conjugate the bilirubin rapidly enough so that it is deposited in the basal ganglia of the brain, causing kernicterus, which results in mental deficiency, spasticity, epilepsy and deafness.

## Treatment

All pregnant women should have their blood grouped and screened for atypical antibodies at the first antenatal visit, and at 24 and 34 weeks' gestation. Atypical antibodies should be identified and monitored. A rising titre of antibodies is an indication for amniocentesis at 28 weeks to determine the degree of fetal jaundice.

Affected babies may be managed by early induction of labour, or if detected at an earlier stage of gestation, then intrauterine transfusion of Rh(D) negative blood may be attempted via the peritoneal route from 24 weeks' gestation, or via the umbilical vein under fetoscopic guidance from 16 weeks' gestation.

After birth, exchange transfusion may be necessary to keep the haemoglobin above 120 g/l and the bilirubin below 240 μmol/l. For less severely affected infants conjugation of bilirubin may be enhanced by phototherapy.

Rh(D) sensitization may be prevented in Rh(D)-negative mothers by injecting 100 μg of anti-D intramuscularily within 36 hours of the birth of an Rh(D)-positive child. The anti-D combines with any fetal red cells which have crossed transplacentally into the mother and prevents them from immunizing her. If more than 4 ml of fetal blood (equivalent to 1:600 fetal:maternal cells) leak into the maternal circulation then a larger dose of anti-D will be required. Anti-D should also be given to Rh(D)-negative women in the case of threatened abortions, haemorrhages and obstetric manoeuvres.

# Incompatible blood transfusion

Transfusion of incompatible blood produces a haemolytic reaction which varies in severity from severe life-threatening intravascular haemolysis to a clinically inapparent shortened survival of transfused red cells.

## AETIOLOGY

Most incompatible transfusions arise from clerical errors. It is extremely important that request forms are filled in completely and accurately and that blood sample tubes are properly labelled. Tests of compatibility involve determination of the blood group of the donor and recipient and screening of the recipient's serum for antibodies to red cells. This is supplemented by the crossmatching of donor cells with the recipient's serum. Agglutination is enhanced by the presence of a low ionic strength medium. In addition, reaction of the cells with IgG in the serum is tested by using an indirect Coombs' test. However, even in the laboratory the commonest errors are clerical ones.

## CLINICAL FEATURES

When there is a major incompatibility, symptoms begin after the transfusion of a few millilitres of blood. The patient complains of restlessness, nausea and back pain, and begins shivering and vomiting. The skin is cold and clammy and may be cyanosed. There is tachycardia, tachypnoea and pyrexia leading to prostration and shock. The features of acute intravascular haemolysis are present and this may give rise to acute renal failure due to acute tubular necrosis.

## DIAGNOSIS

The identification of all samples and of the patient should be checked. The cross-match should be repeated on pre- and post-transfusion samples. The plasma and urine are checked for free haemoglobin. A direct Coombs' test is performed on the post-transfusion sample. Tests for disseminated intravascular coagulation are performed.

## TREATMENT

The object is to maintain blood pressure and perfusion of the kidneys. Intravenous hydrocortisone, saline and frusemide are usually required. Dialysis may be necessary until recovery occurs.

## PREVENTION

The transfusion of blood must not be taken lightly. Check and recheck the identification of patient, sample and blood for transfusion. If in doubt start again. Legal action arising from mistakes cannot be successfully defended.

# Microangiopathic haemolytic anaemia

This is a group of haemolytic anaemias caused by physical damage to the red blood cells. The damage is caused by fibrin strands laid down intravascularly in small blood vessels during various systemic disorders. The commonest of these are septicaemia, accelerated hypertension, eclampsia, the haemolytic uraemic syndrome and thrombotic thrombocytopenic purpura. Because of the nature of these disorders the haemolytic anaemia is usually acute. Damage and fragmentation of red cells also occurs in some patients with prosthetic heart valves.

The diagnosis is made on the blood film which shows fragmented red cells and microspherocytes; these findings give this condition its other name of 'red cell fragmentation syndrome'. Thrombocytopenia is a common accompaniment.

The condition is managed by correcting the anaemia and the thrombocytopenia by transfusion of blood and platelets, respectively, and, in addition, eradicating or minimizing the underlying systemic disorder.

# POLYCYTHAEMIA

Polycythaemia is defined as the presence of a red cell count greater than normal for the age and sex of the patient. It is usually associated with a high haemoglobin and high haematocrit, but to rely on these can be misleading. Some alcoholics have a high haematocrit with a normal red cell count because they have larger than normal red cells, and some patients with polycythaemia who develop an associated iron deficiency are actually anaemic because their red cells are small (Fig. 21.8).

Polycythaemia may be *spurious*, with a normal red cell mass but a decreased plasma volume, or *true* due to an increased red cell mass. The causes of polycythaemia are given in Fig. 21.9.

# Primary proliferative polycythaemia (PPP)

This is one of the myeloproliferative disorders and is due to a clonal proliferation of erythroid progenitor cells. Megakaryocytes and gran-

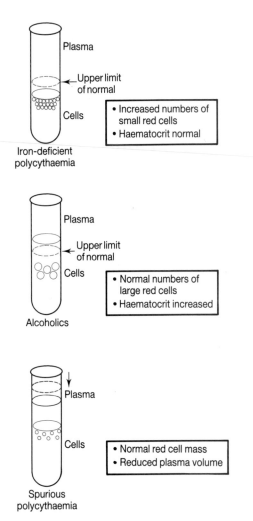

Iron-deficient polycythaemia
- Increased numbers of small red cells
- Haematocrit normal

Alcoholics
- Normal numbers of large red cells
- Haematocrit increased

Spurious polycythaemia
- Normal red cell mass
- Reduced plasma volume

**Figure 21.8** Pitfalls in polycythaemia. Three situations which can mask or mimic polycythaemia.

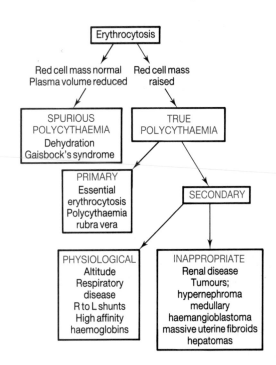

**Figure 21.9** Causes of polycythaemia. R = right. L = left.

ulocyte precursors are frequently involved in the proliferation.

## CLINICAL FEATURES

The symptoms of polycythaemia are a feeling of fullness in the head or headache, shortness of breath, blurred vision, cold hands and feet together with those of any complication of polycythaemia present. Aquagenic pruritis – itching after a hot bath – is typical in PPP. Facial plethora frequently occurs but its appearance can be mimicked by exposure to the weather. Cyanosis, both central and peripheral, may be present because the excess haemoglobin increases the amount of desaturated haemoglobin at any $PaO_2$ level. Splenomegaly is present in at least 75 per cent of patients and hepatomegaly in a third. Hypertension occurs in one-third of patients and small numbers have gout or peptic ulceration.

## DIAGNOSIS

Apart from the rise in Hb, RBC and PCV there may be a low MCV, if iron deficiency has developed during venesection and/or spontaneous bleeding. There is frequently a neutrophil leucocytosis, a raised basophil count and a raised platelet count. The ESR is usually very low (1 mm in the first hour). The leukocyte alkaline phosphatase score is usually high and the serum $B_{12}$ is high in a third of patients. Serum uric acid is often raised. Platelet function may be abnormal leading to bleeding. The bone marrow aspirate is less helpful than the trephine biopsy, which shows hypercellularity with hyperplasia of erythropoiesis, granulopoiesis and thrombopoiesis.

## DIFFERENTIAL DIAGNOSIS

The patient with all of the features of the disease presents little diagnostic problem, but all of the features are seldom present. It is important to estimate the red cell mass and plasma volume to exclude relative or spurious polycythaemia; in primary or secondary polycythaemia the red cell mass is raised and the plasma volume normal. The history and examination should point to underlying diseases of the respiratory or cardiovascular systems and may reveal a tumour. A renal lesion should be excluded by ultrasound, and the arterial oxygen saturation measured to exclude arteriovenous shunting.

## COMPLICATIONS

The most frequent complications are cerebrovascular or peripheral ischaemia caused by the hyperviscosity of the blood. Some patients suffer bleeding manifestations owing to disorders of platelet function. Expistaxis, bruising and gastrointestinal haemorrhages may be seen. Myelofibrosis supervenes in 30 per cent of cases, and transformation to acute leukaemia occurs in 15 per cent.

## TREATMENT

The most important aim of treatment is to lower the viscosity of the blood. This is best done by venesections, at least in the first instance. The aim should be to keep the PCV below 45 per cent (as measured by a centrifugal method). Some authorities prefer to manage the patient in the long term by venesection, relying on the iron deficiency induced to keep the Hb low. Unfortunately, this policy may actually intensify the itching and the platelet count may rise and put the patient at risk from haemorrhage or thrombosis. Long-term low-dose aspirin, 300 mg/day, has been recommended to reduce this risk.

Radioactive phosphorus ($^{32}$P) has been in use for many years. It is a β-emitter which is concentrated in bone and from there irradiates the bone marrow. A single dose produces a remission lasting about 2 years and it may be repeated. There seems little doubt that $^{32}$P increases the risk of leukaemic transformation, although others believe that this feature needs to be weighed against the longer survival in this group of patients compared with those treated by venesection.

Cytotoxic drugs also have their advocates.

Most carry a similar risk of leukaemic transformation as $^{32}$P, although this may not be true for hydroxyurea, 500–1000 mg/day, which is well tolerated, easily reversible and has few side effects.

# Secondary polycythaemia

The control of Hb level depends on oxygen receptors in the juxtaglomerular apparatus of the kidney where hypoxia leads to an increased secretion of erythropoietin. This is entirely appropriate if the hypoxia is caused by anaemia, but of less value in cardiac or respiratory disease and inappropriate when caused by distortion of the renal vasculature as in renal artery stenosis or polycystic kidneys. Inappropriate secretion of erythropoietin may also rarely arise from certain tumours (Fig. 21.9).

Recombinant erythropoietin is now available for treating some anaemias, and is primarily of use in chronic renal failure. It has been abused by some athletes as an undetectable means of raising the haemoglobin so as to produce the same benefit as altitude training. Some professional cyclists have died from cerebral infarction as a consequence.

## TREATMENT

Venesection is often indicated to give symptomatic relief and to reduce the risk of thrombosis, but a balance must be struck between oxygen carriage and viscosity. In patients with right-to-left cardiac shunts haematocrits of 70 per cent or more may occur. However, attempts to reduce viscosity by venesection are limited by symptoms of tissue hypoxia, particularly angina.

# Relative or spurious polycythaemia

Acute dehydration due to burns, vomiting or polyuria will raise the haematocrit. In stress polycythaemia (Gaisbock's syndrome), the plasma volume is chronically reduced for ill-understood reasons. Patients are usually middle-aged men, somewhat overweight, often with hypertension and are usually cigarette smokers. The disease mechanism is obscure but is almost certainly related to cigarette smoking and lack of exercise. Untreated, about half of patients suffer a cardiac or cerebrovascular 'event' within 18 months of diagnosis. The diagnosis is confirmed by measuring the red cell mass and plasma volume, which are normal and low respectively.

## TREATMENT

It is most important to stop smoking. In most patients who are able to stop the plasma volume rapidly returns to normal. The place of regular small-volume venesections is currently being investigated.

# Primary proliferative thrombocythaemia

This condition is closely related to primary proliferative polycythaemia, being a clonal proliferation of stem cells mainly committed to the production of megakaryocytes.

## CLINICAL FEATURES

Many patients are asymptomatic, but both haemorrhagic and thrombotic manifestations occur in cerebral and peripheral circulations. Splenomegaly is rare, possibly because of repeated small splenic infarctions.

## INVESTIGATIONS

The platelet count is usually greater than 1000 $\times$ 10$^9$ per litre. Since platelet function is abnor-

mal, tests for chronic gastrointestinal haemorrhage may be positive and iron deficiency anaemia may be present. Bone marrow shows hypercellularity with increased numbers of megakaryocytes.

## DIFFERENTIAL DIAGNOSIS

The causes of a raised platelet count are given in Table 21.17. It may be difficult to distinguish reactive thrombocytosis from essential thrombocythaemia, but giant platelets and abnormal platelet function are more characteristic of the latter.

**Table 21.17** Causes of a raised platelet count.

**Proliferative**
Primary proliferative thrombocythaemia
In association with other myeloproliferative disorders

**Reactive**
Haemorrhage
Chronic iron deficiency
Chronic infections
Chronic inflammatory conditions (especially
    rheumatoid arthritis and Crohn's disease)
Malignancy
Postsplenectomy
Recovery from
    Megaloblastic anaemia
    Cytotoxic drugs
    Alcohol
Treatment with vinca alkyloids

## TREATMENT

There is no indication to treat asymptomatic patients. Haemorrhagic or thrombotic complications may be controlled or prevented by low-dose aspirin, 300 mg/day. Radioactive phosphorus or hydroxyurea are both effective treatments of the myeloproliferation but there is a small risk of transformation to acute leukaemia. Alpha-interferon or the new agent anegrilide may be effective without this risk. Transformation to acute leukaemia is very rare.

# Myelofibrosis

This condition masquerades under several names, including myelosclerosis, agnogenic myeloid metaplasia and myelofibrosis with myeloid metaplasia (MMM).

## PATHOLOGY

Bone marrow fibrosis may occur in reaction to a number of stimuli, including infiltration with lymphoma, leukaemia or cancer. In the idiopathic type it seems to be in response to a proliferation of haematopoietic stem cells (possibly megakaryocyte precursors). The fibroblasts are not part of the clonal proliferation. Apparently in response to the marrow fibrosis, haematopoietic proliferation occurs in spleen, liver and sometimes lymph nodes.

## CLINICAL FEATURES

Myelofibrosis is a disease of the elderly presenting with the symptoms of anaemia, weight loss, anorexia, night sweats and splenic pain. Bone pain, bruises, bleeding and infections may occur less frequently. There is almost invariably massive splenomegaly.

## DIAGNOSIS

Anaemia is usually present, often with a neutrophil leukocytosis, although neutropenia and thrombocytopenia occur late in the disease. The blood film shows a leukoerythroblastic picture with a characteristic 'teardrop' poikilocytosis. Bone marrow aspirate often yields a 'dry tap', and trephine biopsy shows a hypercellular marrow with increased 'reticulin' demonstrated by silver stains. There is usually increased collagen and often increased bone formation. Megakaryocytes may be prominent.

## TREATMENT

Blood transfusion and folic acid supplements may be all that is required, but the more proliferative cases often benefit from hydroxyurea treatment. Splenectomy is sometimes effective, but choosing when to offer it is difficult. Indications for splenectomy are increasing transfusion requirement, massive splenomegaly causing discomfort, and severe thrombocytopenia. Removing a massive spleen may be difficult (particularly if it has previously been irradiated). Early splenectomy is controversial. After splenectomy the liver often markedly enlarges because of extramedullary haematopoiesis, and this sometimes also causes lymphadenopathy.

## PROGNOSIS

Median survival is 3 years. Fewer than 10 per cent transform to acute leukaemia.

# White cell disorders

## Leukocytosis

Raised numbers of neutrophil granulocytes, eosinophils, monocytes or lymphocytes may all be indicative of either systemic or haematological disease.

## NEUTROPHILIA

This is the commonest abnormality of white blood cells seen in clinical practice. Although neutrophils are characteristically raised in response to bacterial infection, mobilization of the marginated pool and the bone marrow reserve can occur rapidly in response to physiological effects such as exercise and emotion. In infections, as well as increased numbers, the neutrophils show hypolobulation (a left shift), 'toxic' granulation, and bluish cytoplasmic inclusions (Dohle bodies). The causes of neutrophilia are shown in Table 21.18.

**Table 21.18** Causes of neutrophilia.

| Infection | Bacterial |
|---|---|
| Physiological | Exercise, emotion, pregnancy |
| Non-infective inflammation | Burns, surgery, myocardial infarction, rheumatoid arthritis, immune vasculitis |
| Acute blood loss | Haemorrhage, haemolysis |
| Malignancy | Myeloproliferative disorders, other cancers |
| Metabolic | Cushing's syndrome, diabetic ketoacidosis |
| Miscellaneous | Convulsions, postsplenectomy |

## EOSINOPHILIA

The causes of eosinophilia are shown in Table 21.19. Churg–Strauss syndrome is a variant of vasculitis associated with asthma and eosinophilia. Loeffler's syndrome consists of transitory pulmonary shadowing associated with eosinophilia, but other forms of pulmonary eosinophilia are frequently confused with it. Very high eosinophil counts from whatever cause may be associated with endomyocardial fibrosis, and these patients may need to be treated with hydroxyurea to lower the eosinophil count.

## MONOCYTOSIS AND LYMPHOCYTOSIS

Although a monocytosis may be found in a variety of infections and other diseases (Table 21.20), the commonest cause is probably chronic myelomonocytic leukaemia, one of the myelodysplastic syndromes.

**Table 21.19** Causes of eosinophilia.

| Parasites | Filariasis, hookworm, ascariasis, strongyloides, toxocariasis etc. |
|---|---|
| Allergies | Asthma, hay fever, drug reactions, Stevens–Johnson syndrome |
| Skin diseases | Eczema, psoriasis, pemphigus, dermatitis herpetiformis |
| Malignant diseases | Hodgkin's disease, carcinomatosis, angioimmunoblastic lymphadenopathy, chronic granulocytic leukaemia, eosinophilic leukaemia (very rare), melanomatosis |
| Pulmonary eosinophilia | Churg–Strauss syndrome, Löeffler's syndrome |

**Table 21.20** Causes of monocytosis.

| Infections | Tuberculosis, brucellosis, syphilis, typhus, Rocky Mountain spotted fever, leishmaniasis, malaria, trypanosomiasis |
|---|---|
| Gastrointestinal | Ulcerative colitis, Crohn's disease |
| Neoplasms | Hodgkin's disease, carcinomatosis, histiocytic medullary reticulosis, chronic myelomonocytic leukaemia |

Young children respond to most types of infections with a lymphocytosis. Pertussis characteristically produces a very high lymphocyte count. The full list of causes is given in Table 21.21.

# Infectious mononucleosis

In Western Europe and North America infection with the **Epstein–Barr virus** is either subclinical or produces infectious mononucleosis (sometimes known as **glandular fever**). In Africa the same virus is involved in the aetiology of Burkitt's lymphoma and in the Far East it plays a

**Table 21.21** Causes of lymphocytosis.

| Infections | Infectious mononucleosis, rubella, measles, varicella, cytomegalovirus, mumps, infectious hepatitis |
| | Pertussis, tuberculosis, syphilis, brucellosis |
| | Toxoplasmosis |
| Neoplasms | Chronic lymphocytic leukaemia, acute lymphoblastic leukaemia, hairy cell leukaemia, exfoliative lymphomas |

**Table 21.22** Causes of neutropenia.

| Infections | Most viruses can cause mild neutropenia which may persist for 6 weeks or longer |
| | Severe overwhelming infections with Gram-negative bacteria |
| | Typhoid and tuberculosis |
| Drugs | Cytotoxic drugs |
| | Idiosyncratic reactions to many drugs; most important are phenothiazines, phenylbutazone, chloramphenicol, sulphonamides, antithyroid drugs, indomethacin |
| Autoimmunity | Systemic lupus erythromatosus |
| | Felty's syndrome |
| | Autoimmune neutropenia |
| Blood diseases | Megaloblastic anaemia |
| | Aplastic anaemia |
| | Myelodysplastic syndrome |
| | Leukaemia |
| | Lymphoma |
| Splenomegaly | Any cause of a large spleen |

part in the development of nasopharyngeal carcinoma. The incidence of infectious mononucleosis is difficult to calculate, but most adults, when tested, show evidence of previous exposure to the virus.

The condition is discussed further on page 731.

# Neutropenia

Mild neutropenia is one of the commonest findings in the routine blood count. Severe neutropenia (sometimes called agranulocytosis) is very rare and usually of grave significance. The causes of neutropenia are given in Table 21.22.

## PATHOLOGY

The mechanisms of neutropenia are either decreased production or increased destruction. Drugs interact with antibodies and granulocytes in the same way as they react with antibodies and red cells to cause haemolytic anaemias.

## CLINICAL FEATURES

Although the lower limit of normal for neutrophils is $2 \times 10^9$ per litre, infections are unlikely to be more common unless the neutrophil count falls below $1 \times 10^9$ per litre, and unlikely to be life-threatening unless it falls below $0.5 \times 10^9$ per litre. Most of the infections that occur are caused by endogenous organisms, typically Gram-negative coliforms and *Staphylococcus aureus*. Organisms not normally considered patho-

genic, such as *Staphylococcus epidermidis* and *Candida albicans*, cause septicaemias, especially in patients who have already received antibiotics.

## DIAGNOSIS

For mild neutropenia (neutrophils more than $1 \times 10^9$ per litre), a drug history will often reveal the cause. White blood counts performed at weekly intervals will reveal cyclical neutropenia. Tests for neutrophil antibodies and anti-nuclear antibody should be performed. If neutropenia persists more than 6 weeks, then a bone marrow investigation is merited and this should be done at once in severe neutropenia of unknown cause. However, isolated neutropenia is rarely a presenting feature of leukaemia.

## TREATMENT

Definitive treatment is directed at the cause. Mild neutropenia requires no special management. The management of severe neutropenia requires special skills and is dealt with under the management of acute leukaemia.

# The myelodysplastic syndromes (MDS)

In the past these syndromes have been much neglected, mainly because they have gone under so many aliases: refractory anaemia, pre-leukaemia, sideroblastic anaemia, achrestic anaemia, oligoblastic leukaemia etc. They have now been recognized as belonging to a single group of conditions, diagnosable on morphological grounds and surprisingly common in the elderly (a prevalence of 1:1000 in the over-60s).

## PATHOLOGY

Myelodysplastic syndrome is now recognized as a clonal disorder of haematopoietic stem cells which retain the ability to differentiate into end cells, but do so in a disordered manner. All cells deriving from the myeloid stem cell (Fig. 21.1) are involved in the process. The French–American–British (FAB) group have classified the syndrome into five types, which are shown in ascending order of severity in Table 21.23.

The majority of cases of MDS are idiopathic; but with increasing use of cytotoxic drugs and

**Table 21.23** FAB classification of the myelodysplastic syndromes.

| |
| --- |
| Refractory sideroblastic anaemia |
| Refractory anaemia |
| Chronic myelomonocytic leukaemia |
| Refractory anaemia with excess of blasts |
| Refractory anaemia with excess of blasts in transformation |

FAB = French–American–British.

radiotherapy more cases are being seen that are secondary to the use of these agents. Secondary MDS tends to occur in younger people.

## CLINICAL FEATURES

The clinical features are related to anaemia, neutropenia and thrombocytopenia. Since granulocytes and platelets function poorly, infections and bleeding may occur even with relatively normal blood counts.

## DIAGNOSIS

The diagnosis is made on the characteristic appearances of blood and bone marrow, which include dyserythropoiesis, disorders of granulation and nuclear segmentation in white cells and abnormalities of megakaryocytes. Peripheral pancytopenia associated with bone marrow hypercellularity is the rule. Many patients have an abnormal karyotype in bone marrow metaphases.

## DIFFERENTIAL DIAGNOSIS

In the past many cases have been misdiagnosed as aplastic anaemia or megaloblastic anaemia.

## TREATMENT

Supportive care with blood transfusions, antibiotics and platelet transfusions may be required. Aggressive chemotherapy may be offered in young patients, but this is inappropriate for the majority. Low-dose chemotherapy with cytosine arabinoside has been recommended for the treatment of elderly patients. Some specialists recommend the use of growth factors such as G-CSF in neutropenic patients, but these are too expensive at the present time for long-term use.

# THE LEUKAEMIAS

The leukaemias are a group of malignant neoplasms of the bone marrow in which the neoplastic clone replaces the normal tissue, frequently leading to anaemia, neutropenia and thrombocytopenia. Untreated, acute leukaemia is rapidly fatal, but chronic lymphocytic leukaemia is often compatible with a normal life of long duration.

For most leukaemias the cause is unknown, but in a few cases a cause has been determined.

## 1. Radiation

Survivors of the Hiroshima explosion have a twenty-fold increase in most types of leukaemia (but not chronic lymphocytic). Patients with ankylosing spondylitis treated by irradiation of the spine have a six-fold increase in acute myeloid leukaemia. Children whose mothers received diagnostic X-rays in pregnancy have a slight increase in incidence of acute lymphoblastic leukaemia. The evidence does not support direct background radiation as a major cause for leukaemia, but a recent investigation centred on the Sellafield nuclear plant in the UK has suggested irradiation of the father predisposes their progeny to the development of leukaemia.

## 2. Chemicals

Benzene, toluene and related chemicals are leukaemogenic and an environmental hazard in some occupations. Cytotoxic drugs produce leukaemia in a small proportion of patients receiving them. Alkylating agents produce refractory leukaemias associated with deletions of chromosomes 5 and 7, whereas topoisomerase II inhibitors such as doxorubicin and etoposide lead to leukaemias that are more easily treated, and associated with balanced translocations often involving chromosomes 11 and 21.

## 3. Viruses

In cats, mice, cows and sheep leukaemogenic viruses have been identified. In humans, a T-cell leukaemia common in Japan is caused by a retrovirus (HTLVI).

## 4. Congenital factors

There is a high coincidence rate in identical twins. Patients with Downs' syndrome have a twenty-fold increase in incidence of acute myeloid leukaemia.

Leukaemia is classified according to the type of white cell affected and according to the rate of the clinical progression. Greater discrimination is achieved by noting in addition the nature of the cell surface antigens and any karyotypic abnormalities, the so-called MIC classification (morphology, immunology, chromosomes).

## MORPHOLOGY

This is the histological description of the leukaemic cells, with the main classification into myeloid or lymphoid types. Cytochemical techniques also identify cytoplasmic granules.

## IMMUNOLOGY

Cell surface markers can be detected by antibodies. As well as B- and T-cell markers, a marker known as common acute lymphoblastic leukaemia antigen (CALLA) can give prognostic information.

## CHROMOSOMES AND LEUKAEMIA

Acquired chromosomal abnormalities are common in the leukaemias and play an important part in their pathogenesis. The abnormalities are confined to the malignant cells, and as such are clonal markers. Consequently, they have been used to demonstrate that several lineages may be involved within the neoplastic process (e.g. erythroid cells in chronic granulocytic leukaemia). A wide variety of chromosomal abnormalities have been described in association with various leukaemias (Table 21.24), including monosomies, trisomies, deletions and translocations. Increasing chromosomal complexity is associated with increasing malignancy. In many cases the chromosomal abnormality can be shown to give rise to a specific molecular mistake usually involving a cellular oncogene. Of course, similar molecular mistakes can occur without gross changes in chromosomal structure, so that molecular genetic techniques will eventually provide a better means of understanding the neoplastic process.

There are three main ways in which chromosomal abnormalities have been shown to effect molecular events:

### 1. Formation of a conjoint gene

A translocation or internal deletion juxtaposes two separate lengths of DNA. By chance these may be read as a single gene, and translated into a metabolically active protein. The best example is the 9/22 translocation in chronic myeloid leukaemia.

**Table 21.24** Selected chromosomal abnormalities in leukaemias and lymphomas.

| Abnormality | Type of neoplasm | Molecular event |
| --- | --- | --- |
| Trisomy 12 | CLL | ? |
| Trisomy 8 | AML and MDS | ? |
| Monosomy 7 | AML and MDS | ? |
| Monosomy 5 | AML and MDS | ? |
| Del 5q | MDS | Deleted IRF-1 gene |
| Del 13q | CLL | Deleted gene near to Rb |
| t(9;22) | CML | 210 kD chimaeric *bcr/c-abl* protein |
| t(9;22) | ALL | 190 kD chimaeric *bcr/c-abl* protein |
| t(8;14) | Burkitt's lymphoma | IgH promoter gene up-regulates *c-myc* |
| t(14;18) | Follicular lymphoma | IgH promoter gene up-regulates *bcl-2* |
| t(15;17) | AML M3 | Involves retinoic acid receptor gene |

AML = acute myeloblastic leukaemia. ALL = acute lymphoblastic leukaemia. CLL = chronic lymphocytic leukaemia. CML = chronic myeloid leukaemia. MDS = myelodysplastic syndrome. t = translocation.

### 2. Oncogene up-regulation

In a number of lymphoid malignancies the immunoglobulin heavy chain promoter region on chromosome 14 is captured by a translocation and redeployed to enhance the translation of a cellular oncogene. The best known example is the 8/14 translocation in Burkitt's lymphoma.

### 3. Antioncogene deletion

The tumour suppressor genes Rb on the long arm of chromosome 13 and p53 on the short arm of chromosome 17 are deleted in a number of neoplasms.

# Acute myeloid leukaemia

Acute myeloid leukaemia (AML) occurs at any age. It is the commonest type of acute leukaemia in adults and in the first year of life.

## PATHOLOGY

There is a proliferation of the myeloid stem cell, which shows greater or lesser degrees of differentiation that are recognized by the French–American–British (FAB) classification (Table 21.25).

The accumulation of leukaemic cells suppresses the growth of normal cells, leading to pancytopenia which usually occurs before the appearance of a leukocytosis. In the elderly and in patients with secondary acute leukaemia there is often a preceding myelodysplastic phase.

**Table 21.25** FAB classification of the acute myeloid leukaemias.

| | |
| --- | --- |
| M1 | Poorly differentiated myeloblastic leukaemia |
| M2 | Well-differentiated myeloblastic leukaemia |
| M3 | Promyelocytic leukaemia |
| M4 | Myelomonocytic leukaemia |
| M5 | Monocytic leukaemia |
| M6 | Erythroleukaemia |
| M7 | Megakaryoblastic leukaemia |

FAB = French–American–British.

## CLINICAL FEATURES

The clinical manifestations are those of pancytopenia. In M5 particularly there may be infiltrates of the skin and gums. Tender bones are sometimes noted. Splenomegaly and hepatomegaly are rare except in advanced disease.

## DIAGNOSIS

The diagnosis depends on the observation of more than 30 per cent blasts in the bone marrow. Auer rods (long, thin azurophil cytoplasmic inclusions) are characteristic of leukaemic myeloblasts, but cytochemical or immunocytochemical identification of the blasts may be necessary. Some subtypes of AML have a characteristically abnormal karyotype; for example, in M3 a translocation between chromosomes 15 and 17 is almost always seen.

## COMPLICATIONS

In M3 the granules of the promyelocytes contain procoagulant which is capable of inducing disseminated intravascular coagulation (page 645).

## TREATMENT

There are three elements to treatment: remission induction; supportive care; and consolidation and maintenance.

### Remission induction

In patients below the age of 60, complete remission, defined as the return of blood and bone marrow to normal, is achievable in upwards of 70 per cent of patients. However, even in complete remission up to $10^8$ leukaemic cells may remain in the body compared with between $10^{10}$ and $10^{12}$ in the patient with frank leukaemia and marrow failure.

A number of induction regimens are in current use, most involving a combination of daunorubicin, cytosine arabinoside and 6-thioguanine. In M3, the chromosomal translocation involves the gene coding for the retinoic acid receptor. Trans-retinoic acid inhibits clonal growth of the myeloid leukaemia cells and can be used to obtain a remission.

### Supportive care

The induction regimen induces severe pancytopenia which may last for several weeks. Effective supportive care is the cornerstone of successful treatment. Of prime importance is good vascular access. It is usual to introduce a right atrial cannula via one of the subclavian veins. This is left *in situ* for the duration of the induction and consolidation regimen. In order to diminish the risk of cannula-associated infections, the cannula is taken through a subcutaneous tunnel before leaving the skin.

It is essential to have excellent blood product support from the Blood Transfusion Service (Table 21.26). The treatment of anaemia is by red cell transfusion. Prevention of haemorrhage requires platelet transfusions. Most units use platelets prophylactically when the count drops below $20 \times 10^9$ per litre. Some patients become refractory to platelet transfusions owing to the development of isoantibodies. In these, single-

**Table 21.26** Blood product support available from the Blood Transfusion Service.

| Blood product | Use |
|---|---|
| Whole blood | Only for replacement of volume as well as red cells, e.g. acute haemorrhage. Shelf-life 35 days |
| 'Fresh' blood | Mainly required by surgeons for superstitious reasons. Neonates and those with hepatic failure should have blood less than 5 days old |
| Red cell concentrate | Red cells removed from plasma and resuspended in SAG-M solution. The mainstay for red cell replacement. Shelf-life 35 days |
| Filtered blood | Filters deplete 95% of leukocytes. Used for patients with anti-leukocyte antibodies causing febrile reactions or to prevent such antibodies occurring |
| Platelet concentrate | Used to prevent bleeding in severe thrombocytopenia. Prepared by centrifugation of whole blood donations or by apheresis from single donors. Stored at room temperature with agitation for up to 5 days. Maintain ABO and Rh(D) compatibility |
| Fresh frozen plasma | Approximately 200 ml of plasma from one donation, frozen within 6 hours. Used to replenish clotting factors |
| Plasma protein solution | 4.5% solution of plasma proteins (mainly albumin). Free of viral contamination. Used as volume replacement in burns, shock and plasma exchange. Expensive, and can often be substituted by gelatin, starch or dextran solutions |

donor HLA-matched platelets collected on a cell separator are indicated.

Infection is very likely in patients with fewer than $0.5 \times 10^9$ neutrophils per litre. Most infections are with endogenous organisms so that the value of reversed barrier nursing in rooms with laminar flow ventilation is questionable. However, single rooms are preferable to the open ward and reasonable care (such as washing hands between patients) to prevent the spread of infection is essential. Reduction of gut flora by prophylactic oral non-absorbable antibiotics, cotrimoxazole or ciprofloxacin, is practised in many units. Regular cultures of urine, faeces, sputum, and of swabs from the vagina, throat, nose and perineum document the patient's commensal bacteria and their sensitivity to antibiotics.

Fever is the best indication that infection is present and thorough attempts should be made to identify the cause of any organism causing a temperature of 38°C present for 2 hours. At the same time treatment is begun with empirical antibiotics such as a ureido penicillin and an aminoglycoside which will cover likely organisms. If no response occurs the possibility of viral or fungal organisms or *Staphylococcal epidermidis* should be considered. Acyclovir, amphotericin B and teicoplanin are useful drugs in these circumstances. Granulocyte transfusions are now seldom used.

### Maintenance

Remissions are prolonged by two consolidation courses of the induction regimen, but probably not by prolonged treatment with low doses of cytotoxic drugs. Allogeneic **bone marrow transplantation** should be considered in patients aged 50 and under who are in remission and have an HLA compatible sibling. The patient is prepared with total body irradiation and cyclophosphamide which is intended to remove any residual leukaemia. Donor bone marrow drawn from the pelvic bones is filtered and then infused intravenously into the recipient. Recovery of bone marrow function occurs in 2–3 weeks. Bone marrow transplantation remains a hazardous procedure for the recipient. About 25 per cent of patients die from complications of the treatment, and in a further 25 per cent the leukaemia relapses despite the treatment. The major risks are:

1. Infection, particularly with cytomegalovirus (CMV);
2. Graft-versus-host disease (GVHD), an immune attack by immunocompetent leukocytes in the graft on the host causing rash, diarrhoea and hepatitis, as well as increased susceptibility to infection;
3. Interstitial pneumonitis, a usually fatal lung condition possibly related to GVHD, CMV or lung irradiation;
4. Failure of engraftment or rejection of the graft.

The incidence of GVHD may be reduced by depletion of T-cells from the graft or by the immunosuppressive drug cyclosporin A. Bone marrow allografts from HLA-compatible unrelated donors or partially mismatched related donors are experimental procedures.

Bone marrow autografts using bone marrow collected in first remission may have a role in increasing the number of long-term survivors.

## PROGNOSIS

In patients not receiving bone marrow transplants the survival rates for patients under 25 are between 30 and 50 per cent at 5 years. For patients receiving bone marrow transplants, survivals of between 40 and 60 per cent have been achieved.

In older patients the prognosis is much worse. In patients over 60 years, fewer than 60 per cent achieve complete remissions, and these are not usually sustained for much more than 12 months.

# Acute lymphoblastic leukaemia

Acute lymphoblastic leukaemia is the commonest leukaemia of childhood, but it may occur at any age. The most useful classification is according to the cell of origin.

## Common acute lymphoblastic leukaemia

This has a peak incidence between the ages of 2 and 5. It comprises 70 per cent of ALL and has the best prognosis. The cell of origin has recently been identified as a pre-B-cell. Most cases bear the cALLa surface marker (CD10).

## T-cell acute lymphoblastic leukaemia

This is five times commoner in boys than girls and has a peak age of incidence between 10 and 15. It is frequently associated with a mediastinal mass (Sternberg sarcoma).

## B-cell acute lymphoblastic leukaemia

This is very rare (less than 2 per cent of total) and may be regarded as the blood phase of Burkitt's lymphoma.

### CLINICAL FEATURES

These are similar to AML except that tender bones are more common, meningeal involvement (headache, vomiting, diplopia) is much more common, and testicular involvement is a feature. Hepatomegaly and splenomegaly are also more likely to be seen.

### DIAGNOSIS

This is made on bone marrow appearances with the help of immunochemical markers. In 30 per cent of adults with ALL the Philadelphia chromosome is found. Molecular investigation reveals a 190 kD protein product of chimaeric *bcr/c-abl* gene, indicating that these are not lymphoblastic transformations of a silent chronic myeloid leukaemia. The presence of the Philadelphia chromosome carries a poor prognosis.

### TREATMENT

Treatment of ALL, especially in children, is more effective than of AML. Complete remission is achieved in 95 per cent of patients. A combination of drugs is used that always includes vincristine and prednisolone, which are minimally toxic to normal marrow, together with a permutation from asparaginase, daunorubicin, cytosine arabinoside and cyclophosphamide.

Once remission is achieved prophylaxis against meningeal leukaemia is necessary and skull irradiation and intrathecal methotrexate are important adjuncts to treatment. Maintenance chemotherapy with methotrexate and 6-mercaptopurine together is continued for 2–2.5 years with 3-monthly vincristine and prednisolone. Bone marrow transplants are offered to patients in second remission or those in first remission with a poor prognosis.

### PROGNOSIS

Among children the 5-year survival rate is greater than 50 per cent, and many of these may be regarded as cured. Poor prognostic features include a high white count, age greater than 16, chromosomal translocations and T- or B-cell surface markers.

# Chronic myeloid leukaemia

### PATHOLOGY

The disease, which may be seen at any age, has two phases. In the chronic phase there is uncontrolled proliferation of a stem cell which retains the ability to differentiate. Red cells, granulocytes and platelets all derive from the malignant clone which is characterized by an abnormal karyotype. There is a reciprocal translocation between the long arms of chromosome 9 and 22. The small chromosome 22 resulting is known as the **Philadelphia (Ph′) chromosome**. The translocation produces a hybrid gene, *c-abl/bcr*, the product of which is a 210 kD protein which functions as a protein kinase. In most patients, the disorder eventually transforms into an acute leukaemia, on average three years after diagnosis. In 70 per cent of cases this is acute myeloblastic leukaemia and is generally refractory to treatment. In 25 per cent of cases, ALL ensues with a response to treatment typical of other cases of ALL (see above), although remission seldom exceeds 1 year.

## CLINICAL FEATURES

The features of anaemia are usually present together with those of hypermetabolism, weight loss, night sweats and lassitude. In patients with white cell counts greater than $80 \times 10^9$ per litre, splenomegaly is almost always present and it may be massive and associated with pain and discomfort. Bruising and haemorrhage may occur even in the presence of a normal platelet count. A significant number present with gout, neurological symptoms caused by hyperviscosity or priapism.

## DIAGNOSIS

There is usually a leukocytosis with a white blood cell count above $100 \times 10^9$ per litre. A complete range of granulocyte precursors from myeloblasts to metamyeloctyes is seen together with increased numbers of neutrophils, eosinophils and basophils. The bone marrow is hypercellular with a predominance of myeloid precursors. The neutrophil alkaline phosphatase score is zero, serum $B_{12}$ is high and the Ph' chromosome is present in over 95 per cent of cases.

## DIFFERENTIAL DIAGNOSIS

A similar blood picture may be seen in leukaemoid reactions due to infections, marrow infiltration and cancer, myelofibrosis, and in atypical chronic myeloid leukaemia. In all of these the Ph' chromosome is absent. Some cases of Ph'-negative chronic myeloid leukamia behave exactly like Ph'-positive cases. In these the *bcr/c/abl* construct may be found.

## TREATMENT

Busulphan is the drug which has been used most commonly for the chronic phase. It controls the white count, the anaemia and the splenomegaly, but does not delay the onset of the acute phase. Among the side effects are aplastic anaemia, skin pigmentation, lung fibrosis and cataract. Hydroxyurea is equally effective and is easier to control with fewer side effects. Splenic irradiation may be useful in controlling the disease when it becomes refractory to chemotherapy. None of these treatments eliminates the Ph' chromosome. However, in a minority of patients treated with α-interferon the Ph'-positive clone becomes undetectable. Recent randomized controlled trials suggest that interferon treatment leads to longer survival than treatment with either busulphan or hydroxyurea. Bone marrow transplantation may be curative if the criteria of age and availability of an HLA compatible sibling can be fulfilled. Because of the awful prognosis, bone marrow transplantation from a matched unrelated donor can probably be justified. Treatment of the acute phase is disappointing.

## PROGNOSIS

The median survival is 3–5 years, 10 per cent of patients survive 10 years. Bone marrow transplant has improved the survival in younger (<50 years) patients.

# Chronic lymphocytic leukaemia

This is the commonest of the leukaemias. It mainly occurs after the age of 55 and becomes more common in each succeeding decade. The incidence in men at any particular age is twice that of women.

## PATHOLOGY

There is a monoclonal proliferation of early B-lymphocytes which characteristically bear small amounts of surface IgM and IgD, a receptor for mouse red blood cells and the CD5 antigen. The disease apparently starts in the bone marrow and may be non-progressive. If it does progess it involves lymph nodes in the cervical, axillary and inguinal regions, the spleen and the liver. Eventually marrow failure may ensue.

## CLINICAL FEATURES

In one large series from a single centre, over 70 per cent of patients were detected incidentally on routine blood counts. In the remainder the main features were of anaemia, lymphadenopathy and splenomegaly.

## DIAGNOSIS

A lymphocytosis is seen on the blood count or film. Bone marrow trephine may show interstitial, nodular or diffuse infiltration. Cell markers (see above) confirm the diagnosis. Serum immunoglobulins are reduced in over 60 per cent of patients. Staging is according to the Binet system (Table 21.27).

**Table 21.27** Binet staging system for chronic lymphocytic leukaemia.

| | |
|---|---|
| Stage A | <3 involved sites, Hb >100 g/l, platelets >100 × 10⁹/l |
| Stage B | >3 involved sites, Hb >100 g/l, platelets >100 × 10⁹/l |
| Stage C | Hb <100 g/l or platelets <100 × 10⁹/l |

Cervical, axillary, inguinal nodes, spleen and liver each count as one involved site

Hb = haemoglobin.

## COMPLICATIONS

Autoimmune haemolytic anaemia occurs in about 8 per cent of patients. Autoimmune thrombocytopenia is found in 2 per cent. Although transformation does not occur with the same regularity as in CML small numbers of patients develop an aggressive immunoblastic lymphoma which may or may not be clonally related (Richter syndrome). Slightly more common is transformation to prolymphocytic leukaemia. In patients with low serum immunoglobulins infections are common, particularly chest infections and herpes zoster, which occur in about 20 per cent of patients. The latter is often severe, sometimes affecting motor nerve roots and frequently being followed by postherpetic neuralgia.

## TREATMENT

Most patients do not require treatment. Patients with signs of marrow failure and those who have unacceptable organomegaly may be successfully treated by chlorambucil (up to 10 mg/day for 2 weeks every 4 weeks). Prednisolone, 10 mg/day, is often added to this regimen. The new agent fludarabine appears promising in disease resistant to chlorambucil.

Herpes zoster infections should be treated promptly with acyclovir infusions.

# T-cell chronic lymphocytic leukaemia

About 2 per cent of CLL has T-cell markers. Not all T-cell proliferations are neoplastic and clonality can only be determined by the finding of an abnormal karyotype or rearrangement of T-receptor gene. There is a clinical association with rheumatoid arthritis and coeliac disease. Some patients develop pure red cell aplasia which improves with treatment of the leukaemia.

# Prolymphocytic leukaemia

This is a more aggressive variant of CLL almost invariably associated with splenomegaly. Most cases are B-cell in type.

# Hairy cell leukaemia

This variant of CLL is characterized by small numbers of B-cells with filamentous pili protruding from the cytoplasm. There is usually neutropenia and splenomegaly, the bone marrow aspirate showing a 'dry tap' and the trephine a characteristic regular infiltrate. Treatment by splenectomy is often helpful, but more recently very satisfactory remissions in almost all patients have been achieved with either α-interferon or deoxycoformycin therapy.

# Adult T leukaemia lymphoma

This unusual tumour of Japanese and of blacks from the Carribean is caused by infection with the retrovirus HTLV-I. It is generally associated with hypercalcaemia and is refractory to treatment.

# THE LYMPHOMAS

These are divided into two main types: Hodgkin's and non-Hodgkin's lymphoma.

# Hodgkin's disease

First described by Thomas Hodgkin of Guy's Hospital in 1832, this has been one of the greatest successes of modern cancer treatment. There are two peak ages of incidence: between the ages of 20 and 40 and in the over 60s. Although the pathological picture in both is similar the outlook in each is so very different that a different aetiology has been postulated. However, the cause is unknown.

## PATHOLOGY

The characteristic histological abnormality is the Reed–Sternberg cell, a large binucleate cell with acidophilic nucleoli. Just what is the normal counterpart for this cell is vigorously disputed. Reed–Sternberg cells are surrounded by large numbers of T-lymphocytes, plasma cells, neutrophils, monocytes and eosinophils which are not part of the tumour clone, but appear to be the host's defence against the tumour.

Histological grading (Table 21.28) is according to the relative numbers of Reed–Sternberg

**Table 21.28** Histological grading of Hodgkin's disease.

| | |
|---|---|
| Lymphocyte predominant | Increasing malignancy |
| Nodular sclerosing | |
| Mixed cellularity | |
| Lymphocyte depleted | |

cells and host defence cells. In some cases the lymph node is broken into nodules by fibrous tissue.

The disease progresses in a regular fashion from lymph node to contiguous lymph node, usually beginning above the diaphragm. The spleen is always involved before the liver and the bone marrow.

## CLINICAL FEATURES

Most patients present with discrete asymmetrical enlargement of superficial lymph nodes. The nodes are firm and painless. Splenomegaly is present in up to 50 per cent and the liver may be enlarged in more advanced cases. Fever is present in a third of patients. The Pel Ebstein fever (pyrexia alternating with days with a normal temperature) is said to be typical but is rather uncommon. Pruritus and alcohol-induced pain occur in some patients but have no prognostic significance. Weight loss and night sweats are typical in more advanced cases.

## DIAGNOSIS

The diagnosis is made on lymph node biopsy. The blood count may show a neutrophil leukocytosis, sometimes with eosinophilia. Anaemia, lymphopenia and bone marrow failure are evidence of advanced disease. It is important to stage the disease carefully since the success of particular forms of treatment depends on knowing accurately the extent of the disease (Table 21.29). The presence of retroperitoneal lymph nodes is best assessed by lymphography, perhaps supplemented by a computed tomographic (CT) scan.

**Table 21.29** Staging of Hodgkin's disease.

| | |
|---|---|
| Stage 1 | Disease confined to one lymph node site |
| Stage 2 | Disease in more than one lymph node site but confined to one side of the diaphragm |
| Stage 3 | Involvement of lymph nodes and/or spleen on both sides of the diaphragm |
| Stage 4 | Involvement of sites outside the lymphatic system |

**Suffixes**

| | |
|---|---|
| A | Symptom free |
| B | Symptoms present |
| | Loss of more than 10% body weight in 6 months |
| | Unexplained fever above 38°C |
| | Night sweats |
| E | Local extranodal spread within the range of radiotherapy |

Patients for whom radiotherapy is planned (stages I–IIA) have in the past needed to have staging confirmed by laparotomy with specnectomy and lymph node and liver biopsy. With greater experience of CT many doctors feel that laparotomy, with its attendant risks, is unwarranted. Bone marrow trephine shows marrow involvement in 4 per cent of cases.

## COMPLICATIONS

Patients with Hodgkin's disease have deficiencies in cell-mediated immunity. Infections with herpes zoster, cytomegalovirus, Candida and Mycobacteria are common.

## TREATMENT

Patients with stage I or IIA may be cured by radiotherapy alone (4000 rad). A single upper mantle field treats disease above the diaphragm, and below the diaphragm an inverted Y is used. Stages IIB, III or IV should be treated by chemotherapy, for example, MOPP, consisting of mustine, vincristine (Oncovin), prednisolone and procarbazine. The good results obtained with this regimen depend on the recommended dosage being given, but it may be very toxic and regimens with fewer side effects such as ChlVPP (chlorambucil, vinblastine, prednisolone and procarbazine) have been substituted in some centres. Chemotherapy virtually always leads to sterility in males. For this reason males are offered storage of frozen sperm. Patients receiving procarbazine and an alkylating agent have a 5–10 per cent chance of developing secondary acute myeloblastic leukaemia, particularly when these agents are combined with radiotherapy. The risk of radiation-induced carcinomas from radiotherapy is of a similar order. Newer Adriamycin (doxorubicin)-based regimens produce less sterility and less leukaemia.

## PROGNOSIS

Five-year survival rates for stages I and II are 85 per cent, for stage IIIA 70 per cent, for stage IIIB 50 per cent and for stage IV 40 per cent. However, these rates are very age dependent. Young people usually do well; old people less so.

# Non-Hodgkin's lymphoma

The variety of non-Hodgkin's lymphomas is extremely wide and made confusing by the fact that at least six different histological classifications are currently in use.

## PATHOLOGY

The distinction between leukaemias and lymphomas is to some extent arbitrary since many lymphomas involve the blood and many leukaemias involve the lymph nodes and spleen. The differentiation pathways of lymphocytes are complex, and lymphomas may theoretically arise from lymphocytes frozen at any stage of differentiation.

In general, lymphomas with large cells are more malignant than those with small cells, and those with diffuse histology more malignant than those with nodular histology. A recent working formulation recognizes low-grade lymphomas, which have an indolent clinical course, relatively long survival, a non-destructive growth pattern and a tendency to respect privileged sites such as the brain and testes, but which are not curable with chemotherapy; and high-grade lymphomas which have an aggressive clinical course, a short survival without therapy, a destructive growth pattern and a tendency to invade privileged sites but which may be cured by chemotherapy. Low-grade and high-grade lymphomas each comprise about 35 per cent of all lymphomas. Unfortunately a large minority of lymphomas fall into an intermediate group (Table 21.30). In the UK about 20 per cent of lymphomas are of T-cell origin but their classification is unsatisfactory.

**Table 21.30** Classification of non-Hodgkin's lymphomas.

**Low-grade (35%)**
Lymphocytic diffuse (chronic lymphocytic leukaemia)
Lymphoplasmacytic diffuse
Centroblastic/centrocytic nodular

**Intermediate grade (20%)**
Centroblastic/centrocytic diffuse
Centrocytic diffuse

**High-grade (35%)**
Centroblastic diffuse
Immunoblastic diffuse
Lymphoblastic diffuse
Burkitt's lymphoma

**Miscellaneous (10%)**
Mycosis fungoides
Histiocytic
Unclassifiable

## CLINICAL FEATURES

Two-thirds of patients present over the age of 50. Most patients have aysmmetric, painless, superficial lymphadenopathy. Between 5 and 10 per cent have involvement of oropharyngeal lymphoid structures (Waldeyer's ring). Hepatosplenomegaly is more common than in Hodgkin's disease, and massive enlargement of retroperitoneal lymph nodes can sometimes be felt in the abdomen. Extranodal involvement is more common than in Hodgkin's disease, and characteristic lymphomas of skin, stomach, lung and thyroid are recognized.

## DIAGNOSIS

Diagnosis is made by lymph-node biopsy. Eighty-five per cent of patients have disseminated disease. In 50 per cent, tumour cells are detectable immunologically in blood and bone marrow. In the UK most patients have B-cell lymphomas and in these serum immunoglobulins may be low. In about 15 per cent a monoclonal immunoglobulin is detectable in the serum.

## TREATMENT

Radiotherapy is only recommended in the minority of patients (5 per cent) with stage I disease. Low-grade lymphomas should be managed by observation until systemic symptoms, bone marrow failure or uncomfortable or compressive organomegaly ensue. They usually respond to single-agent chemotherapy (e.g. chlorambucil, 10 mg, daily for 2 weeks of every 4 weeks).

High-grade lymphomas should be treated with aggressive chemotherapeutic regimens such as CHOP [cyclophosphamide, Adriamycin (doxorubicin), vincristine and prednisolone]. Experimental treatment includes supralethal chemotherapy with bone marrow allograft or autograft.

## PROGNOSIS

Median survival in low-grade lymphomas is 7 years. In many of these, transformation to high-grade lymphoma occurs. High-grade lymphomas have 'cure' rates of 30 per cent but the majority fail to survive 2 years.

# Burkitt's lymphoma

This is a B-cell lymphoblastic lymphoma, endemic in malarious areas of tropical Africa and New Guinea. Sporadic cases occur elsewhere. It is a disease of children and young people with a peak age of incidence between 4 and 8 years.

Epstein–Barr virus infections are involved in the genesis of the lymphoma, which is almost always associated with a chromosomal translocation between a site on the long arm of chromosome 8 near to the locus coding for the *c-myc* oncogene and a site on the long arm of chromosome 14 near to the locus coding for the heavy chains of immunoglobulin.

The lymphoma involves extranodal sites, particularly the jaws, kidney, adrenals and ovaries. In young women the lactating breast is frequently a site of involvement.

Histologically, there is a characteristic 'starry sky' appearance formed by pale histiocytes in sheets of darkly staining lymphoblasts. Localized tumours respond well to aggressive chemotherapy, but disseminated disease, particularly when it takes the form of a B-cell lymphoblastic leukaemia, has a grave prognosis.

# Mycosis fungoides

This is a low-grade T-cell neoplasm of the skin (and nothing to do with fungus as its name implies). It often begins as an apparent eczema which progresses to erythroderma, or forms plaques or tumours in the skin. The malignant cell is a CD4-positive T-cell which frequently has a bizarre convoluted nucleus. There is a tendency for the disease to become more aggressive and involve liver, spleen, bone marrow and blood. It is then known as Sezary syndrome.

Treatment of mycosis fungoides is by topical steroids or cytotoxics, or by phototherapy (PUVA) or radiotherapy. Sezary syndrome responds for a while to aggressive chemotherapy.

# Angio-immunoblastic lymphadenopathy

This rare condition presents clinically as a systemic disease with pyrexia, weight loss, malaise, pruritus, anorexia, rash, arthralgia, lymphadenopathy, hepatosplenomegaly, eosinophilia and hypergammaglobulinaemia. Histological examination of lymph nodes reveals a pleomorphic proliferation sometimes confused with Hodgkin's disease. Some remain as reactive proliferation but in about 50 per cent a high-grade T-cell lymphoma develops.

# MULTIPLE MYELOMA

Multiple myeloma is a malignant disease of bone marrow plasma cells. Its incidence is 2.6 per 100 000 in the UK.

## PATHOLOGY

The serum immunoglobulins are a mixture of antibody molecules each committed to a different antigen. This commitment occurs as a genetic event in the early B-cell precursors of the plasma cells that secrete immunoglobulin. Neoplastic proliferation begins in one cell and all its progeny secrete one type of immunoglobulin molecule, which is therefore monoclonal. Normal serum electrophoresis demonstrates the immunoglobulins as a broad band towards the cathode, reflecting the molecular heterogeneity.

In myeloma the immunoglobulin has a single molecular structure, and serum electrophoresis therefore demonstrates it as a narrow band (which is sometimes called a paraprotein). In myeloma the majority of tumours produce IgG or IgA. IgD-, IgE- and IgM-producing myelomas are rare. There is usually an excessive production of immunoglobulin light chains and 25 per cent secrete light chains only. About 5 per cent of myelomas are non-secretory, i.e. no paraprotein in the serum. The malignant plasma cells also secrete an osteoclast-activating factor (now known to be 'tumour necrosis factor β') which is responsible for bony destruction around nests of plasma cells and the mobilization of bony calcium.

## CLINICAL FEATURES

Myeloma has a peak incidence between the ages of 60 and 70. The clinical features are wide-ranging. Bone pain is frequently present. Pathological fractures and collapsed vertebrae are not uncommon. Since the axial skeleton is involved, neurological symptoms are common, with severe root pain and paraplegia occurring. Hypercalcaemia causes constipation, vomiting, thirst, polyuria, drowsiness and coma together with renal failure which is usually the result of a combination of causes (Table 21.31). Hyperuricaemia can cause acute renal failure and/or gout.

Bone marrow failure is present in the most advanced cases. Recurrent infections are the consequence of both neutropenia and low levels of normal immunoglobulins. High levels of paraprotein may be associated with the hyperviscosity syndrome, characterized by purpura, haemorrhage, visual defects and heart failure. Fundoscopy reveals dilated veins with a 'string of sausages' appearance.

Amyloidosis may occur leading to macroglossia, carpal tunnel syndrome, purpura, renal failure and cardiomyopathy.

## DIAGNOSIS

The blood count may be normal but frequently shows a degree of anaemia with pancytopenia in the more advanced cases. There is usually rouleaux formation, and the high level of immunoglobulin can often be predicted by a blue background staining. The ESR is frequently greater than 140 mm in the first hour but may be normal in light-chain myeloma. Bone marrow shows increased numbers of plasma cells which may be binucleate or otherwise abnormal, and

**Table 21.31** Causes of renal failure in myeloma (renal failure is usually precipitated by infection and dehydration).

Precipitation of immunoglobulin light chains in renal tubules
Hypercalcaemia
Hyperuricaemia
Amyloidosis
Recurrent urinary tract infections

which on immunostaining show a single heavy- and light-chain type of immunoglobulin.

Serum electrophoresis shows a monoclonal band in 70 per cent of cases, and measurement of specific immunoglobulins shows a rise in one class while the others are depressed. Rarely, all classes are depressed. Urinary electrophoresis may demonstrate a monoclonal band representing free light chains (Bence Jones proteinuria). The test for Bence Jones protein, heating the urine, is now only used to entertain students.

Serum calcium is raised in 45 per cent of cases, but alkaline phosphatase levels are usually normal. Serum uric acid may be raised. Skeletal X-rays show osteolytic areas in 60 per cent of patients or generalized osteoporosis in 20 per cent.

## DIFFERENTIAL DIAGNOSIS

Monoclonal proteins may be found in a number of conditions (Table 21.32). It is important to distinguish myeloma from non-progressive conditions. Two of the following should be present in order to confirm the diagnosis: osteolytic bone disease, paraprotein, and/or more than 10 per cent plasma cells in the bone marrow.

**Table 21.32** Conditions associated with monoclonal immunoglobulins.

Myeloma
Waldenström's macroglobulinaemia
Monoclonal gammopathy of undetermined significance
Cold haemagglutination syndrome
Cryoglobulinaemia
B-cell non-Hodgkin's lymphoma
Chronic lymphocytic leukaemia
Prolymphocytic leukaemia

## TREATMENT

### Acute

Myeloma may be a medical emergency. Renal failure should be treated by rehydration, the correction of hypercalcaemia or hyperuricaemia and the treatment of any infection. Plasmapheresis may be effective in reducing the excretion of immunoglobulin light chains, but early treatment of the myeloma is the ideal way of reducing their production.

Hypercalcaemia should be treated by rehydration, corticosteroids and, if required, one of the biphosphonates, etidronate, pamidronate or clodrinate. Compression paraplegia should be treated by either laminectomy or radiotherapy; whichever can be done the soonest.

Locally painful skeletal lesions require radiotherapy.

### Chronic

For many years the standard treatment has been melphalan, 0.25 mg/kg for 4 days, together with prednisolone, 100 mg/day for four days, repeated every 6 weeks, together with allopurinol. In more than 50 per cent of patients this will alleviate symptoms and halt progression. The paraprotein is seldom abolished but usually plateaus at a lower level, which is a signal for treatment to stop. Remissions last for about 2 years. More intensive regimens produce very little better results with greater side effects. Treatment with high-dose melphalan, 140 mg/m$^2$, produces more complete remissions but they last no longer. Recently there has been a tendency to treat young patients with very high-dose melphalan, 200 mg/m$^2$, or total body irradiation together with a bone marrow allograft, or an autograft of stem cells harvested from the peripheral blood having been propelled there by recombinant GM-CSF.

## PROGNOSIS

The median survival is 2 years. Although there are long-term survivors nobody is cured. Uraemia and anaemia are bad prognostic features, although some patients with irreversible renal damage are suitable for chronic dialysis.

# Waldenström's macroglobulinaemia

This is a malignant tumour of bone marrow composed of lymphoplasmacytoid cells which secrete IgM.

## CLINICAL FEATURES

In many patients it is an incidental finding. When they are present clinical features are related to marrow failure or hyperviscosity, which results in visual disturbances, muscle weakness, confusion, congestive cardiac failure and coma. The retinal changes are characteristic with engorged veins, haemorrhages and exudates and blurred discs.

## DIAGNOSIS

There may be a spurious anaemia owing to increased plasma volume. Rouleaux and a blue background may be seen on the blood film. The features of marrow failure may be present. Bone marrow shows a diffuse infiltrate of small lymphocytes and plasma cells or of lymphoplasmacytoid cells which on immunostaining contain IgM and either $\varkappa$ or $\lambda$ light chains. The ESR is very high. Serum electrophoresis shows a monoclonal protein which may be identified as IgM. Hypercalcaemia and bony disease are not seen.

## TREATMENT

The treatment of hyperviscosity is plasmapheresis supplemented as required by cytotoxic drugs. Chlorambucil and cyclophosphamide are the most widely used drugs.

# Monoclonal gammopathy of undetermined significance

This name is applied to a paraprotein discovered in the serum in the absence of other features of myeloma or Waldenström's macroglobulinaemia (see above). The level of paraprotein is less than 30 g/l and normal immunoglobulins are not suppressed. When followed for 15 years, 30 per cent show signs of myeloma.

# *Smouldering myeloma*

Cases intermediate between multiple myeloma and benign monoclonal gammopathy are sometimes seen. The level of the paraprotein may be greater than 30 g/l, there may be Bence Jones proteinuria or suppression of normal immunoglobulins. There may be increased numbers of plasma cells in the marrow. However, there is no evidence of bony destruction, renal damage or bone marrow failure, nor of progression. In such cases the term 'smouldering myeloma' is sometimes used and the correct management is observation.

# *T*HE HAEMORRHAGIC DISORDERS

As it circulates the blood must remain in a fluid state, yet when the circulation is breached the blood that leaks out must rapidly solidify to staunch the flow. The system of checks and balances that achieves this (Fig. 21.10) is a complex one which is prone to failure. A series of

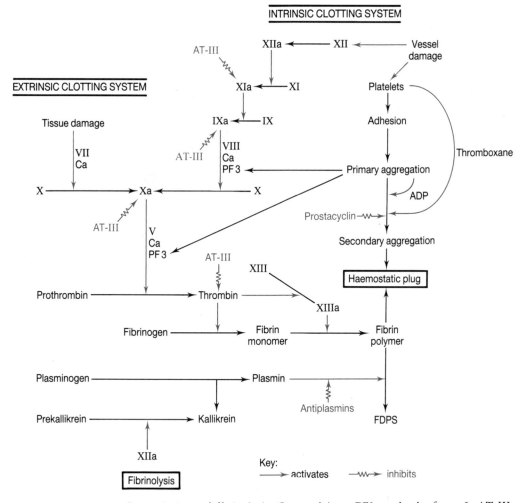

**Figure 21.10** Mechanisms of coagulation and fibrinolysis. Ca = calcium. PF3 = platelet factor 3. AT-III = antithrombin III. ADP = adenosine diphosphate. FDPs = fibrin degradation products.

amplification cascades, designed to ensure that a small stimulus has a large effect, is held in check by a range of inhibitors. A bleeding diathesis may result from disorders of blood vessels, platelets or the coagulation system.

# Disorders of blood vessels

Clinically important disorders of blood vessels are rare and the common ones are clinically insignificant. They are classified in Table 21.33.

**Table 21.33** Disorders of blood vessels.

**Structural malformations**
Hereditary haemorrhagic telangiectasia

Hereditary disorders of connective tissue (Ehlers–Danlos syndrome, pseudoxanthoma elasticum)

Acquired disorder of connective tissue (scurvy, steroids, senile purpura, rheumatoid arthritis, scleroderma, amyloidosis)

**Vasculitis**
Henoch–Schönlein purpura

Drug-induced vasculitis (iodides, quinine, aspirin)

Autoimmune disorders (vasculitis, systemic lupus erythematosus, rheumatoid arthritis, cryoglobulinaemia)

Infections (subacute bacterial endocarditis, meningococcal septicaemia, Rocky Mountain spotted fever)

## HEREDITARY HAEMORRHAGIC TELANGIECTASIA (OSLER–WEBER–RENDU DISEASE)

This rare syndrome is inherited as an autosomal dominant characteristic, the number of lesions increasing with age. Thin-walled dilated capillaries and arterioles may be recognized on skin and mucous membranes, and may characteristically be seen on the lips and tongue. They blanch on compression. Spontaneous epistaxis and gastrointestinal bleeding frequently cause chronic iron-deficiency anaemia. Treatment is difficult, although nasal cautery may be helpful.

Blood loss may be so great that parenteral iron replacement may be necessary to keep up with it.

## HENOCH–SCHÖNLEIN PURPURA

Henoch–Schönlein purpura (page 462) is a vasculitis occurring as an acute disorder, often after an infection, and most commonly in children. Large, often confluent, areas of palpable purpura, accompanied by urticaria, appear on the buttocks and extensor surfaces of the legs. Itching is common. Gastrointestinal involvement may lead to haemorrhage or intussusception; arthritis is common and glomerulonephritis less so. Most cases resolve spontaneously within a few weeks.

# Disorders of platelets (Table 21.34)

Mild thrombocytopenia is a relatively common finding on blood counts and it is usually insignificant. Severe thrombocytopenia may be caused by a failure of production or increased destruction of platelets.

## IMMUNE THROMBOCYTOPENIC PURPURA

Acute immune thrombocytopenic purpura (ITP) is a self-limiting condition seen mainly in children. There may be a history of a recent upper respiratory infection. Chronic ITP is seen more commonly in women than men, particularly between the ages of 20 and 50. An underlying cause (e.g. systemic lupus erythematosus, CLL or drugs) is found in a minority.

### Pathology

Autoantibodies to platelet antigens are produced by the patient, usually for unknown reasons. Sometimes an underlying lymphoid tumour is found or anti-platelet antibodies, as in systemic lupus erythematosus or infectious mononucleosis. Drugs may be implicated in three ways as indicated for autoimmune

**Table 21.34** Disorders of platelets.

**Reduced platelet production**
Selective megakaryocytic suppression
    Congenital (Fanconi's syndrome)
    Drugs (thiazides, sulphonamides)
Part of generalized bone marrow failure
    See Table 21.12

**Increased platelet destruction**
*Immunological causes*
Autoimmune
    Idiopathic
    Drugs
    Systemic lupus erythematosus
    Lymphoid tumours
Isoimmune
    Fetomaternal incompatibility
    Post-transfusion purpura

*Non-immunological causes*
Disseminated intravascular coagulation
Thrombotic thrombocytopenic purpura
Splenomegaly
Dilution by massive transfusion

**Abnormal platelet function**
*Congenital*
Von Willebrand's disease
Glanzman's thrombasthenia

*Acquired*
Aspirin therapy
Myeloproliferative disorders
Paraproteinaemia
Uraemia

haemolytic anaemia (Table 21.16). Antibody-coated platelets are cleared rapidly by the spleen.

## Clinical features

Petechiae and ecchymoses are seen on the skin and mucous membranes. In children with acute ITP serious bleeding is very rare. Chronic ITP is more troublesome with epistaxis, menorrhagia, gastrointestinal haemorrhage and even intracranial haemorrhages occurring. The spleen is not enlarged in primary ITP.

When ITP occurs in pregnancy antibodies can cross the placenta and cause thrombocytopenia in the baby. This is an indication for caesarian section to avoid the risk of cerebral haemorrhage during a normal delivery. Unfortunately, mild to moderate thrombocytopenia is much com-

moner in pregnancy than is ITP, and distinguishing the idiopathic (and harmless) form is sometimes difficult.

## Diagnosis

The platelet count is usually less than $10 \times 10^9$ per litre. On the blood film, platelets frequently appear larger than normal. Bone marrow shows increased numbers of megakaryoctyes which are frequently small with few nuclear lobulations. IgG may be detected on the surface of platelets using a variety of tests which are only available in specialized laboratories. In about 5 per cent of patients an autoimmune haemolytic anaemia is also present (Evans' syndrome).

## Treatment

Acute ITP in children usually recovers spontaneously within 6 weeks to 6 months. Although opinions differ, many authorities prefer to offer no specific treatment but simply to restrict the activities of the children so as to avoid the risk of injury.

In chronic ITP spontaneous remission is rare. Most patients respond to oral prednisolone, 60 mg/day. Gradual reduction of steroid dosage is often possible, but in a large minority relapse occurs while still on an unacceptably high dose. In these patients splenectomy is usually indicated and is successful in restoring a normal platelet count in 75 per cent. Those patients with dangerously low platelet counts despite steroids and splenectomy should be treated with immunosuppressive drugs. Cyclophosphamide and azathioprine have been successfully used, while vincristine is an experimental agent of promise.

High doses of pooled intravenous immunoglobulin, 0.4 g/kg, daily for 4 days has been successfully used. Its action is thought to be by anti-idiotypic antibodies in the pooled gamma-globulin combining with and neutralizing anti-platelet antibodies. In chronic ITP it may be used to restore the platelet count temporarily prior to splenectomy in patients refractory to steroids. In Rh(D)-positive patients moderate (and cheaper) doses of anti-D will have the same effect as high-dose intravenous immuno-globulin.

In post-transfusion purpura in which the patient's own platelets are caught up in an isoimmune reaction against transfused platelets, there is no response to either steroids or splenectomy and high-dose intravenous immunoglobulin is the treatment of choice.

Platelet transfusions are usually ineffective in immune thrombocytopenia since they are themselves destroyed by the immune reaction, but nevertheless they should be used in life-threatening circumstances.

## THROMBOTIC THROMBOCYTOPENIC PURPURA (MOSCHOVITZ DISEASE)

This rare, frequently lethal, condition is characterized by a microangiopathic haemolytic anaemia, severe thrombocytopenia, fever, renal failure and fluctuating neurologic features. In children a similar syndrome is known as the haemolytic uraemic syndrome. The cause of both these disorders is unknown, but abnormalities of prostacyclin metabolism have been found. Treatment is unsatisfactory, but roughly 50 per cent of cases respond to plasma exchange using fresh frozen plasma as the exchange fluid.

## MASSIVE TRANSFUSION SYNDROME

Platelets do not survive in blood stored at 4°C for more than 24 hours. Following transfusion with more than ten units of stored blood in a 24-hour period, a bleeding diathesis is likely. The clotting factors V and VIII also store poorly and bleeding is caused by a combination of deficiencies of these factors and thrombocytopenia. Treatment is by including two units of fresh frozen plasma for every ten units of blood transfused, and platelet transfusion as required.

## HYPERSPLENISM

The normal spleen weighs between 150 and 250 g. The pathological spleen may be up to 20 times larger. In very large spleens 90 per cent of the body's platelets may be pooled in the spleen. This contrasts with red cell pooling which usually accounts for no more than 20 per cent of the red cell mass. On the other hand, normal platelets are not injured by their sojourn in the spleen, whereas red cell life-span is noticeably shortened. The causes of massive splenomegaly are shown in Table 21.35.

**Table 21.35** Causes of massive splenomegaly.

Chronic myeloid leukaemia
Myelofibrosis
Malaria
Primary proliferative polycythemia
Chronic lymphocytic leukaemia
Prolymphocytic leukaemia
Hairy cell leukaemia
Non-Hodgkin's lymphoma
Hodgkin's disease (rarely)
Thalassaemia major
Gaucher's disease
Kala azar
Sarcoidosis (rarely)
Felty's syndrome (rarely)

### Treatment

Thrombocytopenia due to hypersplenism is seldom the cause of bleeding unless platelet function is also abnormal. Splenectomy may be indicated if the hypersplenism is symptomatic.

# Coagulation disorders

Hereditary disorders of each of the coagulation factors have been described. Most are rare, but haemophilia A or B and Von Willebrand's disease are merely uncommon.

## HAEMOPHILIA A AND B

Both types of haemophilia are inherited as X-linked recessive disorders. The diseases are therefore virtually confined to boys. Haemophilia A (factor VIII deficiency) has an incidence of 1 in 100 000 and is five times as common as haemophilia B (factor IX deficiency or Christmas disease).

### Pathology

Both factor VIII and factor IX are essential elements of the intrinsic clotting pathway (Fig. 21.10). Reduced levels of either factor prolongs the time taken for coagulation to occur. Factor VIII is extremely labile with a short half-life. Factor IX is more stable.

## Clinical features

Clinical features are identical in both types of haemophilia. The severity of the disease depends on the levels of the factor concerned (Table 21.36). The most common feature is spontaneous haemarthrosis of knee, ankle, elbow and shoulder. Acutely inflamed joints are immobile, which leads to disuse atrophy of the surrounding muscles. This in turn makes the joints more unstable and increases the risk of further haemoarthroses. A succession of joint bleeds often leads to permanent damage. Bleeding also occurs into muscles; ileopsoas and retroperitoneal bleeds may mimic acute abdominal emergencies. Gastrointestinal haemorrhage is usually consequent on a local lesion. Intracranial bleeds occur mainly in younger haemophiliacs and are usually secondary to trauma. In milder haemophiliacs bleeding is most often related to accidental or surgical trauma. Bleeding is often delayed since the vascular and platelet responses to haemorrhage are normal.

**Table 21.36** Severity of haemophilia related to levels of clotting factors.

| Level of factor VIII or factor IX (% of normal) | Clinical features |
| --- | --- |
| <1 | Severe disease; spontaneous bleeding into muscles and joints every few days from an early age; crippling joint deformities |
| 1–5 | Moderate disease; serious bleeding from trivial operation or injury; occasional spontaneous bleeding |
| 5–20 | Mild disease; serious bleeding after trauma or surgery |
| 25–50 | Subclinical disease; moderate bleeding after surgery; some female carriers fall within this group |

## Diagnosis

The bleeding time is normal in haemophilia. The prothrombin time is normal but the kaolin cephalin clotting time (KCCT) (page 600) is prolonged. Measurement of specific clotting factors VIII and IX will distinguish haemophilia A and B. About 7 per cent of patients with haemophilia A develop antibodies to isologous factor VIII (known as inhibitors). These are detected by the failure of an admixture of normal plasma to correct the KCCT and make management much more difficult.

## Differential diagnosis

The major differential diagnosis is between haemophilia A and Von Willebrand's disease in which factor VIIIC levels (coagulant activity) are also low.

## Treatment

All haemophiliacs should be registered with a Haemophilia Centre which will direct treatment. The basis of treatment is the adequate replacement of the missing coagulation factor. The short half-life and limited availability of factor VIII means that prophylactic treatment is not feasible for any but a selected minority of patients with a history of recurrent severe bleeds. For the rest it is important to treat as early as possible after each bleed.

The haemophiliac himself is usually the best judge of when a bleed is occurring and for this reason most severe haemophiliacs are on home treatment.

For haemophilia A concentrates of factor VIII extracted from donor blood screened for hepatitis B and C and for human immunodeficiency virus (HIV) are available. Those in current use have been heat-treated so as to eliminate as far as possible the risk of virus transmission. For spontaneous joint haemorrhage the aim is to raise the factor VIII level above 20 per cent of normal. For major surgery and post-traumatic bleeding the level should be raised to 100 per cent until haemorrhage has stopped and then maintained above 60 per cent until the risk of haemorrhage has passed. Approximately 0.5 units of factor VIII per kg body weight are required to raise the factor VIII level by 1 per cent. The half-life of factor VIII is only 10 hours so that twice daily treatment is required. Minor surgery such as tooth extraction is usually undertaken under the cover of tranexamic acid which inhibits fibrinolysis and greatly reduces the need for factor VIII. The vasopressin analogue desmopressin (DDAVP) produces an approximately three-fold rise in factor VIII activity, and this may be sufficient to permit surgery in mild haemophiliacs.

Factor VIII concentrates are regarded as safer than cryoprecipitate which is now seldom used. A concentrate which has been affinity purified by immunoabsorption with a monoclonal anti-factor VIII is increasingly favoured, especially for haemophiliacs who have never been previously treated with any other type of concentrate, and also for those who are HIV positive, on the basis that progression to acquired immune deficiency syndrome (AIDS) might be related to the degree of exposure to foreign antigens.

Patients with inhibitors require huge amounts of factor VIII to overcome the antibody and this has only a temporary effect since the immune response is boosted by the infused material. Plasmapheresis to remove the inhibitor may be helpful. Inhibitors do not usually cross-react with pig proteins, and in emergencies porcine factor VIII may be used. Another strategy relies on the presence of activated factor IX in factor IX concentrates to bypass the need for factor VIII in the clotting cascade.

Haemophilia B is treated with factor IX concentrate. This has a longer half-life than factor VIII and may therefore be given less frequently. Cyroprecipitate does not contain factor IX. The days of using crude concentrates which contain many other proteins besides the one that is missing are fast passing. Affinity purified or recombinant clotting factors of all kinds will be available in the near future.

Prevention of crippling joint disease is only achieved by careful attention to detail and prompt treatment. Muscle and joint bleeds are managed by rest for the first 36 hours, splinting sometimes being necessary. Thereafter mobilization under the guidance of a physiotherapist is ideal. Pain relief is usually achievable with paracetamol-based products. Aspirin should be avoided because of its effect on platelets, and strong analgesics carry the real risk of addiction.

## Complications

Owing to virus contamination of clotting concentrates in the past many severely affected haemophiliacs have been exposed to hepatitis B, non-A non-B hepatitis and HIV. Disordered liver function tests are common as are imbalances of T-cell subsets. About 40 per cent have antibodies to HIV; some have already developed AIDS and others are bound to do so. Every Haemophilia Centre has an experienced AIDS counsellor to help with these problems.

Even without the spectre of AIDS many haemophiliacs suffer from psychological problems. The Haemophilia Society provides valuable social and psychological support.

### Screening

Daughters of haemophiliac fathers and mothers of two haemophiliac sons are obligate carriers of the abnormal gene. However, about 30 per cent of cases of haemophilia are thought to arise from new mutations which makes genetic counselling difficult. The detection of haemophilia carriers may be aided by the finding of a disparity between coagulant activity (factor VIII:C) and levels detected by antibody (factor VIII:Ag) in female relatives. Measurement of factor VIII:C in fetal blood and cDNA probes on chorionic villi permit the diagnosis of affected fetuses.

## VON WILLEBRAND'S DISEASE

Von Willebrand's disease (VWD) is an autosomally transmitted deficiency of Von Willebrand's factor (VWF). In most cases the inheritance is dominant, although recessive forms exist. The incidence is 1 in 25 000, although many of these cases are not clinically important. A number of VWD variants exist. Distinction between them is a matter for the expert, but it is perhaps prudent to know that one type (IIB) is associated with moderate thrombocytopenia, and that another (type III) does not respond to treatment with desmopressin (DDAVP).

### Pathology

Von Willebrand's factor is a high molecular weight protein which binds avidly to factor VIII and prolongs its half-life in the circulation. It also binds to platelet membranes and vessel wall collagen and there helps to stabilize the platelet plug. Deficiency of VWF shortens the factor

VIII half-life so that its plasma level falls. In addition, platelet function is impaired.

## Clinical features

The main features are menorrhagia, epistaxis and easy bruising, together with haemorrhage after trauma or surgery. In severe cases, particularly in rare homozygous patients, the factor VIII level may be low enough to lead to muscle and joint bleeds.

## Diagnosis

The bleeding time is prolonged. Clotting tests are also abnormal: the KCCT is prolonged and the factor VIII:C level reduced. Von Willebrand factor, previously known as factor VIII-related antigen factor, is measured immunologically. It is reduced in most forms of VWD, whereas in haemophilia A it is present in close to normal levels. Platelets will normally aggregate in the presence of the antibiotic ristocetin; in VWD they fail to do so.

## Treatment

Desmopressin causes a temporary increase in plasma concentration of Von Willebrand factor and is usually sufficient to cover minor surgery or to stem minor haemorrhage. Major bleeds and major surgery require factor VIII concentrate. An affinity purified VWF will shortly be available.

# Acquired defects of coagulation

## VITAMIN K DEFICIENCY

Vitamin K, a fat-soluble substance obtained from green vegetables, is required by the liver for the formation of factors II, VII, IX and X. Levels are low in the first days of life, especially in premature infants. In adults dietary deficiency is rare, but malabsorption may occur in obstructive jaundice and pancreatic or small bowel disease. In severely affected cases a haemophilia-like syndrome occurs which is on rare occasions fatal. Both the prothrombin time and the KCCT are prolonged. Vitamin K, 1 mg

i.m., is administered prophylactically to all newborn babies (the synthetic vitamin should not be used as it may cause haemolysis and kernicterus). In adults either form given orally or intravenously is satisfactory.

# Liver disease

The bleeding diathesis of liver disease is complex. The component parts are:

1. Malabsorption of vitamin K because of obstructive jaundice;
2. Reduced synthesis of all clotting factors except factor VIII;
3. Production of a functionally abnormal fibrinogen (dysfibrinogenaemia);
4. Hypersplenism due to portal hypertension leading to thrombocytopenia;
5. Low-level disseminated intravascular coagulation.

In addition there is a thrombotic element due to reduced synthesis of antithrombin III.

## DISSEMINATED INTRAVASCULAR COAGULATION (DIC)

The conversion of fibrinogen to fibrin within the circulation leads to the consumption of coagulation factors and platelets and an acute or chronic haemorrhagic state. There are many causes (Table 21.37).

## Pathology

Intravascular coagulation is triggered by the liberation of a thrombogenic substance into the circulation. Platelets and coagulation factors are consumed. A secondary fibrinolysis is induced which further depletes clotting factors. Fibrin degradation products are themselves antithrombins.

## Clinical features

In severe cases there is bleeding from the nose, mouth and venepuncture sites. Petechiae and ecchymoses are found.

**Table 21.37** Causes of disseminated intravascular coagulation.

**Obstetric**
Amniotic fluid embolus
Premature separation of placenta
Septic abortion
Intrauterine death
Eclampsia

**Infection**
Gram-negative shock
Meningococcal septicaemia
*Plasmodium falciparum* malaria
Rocky Mountain spotted fever
Subacute bacterial endocarditis

**Malignancy**
Carcinoma of prostate
Acute promyelocytic leukaemia (M3)
Mucin-secreting adenocarcinoma

**Miscellaneous**
Haemolytic transfusion reaction
Burns
Liver failure
Snake venoms
Hypothermia
Anaphylaxis

*Diagnosis*

The blood film shows anisocytosis, red cell fragments, polychromasia, nucleated red cells and microspherocytes. The platelet count is low and there is prolongation of the prothrombin time, KCCT and thrombin time. The concentration of fibrinogen is reduced. High levels of fibrin degradation products are found in serum and urine.

*Treatment*

It is important to treat the underlying cause. When DIC is severe, replacement therapy with clotting factors and platelet transfusion is necessary. The vogue for using heparin to control the ongoing coagulation seems to have died out except, perhaps, in M3 AML.

## INHIBITORS OF COAGULATION

Inhibitors of coagulation factors are generally antibodies. In congenital clotting factor deficiencies such as haemophilia A and B, antibodies arise in between 5 and 10 per cent of patients against the clotting factor used for treatment; and although they may not cross-react with the patient's own factor VIII or IX, they may be serious barriers to treatment and may need to be lowered by plasmapheresis before clotting factors are given. However, autoantibodies to both factor VIII and VWF may occur in patients with no previous bleeding history. They may be seen *post-partum*, in rheumatoid arthritis and as the antibody activity of the monoclonal protein in Waldenström's macroglobulinaemia. They lead to acquired haemophilia or acquired von Willebrand disease, respectively. Treatment is often difficult, requiring the techniques referred to above for the treatment of haemophilia with inhibitors.

# *T*HROMBOPHILIA

The causes of thrombosis are dealt with in Chapter 11 (page 232), but there are some specifically haematological conditions which give rise to an increased tendency to thrombosis which are collectively known as the thrombophilias (Table 21.38).

Antithrombin III (AT-III) deficiency is rare (0.5 per 1000). It may be congenital or acquired following major surgery or trauma. AT-III is an inhibitor of thrombin and other activated clotting factors, and its absence leads to venous thrombosis, especially when other precipitating factors are present. Treatment of acute thrombosis is with AT-III concentrate followed by long-term warfarin. Heparin is ineffective as it requires AT-III for its anticoagulant activity.

Protein C and protein S are vitamin K-dependent factors produced by the liver which act as inhibitors of coagulation. Deficiency of protein C has a similar prevalence as AT-III but protein S deficiency is rarer. Both lead to recurrent venous thrombosis in a proportion of patients and this is an indication for long-term oral anticoagulation. In protein C defi-

**Table 21.38** Blood diseases associated with risk of thrombosis.

| Disease | Risk factor |
| --- | --- |
| Polycythaemia | Increased haematocrit |
| Chronic myeloid leukaemia | Hyperleucocytosis |
| Myeloma | Hyperviscosity |
| Thrombocythaemia | Platelet aggregation |
| Antithrombin III deficiency | Coagulation inhibitor deficiency |
| Protein C deficiency | Coagulation inhibitor deficiency |
| Protein S deficiency | Coagulation inhibitor deficiency |
| Activated protein C resistance | Coagulation inhibitor deficiency |
| Lupus anticoagulant | Inhibition of protein C? |

ciency a large loading dose of warfarin is likely to lead to skin necrosis.

Recently, it has been established that the commonest type of thrombophilia is congenital resistance to activated protein C. The genetic lesion is a point mutation on factor V and it is found in 50% of patients with familial thromboses.

The lupus anticoagulant is an acquired abnormality in systemic lupus erythematosus, but also in many other conditions, and, indeed, may be an isolated finding. It is an IgG antibody against phospholipid which is often associated with antibodies against cardiolipin and the phosphodiester backbone of DNA. It causes prolongation of the KCCT but is not associated with haemorrhage. Clinically it is associated with a raised incidence of venous and arterial thromboses and recurrent abortions. Treatment of thrombosis is with oral anticoagulants, and prevention of abortions is with steroids and aspirin.

# Anticoagulant drugs

## HEPARIN

Heparin acts by potentiating the inhibitory effects of antithrombin III on activated factors XII, IX, X and thrombin. It is used as a treatment for venous thromboembolism. For preference it should be given as a continuous intravenous infusion. Doses of 30–40 000 units over 24 hours are usually necessary to keep the KCCT in the desired range, 1.5–2.5 times normal. It is frequently used as the initial treatment of venous thrombosis until concurrently administered oral anticoagulants have their maximal effect.

The anticoagulant effect wears off over 6 hours. Overdosage causing bleeding may be

**Table 21.39** Drugs causing serious interactions with oral anticoagulants.

| Potentiation of anticoagulants | Inhibition of anticoagulants |
| --- | --- |
| **Analgesics** | |
| Aspirin | |
| Phenylbutazone | |
| Azapropazone | |
| Indomethacin | |
| Coproxamol | |
| **Antibiotics** | |
| Sulphonamides | Rifampicin |
| Erythromycin | Griseofulvin |
| Metronidazole | |
| Ketoconazole | |
| Miconazole | |
| Latamoxef sodium | |
| Cephamandole | |
| **Hypnotics** | |
| | Barbiturates |
| | Dichloralphenazone |
| **Anticonvulsants** | |
| | Primidone |
| | Carbamazepine |
| **Lipid-lowering agents** | |
| Clofibrate | Cholestyramine |
| Bezafibrate | |
| Dextrothyroxine sodium | |
| **Gastrointestinal drugs** | |
| Cimetidine | Sucralfate |
| **Hormones** | |
| Anabolic steroids | Oestrogens |
| Danazol | |
| **Miscellaneous** | |
| Sulphinpyrazone | |
| Amiodarone | |

reversed by protamine sulphate in a dose of 1 mg for each 100 units of heparin. Heparin is ineffective in antithrombin III deficiency. Low-dose subcutaneous heparin is used for the prophylaxis of venous thrombosis perioperatively and during periods of immobilization. The dose is 5000 units two or three times daily. The calcium derivative is as painful as a bee sting. Complications include rare cases of immune thrombocytopenia (which paradoxically, leads to thrombosis) and osteoporosis with long-term use.

Low molecular weight heparin has recently been introduced. It is obtained by fractionation or depolymerization of standard heparin. While retaining the antithrombotic effect, it is much less likely to cause haemorrhage than standard heparin. It is also very much more expensive.

## ORAL ANTICOAGULANTS

The oral anticoagulants are mainly coumarin derivatives and act as vitamin K antagonists. They inhibit the gamma carboxylation of the terminal glutamic acid residues of factors II, VII, IX and X. These abnormal proteins (known as PIVKAs) have a poor affinity for calcium and thus are poorly able to participate in coagulation. Anticoagulation is controlled using the prothrombin time, results being expressed in a standardized way (the INR) which is comparable between laboratories. An INR of between 2 and 4 is considered to produce a therapeutic effect with little risk of haemorrhage. Almost all patients are treated with warfarin. It is usual to start with 9 mg daily for 3 days, followed by a dose between 1 and 9 mg according to the INR. Anticoagulation is not effective until the third day.

The major cause of lack of control is interaction with other drugs which may potentiate or inhibit the effect of oral anticoagulants (Table 21.39). Overdosage may be reduced by treatment with 1 mg vitamin K, although this should be avoided if possible since the patient is then made refractory to further oral anticoagulants for several days.

A few patients develop skin necrosis on warfarin treatment. Warfarin should not be given during the first and third trimesters of pregnancy as it causes fetal abnormalities and increases the risk of placental haemorrhage. Heparin should be used instead.

## FIBRINOLYTIC AGENTS

Streptokinase and tissue plasminogen activator are enzymes capable of activating the fibrinolytic system. They are used therapeutically for massive pulmonary embolus, for large vessel venous thrombosis and to limit the myocardial damage following coronary thrombosis. Urokinase is used to dissolve thrombus in arteriovenous shunts used for haemodialysis.

# **D**isorders of the Nervous System

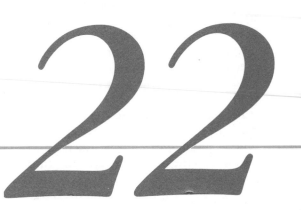

**22**

# *I*NTRODUCTION

Neurology encompasses a very wide range of conditions, from the commonplace such as stroke, to more esoteric syndromes. Because it has a long history of being separate from 'general medicine' it has an aura of being a super-specialty which tends to intimidate a large proportion of practitioners. However, of all the medical specialties it is one of the most logical to study since it can be based on the anatomy of the nervous system. For this reason this chapter follows a different plan to others in this book, following the nervous system through its anatomical structure with descriptions of the diseases within the structural divisions.

Nervous tissue is among the least able to repair itself, and this has proved a therapeutic hurdle for neurologists. Studies of factors controlling and affecting the growth of nervous tissue, although not yet clinically relevant, promise important advances in treatment. By contrast, two areas of study have made great clinical advances in neurology. Genetics has led to improved genetic counselling and understanding of the molecular basis of certain diseases, for example, muscular dystrophy. Secondly, the powerful techniques of imaging such as magnetic resonance imaging and positron emission tomography have allowed precise localization and characterization of lesions affecting some of the most inaccessible parts of the body, such as the brain and spinal cord.

The evaluation and management of neurological problems follows the traditional medical approach of a history, examination and investigation leading to a diagnosis, followed by treatment. The most important part of the initial assessment is the history, the diagnosis being evident in the majority of patients from the history alone. After the initial assessment, the answer to the question 'Where is the lesion?' should be clear. The history sometimes gives a precise answer and nearly always indicates the general area, and the examination provides more precise localization. The answer to the question falls into one of three categories:

1. The history and physical signs can all be explained by a lesion at one location, that is a single focal lesion.
2. It is necessary to postulate more than one focal lesion.
3. It is a system disease.

For example, a patient with a unilateral third cranial nerve palsy and a contralateral hemiplegia need only have a single lesion in the mid-brain at the level of the third cranial nerve nucleus. If this patient also had unilateral amblyopia (loss of visual acuity) with optic atrophy, it would be necessary to postulate at least two lesions, one in the optic nerve and the other in the brain stem. Lesions at two different sites are not necessarily due to the same pathology, as is likely in this example. Common neurological diseases causing multifocal pathology include multiple sclerosis, vascular disease and metastases. Many neurological conditions are neither focal nor multifocal, but affect a whole system, as in motor neurone disease, and these can be conveniently described as system diseases.

Having determined the location of the lesion, the next step is to determine its nature. The history and examination may give the answer and should give a differential diagnosis. Further investigation may be required and the choice of tests depends on the shortlist of diagnostic possibilities. Usually the simpler tests are carried out first and the more complicated tests subsequently until a diagnosis is made or a plan of management determined.

# INVESTIGATIONS

The investigation of neurological problems uses the full range of diagnostic tools available to medicine, but some of the more specialized investigative procedures will be considered here.

## Plain X-rays

### SKULL

Plain skull X-rays have been largely replaced by computed tomography (CT); but where this is not readily available skull X-rays are useful for skull fractures, sinus disease and bony erosions including enlargement of pituitary fossa and the internal auditory meati.

### SPINE

Cervical spine X-rays give valuable information in patients with cervical spondylosis, and it may be necessary to include lateral views in flexion and extension as well as oblique views to show the foraminae. Similar information is available from lumbar and thoracic spinal X-rays. Plain X-rays may also show rib erosions, cervical ribs, congenital fusion of the vertebrae, a narrow spinal canal, Paget's disease (page 505) and metastatic deposits.

## Computed X-ray tomography

The development of CT of the brain has been described as the greatest advance in the use of X-rays since their discovery by Rontgen in 1895. A narrow pulsed beam of X-rays is passed through the brain and a detector records the amount that is transmitted. The X-ray source and its corresponding detector is rotated around the head. From the data obtained the absorption coefficient or X-ray density of small volumes of brain can be computed. The resulting composite picture clearly shows any structure whose X-ray density varies from that of calcium at one extreme to that of fat at the other.

It is therefore possible to delineate tumours, abscesses, haematomas, infarcts and cerebral oedema. The ventricles are clearly seen so it is possible to say whether or not they are dilated or displaced and whether or not there is evidence of cortical atrophy. Tumours that are isodense with brain may not be seen, but their presence may be inferred from distortion of normal structures. Many tumours are enhanced following the intravenous injection of an iodine-containing contrast material, since this makes the blood vessels appear denser than normal and if it extravasates it may increase the apparent density of tumours.

The CT scan is a rapid, accurate, reliable and atraumatic method of visualizing the intracranial contents and a single series is associated with a low radiation dose. The use of these machines has considerably reduced the need for other diagnostic procedures.

## Magnetic resonance imaging

Magnetic resonance imaging (MRI) (also called nuclear magnetic resonance, NMR), provides very detailed images (page 119). The images are constructed by CT techniques from the radiofrequency signal that is emitted as electron orbits return to alignment having been displaced by an electromagnetic force applied to the patient lying in a powerful magnetic field. In the brain, the difference between grey and white matter is particularly well shown and small lesions of white matter are easily seen. The widespread small lesions in multiple sclerosis are particularly well demonstrated. It is possible to reconstruct the image in any plane, and, unlike X-ray CT scans, the image is not distorted by the partial volume effect close to bone and can therefore provide excellent pictures close to the floor of the skull and in the posterior fossa. It has the additional advantage of being non-invasive and does not expose the patient to ionizing radiation. Since good definition of the spinal column and spinal cord can be obtained, this technique has replaced conventional myelography. Good visualization of lumbar roots is obtainable.

Magnetic resonance angiography is now the method of choice for visualization of the dural venous sinuses and developments in technology are already giving arterial angiograms approaching the definition of intra-arterial digital subtraction techniques (see below).

# Cerebrospinal fluid analysis

Lumbar puncture for cerebrospinal fluid (CSF) analysis may be diagnostic in all forms of meningitis and meningoencephalitis. Carcinomatous meningitis may be diagnosed from the morphology of cells obtained by lumbar puncture, and the analysis of CSF proteins, including protein immunoelectrophoresis, may be helpful in the diagnosis of multiple sclerosis.

# Cerebral angiography

The carotid and vertebral arterial system can be visualized by injection of a radio-opaque dye and rapid-sequence X-rays to show the arterial, capillary and venous stages. This is usually done by femoral catheterization and then by selective catheterization of the artery of interest. Angiography is indicated if the CT or MRI scan shows a vascular lesion, particularly a cerebral angioma, or if detailed anatomy of the vascular tree is required by a surgeon planning operative intervention.

Digital computerization of the image from which the digitalized data from a plain skull film can be subtracted produces a subtraction image. This allows visualization of very weak concentrations of contrast medium, so that very high definition films can be obtained following the intra-arterial injection of small volumes of contrast material and this is now the method of choice. Arteries and veins can be seen following intravenous injection, but this opacifies all the vessels and makes interpretation difficult.

# Doppler ultrasonic angiology

This can be used to measure the velocity of red blood cells. It shows the direction of flow and turbulence and is used to assess blood flow in the carotid, vertebral, subclavian and brachial arteries. Transcranial Doppler can measure the velocity of blood in the middle cerebral arteries and basilar artery. B-mode scanning shows an image of the artery so that atheromatous plaques can be directly visualized. It is a valuable non-invasive test for screening patients with vascular disease, particularly for stenoses in the subclavian arteries and the common carotid, internal and external carotid arteries around the bifurcation. Signals can also be obtained from the vertebral arteries, the basilar artery and the first part of the middle cerebral arteries.

# Electroencephalography

Electroencephalography (EEG), a recording of the electrical activity of the brain, provides valuable information in patients with all forms of epilepsy and in many forms of encephalopathy, including toxic, metabolic, inflammatory and degenerative diseases. It is of no value in the assessment of space-occupying lesions.

# Electromyography (EMG)

Surface or needle electrodes record the electrical activity of muscle. This is an important procedure in the evaluation of neuromuscular disease.

# Nerve conduction studies

Measurement of the conduction velocity of peripheral nerves helps to determine the nature of polyneuropathies and locate the site of lesions in peripheral nerve palsies.

# Isotope scans

Isotope brain scans using technetium have been largely replaced by CT scans and MRI. Where these investigations are not available the isotope brain scan may provide useful information in subdural haematoma and multiple metastases. Isotope cisternography may be a useful test in patients with communicating hydrocephalus (page 655).

Single photon emission computed tomography (SPECT) is most often used to measure regional cerebral blood flow. It is a simple technique but with poor resolution.

# Clinical problems

## INTELLECTUAL FUNCTION AND DEMENTIA

## Tests of intellectual function

A formal psychometric analysis of intelligence provides quantitive information and can be used to follow progress. Simple bedside testing provides useful clinical information, but appropriate allowance must be made for educational background. The mini-mental state examination is a convenient screening test for intellectual function.

### ORIENTATION

The patient is asked the day of the week, the date, the month, the year, where he is at the moment and his home address.

### MEMORY

Tests of memory are conveniently divided into three groups:

1. **Immediate recall**: the patient is asked to repeat a sequence of random numbers, first forwards (normal more than six) and then backwards (normal four or more).
2. **The five-minute memory test**: this is usually carried out with a name, an address and a flower. The number of errors and the total number of words should be recorded.
3. **Long-term memory**: questions may include items from the patient's past or items of national importance and should be adjusted to the patient's educational level and social background.

## THE MINI-MENTAL STATE EXAMINATION

### Orientation

Score one point for correct answers to each of the following questions:

What is the time?
    date?
    day?
    month?
    year?     5 points ( )

What is the name of this ward?
    the hospital?
    the district?
    the town?
    the country?   5 points ( )

### Registration

Name three objects. Score up to three points if, at the first attempt, the patient repeats, in order, the three objects you have randomly named. Score two or one if this is the number of objects he repeats correctly. Endeavour, by further attempts and prompting, to have all three repeated, so as to test recall later.

    3 points ( )

### Attention and calculation

Ask the patient to subtract 7 from 100, and then 7 from the result, continue this for five steps, scoring one for each time a correct subtraction is performed.

    5 points ( )

### Recall

Ask for the three objects repeated in the registration test, scoring one for each correctly recalled.

    3 points ( )

### Language

Score one point for two objects (e.g. a pencil and a watch) correctly named.

    2 points ( )

Score one point if the following sentence is correctly repeated. 'No ifs, ands or buts'.

    I point ( )

Score three if a three-stage command is correctly executed, score one for each stage: for example, 'With the index finger of your right hand touch the tip of your nose and then your left ear', or 'Take this piece of paper in your right hand fold in a half and place it on the floor'.

    3 points ( )

On a blank piece of paper write, 'Close your eyes' and ask the patient to obey what is written. Score one point if he closes his eyes.

    I point ( )

Ask the patient to write a sentence. Score one if the sentence is sensible and has a verb and a subject.

    I point ( )

Construct a pair of intersecting pentagons, each side one inch long. Score one if this is correctly copied.

    I point ( )

TOTAL SCORE     (=30) ( )

## LEARNING

The patient should be asked to learn the Babcock sentence ('One thing a nation needs in order to be rich and great is a large, secure supply of wood') by repeating it after the examiner as often as necessary to get it word perfect; this should be achieved in less than five attempts.

## CALCULATION

The patient is asked to subtract 7 from 100 and continue to subtract 7 from the result; the time taken and number of errors should be recorded ('serial sevens').

# Dementia

Dementia (page 876) is a deterioration in the intellectual function of the brain as a result of organic disease. It is a sign and sometimes a symptom, but it is not a diagnosis.

About 50 per cent of elderly patients with dementia have Alzheimer's disease, about 20 per cent have cerebrovascular disease alone and about 20 per cent have a combination of these two degenerative diseases. The remaining 10 per cent are divided among a wide range of conditions, including syphilis, Jakob–Creutzfeldt disease, communicating hydrocephalus. Huntington's chorea, tumours, progressive multifocal leukoencephalopathy, toxic and deficiency diseases, including those involving alcohol, vitamins $B_1$, $B_6$ and $B_{12}$, and myxoedema.

It is usually easy to identify patients with the typical features of the two principal causes of dementia—Alzheimer's disease and vascular disease – but they are not mutually exclusive and in the elderly they often occur together.

## ALZHEIMER'S DISEASE

The cause of this progressive cerebral degeneration is unknown, but cholinergic pathways are the most severely affected. It may occur at any age and is more common in women and in the elderly.

It presents with a very slow insidious onset of mental deterioration, often starting with memory impairment. The presenting features may suggest lateralization to one hemisphere, but focal deficits do not occur and epilepsy is unusual. Alzheimer's disease is the commonest cause of dementia, but in the absence of a specific marker it remains a diagnosis of exclusion in life and can only be diagnosed with certainty on pathological evidence. It has a characteristic pathological appearance with neurofibrillary tangles and argyrophilic plaques. The aetiology is unknown, but has been linked to the deposition of amyloid (page 494) and to aluminium toxicity. About 15% are familial.

## VASCULAR DISEASE

Cerebrovascular disease rarely causes dementia under the age of 60 without clear evidence of generalized vascular disease, particularly systemic hypertension. Dementia may result from strokes and the subsequent deterioration may be stepwise as further infarcts occur. Vascular disease may also cause a more insidious dementia without clinically evident infarcts. Men are much more frequently affected than women and insight is often preserved.

Binswanger's disease is a vascular leukoencephalopathy nearly always associated with hypertension. There is a characteristic appearance on the CT or MRI scan with altered signal in the frontal periventricular white matter.

## COMMUNICATING HYDROCEPHALUS

Formerly called low-pressure hydrocephalus, this is caused by an obstruction of CSF pathways outside the ventricular system, usually at the tentorial hiatus or at the longitudinal sinus. The history of dementia is often short and may be associated with a clearly identifiable cause such as head injury, subarachnoid haemorrhage, meningitis or following surgical intervention in the posterior fossa. The classical triad is dementia with akinesia, incontinence and a gait apraxia. The CT scan shows markedly dilated ventricles including the third and fourth ventricles, and lack of CSF over the surface as the brain is pushed out against the skull. If a suitable isotope is injected into the lumbar theca, it enters the ventricular system and stays there for 48–72 hours, whereas in the normal subject the isotope would be distributed according to the CSF flow over the surface of the brain, to be cleared through the longitudinal sinus. The same test can be carried out using a radio-opaque dye and CT scanning. These patients should show an improvement following withdrawal of CSF by lumbar puncture. Patients who show these characteristic clinical features and investigations, particularly if they have a clear cause for the condition, respond very well to ventriculoatrial or ventriculoperitoneal shunts.

## INVESTIGATION

Although the chances of finding a treatable cause are small, it is important to attempt a precise aetiological or pathological diagnosis and to exclude the treatable conditions, particularly in younger patients.

This should include a search for space-occupying lesions, toxic, metabolic and deficiency states, and tests for syphilis. Special tests should include electroencephalography and a CT scan. Exceptionally a brain biopsy is required to establish a diagnosis. Cerebrospinal fluid analysis may be appropriate in certain cases.

Dementia commonly occurs in the late stages of acquired immune deficiency syndrome (AIDS) and may be a presenting feature.

# THE CEREBRAL HEMISPHERES

## The dominant hemisphere and language

This is the left hemisphere in all right-handed patients and in about 50 per cent of left-handed patients. The dominant hemisphere is concerned with all forms of language.

All language inputs are processed in Wernicke's area, which is at the posterior end of the superior temporal gyrus. It receives input from the primary visual cortex for reading, semaphore and other visual forms of language and from the primary auditory cortex for speech, morse code and auditory forms of language. It may also receive information from the somatosensory cortex for the interpretation of Braille (Fig. 22.1).

A lesion of the primary visual cortex causes blindness, but a lesion of the pathway between the visual cortex and Wernicke's area causes dyslexia; in patients with this condition, comprehension of the spoken word is preserved. Information going initially to the right hemisphere has to cross the corpus callosum to reach Wernicke's area, so that a lesion affecting the left visual cortex and the posterior part of the corpus callosum causes a right homonymous hemianopia and dyslexia because of interruption of information from the right visual cortex to Wernicke's area (Fig. 22.1).

Lesions of Wernicke's area cause loss of ability to understand any form of language input (Wernicke's aphasia; fluent, receptive or sensory aphasia). The patient can still speak clearly and fluently, but since there is no auditory feedback cannot understand what he is saying and is

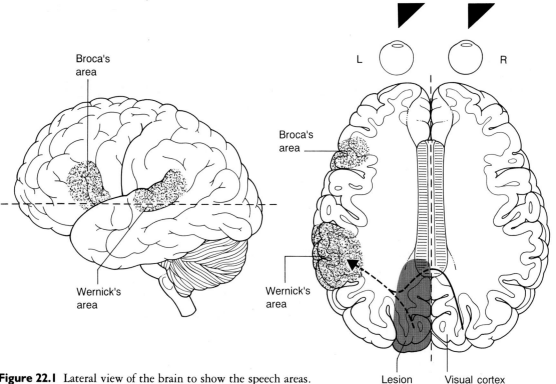

**Figure 22.1** Lateral view of the brain to show the speech areas.

unaware of any errors he may make. This usually produces fluent nonsense (Fig. 22.2).

All language output arises in Broca's area and is then relayed to the motor cortex for speech and writing. If a lesion is confined to Broca's area and Wernicke's area is intact, comprehension is preserved but the patient is unable to express himself (Broca's aphasia; non-fluent, expressive or motor aphasia). If he attempts a word and gets it wrong, he is immediately aware of the error and attempts to correct it. This produces a halting, non-fluent dysphasia, which in mild cases may consist of some hesitation only, while in the more severe cases there may be no speech at all.

Both Wernicke's area and Broca's area, together with their connecting pathways, are supplied by the middle cerebral artery and an infarct in this territory is the commonest cause of dysphasia; tumours are the next commonest cause. Anterior lesions are more likely to cause non-fluent dysphasia and posterior lesions cause fluent dysphasia.

Gerstmann's syndrome is caused by a lesion of the dominant angular gyrus and consists of finger agnosia, right/left disorientation, dysgraphia, dyscalculia and dyslexia.

## THE NON-DOMINANT HEMISPHERE AND SPATIAL ORIENTATION

The non-dominant hemisphere is concerned with spatial awareness, both personal and extrapersonal, at a higher level than the primary sensory cortex which is concerned with vision, hearing and somatosensory information. This is the reason why patients with a right hemisphere

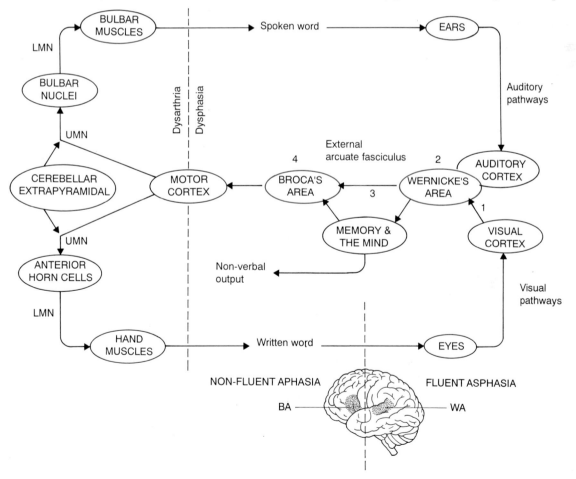

**Figure 22.2** Aphasia. Redrawn from Walton J., *Essentials of Neurology*, 6th ed. (1989) Churchill Livingstone. With permission.

lesion may show a striking neglect of the left side of the body and ignore objects in the left visual field out of proportion to the sensory and visual loss. Lesions of the left hemisphere may cause some sensory extinction, but neglect or denial of the right side of the body is unusual. This loss of spatial orientation causes difficulty in dressing (dressing dyspraxia) and difficulty in finding the way in a familiar environment (topographical amnesia).

## *T*HE CRANIAL NERVES

## *The olfactory nerve (I)*

This is the only cranial nerve in the anterior fossa. Numerous small fibres arising in the mucosa in the roof of the nasal cavity pass through the cribriform plate to reach the olfactory bulb, which is continuous posteriorly with the olfactory tract lying in the olfactory groove. Just above the anterior clinoid processes there is a partial decussation. Lesions behind this decussation cannot cause a unilateral or complete loss of the sense of smell. The sensory cortex for smell is in the uncus on the medial aspect of the temporal lobe.

This pathway serves all smell and this includes all flavour; only the cruder sensations of salt, sweet, bitter and acid are relayed through the chorda tympani and glossopharyngeal nerves.

Apparent loss of the sense of smell may be due to nasal obstruction. It is important, therefore, to determine that the airway is clear before testing smell on both sides separately with a mild non-irritant odour. There may be temporary loss of smell as a result of acute or chronic rhinitis, but the commonest cause is head injury, particularly occipital head injuries. If the penetrating fibres through the cribriform plate are sheared, the loss of smell is permanent. If continuity exists they may recover. Unilateral or bilateral anosmia may be an early sign in tumours in the floor of the anterior fossa, in particular, olfactory groove meningiomas.

## *The optic nerve (II)*

Changes in visual acuity imply some abnormality of macula vision but the lesion could be anywhere in the visual pathway. There may, of course, be a distortion of information reaching the macula due to refractive errors or lens opacities. It is important, therefore, to test visual acuity with the refractive errors corrected. Impairment of visual acuity may also be due to a lesion affecting the macula fibres in the optic nerve. Lesions behind the chiasm always affect the vision in both eyes.

Lesions of the visual pathways causing visual field defects can be accurately localized because of the anatomical arrangement of the visual fibres as they traverse the length of the brain to the visual cortex (Fig. 22.3).

### RETINAL LESIONS

The raised intraocular pressure associated with glaucoma first affects the superficial retinal fibres which come from the periphery, with resultant loss of peripheral vision (tunnel vision). Infarction of small bundles of retinal fibres causes arcuate scotomata.

### LOSS OF ONE VISUAL FIELD

This must be due to disease of the optic nerve. Small lesions cause unilateral scotomata or defects and are best delineated with a small white target; if the scotoma is within 30° of the macula, a small red target is more sensitive. The commonest cause is retrobulbar neuritis.

### LESIONS AFFECTING THE CHIASM

Compression of the chiasma in the mid-line damages the decussating fibres and causes a bitemporal field defect; in the early stages this may be bilateral temporal scotomata, which are often asymmetrical. Later the more typical bitemporal hemianopia develops. The commonest cause is a chromaphobe adenoma of the pituitary. There are usually some features of hypopituitarism or hypothalamic dysfunction, either clinically or on laboratory investigation. Eosinophilic pituitary tumours may also cause chiasmal compression, but the clinical features of acromegaly are usually obvious. Basophil adenomas produce florid Cushing's disease before they become sufficiently large to compress the chiasm. Craniopharyngiomas produce a similar visual field defect; calcification can often be seen in the tumour on plain X-ray and calcification is easily identified on CT scans.

## LESIONS OF THE OPTIC TRACTS, RADIATION AND VISUAL CORTEX

Lesions behind the chiasm cause homonymous hemianopia. The nearer the visual cortex, the more congruous the defect. The fibres of the optic radiation are widely separated shortly after leaving the lateral geniculate ganglion, so that lesions of the temporal lobe may cause an upper quadrantic field defect and lesions above the Sylvian fissure a lower quadrantic defect. Macula sparing may occur in vascular lesions of the cortex because the cortical area concerned with macula vision receives its supply from more than one main cerebral artery.

The retina with its blood supply and the optic disc can be visualized directly by ophthalmoscopy and the cornea, lens, anterior and posterior chambers can be examined.

## DISC SWELLING

The optic disc may be oedematous and appear swollen. If this is due to an inflammatory process of the nerve head (the same pathology as retrobulbar neuritis) it is called **papillitis** and vision is affected early and severely. There are no other retinal changes and no haemorrhages. If the swelling is caused by raised intracranial pressure

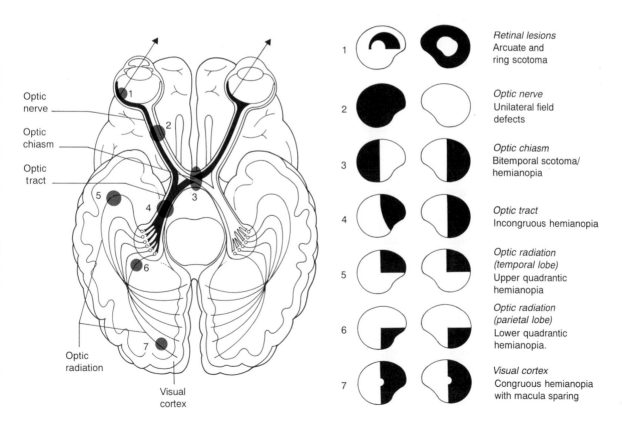

1    *Retinal lesions* Arcuate and ring scotoma

2    *Optic nerve* Unilateral field defects

3    *Optic chiasm* Bitemporal scotoma/ hemianopia

4    *Optic tract* Incongruous hemianopia

5    *Optic radiation (temporal lobe)* Upper quadrantic hemianopia

6    *Optic radiation (parietal lobe)* Lower quadrantic hemianopia.

7    *Visual cortex* Congruous hemianopia with macula sparing

Optic nerve
Optic chiasm
Optic tract
Optic radiation
Visual cortex

**Figure 22.3** Visual pathways.

or systemic hypertension, it is called **papilloedema** and the vision is not affected apart from enlargement of the blind spot. In severe cases of papilloedema the pressure may occlude the arterial supply and cause attacks of amblyopia, which occasionally result in permanent blindness. The presence of hypertensive retinal changes and a markedly elevated systemic blood pressure in the presence of retinal haemorrhages with preservation of vision clearly distinguishes the papilloedema of malignant hypertension from papillitis, but in many patients the appearance of the fundus is indistinguishable. Raised intracranial pressure may be accompanied by headache and vomiting and, if acute, by altered consciousness.

Other local causes of disc swelling include vascular lesions (ischaemic optic neuropathy), infiltration, tumours and benign intracranial hypertension. Occasionally patients are found to have the appearance of papilloedema but with no evidence of raised intracranial pressure (pseudopapilloedema). This may be a congenital abnormality (drusen of the disc). The differentiation from papilloedema may be difficult and many require a CT brain scan and fluorescein angiography.

## OPTIC ATROPHY

Optic atrophy refers to an appearance of the optic disc, which loses its normal pink/yellow colour and assumes a grey/white appearance. There is usually reduced visual acuity or a field defect. The terms primary optic atrophy, secondary optic atrophy and consecutive optic atrophy are purely descriptive and have no pathological connotation. Primary optic atrophy implies a clearly demarcated pale disc with normal retina and blood vessels. It is caused by any lesion of the optic nerve, the commonest of which is retrobulbar neuritis; but it may follow compression by tumours or be the result of toxic (quinine, tobacco, methyl alcohol) or deficiency (vitamin $B_{12}$) states. Secondary optic atrophy implies a pale disc with a hazy outline, which follows swelling of the nerve head (papilloedema or papillitis). Consecutive optic atrophy implies a pale disc where the cause of the atrophy can be seen in the fundus (retinitis pigmentosa, syphilis).

# The oculomotor, trochlear and abducent nerves (III, IV and VI)

Disorders of the oculomotor system can be divided into upper motor neurone lesions (disorders of gaze), lower motor neurone lesions (disorders of the third, fourth and sixth cranial nerves) and internuclear lesions (a mixture of upper and lower motor neurone disorders with vestibular or cerebellar components).

## GAZE PALSIES

Gaze palsies result from upper motor neurone lesions of the oculomotor system and, in common with all upper motor neurone lesions, it is the movement which is affected, not the action of individual muscles – in this case conjugate eye movement. There are centres concerned with gaze both in the cortex and in the brain stem.

### The cortex

There are two cortical gaze centres in each hemisphere. The frontal eye field in the premotor cortex is responsible for scanning and roving eye movements and is the site of conscious voluntary control of eye movement. As with the control of other movements, one hemisphere is responsible for the opposite side of the body and the contralateral extrapersonal space; the left frontal eye field therefore directs eye movement to the right, and vice versa. The effect of destruction and excitation can therefore be predicted:

- **Destruction** (e.g. infarction): transient paralysis of gaze to the opposite side. Occasionally deviation of the eyes to the side of the lesion may be seen.
- **Excitation** (e.g. epilepsy): deviation of the eyes and usually the head to the opposite side (frontal adversive seizure).

Following and reflex eye movements are not affected by lesions of the frontal eye field, and optokinetic nystagmus (page 664) is normal.

The occipital eye field in the visual association

cortex is responsible for following, pursuit and reflex eye movements. It is intimately associated with the visual pathways and lesions in this area are usually associated with a field defect. In destructive lesions (infarction or tumour) there is a full range of voluntary movements but inability to follow or locate objects. Examination is usually complicated by the associated field defect. Optokinetic nystagmus is impaired.

## The brain stem

There are two areas in the brain stem concerned with conjugate eye movements: the upper mid-brain and the pons.

### Upper mid-brain and vertical eye movements

There is no precise centre for vertical eye movement but the pathways concerned must lie at and above the level of the third nerve nucleus in the region of the posterior commissure. Lesions in the pretectal region (e.g. pinealomas) pressing on the superior corpora quadragemini cause defects of upward gaze (Parinaud's syndrome).

### Pons and horizontal eye movements

There are two pontine gaze centres situated close to the sixth nerve nuclei on either side and responsible for gaze to the same side; this function is mediated through the pontine paramedian reticular formation.

Examination for gaze palsies should include both voluntary and following movements as well as tests for optokinetic nystagmus.

Patients should be asked to track a target to both sides, up and down as well as to look in the four cardinal directions, since in some gaze palsies the ability to track a target is preserved, but voluntary gaze is lost.

## LOWER MOTOR NEURONE LESIONS

## Third cranial nerve

The third cranial nerve nucleus lies ventrally in the periductal grey matter in the mid-brain at the level of the superior corpora quadragemini and the red nucleus. It is a large nucleus with clear grouping of nerve cells responsible for the different muscles innervated. Nearby is the Edinger—Westphal nucleus whose parasym-

pathetic fibres run with the third nerve. The nerve runs forwards through the red nucleus and the medial part of the basis pedunculi emerging close to the mid-line in the interpeduncular fossa. The two nerves pass on either side of the basilar artery between the posterior cerebral artery above and the superior cerebellar artery below. The nerve lies just below the posterior communicating artery throughout its length and passes laterally over the internal carotid artery to enter the cavernous sinus where it lies on the lateral wall. It passes through the superior orbital fissure and divides into two main branches – the superior branch to the superior rectus and levator palpebrae superioris and the inferior branch to the medial rectus, inferior rectus and the inferior oblique. The parasympathetic nerves travel with the inferior branch.

A complete third-nerve palsy comprises a fixed dilated pupil due to the unopposed action of the sympathetic, ptosis due to involvement of levator palperbrae superioris, and a fully abducted eye due to the unopposed action of the sixth nerve.

## Fourth cranial nerve

The fourth cranial nerve lies ventrally in the periductal grey matter nearly at the junction of the mid-brain and pons and at the level of the inferior corpora quadragemini. The nerve runs round the aqueduct and decussates in the superior medullary velum. The nerve then passes round the cerebral peduncle below the tentorium, the posterior cerebral artery lying just above the tentorium. Like the third nerve, it passes between the posterior cerebral artery and the superior cerebellar artery, crossing the apex of the petrous temporal bone just above and medial to Meckel's cave, and enters the cavernous sinus lying on the lateral wall below the third nerve. It then passes through the superior orbital fissure to supply the superior oblique muscle.

A fourth-nerve palsy causes vertical diplopia, maximal on downward gaze with the affected eye adducted.

## Sixth cranial nerve

The sixth cranial nerve nucleus lies in the lower pons close to the mid-line and near the floor of the fourth ventricle. The fibres of the seventh nerve are wrapped around the sixth nerve nucleus and this forms a small hump in the floor of the fourth ventricle, the facial colliculus. The nerve runs forward to emerge at the pontomedullary junction near the mid-line. It runs up the clivus in front of the pons parallel to the basilar artery and then at the tentorial hiatus it turns forwards to enter the cavernous sinus where it lies below the internal carotid artery. From the cavernous sinus it passes through the superior orbital fissure to supply the lateral rectus muscle.

A sixth-nerve palsy causes horizontal diplopia, maximal on gaze to the affected side. The affected eye may be adducted.

## LESIONS AND THEIR EFFECTS

All three nerves may be damaged by brain-stem tumours and vascular disease. The extramedullary part of the nerve trunks between the brain stem and the cavernous sinus are vulnerable to granulomatous meningitis (tuberculosis and sarcoid), meningovascular syphilis and nasopharyngeal carcinoma. The intracavernous course of these nerves may be damaged in cavernous sinus thrombosis, carotid aneurysm and pituitary tumours. The superior orbital fissure may be encroached by sphenoidal ridge meningiomas and the nerves may be damaged in the intraorbital part of their course by orbital tumours. In addition the nerves may be damaged by involvement of their vasa-nervorum in diabetes, hypertension and collagen vascular disease (polyarteritis nodosa and giant cell arteritis).

### Lesions of the third nerve

#### Intramedullary lesions

*Nerve nucleus*
Lesions of the nuclei are usually bilateral because they lie close together. The commonest cause is pressure from above by tumours of the pineal gland or gliomas (Parinaud's syndrome).

#### The nerve trunk and red nucleus (Benedikt's syndrome)
The combination of a third-nerve palsy and a contralateral flapping tremor with ataxia of the arm and hand is usually due to vascular disease, disseminated sclerosis or a tumour.

#### Nerve trunk and cerebral peduncle (Weber's syndrome)
A combination of a third-nerve palsy and a contralateral hemiplegia is usually of vascular origin.

*Extramedullary lesions*
Bilateral third-nerve palsies and tetraparesis may result from any large space-occupying lesion in the interpeduncular fossa. The third nerve may be damaged by aneurysm at either end of the posterior communicating artery (page 705).

### Lesions of the fourth nerve
Isolated lesions of the fourth cranial nerve are rare and are usually due to trauma, diabetes, granulomatous meningitis, syphilis or collagen vascular disease.

### Lesions of the sixth nerve
Lesions affecting the nucleus almost always involve the seventh cranial nerve, and since these nerves then follow quite separate pathways, a combination of a sixth and seventh lower motor neurone lesion is likely to be at this level.

Sixth cranial nerve and contralateral hemiplegia (Raymond–Cestan syndrome) is directly analogous to Weber's sydrome.

The nerve trunk is very vulnerable when it crosses the free edge of the tentorium, and it may be damaged here if the brain stem is distorted by a space-occuping lesion in the opposite hemisphere (a false localizing sign) or if there is displacement of the brain stem through the tentorial hiatus (coning).

### Internuclear ophthalmoplegias
A combination of upper motor neurone lesions usually associated with evidence of cerebellar or vestibular involvement (nystagmus) is common because of the wide spatial separation of the third, fourth and sixth nerve nuclei from the upper mid-brain to the lower pons, the separation of mechanisms controlling vertical and horizontal conjugate movement and the intimate relationship of vestibular and cerebellar function to eye movement. There are many

possible combinations; patients may develop a series of different combinations of signs during the course of an illness, particularly in progressive lesions such as pontine glioma. However, there are two principal combinations of signs: anterior and posterior.

*Anterior internuclear ophthalmoplegia (superior or upper, Harris's sign)*

There is normal convergence but a failure to adduct on lateral gaze with nystagmus in the abducting eye. The lesion lies between the fourth and sixth nerve nuclei and involves the medial longitudinal bundle. It is almost always due to disseminated sclerosis.

*Posterior internuclear ophthalmoplegia (inferior or lower)*

This is the opposite of an anterior internuclear ophthalmoplegia, there is failure to abduct on lateral gaze with nystagmus in the adducting eye. The lesion lies at or just below the sixth nerve nucleus.

## Diplopia

The analysis of diplopia depends on a knowledge of the precise actions of the extraocular muscles (Fig. 22.4a). The medial walls of the two orbits are nearly parallel and the lateral walls are roughly at right angles to each other. Since the muscles are inserted into a fibrous ring at the apex of the orbit, the muscle cone is at an angle of about 23° to the optical axis. It is evident, therefore, that the lateral and medial recti only move the eye in the horizontal plane, but the superior and inferior recti only become pure elevators or depressors when the optical axis is the same as the muscle-cone axis, that is, when the eye is 23° abducted, so that the line of pull of the muscle lies over the optical axis of the globe (Fig. 22.4b). Similarly the superior and inferior oblique muscles are only pure elevators or depressors when the eye is adducted since the origin or effective origin of the oblique muscles is anteromedial to the eye (Fig. 22.4c). When the eye is abducted the oblique muscles produce rotation only around the optical axis but little vertical movement, and similarly the superior and inferior recti rotate the eye without much elevation or depression when the eye is adducted.

The reason why patients see double when one muscle is not functioning is that the normal eye moves to keep the image on the macula, but the

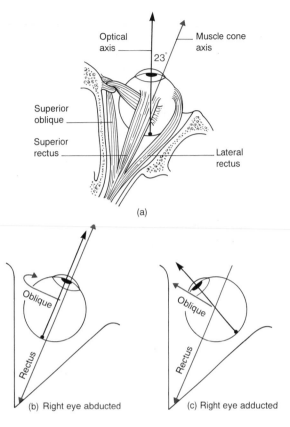

(a)

(b) Right eye abducted    (c) Right eye adducted

**Figure 22.4** Diplopia. Redrawn from Walton J. *Essentials of Neurology*, 6th ed. (1989) Churchill Livingstone. With permission.

image falls progressively further round the retina away from the macula in the palsied eye. The brain projects this false image further away from its true position and the separation of the images is directly proportional to the distance from the macula. It follows, therefore, that the direction of the maximal separation of the images is in the direction of action of the affected muscle, and it also follows that the distal image is always the false one. In this context, distal means further away from a point straight in front of the eyes.

A patient who complains of double vision should be asked the direction in which the separation of the images is maximal and whether the separation is in the horizontal or vertical plane. Since the distal image is always the false one, covering one eye will show which eye is giving rise to the false image. In horizontal diplopia, this will reveal whether the double vision is due to one medial rectus or the other lateral rectus. The situation is complicated in vertical diplopia because two muscles are used to elevate and two to depress the eye. First, determine whether the diplopia is maximal on upward or downward gaze, then determine which eye is responsible for the false image. This reduces the possibility to two muscles, then determine whether the diplopia is maximal with the affected eye abducted (a rectus palsy) or adducted (an oblique palsy). To summarize:

1. The direction of maximal separation of the images is the direction of action of the affected muscle.
2. The peripheral image is always the false one.
3. In vertical diplopia, separation of the images is maximal when the affected eye is adducted in oblique palsies and when abducted with rectus palsies.

The cause of diplopia is often obvious, such as a complete sixth or third nerve lesion. But it may be difficult in partial and multiple lesions without proper examination. The full range of movement should be tested with both eyes open and each eye separately with the cover test to determine which eye is fixing. When the palsy has been present for some time the false image may be suppressed and the patient loses the double vision. When there is already a marked disparity in the visual acuity of the two eyes, the patient may still prefer to fix with the eye with the better visual activity, even if its movement is impaired.

Impairment of eye movement can be recorded qualitatively on a Hess chart, which can then be used to record progress.

## Nystagmus

Nystagmus is the jerky eye movement due to a failure to maintain fixation; the eye drifts away from the object so that a rapid voluntary movement is required to regain fixation.

Accurate and stable eye fixation normally occurs despite constant movement of both the observer and the object. Fixation on a moving object while the observer remains still is achieved by the parieto-occipital eye field and ocular fixation. Compensation for movement of the observer is through a sensitive feedback mechanism from the vestibular system and to a lesser extent from the proprioceptive system via the cerebellum. A lesion affecting any one of these mechanisms, visual fixation, vestibular and cerebellar pathways, can give rise to nystagmus.

### Ocular nystagmus
This is due to a defect of fixation and is, therefore, seen with small central scotomata, general depression of visual acuity (usually congenital), miner's nystagmus and other defects of the macula. It usually takes the form of a fine oscillatory movement without clear fast and slow components; it is present in all directions of gaze, including gaze ahead, and may be only visible on ophthalmoscopic examination as a fine tremor (jelly nystagmus).

### Vestibular nystagmus
Disturbance of the vestibular mechanism is the commonest and most important cause of nystagmus and may be due to a lesion of the vestibular end-organ or its central connections. Nystagmus due to vestibular end-organ disease is always associated with vertigo but within a few weeks disappears due to central compensation. Nystagmus not associated with any other features which persists for more than a few weeks must be due to a central lesion.

### Cerebellar nystagmus
The cerebellum is concerned with the maintenance of ocular fixation. Unilateral lesions of the cerebellum may produce nystagmus, particularly if it affects the deep nuclei. Mid-line and degenerative lesions usually do not cause nystagmus, probably because the balance between the two sides is not disturbed.

### Brain-stem or central nystagmus
Lesions of the vestibular and cerebellar pathways in the brain stem are the commonest cause of nystagmus. This is often lateralized but may be bilateral. Vertical or rotatory nystagmus only occurs in brain-stem lesions.

### Optokinetic nystagmus
This normal effect is seen when telegraph poles are viewed from a moving train and tested in the laboratory by a rotating striped drum.

## Examination
The patient should be asked to follow an object, both vertically and to either side. The object

must be held at or beyond the near point, so that the patient does not have to converge and the extremes of movement should be within binocular vision. Nystagmoid movements of no significance may be seen if these precautions are not followed. The direction of nystagmus is recorded as the direction of the quick component, even though the quick component is the voluntary overriding attempt at fixation and a slow drift to the resting position is the abnormal movement. If nystagmus is not present on gaze ahead but has to be elicited, it is always in the direction of gaze. The degree of nystagmus should be recorded: first-degree nystagmus to the left is nystagmus only on gaze to the left, second-degree nystagmus to the left is nystagmus to the left on gaze ahead and third-degree nystagmus to the left is nystagmus to the left on gaze to the right. In unconscious patients, vestibular lesions or stimulation by caloric testing causes tonic conjugate deviation, because there is no conscious effort to override this.

## The pupil

The pupillary muscles are arranged both concentrically (the sphincter pupilli, which receives its parasympathetic nerve supply from the ciliary ganglion via the short ciliary nerves) and radially (the dilator pupilli, which is innervated by sympathetic fibres via the nasociliary nerve).

The pupil of one eye constricts when that eye is exposed to light (the direct reaction) and at the same time the pupil of the other eye also constricts (the consensual reaction). Dilation occurs in the dark. The afferent pathway is via the optic nerve to the lateral geniculate ganglion and then through the brain stem to the third-nerve nuclei on both sides. The efferent pathway runs from the Edinger–Westphal nucleus via the third nerve to the ciliary ganglion.

Fixation on an object within the near point requires convergence of the optical axes, and this is associated with pupillary constriction. The afferent pathway is with the visual fibres to the occipital cortex, and the efferent pathway is from the Edinger–Westphal nucleus.

### Vascular and hyaline degeneration
This is common in old age and may give rise to pupils which are small, unequal, irregular and relatively immobile.

### The myotonic pupil (Adie's syndrome)
This is dilated and shows a very slow reaction to light and convergence. It may be necessary to keep the patient in the dark for some time before testing the light reflex and to ask the patient to fix on a near object for several minutes to show the contraction with convergence. This condition occurs much more commonly in women and is often of sudden onset. It is thought to be due to a postganglionic lesion in the efferent parasympathetic pathway. The defect is permanent but does not carry any other pathological connotation. The myotonic pupil may be found in conjunction with absence of tendon reflexes (the Holmes–Adie syndrome).

### Horner's syndrome
This consists of pupillary constriction, slight ptosis, and failure to sweat on the same side of the face. The syndrome results from a lesion anywhere in the sympathetic pathway from the hypothalamus down through the lateral part of the pons and medulla, and Clarke's column in the lateral column of the cervical cord. The fibres then emerge at the level of the first thoracic segment to relay in the cervical sympathetic ganglion and then pass up in a plexus on the carotid artery to be distributed throughout the territory of the external and internal carotid arteries. It is, therefore, a poor localizing sign, but a good lateralizing sign because the pathway does remain ipsilateral throughout its course.

### Argyll Robertson pupils
The pupils are small, unequal, eccentric and irregular. They do not react to light but do constrict on convergence. The lesion is thought to affect the afferent pathway in the mid-brain. It is almost always due to syphilis.

### The afferent pupillary defect
This is a useful sign in patients with an optic nerve lesion, such as retrobulbar neuritis. The ipsilateral direct reaction and the contralateral consensual reaction are impaired because of the lesion in the afferent pathway, but the consensual reaction following exposure of the other eye to light is brisk, since the efferent pathway of the affected eye functions normally. If a light is shone alternately into both eyes the affected eye will show only the consensual reaction and, therefore, follows the constriction and dilation

of the normal eye, so that when the light is moved from the normal to the affected eye, the pupil is seen to dilate.

# The trigeminal nerve (V)

The trigeminal nerve has three major peripheral branches. The **ophthalmic** branch supplies the cornea via the nasociliary nerve, the forehead and the scalp as far back as the vertex by the supra-orbital nerve. A small strip extends down the bridge of the nose. The fibres pass back through the roof of the orbit, through the superior orbital foramen, along the lateral wall of the cavernous sinus to reach the gasserian ganglion situated in Meckel's cave at the apex of the petrous temporal bone.

The **maxillary** branch supplies the lower eyelid, the side of the nose, the cheek and the upper lip. It extends laterally only to a line approximately between the outer canthus of the eye and the side of the mouth. The fibres pass through the maxilla and enter the anteromedial aspect of the middle cranial fossa via the foramen rotundum to reach the gasserian ganglion.

The **mandibular** branch supplies the lower lip and chin, a thin strip lateral to the maxillary division but sparing an area of three fingers from the angle of the jaw; it supplies the upper part of the tragus and adjoining parts of the pinna and a variable area of adjacent scalp on the side of the head. The fibres pass back through the pteyrgoid fossa and through the foramen ovale, which lies just below the gasserian ganglion.

The motor division travels with the mandibular branch and supplies muscles of mastication, particularly the lateral pterygoid.

Distal lesions usually affect one branch only because of the wide separation of the three main branches distal to the ganglion. Lesions of the nerve proximal to the ganglion, as it crosses the anterior end of the cerebellopontine angle to enter the mid-pons, affect all three divisions to some extent. The earliest sign of a lesion of the pathway between the gasserian ganglion and the main sensory nucleus is loss of the corneal reflex. Lesions below the mid-pons affect only the descenting tract or its decussating fibres, which relay the sensations of pain and temperature. The arrangement of fibres in the descending tract results in 'onion skin' loss of sensation of the face from compressive lesions, with the snout area nearest the main sensory nucleus and the most peripheral of the 'onion skins' extending down into the upper cervical region. Lesions of the descending tract may cause diminution but not loss of the corneal reflex.

Intramedullary lesions affecting the trigeminal nerve include syringobulbia, demyelinating disease, tumours and infarcts. Extramedullary intracranial causes include lesions in the cerebellopontine angle, such as acoustic neuromas, meningiomas and trigeminal neuromas, granulomatous meningitis (tuberculosis, sarcoid and syphilis) and nasopharyngeal carcinoma eroding the base of the skull.

## PAIN IN THE FACE

There are many causes of facial pain and these need to be differentiated carefully as the treatments are often quite different:

- Idiopathic trigeminal neuralgia
- Symptomatic trigeminal neuralgia
- Atypical facial pain
- Temporomandibular joint dysfunction
- Facial migraine
- Periodic migrainous neuralgia

### Idiopathic trigeminal neuralgia (tic douloureux)

The cause of this condition is unknown. It may occur at any age but becomes more common with increasing age.

#### Clinical features

The pain is always confined to the distribution of the trigeminal nerve, usually affecting either the third or second divisions or both; involvement of the first division alone is rare. Involvement of both sides is quite exceptional.

The pain is paroxysmal and is usually described as a brief, stabbing, lancinating or shooting pain. It is usually extremely severe, lasting for a few seconds only but may be repeated frequently. It is always precipitated and patients may describe a trigger point which is particularly sensitive. Trigger stimuli include touch, washing or shaving, facial movement, eating and drinking hot or cold liquids. During particularly severe bouts, patients may not be able to speak, eat or drink.

Patients usually have frequent stabs of pain over a short period of time and may then have minutes or hours of freedom before the next bout. These paroxysms occur over several weeks before complete remission. The pain always returns but the interval may vary from months to years. The periods of remission tend to become shorter and bouts of pain more severe and longer. A few patients never show remission. The pain always remains paroxysmal and never becomes constant. There are never any abnormal signs.

### Treatment

The only effective medication is carbamazepine and this will control the pain in almost all patients, at least initially. Treatment should be started with 300 mg/day in divided doses and increased as required up to a total dose of 1200 mg/day. The development of a rash (in 3 per cent of cases) is an idiosyncratic side effect and the medication should be stopped. Dose-dependent side effects include unsteadiness, vertigo and nausea and these can be relieved by reducing the dose. In some patients this treatment is ineffective or becomes so with repeated exacerbations. For these reasons, or because the patient is unable to tolerate the medication, it may be necessary to destroy the trigeminal nerve. To be effective the lesion must be at or proximal to the gasserian ganglion as lesions distal to the ganglion cause only temporary relief of symptoms and are usually unsatisfactory. The ganglion may be reached through the cheek and foramen ovale and injected with phenol or alcohol, or destroyed with a radiofrequency probe or cryoprobe. The sensory root may be divided between the ganglion and the pons following craniotomy, in which case an attempt may be made to preserve the corneal reflex by a partial root section. If this is done properly, the analgesia and the relief of pain are permanent. After partial lesions a few patients complain of unpleasant sensations in the face (anaesthesia dolorosa). Most patients quickly become accustomed to a numb face, but they must always exercise great care to prevent corneal ulceration and should wear glasses with a side piece to protect the eye. They should also be warned against nasal ulceration.

## Symptomatic trigeminal neuralgia

This condition may be clinically indistinguishable from idiopathic trigeminal neuralgia with precisely the same features and no detectable neurological deficit. If any abnormal signs are found (usually an impaired corneal reflex) it cannot be idiopathic trigeminal neuralgia and there is an underlying abnormality such as disseminated sclerosis, a congenital vascular anomaly, a neoplasm in the cerebellar pontine angle, or nasopharyngeal carcinoma. Trigeminal neuralgia in a young patient is strongly suggestive of an underlying condition, often multiple sclerosis.

A number of patients have been found to have an aberrant artery which impinges on the trigeminal nerve root. This can be surgically separated and the root decompressed, with relief of symptoms and without damage to the trigeminal nerve. Such patients usually have atypical features such as persisting pain, a pain which is not obviously triggered and some persisting neurological deficit. The absence of these features does not exclude the possibility of an aberrant artery. Younger, fit patients should therefore be offered a posterior fossa exploration, giving consent to division of the nerve root if no structural abnormality is found, since this offers the opportunity to relieve the pain without facial numbness.

## Atypical facial pain

This condition commonly occurs in middle-aged women. The patient complains of constant aching pain, usually in the jaw, which does not vary much throughout the day and persists for months or years. No organic cause is ever found and it is thought to be largely psychosomatic. It is often helped by the use of tricyclic antidepressant drugs.

## Temporomandibular joint dysfunction

This can cause an aching pain in the mandible which is usually worse with chewing, the pain may radiate into the temple.

## Facial migraine

This is a rare manifestation of migraine in which the patient experiences episodic facial pain usually without other migrainous manifestations.

## Periodic migrainous neuralgia

See page 703.

## TRIGEMINAL NEUROPATHY

Patients with this condition develop numbness and often paraesthesiae, which may be confined to one of the divisions of the trigeminal nerve. The motor division is usually spared. The sensory deficit evolves over days or weeks and usually persists. The motor division is rarely involved. In some patients the onset is associated with pain but this does not resemble trigeminal neuralgia. It is important to exclude other causes of trigeminal sensory loss.

**Table 22.1** Facial nerve lesions.

| |
|---|
| **Upper motor neurone lesions** |
| Cerebrovascular disease |
| Space-occupying lesions |
| **Lower motor neurone lesions** |
| Cerebrovascular disease |
| Space-occupying lesions |
| Cerebropontine angle lesions |
|   (a) Space-occupying lesions |
|     Acoustic neuroma |
|     Meningioma |
|     Cholesteatoma |
|   (b) Inflammatory lesions |
|     Sarcoid |
|     Tuberculosis |
| Skull base fractures |
| Guillain–Barré syndrome |
| Bell's palsy |
| Ramsay–Hunt syndrome (herpes zoster) |
| Ear infections |

# The facial nerve (VII)

The facial nerve nucleus lies in the floor of the fourth ventricle in the lower pons; the fibres pass round the sixth nerve nucleus forming a small hump in the floor of the fourth ventricle, the facial colliculus, and then run laterally to emerge from the pons near its lower border (Fig. 22.5). They cross the cerebellopontine angle with the nervus intermedius (secretomotor to the lacrymal gland and taste fibres from the anterior two-thirds of the tongue) and the eighth nerve. All three nerves pass through the internal auditory meatus into the internal auditory canal to the geniculate ganglion. The eighth nerve leaves at this point, and shortly afterwards the chorda tympani and the nerve to stapedius also leave the facial nerve, which finally emerges from the skull through the stylomastoid foramen. It divides in the parotid gland to supply all the muscles of facial expression.

Unilateral upper motor neurone lesions (Table 22.1) of the facial nerve cause quite marked weakness of the lower half of the face with the relative sparing of the upper half. This is because the supranuclear pathways for the muscles of the forehead and around the eyes are bilateral. Upper motor neurone lesions also cause greater impairment of voluntary movement than of involuntary and emotional movement. Strokes and hemisphere tumours are common causes.

Lower motor neurone lesions cause weakness of all facial muscles (Table 22.1). The site of the lesion can often be accurately located because of involvement of associated structures:

1. Lesions of the nuclei are nearly always associated with an ipsilateral sixth-nerve palsy.
2. Lesions in the cerebellar pontine angle are usually associated with eighth-nerve and chorda tympani involvement. In addition the corneal reflex may be absent due to fifth-nerve involvement and there may be cerebellar signs.
3. Lesions in the internal auditory canal as far as the geniculate ganglion may also be associated with lesions of the eighth nerve and chorda tympani, and there may also be hyperacusis due to paralysis of the stapedius muscle.

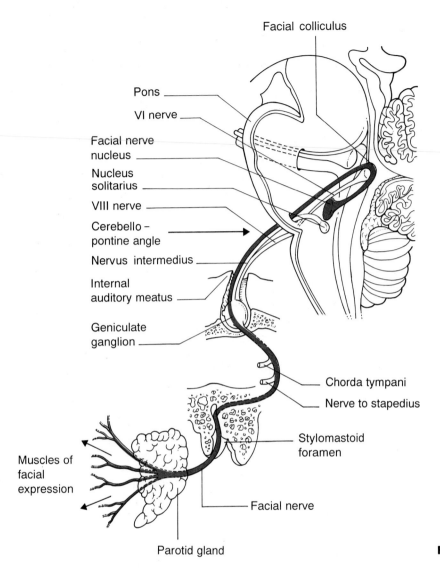

**Figure 22.5** The facial nerve.

If taste is affected and there is hyperacusis, the lesion must be proximal to the middle ear.

In the brain stem, tumours and vascular lesions are the commonest causes of seventh nerve damage. The facial nerve is the most frequently affected cranial nerve in the Guillain–Barré syndrome. It may also be damaged in operations on the parotid salivary gland, and involvement with sarcoidosis may cause bilateral lesions. The commonest cause of a lower motor neurone lesion of the seventh nerve is, however, Bell's palsy.

## BELL'S PALSY

Bell's palsy is an acute lower motor neurone palsy of the facial nerve of unknown aetiology. The occurrence in some patients of hyperacusis or loss of taste on the anterior two-thirds of the tongue implies that the nerve can be involved at different levels within the petrous temporal bone. The onset may be sudden or develop over several hours, rarely more than a day or so. The onset may be associated with some pain in or behind the ear. About 50 per cent of patients make a complete recovery, although this may take weeks or months. Some patients start to improve within a few days but it is possible to make a complete recovery even if the improvement does not start for 6 to 8 weeks. Some estimate of the prognosis can be made from electromyography after 1 month.

Treatment with steroids should be started within 24 hours of the onset of symptoms. Prednisolone, 60–80 mg a day, for 2 or 3 days, followed by a rapidly diminishing dose, is a suitable regimen.

## RAMSAY–HUNT SYNDROME

This is due to infection of the seventh nerve by herpes zoster. The syndrome consists of herpetic vesicles on the soft palate and in the external auditory meatus and may include deafness, facial palsy and trigeminal nerve involvement.

# The acoustic vestibular nerve (VIII)

The acoustic and vestibular parts of the eighth nerve serve quite separate functions. The acoustic nerve arises in the cochlea and the vestibular nerve in the semicircular canals and otolith. Both pass down the internal auditory canal with the seventh nerve and chorda tympani, they cross the cerebellopontine angle and enter the brain stem at the pontomedullary junction. The nuclei are situated in the region of the inferior cerebellar peduncle.

## ACOUSTIC

From the cochlear nuclei some fibres decussate in the trapezoid body and ascend in the lateral lemniscus, and some fibres ascend in the ipsilateral lateral lemniscus, so that there is bilateral representation of hearing at the supranuclear level.

Hearing acuity should be tested and if deafness is found it is then necessary to determine whether this is due to middle-ear disease affecting the ear ossicles (conductive deafness) or whether it is due to a lesion of the nerve (perceptive deafness). Normally air conduction is better than bone conduction and this difference is preserved in perceptive deafness; but in conductive deafness bone conduction appears louder than air conduction because it bypasses the ear ossicles. Perceptive deafness due to intramedullary lesions is unusual and may be associated with other brain-stem or long-tract signs; lesions of the cerebellopontine angle (acoustic neuroma, trigeminal neuroma, meningioma and cholesteatoma) may be associated with fifth- and seventh-nerve palsies and cerebellar signs; lesions in the petrous temporal bone (Paget's disease) may be associated with a facial palsy and impaired taste.

## VESTIBULAR

Vestibular nuclei are connected to the cerebellar hemisphere on the same side, to the third, fourth and sixth nerves via the medial longitudinal bundle, via the vestibular spinal tract to centres in the cord, and via the ipsilateral lateral lemniscus to the thalamus.

Vestibular function is assessed by the caloric test, in which the ear is syringed with water above and below body temperature. This stimulates movements of endolymph in the semicircular canals and causes nystagmus. A standard technique is used and should always be followed. The duration of the nystagmus is timed.

Acute vestibular lesions cause nausea, vomiting, vertigo and disequilibrium. Vertigo which is solely related to changes in position indicates disease of the otolith, although it may occasionally occur in some posterior fossa lesions.

### Vestibular neuronitis

This is an acute vestibular disturbance with nausea, vomiting and unsteady gait, which develops over a few hours and may be completely prostrating for a day or two before passing off over a few more days. Most patients have a liability to vertigo on rapid head movement for several weeks or even months.

### Meniere's disease

Patients with this condition suffer recurrent attacks of vertigo with vomiting and prostration, associated with tinnitus, which persists usually between attacks, and progressive deafness. During the acute attack patients usually have nystagmus, but this disappears during remission. The treatment is symptomatic with intramuscular or oral phenothiazines. The aetiology is unknown.

# The glossopharyngeal nerve (IX)

This is a mixed motor and sensory nerve which arises in the medulla and leaves the skull through the jugular foramen with the vagus and the spinal accessory nerves and supplies the stylopharyngeus muscle. Sensory fibres carry all forms of sensation, including taste, from the posterior third of the tongue, the tonsillar fossa and the pharynx. Parasympathetic fibres from the inferior salivary nucleus also travel with the glossopharyngeal nerve but leave it within the skull to supply the parotid gland via the otic ganglion.

Isolated lesions of the glossopharyngeal nerve are rare; lesions at the jugular foramen also involve the vagus and accessory nerves.

## GLOSSOPHARYNGEAL NEURALGIA

This is a condition similar to trigeminal neuralgia (page 666) but the pain is felt in the distribution of the glossopharyngeal nerve and is precipitated by eating and swallowing. Pain may also be felt deep in the ear. The treatment is also with carbamazepine. If this fails to control the pain, the nerve should be surgically divided.

# The vagus (X)

The nuclei of this motor and sensory nerve are situated in the medulla. The nerve leaves the skull through the jugular foramen and it lies in the carotid sheath in the neck. It is the motor supply to the pharyngeal and laryngeal muscles and it carries the parasympathetic supply to the thoracic and abdominal viscera. Sensory fibres carry sensation from the larynx. Lesions of the vagus nerve result in paralysis of the soft palate, the pharynx and the larynx causing dysphonia

and dysphagia, with a curtain movement of the uvula away from the side of the lesion on phonation. There are no clinical consequences from viscera supplied by the vagus.

# The spinal accessory nerve (XI)

The nuclei of this motor nerve lie in the lower medulla and upper part of the spinal cord. The nerve emerges from the medulla and spinal cord in a continuous line of rootlets. The spinal rootlets unite to form a trunk which ascends through the foramen magnum to join the cranial rootlets. The nerve leaves the skull through the jugular foramen with the vagus. The cranial fibres are distributed to the pharynx and larynx. The spinal fibres descend to supply the sternomastoid and the upper fibres of trapezius. The nerve may be damaged in operations on cervical glands or injury to the neck producing weakness of sternomastoid movement and shoulder elevation.

# The hypoglossal nerve (XII)

The nucleus lies in the dorsal part of the lower medulla and the nerve leaves the skull through the hypoglossal foramen and supplies the muscles of the tongue.

Lesions of the twelfth nerve cause wasting, fasciculation and weakness of the ipsilateral side of the tongue, and the tongue deviates to the affected side on protrusion.

# Dysarthria

Dysarthria is a disorder of articulation. In contrast, aphasia/dysphasia is an abnormality in language function caused by brain damage.

Dysarthria may occur in any lesion of the motor pathway to the bulbar muscles. Because the pathways are bilateral above the bulbar nuclei, a unilateral upper motor neurone lesion only causes temporary dysarthria. Dysarthria occurs in pseudobulbar palsy (upper motor neurone lesions) and in bulbar palsies (lower motor neurone lesions). Dysarthria may also occur in extrapyramidal and cerebellar lesions, myasthenia gravis and in some diseases of muscle.

It is necessary only to determine that the patient has dysarthria, since the physical signs will indicate the cause.

# Bulbar and pseudobulbar palsies

The lower cranial nerves (IX–XII) arise from a chain of motor nuclei in the medulla and emerge as an almost continuous line of rootlets. The ninth, tenth and eleventh nerves all leave the skull through the jugular foramen. This anatomical arrangement means that these nerves are usually affected together.

A bulbar palsy is a lower motor neurone lesion affecting the cranial nerves whose nuclei lie in the bulb (the medulla). The commonest causes include syringobulbia, motor neurone disease and vascular lesions. The nerves may be affected outside the medulla in diphtheria and the Guillain–Barré syndrome. Tumours in the region of the jugular foramen may affect the ninth, tenth and eleventh nerves, and these include nasopharyngeal carcinoma, meningioma and glomus jugulari tumours.

Patients with bulbar palsy complain of dysarthria and dysphagia, and fluids may regurgitate through the nose when they attempt to swallow. Signs include loss of taste and sensation on the posterior third of the tongue and in the tonsillar fossa (IX), paralysis of the vocal cords (X), weakness of the sternomastoid and upper fibres of trapezius (XI) and, if the twelfth cranial nerve is involved, there may be wasting and fasciculation of the tongue.

Patients with pseudobulbar palsy have the same complaints and difficulties as patients with a bulbar palsy, but it is due to an upper motor neurone lesion of the bulbar muscles. The upper motor neurone pathway must be affected on both sides because the pathways are bilateral. Causes include motor neurone disease, vascular lesions (usually associated with hypertension) and multiple sclerosis. Signs include a brisk jaw jerk and a slow-moving spastic tongue. The plantar responses are usually extensor.

# $T$HE MOTOR SYSTEM

The motor system comprises the upper motor neurone pathway, the lower motor neurone, the myoneural junction and muscle.

## Cortex

The upper motor neurone pathway arises in the precentral gyrus. Lesions strictly confined to the motor cortex give rise to a characteristic pattern of motor deficit. There is weakness of all movements of the affected part and there may be some wasting, but there is no tone or reflex change (cortical pattern of motor deficit). Because of the wide extent of the motor cortex with the face/hand area laterally and the foot area medially, a single lesion only produces these signs in a relatively small part of the body, perhaps the hand or the foot. Large lesions necessarily involve subcortical structures and this produces a different pattern.

## The pyramidal tract

The upper motor neurone pathway descends from the precental gyrus gathering into a compact bundle at the internal capsule, so that lesions at this level tend to produce a complete hemiplegia, including the face. Any lesion above the mid-brain will affect the cranial nerves on the same side as the hemiplegia. Some fibres cross the mid-line in the mid-brain, pons and upper medulla to supply the contralateral cranial nerve nuclei. A lesion, therefore, of a cranial nerve on one side, together with a hemiplegia on the other side, accurately locates the site of the lesion to the level of that cranial nerve nucleus. In the lower part of the medulla, just above the level of the foramen magnum, the pyramidal tract decussates from its anterior position in the brain stem to the lateral column of the cord on the opposite side.

Lesions of the pyramidal tract cause spasticity, which is an increase in muscle tone that is not uniform throughout the range of movement and does not affect both directions of movement equally. There may be flaccidity after an acute pyramidal tract lesion due to 'spinal shock', and spasticity may only develop later. Conversely, marked spasticity without much weakness is a sure sign of chronicity.

Lesions of the pyramidal tract cause a characteristic distribution of muscle weakness. All the muscles may be weak on the affected side, but in the upper limb the extensors are much more affected than the flexors and in the lower limb the flexors are much more affected than the extensors. Shoulder abduction, elbow extension, wrist and finger extension and finger abduction in the upper limb, and hip flexion, knee flexion and ankle dorsiflexion in the lower limb are always weaker than their antagonists.

The reflexes are all pathologically brisk. Reflexes that are normally only just obtainable may be very brisk, such as the digital reflex, and there may be clonus, particularly at the ankle. Clonus is the rhythmic contraction and relaxation of opposing groups of muscles at a joint; it occurs spontaneously or is elicited by firm and sudden flexion, for example, of the ankle. The cutaneous reflexes (the abdominal and cremasteric reflexes) are reduced or abolished on the affected side and the plantar response is extensor.

# The lower motor neurone

The lower motor neurone, arising in the anterior horn cells of the spinal cord, is the final common pathway to muscle. Lesions anywhere in this pathway cause wasting and weakness. The reflexes are absent due to disruption of the efferent limb of the reflex arc. The nearer the lesion is to the spinal cord, the more likely is fasciculation to be found in the affected muscles. It is, therefore, very common in anterior horn cell lesions, frequently seen in root lesions and rare in peripheral nerve lesions (see disorders of the peripheral nervous system).

## MOTOR NEURONE DISEASE

This is a progressive degeneration of the motor pathways in the central nervous system. It may affect any part of the pathway from the motor cortex to the anterior horn cells. It usually occurs between the ages of 50 and 70 and is extremely rare before the mid-thirties. Men are affected more often than women. The clinical signs are strictly confined to the motor system and there are never any sensory signs or sphincter disturbance. The disease usually presents with one of three groups of symptoms – progressive bulbar palsy, amyotrophic lateral sclerosis or progressive muscular atrophy – but any combination may occur and eventually all these features are usually present. A pure upper motor neurone syndrome, either with a spastic quadraparesis or sometimes a pure pseudobulbar palsy, occasionally occurs.

The diagnosis is often clear on clinical grounds alone but it may be confirmed by electromyography (EMG). No treatment is known to influence the course of the condition.

### Progressive bulbar palsy

This is progressive degeneration of the motor nuclei in the medulla, causing a lower motor neurone bulbar palsy (page 672). A wasted fibrillating tongue is the most important sign. This is the form with the worst prognosis and patients seldom survive more than 18 months after the diagnosis is made.

### Amyotrophic lateral sclerosis

This is the most common presentation of motor neurone disease and, as the name implies, it is due to a combination of wasting and weakness, obvious in the hands, and pyramidal tract involvement, often most prominent in the legs. The finding of upper motor neurone signs with widespread fasciculation is a characteristic feature. The survival from diagnosis is usually less than 5 years and this is largely determined by the development of bulbar signs.

### Progressive muscular atrophy

In this form of motor neurone disease there is a slowly progressive lower motor neurone involvement of the arms and legs with wasting and weakness. This is the form with the best prognosis and patients may survive from 5 to 15 years; again, the length of survival depends largely on whether or not the bulbar muscles become involved.

## SPINAL MUSCULAR ATROPHY

There is a group of genetically determined degenerations of the lower motor neurone which produce wasting and weakness of muscles, often wth fasciculation.

### Werdnig–Hoffman disease

This is the commonest form and occurs in infancy. Survival is usually a matter of months.

### Kugelberg–Welander syndrome

This presents at any age with wasting and weakness of the arms and legs and is slowly progressive. It appears to be inherited by an autosomal recessive mechanism. The condition probably accounts for most patients previously thought to have a 'limb girdle dystrophy' (page 676). Some patients show widespread fasciculation. The diagnosis can be confirmed by EMG and muscle biopsy, but the interpretation may be complicated by the fact that secondary myopathic change commonly occurs.

# The neuromuscular junction

The arrival of a nerve impulse at the neuromuscular junction causes the release of acetylcholine. The acetylcholine crosses the cleft between nerve and muscle and becomes attached to the acetylcholine receptor in the motor end-plate, causing depolarization and subsequent contraction of the muscle. The acetylcholine is rapidly destroyed by cholinesterase or taken up by nerve endings, and the motor end-plate repolarizes.

Procaine and botulinus toxin inhibit the release of acetylcholine, whereas guanidine increases the release of acetylcholine. Physostigmine, neostigmine and pyridostigmine inhibit cholinesterase and allow the acetylcholine to accumulate, perpetuating its action. Curare, tubocurarine and galamine act as competitive inhibitors by reacting with the acetylcholine receptors on the end-plate, producing a conduction block.

## MYASTHENIA GRAVIS

Myasthenia gravis is an immunological disease with damage of the acetylcholine receptors by antibody, which not only blocks the receptor sites but also causes degeneration of the receptors. The characteristic feature of this disease is abnormal fatiguability of striated muscle with rapid recovery after rest.

It may occur at any age but most commonly affects women in the second and third decades. Children born of myasthenic mothers may show evidence of myasthenia for some days after birth because the mother's antibodies cross the placenta. There is an increased incidence of thyrotoxicosis in patients with myasthenia. Thymomas may occur in association with myasthenia; a minority are malignant.

### Clinical features

The condition does not affect all striated muscle equally and, although electromyography may show evidence of widespread disease, it may be quite localized clinically. It commonly affects the external ocular, bulbar, neck and limb girdle muscles. The onset is often gradual and fluctuating. Patients may complain of diplopia, dysphagia, dysarthria and difficulty in chewing, and these symptoms may all show marked variability. Patients, for example, may have difficulty in completing a meal or only develop ptosis and diplopia in the evening.

Examination shows no wasting or fasciculation. The most striking feature is undue fatiguability, which can be shown by asking the patient to raise the arm above the head 20 times and demonstrating the development of weakness as a result. Normal power returns after a few moments of rest. Patients with bulbar symptoms should be asked to start counting and after a variable time they develop dysarthria.

## Diagnosis

The diagnosis can be confirmed by intravenous edrophonium. This is a short-acting anticholinesterase drug which may give a dramatic response for up to 2 or 3 minutes. Atropine should be administered first to block stimulation of muscurinic receptors, followed by a test dose of 1 mg of intravenous edrophonium; if no undue reaction occurs, a further 9 mg may be injected.

The response to edrophonium is often disappointing in ocular and bulbar myasthenia and a negative test does not exclude these varieties of myasthenia. Confirmation of the diagnosis may be obtained from electromyography, which shows the characteristic decrease in evoked response with faradic stimulation. Single-fibre recording shows an increase in jitter, demonstrating instability of neuromuscular junctions within one motor unit. Thyroid function tests should be carried out because of the association with thyrotoxicosis, and it is important to look for an associated thymoma with chest X-ray and CT of the mediastinum.

Skeletal muscle antibodies may be elevated, and are almost always elevated if there is an underlying thymoma. Acetylcholine receptor antibody is usually elevated, but the level does not show an obvious relationship to the severity of the disease.

## Treatment

Anticholinesterase drugs have been the basis of treatment since their use was first described in 1934 and remain the initial treatment of choice for limb myasthenia. Treatment should be started with pyridostigmine, 60 mg three times a day, and increased as necessary. Some patients require up to 600 mg a day. The half-life of pyridostigmine is about 4 hours. It may be helpful occasionally to use the shorter acting neostigmine bromide with a half-life of 1.5 hours when a short-lived boost is required, such as just before a meal in patients with bulbar

myasthenia, but it is usually easier to stabilize the patient on pyridostigmine alone.

Although increasing the dose results in increasing strength initially, a plateau is soon reached and further increase results in progressive weakness due to conduction block. A patient who deteriorates while on treatment may be having either a myasthenic or a cholinergic crisis. These can be distinguished by intravenous edrophonium, which can also be used to determine whether a patient is on an optimal dose of drugs.

Ocular and bulbar myasthenia often respond poorly to anticholinesterase drugs and in these patients steroids are the treatment of choice. In contrast to the usual use of steroids, it is important to start with a small dose and make gradual increments until a therapeutic effect is achieved. Large doses given initially may precipitate a myasthenic crisis. It is usually possible to control symptoms satisfactorily with a modest dose of steroid, which should be given on alternate days to minimize the long-term side effects.

If these measures fail to control the patient's symptoms, thymectomy should be considered; and it is better to carry out this procedure sooner rather than later, particularly if immunosuppresive drugs are to be used in the treatment of limb myasthenia. Patients with a thymoma or thymic hyperplasia have a worse prognosis than those with a normal thymus. Thymectomy appears to make patients more responsive subsequently to anticholinesterase drugs and immunosuppression, and this may be related to a reduction in the amount of circulating antibody. The amount of circulating antibody can be temporarily reduced by plasmapheresis and this may be helpful as a short-term measure while awaiting a response from immunosuppression. It may, for example, be enough to keep a patient off a ventilator during a critical time. If large doses of steroids are required to keep control or it is likely that this treatment would need to be continued for a long time, the steroid should be combined with an immunosuppressive drug such as azathioprine.

## MYASTHENIC SYNDROME

This condition (the Eaton–Lambert syndrome) usually complicates small-cell carcinoma of the bronchus (page 307), but it has been described with other tumours. The weakness may precede clinical evidence of the carcinoma by months or years. The patient complains of weakness after exertion, but examination shows weakness of proximal limb girdle muscles which improves after exercise. The reflexes are almost always depressed or absent, unlike true myasthenia. The edrophonium test is usually positive but anticholinesterase drugs given therapeutically have little or no effect. The diagnosis can be confirmed by electromyography. The condition responds to guanidine hydrochloride or 3–4 diaminopyridine.

# DISEASES OF MUSCLE

Diseases of muscle may be conveniently divided into the genetically determined abnormalities, which carry the generic name of muscular dystrophy, and acquired diseases.

# Muscular dystrophies

These are classified according to their clinical picture and mode of inheritance.

## SEX-LINKED PSEUDOHYPERTROPHIC MUSCULAR DYSTROPHY (DUCHENNE AND BECKER DYSTROPHY)

This is due to a sex-linked recessive gene, although there is a high rate of new mutations. The abnormality becomes apparent at about the age of 3, with difficulty in walking and climbing stairs owing to proximal leg weakness. Some pseudohypertrophy is very common and principally affects the calf muscles. Although termed pseudohypertrophy, there is, in fact, enlargement of individual muscle fibres. The condition is slowly progressive, patients become chairbound between the ages of 8 and 10 and die at around the age of 15, usually from respiratory causes related to aspiration and hypoventilation and from cardiac causes due to heart muscle involvement. During the later years of his life the patient suffers progressive deformity, particularly of the chest. There is no treatment. Female carriers can often be identified and, if they become pregnant, the sex of the child can be determined by amniocentesis. Some mothers choose a termination if the child is male.

The Becker type of muscular dystrophy is a more benign form of the Duchenne type and constitutes about 10 per cent of cases. The condition may develop at any age up to about 25 and patients may not become chairbound for another 25 years.

Both Duchenne and Becker dystrophies are caused by deletion at a gene on the X chromosome. Several different deletions have been described. The gene product, dystrophin, is absent in Duchenne dystrophy and partially absent in Becker dystrophy. It is a cytoskeletal protein associated with the sacrolemmal membrane, but its precise function is unknown.

Definition of the gene deletion has enabled precise diagnosis in males and detection of the carrier state in females.

## AUTOSOMAL DOMINANT FACIOSCAPULOHUMERAL MUSCULAR DYSTROPHY

This condition affects both sexes equally and usually presents in adolescence with facial involvement, followed shortly by weakness of the shoulder girdle muscles. It may follow a very prolonged, indolent course and the patients may never become chairbound.

## LIMB GIRDLE DYSTROPHY

This is not a single clinical entity. A number of conditions can cause a slowly progressive symmetrical proximal limb girdle weakness and many patients with this clinical picture have the Kugelberg–Welander syndrome (page 674).

# MITOCHONDRIAL MYOPATHY

Mitochondrial abnormalities can produce a wide range of clinical conditions (mitochondrial cytopathy) including a myopathy associated with a characteristic muscle biopsy. This condition may present as a pure ocular myopathy. The patients usually present with ptosis and subsequently develop a bilateral external ophthalmoplegia over many years. Although the condition may be confined to the ocular muscles, some patients show weakness of facial and shoulder girdle muscles and others show evidence of degeneration in other parts of the nervous system.

# MYOTONIC SYNDROMES

Myotonia is the persistence of muscle contraction after voluntary effort has ceased and is well demonstrated by difficulty in relaxing the grip after vigorous contraction. Percussion of a muscle belly causes a localized area of contraction, which relaxes slowly (myotonic dimpling).

## Dystrophia myotonica

This is a widespread dystrophic condition, not only affecting muscle. There is an autosomal dominant inheritance with onset usually in adolescence and early adult life. It shows the phenomenon of anticipation within a family, with each succeeding generation showing more widespread abnormalities (page 59). The first member of the family to be affected with this condition may have cataracts alone and the fully developed picture may not present for two or three generations. However, this may be an artefact because careful examination of all members of an affected family may show mild or partial expressions of the disease in asymptomatic subjects.

The fully developed syndrome consists of frontal baldness, wasting of the masseter, temporal and sternomastoid muscles, facial weakness with ptosis, posterior capsular cataracts and a distal myopathy with wasting and weakness, starting in the hands and later involving the feet, gonadal atrophy – as shown by small testes in the male and menstrual irregularity in the female – and impaired production of thyroid hormone and insulin. There is no treatment for the underlying disease but myotonia can be relieved by a variety of drugs, for example, procainamide, quinine, phenytoin and corticosteroids.

## Myotonia congenita (Thomsen's disease)

Patients show widespread myotonia from birth. The other features of dystrophia myotonica are absent. There is usually hypertrophy of muscles, giving the appearance of a 'Little Hercules'. The condition is usually dominantly inherited.

# Acquired disorders of muscle

These can be conveniently divided into primary inflammatory disorders of muscle (polymyositis) and those myopathies which complicate systemic disease, although this may be an artificial distinction.

## POLYMYOSITIS

This is a group of conditions associated with weakness of proximal muscles and is probably due to an autoimmune mechanism. One muscle group constantly affected in polymyositis, which may be spared in other myopathies, are the neck extensors. It may occur at any age and usually follows a very prolonged relapsing and remittent course. Raynaud's syndrome is a common association in younger patients, and there may be a characteristic rash (dermatomyositis). There is an association with occult neoplasm and this increases with age; there is usually a loss of reflexes in these patients. The diagnosis is made by the characteristic clinical picture, EMG and muscle biopsy. The erythrocyte sedimentation rate (ESR) is usually raised, as are the muscle enzymes such as creatin phosphokinase (CPK).

The majority of patients respond to steroids, which may need to be continued for several years. Patients who require continued high-dose steroid medication may benefit from an alternate-day regimen or the addition of immunosuppressive drugs, such as azathioprine.

## MYOPATHIES COMPLICATING SYSTEMIC DISEASE

Inflammatory conditions of muscle may complicate sarcoidosis, rheumatoid arthritis, vasculitis, systemic lupus erythematosus and scleroderma.

A proximal limb girdle myopathy may complicate steroid therapy, thyrotoxicosis and occasionally myxoedema. Diabetic amyotrophy is not a myopathy but describes the wasting that follows a neuropathy principally affecting the femoral nerve.

Polymyalgia rheumatica is described on page 586.

# *T*HE BASAL GANGLIA AND EXTRAPYRAMIDAL SYSTEM

There are two principal non-pyramidal systems concerned with control of movement: the cerebellum and the extrapyramidal system. Disorders of the basal ganglia and extrapyramidal system can cause a wide variety of movement disorders.

# *Parkinson's disease*

## CLINICAL FEATURES

James Parkinson first described paralysis agitans in 1817. Its three principal characteristics are an increase in muscle tone (**rigidity**), slowness of movement (**bradykinesia**) and a characteristic **tremor**.

1. *Rigidity*
   This form of hypertonus must be distinguished from spasticity (page 673). In rigidity the increase in tone is present throughout the range of movement and equally in both directions. It is easily enhanced by alternating movements of the opposite limb. The rigidity becomes regularly increased and decreased when tremor coexists to give a typical 'cogwheel' rigidity.
2. *Bradykinesia*
   The slowness of voluntary movement is out of proportion to the degree of rigidity and patients have difficulty in initiating, and are slow to carry out, coordinated movements.

3. *Tremor*
   This is present at rest and inhibited by movement. It is absent during sleep and may also be temporarily inhibited by conscious effort. In the hand regular pronation/supination of the wrist with flexion/extension of the fingers gives the 'pill-rolling' appearance of the fingers and thumb.

Parkinson's disease may develop at any age but is much commoner after the fifth decade. The patient may present either with rigidity and bradykinesia and little or no tremor, or with an obvious tremor which may be confined to one limb with little or no rigidity and bradykinesia. All three features eventually develop. The condition is slowly progressive over many years. Early features include loss of facial expression, a monotonous speech and loss of associated movements, such as swinging the arms when walking.

The disease is caused by the degeneration in the substantia nigra with subsequent involvement of the dopaminergic pathways to the basal ganglia, principally the globus pallidus. These structures are found to be relatively deficient in dopamine in patients with Parkinson's disease. The characteristic pathological appearance is the presence of Lewi bodies, although these are found in other degenerative conditions.

## TREATMENT

The aim of treatment is to increase the dopamine levels in the brain (Fig. 22.6). Dopamine cannot

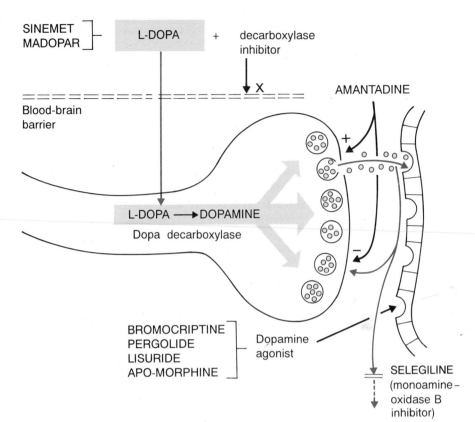

**Figure 22.6** Drugs in Parkinson's disease.

be given orally because it does not cross the blood–brain barrier. Dopa is its immediate precusor but only the laevo form (**levodopa**) crosses the blood–brain barrier. More than 90 per cent of an orally administered dose of dopa is destroyed outside the brain by dopa decarboxylase. It is usual, therefore, to administer levodopa, together with a proportionate amount of decarboxylase inhibitor, which itself does not cross the blood–brain barrier but inhibits the extracerebral decarboxylation of levodopa. This combination makes more levodopa available in the brain and considerably reduces systemic side effects.

When using lower doses of levodopa it is usually necessary to use a preparation with a 4:1 levodopa:decarboxylase inhibition ratio in order to achieve satisfactory peripheral decarboxylase inhibition, which needs a dose of 70–100 mg of inhibitor a day. A 10:1 ratio gives a satisfactory inhibition in the majority of patients at higher dose levels. Treatment should be gradually increased according to response. Since the half-life of levodopa is only about 4 hours, a smoother response is obtained with multiple divided doses.

The response to levodopa is often dramatic and the patients may be able to return to a relatively normal life. It does not, however, alter the long-term prognosis and over the years it tends to become less effective, often producing unacceptable side effects at a lower dosage. The principal dose-limiting side effect is orofacial dyskinesia and other dystonic movements affecting the limbs. This is dose dependent and disappears with reduction in dosage. The reduction of the effect of levodopa with time may be partly due to the loss of the enzyme which converts dopa to dopamine. This loss of response may occur after 3–10 years of treatment with levodopa and has led to the suggestion that treatment in younger patients should be initiated with anticholinergic drugs and only changed to levodopa when these become ineffective. In this way the problems associated with long-term levodopa therapy may be postponed.

Normally the dopaminergic pathways are in balance with the cholinergic pathways. If a satisfactory response cannot be obtained by increasing the dopa levels in the brain the balance between these two systems may be restored by inhibition of the cholinergic system. The use of **anticholinergic drugs** is well established and was the mainstay of treatment before the advent of levodopa. The most effective is benzhexol which is available in tablets containing 2 and 5 mg. It may be given in addition to levodopa in a dose of between 6 and 15 mg a day. Orphenadrine may be better tolerated. Benztropine, methixene and procyclidine have similar properties. Side effects include dry mouth, blurred vision and, commonly in older patients and those with advanced disease, confusion and hallucinations.

The biggest problem in the management of Parkinson's disease now is dealing with patients who no longer respond to levodopa. Problems include hallucinations and confusion, unacceptable dyskinesia, wide fluctuations in performance from gross dyskinesia to akinesia (the on–off phenomenon), as well as painful dystonic movements. The first step is to try and smooth out the levodopa dosage with multiple divided doses throughout the day, keeping the total dose to a level which does not cause confusion and hallucinations. The next step is to add the monoamine oxidase B inhibitor **selegiline**; this inhibits the clearance of dopamine and, because of its long effect, can be given as a single daily dose of either 5 or 10 mg. A useful response may also be obtained from amantadine which appears to promote the release of levodopa from the synaptic vesicles. The dose is 100 mg twice a day. Unfortunately many patients find the beneficial effect of amantadine to be short lived.

It may be possible to postpone starting levodopa therapy by the use of selegiline or amantadine. There is some controversy over delaying the onset of levodopa therapy, and some authorities think that the development of intolerance to levodopa is related to the severity of the disease and not necessarily to the duration of treatment. Until this point has been determined it seems sensible to postpone the onset of levodopa therapy in younger patients by using alternative medication, but not to deny the patient the benefit of levodopa unreasonably; there is no need to do this with older patients.

Some additional response may be obtained by using a dopamine agonist acting directly on dopaminergic receptors. Bromocriptine has a half-life of about 8 hours and may therefore be used to provide a background dopamine stimulation to which a suitable amount of levodopa can be added. The initial dose is 2.5 mg twice a day, which may be increased slowly to 40–60 mg a day according to response. Occasionally marked postural hypotension occurs after the smallest dose so that a test dose of 1.75 mg should be given in the evening before starting treatment.

**Lysuride**, like bromocriptine, is a predominantly $D_2$ dopamine agonist but with a greater affinity for these receptors than bromocriptine. Hypotensive reactions may also occur. The initial dose is 200 μg at night, increasing by 200 μg every week to a maximum of 5 mg in divided doses. **Pergolide** is a $D_1$ and $D_2$ receptor agonist and again hypotensive reactions may occur. The initial dose is 50 μg daily increasing every few days to a maintenance dose of 3 mg a day.

**Physiotherapy** can often result in considerable improvement in the performance of patients with Parkinson's disease; and when it is combined with help and advice from occupational therapists, patients are often able to continue to lead an independent existence where this might otherwise not be possible.

Stereotactic **thalamotomy**, once commonly performed, is now rarely necessary in view of the response of Parkinson's disease to levodopa. However, it remains suitable for younger patients who have a unilateral tremor and little in the way of bradykinesia and rigidity and in whom there are no general medical contraindications to surgery, such as hypertension. Surgery does not affect the subsequent response to levodopa.

## OTHER CAUSES OF THE PARKINSONIAN SYNDROME

In the 1920s there was a pandemic of encephalitis thought to be of viral origin, although a virus was never isolated (**encephalitis lethargica**). This resulted in a very large number of patients with a parkinsonian syndrome, postencephalitic Parkinson's. These patients had all the characteristic features of Parkinson's disease; in addition there was usually evidence of cortical damage from the encephalitis, and this seems to make these patients peculiarly susceptible to levodopa preparations, so that very small doses cause unacceptable mental confusion. They were also subject to oculogyric crises. Since no authenticated cases of this encephalitis have occurred since the 1920s, the condition is extremely rare.

Vascular disease does not cause a true parkinsonian syndrome, but extrapyramidal signs may occur in patients with vascular disease, often associated with pseudobulbar palsy.

# *Chorea*

Choreiform movements are involuntary movements which resemble part of a coordinated intended movement, and patients may be able to disguise the fact that movement is involuntary.

## SYDENHAM'S CHOREA

This occurs in children in association with rheumatic fever (page 189). It is usually a benign condition and most patients recover within a few weeks.

## CHOREA GRAVIDARUM

A similar clinical picture may occur during pregnancy and some patients develop chorea on the contraceptive pill.

## CHOREA FOLLOWING STROKE

Choreiform movements may occur after cerebrovascular lesions, particularly in the elderly. There may be an obvious association with a stroke or the chorea may develop without such an obvious cause. The onset is sudden and unilateral. The chorea may persist but does not progress. Particularly violent movements (hemiballismus) may follow infarction of the subthalamic nucleus.

## HUNTINGTON'S CHOREA

This condition is inherited as an autosomal dominant trait and is characterized by chorea and progressing dementia. The gene has been mapped to chromosome 4. Linkage analysis can predict the occurrence of the disease in affected individuals before symptoms develop (page 58). The new mutation rate is very low so that a positive family history is usually obtainable. Although evidence of the disease may appear at any age it is most common in middle age and usually after the reproductive period, so that patients often have had children and grandchildren before the diagnosis is made. In children it may present with widespread rigidity mimicking an extrapyramidal disorder (rigid Huntington's).

The condition may present with either involuntary movements or with dementia, but the former is more common. The combination of involuntary movement and dementia is strongly suggestive of this condition. If the family history is known to the patient, the depression associated with the development of involuntary movements is often mistaken for dementia. The diagnosis is confirmed by obtaining a positive family history and finding the specific genetic abnormality. There are no specific investigations but the CT brain scan and MRI shows a characteristic dilation of the lateral ventricles due to atrophy of the caudate nuclei. Tetrabenazine may be effective in reducing the abnormal movements.

## TORSION DYSTONIA

This is a disorder of the basal ganglia of unknown aetiology. The onset is usually gradual, starting at any age, and the characteristic features are strong intermittent uncontrollable contractions of voluntary muscle. There is a wide spectrum of presentation, from dystonia musculorum deformans presenting in childhood and resulting in considerable deformity over the years, to fragmentary forms, including spasmodic torticollis and writer's cramp. Anticholinergic drugs may be of some benefit, and patients may tolerate quite high doses if the dose is increased slowly. Benzhexol should be started in a dose of 2 mg three times a day and gradually increased up to 30–40 mg a day, the result is often disappointing and the side effects may be unacceptable. The local injection of botulinus toxin into the motor end-plate of the principally affected muscles temporarily paralyses the muscle and can result in considerable clinical improvement. The effect usually wears off after some months, but can easily be repeated.

## *T*HE CEREBELLUM

The cerebellar hemispheres are concerned with coordination of movement on the same side of the body. Coordination depends on the smooth contraction of one group of muscles (agonists), the equally smooth relaxation of the opposing muscles (antagonists) and the maintained contraction of other muscles to support the part of the body concerned. The central part of the cerebellum, the vermis, is concerned with equilibrium and maintains balance when the centre of gravity changes.

### SIGNS OF CEREBELLAR DISEASE

#### Nystagmus

See page 664.

#### Dysarthria

The coordination of the muscles of speech are affected (page 671).

#### Intention tremor

Attempts at fine coordinated movement produce a tremor, which is worse at the completion of the movement and may be demonstrated by the finger/nose test and the heel/knee/shin test. Occasionally there may be a flapping tremor at rest, or on maintained posture. This is often called a red nucleus tremor but is due to a lesion anywhere in the pathway from the dentate nucleus via the superior cerebellar peduncle to the red nucleus and on the thalamus.

#### Disequilibrium

This is caused by a lesion of the vermis or bilateral cerebellar hemisphere disease. There may be a marked disturbance of gait without any evidence of ataxia or other physical signs.

## Lesions of the cerebellum and its connections

The cerebellar pathways are frequently affected in disseminated sclerosis. Space-occupying lesions of the posterior fossa usually cause some cerebellar signs and there may also be involvement of the brain stem. The volume of the posterior fossa is relatively small, so that small lesions may obstruct CSF pathways and produce hydrocephalus.

The patient presenting with the slow insidious onset of a cerebellar syndrome may have a cerebellar degeneration. Usually no cause is found, but it may be a complication of myxoedema, alcoholism, some drugs (e.g. phenytoin) and as a non-metastatic manifestation of an occult neoplasm when Purkinje cell antibodies may be found in the peripheral blood.

# THE SENSORY SYSTEM

Pathways for the different modalities of sensation have separate courses in different parts of the nervous system, so that lesions at various levels produce characteristic patterns of sensory deficit.

## Peripheral nerve lesions

The area of sensory loss in a peripheral nerve lesion is fairly constant. It may be associated with dysaesthesia, such as pins and needles, tingling or burning sensations. The triple response – a wheal, erythema and flare induced by intracutaneous histamine – is abolished.

## Root lesions

The autonomous area of skin supplied by a single root may be extremely small, so that even a complete lesion may not produce any detectable sensory loss; this is because of overlap from adjacent dermatomes. Conversely, the rash of herpes zoster may be found over a relatively large area, since vesicles occur where there is any contribution from one nerve root.

## Sensory pathways in spinal cord to the thalamus and cortex

After entering the spinal cord through the dorsal root, there is a separation of fibres, with those responsible for pain and temperature crossing the mid-line to reach the contralateral spinothalamic tract in the anterior white matter of the cord, and those fibres concerned with touch and position sense travelling in the ipsilateral posterior columns to the gracile and cuneate nuclei in the lower medulla. Fibres from these nuclei decussate to form the medial lemniscus and lie in close association with the spinothalamic tract so that the pathways for all sensation lie on the same side of the brain stem. These pathways are joined by the fibres from the fifth-nerve nucleus, the quintothalamic tract. The sensory pathways then pass up to the thalamus, where all sensory information from one half of the body is relayed to the cortex. The pain pathways above the thalamus are very extensive, so that localized lesions of the main sensory radiation cause marked loss of light touch and position sense with relative preservation of pain.

# THE SPINAL CORD

The spinal cord is a segmental structure. The location of a lesion within the cord can be determined by finding the highest affected segment. This level may be motor, sensory or reflex.

- A **motor level** would give lower motor neurone signs at the affected segment due to involvement of the anterior horn cells and the emerging motor root, and upper motor neurone signs below this on the same side.

- A **sensory level** would give loss of all forms of sensation at the affected level due to involvement of the dorsal root and its entry zone, impairment of pain and temperature sense below this level on the opposite side due to involvement of the crossed spinothalamic tract, and impairment of light touch and joint position sense on the same side due to involvement of the uncrossed posterior columns.
- A **reflex level** is the absence of a reflex at the level of a lesion due to interruption of

the reflex arc and brisk reflexes below this on the same side with an extensor plantar response due to involvement of the pyramidal tract.

Hemisection of the cord would, therefore, produce lower motor neurone weakness, absent reflex and impairment of all forms of sensation at the level of the lesion on the same side. Below this level there would be ipsilateral pyramidal tract signs with brisk reflexes and impairment of touch and proprioception, while on the contralateral side there would be impairment of pain and temperature appreciation. This is the **Brown-Sequard syndrome** and is seldom seen in its complete form. Partial forms due to compression are quite common and usually associated with bilateral pyramidal involvement, often asymmetrical (Fig. 22.7).

The causes of focal disease of the spinal cord may be conveniently divided into extradural and intradural (Table 22.2). Intradural lesions are either extramedullary or intramedullary.

## MANAGEMENT OF SPINAL CORD LESIONS

Any patient developing a focal lesion of the spinal cord must be assumed to have cord compression until proved otherwise. The patient should be investigated as a matter of urgency. Plain X-rays should be followed by myelography or spinal MRI, and this is preferably carried out in a neurosurgical unit so that decompression can follow the investigation immediately if a compressive lesion is found. In many patients a good recovery will occur if surgery is performed without delay.

# *Syringobulbia, syringomyelia and hydromyelia*

The majority of patients with syringomyelia (Fig. 22.8) have a developmental abnormality in the region of the foramen magnum with pro-

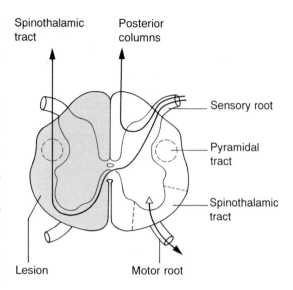

**Figure 22.7** Brown–Sequard syndrome and central cord lesions.

|  | IPSILATERAL | CONTRALATERAL |
|---|---|---|
| At the level of the lesion | Lower motor neuron signs. Impairment of all forms of sensation. Absent reflex. | Nil |
| Below the level of the lesion | Impaired light touch and joint position sense. Upper motor neurone weakness and spasticity. Increased reflexes. Extensor/plantar response. | Impairment of pain and temperature sensation. |

lapse of the cerebellar tonsils through the foramen magnum (tonsillar ectopia), with obstruction of the normal outflow of CSF from the fourth ventricle. This may be associated with adhesions which further impede the flow of CSF. The upper end of the central canal of the cord is kept patent by the normal pulse pressure waves in the ventricular system, and dilates. Eventually, the ependymal lining of the central canal ruptures and there is an extravasation of the CSF into the surrounding central grey matter. These outpouchings dissect up and down to produce the typical syrinx seen on cross-section which

**Table 22.2** Acquired lesions affecting the spinal cord.

1. Extradural lesions: these lesions may compress the spinal cord
   Metastases – lung, breast, prostate
   Intervertebral disc prolapse
   Epidural abscess, including tuberculosis
   Chordoma
   Myeloma
   Cord contusion due to injury

2. Intradural extramedullary lesions: these lesions lie within the theca but outside the spinal cord
   Meningioma
   Neurofibroma
   Dural arteriovenous malformation
   Lipoma
   Arachnoid cysts
   Meningitis, including tuberculosis, syphilis, sarcoidosis and carcinomatous meningeal deposits

3. Intramedullary lesions: these lesions lie within the spinal cord itself and may be:
   (a) Space-occupying lesions
       Ependymoma
       Intramedullary arteriovenous malformations
       Glioma
       Lipoma
   (b) Non space-occupying lesions, and this is known as a 'transverse myelopathy'
       Multiple sclerosis
       Viral infections
       Postvaccination
       Postinfective
       Vascular
       Radiation
       Syringomyelia

4. System diseases: a number of other conditions can affect different cell groups or anatomical pathways in the spinal cord
   (a) The pyramidal tracts
       Motor neurone disease, subacute combined degeneration of the cord, hereditary spastic paraparesis, HTLVI infection (tropical spastic paraparesis)
   (b) Anterior horn cells
       Polio, motor neurone disease, spinomuscular atrophy
   (c) Posterior columns
       Tabes dorsalis, subacute combined degeneration

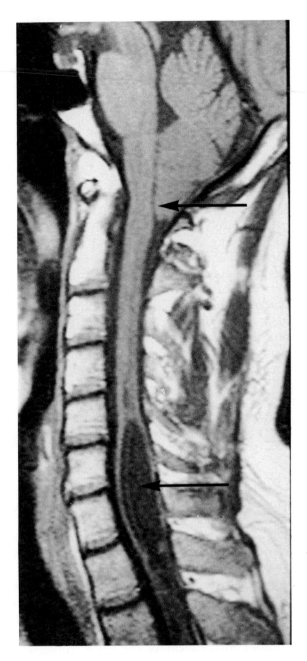

**Figure 22.8** Syringomyelia. Sagittal T1 weighted magnetic resonance image showing tonsillar ectopia (upper arrow) and a syrinx below C5 (lower arrow).

may not obviously show a connection with the central canal. The first symptoms and signs are nearly always in the cervical cord and the condition may remain localized, but the whole cord may become affected. Rarely a syrinx will develop as a result of trauma to the cord and dissection occurs up or down from the level of the lesion.

## CLINICAL FEATURES

The early involvement of the central grey matter interrupting the decussating pain and temperature fibres and the reflex arc determines the cardinal signs of syringomyelia, which are:

1. Dissociated cutaneous loss: loss of pain and temperature sensation with preservation of touch
2. Loss of reflexes.

As the lesion becomes more extensive, so there may be involvement of the anterior horn cells with wasting of the small hand muscles, involvement of the pyramidal tracts with development of upper motor neurone signs in the legs, involvement of Clarke's column with a Horner's syndrome and finally, in the late stages, involvement of the posterior columns. Syringomyelia is probably the commonest cause of neuropathic joints (Charcot's joints) in the upper limbs whereas diabetes is commonest in the lower limbs. The arthropathy itself is painless. It is due to loss of pain appreciation and results in gross disorganization of joints. Despite this, pain is not an uncommon symptom in syringomyelia.

Upward dissection of a syrinx may extend into the medulla (syringobulbia) causing a bulbar palsy (page 672).

## TREATMENT

Although syringomyelia is usually progressive, it need not be so and it may follow a very indolent course. If there is no evidence of progression then intervention is not indicated. If tonsillar ectopia can be demonstrated by myelography, CT or MRI and there is no evidence of adhesions, the treatment of choice is decompression by enlargement of the foramen magnum and a laminectomy of C1 and C2. The presence of adhesions is a contraindication to this procedure. Occasionally a syrinx may be drained by a shunt.

# SPINAL ROOT AND PERIPHERAL NERVE LESIONS

Lesions at different levels in the lower motor neurone produce characteristic patterns of neurological deficit.

The *motor distribution* of peripheral nerves is very constant, so that a lesion of one nerve causes weakness in a particular and specific combination of muscles. The level of the lesion can be predicted from the muscles affected and a knowledge of the levels at which the main branches arise; these may, of course, be affected without involvement of the main trunk. The motor distribution of roots is much less specific and most muscles receive some contribution from several roots; it is, however, important to know the principal contribution.

The *cutaneous distribution* of peripheral nerves (Fig. 22.9) is also fairly specific, although there is some variability and overlap. The cutaneous distribution of roots is extremely variable and there is considerable overlap. The autonomous area for a single root may be so small that a complete lesion may not cause any detectable sensory loss; whereas the rash of herpes zoster, which occurs wherever there is any contribution from the affected root, involves a relatively large area (Fig. 22.9).

# Root lesions

## INTRAVERTEBRAL DISC PROLAPSE AND OSTEOPHYTES

A nerve root may be affected in the spinal canal by a lateral disc protrusion or as it enters the exit foramina by osteophytes, and these are usually associated with chronic disc degeneration and a narrow disc space. These lesions occur at sites of greatest spinal mobility and are, therefore, frequently found in mid-cervical and lower lumbar regions. Thoracic disc prolapse is a rare cause of spinal cord compression and is always associated with plain X-ray changes. In the cervical spine the root emerges above the vertebral body of the

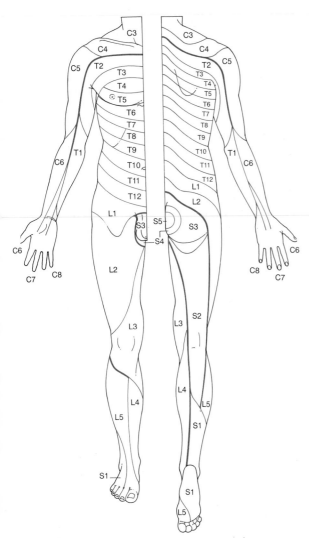

**Figure 22.9** Cutaneous distribution of peripheral nerves, dermatomes. Redrawn from *Aids to the Examination of the Peripheral Nervous system* (1986) Baillière Tindall. With permission.

same number and is affected by disc prolapse at the same level. For example, the C7 root is affected by the C6/7 disc. Since there are eight cervical roots and only seven cervical vertebrae, this relationship changes below C7, and in the thoracic and lumbar spine the root emerges below the corresponding vertebral body. In the lumbar spine a root is affected by the disc at one level above its exit. For example, the L5 root is affected by disc protrusion between L4 and L5, although it emerges between L5 and S1.

Disc herniation causing root compression may occur at any age and usually presents acutely with pain, which may be severe. The pain of a root lesion is felt in the myotome and not in the dermatome, so that the pain of a C7 root lesion is felt in triceps and in the forearm extensors and sometimes in pectoralis major. Numbness and dysaesthesia is felt in the dermatome, so that tingling and numbness in a C7 root lesion is usually maximal in the middle finger. Depression or loss of a reflex at the appropriate level is an early sign in root lesions (Table 22.3).

**Table 22.3** Principal 'root values' of selected muscles in the arms and legs.

| Root | Muscle | Reflex |
|------|--------|--------|
| C5 | Deltoid | |
| C5/6 | Biceps | + |
| C6 | Brachioradialis | + |
| | Extensor carpi radialis | |
| C7 | Triceps | + |
| | Extensor digitorum | + |
| C8 | The finger flexors | + |
| T1 | The small hand muscles | |
| L1/2 | Iliopsoas | |
| L2/3 | Adductors | + |
| L3/4 | Quadriceps | + |
| L4 | Tibialis anterior | |
| L4/5 | Tibialis posterior | |
| L5 | Extensor hallucis longus | |
| L5/S1 | Peronei · | |
| S1/S2 | Gastrocnemius and soleus | + |

Radiography of the spine may show narrow disc spaces, osteophytes, subluxation or vertebral collapse, although the plain X-ray changes often do not accord with clinical evaluation or with the level of maximal compression as determined by myelography. In younger patients with acute disc prolapse, X-rays are usually normal. Myelography is only indicated if the diagnosis is in doubt or if surgery is contemplated. Surgery is indicated for pain or increasing neurological deficit. Painless stable deficit seldom improves after surgery.

## HERPES ZOSTER (SHINGLES)

See page 729.

## TUMOURS

Tumours affecting the cervical roots are rare. Neurofibromata (page 712) may occur and produce a characteristic enlargement of the foramina on plain X-rays.

## TRAUMA

Cervical roots may be avulsed from the spinal cord by traction and the commonest cause of this is motorcycle accidents. If the roots are completely avulsed, there is a characteristic myelographic appearance and recovery does not occur. If continuity of the roots is preserved, some recovery is possible.

# Plexus lesions

## BRACHIAL PLEXUS

### Trauma

Any part of the plexus may be damaged by trauma. Lesions of the upper part of the brachial plexus (C5, C6 and the upper trunk) are nearly always traumatic, but lesions of the lower part of the plexus (C8, T1 and the lower trunk) are less often due to trauma and are usually due to malignant infiltration or to the thoracic outlet syndrome (see below).

### Ruck sack palsy

This is due to traction on the upper trunk (C5/6) from heavy and badly adjusted backpacks. The nerves remain in continuity and recovery is usually complete.

### Malignant infiltration

This may be due to apical lung carcinoma (Pancoast's tumour) or to local metastatic spread from mammary carcinoma. A slowly progressive weakness develops in the small hand muscles (T1) and spreads to involve the finger flexors (C8). There is usually pain and sensory loss in the medial aspect of the forearm (T1). Horner's syndrome commonly occurs by involvement of the cervical sympathetic ganglia (page 665).

### Thoracic outlet syndrome

The lower trunk of the brachial plexus may be angulated over a **cervical rib**, together with the subclavian artery. Patients may present with a neurological deficit or with vascular symptoms or both. Neurological signs and symptoms predominate with the small rudimentary ribs which continue into a fibrous band, and vascular features predominate in the large well-formed bony cervical ribs.

Cervical ribs are quite common and only rarely cause symptoms. Neurological features commonly present in young women with the insidious onset of wasting and weakness of the small hand muscles, often accompanied by pain; a bruit may be heard over the subclavian artery. Other causes of a thoracic outlet syndrome include compression of the neurovascular bundle between scalenus anterior and the first rib. Investigations should inclue plain X-rays with oblique views of the lower cervical spine to show cervical ribs, electromyography to show involvement of the medial cord of the brachial plexus and ultrasonic angiology of the subclavian arteries.

### Neuralgic amyotrophy (brachial neuralgia)

This is an inflammatory neuropathy principally affecting branches of the brachial plexus. A characteristic feature is the dense involvement of some muscles and sparing of others within the same myotome. It commonly occurs in young adults and pain is usually a prominent feature at onset. It is soon followed by weakness and later there may be quite marked wasting. The pain usually subsides in a week or so, but the weakness may persist for months, often with incomplete recovery, so that some wasting may be permanent.

## LUMBOSACRAL PLEXUS

Malignant infiltration is by far the commonest cause, often due to spread from carcinoma of the cervix or uterus. It may also occur in the lymphomas. A radiculogram may be necessary to distinguish these conditions from intraspinal lesions. Lesions of the lumbosacral plexus are best demonstrated by a CT scan or MRI.

# Peripheral nerve lesions

A mononeuropathy is a lesion of a single peripheral nerve. Mononeuritis multiplex is involvement of more than one peripheral nerve and may be due to trauma but should always raise the possibility of an underlying systemic disease such as vasculitis, amyloid, systemic lupus erythematosus and rheumatoid arthritis. Polyneuropathy (page 691) is symmetrical involvement of all peripheral nerves.

Peripheral nerves may be damaged by external compression or by internal entrapment. Other causes include trauma, fractures, operations, penetrating injuries and injections.

Compression usually occurs where a nerve lies between skin and bone, unprotected by soft tissue; for example, the ulnar nerve at the elbow and the common peroneal nerve at the head of the fibula. This anatomical arrangement means that some nerves are particularly prone to damage at certain sites, particularly if pressure is maintained for long periods without change in posture.

Entrapment usually occurs where a nerve passes through a fascial plane or down a fibro-osseous tunnel; for example, the median nerve in the carpal tunnel.

Electromyography and nerve condition studies may be helpful to localize the precise site of the lesion and quantify the severity of the lesion.

## THE MEDIAN NERVE

The carpal tunnel syndrome is the commonest mononeuropathy and is due to compression of the median nerve as it passes through the carpal tunnel in the flexor retinaculum. There is usually no associated systemic disease, but the carpal tunnel syndrome may occur in rheumatoid arthritis, myxoedema, acromegaly, oedema, pregnancy and obesity. It is much more common in women and usually affects the dominant hand first. Patients complain of pain and paraesthesia which may wake them at night and they may shake the hand out of bed to obtain relief. Symptoms are brought on or aggravated by use, particularly activities which require gripping. In the early stages there may be no detectable deficit but, as the condition progresses, weakness of abductor pollicis brevis may develop with difficulty in fine manipulation and the wasting of the thenar eminence. The earliest sensory deficit is usually widening of two-point discrimination followed by loss of superficial sensation in the thumb, index and middle fingers and lateral half of the ring finger. Abnormal signs are strictly confined to median nerve territory, but symptoms may occur in all digits and there may also be pain in the forearm. Percussion over the carpal tunnel may produce paraesthesiae in the distribution of the sensory loss (Tinel's sign).

Splinting, diuretics and local steroid injections may relieve the symptoms and may be the only treatment necessary for self-limiting conditions, such as pregnancy. In more severe cases, particularly if there is sensory loss or progressive weakness, surgical decompression is necessary. Pain and intermittent symptoms are relieved immediately, and the continuous symptoms may resolve with time, but wasting of abductor pollicis brevis may never recover.

A lesion of the anterior interosseus nerve produces weakness of the flexor pollicis longus, flexor digitorum profundus 1 and 2 and pronator quadratus. There is no sensory loss. Spontaneous recovery usually occurs, but the nerve should be explored if recovery is delayed beyond 3 months. It is usually due to an entrapment neuropathy of a nerve as it descends through the two heads of pronator teres alongside the main trunk of the median nerve, which may also be affected in this situation (the pronator syndrome).

## THE ULNAR NERVE

Lesions of the ulnar nerve (Fig. 22.10) occur at four sites: behind the medial epicondyle, in the cubital tunnel, at the wrist and in the hand.

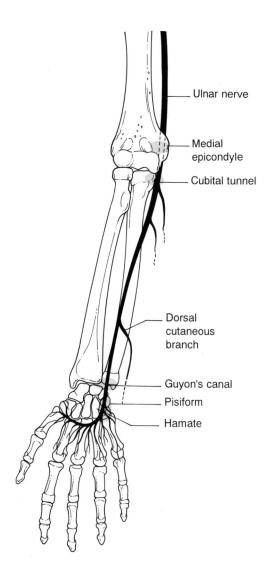

**Figure 22.10** Ulnar nerve lesions.

1. The elbow is a classic site for a compression lesion. Damage occurs if the groove is shallow and particularly if there has been damage to the elbow joint by a previous fracture. Sometimes the nerve may override the medial epicondyle in full flexion. These patients present with a slowly progressive deficit which may be predominantly motor or sensory. The nerve is usually thickened. Involvement of the ulnar innervated long flexors (flexor digitorum profundus 3 and 4) is rather variable; but if affected, the lesion must be at the elbow.

The hypothenar eminence, interossei and medial part of thenar eminence waste with a typical 'claw' hand. There is sensory loss of the medial one-and-a-half fingers and medial dorsal and palmar surfaces of the hand.

In mild cases it may be sufficient to advise against full elbow flexion and leaning on the elbow. In more severe cases, or where the lesion is clearly progressing it may be necessary to transpose the nerve anteriorly. Medial epicondylectomy has been widely used, it has the advantage that it is not necessary to mobilize the ulnar nerve and reduces the risk of damage to the nerve, but following operation the ulnar nerve remains superficial.

2. The cubital tunnel syndrome is an entrapment neuropathy of the ulnar nerve in the forearm flexor group. Clinically it is similar to the lesion at the elbow. Simple decompression is all that is necessary.

3. At the wrist the nerve may be compressed by a ganglion in Guyon's canal. Since the dorsal cutaneous branch arises several centimetres above the wrist, lesions of Guyon's canal do not affect this branch and sensation is spared on the dorsum of the hand.

4. In the hand the deep motor branch may be compressed against the pisiform and the hamate if the hand is used as a mallet. The sensory branches are always spared and the motor supply to the hypothenar eminence may also be spared or less affected than the other ulnar innervated small hand muscles.

## THE RADIAL NERVE

The commonest sites for radial nerve lesions are in the arm and in the extensor muscles affecting the posterior interosseus branch.

Crutch palsy is due to compression of the radial nerve above the spiral groove by long crutches when the weight is taken in the axilla. Saturday-night palsy is due to compression of the radial nerve in the upper part of the arm and is caused by resting the arm against a sharp edge for a prolonged period; triceps is spared. Both these lesions produce weakness of brachioradialis, wrist and finger drop and weakness of the long thumb extensors and abductor. There may be dysaesthesia in the distribution of the superficial radial nerve.

Posterior interosseus palsy is caused by entrapment of the posterior interosseus nerve in the forearm extensor group. It presents with weakness of finger and thumb extension but the radial wrist extensor and brachioradialis is spared and there is no sensory loss. These lesions usually do not recover spontaneously and should be explored without delay.

## LATERAL CUTANEOUS NERVE OF THE THIGH

In **meralgia paraesthetica** the lateral cutaneous nerve of the thigh may be trapped under the lateral end of the inguinal ligament. Patients complain of an area of pain and paraesthesia with numbness on the lateral aspect of the thigh just above the knee. The area never extends across the mid-line anteriorly or below the knee or posterior to the hamstring tendons. It is more likely to occur in obese, middle-aged patients and weight reduction may be the only treatment necessary. Local steroid injections are sometimes effective; decompression is occasionally required.

## FEMORAL NERVE

A localized lesion of the femoral nerve may occur following trauma, during operations and in diabetes (**diabetic amyotrophy**). Apparently spontaneous haematomas may also affect the femoral nerve, and this occurs in patients with bleeding diathesis or in patients who are on anticoagulant treatment. The result is wasting of the quadriceps, weakness of knee extension, absent knee jerk and sensory impairment over the front of the thigh and medial side of the leg.

## SCIATIC NERVE

The sciatic nerve may be damaged by trauma, pelvic tumours, spontaneous haematomas and misplaced injections. The characteristic lesions are foot drop, anaesthesia over the foot and an absent ankle jerk.

The common peroneal nerve is relatively un-protected as it traverses the lateral aspect of the head of the fibula and may be compressed at this site. Patients present with a painless foot drop and may complain of numbness or paraesthesia on the lateral aspect of the foot (**common peroneal palsy**). Examination shows weakness of dorsiflexion and eversion of the foot and weakness of extensor hallucis longus. Inversion and plantar flexion are normal and the ankle jerk is preserved. In the majority of patients, where the lesion is due to simple compression, recovery occurs within a few weeks. If the weakness progresses or fails to resolve in a month or two or if there is any obvious local lesion, surgical exploration may be required.

# *Polyneuropathy*

Polyneuritis or polyneuropathy (Table 22.4) is the term used to describe symmetrical involvement of all the peripheral nerves. The longest nerves are affected first so that signs and symptoms start in the feet and progress proximally, later involving the hands. The majority of patients have both motor and sensory signs and symptoms but some neuropathies are predominantly motor and others predominantly sensory.

The earliest symptoms are usually persistent tingling and numbness of the hands and feet, accompanied by peripheral weakness. The signs accord with the symptoms with uniform distal weakness, absent reflexes and a characteristic 'glove-and-stocking' sensory impairment. In some patients the weakness is more proximal. Pathologically there are two main groups, the demyelinating neuropathies and the axonal neuropathies.

**Table 22.4** Causes of polyneuropathy.

| | |
|---|---|
| Infection | Leprosy |
| Immunological | Guillain–Barré syndrome |
| Metabolic | Diabetes, uraemia, amyloid, porphyria |
| Deficiency states | Vitamins $B_1$, $B_6$ and $B_{12}$ |
| Toxic | Diphtheria, alcohol, heavy metals, drugs and industrial toxins |
| Vascular | Collagen vascular disease, systemic lupus erythematosis and vasculitis |
| Genetic | Hereditary motor and sensory neuropathy (HMSN) and metachromatic leukodystrophy |
| Malignancy | Non-metastatic paraneoplasia |

692 PRINCIPLES OF CLINICAL MEDICINE

The striking feature of demyelinating neuropathies is the slowing of conduction velocity. Causes include diabetes, the Guillain–Barré syndrome, carcinomatous neuropathy, hypertrophic neuropathy, metachromatic leukodystrophy and diphtheria.

Nerve conduction velocity may be relatively preserved in the early stages of an axonal neuropathy due to normal conduction in unaffected fibres. Causes include alcoholism, porphyria, isoniazid, vincristine and thalidomide.

This differentiation is only valid in the early stages and eventually both myelin and axons are affected. This mixed pattern is commonly seen in diabetes.

## ACUTE INFECTIVE POLYNEUROPATHY (GUILLAIN–BARRÉ SYNDROME)

This predominantly motor demyelinating neuropathy usually follows an upper respiratory tract infection by a week or so. The infection may be due to a wide range of organisms, including *Campylobacter jejuni*, glandular fever, cytomegalovirus infection and Mycoplasma infection. It may occur in either sex and at any age. It develops rapidly from onset, reaching its maximum within a few days. The paralysis may affect all four limbs and endanger respiration. Facial weakness occurs in most patients but any of the cranial nerves may be involved.

Autonomic involvement is common with labile blood pressure and cardiac involvement. Since this is the cause of death in a number of patients with this condition, cardiac monitoring is essential in the acute phase of the disease.

It is unlikely that this is a single disease entity, but the diagnosis can be made on clinical grounds and supported by the demonstration of marked slowing of peripheral nerve conduction. Anlaysis of the CSF shows characteristic changes with a markedly elevated CSF protein, due to involvement of the spinal roots, with a normal cell count. Even in severe cases, it is not usually necessary to ventilate the patient for more than 2 or 3 weeks. With modern methods of artificial ventilation there is no reason why patients should not survive this critical period. Recovery can be quite prolonged, extending from 6 months to 2 years, but this is not incompatible with a complete restoration of function. Nerve conduction abnormalities usually persist, but a residual deficit detectable clinically only occurs in around 30 per cent of cases and this is usually not of great significance. Temporary relapses may punctuate return to activity.

Patients still progressing in the early stages must be transferred immediately to a unit where ventilation and cardiac monitoring is available. Plasmapheresis is of benefit in the acute stages and may produce sufficient benefit to keep a patient off a ventilator. Steroids are now known to be of no benefit and there is some evidence that they may actually retard progress, although they are of value in chronic idiopathic demyelinating polyneuropathy.

# INFECTIONS

Infections of the nervous system may be divided into acute and chronic infections of the meninges (meningitis) and of the brain parenchyma (encephalitis) and further divided into the bacterial, pyogenic infections, fungal and viral infections.

## Chronic meningitis

Tuberculosis, syphilis and the Cryptococcus are important causes but many organisms can cause a subacute or chronic meningitis and this may also be the consequence of inadequate treatment of organisms usually associated with acute meningitis.

## TUBERCULOUS MENINGITIS

In most patients this is the consequence of rupture of a small tuberculous brain abscess, which in turn is the result of blood-borne infection. A chronic granulomatous basal meningitis develops. Most patients have evidence of tuberculosis elsewhere, usually in the lung. Dissemination may occur spontaneously or the organism may be released by the use of systemic steroids. The onset is insidious, often with several weeks of vague ill health, sometimes with confusional episodes. Because of this the diagnosis is often delayed. Eventually the patient develops headache, often with vomiting, convulsions may occur and the patient becomes drowsy or even delirious. There is usually a low-grade fever. Papilloedema is a late development but choroidal tubercles may be seen quite early in the course of the illness. Cranial nerve palsies are quite common.

Lumbar puncture shows CSF under increased pressure; it is usually clear initially but on standing may develop a fine 'cobweb clot'. Analysis shows a lymphocytosis with increased protein and a reduced glucose level. In the more acute forms there may be an initial polymorphonuclear leukocytosis, but this changes to a predominant lymphocytosis. A low CSF chloride, once thought to be characteristic of this condition, is a measure of the amount of vomiting. The tubercle bacilli may be found by direct staining in about 25 per cent of cases from a single CSF sample, but this can rise to 75 per cent with repeated lumbar punctures. This, of course, confirms the diagnosis; but in the majority of cases the organism is not seen and the culture may not be positive for several weeks, which often results in further delay in diagnosis and treatment.

It is usually necessary, therefore, to start treatment on the basis of a high index of clinical suspicion, rather than on a confirmed diagnosis. The difficulty with antibiotic treatment is the poor penetration of the most suitable agents into the CSF. Isoniazid in doses of 300–450 mg/day combined with pyridoxine 10 mg daily to avoid polyneuritis, is the most useful drug. This may be combined with rifampicin, 450–600 mg/day, and pyrazinamide, 1.5–2 g/day, orally. The latter penetrates well into the CSF. In addition, oral ethambutol or intramuscular streptomycin may be given initially. Prednisolone is often given for the first few weeks of treatment to minimize reactive fibrosis in the meninges.

## CRYPTOCOCCAL MENINGITIS

*Cryptococcus neoformans* is a fungus which may cause a chronic meningitis particularly in patients with AIDS (page 762). This may escape detection unless special stains are requested. Amphotericin B and 5-flurocytosine are effective treatments followed by maintenance treatment with flucanazole to prevent relapse.

Sarcoidosis (page 314), syphilis (page 758) and carcinoma may all cause a chronic basal meningitis.

# *Acute meningitis*

## ACUTE VIRAL MENINGITIS (LYMPHOCYTIC MENINGITIS)

Viral infections are seldom confined to the meninges and usually cause a meningoencephalitis. This may be produced by a wide variety of organisms including mumps, glandular fever, some Coxsackie and Echo viruses, poliomyelitis and the virus of acute lymphocytic choriomeningitis. The clinical picture is similar with acute or subacute onset of meningitis. In the early stages CSF analysis shows both polymorphs and lymphocytes but, after a few days, it becomes purely lymphocytic and this is associated with a normal glucose level. There may be diagnostic difficulty in distinguishing this from tuberculous meningitis, when acid-fast bacilli have not been found in the CSF. The CSF sugar is not a reliable distinguishing feature. There may be other signs which help with the diagnosis, such as pharyngitis and lymphadenopathy in glandular fever and swelling of the salivary glands with mumps. There is no specific treatment, the prognosis is good with the majority of patients making a complete recovery.

## ACUTE BACTERIAL MENINGITIS

This is discussed on page 745.

# Pyogenic encephalitis (brain abscess)

Intracranial abscess may be extradural and secondary to osteitis of the skull or intracerebral, usually as a result of blood-borne infection. Subdural and subarachnoid abscesses are rare. Cerebral abscess due to spread of infection from middle-ear disease was once common, but with effective early control of this condition, cerebral abscess is now a rare complication.

A cerebral abscess starts as a localized area of cerebritis, which later breaks down with pus formation. An encapsulated abscess then develops and may go on to act as a progressive space-occupying lesion.

Causes include spread from middle-ear disease, septicaemia, particularly in patients on steroids and immunosuppressive drugs, acute infective endocarditis and fractures of the skull. If the intracranial abscess is secondary to infection elsewhere, this is usually in the lungs. The onset may be acute or chronic, there is often evidence of infection elsewhere, there may be focal signs, there is usually headache and fever and there may be papilloedema. Most patients have a leukocytosis and the organism may be cultured from the blood. Patients may rapidly deteriorate and investigation and treatment is, therefore, a matter of some urgency. Lumbar puncture should be avoided because of the risk of herniation. The EEG is always abnormal and usually shows high-amplitude slow activity over the abscess. Computed tomography is the definitive investigation. The treatment is neurosurgical.

# Acute viral encephalitis

A wide range of both DNA and RNA viruses may cause encephalitis. The onset may be acute or subacute with confusion, drowsiness, hallucinations and abnormal movements suggesting basal ganglia involvement. The EEG is always abnormal. The CSF may be either normal or show a lymphocytosis. The causative agent is identified by a rising antibody titre; some viruses can now be detected very early by polymerase chain reaction (PCR) techniques.

## HERPES SIMPLEX ENCEPHALITIS

Herpes simplex (page 729) may cause an acute necrotizing encephalitis which usually starts in one temporal lobe and a few days later affects the other temporal lobe. It is the commonest cause of severe encephalitis in the UK. Epilepsy may be a presenting feature. The patient is usually seriously ill within a few days. The EEG is abnormal in the early stages and between the second and the twelfth day may show periodic complexes with relative attenuation of activity between; in severe cases this precedes marked flattening of the record on that side. Changes in the other temporal lobe follow the first affected side by a few days. The CT scan shows low-density areas in the temporal lobe, indicative of oedema. The diagnosis can be confirmed by biopsy and the virus identified by PCR, immunofluorescence, electron microscopy and culture and also by the demonstration of a rising antibody titre, although this takes longer.

Treatment should be started as soon as possible with systemic acyclovir, and it may also be necessary to give corticosteroids to reduce cerebral oedema. It was once thought that herpes simplex encephalitis was uniformly fatal, but it is now clear that milder cases do occur and the course of the illness may be modified by treatment. Patients are often left with a dense memory defect and dysphasia.

## POLIOMYELITIS

The development of polio vaccines has dramatically altered the incidence of this disease, but outbreaks still occur from time to time (page 719). The portal of entry is thought to be the nasopharynx and there is an incubation period of about 2 weeks. In epidemics there is evidence that many patients are infected and have only a mild 'flu-like' illness; only a small proportion of patients develop paralysis, which usually progresses rapidly over a few days. The extent and the degree of the paralysis are extremely variable. The commonest cause of death is from respiratory paralysis, either as a consequence of bulbar nuclei involvement or from paralysis of the muscles of respiration. The mortality decreased considerably with the introduction of better methods of artificial respiration. Some recovery usually occurs but this is often incomplete.

## RABIES

Infection by the rabies virus (page 747) may follow the bite of an infected animal because the virus is found in large quantities in the saliva and a bite is an effective innoculation. The disease is endemic in many parts of the world, including most of the continent of Europe. Although widespread among wildlife, most cases of human infection are due to dog bites. The virus travels to the brain along nerve trunks, so that the incubation period depends on the distance from the bite to the brain (usually between 1 and 2 months). An early symptom is pharyngeal spasm brought on by drinking and this seems to lead to marked hydrophobia. The disease is almost invariably fatal. No cases of infection between human contacts have been reported.

The use of modern diploid vaccines is very effective in treating patients who have been infected. The vaccination should be given as soon as possible after exposure to the virus.

# Chronic viral encephalopathies

## SUBACUTE SCLEROSING PANENCEPHALITIS

This disease is due to the measles virus and may develop months or even years after an attack of measles. It is slowly progressive over months or years and is nearly always fatal. Initially, there are signs of intellectual deterioration, accompanied by myoclonic jerks and occasionally by fits. The patient gradually becomes more demented. The EEG may show a repetitive burst suppression pattern. The diagnosis can be confirmed by finding an elevated measles antibody titre in the CSF.

## PROGRESSIVE MULTIFOCAL LEUKOENCEPHALOPATHY

This is an opportunistic viral encephalopathy caused by a papovirus which occurs in patients whose immunological competence is impaired. Associated conditions include the reticuloses, sarcoidosis and AIDS. The infection causes foci of demyelination in the white matter of the brain. The clinical course is one of progression over months and the disease is usually fatal. Occasionally, patients survive for some years. The CT scan shows a characteristic appearance and the diagnosis can be confirmed by cerebral biopsy. Antiviral agents may be of value if given early.

# Prion protein disease (slow viruses)

## JAKOB–CREUTZFELD DISEASE (SUBACUTE SPONGIFORM ENCEPHALOPATHY)

This is due to a slow virus whose transmissability has been demonstrated in humans. The source cannot be traced in most patients. Some have been due to the use of growth hormone derived from human pituitary glands removed at *post-mortem* and given to patients with growth hormone deficiency, this practice ceased several years ago because a synthetic growth hormone was developed, others to corneal transplants and the use of infected instruments. The incubation period is several years. Patients present with a rapidly developing dementia, associated with extrapyramidal features and myoclonus. The EEG is abnormal and may show a burst–suppression pattern. The condition is invariably fatal, usually within 6 months.

# Neurosyphilis

The nervous system is involved in secondary syphilis. Invasion of the meninges by the spirochaete produces the symptoms of meningitis. Examination may show papilloedema and neck stiffness. These symptoms resolve, together with the other features of secondary syphilis, and there may be no further clinical manifestation. Fewer than 10 per cent of patients later develop tertiary neurosyphilis and this may follow the original infection by many years.

Tertiary neurosyphilis classically presents as one of three clinical syndromes: meningovascular syphilis, tabes dorsalis or general paralysis of the insane (GPI). In addition there may be gumma formation and optic atrophy. These typical and well-known presentations are relatively rare now and this may be because of the widespread use of penicillin. It is now more common to find positive serological tests for syphilis in patients with a wide variety of neurological signs and symptoms which are not immediately suggestive of this disease. It is important to carry out these tests in all patients with otherwise unexplained central nervous system disease, particularly as it is treatable.

## MENINGOVASCULAR SYPHILIS

This is due to an endarteritis affecting meningeal vessels and cerebral vessels. It may present as a basal granulomatous meningitis with cranial nerve palsies and obstruction to CSF pathways. A local syphilitic granuloma (gumma) may present as a space-occupying lesion either in the subarachnoid space or in the brain itself.

Meningovascular syphilis affecting the spinal cord can cause a transverse myelitis. The CSF is abnormal with a raised protein and an increased immunoglobulin fraction, lymphocytosis and positive serological tests for syphilis.

## TABES DORSALIS

In this form of neurosyphilis there is progressive demyelination and atrophy of the posterior roots, the root entry zone and the posterior columns. The decussating pain and temperature fibres are also involved but the spinothalamic tracts do not show demyelination because they comprise second-order neurons.

The presenting symptoms include pain, paraesthesia, sensory ataxia and bladder disturbance. In more advanced cases there may be rectal incontinence, impotence, neurogenic ulcers and neuropathic joints (Charcot joints, page 589).

Lightning pains are common and characteristic. They occur without obvious provocation and are described as momentary sharp stabs of pain affecting one spot, as if stabbed by a knife. The affected spot is usually in the thigh, calf or ankle.

The pupils are usually small, irregular in outline and unreactive to light, but contract normally on convergence (**Argyll Robertson pupils**). Cutaneous hypoalgesia is often found in the legs and over the trunk anteriorly and down the medial aspects of both arms, as well as across the nose. The deep tendon reflexes are absent, there is loss of light touch, vibration and position sense, particularly in the legs, loss of deep pain appreciation and impairment of pain sensation, often accompanied by a prolonged delay in appreciating stimuli. The proprioceptive sensory loss leads to a characteristic high-stepping gait.

There may be trophic ulcers on the feet and neuropathic joints may develop due to loss of sensation; the shoulders, spine, hip, knees and ankles are commonly involved. There is gross disorganization of the joint, which is nearly always painless. The CSF is usually abnormal.

## GENERAL PARALYSIS OF THE INSANE

This is a chronic spirochaetal meningoencephalitis, and the spirochaete may be isolated from the brain. The presenting features are those of dementia and personality change, and epilepsy may be an early symptom. Examination shows the features of dementia, often associated with a dysarthria, tremors of the hands, lips and tongue, a spastic paraparesis with extensor plantar responses, optic atrophy and Argyll Robertson pupils. The CSF is abnormal.

## SYPHILITIC OPTIC ATROPHY

This may occur as an isolated manifestation of neurosyphilis or it may accompany any of the other clinical syndromes. The funduscopic appearance may be that of a primary optic atrophy or there may be evidence of syphilitic choroidoretinitis.

## TREATMENT

The treatment of all forms of neurosyphilis is by intramuscular procain penicillin, 1 g daily, for 3 weeks. A Herxheimer reaction (page 760) is rare but can be prevented by covering the first few days of treatment with oral steroids.

# *Acquired immune deficiency syndrome*

A very wide range of neurological abnormalities has been described in patients with AIDS (page 762), extending from an encephalopathy to a peripheral neuropathy. In addition, patients with AIDS are particularly prone to opportunistic infections which may affect the nervous system such as Cryptococcus, Toxoplasma, Cytomegalovirus and Mycobacteria. The diagnosis should be considered in all patients presenting with atypical syndromes, particularly in those groups known to be at risk. Progressive dementia is a common late phenomenon in AIDS.

# *S*ARCOIDOSIS

Sarcoidosis may affect any part of the nervous system but the meninges and peripheral nerves are the most frequently involved. Sarcoid may cause a chronic granulomatous basal meningitis often associated with cranial nerve palsies. There may be hypothalamic, pituitary and chiasmal involvement.

Intracranial sarcoid granulomas are rare and tend to occur in the hypothalamus. Involvement of the meninges may result in obstruction of CSF pathways with raised intracranial pressure and papilloedema. There may be direct involvement of the optic nerve as well as retinal lesions and uveitis. The peripheral nervous system may also be affected with polyneuritis and there may be direct involvement of muscle (sarcoid myopathy).

Although neurological sarcoid is usually associated with evidence of sarcoidosis elsewhere, it may be confined to the nervous system. The CSF is usually abnormal, often with a markedly raised protein and a few lymphocytes.

The condition usually runs a fluctuating low-grade course and may be modified by steroids.

# *E*PILEPSY

Epilepsy is the clinical manifestation of a paroxysmal electrochemical disturbance in the brain. The attacks are of sudden onset and brief duration. Heredity is an important factor and it may be that what is inherited is the epileptic threshold. Patients with the lowest threshold would be prone to spontaneous attacks and show the features of idiopathic (generalized, centrencephalic or major) epilepsy (see below). Those with a slightly higher threshold would only develop epilepsy if the brain was damaged by birth trauma, tumours, angiomas, head injury, infections, vascular disease, poisons and drugs, anoxia, congenital abnormalities, degenerative conditions and inborn or acquired errors of metabolism. The higher the threshold, the less likely that these conditions would cause epilepsy. Patients with the highest thresholds would be unlikely to develop epilepsy whatever the cerebral insult. This concept explains why some patients develop epilepsy and others with apparently similar conditions do not.

It is convenient to divide epilepsy in adults into two main groups, the generalized and the focal. This also applies to children, but there are many other factors to consider in children, partly because the maturing brain reacts differently from the adult brain and partly because children are subject to different diseases and hazards.

# Focal epilepsy (simple and complex partial seizures)

The term implies that the attacks arise from a focal discharge. The attack may take any form from a brief focal event to a major convulsive seizure (see below), and this is a continuum.

## AURA

A focal discharge may cause a brief focal disturbance usually called an aura, although it need not proceed any further. The nature of the attack depends on the location of the focus. Examples include a curious smell, usually unidentifiable and often unpleasant (uncinate attacks), a brief flash of light, a formed visual hallucination, auditory hallucination, *déjà vu* experiences, twitching of the thumb and index finger, abdominal sensations, feelings of fear and panic, and numerous others. Nothing else develops and consciousness is preserved. The commonest form of focal epilepsy originates in the temporal lobe. Common features of temporal lobe epilepsy are facial grimacing, abdominal discomfort and the abnormal perceptions of hallucinations and *déjà vu*.

## EPILEPSIA PARTIALIS CONTINUA

Rarely a persisting focal discharge may cause a focal attack which continues for hours or days.

## JACKSONIAN MARCH

A focal disturbance causing symptoms, such as twitching of the thumb and index finger, may spread across the cortex, causing twitching of the hand, face and arm in sequence. Consciousness need not be lost.

## LOSS OF CONSCIOUSNESS

If the disturbance becomes generalized, consciousness may be lost. This is often very brief and not associated with any convulsive features. Sudden loss of consciousness without a clinically identifiable aura does not exclude the presence of a focus, since the focal event may have been too brief to identify or have occurred in a part of the brain which is not symptomatically eloquent.

## LOSS OF CONSCIOUSNESS AND CONVULSIVE SEIZURE

The sequence outlined so far may finish with a major tonic–clonic seizure. In a major convulsive seizure a phase of rigidity (tonic phase) is followed by repetitive violent movements (clonic phase). Incontinence of urine is common. Trauma may occur during the seizure through biting of the tongue, injuries on falling or during clonic movements, or fractures through intense muscle contraction.

## TREATMENT

Treatment is effective in controlling the later stages of this progression, the initial focal event itself being the most refractory. The specific drugs are described below.

# Generalized epilepsy

In patients with a low epileptic threshold, the whole brain may discharge synchronously and the EEG shows a characteristic spike and wave pattern. This is not necessarily associated with loss of consciousness unless it lasts for several seconds. The clinical manifestations range from a brief absence to a major convulsive seizure (*grand mal*). Many patients diagnosed as having *petit mal* suffer from a minor form of generalized epilepsy. The term *petit mal* should either be abandoned or reserved for the classical absence attacks of adolescence associated with three per second spike and wave in the EEG. In an absence attack the child is unaware of the surroundings for a few seconds, stopping what they are doing and staring ahead. The differentiation is important because the true *petit mal* requires different medication.

## DIAGNOSIS

The diagnosis of epilepsy is made on the history alone. The account of a witness is often helpful since there are usually no abnormal signs. In developing focal lesions, such as a brain tumour, persisting signs may not appear for several years. Occasionally focal signs, usually paresis of a limb or limbs persist after the attack – **Todd's paralysis** – but this term should only be used when the signs resolve within 24 hours. In adults this strongly implies an underlying structural lesion.

## INVESTIGATION

In addition to a full clinical examination, all patients with epilepsy should have an EEG and a screen for biochemical abnormalities. When epilepsy develops later in life and in patients with focal features, either clinically or on the EEG, further investigation is necessary and a CT or MRI scan is the most appropriate.

## TREATMENT

The object of treatment is to control the attacks so that the patient may lead a normal life and this can be achieved in 80 per cent of patients with a single drug.

A major advance in recent years has been the development of methods of measuring antiepileptic drug blood levels, and this has profoundly affected the management of patients with epilepsy. The blood level cannot be predicted from the oral dose. The therapeutic range is arbitrarily derived; levels below the lower limit usually have little effect and levels above

the upper limit are often associated with signs of toxicity; although it is, of course, the patient who requires treatment and not the blood level.

Drug treatment, however successful, is not a cure and patients may have to continue regular medication for many years. Since there may be no immediate consequence if a dose is missed, compliance is often poor. Medication given in one or two doses a day considerably improves compliance. Three doses a day necessitates taking tablets to school or work and is to be avoided. Dose frequency depends on the biological half-life of the drug, and all the major anticonvulsants have half-lives long enough to allow a twice-daily regimen.

Drug interactions are particularly important for patients on long-term treatment, and it may be necessary to advise patients accordingly. For example, enzyme-inducing antiepileptic drugs such as phenytoin, carbamazepine and phenobarbitone considerably reduce the blood levels of hormones derived from the oral contraceptive pill, so that ovulation may not be inhibited. These patients should take a larger dose of oestrogen. Drug combinations in a single preparation should not be used, since it is not possible to vary the doses independently.

Some basic data about the more commonly used drugs are given in Table 22.5. Patients should be started on one drug in moderate dose (for example, the initial figure in the table under 'Usual daily dose range'). If the attacks are controlled, no further action is required. If attacks continue, the blood level should be measured and the dose adjusted, bearing in mind that it takes 2–3 weeks for most drug blood levels to stabilize. If attacks continue despite a blood level in the upper part of the therapeutic range, a different drug should be either substituted or added and the process repeated.

### Phenytoin

Hydroxylation of phenytoin in the liver is a saturable process, so that a small dose increment can result in a considerable rise in blood level. It is unwise, therefore, to increase the dose of phenytoin by more than 25 or 50 mg when the daily dose exceeds 300 mg. The long half-life of phenytoin means that it need be given only once a day.

**Table 22.5** Antiepileptic drugs.

| Preparations | Tablet or capsule size (mg) | Usual daily dose range (mg) | Therapeutic range (mg/l) | Approximate half-life (hours) | Usual dose frequency |
|---|---|---|---|---|---|
| Phenytoin | 25 50 100 300 | 200–400 | 7–17 | 12–40 | Twice daily or daily |
| Carbamazepine | 100 200 400 | 400–1200 | 4–14 | 9–20 | Twice daily |
| Sodium valproate | 200 500 | 600–2500 | 40–100 | 7–9 | Twice daily |
| Primidone | 250 | 500–1500 | <14 | 5–15 | Twice daily |
| Phenobarbitone | 15 30 60 100 | 30–120 | 9–25 | 75–108 | Daily |
| Clonazepam | 0.5 & 2 | 1–6 | | | Twice daily |
| Clobazam | 10 | 20–30 | | | Twice daily |
| Vigabatrin | 500 | 1000–3000 | | | Twice daily |
| Lamotrigine | 50 100 | 100–400 | | | Twice daily |
| Gabapentin | 100 300 400 | | | | 3 × day |

Dose-related side effects include nystagmus, ataxia and dysequilibrium. Gingival hyperplasia may occur in children, and hirsutism may be a problem in young women. Some patients are allergic to the drug and develop a rash.

## Sodium valproate

This drug has a short blood half-life of about 8 hours, but it is reasonable to give the drug twice a day since the anticonvulsant effect lasts much longer. The short half-life also makes blood level measurements difficult to assess, unless taken at a fixed time after a dose (perhaps 2 hours).

It is the drug of choice for generalized epilepsy, photosensitivity and myoclonus. Gastrointestinal upset is a common early side effect but often improves with continuing medication. Hair loss occasionally occurs, and some patients develop a fine tremor. Weight gain may be a problem.

## Carbamazepine

This drug is probably the treatment of choice for focal epilepsy and in women of child-bearing age or who are likely to enter the child-bearing age during the course of treatment, as it is the least likely to be associated with fetal abnormalities. A rash is an idiosyncratic side effect that occurs in 3 per cent of patients. Toxic side effects include unsteadiness, sedation and headache.

## Clonazepam and clobazam

These two benzodiazepines are effective anticonvulsants particularly for myoclonus, but they may show drug fatigue which limits use, and both drugs cause sedation.

## Primidone

A variable proportion of an oral dose of primidone is converted into phenobarbitone. There is, therefore, no reason to use a combination of primidone and phenobarbitone. Patients who are stabilized on primidone alone show a ratio of phenobarbitone to primidone which exceeds 2:1. If the primidone level exceeds the phenobarbitone level, it can be concluded that compliance is poor.

The dose of primidone must be gradually increased, starting with 125 mg at night and increasing every 3 or 4 days to a therapeutic dose. If this is not done a number of patients will develop acute nausea, vomiting and unsteadiness which may also occur as toxic side effects.

### Phenobarbitone

Although still very widely used, phenobarbitone is no longer a treatment of first choice in adult patients with epilepsy. It may cause behavioural disturbance in children, the sedation is unacceptable to young adults and it may contribute to depression in the middle aged. Blood levels should not normally exceed 25 mg/l, especially in children, but many patients who have been stabilized on this drug for many years tolerate much higher levels without signs of toxicity. Withdrawal of the drug should be gradual because of the risk of precipitating fits.

### Vigabatrin, lamotrigine and gabapentin

Vigabatrin, lamotrigine and gabapentin are recently introduced antiepileptic drugs which are currently being used as add-on therapy in patients with intractable epilepsy.

### Surgery

Surgery is occasionally used for refractory epilepsy especially focal seizures arising in the temporal lobe.

# Status epilepticus

Status epilepticus is a series of major attacks without full recovery between seizures. This is a dangerous condition with a high mortality and requires urgent treatment.

The priority is to stop the attack, and this is best done with an intravenous injection of diazepam, 10–20 mg, or clonazapam, 1–2 mg. It should not be given intramuscularly or diluted in intravenous infusion fluids. The diazepam injection may be repeated and is often all that is necessary.

Control must be maintained; if attacks recur less than an hour or two after two injections of diazepam, the patient must be transferred to an intensive care unit where methods of artificial ventilation are available. Chlormethiazole may be used by slow intravenous infusion, and this may be combined with paralysis and ventilation. While paralysed and ventilated the patient's brain activity may be monitored by EEG.

# Epilepsy in pregnancy

Phenytoin and carbamazepine are powerful liver enzyme inducers and when used in patients on the combined contraceptive pill it is necessary to prescribe a preparation containing at least 50 μg oestrogen.

There is an increased risk of fetal abnormalities in children of patients with epilepsy and this risk is increased by medication, particularly combinations of drugs. There is about fivefold increase in the risk of cleft palate and cardiac abnormalities in children born to mothers with epilepsy on phenytoin; carbamazepine may be a safer drug to use in pregnancy. Phenobarbitone should be avoided, and sodium valproate has been associated with neural tube defects.

In the majority of patients with epilepsy it is important to maintain their medication during pregnancy. As pregnancy advances the blood levels of most antiepileptic drugs fall; this is partly dilutional and partly due to more rapid clearance. It is, however, very rarely necessary to increase the dose during pregnancy, but if this is done, the dose must be reduced after delivery.

Most antiepileptic drugs are excreted in small quantities in breast milk; but breast feeding is not contraindicated except for patients on phenobarbitone, which tends to cause drowsiness in the infant.

The risk of a child born to a patient with epilepsy of developing the same condition is only slightly greater than chance. If there is also a history of epilepsy in the father's family, the risk rises considerably.

## EPILEPSY AND DRIVING

A single epileptic attack does not constitute epilepsy, which is by definition a liability to attacks. The law in the UK does not allow patients who have had more than one attack to drive until they have been attack-free for more than 2 years. A single attack of epilepsy with an abnormal EEG is considered to indicate a liability to epilepsy.

If the attacks are nocturnal (i.e. while asleep) and continue to be solely nocturnal for more than 3 years, then a driving licence is allowed.

The regulations are much stricter for heavy goods and public service vehicle licences.

# MIGRAINE

## CLINICAL FEATURES

Migraine is a paroxysmal headache which may be clearly lateralized, but not necessarily always to the same side, or it may be generalized. The headache may be preceded by an 'aura' which can take many forms, the most common of which are a variety of visual disturbances such as fortification spectra (shaped like the battlements on forts), flashing lights (teichopsia) or hemianopic defects. There may be numbness or tingling of the face and arms, weakness of one side of the body and, occasionally, dysphasia. These symptoms usually evolve over a few minutes and last for between 15 and 25 minutes. The headache starts towards the end of the aura and usually builds up to a maximum over an hour or so. It may remain severe for several hours and the whole attack is over in 6–12 hours; occasionally, attacks last a day or two. The headache is often accompanied by nausea and vomiting, photophobia and noise intolerance. The frequency of migraine is very variable, ranging from weekly to yearly; but about once a month is common and attacks are often related to menstruation.

## PATHOPHYSIOLOGY

The aura stage of migraine is associated with cerebral vasoconstriction, the headache stage is associated with non-cerebral cranial vasodilation but these vascular changes may be the result of some other process rather than the cause of the condition. The cause of migraine is unknown, but there is probably a genetic factor because there is often a family history.

## TREATMENT

### Avoidance of aggravating or precipitating factors

Some patients are able to identify a major aggravating or precipitating factor and it is much better to avoid this than to take medication. Only a few patients are sensitive to food substances and these include cheese, chocolate, citrus fruits, caffeine-containing drinks and alcohol, particularly red wine and the fortified wines. The contraceptive pill usually aggravates migraine. Though it may be reasonable to take simple treatment for the migraine, if severe attacks persist then alternative methods of contraception should be used. The contraceptive pill is contraindicated in patients who repeatedly have the same aura. The commonest cause of an aggravation of migraine in middle age is the development of hypertension. The menopause is often associated with a change in the pattern of attacks. Other aggravating factors include stress and anxiety, relaxation (weekend migraine) and the menstrual cycle.

### Treatment of the acute attack

The simplest treatment for an attack of migraine is a combination of soluble aspirin or an equivalent mild analgesic, taken together with metoclopramide, 10 mg. The metoclopramide promotes the absorption of aspirin and is useful for its antiemetic effect. Some patients benefit from the use of a mixture of analgesics and an antiemetic. If these measures fail, an ergotamine preparation may be used and these are available either sublingually, to swallow, by inhalation or by suppository. The 5-hydroxytryptamine antagonist sumatriptan, given by subcutaneous injection or orally at the onset of an attack, is often very effective.

## Prophylaxis

This is the most effective form of treatment for patients who have frequent attacks and may, of course, be combined with treatment for the acute attack; a number of drugs are effective:

- On vascular innervation: propranolol starting with 10 mg three times a day
- By serotonin antagonism: pizotifen up to 3 mg a day
- On psychological factors: tricyclic antidepressants (amitriptyline, 25–50 mg, at night)

# MIGRAINOUS NEURALGIA

This is a paroxysmal vascular headache but is otherwise different from migraine. It is much more frequent in men than in women and the attacks are not preceded by an aura. Attacks occur in clusters (hence 'cluster headache'), the patient usually having one or two attacks a day for several weeks before remission, which may last for months. The attacks are sharply localized to one supra and retro-orbital region and it may spread to the cheek. The pain is very intense and lasts for about an hour. The attack is associated with watering of the eye and blocking of the nose on the same side; subsequently the nose runs. In severe attacks there may be a Horner's syndrome (ptosis and a small pupil, page 665), and this occasionally persists between attacks. The attacks often occur at the same time every day and may waken the patient from sleep.

β-Blockade with propranalol and the serotonin antagonist methysergide may also be effective prophylaxis in some patients. Individual attacks may respond to the inhalation of oxygen, or an ergotamine suppository containing 2 mg either daily or twice a day up to 5 suppositories weekly, or an injection of sumatriptan. Alcohol should be avoided as this often precipitates attacks during clusters.

# CEREBROVASCULAR DISEASE

## *Intracranial haemorrhage*

### EXTRADURAL HAEMORRHAGE

This may occur after head injury and is due to the fracture line crossing a meningeal artery, usually the middle meningeal artery. The initial head injury is of sufficient severity to cause loss of consciousness, from which the patient often recovers. The bleeding is arterial, so that the haematoma forms over several hours, causing gradually increasing coma and in the later stages progressing to hemiplegia with fixed dilated pupils. Removal of the haematoma is lifesaving.

There may be no lucid interval if the initial injury is particularly severe. In suspected cases burr-holes should be made as a matter of urgency. The prognosis is related to the promptness of treatment, which should not be postponed until the patient is transferred to a neurosurgical unit if this is likely to result in undue delay. The haematoma can be demonstrated by a CT scan.

### SUBDURAL HAEMORRHAGE

Subdural haematomas also follow head injuries but the injury may be quite slight and the history of trauma may be unobtainable. The haematoma is due to venous bleeding and it may take days or weeks to form. It usually occurs in the young and elderly. The presenting feature may be headache or epilepsy. Later there are periods of fluctuating drowsiness leading to coma, and there may be clear lateralizing signs or evidence of brain-stem compression. The haematoma may be demonstrated by a CT scan (Fig. 22.11), although there is a stage at which the haematoma is isodense with brain. If unilateral, there will be displacement of the ventricles but, if bilateral, there may be no shift of mid-line structures. However, in such patients, the ventricles appear unusually small and the cerebral sulci are not prominent.

Small subdural collections, in the absence of any physical signs or symptoms or evolving clinical picture, may be left to resolve; otherwise the treatment is by surgical evacuation of the clot.

## SUBARACHNOID HAEMORRHAGE

This is usually due to the rupture of a **berry aneurysm** or bleeding from an arteriovenous malformation, and it most commonly occurs in middle life. The onset is usually abrupt with severe headache and often with loss of consciousness. Subsequently, the patient complains of severe occipital headache and this is often accompanied by vomiting. Examination of the fundi may show subhyaloid haemorrhages which are posterior to the hyaloid membrane with the distinctive appearance of a fluid level at the upper edge when the patient is upright and there is marked neck stiffness. Focal signs, such as aphasia, a visual field defect or hemiparesis may occur either because the bleeding is partly subarachnoid or because of associated spasm of major cerebral arteries. The clinical diagnosis can be confirmed by a CT brain scan which may show blood in the ventricles or in the subarachnoid spaces if it is carried out within a week of the bleed and may also show the aneurysm if this is large enough (Fig. 22.12). If this investigation is not available, lumbar puncture may show CSF under pressure and a diagnostic feature is xanthochromia, which may persist for up to 3 weeks.

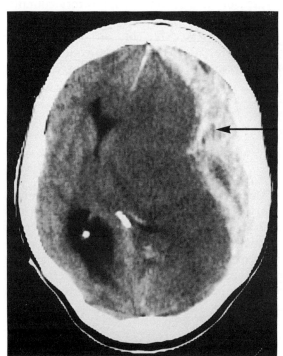

**Figure 22.11** Subdural haematoma. Axial unenhanced computed tomographic scan showing a left subdural haematoma of mixed density; there is oedema of the underlying hemisphere and mid-line shift. The arrow indicates subdural collection.

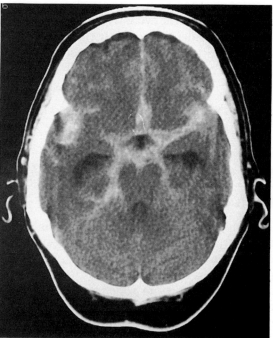

**Figure 22.12** Subarachnoid haemorrhage. Axial unenhanced computed tomographic scan showing blood in the basal systems and Sylvian fissures with dilation of the temporal horns indicating hydrocephalus.

## Cerebral aneurysm

There are several different sorts of cerebral aneurysm, but the one most likely to cause subarachnoid haemorrhage is a berry aneurysm (Fig. 22.13), which is due to a congenital defect of the arterial wall at major branches. Berry aneurysms are commonly found around the Circle of Willis, particularly on the internal carotid artery at the origin of the posterior communicating artery. Other common sites are on the anterior communicating artery and at the trifurcation of the middle cerebral artery. Aneurysms at either end of the posterior communicating artery may be associated with a third nerve palsy.

The fusiform aneurysms associated with degenerative vascular disease and hypertension and large saccular aneurysms seldom rupture and usually present with compression of cranial nerves.

Mycotic aneurysms may complicate bacterial endocarditis and are the result of embolization of a cerebral artery with infected material.

## Cerebral angioma

This is a congenital arteriovenous malformation (Fig. 22.14) which, although present from birth, may not give rise to symptoms until the second or third decade.

Patients may present in several ways:

- Headache, which is usually worse with exercise
- Subarachnoid haemorrhage, in which case the bleeding is usually less than occurs with the rupture of a berry aneurysm and recurs
- Epilepsy, which is usually focal
- Slowly progressive neurological deficit

A bruit may be heard over the mastoids or orbits and a venous hum may be heard in the neck.

## Investigation

If a patient survives the rupture of a berry aneurysm, investigations to find the source of the bleeding should be undertaken as soon as the patient has made a reasonable recovery. Patients

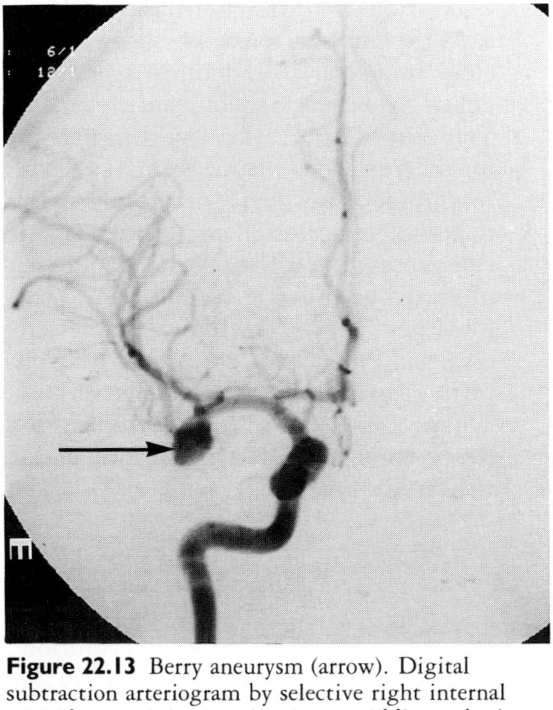

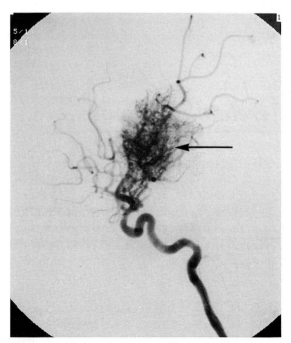

**Figure 22.13** Berry aneurysm (arrow). Digital subtraction arteriogram by selective right internal carotid artery injection showing a middle cerebral bifurcation berry aneurysm.

**Figure 22.14** Arteriovenous malformation (arrow). Lateral digital subtraction arteriogram with selective internal carotid artery injection showing an arteriovenous malformation in the Sylvian fissure.

are at risk from rebleeding at any time and there is no safe period. Bilateral carotid and vertebral angiography should therefore be undertaken as soon as possible with a view to a surgical approach to the aneurysm, if such be found. No cause for the subarachnoid haemorrhage is found in about 20 per cent of cases.

# Intracerebral haemorrhage

This is nearly always associated with systemic hypertension and the commonest cause is the rupture of a **Charcot–Bouchard aneurysm**. These microaneurysms occur on the short perforating arteries arising from the Circle of Willis and the lenticulostriate arteries. For this reason cerebral haemorrhage usually occurs in the internal capsule, corpus striatum, upper brain stem and thalamus. The onset is usually abrupt and the rapidly expanding lesion may cause loss of consciousness either at or shortly after onset. The destruction of brain tissue and the site of the lesion usually results in severe deficit and recovery is often poor. It is not uncommon for the haemorrhage to rupture into the lateral ventricles. Surgical evacuation of the clot is usually disappointing.

# Cerebral ischaemia

Cerebral ischaemia or infarction occurs when a cerebral artery is occluded by thrombus or embolus.

Overall cerebral thrombosis accounts for 80–85 per cent of strokes. A cerebral thrombosis is unusual in young patients and in premenopausal women. If a stroke occurs in these two groups, it is likely either to be an embolism from the heart or in association with one or more major risk factors and the screening of these patients should include estimates of protein C, protein S (page 647) and lupus anticoagulant (page 647). Risk factors need to be assessed in all patients with stroke and, if found, treated accordingly. Major treatable risk factors include smoking, hypertension, diabetes, hypercholesterolaemia and cardiac conditions especially atrial fibrillation.

## CEREBRAL THROMBOSIS

The onset is usually less abrupt than cerebral haemorrhage and the neurological defect may take several hours to evolve. This often occurs overnight and the patient wakes with a completed stroke. Occlusion is due to the formation of clot at a site where the artery is already narrowed by an atheromatous plaque. Occasionally a thrombus forms in a segment of inflamed artery (arteritis) and causes include giant-cell arteritis, syphilis, vasculitis and systemic lupus erythematosus.

## CEREBRAL EMBOLISM

Emboli to the brain may arise from any part of the vascular tree from the heart to the major cerebral vessels. The commonest sites are the heart and the carotid bifurcation.

1. Emboli from the heart may arise from mural thrombi which form as the result of myocardial infarction or in the atria in association with atrial fibrillation. In both cases the embolus consists of formed blood clot. In bacterial endocarditis, infected debris may cause a myotic aneurysm.
2. The carotid bifurcation is a common site for atheromatous plaque formation. This may produce any degree of carotid stenosis to complete occlusion and at any stage in this process the surface of the plaque may ulcerate, giving rise to emboli of atheromatous debris, including cholesterol crystals. Platelets aggregate on the raw surface and may form platelet emboli. This process may also occur at the origin of the cerebral arteries from the aorta and in the carotid syphon.

Whatever the source of the embolus, the onset is abrupt, though the deficit may subsequently increase or repeated emboli may give rise to a 'stuttering hemiplegia' or 'stroke in evolution'. If an embolus impacts in a cerebral artery and subsequently fragments, the resulting transient neurological deficit is called a **transient** ischaemic attack (TIA) and is usually due to a platelet embolus. By international convention, TIAs resolve completely in less than 24 hours. Any attack which results in permanent neurological deficit is known as a completed stroke. If the deficit lasts longer than 24 hours but recovers completely, it is known as reversible ischaemic neurological deficit (RIND).

The clinical syndrome that results from cerebral embolism depends on which artery is involved, and for descriptive purposes the area of brain involved is identified by its feeding artery. Occlusion of the main trunk of the middle cerebral artery causes damage in its entire territory, with motor and sensory deficit on one side of the body associated with aphasia if the dominant hemisphere is affected, and a homonymous hemianopia due to involvement of the optic radiation. Fragmentary forms of this syndrome occur with embolization of more distal branches.

The carotid artery syndrome consists of attacks of ipsilateral visual loss (amblyopia) and attacks with contralateral long tract signs. It is due to emboli from the carotid artery to the ophthalmic artery and middle cerebral artery. The emboli may be seen traversing the retinal circulation. If the eye and the brain are affected at the same time, the cause is more likely to be a perfusion failure due to a tight carotid stenosis or occlusion.

About 30 per cent of patients who have TIAs develop a completed stroke within 3 years and this may occur after only a few attacks. These patients should be investigated with a view to endarterectomy if a surgically treatable lesion is found. Recent trials have conclusively shown that endarterectomy is better than best medical care for stenoses greater than 70 per cent, but that the surgical risk outweighs the benefit if the lesions are less than 30 per cent. The role of surgery for lesions between 30 and 70 per cent has yet to be determined. Vertebrobasilar TIAs should be managed conservatively since they have a better prognosis than those in carotid territory and most of the vertebrobasilar system is not accessible for surgery. A bruit over the appropriate carotid bifurcation is a strong indication of stenosis of the artery at that site and considerably increases the chances of finding an operative lesion. Initial screening may be carried out with Doppler

ultrasonic angiology. Useful information may also be obtained from digital subtraction angiograms following intravenous injection of contrast medium, but the definitive investigation is ateriography preferably with digital subtraction, usually performed by femoral catheterization and subsequent selective catheterization of the appropriate vessels.

If emboli are thought to arise in the heart, the patient should be anticoagulated. Emboli arising more distally in patients not suitable for surgery may be treated with antiplatelet drugs, such as aspirin, 300 mg, daily.

Any consideration of surgery must take account of the operative mortality and morbidity of carotid endarterectomy. It is doubtful if the operation should be performed if the combined mortality and morbidity exceeds 5 per cent and good centres achieve less than 3 per cent.

### Management of a completed stroke

About 50 per cent of patients who have a hemiplegic stroke make a good recovery, about 25 per cent die within the next month and the remainder are left severely disabled.

The immediate treatment consists of good nursing care with particular attention to the avoidance of chest infection and the management of urinary retention if it occurs. Although the blood pressure may be quite high in the hours after a stroke, it usually settles in a few days and treatment which causes a precipitous fall in pressure should be avoided. Dehydration must be prevented as it increases the tendency to thrombosis. Rehabilitation by physiotherapists and, if necessary, speech therapists should be commenced as soon as possible, as vigorous early treatment probably decreases subsequent disability.

# Venous sinus thrombosis

This usually results from spread of infection from the middle ear, mastoid or air sinuses. It may be associated with cerebral abscess. Venous sinus thrombosis also occurs in association with pregnancy and may result from a head injury associated with skull fracture. Magnetic resonance angiography is the investigation of choice. These patients should be anticoagulated, even if the CT scan shows evidence of some leakage of blood, since it has been shown that the prognosis without anticoagulation is poor and the risk of more extensive bleeding is very small.

# INTRACRANIAL TUMOURS

Any of the intracranial structures may give rise to tumour. Table 22.6 lists some of the common tumours.

**Table 22.6** Common intracranial tumours.

| Site/cause | Tumour |
| --- | --- |
| Meninges | Meningioma |
| Brain parenchyma | Gliomas |
| Cranial nerves | Optic nerve glioma, neurofibromas (acoustic and trigeminal) |
| Endocrine | Pituitary and pineal |
| Congenital | Craniopharyngioma, chordoma |
| Blood vessels | Angioma, haemangioblastoma |
| Granulomas | Tuberculosis, sarcoid and syphilis |
| Metastatic tumours | Usually from lung or breast |

In adults the most common neoplasms are supratentorial gliomas and metastatic tumours. In children, posterior fossa tumours are more common and they are usually medulloblastomas or astrocytomas.

## CLINICAL FEATURES

The presentation of an intracranial tumour depends very much on its location and speed of growth. The majority of supratentorial tumours present with steadily progressive neurological deficit. A tumour in the frontal lobe may present with personality changes and dementia. If slightly more posterior, it may present with a slowly progressive hemiplegia and there may be speech involvement if it affects the dominant hemisphere. The earliest features of a temporal lobe tumour are facial weakness, slight drift of the outstretched arm and an upper quadrantic hemianopia. Parietal lesions often cause hemianopia and may be associated with receptive speech difficulty in the dominant hemisphere or difficulties with spatial orientation in the non-dominant hemisphere.

Epilepsy may be the earliest symptom, and this implies involvement of the cortex. In some very slowly growing tumours, such as meningiomas, the epilepsy may precede the development of other focal signs by many years.

Posterior fossa tumours usually present in a slightly different way. There is comparatively little space in the posterior fossa, so that a relatively small tumour quickly obstructs CSF pathways; headache, vomiting and papilloedema may occur early and there may be signs of brainstem compression.

## INVESTIGATION

A CT brain scan (Fig. 22.15), MRI, plain skull films and cerebral angiography may all be re-

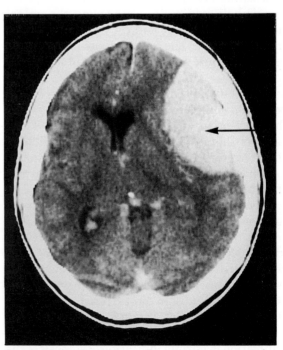

**Figure 22.15** Meningioma (arrow). Axial computed tomographic scan showing a large left enhancing extrinsic mass lesion causing compression of the hemisphere and middle shift.

quired to determine the precise location and likely nature of an intracranial tumour.

## TREATMENT

Treatment of intracranial tumours depends entirely on their nature and their situation. An attempt should be made to remove benign tumours, such as pituitary adenomas, acoustic neuromas and meningiomas, except where to do so would leave unacceptable deficit. Malignant gliomas are, on the whole, not removable, although if confined to the anterior part of the frontal lobe or the anterior part of the temporal lobe, it may be possible to carry out a radical resection. Otherwise, the nature of the tumour should be determined by biopsy and consideration given to the possibility of X-ray therapy. Metastatic tumours, if solitary and near the surface, can often be removed entirely. Chemotherapy has so far proved disappointing. Many cerebral tumours, particularly metastases and meningiomas, are associated with extensive white-matter oedema. This can be effectively treated with dexamethasone, 16 mg a day initially, and this treatment will often result in a dramatic improvement in the patient's condition.

# MULTIPLE SCLEROSIS

In this condition patches of demyelination occur at different times scattered throughout the central nervous system. These 'plaques' evolve and resolve to give the characteristic episodes of neurological dysfunction, from which there may be complete clinical recovery, although pathologically they leave small scars in the white matter.

## AETIOLOGY

The cause is unknown. There are features which suggest a genetic or an immunological mechanism, perhaps with an infective agent, and these possibilities are not mutually incompatible. In addition there is evidence that the composition of myelin in patients with multiple sclerosis is slightly different from normal subjects.

## EPIDEMIOLOGY

The disease seems to be much more common in temperate climates and is comparatively rare in equatorial countries. There is some evidence that migration from a high-risk area to a low-risk area or vice versa only changes the risk for an individual if this migration takes place before adolescence. These geographical features have been disputed.

About 60 per cent of patients have their first attack between the ages of 20 and 40, and a first attack below the age of 15 or over the age of 50 is rare. In the UK women are affected more than men in a ratio of 2:1.

## CLINICAL FEATURES

The signs and symptoms of multiple sclerosis depend entirely on the site of the lesions but it is confined to the central nervous system. Although cranial nerve palsies occur, lower motor neuron signs in the limbs do not. Unilateral retrobulbar neuritis is often an early feature with the rapid progression of visual impairment, usually due to a central scotoma, associated with pain on eye movement. An afferent pupillary defect is a characteristic feature (page 665).

Vision may remain unchanged for days or a few weeks and then gradually improve. The disc may show swelling (papillitis) initially and later optic atrophy. Involvement of cerebellar pathways in the brain stem is common and results in nystagmus, internuclear ophthalmoplegia, dysarthria, ataxia and disequilibrium. Spinal cord involvement is also common affecting the pyramidal tracts and posterior columns. Sphincter disturbance is an early feature with spinal cord involvement.

These features usually evolve over a few days, last a few weeks and resolve over weeks or months. There may be complete remission of all signs and symptoms after the first episode and recurrence may not occur for many years. Often recovery is incomplete if the relapses are frequent, causing increasing permanent disability. It is not possible to predict the outcome of the disease in the early stages, but the state of the patient 5 years after the first attack is some guide to prognosis. In some patients, particularly the young, the disease shows wide fluctuations between exacerbations and remissions whereas others, particularly the older patients, may show a very slow progressive course over many years without obvious remissions.

## DIAGNOSIS

The diagnosis depends on the demonstration of multiple lesions within the nervous system and documented evidence of multiple lesions in time (definite multiple sclerosis). The demonstration of a single focal lesion for which no other cause can be found, with a history suggestive of other lesions, is usually designated 'probable multiple sclerosis', whereas a single lesion without any evidence of other lesions, but no alternative diagnosis, may be called 'possible multiple sclerosis'. It is, of course, necessary to exclude focal lesions due to some other cause. This difficulty often occurs with a slowly progressive spinal cord lesion in middle age with no other features, in which case a compressive lesion must be excluded by myelography or MRI.

## INVESTIGATION

### Cerebrospinal fluid

Analysis of the CSF may show a slightly raised CSF protein with a disproportionate increase in the amount of the immunoglobulin IgG. This is usually expressed as the IgG:albumin ratio. A more accurate test compares the relative amount of IgG to albumin in CSF to the same measurement in the blood and, by this means, it can be demonstrated that the immunoglobulin is produced on the brain side of the blood–brain barrier. The abnormal IgG is oligoclonal and this can be demonstrated by immunoelectrophoresis.

### Evoked responses

In patients with a single focal lesion both clinically and historically, additional focal lesions within the nervous system may be demonstrated by measurement of central conduction velocities. For visual evoked responses, the patient is asked to look at a black and white checkerboard pattern, which flashes black and white alternately. This produces a time-locked response in the visual cortex which can be recorded by surface electrodes. The amplitude is much less than that of the EEG so that an averager is required. Delayed conduction from one eye compared with the other or to normal values indicates a lesion of the optic nerve on that side.

A similar technique can be used to measure central conduction velocities in the auditory system (auditory evoked responses and crossed acoustic response) and in the sensory system (somatosensory evoked responses).

### Magnetic resonance imaging

Magnetic resonance imaging is a particularly sensitive technique for showing the multiple periventricular plaques in multiple sclerosis and lesions in the corpus callosum are almost pathognomonic (Fig. 22.16).

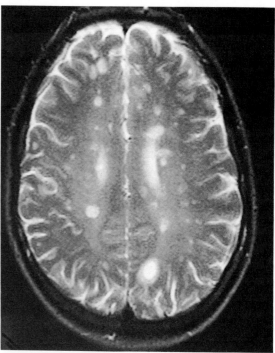

**Figure 22.16** Multiple sclerosis. Axial T2 weighted magnetic resonance image showing multiple plaques of demyelination in the periventricular and subcortical white matter and in the corpus callosum.

## TREATMENT

There is no specific treatment which influences the course of the disease. There is some evidence that a short course of high-dose steroids given during the acute attack induces a remission earlier and with less deficit than might otherwise have occurred. This is presumably by an effect on the oedema and inflammation of an evolving plaque. There is no case for continued treatment with steroids.

# Neuromyelitis optica (Devic's disease)

This condition is closely related to disseminated sclerosis but it tends to develop earlier, usually affecting adolescents. The clinical picture is that of bilateral retrobulbar neuritis occurring either simultaneously or consecutively and associated with a transverse myelitis which results in a spastic paraplegia or quadriplegia. The pathological changes are similar to disseminated sclerosis. Recovery is often poor but relapses are rare. The treatment is with steroids.

# HEREDITARY SPINOCEREBELLAR DEGENERATIONS

Any part of the neuraxis may be affected by genetically determined degenerative processes. The most common parts of the nervous system to be involved are the cerebellum, the spinal cord and the peripheral nerves. The extent to which these structures are involved varies from family to family but tends to breed true within a family. Although there is a continuum from a pure cerebellar degeneration to pure peripheral nerve involvement, some combinations of signs are much commoner than others and these were recognized early; an eponymous nomenclature has continued.

# Friedreich's ataxia

This is the commonest form of this group of degenerative disorders and is the result of degeneration in the cerebellum, posterior and lateral columns of the cord and less severe involvement of the optic nerves and peripheral nerves. The inheritance is autosomal recessive. The onset is usually in the first or second decade with unsteadiness of gait followed by clumsiness of the hands. The cerebellar degeneration results in nystagmus, dysarthria and ataxia. Spinal cord involvement results in pyramidal weakness of the legs with extensor plantar responses, but the knee and ankle reflexes are usually absent because of the associated peripheral neuropathy. The condition is associated with pes cavus, which may be found in unaffected members of the family, and there may be cardiac changes.

# Hereditary motor and sensory neuropathy

**Peroneal muscular atrophy**, or **Charcot–Marie–Tooth disease** is characterized by pes cavus with wasting and weakness of the muscles which begins in the peronei and progresses proximally, later involving the hands. The wasting seldom progresses above mid-thigh to give an 'inverted champagne bottle' appearance to the legs. It is a degenerative disease predominantly of the peripheral nerves, but there is evidence of anterior horn cell involvement and sometimes of cord involvement. There are two principal types, one usually presents in the first decade [dominant inheritance and demyelinating; hereditary motor and sensory neuropathy (HMSN) type 1] and the other often presents later (dominant and axonal; HMSN type 2). Recessive forms of both types occur.

# *Hypertrophic interstitial neuropathy*

Dejerine–Sottas disease (HMSN type 3) is inherited as an autosomal dominant and affects peripheral nerves with marked thickening due to Schwann cell proliferation. There is marked slowing of peripheral conduction. The disease is slowly progressive, usually presenting in adolescence. If it starts in the first decade, marked kyphoscoliotic deformities may develop. The CSF protein is always raised because the roots are consistently involved.

## NEUROFIBROMATOSIS

Two genetically distinct forms of neurofibromatosis exist: neurofibromatosis I or **Von Recklinghausen's disease** is a congenital ectodermal abnormality inherited as an autosomal dominant (Fig. 22.17). Both the central and peripheral nervous system may be involved with multiple neurofibromas. The most striking feature is multiple tumours of the cutaneous nerves, which present as subcutaneous nodules of varying size which may be pedunculated. Patchy cutaneous pigmentation is almost invariably present; these too may vary in size from a few millimetres to several centimetres. They are usually described as **café au lait spots** and more than five are required for the diagnosis. Phacomas may be found in the retina and there may be small depigmented areas seen in the iris (Lisch nodules). There are often congenital abnormalities of the skeleton. The condition may be confined to the peripheral nervous system. Axillary freckling is said to be a reliable marker of central involvement.

Neurofibromas of the cranial nerves, particularly of nerves V, VIII and IX, may occur in association or as an isolated occurrence (neurofibromatosis 2). Similarly, isolated neurofibromas of spinal roots may occur and these give rise to wasting, weakness and pain in the myotome affected as well as causing a characteristic enlargement of the intervertebral foramen. The tumour assumes a dumb-bell appearance on either side of the foramen, and cord compression often occurs. Central nervous system neuro-

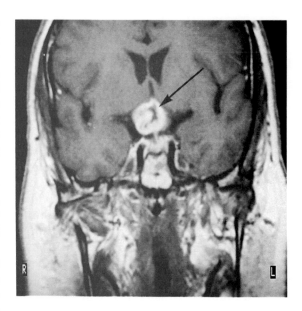

**Figure 22.17** Neurofibromatosis. Coronal T1 weighted magnetic resonance image showing a suprasellar–hypothalmic mass lesion. This is an optic nerve glioma (arrow) in a patient with neurofibromatosis.

fibromas are almost invariably associated with a markedly elevated CSF protein.

### COMPLICATIONS

There is a high incidence of glioma, particularly of the optic nerve, ependymoma and meningioma in association with neurofibromatosis. Occasionally, a neurofibroma may become sarcomatous.

# DEFICIENCY STATES

See Chapter 16.

## Vitamin B₁ deficiency

Thiamine deficiency may present as a peripheral neuropathy (beri-beri) or as one of two forms of encephalopathy (Korsakoff's psychosis and Wernicke's encephalopathy).

### BERI-BERI

This presents with pain and paraesthesia in the hands and feet, followed later by weakness. Examination shows wasting and weakness of the small hand muscles and the feet, absent reflexes and 'glove and stocking' cutaneous sensory loss. If there is associated cardiac failure with oedema, the condition is known as wet beri-beri.

### KORSAKOFF'S PSYCHOSIS

This is often associated with polyneuritis. The syndrome is characterized by confusion, disorientation and striking loss of recent memory with a tendency to confabulate.

### WERNICKE'S ENCEPHALOPATHY

This too may be associated with Korsakoff's psychosis and polyneuritis. The characteristic features are vertigo, nystagmus, ocular palsies, ataxia and drowsiness.

These clinical manifestations of thiamine deficiency are usually associated with chronic alcoholism but may be due to malnutrition. Wernicke's encephalopathy is a rare complication of hyperemesis gravidarum.

Treatment is a matter of urgency and as soon as the diagnosis is made the patient should be given large doses of thiamine intravenously. Since thiamine deficiency is often associated with deficiency of other vitamins, it is usual to give a preparation containing other vitamins of the B complex and vitamin C.

## Vitamin B₁₂ deficiency

Deficiency of vitamin $B_{12}$ (page 604) may give rise to a macrocytic anaemia, subacute combined degeneration of the cord associated with a mild peripheral neuropathy, dementia and optic atrophy.

The lower limit of normal serum vitamin $B_{12}$ in most laboratories is around 200 mg/l. Macrocytosis may develop at levels below this but neurological complications are rare if the level exceeds 100. Neurological complications are virtually unknown in the presence of a normal blood picture.

**Subacute combined degeneration of the cord** is so called because of the combined involvement of the posterior and lateral columns of the cord. This gives rise to impairment of touch, vibration and joint position sense, together with pyramidal tract signs, which always involve the legs first. Patients complain of paraesthesia in the hands and feet, followed by increasing numbness and sensory ataxia. The knee and ankle jerks are absent because of the associated peripheral neuropathy but the plantar responses are extensor. Mental symptoms may accompany this condition but may rarely appear alone. Optic atrophy occurs in about 5 per cent of cases.

Treatment is by intramuscular injection of hydroxycobalamin, 1 mg, six doses over 2 weeks and then at increasing intervals to a maintenance dose of 1 mg every 3 months. This treatment must be continued for life.

# NON-METASTATIC NEUROLOGICAL COMPLICATIONS OF CARCINOMA

Any part of the neuraxis may degenerate in the presence of a carcinoma elsewhere, usually an small-cell carcinoma of the lung (page 308). The commonest manifestation is a mixed motor and sensory polyneuropathy, but dementia, cerebellar atrophy and myelopathy may also occur.

These conditions may occur in association with myeloma and the lymphomas. Unfortunately the neurological complications often fail to improve with treatment of the underlying neoplasm.

# Infectious and Tropical Diseases

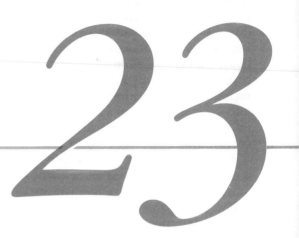

# INTRODUCTION

The term 'infectious disease' might be applied to any illness in which micro-organisms play a causative role. The term is sometimes limited to diseases which are caused by extraneous organisms (those not part of the indigenous flora of the body) that spread from person to person. This chapter deals mainly with such diseases but also includes some infections that do not fit easily into other chapters on specific systems. Other infections have been dealt with under the relevant system and are not covered here.

Every day we come into contact with various types of micro-organisms in the environment. In most cases the protective mechanisms discussed below ensure that no harm comes from this contact. Infections occur with virulent unusual organisms, when protective barriers are breached or when we encounter common organisms before immunological resistance has been developed naturally or by immunization.

In developed countries infections are particularly common in children. Many of the common viral infections of children are managed by general practitioners and are rarely seen in hospital. The emergence of human immunodeficiency virus (HIV) infection has produced a remarkable change in our infectious disease experience in the UK. It has provided a reminder of the potential dangers from organisms which change their genetic content, encounter a population or develop a new method of transmission.

In developing countries, particularly tropical areas, infections have a much more prominent place, often as the major cause of death. This is related to the climatic conditions, nutrition and poor sanitation. In some of these areas the number of people infected with HIV will produce an enormous health and economic problem over the next 10 years.

Advances in the field of infectious diseases have come in the understanding of immune responses and other protective mechanisms. The approach to diagnosis is changing with the ability to detect small quantities of microbial DNA by techniques such as polymerase chain reaction (PCR). In conditions such as malaria there is a continuing battle to keep ahead of changes in resistance while the search for an effective vaccine continues. The onset of HIV infection has provoked great interest in research into treatment and prevention of viral infection which hopefully will prove beneficial in HIV and other infections in the future.

# INFECTION AND IMMUNITY

Infection can be defined as the process by which organisms invade the tissues or organs of the body and cause injury. The development and outcome of infection depend upon three requirements: invasion, injury and reaction on the part of the host. Only a small fraction of the enormous numbers of environmental micro-organisms to which humans are continually exposed are pathogenic, i.e. capable of satisfying the requirements of invasion and production of injury to the host tissues. The virulence of an organism is the degree of pathogenicity shown for a particular host species. Determinants of virulence differ from one organism to another and include the ability to attach to and invade cells, the production of toxins that may interfere with cellular functions either locally or at a distance (after blood-borne spread), and the ability to multiply intracellularly (and hence avoid humoral immune mechanisms).

The initial step in invasion is adherence of the organism to the surface tissues. This is a complex process mediated by either specific molecules on the viral or bacterial cell surface (adhesins) or adhesive organelles called fimbriae or pili that project from bacterial surfaces. The specificity of adhesins for different cells explains the propensity of different strains of bacteria to cause disease at particular sites. Once an organism is attached to a mucosal surface there are two pathophysiological mechanisms by which it may cause invasion. Bacteria may produce toxins, which can either be part of the bacterial structure (endotoxins) and perhaps only be released when the organism is lysed, or are exotoxins that are released into the surroundings during growth of the bacterium. Some of these exotoxins (such as diphtheria toxin, botulinum toxin and cholera toxin) are totally responsible for the manifestations of the disease process, whereas others have less clear-cut roles. The other pathophysiological mechanism (the ability of the microbe to invade cells or penetrate tissues) requires less well-clarified virulence factors.

The host defences that a virulent microorganism must overcome comprise both the various components of 'natural immunity' and the body's adaptive immune system (see Chapter 8).

# Natural immunity

The natural defences of the host are composed of the first-line anatomical barriers that block access of organisms to the body together with a series of non-specific processes including the inflammatory response and phagocytosis. The intact surface of the skin is very resistant to penetration by most micro-organisms; only certain viruses, for example, wart viruses, and the larvae and intermediate forms of some parasites such as hookworms, can breach this barrier. The skin barrier is overcome by lacerations, puncture wounds and bites from animals or insect vectors. Entry of organisms is easier through the intact mucosa of the respiratory, genitourinary or gastrointestinal tract but here too there are efficient natural defences. There are a number of secretions produced at these body surfaces that play an important role in the prevention of infection. Cervical mucus, prostatic secretions and tears all have potent antibacterial properties. The mucus layer of the respiratory tract traps inhaled organisms and the epithelial cilia move the mucus up through the larynx to be swallowed. The acid pH of the gastric acid, the vaginal secretions and urine is lethal to many bacteria, and digestive enzymes in bile and pancreatic secretions also destroy many ingested organisms. Gastrointestinal peristalsis is also an important line of defence.

Many areas of the body contain normal indigenous microflora that protect the host from pathogenic microbes by competition for space or nutrients. Alterations in these microflora (known as commensal organisms) can lead to overgrowth with pathogenic organisms or suprainfection with normally commensal organisms such as *Candida*.

Once a micro-organism has breached the surface epithelial barrier it must overcome the inflammatory response. Inflammation has the function of increasing the immune response at the particular site and the response can be divided into three categories: increased blood supply, increased capillary permeability and migration of phagocytic cells into the tissues. The inflammatory response is initiated by the release of histamine, lysosomal enzymes, kinins and various prostaglandins and other derivatives of arachidonic acid. The various phagocytic cells engulf particles, including infectious agents, and then destroy them. The circulating phagocytes, i.e. polymorphonuclear granulocytes (neutrophils or eosinophils) and monocytes can leave the circulation and enter tissues during the inflammatory response. Some pathogenic bacteria have polysaccharide capsules that reduce phagocytic efficacy and others are able to survive the phagocytic process, multiply and be carried to sites such as regional lymph nodes.

# Cytokines

Cytokines are polypeptides produced by macrophages and lymphocytes during initial exposure to an infectious agent. A growing number of different cytokines are recognized and each usually has a variety of biological functions (see Table 8.1, page 80). The best understood of these substances are interleukin-1, tumour necrosis factor, interferons and various colony-stimulating factors. The interplay between these cytokines is very complex but the net result of this so-called cytokine cascade is an increase in both the non-specific defences and the specific immune responses against pathogenic micro-organisms through antibody-mediated and cellular immunity (see Chapter 8).

# *Fever*

Normal body temperature is kept within a stable range by the thermoregulatory centre in the hypothalamus. Stability of body temperature is achieved by the autonomic nervous system adjusting the level of heat conservation via sweating, skin perfusion and involuntary muscular activity (shivering). Fever occurs as the result of raising the temperature set-point. Microbial products and other biological agents (exogenous pyrogens) induce the release of macrophage cytokines (endogenous pyrogen) which act via prostaglandins upon the thermoregulatory centre in the hypothalamus to alter the set-point (Fig. 23.1).

Many micro-organisms and microbial products are capable of inducing pyrogen release from macrophages and other host cells. Such inducers include endotoxins from Gram-negative bacteria, exotoxins, breakdown products of bacterial cell walls (peptidoglycans), tuberculin, polysaccharides (from fungi and yeasts), interferons and complement fragments.

Endogenous pyrogen comprises several polypeptides with the ability to interact with the

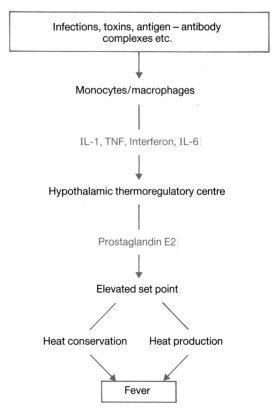

**Figure 23.1** Pathogenic mechanisms responsible for fever. IL = interleukin. TNF = tumour necrosis factor.

thermoregulatory mechanisms; these include interleukin-1, interferon-α and tumour necrosis factor. Why some fevers should return to 37°C (intermittent) whereas others fluctuate above normal (remittent) or remain constantly elevated (sustained) is not understood. Generally, the patterns of fever are of little help in determining aetiology.

# *I*MMUNIZATION

Immunization can be active, with stimulation of the body's immune system by administration of an antigen, or passive, through administration of serum containing preformed specific antibodies.

Active immunization can be given with vaccines containing live attenuated (avirulent) forms of the organism, killed or inactivated organisms or toxoids (inactivated but immuno-

genic bacterial toxins). Live vaccines tend to produce more rapid immunological responses but can result in disease from the vaccine itself in immunocompromised individuals or in pregnancy.

The immunogenicity of some vaccines is improved by the use of 'adjuvants', which act upon macrophages and improve antigen presentation to T-cells. Polysaccharide antigens, such as those of the capsular material of some bacteria e.g. *Haemophilus influenzae* and pneumococci, are poor at inducing T-cell help and fail to elicit adequate antibody responses in children under 2 years old. If such vaccines are to be used in children the polysaccharide is combined with a carrier protein which provides effective T-cell help to B-cells and enables the polysaccharide to produce good antibody responses.

Passive immunization provides temporary protection, which disappears as the antibodies are broken down. Animal antisera carry the risk of hypersensitivity reactions and anaphylaxis, and have been largely superseded by human immunoglobulin preparations. Normal serum immunoglobulin is produced from a large pool of blood donors and contains antibody to many naturally occurring diseases but hyperimmune globulins are obtained from humans who have recovered from a specific disease.

The scheme of prophylactic immunizations given in the UK is in Table 23.1.

## Primary course

Triple vaccine (diphtheria toxoid, pertussis (whooping cough) vaccine and tetanus toxoid) is given together with oral polio vaccine. The course is now commenced at 2 months of age in order that the primary course of three doses can be completed at an early age to provide protec-

tion against whooping cough in those most at risk of severe disease (the child under 6 months old). If the primary course is interrupted, it should be resumed but not repeated.

Worries about the safety of pertussis vaccine led to a fall in vaccination rates to about 30 per cent in the 1970s but the rarity of severe neurological reactions to the vaccine has now been confirmed and acceptance rates are again about 90 per cent. Encephalopathy due to pertussis vaccine probably occurs after 1/300 000 injections. The only absolute contraindications to pertussis vaccine are severe local or general reactions to a preceding dose. Contraindications are an evolving neurological disease or history of convulsions in the child or idiopathic epilepsy in the parents or siblings. Allergy or stable neurological conditions such as spina bifida or cerebral palsy are not contraindications.

## Hib immunization

Vaccination against *Haemophilus influenzae* type b disease became part of the primary course of vaccines in the UK in October 1992. The conjugate vaccine is given into a different site to that used for triple vaccine. A 'catch-up' programme is operating for children between 5 months and 4 years of age. Minor local reactions occur in less than 10 per cent of children. No booster dose is necessary.

**Table 23.1** Recommended schedule for active immunization of infants and children in the UK.

| Vaccine | Age | Notes |
|---|---|---|
| DTP, oral polio and Hib | | |
|   1st dose | 2 months | |
|   2nd dose | 3 months | Primary course |
|   3rd dose | 4 months | |
| Measles, mumps and rubella (MMR) | 12–18 months | Can be given at any age over 12 months |
| Booster DT and polio | 4–5 years | |
| Rubella | 10–14 years | Girls only |
| BCG | 10–14 years | Leave interval of 3 weeks between rubella and BCG |
| Booster tetanus and polio | 15–18 years | |

DTP = Diphtheria, tetanus and pertussis. DT = Diphtheria and tetanus. BCG = Bacille-Calmette-Guérin (for immunizing against tuberculosis). Hib = *Haemophilus influenzae* type b.

# Measles, mumps and rubella vaccine

This live attenuated combined measles, mumps and rubella (MMR) vaccine was introduced in the UK in 1988. It is given to children over 12 months of age irrespective of a history of natural infection. A mild attack of rash, fever and malaise may occur 1 week after the vaccination and about 1 per cent of vaccinees develop parotid swelling after about 3 weeks. These complications are not infectious.

## RUBELLA

Because of the complications of rubella in pregnancy (see below), girls aged 10–14 years are given rubella vaccination, unless there is documented evidence of prior MMR vaccination, to maintain a high proportion of women with rubella antibody. Screening of women during pregnancy is also undertaken and those found negative should be vaccinated after delivery and before the next pregnancy.

# Bacillus Calmette–Guérin vaccine

Bacillus Calmette–Guérin (BCG) vaccine is a live attenuated *Myobacterium bovis* strain given intradermally to those who have a negative response to intradermal tuberculin at the age of 10–14 years. It is also administered to neonates of immigrants from areas of high prevalence of tuberculosis. It induces a hypersensitivity reaction manifest as a small papule or ulcer at the site.

Tuberculosis is discussed on page 302.

# TRANSMISSION

There are four main routes of transmission of infection: contact (direct, indirect or via droplets), common vehicle (e.g. food or water), airborne and vectorborne. Direct contact or person-to-person transmission follows physical contact between the source and the host and may involve touch, kissing or sexual activity. Indirect contact involves transmission of the organism from one individual to another on an inanimate object. Droplets, which are usually produced by sneezing or coughing, are also a form of contact transmission since these particles travel for only very short distances (approximately 1 m).

Airborne spread occurs when micro-organisms are contained in droplet nuclei (small particles that remain after evaporation of droplets) or dust particles that are capable of travelling great distances in currents of air.

If spread by a common vehicle, many hosts can become infected as a result of microbial contamination: food, water, blood and intravenous fluids can each act as a common vehicle for spread.

Insects are the source of vectorborne infections. In some of these the insect merely acts as a carrier of organisms from one host to another, for example, typhus, whereas in others the micro-organism undergoes a stage of its life cycle within the vector, for example, in malaria.

# *I*NCUBATION PERIOD

This is the interval between exposure of the tissues of a susceptible host to the organism and the onset of the first symptoms of disease. During this period the organism is multiplying and often spreading throughout the body, before causing damage to specific target tissues. The incubation periods of most infectious diseases remain fairly constant and some are shown in Table 23.2. The latent period of an infection is the period between exposure and shedding of the organism (Fig. 23.2).

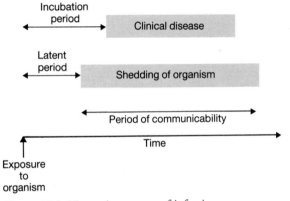

**Figure 23.2** The various stages of infection.

**Table 23.2** Incubation periods of common infectious diseases.

| | |
|---|---|
| Less than 7 days | Bacillary dysentery (1–7 days) |
| | Meningococcaemia (2–4 days) |
| | Diphtheria (2–5 days) |
| | Cholera (few hours–5 days) |
| | Scarlet fever (1–3 days) |
| 7–14 days | Measles (7–14 days) |
| | Pertussis (7–10 days) |
| | Typhoid (7–14 days) |
| | Poliomyelitis (3–14 days) |
| 14–21 days | Mumps (16–21 days) |
| | Chickenpox (14–21 days) |
| | Rubella (14–21 days) |
| | Amoebiasis (14–28 days) |
| >21 days | Hepatitis A (2–6 weeks) |
| | Hepatitis B (6 weeks–6 months) |
| | Brucellosis (days–months) |
| | Leprosy (months–years) |

# *Clinical problems*

# *C*HILDHOOD VIRAL INFECTIONS

# *Measles*

Measles virus is an RNA-containing enveloped paramyxovirus with a worldwide distribution. The virus is transmitted by droplets of respiratory secretions and, in temperate countries, measles tends to be a winter disease. A patient is infectious for about 7 days from the onset of symptoms. The disease is highly communicable and epidemics tend to occur every 2–5 years in young children in countries where there is not widespread uptake of measles vaccine.

## CLINICAL FEATURES

The incubation period ranges from 7 to 14 days and is followed by a prodromal phase, which corresponds to the viraemic period. The prodromal symptoms are cough, coryza, conjunctivitis, fever and anorexia and last normally for 2 to 4 days. During this period the patients are at their most infectious (Fig. 23.3).

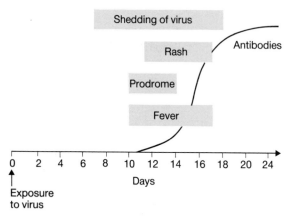

**Figure 23.3** Diagram of the natural history and period of virus shedding in measles.

**Koplik's spots** are found towards the end of the prodrome: this pathognomonic sign of measles can be seen as minute bluish white spots, resembling grains of salt, on a red background of the buccal mucosa. They are often particularly seen inside the cheeks opposite the molar and premolar teeth. The exanthem (rash) of measles appears first as pink macules behind the ears, then spreads rapidly over the face and onto the trunk and limbs. Individual spots are irregular and of variable size and, as it progresses, the rash often coalesces into large, blotchy, darker red areas on the face and upper trunk. In black skins the rash consists of paler follicular dots on a dark background.

After a few days of measles, the fever subsides and the rash fades. Transient brown staining of the skin may occur in the distribution of the rash.

## COMPLICATIONS

The complications of measles are:

1. Bacterial superinfection of the respiratory tract (particularly bronchopneumonia and otitis media) is the most common complication.
2. Bronchiectasis (page 293).
3. Croup.
4. Postinfectious hypersensitivity encephalitis which complicates about 1 in 1000 cases of measles. About 10 per cent of these children die and another 20 per cent are left with neurological sequelae.
5. Malnourished children in the tropics often have very severe measles, which is frequently complicated by corneal ulceration and blindness.
6. In patients with defective cellular immunity, measles can be a very severe illness: a viral pneumonia may develop without any evidence of a rash.
7. Subacute sclerosing panencephalitis (SSPE) occurs several years after measles in about 1 in 100 000 cases (page 695).

## ATYPICAL MEASLES

A severe and unusual form of measles may occur in patients infected several years after having received killed measles vaccine. The rash often starts peripherally and may be vesicular, urticarial or haemorrhagic. Viral pneumonia is invariable and the illness is often prolonged.

## DIAGNOSIS

Classical measles is usually easy to diagnose clinically but laboratory methods may be needed for atypical cases. A rapid diagnosis can be made by detection of measles antigens in nasopharyngeal cells by direct immunofluorescence but the usual laboratory method is serological by the demonstration of measles antibody by the haemagglutination inhibition test.

## TREATMENT

No specific antiviral treatment for measles is available but vitamin A has been shown to prevent many of the complications in malnourished children.

## PREVENTION

Active immunization with a single dose of live measles vaccine confers probable life-long immunity. In the UK it is given as part of the MMR (see above) vaccine at 15–18 months of age. In the developing world the World Health Organization (WHO) recommends vaccination against measles at 9 months of age.

Passive immunization with normal human immunoglobulin is recommended for exposed susceptible patients who are at high risk of severe infection (children with cell-mediated immunity defects or malignancy). The immune globulin should be given within 6 days of exposure to measles.

# Rubella (German measles)

Rubella virus is an enveloped RNA virus in the togavirus family. It is spread by respiratory droplets and is moderately infectious from 7 days before to 4 days after the onset of the rash. Infection is usually seen in primary school children and is most frequent during the spring. The large epidemics of infection that previously occurred every 5–10 years have been prevented by widespread vaccination. Intrauterine infection via transplacental spread is the major complication.

## CLINICAL FEATURES

The incubation period of rubella averages 18 days with a range of 12 to 23 days (Fig. 23.4). The clinical features vary markedly with age. Children tend to have mild disease and do not usually have prodromal symptoms: adults may have several days of malaise and fever before lymphadenopathy and rash appear. The rash of rubella consists of generalized, discrete, pink, macules which are often most marked on the face and trunk on the first day. It lasts for only 1 to 3 days. In black children the rash is extremely difficult to detect. The lymphadenopathy may be generalized, but the posterior cervical and suboccipital lymph nodes are characteristically enlarged. It may last for several weeks. Other common features of rubella are mild conjunctival infection, pharyngeal infection and petechial lesions (Forscheimer spots) on the palate. Subclinical infection is very common in children.

## COMPLICATIONS

The most common complication of rubella is arthralgia or overt arthritis, affecting both small and large joints; this occurs most frequently in adult women. Rarer complications are thrombocytopenia or encephalitis. The major importance of rubella is the effect it may have upon the fetus if the woman contracts infection during the first 4 months of pregnancy. The congenital rubella syndrome causes intrauterine growth retardation, cardiac defects, especially ventricular septal defect and patent ductus arteriosus, ocular problems (especially cataracts), deafness and microcephaly. The earlier in pregnancy the mother contracts rubella, the more likely it is that the fetus will be affected and the more severe will be the defects. Overall, about 70 per cent of the fetuses of women who contract rubella in the first 12 weeks of pregnancy will have some handicap, often involving cardiac, ocular and auditory damage. Infection in weeks 13 to 16 causes less severe damage to about 30 per cent of infants and infection after 18 weeks is most unlikely to cause congenital defects, although some infected babies appear normal at birth, only to develop deafness several months or years later.

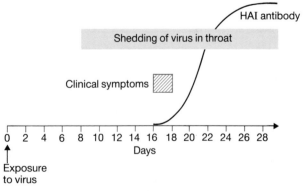

**Figure 23.4** Diagram of the natural history and period of viral shedding in rubella. HAI = haemagglutination inhibiting.

## DIAGNOSIS

The diagnosis of rubella is confirmed serologically. The haemagglutination-inhibition (HAI) technique has now been superseded by several simpler methods, including passive latex agglutination, enzyme-linked immunosorbent assay (ELISA) and radial haemolysis. IgM antibodies to rubella can be distinguished and an acute infection confirmed within a few hours.

## TREATMENT

There is no specific therapy for rubella.

## PREVENTION

Live vaccines are used to prevent congenital rubella. Live attenuated rubella vaccine is given to young children as part of the MMR vaccine and, in the UK, to girls between the ages of 11 and 14 years. Susceptible women are also vaccinated just after delivery of an infant. The use of the vaccine is contraindicated in immuno-compromised patients and in pregnancy (even though the risks of complications following vaccination in early pregnancy are extremely low and if a pregnant woman is vaccinated inadvertently, termination does not need to be offered routinely). Despite specific immunity, reinfection with rubella virus is now known to occur and viraemia (and hence clinical illness and transmission of virus to the fetus) can occasionally result.

# Erythema infectiosum

This common infection (also known as fifth disease as it was considered to be the fifth of the common infectious diseases of childhood after measles, rubella, scarlet fever and a condition known as epidemic pseudoscarlatina or Duke's disease which is no longer thought to be a distinct entity) in primary school children is caused by human parvovirus type B19, a small DNA-virus. Infection sometimes occurs in small epidemics during the winter or spring. The incubation period is 4 to 14 days. A short

non-specific respiratory illness with fever is a common manifestation of parvovirus infection in children and adults but the rash of erythema infectiosum is the most characteristic clinical manifestation. The rash has three stages; the first is a confluent indurated rash on the face, giving the 'slapped cheeks' appearance. A variable, often lace-like rash appears on the limbs a day or so later and may last for a week or so. During the third stage, this peripheral rash may recur over a period of weeks in response to heat, exercise or emotion. Fever, adenopathy and gastrointestinal symptoms are rare. Arthralgia and arthritis occur in some children and in 80 per cent of adult females with parvovirus B19 infection, sometimes in the absence of a rash. After acute infections adults are likely to remain fatigued and depressed for several weeks. Parvovirus-specific IgM can be detected and used as a diagnostic test.

In certain groups of individuals parvovirus may cause other, more dramatic illnesses:

1. Aplastic crises: during infection with parvovirus B19 there is often a fall in haemoglobin concentration. This is due to an inhibition of the bone marrow erythroid precursors by the virus. It is of little consequence in normal individuals but in patients with a variety of chronic haemolytic anaemias, including sickle cell disease and hereditary spherocytosis, infection with parvovirus B19 is responsible for severe aplastic crises.
2. In patients with defective immunity, for example, those with human immuno-deficiency virus (HIV) or congenital combined immunodeficiency, chronic relapsing anaemia and bone marrow suppression can occur.
3. Parvovirus infection in pregnancy may cause anaemia in the fetus and lead to spontaneous abortion or hydrops fetalis.

# Chicken pox (varicella)

Varicella-zoster virus is morphologically indistinguishable from herpes simplex virus. It is transmitted from person-to-person by the respiratory route and causes chickenpox as a primary infection. Chickenpox is a highly contagious disease with attack rates of more than 90 per cent in susceptible household contacts of an index case. The patient becomes infectious 5 days before the rash and remains so until 6 days after the last crop of spots appears. After primary infection, the virus then lies dormant in dorsal root ganglia, from where it may later become reactivated to cause herpes zoster (shingles, page 729). Reinfections with varicella-zoster virus can occur; these are often subclinical but second attacks of chickenpox in normal children have been well documented.

## CLINICAL FEATURES

Chickenpox is most frequent in the winter and early spring and 90 per cent of infections occur before the age of 10 years. The incubation period is usually 14 or 15 days with a range of 11 to 20 days. In children a prodromal illness is rare and fever and rash, often starting on the scalp, are the initial signs of infection. Adults more commonly have myalgia, arthralgia, fever and chills for 2–3 days before the rash appears. The rash is discrete, varying in severity from less than 20 to more than 500 individual lesions. Each lesion begins as a small macule which rapidly becomes papular and then vesiculopustular. The vesicles are very superficial and pruritic. Within 1 or 2 days, the lesion is scratched or becomes inspissated: in either case the lesion becomes scabbed. Within a few more days the scabs separate, leaving small, often oval, scars and, in dark skins, temporary depigmentation at the site of each lesion. It is characteristic of chickenpox that the eruption appears in crops over a period of about 4 days, so that lesions at different stages of evolution are to be seen. The distribution of the rash is central, i.e. the rash is more dense on trunk and face than on the periphery. Lesions are often found on the mucous membranes of the conjuctivae or mouth.

## COMPLICATIONS

The complications of chickenpox depend upon age and host immunity. In the normal child secondary infection of the lesions with sta-phylococci or streptococci is the only frequent complication although haemorrhagic chickenpox with disseminated intravascular coagulation and pneumonitis occasionally occurs. Central nervous system involvement causing cerebellar ataxia, generalized encephalitis or other neurological complications occurs in about 0.1 per cent of older children (page 694). The disease is more severe in adults, because of pneumonitis, the commonest complication. This presents as cough, chest pain, shortness of breath and sometimes haemoptysis.

Pneumonitis may be severe and may lead to permanent calcified lesions on the chest X-ray. In the immunocompromised individual (usually a child), the rash is more extensive and the individual lesions are often haemorrhagic and necrotic. The lesions continue to crop for more than 1 week and visceral involvement (particularly of the lungs, liver and central nervous system) is frequent. Chickenpox may also be severe in the perinatal period if the baby is born within 5 days of the onset of varicella in the mother.

## CONGENITAL VARICELLA

Maternal chickenpox during the first 20 weeks of pregnancy is uncommon but may result in skin scarring (often of a dermatomal distribution), eye abnormalities, hypoplastic limbs and neurological damage in the fetus.

## DIAGNOSIS

The diagnosis of varicella is readily made clinically. If laboratory assistance is required then virus can be found in the vesicular fluid by electron microscopy within an hour or so. In the normal individual the virus is present in the vesicle for about 3 days but this may be prolonged for 10 days or more in the immunocompromised. Serological tests are also available.

## TREATMENT

Severe varicella in the immunocompromised individual should be treated with intravenous acyclovir. Uncomplicated chickenpox in normal children is treated symptomatically with antipruritics such as calamine lotion or anti-histamines. Oral acyclovir shortens the duration of the rash and fever by a day or two but such treatment is probably only cost-effective in those with very severe disease and/or adults, when there is a significant risk of pneumonitis.

## PREVENTION

Specific varicella-zoster immunoglobulin (VZIg) administered within 72 hours of exposure can ameliorate disease in susceptible patients at risk of serious complications. A live-attenuated vaccine for varicella is now available and may become used to prevent chickenpox in the UK. It has been safely used to prevent varicella in immunocompromised children.

# Enteroviral infections

Enteroviruses are spread by direct or indirect faecal–oral contamination. Infection is very common but many infections are asymptomatic. Epidemics of infection due to different serotypes emerge from year to year. Enteroviruses chiefly comprise polioviruses, coxsackie viruses and echoviruses; the last two cause a variety of clinical symptoms, ranging from the insignificant to the lethal (Table 23.3). The viruses are very small RNA viruses with a worldwide distribution.

## CLINICAL FEATURES

Aseptic meningoencephalitis is the most important clinical manifestation of enterovirus infections and this is dealt with elsewhere (page 693). Coxsackie B viruses also cause about 50 per cent of cases of acute pericarditis and myocarditis (page 186).

The skin and mucous membrane manifestations of enteroviral infection are very variable but a number of specific syndromes stand out.

1. The most common form of rash resembles that of rubella. It is pink and always affects the face (where the rash may sometimes be more blotchy than rubella); lymphadenopathy is most unusual and this, together with its summer occurrence, is useful in distinguishing it from true rubella.
2. Hand, foot and mouth disease, usually caused by coxsackie A16 (occasionally by A5 and A10) is characterized by small vesicles within an erythematous margin on the hands and feet together with painful ulcers within the mouth. It is usually seen in children under 10 years old and is accompanied by fever and sore throat. Sometimes vesicles are seen elsewhere on the body.
3. Herpangina is a vesicular and ulcerating eruption on the fauces, tonsils and palate that is caused by several types of coxsackie A viruses. It is mild and self-limiting.

**Table 23.3** Clinical syndromes and the common coxsackie and echovirus serotypes.

| Syndrome | Coxsackie viruses | | Echoviruses |
| | Group A | Group B | |
| --- | --- | --- | --- |
| 1. Neurological | | | |
|    Meningoencephalitis | Types 7,9 | Types 2–5 | Types 4,6,9,11,16,30 |
|    Paralysis | Types 7,9 | | Enterovirus 71 |
| 2. Pericarditis and myocarditis | Types 4,16 | Types 2–5 | Uncommon |
| 3. Skin and mucous membranes | | | |
|    Hand, foot and mouth disease | Type 16 (also 5,7,9) | Uncommon | |
|    Herpangina | Types 1–10,16,22 | Uncommon | Uncommon |
|    Rubelliform | Type 9 | Uncommon | Types 9,11,16 |
| 4. Myositis (Bornholm disease) | Uncommon | Types 1–5 | Uncommon |
| 5. Generalized disease (in infants) | | Types 2–5 | Type 11 |

4. Epidemic myalgia (Bornholm disease or pleurodynia) is manifest as fever and sudden severe upper abdominal or lower thoracic pain, often aggravated by breathing or movement. It may last for 2 weeks and is caused by coxsackie B viruses. It may be confused clinically with pneumonia or pulmonary embolism.

# Mumps (epidemic parotitis)

Mumps is a paramyxovirus restricted to a human reservoir and spread by the respiratory (droplet) route. The highest frequency of infection is in the 5–15 year age group and the highest incidence of infection is in the late winter and spring. The infectious period lasts from 3 days before to 7 days after the salivary gland swelling, but up to 40 per cent of infections are asymptomatic.

## CLINICAL FEATURES

After an incubation period of 2 to 4 weeks (average 16–18 days) symptomatic patients develop fever, malaise and painful swelling of the salivary glands (usually the parotids but sometimes the submandibular glands only). Parotid swelling can be distinguished from lymph-node enlargement in that it fills in the hollow between the angle of the mandible and the mastoid process and may also elevate the ear lobe. The swelling may be unilateral or bilateral and the affected glands are tender. The glands reach their maximum size within 3 days and the fever and glandular enlargement last for about 1 week.

## COMPLICATIONS

There are a number of complications of mumps, many of which can occur without parotitis:

1. Meningitis is clinically evident in only 10 per cent of infected patients although a pleocytosis is present within the cerebrospinal fluid (CSF) of almost all cases of mumps. It is usually a mild form of aseptic meningitis (page 693).
2. Encephalitis is much less common and much more severe with a significant mortality.
3. Deafness, which may be permanent, is occasional.
4. Orchitis is seen in about 25 per cent of infected postpubertal males. It is usually unilateral and causes some degree of testicular atrophy. Even when bilateral, however, the degree of atrophy is rarely sufficient to produce sterility.
5. Oophoritis is less common and causes lower abdominal pain.
6. Pancreatitis causes upper abdominal pain, vomiting and fever.
7. Other complications include mastitis, inflammation of other salivary glands, myocarditis, thyroiditis and thrombocytopenia.

## DIAGNOSIS

In clinically doubtful cases, mumps can be diagnosed by isolation of virus from the saliva or urine or by direct detection of mumps antigen in nasopharyngeal cells by direct immunofluorescence. Serological tests will confirm a rising antibody titre in acute and convalescent specimens. The serum amylase is raised in salivary gland swelling and pancreatitis should not be assumed to be present on this basis alone.

## TREATMENT

No specific therapy is available for mumps. The pain of mumps orchitis can be ameliorated by a scrotal support and a course of oral prednisolone, 40 mg/day, for 5 days but this does not prevent occasional testicular atrophy.

## PREVENTION

A live attenuated mumps vaccine is highly effective and is given as a component of the MMR vaccine in the second year of life. Occasionally vaccination is followed by mild parotid swelling and fever.

# $S$KIN INFECTIONS

# *Herpes simplex*

Herpes simplex virus (HSV) is a large DNA virus consisting of a nucleocapsid containing the viral DNA surrounded by protein and then a trilaminar outer envelope. Two distinct antigenic types of HSV exist (HSV-1 and HSV-2). Each is transmitted principally by intimate contact. Following primary infection HSV induces life-long latent infection in sensory nerve ganglia and recurrent infection occurs frequently. The factors that precipitate recurrences differ between individuals but include menstruation, fever, ultraviolet light, trauma and emotional stress. Herpes simplex type 1 is the chief cause of most non-genital HSV infections, whereas most cases of genital herpes (page 758) are due to HSV-2.

## CLINICAL FEATURES

Primary infection with HSV-1 is often asymptomatic. The commonest clinical manifestation is gingivostomatitis in a 1–5 year old child and is probably transmitted by kissing. There are vesicles or ulcers on the tongue, buccal mucosa, gingiva, lips and pharynx, and the child is feverish and irritable. The lesions are painful and there is cervical lymphadenopathy. The illness lasts for 1 to 2 weeks. In young adults primary infection often presents as an ulcerative pharyngitis.

Reactivation of HSV causes recurrent attacks of cold sores or herpes labialis. There is usually tingling in the skin followed by a crop of vesicles at the mucocutaneous junction of the lips or elsewhere around the mouth or nose. The vesicles only last for 1–2 days and then leave shallow ulcers. Systemic symptoms are rare and the illness only lasts for a few days.

Primary HSV skin infections may occur at any site as a result of direct inoculation of the virus through traumatized skin. This may occur as a result of wrestling (herpes gladiatorum) or other contact sports or by transfer of infection from the mouth to other areas via the fingers. Herpes simplex may infect the finger pulp after inoculation of HSV through a small skin abrasion. The resulting painful, deep, vesiculopustular lesions (herpetic whitlow) often recur.

Patients with defective cellular immunity, such as those with haematological or lymphoreticular malignancies, those taking immunosuppressive drugs and patients with acquired immune deficiency syndrome (AIDS), are at increased risk of severe cutaneous HSV. The other group of people who develop severe HSV skin infection are those with eczema, especially if they have been using topical steroid preparations: widespread cutaneous HSV results – a condition termed Kaposi's varicelliform eruption or eczema herpeticum.

The virus can also be inoculated into the eye to cause conjunctivitis and branching corneal ulcers (dendritic ulcers). Recurrent ocular lesions may involve deeper layers of the cornea (stromal keratitis).

The encephalitis that sometimes results from HSV infection is dealt with on page 694.

## DIAGNOSIS

Herpes simplex infection is usually clinically obvious but can be confirmed by electron microscopy of vesicular fluid or by growing the virus in tissue culture. Monoclonal antibodies are available to distinguish HSV-1 and HSV-2.

## TREATMENT

The treatment of HSV is with acyclovir, a thymidine analogue that selectively inhibits viral replication without any significant toxicity. Acyclovir needs to be phosphorylated before it has any antiviral activity and the first step in phosphorylation is dependent upon a herpes virus-encoded enzyme, thymidine kinase. Thus the drug is only active in virally infected cells and this accounts for its great therapeutic safety margin. The various HSV infections are treated with different formulations and dosages of acyclovir (Table 23.4).

**Table 23.4** Treatment of mucocutaneous herpes simplex infections.

| Gingivostomatitis | Acyclovir suspension, 200 mg, five times daily for 5 days |
|---|---|
| Herpes labialis | Patient-initiated 5% acyclovir cream or oral acyclovir tablets, 200 mg, five times daily for 5 days. Doses of 400 mg five times daily may be needed in immunosuppressed hosts. Acyclovir, 400–800 mg/day, can be used as prophylaxis for those with frequent attacks |
| Herpetic whitlow | Acyclovir 200–400 mg five times daily for 5–7 days |
| Eczema herpeticum | Severe cases may need i.v. acyclovir, 5 mg/kg, three times daily. Others can be given oral acyclovir, 200–400 mg, five times daily for 7 days |
| Corneal ulcers | 3% acyclovir eye ointment five times daily |

# Herpes zoster (shingles)

Following an initial infection with varicella-zoster virus (VZV) (chickenpox, page 724), the virus remains latent in the dorsal root ganglia. If the virus reactivates it causes pain and a rash in a sensory nerve distribution. Zoster can occur at any age but in normal individuals it is much more common in the elderly. Anything that depresses cellular immunity allows the virus to reactivate so that it is also common in patients with lymphoreticular malignancies, and those taking immunosuppressive drugs, and is being seen increasingly in young persons infected with HIV.

## CLINICAL FEATURES

The illness usually begins with pain in the area supplied by the affected sensory nerve, followed by the rash. The rash is unilateral and begins as a faint erythema on which the typical vesiculopustular eruption develops. Any dermatome may be involved although most cases are on the face or trunk. New lesions appear within the affected dermatome for several days and the eruption gradually scabs over 2 to 3 weeks. Herpes zoster is often much more severe in the immunosuppressed individual, in whom new lesions can continue to appear for several weeks.

## COMPLICATIONS

The complications of herpes zoster include:

1. Encephalitis (page 694).
2. Muscle weakness due to motor nerve involvement. The **Ramsay Hunt syndrome** is a combination of a lower motor nerve facial palsy and vesicles in or on the external ear. The weakness usually resolves after a few weeks.
3. Ocular problems after trigeminal involvement. The complications range from superficial keratitis to uveitis and secondary glaucoma. Patients with a red eye and ophthalmic zoster should be seen by an ophthalmologist.
4. The most frequent problem is postherpetic neuralgia, the pain persisting for months, and occasionally years, after the vesicles heal. This occurs in about 10 per cent of individuals but is much more common in the elderly. The pathogenesis of this pain is not fully understood.

## TREATMENT

Herpes zoster in the immunocompromised individual is treated with parenteral acyclovir. In the normal host either acyclovir, given either parenterally or in high doses orally, or oral famciclovir, a similar antiviral drug, will reduce the severity of the acute illness and are of some benefit in preventing postherpetic neuralgia.

# *Molluscum contagiosum*

Molluscum contagiosum is a benign disease caused by a poxvirus. The lesions are characteristic firm white cutaneous nodules, often with central umbilication. They vary greatly in number and tend to persist for a period of weeks to months. In patients with AIDS, the lesions may not resolve but continue to spread and enlarge: the diagnosis may be made by biopsy or electron microscopy. Physical stimulation of individual lesions by enucleation or application of silver nitrate may speed up healing.

# *Orf*

Orf virus is a poxvirus of sheep and goats which accidentally infects humans at the site of an abrasion or bite. Each lesion is a reddish papule that becomes a large haemorrhagic pustule on a red base. The lesions are usually on the hands. The pustule may rupture to leave an ulcerated nodule with a grey crust. The diagnosis is usually made clinically but can be confirmed by electron microscopy.

# *U*PPER RESPIRATORY TRACT INFECTIONS

# *Streptococcal sore throat*

Pyogenic streptococci are classified into groups by the presence of Lancefield cell wall polysaccharide antigens. Group A streptococci or *Streptococcus pyogenes* produce a clear zone of haemolysis (β-haemolysis) on blood agar, and are the species responsible for both acute pyogenic infections and the non-suppurative poststreptococcal sequelae of acute rheumatic fever and glomerulonephritis (pages 189 and 455). Some group A strains also produce erythrogenic toxin which is responsible for the rash of scarlet fever. Pharyngitis is one of the most common infections caused by *S. pyogenes*; other infections caused by this bacterium include otitis media, sinusitis and cellulitis.

## CLINICAL FEATURES

Streptococcal pharyngitis is most common between the ages of 5 and 15 years. After 2 or 3 days' incubation, acute sore throat, fever and headache develop. The fauces, uvula and soft palate are red and swollen and the tonsils enlarged with a yellow-white exudate. Local lymph nodes becomes enlarged and tender. The fever settles after a day or two. Sometimes infection spreads beyond the pharynx to cause an abscess in the peritonsillar soft tissues (a quinsy) or a retropharyngeal abscess, otitis media, sinusitis or suppurative lymphadenopathy.

# *Scarlet fever*

If the streptococcus produces erythrogenic toxin and the individual has no circulating antibody to the toxin, then the signs of scarlet fever may also be present. A punctate, erythematous rash that blanches on pressure appears on the upper chest on the second day of the illness and spreads to become generalized. The skinfolds in the axilla, groin and neck become darker pink or red (Pastia's lines). The skin often feels like fine sandpaper and the face is deep red with characteristic circumoral pallor. The tongue is covered with a white coating through which the red papillae are prominent (strawberry tongue). After about a week extensive desquamation of the skin occurs.

## DIAGNOSIS

Streptococcal sore throat can not be distinguished from viral pharyngitis on the basis of clinical features. The organism may be grown from throat swabs although it may also be found in asymptomatic subjects. More rapid diagnostic tests detect group A antigens in throat swab material by latex agglutination or enzyme techniques. Infection can also be diagnosed by determining the antibody response to various enzymes produced by the streptococcus: the anti-streptolysin O titre (ASOT) and anti-DNAase B titre are particularly valuable.

## COMPLICATIONS

### Rheumatic fever

This non-suppurative complication may follow 1–5 weeks after a group A streptococcal infection and is due to an autoimmune cross-reaction between streptococcal and human tissue antigens. The clinical features are described on page 189.

### Acute glomerulonephritis

This may follow either pharyngeal or cutaneous infection with a limited number of strains of group A streptococci (page 455).

## TREATMENT

Group A streptococci are always highly susceptible to penicillin. Therapy only has a minor effect upon the duration of the pharyngitis and is primarily given to prevent rheumatic fever. Mild disease is treated with oral penicillin (phenoxymethyl penicillin, 125–250 mg four times daily) for 10 days (shorter courses do not reliably eradicate the organism from the throat). Parenteral penicillin may be needed for more severe infections. A macrolide, such as erythromycin or clarithromycin, or clindamycin can be used in individuals allergic to penicillin.

# Infectious mononucleosis

Infectious mononucleosis (glandular fever) is caused by primary infection with Epstein–Barr virus (EBV), a herpes virus that occurs worldwide. In young children primary infection is usually asymptomatic but in adolescents and young adults about 50 per cent of infections result in infectious mononucleosis. Following primary infection the virus becomes latent in lymphocytes and virus is continually excreted in small amounts in the oropharyngeal secretions. The virus is of relatively low infectivity and is probably transmitted by saliva during kissing or the sharing of drinking vessels.

## CLINICAL FEATURES

The incubation period is several weeks. Epstein–Barr virus can infect B lymphocytes and cause them to undergo blast transformation and produce antibody. There is thus a polyclonal increase in immunoglobulins. The stimulation of B-cells provokes a vigorous T-cell response and it is the self-limited proliferation of T-cells that causes many of the clinical features of infectious mononucleosis. The characteristic symptoms are persistent fever, lassitude, malaise and sore throat. The tonsils are enlarged and covered with a white exudate, there is superficial lymphadenopathy in the neck and sometimes elsewhere, and about half the patients have palpable splenomegaly. A mild hepatitis is common but clinical hepatomegaly and jaundice are infrequent. Some patients have a transient macular rash and palatal petechiae are common but not pathognomonic.

## COMPLICATIONS

Complications of infectious mononucleosis include myocarditis, aseptic meningitis, transverse myelitis, haemolytic anaemia, thrombocytopenia, respiratory obstruction from tonsillar enlargement and faucial oedema, and splenic rupture. Almost all patients with infectious mononucleosis will develop an allergic rash if given ampicillin or amoxycillin: this does not mean that future use of penicillins must be avoided. Convalescence from infectious mononucleosis is often prolonged.

Separate from its link to infectious mononucleosis, EBV is also associated as a cofactor in several malignancies, including African Burkitt's lymphoma, nasopharyngeal carcinoma and possibly Hodgkin's disease and lymphomas in patients with AIDS.

## DIAGNOSIS

The blood film shows an absolute lymphocytosis with a large number of 'atypical' mononuclear cells. These T-lymphocytes are large cells with plentiful basophilic cytoplasm. Mild thrombocytopenia and alterations of liver function tests are common. In most cases of infectious mononucleosis the polyclonal immunoglobulin response includes antibodies capable of agglutinating sheep, horse and ox red blood cells (heterophile antibodies). These are detected by the Paul–Bunnell test (Table 23.5) or one of the rapid screening slide tests derived from it (such as the Monospot test). The test may remain positive for up to a year. If the Paul–Bunnell test is negative, as it is in around 20 per cent of cases, then the possibility of cytomegalovirus infection or toxoplasmosis needs consideration. In doubtful cases EBV infection can be confirmed by the detection of IgM antibodies against the viral capsid antigen (VCA). IgG antibodies to VCA merely indicate past infection, as do antibodies to EBV nuclear antigens (EBNA).

## TREATMENT

There is no specific treatment for infectious mononucleosis. Corticosteroid therapy is used for haemolytic anaemia and for thrombocytopenia: there is no clear evidence of the efficacy of steroids for those with neurological complications.

# Diphtheria

This infection is now rare in Western countries, but can easily return in the unimmunized population if hygiene and nourishment are poor as occurred in Russia during 1993.

*Corynebacterium diphtheriae* is a Gram-positive bacillus that may produce a potent exotoxin that inhibits protein synthesis in cells. The ability to produce toxin is contained in a bacteriophage and the amount of toxin produced by different strains of the bacterium varies markedly. Non-toxigenic strains of *C. diphtheriae* can produce pharyngitis but not diphtheria.

## CLINICAL FEATURES

After an incubation period of 2–4 days the clinical features depend upon the site of infection and the amount of toxin released.

1. Faucial diphtheria is the most common variety. There is pharyngitis and tonsillitis, malaise and fever, and a grey-white membrane adherent to the underlying mucous membrane. This membrane varies in extent from a small patch on the tonsils to involvement of the entire oropharynx. Regional lymphadenopathy and oedema produce a 'bullneck' appearance.
2. Nasal diphtheria tends to occur in young infants and resembles the common cold with a serosanguinous discharge.
3. Laryngeal diphtheria results if the membrane extends from the oropharynx to the larynx and trachea. Cough, dyspnoea and respiratory obstruction result.
4. Cutaneous diphtheria is most common in the tropics and causes a chronic shallow, punched out, skin ulcer. There is usually little toxin absorption from cutaneous infections.

**Table 23.5** Differentiation of heterophile antibody produced in infectious mononucleosis from the Forssman antibody (found in normal serum) and similar antibodies found in serum sickness. This is the basis of the Paul Bunnell test. The + signs indicate the degree of agglutination of sheep red cells by the serum.

| Source of serum | Unabsorbed | After absorption with | |
| --- | --- | --- | --- |
| | | Guinea-pig kidney | Ox red cells |
| Infectious mononucleosis | ++++ | +++ | 0 |
| Serum sickness | +++ | 0 | 0 |
| Forssman antibody | + | 0 | + |

# COMPLICATIONS

Respiratory obstruction may result from local oedema and membrane formation. The other complications of diphtheria are due to the systemic effects of toxin absorbed from the site of infection. Myocarditis appears during the second week and may result in arrhythmias and fatal circulatory failure. Neurological damage can result in palatal and other cranial nerve palsies, peripheral neuropathy and, rarely, paralysis of limbs and respiratory muscles, occurring in that order over the 7 weeks after acute infection. Tracheostomy and artificial ventilation may be necessary.

# DIAGNOSIS

Diagnosis of diphtheria is initially clinical since therapy must be started without delay. Confirmation of the diagnosis can be made by isolation of the bacterium and demonstration of its ability to produce toxin.

# TREATMENT

Treatment is primarily aimed at neutralization of the toxin. Diphtheria antitoxin (produced in horses) is given with due caution against anaphylaxis. The dose is in proportion to the severity of the local membrane formation. Benzylpenicillin or erythromycin will eliminate the organism and prevent further toxin production. The complications may require intensive care.

# PREVENTION

The mainstay of diphtheria prevention is immunization with toxoid in childhood. This is highly effective and booster doses every 10 years will maintain immunity. In persons over the age of 10 years, low-dose diphtheria vaccine is used to prevent the severe reactions that sometimes result from normal strength vaccine. Contacts of a case of diphtheria should have nose and throat swabs taken. Carriers should be treated with oral erythromycin and eradication confirmed by further swabs.

# Pertussis (whooping cough)

Whooping cough is an infection of the respiratory tract caused by *Bordetella pertussis* (or very occasionally *B. parapertussis*), small Gram-negative coccobacilli. The organisms produce exotoxins that damage the respiratory mucosa and stimulate lymphocytosis. *Bordetella pertussis* is highly transmissible by respiratory droplets and infection occurs worldwide, often in 4-yearly epidemic cycles.

## CLINICAL FEATURES

Infants receive no passive immunity from the mother and are susceptible to pertussis from birth. The most severe cases and 70 per cent of deaths occur in the first year of life: almost all cases occur in children under 5 years old. After an incubation period of 7–14 days (range 3–21 days), the clinical features of pertussis occur in three stages:

1. In the catarrhal stage the child has what appears to be an ordinary cold with profuse rhinorrhoea and malaise that persists for about 1 week. This is the period of extreme infectivity.
2. The paroxysmal stage is characterized by the development of episodes of paroxysmal coughing, occurring many times each day. Each paroxysm consists of a rapid series of explosive coughs during which the child may become cyanosed. Vomiting often follows the coughing. The attack may end with the characteristic inspiratory whoop as air is drawn in through the narrowed glottis. Paroxysm after paroxysm renders the child miserable and exhausted. There is a marked lymphocytosis during this stage of the illness which lasts for 2–4 weeks. Partially immune subjects and young infants may not have the typical paroxysms of coughing or lymphocytosis. Complications at this stage include pneumonia (saliva and vomitus may be inhaled during the whoop) and atelectasis, traumatic ulcers

on the frenum of the tongue, conjunctival haemorrhages and rectal prolapse from the force of the coughing. Cerebral anoxia and convulsions can occur.

3. During the convalescent stage, which lasts 3–4 weeks, the paroxysms gradually become less severe and frequent. The prolonged illness may cause nutritional problems and exhaustion of the parents as well as the child. Atelectasis and plugging of small airways can result in bronchiectasis as a late complication of pertussis.

## DIAGNOSIS

The clinical diagnosis of whooping cough can be supported by the finding of an absolute lymphocytosis and confirmed by isolation of *B. pertussis* from a pernasal swab. Unfortunately the diagnosis is often not considered until the paroxysmal stage, when the chances of bacterial isolation are considerably diminished.

## TREATMENT

Erythromycin, if given during the catarrhal stage, will limit the severity of the infection but, once the paroxysmal stage has become established, antibiotics do not influence the disease. At this stage treatment is supportive. Very young infants should be admitted to hospital for vigilant nursing care and prevention of aspiration pneumonia.

## PREVENTION

Active immunization is effective in preventing pertussis and the triple vaccine (diphtheria, tetanus and pertussis) is given as early in life as possible because of the risks of pertussis in infancy. The risks of pertussis immunization have been greatly exaggerated: it should be advised for all infants except those with progressive neurological diseases or a history of severe reactions to previous pertussis immunization (page 718). New vaccines with increased immunogenicity and even lower complication rates are being introduced.

# Influenza

Influenza viruses, of which there are three types – A, B and C – are RNA-containing orthomyxoviruses. The viruses have an outer envelope studded with two glycoprotein antigens, haemagglutinin and neuraminidase (Fig. 23.5). Each of these antigens can exist in a variety of subtypes (shifts) and within each subtype there are other minor antigenic differences (drifts). Major antigenic shifts often result in severe epidemics or pandemics of influenza since the population has little or no immunity against the new subtype, whereas minor antigenic drift causes less severe outbreaks of infection because subtype-specific immunity is still present and offers partial protection.

Major outbreaks of influenza A tend to occur every 2–3 years and influenza B every 4–5 years; influenza C rarely produces disease in humans.

## CLINICAL FEATURES

The incubation period is 1–3 days. Onset is abrupt with fever, chills, myalgia and headache developing over a few hours. Dry cough and sore throat develop and the illness persists for up to 1 week. In some patients convalescence is prolonged for several weeks.

## COMPLICATIONS

Complications of influenza include viral pneumonitis, secondary bacterial pneumonia, particularly caused by *Staphylococcus aureus*, myocarditis and encephalitis.

## DIAGNOSIS

Influenza virus can be isolated from the respiratory tract during the acute illness but a more rapid procedure is the direct immunofluorescent detection of influenza antigen in cells from a nasopharyngeal aspirate. Serological diagnosis is chiefly of epidemiological interest.

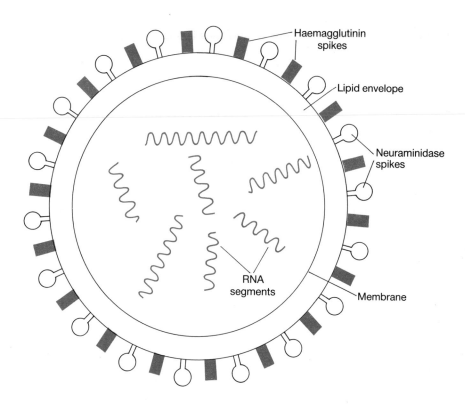

**Figure 23.5** Structure of influenza virus.

## TREATMENT

Symptomatic management with analgesics and antipyretics is usually combined with bed rest. Antibiotics are used for bacterial superinfection: an antistaphylococcal antibiotic should be included in the empirical therapy of severe pneumonia occurring in an influenza epidemic.

Amantadine hydrochloride therapy is moderately effective for influenza A infections but needs to be given early in the illness and is of no help in influenza B or C infections.

## PREVENTION

Immunization with killed virus vaccines offers about 70 per cent protection against infection. New vaccines have to be prepared and administered each year to provide protection against the antigenic drifts of influenza virus. Vaccination is directed primarily against those with chronic cardiorespiratory disease, the elderly and those working in the health service. Amantadine given daily, offers short-term protection against influenza A and may be useful in controlling epidemics amongst non-immunized populations.

# GASTROINTESTINAL INFECTIONS

## Viral gastroenteritis

Infective diarrhoea is one of the major causes of death in children in the developing world and even in Britain it is one of the ten most common causes of hospital admission in children. Viruses are now known to be the most common cause of severe diarrhoea in infants and young children, accounting for 40 per cent or more of cases. The

**Table 23.6** Characteristics of viruses causing diarrhoea.

| Virus | Nucleic acid |
| --- | --- |
| Rotavirus | Double-stranded RNA |
| Adenovirus | DNA |
| Norwalk virus | RNA |
| Caliciviruses | Single-stranded RNA |
| Astroviruses | RNA |
| Coronaviruses | Single-stranded RNA |

viruses responsible include rotaviruses, adenoviruses, astroviruses, caliciviruses, coronaviruses, Norwalk virus and other small, round viruses (Table 23.6).

## ROTAVIRUSES

Rotaviruses are named after their structural resemblance to a spoked wheel. They are responsible for about half the cases of watery diarrhoea in infants and young children worldwide. The greatest incidence is between 3 and 15 months of life and the peak prevalence of infection is in the winter and early spring. The initial symptoms are often respiratory with cough and runny nose, followed by fever, vomiting and watery diarrhoea lasting for 5–7 days. The virus is found in large quantities in the faeces and a number of antigen assays are available. Treatment is symptomatic. An oral rotavirus vaccine is under development.

## ADENOVIRUSES

Enteric adenoviruses (types 40 and 41) cause gastroenteritis predominantly in children aged less than 2 years. The illness is typically longer lasting but milder than that caused by rotaviruses, and respiratory symptoms are rare.

## NORWALK VIRUS

This agent is the cause of outbreaks of gastroenteritis that occur in all age groups, often as a result of eating inadequately cooked shellfish harvested from sewage-polluted water. Person-to-person spread may occur by the airborne route (probably from aerosols generated by vomiting). The incubation period is 12–48 hours and then there is malaise, anorexia, abdominal cramps and headache. Vomiting, often copious and projectile, and/or watery diarrhoea lasts for 1 to 2 days.

## OTHER ENTERIC VIRUSES

A number of other viruses (Table 23.6) are now recognized as causing diarrhoea, particularly in childhood. They are all diagnosed from electron microscopical examination of the stools.

# Cholera

*Vibrio cholerae* is a comma-shaped Gram-negative organism that only infects humans. Cholera is primarily spread via contaminated water supplies as the classical studies of John Snow demonstrated in the streets of London's Soho in the middle of the last century. Over the past few decades the geographic distribution of the disease has spread to involve much of Asia, Africa and, recently, South America. The vibrios produce a toxin which stimulates cyclic adenosine monophosphate activity in the small intestine and this in turn results in massive secretion of chloride and inhibition of sodium and water absorption.

## CLINICAL FEATURES

The incubation period is often only a few hours before abdominal fullness and profound watery diarrhoea develop. The stools are watery, odourless and contain flecks of mucus ('rice-water' stools). If fluid and electrolyte replacement is inadequate then hypovolaemia, shock, renal failure, acidosis and ultimately intracellular dehydration and death follow.

## TREATMENT

Rehydration is the mainstay of treatment of cholera and this can usually be achieved orally, although occasionally intravenous administration of fluid is necessary. In order to absorb sodium (and hence water) from oral rehydration solutions, glucose, sucrose or starch must be

**Table 23.7** Features of intestinal infections caused by *Escherichia coli*.

| Feature | ETEC | EPEC | EIEC | EHEC |
|---------|------|------|------|------|
| Pathogenesis | Enterotoxins | Unknown | Invasion | Cytotoxin |
| Site of infection | Small intestine | Small intestine | Colon | Colon |
| Epidemiology | Travellers' diarrhoea | Infant diarrhoea | Foodborne outbreaks | Sporadic or foodborne outbreaks |
| Type of diarrhoea | Watery | Watery | Dysenteric | Dysenteric |

ETEC = enterotoxigenic *E. coli*. EPEC = enteropathogenic *E. coli*. EIEC = enteroinvasive *E. coli*. EHEC = enterohaemorrhagic *E. coli*.

added since sodium absorption is linked to absorption of these other substances and this is not inhibited by cholera toxin. Antibiotics (e.g. tetracycline) will reduce the length of the illness.

## PREVENTION

The current parenteral cholera vaccine provides poor protection and is not recommended. Oral cholera vaccines consisting of live, non-toxin-producing strains of *V. cholerae* (often combined with the binding subunit of cholera toxin) have been developed and are effective.

# *Escherichia coli intestinal infections*

*Escherichia coli* produce diarrhoea by several different pathogenic mechanisms (Table 23.7).

1. Enterotoxigenic *E. coli* (ETEC) are responsible for at least 50 per cent of cases of travellers' diarrhoea but are uncommon causes of diarrhoea in industrialized countries. They produce two distinct enterotoxins that act in a similar way to cholera toxin. The organisms are spread via faecally polluted food or water and the incubation period is 12 to 72 hours. The illness consists of a few days of watery diarrhoea with some abdominal cramps and nausea but little or no fever. Often oral rehydration is all the treatment that is needed but the more severe cases may need

antibiotic therapy: a quinolone is probably the best available choice.
2. Enteropathogenic *E. coli* (EPEC) adhere to small bowel cells and produce 1 to 2 weeks of diarrhoea in young infants. The mechanism is not clearly understood.
3. Enteroinvasive *E. coli* (EIEC) produce a dysenteric illness similar to *Shigella* (see below).
4. Enterohaemorrhagic *E. coli* (EHEC) adhere to the mucosa of the distal ileum and proximal colon and produce a powerful cytotoxin (verotoxin). The incubation period is more than 1 week and there is severe abdominal pain, distention and tenderness associated with diarrhoea that may contain blood. In about 10 per cent of cases systemically absorbed verotoxin leads to intravascular haemolysis which in turn leads to the haemolytic uraemic syndrome. These infections may be associated with the consumption of poorly cooked beef (particularly hamburgers) but person-to-person spread also occurs.

# *Shigellosis (bacillary dysentery)*

There are four species of *Shigella* (*S. sonnei*, *S. flexneri*, *S. boydii* and *S. dysenteriae*). The infective dose is very small and infection is usually spread from person-to-person by the faecal–oral route. Infection is found worldwide. In developing tropical countries most cases are due to *S. dysen-*

teriae and *S. flexneri*: in the UK outbreaks of *S. sonnei* infection occur in conditions of poor hygiene such as nursery schools, prisons, mental hospitals etc.

## CLINICAL FEATURES

Bacillary dysentery has an incubation period of 2–3 days and is characterized by severe lower abdominal pain, bloody mucoid stools, fever, systemic toxicity and tenesmus. In young children, hyperpyrexia and convulsions may occur. The severity of the disease is very variable: *S. sonnei* infection is generally mild and lasts only a few days, *S. flexneri* and *S. boydii* cause more severe illnesses lasting for a week or more and epidemics of *S. dysenteriae* infection are associated with an appreciable mortality.

Reiter's syndrome (page 570) may follow dysentery.

## DIAGNOSIS

The definitive laboratory test is stool culture: organisms may be excreted in the bowel for a few weeks after recovery.

## TREATMENT

Well-absorbed oral antibiotics to which the organism is sensitive shorten the duration and reduce the severity of the illness. Treatment can also be used to eradicate the organisms from the bowel and render the patient non-infectious in conditions of poor hygiene. Resistance to ampicillin, cotrimoxazole and tetracyclines is now very common among *Shigella*. Quinolones are probably the best first-line agents in adults. Antimotility agents should not be used as they prolong the illness.

# Salmonellosis

*Salmonella typhi*, the cause of typhoid (page 752), is a strict human pathogen but the more than 2000 other strains of salmonellae are ubiquitous intestinal parasites of most domestic and wild animals. Most are strains of *S. enteritidis* that cause an acute enterocolitis after accidental transmission to humans, usually as a result of poor food hygiene. Poultry and egg products account for the majority of cases: there has been an epidemic of infection in Britain in recent years caused by a strain of *S. enteritidis* that can spread transovarially in chickens and is hence present within egg yolks. One infected egg is capable of contaminating large batches of mayonnaise or other uncooked egg-based products.

## CLINICAL FEATURES

Infection with salmonellae begins with diarrhoea, abdominal pain, fever, nausea and vomiting 12 to 48 hours after ingestion. The illness usually resolves within 4 or 5 days although sufferers may continue to be asymptomatic and excrete the organism in their stools for several months. More severe illness and septicaemia is seen in very young or elderly persons. It is also a particular problem in individuals with AIDS, in whom recurrences of septicaemia are likely to occur. These illnesses are similar to typhoid (page 752). Following bloodborne spread salmonellae may cause focal infections including osteomyelitis, meningitis and abscesses.

## DIAGNOSIS

Salmonellae can be cultured from the stools and from the blood in more severe cases.

## TREATMENT

Uncomplicated enterocolitis usually only requires fluid replacement. Antibiotic therapy with chloramphenicol, trimethoprim, ampicillin or a quinolone may be used for bacteraemic and localized infections. The use of antibiotics in uncomplicated salmonella enterocolitis has not been encouraged since older agents did not influence the acute illness and may have prolonged the period of chronic carriage of salmonellae. Ciprofloxacin and other fluoroquinolone agents, however, may be beneficial in treating salmonella enterocolitis and do not seem to lead to increased carriage (indeed they may reduce the frequency of chronic carriage).

# Campylobacter enteritis

*Campylobacter jejuni* is a spiral Gram-negative rod that is one of the most common causes of acute enterocolitis in the UK. It is found in the gut of many animals and birds. Most human cases are sporadic and are transmitted via undercooked meat or poultry, milk or water.

## CLINICAL FEATURES

The incubation period ranges from 1 to 7 days and there may be a non-specific prodrome of fever and malaise for a few hours before diarrhoea and severe, cramping abdominal pain start. The clinical features of infection are indistinguishable from those of salmonella food poisoning or *Shigella* dysentery, although the abdominal pain tends to be more severe and prolonged. Most cases resolve within a week although excretion of the organism in the faeces can persist for several weeks.

## COMPLICATIONS

Septicaemia is rare and complications infrequent: reactive arthritis (as with all forms of infective colitis) and the Guillain–Barré syndrome may occur a week or two later.

## TREATMENT

If therapy is commenced early enough, erythromycin or ciprofloxacin may shorten the duration of diarrhoea.

# Yersinia infections

Most human infection with the zoonotic pathogens *Y. enterocolitica* and *Y. pseudotuberculosis* follow ingestion of contaminated food, water and milk.

## CLINICAL FEATURES

The incubation period is a few days. In young children the illness is an enterocolitis lasting for 1–2 weeks, whereas in older persons there is terminal ileitis and mesenteric adenitis with features that mimic acute appendicitis. Erythema nodosum may occur.

## COMPLICATIONS

Bacteraemia and focal abscesses may complicate the illness in adults.

## TREATMENT

Enterocolitis does not require antibiotic therapy as it settles spontaneously in 1–2 weeks. Septicaemic illnesses and focal abscesses respond to tetracycline, cotrimoxazole, third generation cephalosporins and aminoglycosides.

# Food poisoning

Salmonellosis, yersiniosis and campylobacteriosis are three forms of food poisoning. Other bacterial causes, either intoxications or infections, are shown in Table 23.8.

# Antibiotic-associated colitis

Antibiotic-associated colitis (AAC) is caused by cytotoxins produced by *Clostridium difficile*. In the more severe cases there is formation of a pseudomembrane over the colonic mucosa (**pseudomembranous colitis**). It may follow administration of any antibiotic (which induce *C. difficile* to produce increased amounts of toxin).

## CLINICAL FEATURES

Antibiotic-associated colitis typically starts 4–10 days after commencement of antibiotic administration with sudden watery, foul smelling, green, non-bloody diarrhoea associated with abdominal cramps, leukocytosis and fever.

**Table 23.8** Features of bacterial causes of food poisoning.

| Organism | Source | Incubation period | Symptoms |
|---|---|---|---|
| **Toxins** | | | |
| *Bacillus cereus* (type 1) | Rice | 1–6 hours | Vomiting |
| *Bacillus cereus* (type 2) | Meat, dried foods and dairy products | 6–24 hours | Watery diarrhoea |
| *Staphylococcus aureus* | Meats, salads and cream | 2–4 hours | Vomiting |
| *Clostridium botulinum* | Preserved and tinned vegetables, meat and fish | 18–36 hours | Neuromuscular paralysis |
| *C. perfringens* | Meat | 8–20 hours | Watery diarrhoea |
| **Infections** | | | |
| Salmonella | Poultry, eggs and meat | 8–48 hours | Watery or bloody diarrhoea |
| *Campylobacter jejuni* | Poultry, water and milk | 48–96 hours | Watery or bloody diarrhoea |
| *Vibrio parahaemolyticus* | Shellfish | 10–24 hours | Watery diarrhoea |
| *Yersinia enterocolitica* | Meat, water and milk | 1–10 days | Watery or bloody diarrhoea; mesenteric adenitis |

If the antibiotic is stopped then the illness usually settles within a week. More severe cases have mucosal oedema and necrosis and a yellowish pseudomembrane visible over the mucosa at sigmoidoscopy. Toxic megacolon and perforation may occur.

## DIAGNOSIS

The diagnosis is made by culture of the organism and cytotoxin assay from the stools.

## TREATMENT

Specific treatment is needed for the more severe cases and treatment is with oral vancomycin or metronidazole for 7–14 days: this gives an initial cure rate of more than 90 per cent. Relapses are not infrequent – possibly due to sporulation and persistence of the bacteria throughout therapy.

# Giardiasis

*Giardia lamblia* is a flagellate protozoan which is a major cause of diarrhoeal infection in the world. The organism lives as a trophozoite form, attached by a sucking disc to the mucosa, in the small intestine and produces thin-walled cysts.

These are passed in the faeces and infect others via faecally contaminated water (the cysts can survive chlorination of drinking water). Infection is sometimes found among homosexual men and children in daycare and is frequent among travellers.

## CLINICAL FEATURES

Many infections remain asymptomatic but in some, after an incubation period of 1–3 weeks, diarrhoea, abdominal distension and flatulence develop. Malabsorption may result from villus damage in the small intestine and lead to frothy, greasy stools and weight loss. Most patients recover spontaneously over weeks or months. Severe infections occur in patients with hypogammaglobulinaemia.

## DIAGNOSIS

Microscopical examination of the stools may reveal the cysts but even after three specimens the detection rate is not 100 per cent; duodenal aspiration or biopsy to find the trophozoites may be needed.

## TREATMENT

Therapy for giardiasis is with metronidazole, 2 g, once daily for 3 days.

# Cryptosporidiosis

This protozoan is found in many domestic and wild animals and is a relatively common cause of transient watery diarrhoea and fever, especially in young children and visitors to countries which have water supplies contaminated from animal sources. It is also a major cause of devastating watery diarrhoea and malabsorption in persons with AIDS. Involvement of the biliary tract also sometimes occurs in patients with AIDS.

## DIAGNOSIS

Diagnosis is made by visualization of the 2–4 μm cysts by a modified acid-fast or iodine stain of the stool.

## TREATMENT

There is no effective therapy for this infection, although a number of antibiotics are being tested in patients with cryptosporidiosis and AIDS.

# Amoebiasis

*Entamoeba histolytica* exists as a trophozoite that dwells in the lumen and on the wall of the human colon, particularly the ascending colon, and feeds upon bacteria and tissue cells. As the faeces become more solid the amoebae encyst and the cysts are passed in the stool. Transmission to a fresh host is via contaminated water or vegetables (or occasionally by direct faecal–oral spread). Incidence of infection is very high in many areas of the world. In the UK it is particularly common in immigrants and homosexual men. Asymptomatic infection is common and even those with illness often only have mild, chronic, intermittent diarrhoea and abdominal pain. Occasionally, for reasons that are poorly understood, trophozoites invade the colonic tissues and produce dysenteric symptoms (which are often less florid than those in bacillary dysentery). Spread of trophozoites to the liver via the portal vein may occur.

## CLINICAL FEATURES

Most patients with amoebiasis have intermittent complaints of diarrhoea, abdominal pain and flatulence over many months or years. During the episodes of diarrhoea the stools are foul-smelling and contain some mucus and blood. Systemic symptoms are limited to general malaise. Acute amoebic colitis occurs more often in debilitated or pregnant women or those receiving corticosteroids. The patient has an abrupt high fever, abdominal cramps and profuse bloody stools. There is marked abdominal tenderness and often liver tenderness also. There is usually a polymorphonuclear leukocytosis.

## COMPLICATIONS

Complications of acute amoebic dysentery are:

1. Fulminant colitis with toxic megacolon
2. Bowel perforation
3. Massive haemorrhage
4. A tumour-like mass of granulation tissue (amoeboma) in the colon
5. Colonic strictures.

Patients with amoebic liver abscesses often give no history of amoebic dysentery but present with fever and tender hepatomegaly. The abscess is usually single and more often in the right lobe of the liver. There is often a specific point of maximal tenderness over the abscess and the chest X-ray shows a raised right hemidiaphragm. Liver transaminase levels are usually well preserved but the alkaline phosphatase is often elevated. The presence of an abscess cavity will usually show on ultrasound scan and if the abscess is aspirated the necrotic liver tissue obtained has an appearance classically likened to anchovy sauce. If not treated a liver abscess is likely to rupture into any contiguous structure leading to empyema, pneumonia, pericarditis, peritonitis or, rarely, a subcutaneous abscess and ulceration.

## DIAGNOSIS

Amoebiasis is diagnosed by finding cysts or trophozoites in the stools or in rectal mucus obtained at sigmoidoscopy. The trophozoites can be distinguished from commensal, non-pathogenic species of amoebae by the presence of ingested red cells.

Amoebic infection can also be diagnosed by the amoebic fluorescent antibody test (FAT), which is positive in most patients with symptomatic intestinal disease and almost all those with liver abscesses. In those with asymptomatic cyst excretion the serological tests are often negative.

## TREATMENT

Invasive colitis and amoebic liver abscesses can be treated with oral metronidazole, 800 mg, 8-hourly given for 5 days for intestinal infections and for 10–14 days for hepatic or other extraintestinal spread, but this is primarily a tissue amoebicide and is less effective against organisms in the gut lumen. It should be followed, therefore, by 5–10 days of diloxanide furoate, which is a luminal amoebicide. Diloxanide furoate alone will cure asymptomatic intraluminal infections and eliminate cysts.

# *I*NTESTINAL NEMATODES

Several roundworms live within the human bowel. Most do not cause very severe symptoms and their major impact is often psychological rather than medical. They are contracted either by the faecal–oral route (usually in under-developed communities) or via larval forms which penetrate the skin (Table 23.9). Most are diagnosed by microscopic examination of the stools for their ova. Prevention of most roundworm infections depends upon adequate sanitation.

## *Enterobiasis*

*Enterobius vermicularis*, the common threadworm or pinworm, is the only worm commonly found in the UK in those who have never been abroad. It is especially prevalent among school children. The adult worms live in the colon and the females migrate at night to lay eggs upon the perianal skin. The eggs are then transferred on fingers to the mouth to autoinfect the host or to transmit the infection to others. The only symptom is intense perianal itching, particularly at night. The adult worms can sometimes be seen in the stools and the diagnosis can be confirmed by applying clear adhesive tape to the perianal region and then examining the tape microscopically for adherent eggs. Treatment should be administered to the entire family. A single dose of mebendazole, pyrantel pamoate or piperazine, repeated 2 weeks later is effective.

## *Trichuriasis*

*Trichuris trichiura* (whipworm) is a very common infection in tropical countries. The adults are 3–5 cm long and live attached to the mucosa of

**Table 23.9** Intestinal nematodes and clinical features.

| Worm | Mode of infection | Site of infection | Clinical features |
|------|-------------------|-------------------|-------------------|
| *Ascaris lumbricoides* | Faecal–oral | Small bowel | Intestinal obstruction; malabsorption |
| Hookworms (*Necator americanus, Ancylostoma duodenale*) | Larval skin penetration | Small bowel | Iron-deficiency anaemia |
| *Trichuris trichiura* | Faecal–oral | Large bowel | Dysentery, rectal prolapse |
| *Enterobius vermicularis* | Faecal–oral | Rectum/colon | Anal pruritus |
| *Strongyloides stercoralis* | Larval skin penetration | Small bowel | Malabsorption |

the large bowel. The eggs are excreted in the faeces and develop further in moist soil. Infective eggs are ingested by another human host, thus completing the life-cycle. Most infections are asymptomatic but heavy infections can cause mucosal damage and bloody diarrhoea. Rectal prolapse can be caused by very heavy worm loads. Mebendazole is effective therapy for symptomatic infections.

# Ascariasis

Infection with *Ascaris lumbricoides* is very common worldwide, particularly in tropical countries. The worm is about the same size and shape as the common earthworm but is cream in colour. The life-cycle is shown in Fig. 23.6. Large numbers of larvae migrating through the lungs can produce an allergic pneumonitis in persons with hypersensitivity from a previous infection. Cough, wheeze and flitting pulmonary infiltrates are common and the larvae may be found in the sputum. Light infections with adult worms are usually asymptomatic but large numbers of adult worms can cause abdominal

pain and interfere with small bowel absorption. A bolus of worms can cause intestinal obstruction and single worms can migrate to block the bile duct or appendix. Mebendazole is the most effective therapy.

# Hookworm

Infection with one or other of the two species of human hookworm affects more than 25 per cent of the world's population in subtropical and tropical climates. The adults are about 1 cm in length and live attached to the mucosa of the small bowel. They suck blood, each *Ancylostoma* ingesting up to 0.2 ml every day: heavy infections and the 2–10 year life-span of the hookworms eventually lead to iron-deficiency anaemia and hypoalbuminaemia. The eggs develop into larvae in warm, moist soil and these larvae are capable of penetrating intact human skin. The full life-cycle is shown in Fig. 23.7. Mebendazole given twice daily for 3 days is effective in both types of hookworm.

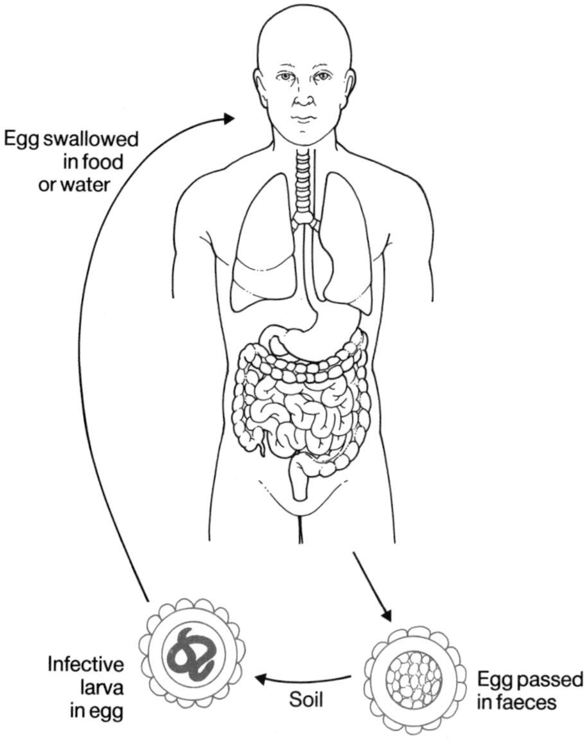

**Egg swallowed in food or water**

**Infective larva in egg**

**Soil**

**Egg passed in faeces**

**Figure 23.6** Life-cycle of *Ascaris lumbricoides*.

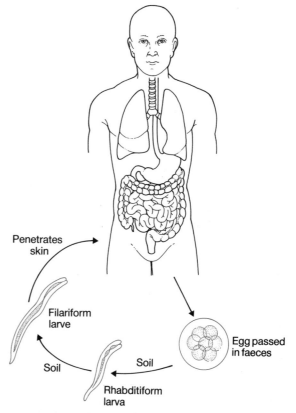

**Penetrates skin**

**Filariform larve**

**Soil**

**Rhabditiform larva**

**Soil**

**Egg passed in faeces**

**Figure 23.7** Life-cycle of hookworm.

# *Strongyloidiasis*

Infection with *Stronglyoides stercoralis* is not common but has important implications. One is that autoinfection can occur so that infection can persist for several decades. The other is that generalized and sometimes fatal infections can occur in immunosuppressed individuals. *Strongyloides* infections are particularly common in former Far East prisoners of war who worked on the infamous Burma–Thailand railway. The life-cycle is shown in Fig. 23.8. The adult females live and lay their eggs in the duodenal mucosa. The eggs hatch into rhabdiform larvae which are usually passed in the faeces. Sometimes these larvae can develop into infective filariform larvae which can penetrate the perianal skin leading to autoinfection. As larvae migrate through the body they can produce a characteristic, rapidly elongating (about 1–2 cm/hour) pruritic skin rash. This settles after a day or so, only to reappear at intervals over many years. Infections with adult worms are often asymptomatic but can cause abdominal pain similar to that of a peptic ulcer, diarrhoea and weight loss. There is usually an eosinophilia. Massive hyperinfection with enterocolitis and malabsorption can occur in the immunocompromised patient.

*Strongyloides* infections can be diagnosed by finding larvae in the faeces or duodenal fluid or by serological tests for antibodies. Immigrants and others in whom infection is possible need to be carefully screened prior to organ transplantation or other forms of immunosuppression. Treatment is with thiabendazole which must be given for 1 to 2 weeks in the hyperinfection syndrome.

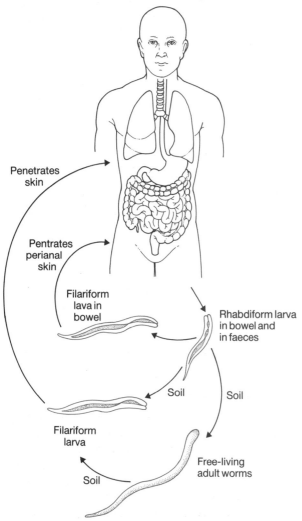

**Figure 23.8** Life-cycle of *Strongyloides stercoralis.*

# *Tapeworm infections*

Tapeworms have both definitive hosts, in which the adult worms inhabit the bowel, and intermediate hosts, which harbour the larval forms. Humans are the definitive host for four tapeworms:

1. *Taenia saginata* (beef tapeworm)
2. *T. solium* (pork tapeworm)
3. *Diphyllobothrium latum* (fish tapeworm)
4. *Hymenolepis nana* (dwarf tapeworm)

Taeniasis is acquired by eating undercooked beef (*T. saginata*) or pork (*T. solium*) which harbours the encysted larvae. The adults are several metres in length and the terminal segments containing eggs are shed in the faeces to be eaten by cattle or pigs, which serve as intermediate hosts. The pork tapeworm is particularly dangerous to humans in that the eggs, after ingestion via the faeco–oral route, can develop into larvae and encyst, producing mass lesions in almost any part of the body (cysticercosis).

*Diphyllobothrium latum* is acquired from eating raw fish: the adult worm competes with the host for vitamin $B_{12}$ and megaloblastic anaemia can occur.

Tapeworms are diagnosed by finding proglottides (segments of the adult worm) in the faeces and all can be treated with praziquantel or niclosamide.

# NEUROLOGICAL INFECTIONS

See also page 694 for poliomyelitis.

# Bacterial meningitis

Many bacteria are capable of causing inflammation of the meninges but most cases of acute pyogenic meningitis are caused by one of a small number of important pathogens. Neonatal meningitis is usually caused by Gram-negative bacilli, group B streptococci or *Listeria monocytogenes*. In older children and adults, *Neisseria meningitidis, Streptococcus pneumoniae* and type b *Haemophilus influenzae* (the latter almost exclusively in preschool age children) are the three commonest pathogens. *Staphylococcus aureus* may cause meningitis in association with trauma, endocarditis and neurosurgery.

## CLINICAL FEATURES

Symptoms and signs of bacterial meningitis are caused by meningeal inflammation, raised intracranial pressure, cerebral ischaemia and disturbance of cerebrospinal fluid circulation. Characteristic features are fever, headache, photophobia, neck stiffness and a positive Kernig sign (hamstring spasm and inability to extend the knee passively with the patient supine and the hip flexed to 90°). These features of meningeal irritation (meningism) may be combined with vomiting, confusion, depression of consciousness and cranial nerve palsies. The specific signs of meningism may be absent in very young or very old patients. Bacterial meningitis often progresses very rapidly and its recognition requires a constant level of awareness.

Various forms of bacterial meninigitis may have more specific features.

## Neisseria meningitidis (meningococcus)

This condition is most common in young children and may occur in sporadic or epidemic form. The organism is a Gram-negative diplococcus that is often carried asymptomatically in the oropharynx. Meningitis is often accompanied by septicaemia with a petechial or purpuric rash, septic shock and disseminated intravascular coagulation (DIC) (page 645) leading to haemorrhagic infarction of the adrenal glands and other organs (Waterhouse–Friderichsen syndrome). A fulminant infection with coma and death within a few hours can occur.

## Streptococcus pneumoniae (pneumococcus)

The pneumococcus is a Gram-positive diplococcus that causes meningitis particularly in the very young and the elderly and in individuals with predisposing factors such as sickle cell disease, asplenism, alcoholism, multiple myeloma or fractures in the base of the skull. Half the cases are accompanied by sinusitis, otitis media or pneumonia. Hydrocephalus, convulsions and permanent neurological sequelae are more common than with other forms of meningitis.

## Haemophilus influenzae

This small Gram-negative coccobacillus rarely causes meningitis in those over 6 years old, yet it was still the most common form of bacterial meningitis in the UK prior to the introduction of *H. influenzae* vaccination. The onset may be more subacute than in other forms of meningitis and often follows symptoms of an upper respiratory tract infection.

## DIAGNOSIS

Whenever meningitis is suspected it is essential to perform a lumbar puncture and to examine the CSF biochemically and microbiologically in order to distinguish acute bacterial from viral or tuberculous infections. The typical features of the various forms of meningitis are shown in Table 23.10. The yield of microbiological investigations may be reduced by prior antibiotic therapy but various antigen detection techniques can be used upon the CSF to provide a specific aetiological diagnosis.

## COMPLICATIONS

Focal or generalized seizures may occur. Focal neurological signs can be related to cranial nerve involvement from the inflammation of the basal meninges or arteries. Infection or infarction of the cerebral cortex can also cause neurological deficit. A brain abscess or subdural collection of pus may result in papilloedema from raised intracranial pressure. Septic shock and DIC are other acute complications.

## TREATMENT

Bacterial meningitis is a true medical emergency and antibiotic therapy should be started as soon as possible, if necessary before the precise aetiology has been confirmed. Suitable antibiotic regimens are shown in Table 23.11. Treatment for shock and DIC (page 645) should

**Table 23.11** Antibiotic treatment of bacterial meningitis.

| | |
|---|---|
| Meningococcal | Intravenous benzylpenicillin, 150 mg/kg/day, given 4-hourly for 5–7 days. Chloramphenicol, 100 mg/kg/day, or cefotaxime, 150–200 mg/kg/day, for penicillin-allergic patients |
| Pneumococcal | As above, except that treatment should be continued for 10–14 days |
| *Haemophilus influenzae* | Cefotaxime, 150–200 mg/kg/day, given 6-hourly for 7–10 days. Chloramphenicol or ampicillin may be used once the organism is known to be sensitive |
| Neonatal meningitis | Ampicillin, 300 mg/kg/day, given 4 hourly plus an aminoglycoside, given for 2–3 weeks |
| Organism unknown | |
|   Child under 6 years | As for *H. influenzae* above |
|   Patient over 6 years | As for meningococcal above |

**Table 23.10** The cerebrospinal fluid changes in various forms of meningitis.

| | Normal | Pyogenic bacteria | Viral meningitis | Tuberculous meningitis |
|---|---|---|---|---|
| Appearance | Clear | Turbid/purulent | Clear/opalescent | Clear/opalescent |
| White cells/mm³ | 0–5 | 5–5000 | 5–500 | 5–2000 |
| Predominant cell type | Lymphocytes | Neutrophils | Lymphocytes | Lymphocytes |
| Glucose (% of blood concentration) | 2.2–3.3 mmol/l (>60) | Very low (<45) | Normal* (>60) | Low (<45) |
| Protein (mg/l) | <400 | >600 | 400–800 | >600 |
| Other tests | | Bacteria on Gram stain | | Bacteria on Ziehl–Neelson stain or fluorescent antigen detectable |

*Occasionally low in mumps meningitis.

be instituted if necessary. Many of the complications of bacterial meningitis are consequent upon the release of tumour necrosis factor and other cytokines by bacterial products. Attempts to counter the release of these by treatment with monoclonal antibodies are under investigation. The only form of adjunctive therapy of proven benefit in meningitis is corticosteroids administered with the initial antibiotic therapy. This has been shown to reduce the risk of deafness as a complication of meningitis in children; it is still not clear whether corticosteroids should be used in adults with meningitis.

## PREVENTION

The risk of secondary cases of meningococcal meningitis can be reduced by giving rifampicin, 600 mg, orally bd for 2 days, to family and/or nursery school contacts of an index case. Prophylaxis is also given to all family contacts of cases of *H. influenzae* meningitis, (or other invasive type b *H. influenzae* disease), if there is another child under 4 years old within the family. Rifampicin, 600 mg, daily for 4 days is used.

Vaccines are available against meningococci in groups A, C, Y and W135 and the use of vaccine is advocated for some travellers and if there is an outbreak of meningitis caused by one of these strains. There is, however, no vaccine for group B strains, which are the most common strains in the UK. Conjugate vaccines against *H. influenzae* type b are now available for administration to young children.

# Rabies

Rabies is caused by a bullet-shaped rhabdovirus. It results in a severe encephalomyelitis which is almost inevitably fatal. The virus can infect any mammal and rabies is widespread throughout most of the world, although the UK and some other countries that are geographically isolated have been able to eradicate rabies by the adoption of animal quarantine practices. Most cases of human rabies result from bites, scratches or licks from infected animals, particularly dogs or

certain wild animal species such as foxes, skunks, wolves or bats. Occasional cases have occurred from inhalation of aerosolized virus or from corneal transplantation from a donor with unsuspected rabies.

## CLINICAL FEATURES

The incubation period varies from a few days to several years but is usually between 1 and 3 months. The initial symptoms consist of pain or paraesthesia at the site of inoculation together with fever, malaise and headache. The disease then follows one of two courses:

1. In furious rabies, within a few days there is anxiety, agitation, hallucinations, bizarre behaviour and painful spasms of the pharynx and larynx in attempting to eat or drink (hydrophobia). On examination there is spasticity, hyperexcitability in response to noise and sympathetic overactivity.
2. Dumb or paralytic rabies typically causes a symmetrical ascending paralysis.

Only a handful of patients have ever survived rabies; all others have died within 10 to 14 days from convulsions, respiratory paralysis or cardiac arrhythmias, even with full intensive care.

## DIAGNOSIS

A history of exposure and the clinical picture are usually sufficient to make the diagnosis. Viral antigens can be detected in saliva, skin biopsies or corneal impressions by fluorescent antibody tests and eosinophilic cytoplasmic inclusions (Negri bodies) can be found within brain cells at *post-mortem*.

## TREATMENT

Patients should be sedated, given intensive care, and nursed in a quiet, darkened room. However, the prognosis is virtually hopeless.

## PREVENTION

Prevention of rabies largely depends upon postexposure prophylaxis with prompt cleansing of potentially infected wounds, active immunization with human diploid cell rabies vaccine and passive protection with human rabies immunoglobulin. Each instance of exposure to a potentially rabid animal needs to be carefully evaluated and advice from experts should be sought. If vaccination is advised, the vaccine course is given by intramuscular injections on days 0, 3, 7, 14 and 28. If the animal responsible for the bite is *known* to be still alive 10 days later it is extremely unlikely to have been rabid and the immunization course can be terminated.

Individuals whose occupation puts them at high risk of rabies exposure, for example, workers in quarantine kennels or laboratory workers, can be given pre-exposure prophylaxis with three doses of vaccine on days 0, 7 and 21 or 28.

# Tetanus

*Clostridium tetani* is a strictly anaerobic Gram-positive bacterium, the spores of which are widespread in the environment, particularly in manured soil. If spores are introduced into wounds and conditions are favourable, the organisms germinate and a powerful neurotoxin, tetanospasmin, is produced. Tetanus results from the actions of tetanospasmin. The toxin is produced locally at the site of the wound and is taken up by neuromuscular junctions, both locally and following bloodstream dissemination. It ascends to the central nervous system where it blocks the inhibition of motor reflexes and the sympathetic nervous system. Muscle spasms and autonomic dysfunction result.

## CLINICAL FEATURES

The incubation period of tetanus is from a few days to several weeks. In general, shorter incubation periods are associated with more severe disease. Although tetanus may be localized to the muscles in the region of the wound, most cases are generalized. The first symptom is often increased tone and spasm in the masseter muscles causing trismus or 'lockjaw'. Muscular

rigidity spreads and within a day or so reflex spasms occur and may become generalized. The longer the delay in the appearance of spasms, the better the prognosis. Spasm of the facial muscles in conjunction with trismus causes the classical risus sardonicus (sardonic smile) where the lips are separated but the teeth are clenched.

Spasms are triggered by stimuli such as noise, clinical examination or even bright light. In a spasm the whole body becomes rigid with extension of the limbs and clenching of the teeth. Opisthotonos may result from spasm of the spinal muscles. Laryngeal and oesophageal spasm cause respiratory difficulty and dysphagia. Autonomic dysfunction may produce tachycardia, labile blood pressure, arrhythmias and sweating. Consciousness is not disturbed.

## DIAGNOSIS

The diagnosis of tetanus is a clinical one. In most cases *C. tetani* will not be isolated from cultures of the wound.

## TREATMENT

Optimal treatment of tetanus involves a number of measures:

1. Human tetanus immunoglobulin should be given intramuscularly to neutralize any toxin which has not yet entered the nervous system.
2. After the immunoglobulin has been given, the wound should be debrided or excised.
3. Benzyl penicillin or metronidazole therapy eradicates any remaining *C. tetani*.
4. The patient should be nursed in a quiet, shaded room with minimal stimulation. Diazepam given intravenously prevents spasms and provides sedation. In severe cases respiratory paralysis, tracheostomy and ventilatory assistance are required.
5. Autonomic dysfunction may require β-blockade.
6. Since disease confers incomplete immunity a course of tetanus toxoid should be initiated during recovery.

With these measures the overall mortality from tetanus has now been reduced to 10–20 per cent.

## PREVENTION

Routine active immunization with tetanus toxoid, given either as a single agent or combined with diphtheria toxoid and/or pertussis vaccine, can completely prevent the disease. Booster injections every 10 years will ensure maintenance of immunity.

Non-immunized individuals with tetanus-prone wounds should be given passive immunity with human tetanus immunoglobulin as soon as possible. At the same time a course of active immunization should be initiated. In the previously immunized patient, a booster dose of toxoid is indicated:

1. After all wounds for those whose last booster was more than 10 years previously, and
2. For those with tetanus-prone wounds and no booster within the past 5 years.

# GENERAL INFECTIONS

A number of infections can involve multiple symptoms. They may present with predominant effects on one system but are included in this section because of their ability to affect various organs alone or in combination.

# Cytomegalovirus

Human cytomegalovirus (CMV) is a herpesvirus that is found worldwide and infects about 80 per cent of the world's population. It can cause a number of clinical syndromes but frequently primary infection is asymptomatic; reactivation of latent virus commonly leads to opportunistic infection in immunocompromised individuals. The virus can be found in saliva, semen and female genital secretions, urine and white cells. Primary infection is common during preschool life and there is a second peak in young adulthood, probably related to sexual transmission.

## CLINICAL FEATURES

The clinical syndromes associated with CMV depend upon the age and immune status of the patient.

1. Congenital infection results from maternal infection early in pregnancy. About 1 per cent of infants are excreting the virus at birth but only about 10 per cent of these infected neonates have some or all of the following abnormalities: jaundice, hepatosplenomegaly, encephalitis, microcephaly, chorioretinitis, anaemia, thrombocytopenia. Ninety per cent of infants infected *in utero* appear normal at delivery but some of these will go on to develop sensorineural deafness or mental retardation.
2. Acquired infection, whether acquired neonatally, in childhood or as an adult, is usually totally asymptomatic. Some young adults develop an infectious mononucleosis-like syndrome with a negative Paul–Bunnell test (page 732). Others have a hepatitic illness.
3. In immunosuppressed individuals reactivation of latent CMV can cause severe disease. Interstitial pneumonitis is especially common in bone marrow transplant recipients, while in patients with AIDS, a severe necrotizing retinitis is a major manifestation of CMV disease. Alternatively CMV may just produce a temporary rise in liver enzymes with fever in some transplant patients.

## DIAGNOSIS

Laboratory diagnosis of CMV infection depends upon finding characteristic intracellular inclusion bodies ('owl's eye' inclusions) in tissue biopsy specimens, detecting viral antigens with monoclonal antibodies, culturing the virus from blood or detecting specific IgM antibodies in the serum. The polymerase chain reaction (PCR) may be used to detect CMV DNA in various body fluids.

## TREATMENT

No specific therapy is needed for acquired infection which resolves spontaneously. In the immunocompromised host where infection can be life- or sight-threatening, intravenous ganciclovir or foscarnet are effective. These drugs are toxic and cannot be used in pregnant women to prevent congenital infections.

# Leptospirosis (Weil's disease)

*Leptospira* are fine spirochaetes with hooked or bent ends. Free-living saprophytic strains are a separate species and disease is due to a single species of spirochaete, *Leptospira interrogans*. Within this species there are several serogroups and numerous serotypes. Pathological serogroups include: *L. icterohaemorrhagiae, L. hardjo* and *L. canicola*. Leptospirosis is a zoonosis with different serogroups tending to have different animal reservoirs. Thus infection with canicola relates to dogs, hardjo to cattle and classical icterohaemorrhagiae to rats. Animals excrete the organisms in the urine for a long time without any evidence of disease and humans become infected via direct or indirect contact with urine from a reservoir animal. The leptospires gain access through ingestion, mucous membranes or skin abrasions. In the UK leptospirosis is mainly a disease of certain groups whose occupational or leisure activities bring them into close contact with animals or water polluted with animal urine.

## CLINICAL FEATURES

The incubation period ranges from 2 to 20 days. Subclinical infection is common and of those who are ill, only about 10 per cent have severe disease. The illness is often biphasic (Fig. 23.9). The initial clinical symptoms are influenza-like with fever, headache, myalgia, anorexia, rash and conjunctival infection. This initial phase of the illness lasts for 5–7 days and complete or partial recovery then occurs. In some cases the second phase never occurs but, in most, a day or two later a severe headache with meningism or a more generalized disease with myalgia, rash, splenomegaly, and abnormal renal and kidney function occurs. In the most severe forms (Weil's disease), usually caused by *L. icterohaemorrhagiae*, there is jaundice, renal failure, haemorrhage and vascular collapse. The jaundice is usually not associated with marked

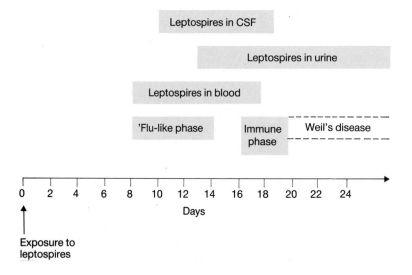

**Figure 23.9** Diagram of clinical features of leptospirosis. The second 'immune' phase is often mild and short lived but sometimes jaundice, renal impairment and bleeding (Weil's disease) occurs. CSF = cerebrospinal fluid.

hepatocellular damage. The urine contains blood and protein. Such cases still have an appreciable mortality.

## DIAGNOSIS

Direct dark-ground microscopy or culture of blood specimens may identify the leptospires during the first phase of the illness but the second phase is immunologically mediated and serology is more helpful at this stage. Specific IgM antibodies should be sought.

## TREATMENT

Antibiotic therapy with either intravenous penicillin or ampicillin given within a few days of the onset of symptoms is effective. Less severely ill patients should be given oral doxycycline or amoxycillin. The contribution of antibiotics to the resolution of the second, immune phase of leptospirosis is less clear.

## PREVENTION

Vaccines are not available for human use. Prevention primarily relies upon avoiding contamination but prophylactic doxycycline has been successfully used.

# Lyme disease

Lyme disease (named after a town in the USA) (page 583) is a multisystem disorder that is now known to be caused by the tick-transmitted spirochaete *Borrelia burgdorferi*. The infection occurs in many parts of the world and the onset of the illness is generally between May and November, when the ticks bite. Ticks are found on deer, dogs and, in the USA, racoons.

## CLINICAL FEATURES

The first stage of the illness is a characteristic skin rash called erythema chronicum migrans (ECM) which begins within a few weeks at the site of the tick bite. Erythema chronicum migrans starts as a small indurated red macule that

progresses to form an annular plaque with a clear centre that steadily expands in diameter up to 50–60 cm. During this first stage of Lyme disease, patients may also have intermittent fever, headache, stiff neck and meningism, musculoskeletal pains, fatigue and malaise. The skin lesions tend to last for several weeks.

## COMPLICATIONS

Weeks or months after the first stage some patients develop cardiac (myocarditis), neurological (meningoencephalitis, cranial nerve palsies and painful peripheral neuropathies) and rheumatological (recurrent arthritis) complications.

## DIAGNOSIS

Although the organism may be isolated from blood, CSF, skin or synovial fluid at various stages of Lyme disease, the diagnosis often relies upon serological techniques. IgM titres rise within 2 to 6 weeks, whereas IgG titres may take months to peak. The initial antibody response seems to be directed at one of the flagellar antigens of the spirochaete whereas later responses are to other components of the organism.

## TREATMENT

The treatment for ECM and the early stages of Lyme disease is probably best given with amoxycillin and probenecid or with doxycycline for at least 10 days. For late complications a third generation cephalosporin seems to be more effective than penicillin.

# Brucellosis (undulant fever; Malta fever)

Three species of *Brucella*, Gram-negative coccobacilli responsible for genitourinary infection and abortion in animal hosts, are pathogenic for humans. *Brucella abortus* is acquired from cows by the ingestion of infected milk, milk products and aerosol inhalation. *Brucella melitensis* comes from goat's milk products and causes disease in Mediterranean and African countries and *B. suis* is transmitted by direct contact with infected carcasses of pigs. The disease has now been eradicated from cattle within the UK.

Following entry to the body, brucellae are phagocytosed but are capable of remaining viable within mononuclear cells of the reticuloendothelial system. This results in granuloma formation in several organs.

## CLINICAL FEATURES

The clinical features of brucellosis are very variable, depending upon the host's immunity and the species involved: *B. melitensis* and *B. suis* cause more serious disease than *B. abortus*. There is an incubation period from 7 to 21 days and then the illness may be acute or subacute in onset. Only a third have drenching sweats and high fever. In the remainder the fever, when present, is low grade. Episodes of fever may recur for weeks or months (undulant fever). The patient often has considerable anorexia, lethargy, muscle and joint pains and the spleen, liver or lymph nodes may become palpable. The blood count usually shows a leukopenia and mild anaemia.

## COMPLICATIONS

In a few patients acute brucellosis is complicated by localized infection affecting almost any organ system. Skeletal involvement is most common with arthritis, affecting the spine and large joints, being particularly common. Other complications include endocarditis, hepatitis, haemolytic anaemia, epididymo-orchitis, meningoencephalitis, myelitis and depression.

Re-exposure to *Brucella* in seropositive persons (particularly in veterinary surgeons or laboratory workers) may cause hypersensitivity reactions which mimic acute brucellosis.

## DIAGNOSIS

Cultural isolation of *Brucella* from the blood and bone marrow is often technically difficult and serodiagnosis provides the usual confirmation. In the acute phase both IgM and IgG antibodies

are usually present: with adequate treatment IgG disappears or decreases to very low levels. In the chronic phase or with exacerbation or reinfection IgG antibodies rise again.

## TREATMENT

A combination of rifampicin, 600–900 mg/day, with doxycycline, 200 mg/day, for 6 weeks is currently considered the treatment of choice. Tetracycline with intramuscular streptomycin is cheaper but more difficult to administer. Endocarditis requires prolonged treatment with additional cotrimoxazole.

## PREVENTION

Vaccinating cattle and goats, and pasteurizing milk and dairy products, have largely eliminated brucellosis in countries with organized agriculture. Human vaccines are not widely available or reliably protective.

# Typhoid and paratyphoid (enteric fever)

*Salmonella typhi* differs from the food-poisoning strains of salmonellae (page 738) in that it is an exclusively human pathogen. Infection is transmitted by food or water contaminated by excreta from carriers or patients with the disease.

## CLINICAL FEATURES

The incubation period is generally 10–14 days before the gradual onset of headache, myalgia, cough, constipation, tiredness and fever, which is remittent and typically rises in 'step-ladder' fashion to 39–40°C over 3–4 days (Fig. 23.10). During this stage there is a relative bradycardia and at the end of the first week the characteristic rash may become visible on the trunk. It consists of crops of 1–2 mm pink macules which blanch on pressure; each only lasts for a day or so. The spleen also becomes palpable at about this time. The fever remains at a high level and initially is accompanied by bradycardia and constipation.

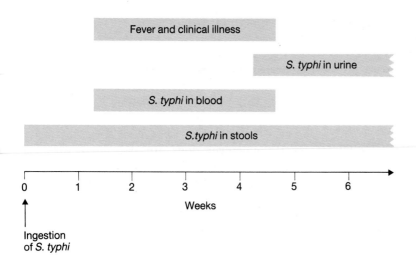

Fever and clinical illness

S. typhi in urine

S. typhi in blood

S.typhi in stools

0  1  2  3  4  5  6

Weeks

Ingestion
of S. typhi

**Figure 23.10** Diagram of the course of untreated *Salmonella typhi* infection.

Greenish watery diarrhoea starts during the second week of the illness. By this time the patient is very unwell. After 3–4 weeks the patient usually gradually improves although complications also tend to occur during this period of the illness. The most common problems are perforation of the ileum and haemorrhage from the bowel, either of which may prove fatal.

Paratyphoid, caused by *S. paratyphi* A, B or C is a similar but less severe illness.

Following acute infection some individuals continue to excrete salmonellae in the faeces for many months or years. The persistent infection is often in the gall bladder.

## DIAGNOSIS

There is usually a leukopenia. Blood culture is the best means of establishing the diagnosis, but the rate of positivity drops as the disease progresses beyond the second week. Cultures of urine, stool and bone marrow may also be positive. Serological tests are less helpful but the Widal reaction, which measures serum agglutinins against the O and H antigens of *Salmonella* species, is sometimes useful.

## TREATMENT

The antibiotic therapy of typhoid is best given with an antibiotic that penetrates well intracellularly (where the salmonellae replicate) and to which the bacteria remain sensitive. Chloramphenicol, cotrimoxazole and ampicillin are effective but resistance to these agents is spread-

ing. A fluoroquinolone seems the best empirical choice for most patients at present. Eradication of the carrier state can be difficult. High-dose ampicillin, sometimes combined with cholecystectomy, is occasionally effective but fluoroquinolones seem to show more promise.

## PREVENTION

A two-dose course of immunization with the parenteral inactivated vaccine gives relatively good protection against typhoid for 3 years. An oral vaccine containing an attenuated strain of *S. typhi* is now available in the UK.

# Actinomycosis

*Actinomyces* are Gram-positive branching bacteria that are normal inhabitants of the mouth and gastrointestinal tract. They produce chronic infections in three different areas of the body: the jaw, the abdomen and the lung.

## CLINICAL FEATURES

1. Actinomycosis of the jaw is the most common site of infection and usually follows dental extraction. It is indolent and the organism gradually spreads through the tissues of the mandible and overlying skin ('woody jaw'). Multiple discharging sinuses develop. There is little pain or

constitutional upset and lymphadenopathy is uncommon.

2. Abdominal actinomycosis may involve the ileocaecal region causing a chronic enlarging mass in the right iliac fossa, or pelvic disease, often secondary to the use of intrauterine contraceptive devices.

3. Actinomycosis of the lung is usually secondary infection of previously damaged tissues. Fever, haemoptysis and chest pain may suggest tuberculosis. In many patients the disease spreads to the pleura causing empyema.

## DIAGNOSIS

In actinomycosis, the pus contains visible colonies of the organism which appear as 'sulphur granules'. The branching bacteria can be identified microscopically.

## TREATMENT

The treatment usually involves surgery in combination with prolonged penicillin therapy. Tetracyclines can be used for penicillin-allergic patients.

# Hydatid disease

Hydatid disease results from the development in humans of the intermediate form of the dog tapeworm, *Echinococcus granulosus*. The normal host for this stage of the tapeworm is sheep, cattle or pigs. Disease occurs throughout the world wherever dogs are associated with the raising of sheep and other livestock. Human infection occurs when people ingest vegetables contaminated with canine faeces or from eggs adhering to the hands after contact with a dog. The life-cycle of the parasite is shown in Fig. 23.11.

## CLINICAL FEATURES

Most cysts develop within the liver but they may also grow within the lung, kidneys, bone or central nervous system. In the liver the lesion is usually within the right lobe. Cysts are often asymptomatic, merely producing slowly progressive pressure symptoms. Occasionally cysts rupture into the peritoneum or pleural cavity. There is sometimes an eosinophilia.

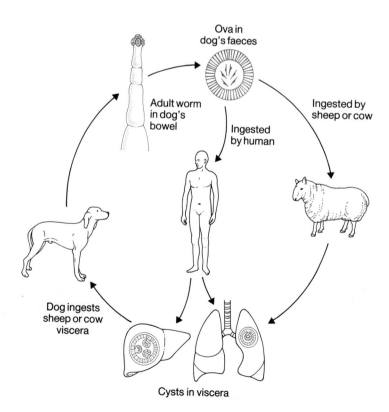

Ova in dog's faeces

Adult worm in dog's bowel

Ingested by sheep or cow

Ingested by human

Dog ingests sheep or cow viscera

Cysts in viscera

**Figure 23.11** Life-cycle of *Echinococcus granulosis*.

## DIAGNOSIS

A calcified round lesion in the liver or lung may be seen on routine radiological examination. Ultrasound and CT scans are helpful and may show the presence of daughter cysts within the cavity. Serological tests detecting antibody are available; the most useful are the complement fixation and the immunoelectropheresis tests. Aspiration of fluid from a suspected hydatid cyst should not be undertaken as it may spread daughter cysts and cause fatal anaphylaxis.

## TREATMENT

Therapy is now usually given with albendazole or praziquantel followed if necessary by removal of the cyst if it is producing symptoms. If possible the cyst should be removed intact.

# Toxoplasmosis

The protozoan *Toxoplasma gondii* undergoes sexual reproduction in the gastrointestinal tract of cats and oocysts are passed in the cat faeces (Fig. 23.12). Ingestion of these cysts by other warm-blooded animals results in the release of trophozoites which then are disseminated throughout the body and encyst to form long-lived tissue cysts. Humans become infected from eating either food contaminated with cat faeces or undercooked meat containing tissue cysts. Congenital infection also occurs. The disease has a worldwide distribution and in the UK serological studies show an infection rate of 10–20 per cent in children and young adults, and up to 50 per cent in middle-aged adults.

## CLINICAL FEATURES

The vast majority of patients infected with *T. gondii* remain completely asymptomatic. Clinical symptoms may occur and depend upon the type of host involved.

1. Congenital toxoplasmosis usually follows acute infection of the mother in the first trimester of pregnancy. Chorioretinitis, hydrocephalus, intracranial calcification, convulsions and mental retardation result. Some children appear normal but develop neurological problems months later. Chorioretinitis can present in later childhood or early adult life.

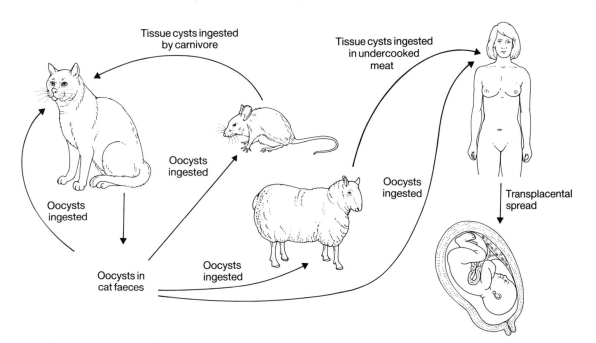

**Figure 23.12** Life-cycle of *Toxoplasma gondii*.

2. Acute toxoplasmosis in the normal host may result in localized lymphadenopathy, occasionally with symptoms and haematological changes suggestive of glandular fever. The diagnosis may be established by biopsy of a lymph node.

3. In the host with cellular immunodeficiency, primary infection can result in a disseminated infection with pneumonitis and encephalitis. More commonly, reactivation of tissue cysts causes encephalitis and single or multiple focal mass lesions. This is invariably fatal if untreated and is seen in up to a quarter of patients with AIDS.

## DIAGNOSIS

Serological tests are the primary means of diagnosing acquired infection. Tests for IgG (including the dye test) and IgM antibodies are available. Unfortunately patients with AIDS often do not mount an acute antibody response following reactivation of latent cysts and biopsy of the cerebral lesions may be necessary for diagnosis.

## TREATMENT

No therapy is needed for most patients. Immunocompromised patients and those with ocular disease are given pyrimethamine plus a sulphonamide or clindamycin. Pyrimethamine is teratogenic and toxoplasmosis in the first trimester of pregnancy should be treated with spiramycin. In AIDS the problems usually recur if suppressive treatment is stopped.

# Cat-scratch fever

This disease is caused by a recently described Gram-positive bacillus (*Rochalimaea henselae*) transmitted by the scratch of apparently healthy cats. A small papule or ulcer may develop at the site of the scratch, followed by tender regional lymphadenopathy. The glands may become fluctuant and remain swollen for several months. Encephalitis, hepatitis and bone lesions are rare complications. Diagnosis is by biopsy of a gland which shows granulomas and eosinophilic microabscesses. The bacterium is sensitive to aminoglycosides and some cephalosporins but most cases resolve spontaneously.

# INFECTIONS OF THE GENITAL TRACT

# Gonorrhoea

There was a steady increase in the incidence of gonorrhoea over the three decades before 1985. The number of new cases then declined once awareness of the AIDS epidemic led to changes in sexual behaviour although recently numbers are increasing again. *Neisseria gonorrhoeae* is a Gram-negative, kidney-shaped diplococcus that is seen intracellularly in clinical specimens. Gonococcal infection is almost always transmitted sexually. Asymptomatic infection occurs in up to 50 per cent of females and in 5–25 per cent of males. These asymptomatic individuals are the major source of disease transmission.

## CLINICAL FEATURES

The most common manifestations of gonococcal infection are urethritis in either sex and cervicitis in women. Symptoms begin 2–5 days after infection and consist of dysuria and urinary frequency followed by a purulent urethral or vaginal discharge. In men, the meatus is inflamed and, in women, the cervix is red and friable. Anorectal infection is often asymptomatic although anal irritation, pain, bleeding and mucopurulent discharge may occur. Oropharyngeal infection also rarely causes symptoms.

## COMPLICATIONS

Local complications of gonorrhoea are relatively uncommon. In the male the most common complication is epididymitis; prostatitis, infection of the seminal vesicles and periurethral abscesses also occur. Stricture formation may follow gonococcal urethritis. In 10–15 per cent of females infection spreads upwards to the endometrium, fallopian tubes and then may extend to cause tubo-ovarian or pelvic abscesses. Gonococcal pelvic inflammatory disease causes lower abdominal pain, fever and adnexal tenderness. Disseminated gonococcal infection occurs very rarely and produces a pustular rash on the extremities, asymmetric tenosynovitis and septic arthritis.

## DIAGNOSIS

In infected males Gram stain and microscopy of a urethral smear usually reveals intracellular Gram-negative diplococci. Only 50 per cent of symptomatic females, however, give a positive result on Gram stain of endocervical exudate. Cultures are therefore necessary and in women and homosexual men rectal swabs should also be cultured routinely. Pharyngeal swabs should also be cultured. Other sexually transmitted diseases should be sought.

## TREATMENT

The treatment of gonorrhoea has undergone change since the emergence of penicillin resistance in *N. gonorrhoeae*. Some of these strains produce a penicillinase (β-lactamase) and are known as PPNG (penicillinase-producing *N. gonorrhoeae*). In others the resistance is not due to β-lactamase production: these strains are also resistant to tetracyclines. The choice of therapy depends upon the site of infection, any history of penicillin allergy and the prevalence of penicillin-resistant strains in the community where the infection was acquired. Penicillinase-producing *N. gonorrhoeae* strains are particularly prevalent in the Far East and parts of Africa. For uncomplicated gonococcal urethritis, cervicitis or rectal infection, therapy with a single dose regimen is adequate. When the infection is known for certain to be caused by penicillin-sensitive gonococci, either oral amoxycillin, 3 g,

or intramuscular procaine penicillin, 2.88 g (4.8 megaunits), combined with probenecid may be used. Otherwise the recommended therapy is intramuscular spectinomycin, or oral cefuroxime axetil plus probenecid, cefixime or a quinolone such as ciprofloxacin, any of which will deal with PPNG strains. In pharyngeal gonorrhoea spectinomycin is unreliable: procaine penicillin, a quinolone or a week of oral tetracycline are used. There is coexistent chlamydial infection in up to half the cases of gonorrhoea and treatment should, therefore, be followed by a course of therapy for *Chlamydia trachomatis* infections.

Contacts should be traced and treated if necessary.

# Chlamydia trachomatis infections

Non-specific or non-gonococcal urethritis (NSU; NGU) and cervicitis have also become much more frequent and are the most common sexually transmitted diseases in the West. The D-K serovars of *C. trachomatis* are the most important cause and can be found in about half the cases of NSU in men: two-thirds of the female partners of these culture-positive cases will have chlamydial endocervicitis. Non-specific urethritis in men produces a mucoid urethral discharge and dysuria. Symptomatic urethritis may occur in women but, *C. trachomatis* more often causes asymptomatic endocervicitis. Asymptomatic women are an important reservoir of infection, transmitting infection to their sexual partners and to their neonates, producing neonatal ophthalmia and pneumonia. Untreated NSU in men may lead to prostatitis or epididymitis and strains of *C. trachomatis* have been isolated from many female patients with chronic pelvic sepsis and constitute an important cause of infertility.

## DIAGNOSIS

Examination of the urethral or endocervical discharge reveals pus cells but no evidence of intracellular gonococci (although concurrent infections may occur). Inclusion bodies may be detected by means of Giemsa or Wright's staining of smears but diagnosis is now chiefly undertaken by detection of chlamydial antigens by direct immunofluorescence using a monoclonal antibody test or an enzyme-linked immunosorbent assay (ELISA).

## TREATMENT

Traditionally, NSU was treated with doxycycline, 100 mg every 12 hours, or erythromycin for 14 days. A single 1 g dose of azithromycin has now been shown to be equally effective. Control cannot be expected unless sexual partners are traced and treated concurrently.

# Herpes genitalis

Genital herpes has markedly increased in incidence in developed countries over the 1970s and early 1980s. It is caused by either type 1 or type 2 herpes simplex viruses (HSV-1 and HSV-2), although type 2 accounts for about 80 per cent of genital infections. Transmission is by sexual or other physical contact.

## CLINICAL FEATURES

Primary infection produces lesions 2–4 days after exposure. It results in clusters of painful vesicles or ulcers on the skin or mucous membranes of the penis, labia, introitus, or anorectal and adjacent areas; the cervix is commonly involved. The lesions and shedding of virus last about 10 days and complete healing may take 3 weeks. Viraemia and systemic symptoms are common in primary infection: depending upon the site involved, inguinal lymphadenopathy, discharge from the urethra, vagina, cervix or anus, urinary retention, tenesmus and constipation may also occur. Rarely there is a meningitis or sacral nerve involvement.

Following primary infection HSV becomes latent in the sacral ganglia and reactivates to cause recurrent episodes of genital herpes at intervals. Recurrent episodes are much less severe. The precipitating factors for recurrences are poorly understood but may include menstruation, sexual intercourse and stress. Extensive perianal herpes and HSV proctitis may be seen in patients with AIDS.

Infection of the neonate with HSV may occur following vaginal delivery in women with active genital herpes: most cases, however, result from asymptomatic HSV shedding from the cervix. Caesarian section should be considered if the mother has evidence of genital lesions at or near the time of delivery.

## DIAGNOSIS

The diagnosis of genital herpes may be made on clinical grounds but can be confirmed by viral isolation or direct immunofluorescence or Giemsa staining of smears from the lesions.

## TREATMENT

A patient with genital herpes is often apprehensive and in need of reassurance and explanation about the risks and consequences of the infection. In primary episodes of genital herpes, oral acyclovir, 200 mg, five times daily for 7–10 days is the best management. In recurrent herpes genitalis the clinical benefits of acyclovir therapy are only marginal. For the patient with frequent recurrences, prophylactic acyclovir is helpful.

# Syphilis

Syphilis declined markedly following the development of improvements in therapy after the second world war, but began to rise again in developed countries in the mid-1960s: these infections were chiefly in homosexual men. After the recognition of the AIDS epidemic, there was a change in sexual practices among these men and cases of syphilis declined again. In the developing world and in deprived communities in the West, however, syphilis still constitutes a major health problem.

The causative organism is *Treponema pallidum*, a spirochaete 6–14 μm long and 0.5 μm wide.

Nearly all cases of acquired syphilis are transmitted by sexual contact, although transmission may occur via blood transfusions. Congenital syphilis is transmitted transplacentally during the later stages of pregnancy.

## CLINICAL FEATURES

The manifestations of acquired syphilis are diverse. Early disease is divided into primary and secondary stages and is characterized by mucocutaneous lesions. There is then a period of latent infection sometimes followed by the tertiary stage, typified by progressive lesions of the nervous, cardiovascular and musculoskeletal systems.

### Primary syphilis

After an incubation period of 2–4 weeks, the primary lesion (occasionally multiple lesions) appears at the site of infection. The **primary chancre** begins as a papule which becomes a well-defined, painless, indurated ulcer about 1 cm in diameter. Most chancres are on the external genitalia, in the anorectal area, on the fingers, in the oral cavity or on the lips. Chancres at any site are accompanied by discrete painless enlargement of the regional lymph nodes. The chancre heals over 2–8 weeks if untreated.

### Secondary syphilis

Secondary syphilis develops about 6–8 weeks after the appearance of the primary lesion, which may not have yet healed. It is characterized by:

1. A generalized rash (syphilide). Rashes vary greatly in appearance but generally include the palms and soles, but not the face, and are non-irritant.
2. Generalized non-tender lymphadenopathy.
3. Non-specific systemic symptoms such as fever, aching limbs, anorexia, headache and arthralgia.
4. Mucous patches: these oval, shallow erosions may be anywhere in the mouth or throat.
5. Condylomata lata which may be seen in any warm and moist area, especially round the anus. They consist of papular lesions which have enlarged to form pink warty, erosions.

### Latent syphilis

Early syphilis, even if untreated, tends to resolve after many weeks or months. Thereafter, infection remains latent and may be revealed only by a chance blood test, during pregnancy for example.

### Tertiary syphilis

Clinical tertiary lesions appear after 5–20 years in about one-third of patients with untreated latent syphilis. Cardiovascular syphilis and neurosyphilis are described elsewhere (page 201 and 695). Localized swellings termed **gummas** also occur. Almost every organ of the body can be affected by gummas but lesions are most often seen in skin, mucous membranes, bones and joints. If the centre of a gumma breaks down then a punched out ulcer develops. This can cause perforation of the nasal septum or hard palate.

### Congenital syphilis

Transplacental spread of *T. pallidum* may result in fetal death, prematurity or congenital syphilis. Congenital syphilis occurs when *T. pallidum* spreads to the fetus after the fourth month of gestation. The features of the early syndrome may not be present at birth, only becoming apparent during the subsequent 4 weeks. There is failure of the baby to thrive and usually a generalized eruption that resembles those of acquired secondary syphilis. There are also mucosal lesions, those of the nasal mucosa giving rise to syphilitic rhinitis (snuffles). Enlargement of the liver, spleen and lymph nodes is common but many other organs may be involved. After a year or two, late congenital syphilis may develop: this involves the eyes, giving interstitial keratitis, as well as the skin, bones and joints (characterized by metaphyseal perichondritis and osteitis) and central nervous system. Other residual stigmata that develop are:

1. Hutchinson's teeth. These are abnormal permanent incisors, smaller than usual with the sides converging towards the cutting edge, which often shows a notch.

2. Syphilitic 'saddle nose'. This is a flattened bridge due to poor development resulting from syphilitic rhinitis.

## DIAGNOSIS

*Treponema pallidum* can be seen by dark ground examination of material from the cutaneous lesions of primary or secondary syphilis, which are highly infectious. The motile spirochaetes are looked for by dark ground microscopy of a drop of serous fluid expressed from a lesion. Any suspicious lesion should be re-examined serially if the initial test is negative.

Serological tests for syphilis are not of help in primary syphilis but are useful for the diagnosis of secondary, latent and tertiary disease and for the assessment of response to treatment. There are two types of tests:

1. Non-specific tests, such as the Venereal Disease Research Laboratory (VDRL), or rapid plasma reagin (RPR) which employ a cardiolipin antigen. The reaginic antibody tests are useful as screening tests or for measuring the response to treatment. False positive results occur so any positive result requires confirmation.
2. Specific anti-treponemal antibody tests such as the *T. pallidum* haemagglutination test (TPHA), the fluorescent treponemal antibody absorption test (FTA-Abs) and the *T. pallidum* immobilization test (TPI). The FTA-Abs is the standard specific test used.

The rates of positive tests in untreated syphilis at various stages are summarized in Table 23.12.

**Table 23.12** Frequency (%) of positive serological tests in untreated syphilis.

| Stage of disease | VDRL | FTA-Abs |
|---|---|---|
| Primary | 50–75 | 70–85 |
| Secondary | 99 | 99 |
| Latent | 75 | 98 |
| Tertiary | 70 | 98 |

VDRL = Venereal Disease Research Laboratory test. FTA-Abs = fluorescent treponemal antibody absorption test.

Congenital syphilis is diagnosed by finding passively transferred maternal serological reactivity or by measuring specific IgM by a FTA test. A positive VDRL from the CSF is diagnostic of neurosyphilis. A positive FTA-Abs is diagnostic of infection but remains positive for life, with or without treatment, so it cannot be used to monitor the efficacy of therapy.

## TREATMENT

Penicillin is the drug of choice for the treatment of all stages of syphilis. The recommended regimens and follow-up are summarized in Table 23.13.

The Jarisch–Herxheimer reaction may occur 2–24 hours after treatment for syphilis is begun. It is manifest as fever, chills, general malaise and headache, lasting for a few hours, and is caused by release of endotoxin as large numbers of spirochaetes are killed. It is particularly likely in secondary syphilis. Particularly severe reactions can occur in tertiary syphilis and prednisolone should be given prior to penicillin therapy in such patients.

# *Lymphogranuloma venereum*

This uncommon infection is caused by the L-1, L-2, and L-3 serovars of *Chlamydia trachomatis*. It is uncommon in the West – most cases arise in subtropical and tropical countries.

## CLINICAL FEATURES

The primary lesion is a painless non-indurated vesicle or papule which develops on the genitalia 1–4 weeks after infection. This heals quickly and is often unnoticed. Regional lymphadenopathy, with stretched and discoloured overlying skin and systemic symptoms follow a few days later. The lymph nodes become matted and fluctuant (buboes) with multiple abscesses and sinus formation. In males the inguinal glands are most commonly involved but in females and homosexual males the perirectal

**Table 23.13** Treatment and follow-up of various stages of syphilis.

| Stage | Treatment | Follow-up |
|---|---|---|
| Primary, secondary or latent syphilis of less than 1 year's duration | Benzathine penicillin, 2.4 million units (1.44 g) i.m. once or penicillin G, 600 000 units (0.36 g)/day for 10 days | 1, 3, 6 and 12 months |
| Latent syphilis of more than 1 year's duration or cardiovascular syphilis | Benzathine penicillin as above, weekly for 3 weeks | Above, then at 18 and 24 months |
| Neurosyphilis | Penicillin G, 12–24 million units (7.2–14.4 g)/day i.v. for 10 days followed by benzathine penicillin 2–4 million units i.m. weekly for 3 weeks | As above, then at 30 and 36 months: plus cerebrospinal fluid examination every year for 3 years |
| Congenital | Procaine penicillin, 50 000 units/kg (30 mg/kg), i.m. daily for 10 days or penicillin G, 100 000–150 000 units/kg/day, i.v. for 10–14 days | 1, 3, 6 and 12 months |
| **Penicillin-allergic patients** | | |
| 1. Primary, secondary or latent syphilis of less than 1 year's duration | Tetracycline or erythromycin, 500 mg po, 6 hourly for 15 days | |
| 2. Latent syphilis of more than 1 year's duration or cardiovascular syphilis | Tetracycline or erythromycin, 500 mg po, 6 hourly for 30 days | |
| 3. Neurosyphilis or congenital syphilis | Skin-testing with desensitization to penicillin recommended | |

glands suppurate and may be associated with painful proctitis and bloody anal discharge. Unless treated, perirectal abscesses and fistulas, or elephantiasis of the genitalia may follow.

## DIAGNOSIS

Diagnosis is usually made by serological means (complement fixation and microimmunofluorescence) but *C. trachomatis* can be cultured from aspirates of the suppurative lymph nodes or abscesses. The organism can also be detected in smears or other specimens by direct immunofluorescence with monoclonal antibodies.

## TREATMENT

Tetracyclines or sulphonamide treatment during the acute phase will prevent the subsequent chronic changes but, once these have developed, antimicrobial agents have little effect. Fluctuant buboes should be aspirated.

# Chancroid

Now becoming more common in the developed world, chancroid or soft chancre is frequently seen in the tropical countries of S.E. Asia, Africa and South America. It is caused by *Haemophilus ducreyi*. The incubation period is 4–10 days, after which one or more red genital papules appear and, within a few days, break down to form ragged ulcers. The ulcers may be extremely painful. Many patients have unilateral or bilateral painful lymphadenopathy – without effective treatment buboes may occur and suppurate.

## DIAGNOSIS

Chancroid can be distinguished from syphilis by finding *H. ducreyi* in a Gram-stained smear of material from a genital lesion or by culturing the organism on special media.

## TREATMENT

Oral cotrimoxazole, erythromycin or a quinolone such as ciprofloxacin usually results in healing within 1 or 2 weeks. More prolonged courses may be needed for those with underlying HIV infection.

# Granuloma inguinale

This uncommon, sexually transmitted condition is seen mainly in S.E. Asia, the Caribbean and Southern India. Infection is caused by *Calymatobacterium granulomatosis*, a small Gram-negative intracellular bacterium.

## CLINICAL FEATURES

Papules appear 1–12 weeks after exposure on the genitalia, perineum, groin or occasionally at other sites; these break down into progressively enlarging ulcers. The granulomatous mass spreads and the slowly progressive destruction may cause considerable disfigurement. Regional lymphadenopathy does not usually occur, although the enlarging granulomatous process may mimic a bubo, and systemic symptoms are rare.

## COMPLICATIONS

Complications include stenosis of the urethral, vaginal or anal orifices, and massive elephantoid oedema.

## DIAGNOSIS

*Calymatobacterium granulomatosis* can not be cultured on ordinary laboratory media. Diagnosis is confirmed by finding Donovan bodies (stained organisms within macrophages) in a biopsy of a piece of granulation tissue from the edge of the lesion.

## TREATMENT

The drugs of choice for treatment are tetracycline, streptomycin or cotrimoxazole given until healing has occurred (usually 2–3 weeks).

# $H$IV INFECTION AND AIDS

The acquired immune deficiency syndrome (AIDS) was first described in 1981 and, a few years later, the viral cause of the syndrome was discovered and termed human T-lymphotropic virus, type 1 (HTLV-1). Subsequently the virus was renamed human immunodeficiency virus (HIV). Human immunodeficiency virus is a member of the lentivirus subfamily of retroviruses, which are RNA viruses that replicate through a unique mechanism involving a reverse transcriptase enzyme. This transcribes the viral RNA to DNA which is then integrated into the host cell genome. Once integrated into host DNA, the virus is capable of replication whenever certain promotor genes are activated. Two distinct forms of HIV (HIV-1 and HIV-2) have been described: their replication and effects are virtually indistinguishable.

The structure of HIV is shown in Fig. 23.13. The virus has an envelope through which projects a structural glycopeptide gp41 and a major surface glycopeptide, gp120. The central core consists of a protein, p24, surrounding the RNA and reverse transcriptase molecules.

## IMMUNOLOGY

The gp120 glycopeptide of HIV binds to cells that express the CD4 protein molecule upon

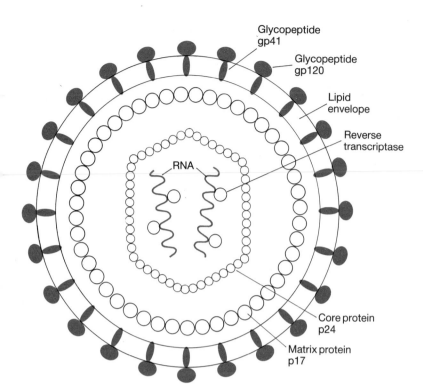

Glycopeptide gp41

Glycopeptide gp120

Lipid envelope

Reverse transcriptase

RNA

Core protein p24

Matrix protein p17

**Figure 23.13** Structure of human immunodeficiency virus (HIV).

their surface. This includes the T4 (helper-inducer) subset of T-lymphocytes, the macrophage–monocyte cell line and glial cells within the central nervous system. After binding HIV enters the cell. Once infected, cells may be destroyed by the replication and budding of new HIV virions or by immune-mediated mechanisms which recognize viral antigens expressed on the surface of the cells. The end result is a striking depletion of T4-lymphocytes. These cells play a pivotal role in virtually all immune responses and depletion of T4 cells renders the individual highly susceptible to certain opportunistic infections and secondary neoplasms. Destruction of CD4-positive cells within the central nervous system causes progressive neurological dysfunction. Once certain opportunistic infections, neoplasms or other defined manifestations (Group IV manifestations, see below) have developed then the patient is defined as suffering from the acquired immune deficiency syndrome (AIDS), which is the final stage of HIV infection.

## EPIDEMIOLOGY

The transmission of HIV is by sexual contact, by blood or vertically from mother to child either congenitally, during delivery or during breast feeding. Although HIV is found in a wide range of secretions and fluids of infected individuals it is not transmitted by social, non-sexual contact. Sexual transmission is the predominant route: bidirectional transmission may occur during homosexual or heterosexual sexual intercourse. Transmission during vaginal intercourse seems more likely to occur from an infected male to the female. The transmission of infection depends upon the stage of disease in an individual (higher rates being found in the later stages of HIV infection), and the presence of genital ulceration, which promotes transmission of HIV. Spread of infection in the community depends upon the number of sexual partners an individual has. Among intravenous drug users the sharing of needles and other equipment used for injection is the major risk factor. A small number of cases have been transmitted to health workers from needle-stick exposure. Vertical transmission occurs in 20–50 per cent of deliveries from HIV-infected mothers. A second strain of HIV, HIV-2, has been reported in parts of West Africa.

Three broad epidemiological patterns of HIV and AIDS are found in different parts of the world:

1. *UK/Western Europe, North America, and Australasia*

   There is considerable variation in the levels seen in different countries but most cases are found in homosexual/bisexual men or intravenous drug abusers (Table 23.14). In the UK cases of HIV attributable to heterosexual intercourse are increasing in both absolute terms and as a proportion of the total.

2. *Sub-Saharal Africa, South America*

   There is a major epidemic with most cases in heterosexuals of either sex, particularly those with multiple sexual partners, e.g. prostitutes, and children (as a result of vertical spread).

3. *Rest of the world*

   The incidence is still low but spreading as a result of drug abuse, contaminated blood transfusions or sexual transmission.

**Table 23.14** AIDS cases in the UK by exposure category (January 1993).

| | |
|---|---|
| Homosexual or bisexual men | 5333 |
| Intravenous drug users (IVDU) | 321 |
| Homosexual/bisexual men and IVDU | 115 |
| Haemophiliacs | 342 |
| Heterosexual men and women | 675 |
| Recipients of infected blood/organs | 83 |
| Children whose mothers have HIV | 81 |
| Undetermined | 95 |
| Total | 7045 |

The number of cases of HIV infection worldwide is estimated to be at least 8–10 million with the highest prevalence of infection in parts of East and Central Africa. In the UK over 8000 AIDS cases had been reported by September 1993, but no accurate prevalence data are available for HIV infection.

## STAGES OF INFECTION

The clinical spectrum of HIV infection ranges widely and is classified by a number of different systems, dependent upon the availability of laboratory investigations and either the clinical features or the CD4-positive T-lymphocyte count in the blood. The classifications used most frequently in the UK for adults and children are those of the US Centers for Disease Control shown in Tables 23.15 and 23.16.

The rate of decline of immune function in HIV infection differs markedly between individuals. In general the rate of decline is most rapid in children and in the elderly but the factors responsible for the variation between individuals are unclear. The median time between infection with HIV and development of AIDS is 10–11 years; the rate of progression is low initially but increases progressively with duration of infection.

### Stage I: acute seroconversion syndrome

In about one-half of individuals acquisition of HIV is followed within 4 to 6 weeks by a glandular fever-like syndrome (fever, malaise, myalgia, oral ulcers, rash, meningism and

**Table 23.15** Centers for Disease Control (USA) Classification of HIV infection in adults.

| Group | | Clinical features |
|---|---|---|
| Group I | | Acute seroconversion syndrome |
| Group II | | Asymptomatic infection |
| Group III | | Persistent generalized lymphadenopathy |
| Group IV | A | Chronic constitutional disease |
| | B | Neurological disease due to HIV |
| | C | Specified opportunistic infections |
| | D | Specified secondary malignancies |
| | E | Other conditions, e.g. thrombocytopenia |

**Table 23.16** Centre for Diseases Control classification of HIV infection in children under 13 years old.

| | | |
|---|---|---|
| Class P-0 | | Indeterminate infection |
| Class P-1 | | Asymptomatic infection |
| | Subclass A | Normal immune function |
| | Subclass B | Abnormal immune function |
| Class P-2 | | Symptomatic infection |
| | Subclass A | Non-specific findings |
| | Subclass B | Progressive HIV-related neurological disease |
| | Subclass C | Lymphoid interstitial pneumonitis |
| | Subclass D | Opportunistic infections |
| | Subclass E | Secondary neoplasms |

lymphadenopathy) or an acute reversible encephalopathy. There may be elevation of transaminase levels. There is a viraemia and p24 antigen is detectable in the serum. Anti-gp41 and anti-p24 antibodies first appear some weeks later. Symptoms settle within a week or two.

## Stage II: asymptomatic period

During the asymptomatic period p24 antigen is not detectable in the serum but the presence of anti-p24 enables the diagnosis of HIV infection to be made (Fig. 23.14). During this period there is usually a progressive decline in the CD4-positive lymphocyte count in the peripheral blood. After a number of years the antibody levels decline and p24 appears again in the blood.

## Stage III: persistent generalized lymphadenopathy (PGL)

In one-third to one-half of the patients with HIV infection, symmetrical rubbery lymphadenopathy involving two or more extrainguinal sites develops and persists for more than 3 months. The nodes show non-specific follicular hyperplasia if biopsied.

During stages II and III of HIV infection a number of dermatological problems, both infective and non-infective, are more common. These include seborrhoeic dermatitis, psoriasis, acne, folliculitis, herpes simplex and zoster, dermatophytes and molluscum contagiosum. They are often more resistant to therapy than similar problems in non-HIV-infected persons.

## Stage IVA: constitutional disease

This stage of infection is also called the AIDS-related complex (ARC) and consists of fever, night sweats, weight loss, oropharyngeal candidiasis, chronic diarrhoea and herpes zoster. Hairy leukoplakia, a ridged raised white lesion of the oral mucosa and tongue, related to Epstein–Barr virus replication, may also occur. The appearance of ARC heralds the development of AIDS in many patients.

## Group IVB: neurological manifestations of HIV

More than 90 per cent of patients with AIDS have clinical evidence of HIV infection of the CNS. This may be subtle and sometimes appears before the other features of AIDS. Cognitive dysfunction, behaviour change and pyschosis, with or without motor changes and spastic paralysis occur. There is cerebral atrophy on computed tomographic scans (CT) or magnetic resonance images (MRI) and the CSF shows a normal cell count and a raised protein concentration. The pathology of the myelopathy is vacuolation of the posterior and lateral columns. Between one-third and one-half of patients progress to a severe global dementia.

## Group IVC: opportunistic infections

The development of certain specified opportunistic infections (Table 23.17), indicative as they are of severe immunological dysfunction, is the most common AIDS-defining condition.

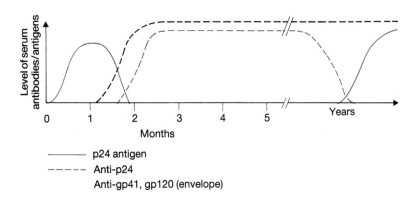

**Figure 23.14** Time course of serological response to HIV infection.

The most frequently reported opportunistic disease is *Pneumocystis carinii* pneumonia, followed by oesophageal candidiasis, cryptococcosis, toxoplasmosis and cytomegalovirus infection. The common sites of infection with the various opportunistic pathogens are given in Table 23.18 and the chief causes of the most common clinical syndromes seen in AIDS are given below.

## Group IVD: malignancies

Kaposi's sarcoma, a tumour of spindle-shaped vascular endothelial cells, is frequent in homosexual men with HIV infection but is less common in intravenous drug abusers. It is commonly multifocal and is seen on the skin, in the mouth, within the bowel and in the lungs. Lesions are raised violaceous nodules and plaques 2–50 mm in diameter. Non-Hodgkin's lymphoma (intracerebral or peripheral) is another malignancy recognized as related to HIV infection.

## CLINICAL FEATURES OF AIDS

Most patients with AIDS will have a number of different clinical, social and psychological problems related to their infection. The chief clinical syndromes with which AIDS may present or which need investigation and treatment are the following.

## Lung disease

Patients present with respiratory illness or are found to have chest X-ray abnormalities incidentally or while under investigation for fever or other systemic symptoms. The list of possible causes is very long but the most common diagnoses are:

1. *Pneumocystis carinii* pneumonia (page 300)
2. Mycobacterial infection – either *Mycobacterium tuberculosis* (page 302) or *M. avium-intracellulare*
3. Bacterial pneumonia
4. Fungal infections
5. Cytomegalovirus pneumonia
6. Kaposi's sarcoma
7. Lymphocytic interstitial pneumonia is common in paediatric AIDS

**Table 23.17** Opportunistic infections diagnostic of AIDS in an HIV-infected individual over 1 month of age.

*Pneumocystis carinii* pneumonia
Disseminated atypical mycobacterial infection
Toxoplasmosis of the brain
Oesophageal or pulmonary candidiasis
Cryptosporidiosis or isosporiasis with diarrhoea of >1 month's duration
Cytomegalovirus infections outside the reticuloendothelial system
Extrapulmonary cryptococcosis
Progressive multifocal leukoencephalopathy
Non-cutaneous herpes simplex infection
Disseminated histoplasmosis or coccidioidomycosis
Non-pulmonary tuberculosis
Recurrent salmonella septicaemia

**Table 23.18** The principal clinical syndromes caused by the major opportunistic pathogens in HIV-infected persons.

Candida
    Oropharyngeal disease
    Oesophageal infection

*Pneumocystis carinii*
    Pneumonia

*Mycobacterium tuberculosis*
    Pulmonary disease
    Meningitis

Herpes simplex
    Oral and oesophageal disease
    Anal and genital lesions

Cytomegalovirus
    Retinitis
    Colitis
    Adrenal infection
    Biliary tract infections
    Encephalitis

*Cryptosporidium parvum*
    Enterocolitis
    Biliary tract disease

*Mycobacterium avium-intracellulare*
    Fever and weight loss
    Pulmonary disease

*Cryptococcus neoformans*
    Meningitis

*Toxoplasma gondii*
    Brain abscesses

## Neurological manifestations

About 10 per cent of AIDS patients present with neurological disease and about one-half will have CNS disease other than HIV-related encephalopathy at some stage or other.

The most common cause of meningitis is *Cryptococcus neoformans*, which often presents insidiously. The chief causes of space-occupying cerebral lesions are toxoplasmosis, lymphomas, progressive multifocal leukoencephalopathy (a papovavirus infection) and fungal abscesses. Peripheral neuropathies of several types also occur.

## Gastrointestinal disease

Opportunistic infections and secondary neoplasms may involve any part of the gastrointestinal tract. The oropharynx is often infected with *Candida* and the palate is an early site of Kaposi's sarcoma lesions. Dysphagia may be caused by the spread of *Candida* down the oesophagus. Chronic diarrhoea is common but it can be very difficult to find any infective cause. Infections with *Cryptosporidium, Isospora, Salmonella* and *Campylobacter* are common. A malabsorptive syndrome can be caused by *M. avium-intracellulare* (MAI) which can be detected inside macrophages throughout the small bowel. Colitis may be caused by several of the above organisms and also by cytomegalovirus and herpes simplex virus. Kaposi's sarcoma is often present throughout the entire bowel and can cause obstruction, bleeding or a protein-losing enteropathy.

Overall about 50 per cent of patients are dead within 2 or 3 years of the diagnosis of AIDS. Children and elderly patients have a worse prognosis.

## DIAGNOSIS

The diagnosis of HIV infection is usually made by detecting specific antibodies to the p24 antigen by an enzyme immunoassay (EIA). The EIA can be confirmed by the highly specific Western blot test. Direct detection of viral antigens and viral culture are also possible but not routinely performed. The changes in p24 and anti-p24 levels in the blood are shown in Fig. 23.14. Progression of the disease can also be monitored by measuring the CD4-positive lymphocyte count. Appropriate counselling should take place before and after HIV testing.

## TREATMENT

There is no cure for HIV infection. Certain drugs particularly zidovudine (AZT), zalcitabine (dideoxycytosine; ddC) and didanosine (dideoxyinosine; ddI) inhibit the reverse transcriptase of HIV and slow progression of the disease. AZT is now offered to patients with AIDS and to individuals when their peripheral blood CD4-positive lymphocyte count falls below $200/mm^3$ or higher levels if associated with symptoms. Studies are underway to determine whether combinations of AZT with ddI or ddC will be more effective or less toxic than AZT alone, which is myelotoxic and can cause myopathy. Primary prophylaxis against *P. carinii* pneumonitis is started if the CD4-positive lymphocyte count falls below $250/mm^3$. Cotrimoxazole is the usual prophylaxis; dapsone plus trimethoprim and nebulized pentamidine are alternatives. After clinically apparent opportunistic infections, secondary prophylaxis has to be given lifelong to prevent reactivation of the particular pathogen.

## PREVENTION

In the absence of vaccines, prevention of HIV infection can only be based upon safer sexual practices (condoms, non-penetrative sex and reduction in number of sexual partners), screening of blood products and organ transplantation donors, and strategies to limit intravenous drug abuse and perinatal spread of infection from HIV-positive mothers. Sensible precautions regarding injuries from 'sharps' and the disinfection of equipment need to be implemented in hospitals but there is no need for the isolation of HIV-infected individuals. The place for AZT or other antiviral drugs given to health workers as prophylaxis after needle-stick injuries from infected patients is still to be clarified.

## *T*ROPICAL DISEASES

# *Malaria*

The distribution of malaria worldwide is between the latitudes of 40° north and 30° south, generally at altitudes below 2000 m (Fig. 23.15). About 100 million people are affected and about 1 million, primarily African children, die of the disease each year.

Four species of *Plasmodium* infect humans. *Plasmodium vivax* and *P. ovale* are the cause of benign tertian malaria, *P. falciparum* is the cause of malignant tertian and *P. malariae* the cause of quartan malaria. Infections due to *P. vivax* and *P. falciparum* are much more common than those due to the other two species.

## LIFE-CYCLE OF THE *PLASMODIUM* PARASITE

The life-cycle of malaria parasites consists of an asexual cycle in humans and a sexual cycle in a female *Anopheles* mosquito (Fig. 23.16). Sporozoites are injected ino the human when the mosquito bites and within an hour enter the parenchymal cells of the liver. In *P. vivax* and *P. ovale* infections some of the sporozoites remain in a latent form and are termed hypnozoites. Within the hepatocytes each of the remaining sporozoites multiplies to form a tissue schizont containing several thousand merozoites. One to two weeks later the schizonts rupture and the merozoites are released into the circulation. The merozoites attach to specific receptors (a dif-

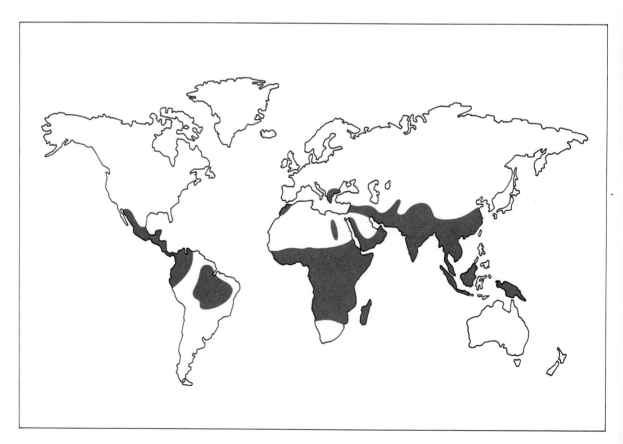

**Figure 23.15** Distribution of human malaria.

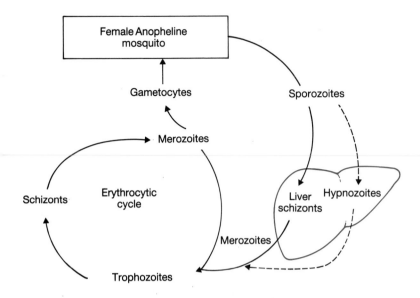

Plasmodium vivax

**Figure 23.16** Life-cycle of *Plasmodium* parasites.

ferent receptor for each species of *Plasmodium*) on the red cell surface and enter the red cells. The intracellular parasites then develop to form ring-shaped trophozoites and then multinucleated schizonts. In turn these rupture to release more merozoites which reinvade red blood cells. Within a few cycles within the red cells the release of merozoites becomes synchronized (approximately every 48 hours for *P. falciparum, P. vivax* and *P. ovale* and 72 hours for *P. malariae*). After several cycles some of the merozoites do not attach to red cells but develop into sexual forms or gametocytes which continue to circulate until ingested by a biting mosquito. The male and female gametocytes replicate in the sexual cycle to form sporozoites which enter the mosquito salivary glands ready to be transmitted to the next host.

Malaria is occasionally transmitted by blood transfusion or transplacentally.

## CLINICAL FEATURES

The incubation period of malaria is usually 10–14 days and the most common presentation is with fever. This is initiated by the release of each generation of merozoites into the circulation and hence starts irregularly but typically, within a few days, settles into a pattern of paroxysms at intervals of 48 or 72 hours. The paroxysms begin with a feeling of intense cold and rigors followed by a rapid rise in temperature. After an hour or so there is a phase of delirium and hot skin lasting for several hours which is ended after several hours by intense sweating, exhaustion and return of the temperature to normal.

Hepatosplenomegaly and anaemia, largely due to haemolysis, are usually also present. Thrombocytopenia is common. The major clinical features of malaria are those of the complications: these are particularly associated with *P. falciparum* infections.

### Plasmodium falciparum

This is the most severe form of malaria. The parasite is capable of invading red blood cells of whatever age and can produce very high levels of parasitaemia. The infected red cells also become morphologically altered and adhere more easily to vascular endothelium. The adherent cells then cause vascular occlusion and tissue hypoxia. Almost any organ can be damaged or fail but a number of serious complications are common:

1. Cerebral malaria (when the central nervous system is involved) is characterized by, often sudden, deterioration in consciousness, convulsions, paralysis and death.

2. Pulmonary involvement with cough, haemoptysis, and shock lung.
3. Splanchnic ischaemia with abdominal pain, vomiting and bloody diarrhoea.
4. Acute tubular necrosis.
5. Jaundice due to haemolysis and/or hepatocellular dysfunction.
6. Haemoglobinuria and dark urine (black-water fever) due to massive haemolysis.
7. Hyponatraemia and hypoglycaemia can be severe and fatal.

The speed of development of *P. falciparum* infection means that the periodicity of fever paroxysms may never become established.

Individuals with heterozygous sickle cell trait, thalassaemia and glucose-6-phosphate dehydrogenase deficiency (G6PD) are partially protected from *P. falciparum* infection. Continual exposure to falciparum malaria in childhood produces partial immunity and hence many adult Africans have only mild illnesses when infected. This immunity is lost after a year or so of residence outside a malarious area.

### *Plasmodium vivax and Plasmodium ovale*

Individuals lacking the Duffy blood group antigen are naturally immune to *P. vivax* infection, since they also lack the specific receptor for merozoite attachment.

These forms of malaria are rarely severe since the parasites only attack immature red blood cells. Parasitaemia is rarely above 1 or 2 per cent of the red cell population. Merozoites may also be released from long-term hypnozoite forms of these parasites within the liver and benign tertian malaria can appear for the first time or relapse may occur several months after leaving a malarial area.

### *Plasmodium malariae*

This is an uncommon form of malaria. The parasite only infects senescent red blood cells but the infection can run a chronic course with low-grade fever for many years. The chronic immunological stimulation can lead to nephrotic syndrome.

### DIAGNOSIS

Diagnosis relies upon detection and identification of the different malarial parasites in smears of peripheral blood stained with Wright or Giemsa stain. If parasites are seen in more than 10 per cent of erythrocytes the prognosis is poor.

### TREATMENT

Treatment of malaria requires killing of the erythrocytic stages of the parasite in order to terminate the acute attack, together with eradication of any hepatic schizonts to prevent relapses.

1. Several drugs can destroy asexual stages of the parasites (Table 23.19). Chloroquine is the most suitable drug for all forms other than falciparum malaria. Falciparum strains resistant to chloroquine are now widespread in Africa, South America and Asia. Almost all patients with falciparum infection (the exception being those from Central America or the Arabian Gulf area) should be treated with quinine sulphate, mefloquine or a derivative of qinghaosu (e.g. artemether).
2. Chloroquine will not eradicate hepatic schizonts and to prevent relapse of vivax or ovale infections a course of primaquine needs to follow the chloroquine. Primaquine causes haemolysis in those with G6PD deficiency and the patient's blood needs to be checked before primaquine is given.
3. Exchange blood transfusion can be used in severe parasitaemia (>10 per cent of infected erythrocytes).

Monitoring for complications and supportive measures are essential for the care of patients with severe (more than 5 per cent parasitaemia) falciparum infections.

### PREVENTION

Persons travelling to malarial areas must be protected against malaria. Mosquito contact can be minimized by the use of mosquito nets around beds, insect repellents and the wearing of trousers and avoidance of short-sleeved shirts. Chemoprophylaxis should also be given but the widespread distribution and changing patterns of resistance among *P. falciparum* strains makes

**Table 23.19** Drug therapy for malaria.

| Drug | Clinical purpose | Dose |
|---|---|---|
| Chloroquine | Treat acute attack of vivax, ovale, malariae and (rarely) falciparum | Oral 600 mg chloroquine base initially, followed by 300 mg after 6 hours and then 300 mg daily for 3 days |
| Quinine | Treat acute attack of chloroquine-resistant falciparum malaria | Intravenous 10 mg/kg in saline as a 4-hour infusion 8–12 hourly or oral 600 mg every 8 hours for 5 days |
| Pyrimethamine and sulphadoxine | Final eradication of falciparum parasites | Oral single dose of Fansidar (3 tablets) after the quinine course has ended |
| Artemether | Treat acute attack of chloroquine-resistant falciparum malaria | Intramuscular 3–4 mg/kg initial dose, then 1–2 mg/kg/day |
| Tetracycline | Final eradication of falciparum parasites | Oral 500 mg qds for 1 week after the quinine course has ended |
| Primaquine | Eradication of liver schizonts in vivax and ovale infections | Oral 15 mg daily for 2 weeks (3 weeks for those from S. Asia or the Pacific Islands) |

detailed recommendations unwise. Up-to-date advice should be sought and travellers may need to be warned that no prophylactic regimen is certain to provide protection and that they should seek urgent medical advice if they develop a feverish illness while abroad or within 2 months of their leaving a malarial area (when the risk of life-threatening falciparum infection still needs considering). An effective vaccine is awaited.

# Trypanosomiasis

Trypanosomes are flagellated protozoa. Two main forms of disease occur in humans: African trypanosomiasis (sleeping sickness) and American trypanosomiasis (Chagas' disease) (Fig. 23.17).

## AFRICAN TRYPANOSOMIASIS (SLEEPING SICKNESS)

This highly lethal form of meningoencephalitis, transmitted by the bites of infected tsetse flies,

exists in two forms. Gambian sleeping sickness is caused by *T. brucei gambiense* and is a slowly developing illness found in West and Central Africa (Fig. 23.17). Rhodesian sleeping sickness is a much more acute form that is found in southeast Africa and is caused by *T. brucei rhodesiense*.

## Clinical features

After injection into the skin the trypanosomes multiply and a small nodule (trypanosomal chancre) forms at the site. A few weeks later there is parasitaemia and the patient develops recurrent bouts of fever, generalized, rubbery lymphadenopathy, general malaise, tachycardia, headache and hepatosplenomegaly. In the Rhodesian form, myocarditis and central nervous system involvement begin within a few weeks and death follows within a few months. The Gambian form progresses very much more slowly and causes headache, intellectual deterioration, apathy and disturbance of sleep pattern. The patient eventually becomes stuporose and needs to be roused to eat: death often results from intercurrent infection.

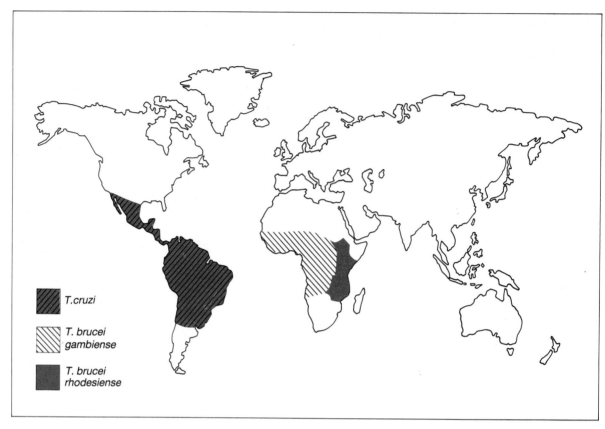

**Figure 23.17** Distribution of various species of trypanosomes.

## Diagnosis

The diagnosis is usually made by demonstration of trypanosomes in blood, lymph node aspirates or CSF. Serological tests are not very useful but newer tests using DNA hybridization probes are being developed.

## Treatment

Suramin is the drug of choice for the treatment of the early stages of trypanosomiasis; pentamidine will also work in the Gambian form. Neither drug crosses the blood–brain barrier, however, and for the late, neurological stages the traditional therapy is with the toxic arsenical drug melarsoprol. Recently a new drug, eflornithine, has shown some promise.

## AMERICAN TRYPANOSOMIASIS (CHAGAS' DISEASE)

Chagas' disease occurs widely in South and Central America (Fig. 23.17). It is caused by T. cruzi, transmitted to humans in the faeces of triatomid or reduviid bugs which live in the walls and roofs of primitive wood and mud houses. As the bug feeds it defecates and the organisms are inoculated when the host scratches the site of the bite or rubs the faeces onto a mucosal surface such as the conjunctiva.

## Acute disease

A small area of local inflammation develops at the site of inoculation and is accompanied by fever and regional lymphadenopathy. If the portal of entry is the conjunctiva, there is unilateral periorbital oedema (Romanas' sign). Occasionally there is a degree of myocarditis or meningoencephalitis but most ·atients recover completely within a few weeks

## Chronic disease

Many years later, chronic Chagas' disease may develop. It is an autoimmune reaction directed against the myocardium accompanied by degeneration of the autonomic nervous system in the gut. There is dilation and dysfunction of the heart and mural thrombi may develop with subsequent embolization. The complications of mega-oesophagus (dysphagia and aspiration pneumonia) and mega-colon (constipation and abdominal distension) may also be present.

## Diagnosis

During the acute phase trypanosomes may be detected in the peripheral blood but the diagnosis of chronic Chagas' disease relies upon epidemiological and serological findings.

## Treatment

No completely satisfactory treatment for Chagas' disease is available, although nifurtimox and benznidazole are useful in the acute phase.

# Leishmaniasis

Leishmaniasis is caused by protozoa of the genus *Leishmania* which have an asexual life-cycle in vertebrate hosts. Sandflies feed on the infected animal and ingest the parasites. They then undergo a sexual replication in the sandfly and are inoculated into another host when the sandfly next feeds. The many strains of *Leishmania* that are capable of causing infection in humans are divided into four groups (Fig. 23.18): *L. tropica* in the Old World and *L. mexicana* in the New World produce localized forms of cutaneous disease; *L. braziliensis* is the cause of an aggressive form of cutaneous disease termed espundia; and *L. donovani* is the aetiological agent of visceral leishmaniasis or kala-azar.

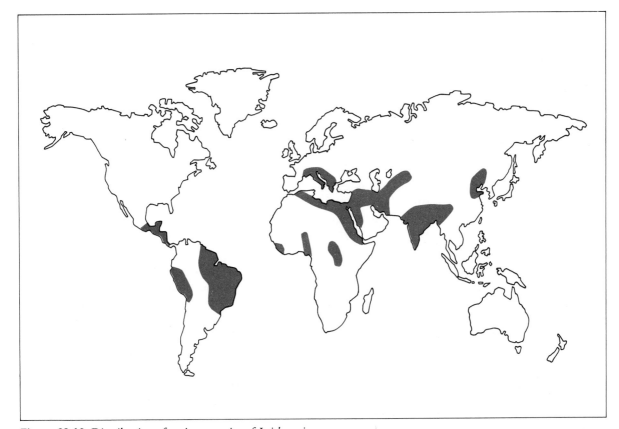

**Figure 23.18** Distribution of various species of *Leishmania*.

## CUTANEOUS LEISHMANIASIS

In Mediterranean countries, the Middle East through to India and in Central Asia and China, *L. tropica* causes a slowly growing red papule which develops into a shallow ulcer with a granulating base (oriental sore or Delhi boil) at the site of the bite. This eventually heals spontaneously leaving an atrophic scar. Treatment with pentavalent antimonials such as sodium stibogluconate speeds healing.

Similar disease caused by *L. mexicana* may be seen in South America. If the infection involves the cartilage of the ear, however, then a chronic destructive lesion occurs (chiclero's ulcer). This can be treated with intramuscular cycloguanil pamoate.

Infection with *L. braziliensis* is found in areas of South America. The initial lesions are similar to those described above but several weeks or years later, sometimes after healing of the skin, secondary or metastatic lesions develop at mucocutaneous junctions of the nose and mouth. This mucocutaneous disease is progressive and leads to nasal obstruction, ulceration, destruction of the nasal septum and eventually to destruction of the entire front of the face. Death results from aspiration and secondary infection. Treatment is also with pentavalent antimonials.

Diffuse cutaneous leishmaniasis with massive dissemination of skin lesions occurs with some strains of *Leishmania*.

### Diagnosis

Diagnosis of cutaneous leishmaniasis is established by demonstrating forms of the parasite (Leishman–Donovan bodies) in histological samples. There is a vigorous cellular immune response and a positive leishmanin skin test.

## VISCERAL LEISHMANIASIS (KALA-AZAR)

Visceral leishmaniasis occurs in the Mediterranean and Middle East, Asia, Africa and South America and is caused by strains of *L. donovani*. In most parts of the world the reservoir is domestic dogs and wild canines but in India, humans are the only known host. Transmission is by *Phlebotomus* sandflies and after inoculation into the host the parasites disseminate throughout the reticuloendothelial system. Kala-azar is a risk to patients with depressed cellular immunity: it is increasingly seen in patients with AIDS who live in or travel to endemic areas.

### Clinical features

After an incubation period of 2–12 months, fever develops and is intermittently present throughout the illness. Diarrhoea, malabsorption and weight loss associated with hepatosplenomegaly and lymphadenopathy are the principal features. The spleen can be massively enlarged and contributes to the pancytopenia which is found in advanced cases. The skin may become pigmented and this gives the disease its name (kala-azar is Hindi for black disease). Without therapy the disease is 70–90 per cent fatal.

### Diagnosis

There is anaemia and leukopenia, and a marked elevation of IgG levels. The diagnosis is confirmed by finding numerous Leishman–Donovan bodies within the macrophages in aspirates of liver, bone marrow, lymph nodes or spleen. Serological tests are also available.

### Treatment

Treatment is with pentavalent antimonial drugs given for several weeks. Amphotericin, pentamidine and interferon-γ can be used in cases that either fail or relapse after initial therapy.

# Schistosomiasis

The schistosomes are a group of parasitic flukes that inhabit the blood stream. Three species, *Schistosoma mansoni*, *S. haematobium* and *S. japonicum*, together infect more than 200 million people worldwide (Fig. 23.19). The adult worms of *S. mansoni* and *S. japonicum* inhabit the portal and mesenteric veins while *S. haematobium* inhabits the veins of the bladder and pelvis. Each female worm deposits several hundred eggs each day throughout its life. Some of these eggs rupture into the lumen of the bowel or bladder

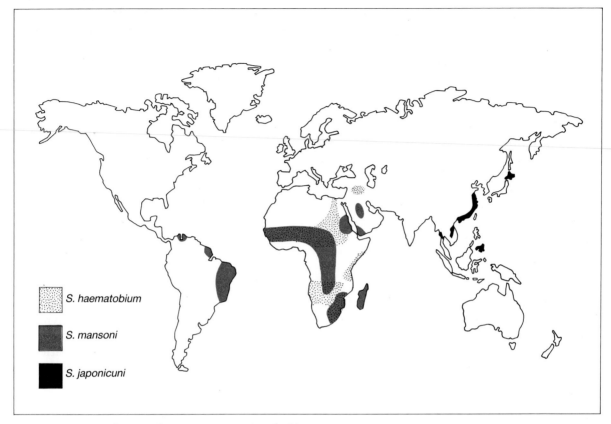

**Figure 23.19** Distribution of three human species of schistosomes.

and are excreted. The eggs of the various species can be distinguished morphologically: those of *S. mansoni* are oval with a lateral spine, *S. haematobium* have a terminal spine and those of *S. japonicum* are round with a tiny lateral spine.

In fresh water the eggs hatch into miracidia which invade their intermediate snail host. Within the snail thousands of cercariae develop and emerge within a few weeks. These cercariae penetrate human skin and develop over a few months into adult flukes.

## CLINICAL FEATURES

Schistosomes cause three distinct syndromes:

1. Swimmer's itch
2. Katayama fever
3. Chronic schistosomiasis

Swimmer's itch is a papular skin rash occurring within a few hours of cercarial penetration. It is a hypersensitivity reaction to the parasites. Within a few weeks of heavy infections there is a serum sickness-like syndrome called Katayama fever. There is fever, cough, urticaria, eosinophilia, diarrhoea, lymphadenopathy and hepatosplenomegaly. The illness usually resolves within a few weeks.

Chronic schistosomiasis is caused by the inflammatory response to those eggs which are retained in host tissues. The antigens induce granuloma formation, vascular obstruction and fibrosis, the degree of tissue damage depending upon the total number of retained eggs.

### Schistosoma mansoni and Schistosoma japonicum

Patients suffer a chronic dysenteric illness with abdominal pain and bloody diarrhoea. Colonic polyps may occur. Some eggs are carried to the liver where they cause periportal fibrosis and portal hypertension with ascites, splenomegaly and bleeding from oesophageal varices. Occasionally eggs bypass the liver and are deposited in the lungs, spinal cord or brain.

### Schistosoma haematobium

The fibrous tissue and scarring around retained eggs lead to urinary obstruction and irregularity of the bladder wall, which may eventually calcify. Persons infected with *S. haematobium* usually have terminal haematuria and dysuria, other symptoms resulting from obstruction or recurrent urinary infections. Chronic *S. haematobium* infection is associated with carcinoma of the bladder. A definitive diagnosis can be made by finding schistosome eggs in the urine, best collected in the early afternoon.

## TREATMENT

This is now best given with a single oral dose of praziquantel, 40 mg/kg body weight, which is effective against all human schistosomes and is remarkably free of serious side effects.

# TISSUE NEMATODES

There are a number of roundworms that produce diseases as a result of their presence in human tissues (Table 23.20).

# Filariasis

There are several different types of filariasis caused by members of the superfamily *Filarioidea*. Their worldwide distribution is shown in Fig. 23.20. The adult worms produce larvae called microfilariae which are transmitted by a variety of biting insect vectors.

## LYMPHATIC FILARIASIS

The two organisms commonly causing lymphatic filariasis are *Wuchereria bancrofti* and *Brugia malayi*. The former is found in Africa, Latin America, the Pacific Islands, northern Australia and India and the latter in coastal areas of Asia and the South Pacific. Both are transmitted by mosquitoes. The adult worms lie in the lymphatics and cause inflammation and fibrosis. The microfilariae travel from the lymphatics to the blood but produce no symptoms. During the day they spend their time in the pulmonary circulation but in the late evening (when the mosquito vectors are biting) they are released into the peripheral circulation.

## CLINICAL FEATURES

After an incubation period of 8–12 months the adult worms cause attacks of fever, lymphangitis and lymphadenitis, particularly in the groin. The lymphatics of the spermatic cord may also be inflamed. After repeated attacks (the adults live many years) there is chronic fibrosis and lymphatic blockage. Hydrocoeles and elephantiasis (chronic oedema of the scrotum or legs) may develop. Eosinophilia is usually present but

**Table 23.20** Characteristics of tissue nematodes.

| Parasite | Site of infection | Disease | Source of infection |
|---|---|---|---|
| *Wunchereria bancrofti* | Lymphatics | Lymphatic filariasis (elephantiasis) | Mosquitoes |
| *Brugia malayi* | | | |
| *Onchocerca volvulus* | Subcutaneous tissues | Onchocerciasis (river blindness) | Blackflies |
| *Loa loa* | Subcutaneous tissues | Loiasis (Calabar swellings) | Deerflies |
| *Toxocara canis* | Eyes | Toxocariasis (visceral larva migrans) | Ova in dog faeces |
| *Trichinella spiralis* | Muscles | Trichinosis | Inadequately cooked pork |

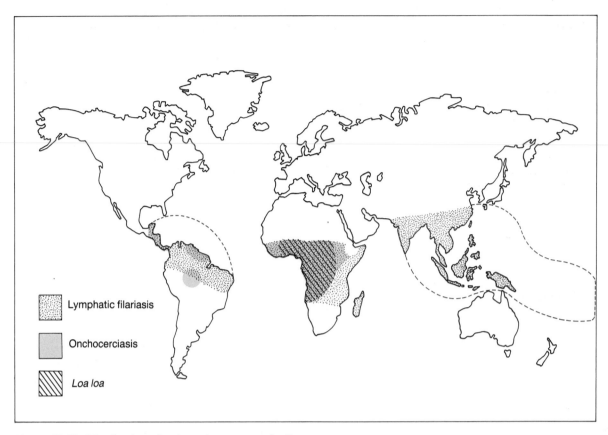

**Figure 23.20** Distribution of various tissue nematode diseases.

the diagnosis can only be confirmed by identification of microfilariae in the blood: nocturnal samples should be taken. The serological tests are sensitive but not very specific among the filarial group. Treatment is with diethylcarbamazine (DEC).

Tropical eosinophilia (page 623) is due to a hypersensitivity reaction to lymphatic filariae. There is cough, bronchospasm, pulmonary infiltrates and a very high eosinophilia.

## Onchocerciasis

Ochocerciasis or river blindness occurs in tropical Africa and in some areas of Latin America. The adult worms lie in subcutaneous nodules, 2–3 cm in diameter, situated particularly on the trunk and legs. The microfilariae are in the skin and eyes. In the skin the inflammation causes intense itching, lichenification and atrophy. In the eye there is keratitis, iritis and chorioretinitis ultimately causing loss of visual acuity. In certain parts of Africa onchocerciasis is a major cause of blindness. The microfilariae can be seen in snips of skin. Treatment is with DEC or ivermectin which have to be given repeatedly as neither kills the adult worms.

## Loaisis

*Loa loa* infections only occur in West Africa. The adult worms migrate continuously in the subcutaneous tissues at about 1 cm per hour. Calabar swellings are egg-sized lesions that occur on the skin as worms are passing: the worm can also occasionally be seen crossing the conjunctiva. The microfilariae are found in the blood during the day and their discovery confirms the diagnosis. There is an eosinophilia. Treatment is with ivermectin or DEC.

## Toxocariasis

Toxocara canis and T. cati are roundworm parasites of dogs and cats, thus making the distribution of the disease worldwide. Humans (usually children) become infected by ingestion of animal faeces and the larvae leave the bowel and encyst in the tissues. Most infections are asymptomatic but occasionally fever, skin rash and dysfunction of a variety of organs occurs (visceral larva migrans). Ocular invasion by larvae causes a granulomatous chorioretinitis and visual loss. Eosinophilia may be present in the acute phase

and serological tests are available. The efficacy of treatment with thiabendazole is still uncertain.

## Trichinosis

Trichinosis caused by Trichinella spiralis is acquired by eating the undercooked flesh of pigs and other carnivores. The adult worms in the bowel cause diarrhoea and abdominal pain and the larvae, after penetrating the bowel wall, migrate and encyst in muscles. In heavy infections there is fever, muscle weakness and tenderness, and periorbital oedema. Eosinophilia is pronounced. Serology and muscle biopsy confirm the diagnosis but the value of anthelminthic therapy is uncertain.

# CUTANEOUS WORMS

## Cutaneous larva migrans

Also known as creeping eruption, this migratory, intensely itchy, serpiginous eruption is the result of infestation with larval nematodes of various species, usually dog or cat hookworms of low human pathogenicity. Animal hookworms produce eggs which are then shed with the faeces, often on beaches or other sandy areas. The larvae hatch and are able to penetrate human skin: the track marks the route of the parasite as it wanders aimlessly in the skin. Without treatment the lesions gradually disappear, but topical or systemic thiabendazole leads to more rapid resolution.

## Dracunculiasis (Guinea worm infection)

Estimates of the number of people infected with Dracunculus medinensis in Africa, the Middle East, India and other tropical areas range from 50 to 150 million. Infection is acquired by ingesting water containing tiny infected crustaceans of the genus Cyclops. Larvae leave the stomach and develop into adults. After fertilization the female worm migrates to the subcutaneous tissues, usually in the legs. A painful papule develops and eventually ulcerates, exposing the end of the worm. When this area comes in contact with water, large numbers of larvae are released and are ingested by Cyclops to complete the life-cycle.

Secondary bacterial infection of the ulcers is common. Treatment with niridazole or thiabendazole reduces the inflammation and enables the worm to be removed by gently rolling it around a small stick.

# LEPROSY

Leprosy is still one of the most important infectious diseases, affecting many millions of persons worldwide. The organism responsible, *Mycobacterium leprae*, invades skin and peripheral nerves and is probably spread by nasal secretions of patients with very bacilliferous forms of the disease.

## CLINICAL FEATURES

Essentially the clinical presentation of leprosy depends on the host's immune response to infection with *M. leprae* and the form of disease also determines infectivity and the likelihood of neurological damage. Two major forms of the disease are recognized, although intermediate forms also occur. The type of disease can be assessed either clinically or histologically.

### Lepromatous leprosy

The cellular immune response is not activated in individuals with the lepromatous form of the disease, which is characterized by widespread skin lesions and by the presence of large numbers of organisms. These can be demonstrated in nasal smears or in skin biopsy specimens. Skin lesions are erythematous or brown, papular or nodular and are not anaesthetic. As the disease extends, the skin of the face, especially the nose and ear lobes become thickened producing a typical leonine facies. Rhinitis, testicular atrophy and ocular damage are common.

### Tuberculoid leprosy

Patients with an effective cellular immune response to *M. leprae* have fewer skin lesions but suffer damage to peripheral nerves mediated by delayed-type hypersensitivity reactions. This form of disease is characterized by a limited number of erythematous or hypopigmented skin lesions which may be macular or annular with a raised edge and an anaesthetic, dry and hairless centre. The nerves near the skin lesions are damaged and feel thickened. The neuropathy of leprosy leads to palsies and the anaesthesia to ulceration and loss of tissue. Histology of the skin in tuberculoid leprosy shows granulomas and absent or scanty bacilli.

### Borderline leprosy

Borderline leprosy occupies a halfway position between lepromatous and tuberculoid forms. It is clinically unstable and patients tend to move towards one of the polar forms of the disease. The skin lesions of borderline leprosy are variable and nerve damage is common.

## TREATMENT

Combination therapy with rifampicin, dapsone and clofazimine for at least 2 years is recommended for lepromatous leprosy. For paucibacillary forms, such as tuberculoid leprosy, daily dapsone and monthly rifampicin is given for 6 months. Contacts of highly infective cases can be given prophylaxis with dapsone.

# RICKETTSIAL INFECTIONS

Rickettsiae are small, obligatory intracellular bacteria. Almost all the major human rickettsial diseases are zoonoses and are spread to humans by arthropod vectors (Table 23.21). The predominant pathology of rickettsial diseases involves infection and damage to the vascular endothelial cells, resulting in a vasculitis.

## Epidemic typhus

Louse-borne typhus is not a tropical disease: it has been more prominent in Europe and Asia during periods of war and social upheaval. There is no zoonotic reservoir and the human body

**Table 23.21** Rickettsial diseases.

| Disease | Organism | Reservoir | Vector | Distribution |
|---|---|---|---|---|
| Epidemic typhus | R. prowazeki | Humans | Lice | Africa, Asia, Central and South America |
| Endemic typhus | R. mooseri | Rats | Fleas | Africa, Central America, S.E. Asia |
| Rocky Mountain Spotted Fever | R. rickettsiae | Rodents | Ticks | North and South America |
| Scrub typhus | R. tsutsugamushi | Rodents | Mites | Asia |
| Rickettsial pox | R. akari | Mice | Mites | Asia, Africa, N. America |
| Q fever | Coxiella burnetii | Cattle | Ticks, dust | Worldwide |

louse is the vector. It is the louse faeces that are infectious and these either enter through contaminated skin abrasions or are inhaled.

The incubation period is 1–3 weeks followed by unremitting fever, severe headache and myalgia. After several days there is a pink macular rash over the whole body: the rash later becomes petechial or frankly haemorrhagic. Complications include meningoencephalitis, hepatitis, bronchitis and myocarditis. The fever settles in about 2 weeks but there is often considerable postinfectious fatigue, which can last for months. Untreated, the mortality may be 25 per cent or more.

Late relapses of the original *R. prowazeki* infection may ensue; these are attributed to diminishing immunity and stress and are termed Brill–Zinsser disease.

# Endemic murine typhus

Murine typhus is caused by *R. typhi* and is spread by the faeces of the rat flea. The clinical illness is similar to louse-borne typhus but somewhat less severe.

# Rocky Mountain spotted fever

Rocky Mountain spotted fever (RMSF) is caused by *R. rickettsii* which is transmitted to humans by the bite of hard ticks, often the dog tick. It is not limited to the Rocky Mountain states of the USA but is found in both North and South America. Most cases occur in children. The incubation period is about 1 week and the onset is sudden with fever, chills, myalgia and headache. The rash appears within 3–5 days of the fever: initial lesions are on the extremities and are maculopapular, later spreading to the trunk and becoming petechial and purpuric. Neurological, renal and cardiovascular complications are common and death occurs in about 5 per cent of cases.

# Other tick-borne spotted fevers

There are a variety of other tick-borne rickettsial illnesses in the eastern hemisphere. Marseilles fever, South African tick typhus, Mediterranean fever (*fièvre boutonneuse*) are all caused by varieties of *R. conori*, Asian tick typhus by *R. siberica* and Queensland tick typhus by *R. australis*. In most clinical respects these illnesses resemble RMSF. An important feature, however, is the presence of an eschar at the site of the tick bite. This is a small painless ulcer with a central black necrotic area resulting from the endothelial damage caused by the rickettsiae.

# Scrub typhus

Scrub typhus is caused by *R. tsutsugamushi* which is transmitted by larval mites (chiggers) in the

Far East. Following infection there is local multiplication and formation of an eschar with local lymphadenopathy. The incubation period is 10 to 14 days and the clinical illness later resembles that of epidemic typhus.

## DIAGNOSIS

Diagnosis of rickettsial illnesses during the acute phase must normally be clinical, although direct immunofluorescence of skin biopsies from the rash can be undertaken at reference laboratories. Serological methods can be used for retrospective confirmation of the diagnosis. The non-specific Weil–Felix reaction which depended upon the agglutination of various strains of *Proteus vulgaris* by rickettsiae, has been largely superseded by specific complement fixation tests.

## TREATMENT

Rickettsial infections respond to oral tetracycline, doxycycline or chloramphenicol therapy. The response is usually rapid and therapy can be discontinued a day or two after the fever has settled.

# Relapsing fever

There are two forms of relapsing fever, one caused by the spirochaete *Borrelia recurrentis* which is spread by body lice and one by *B. duttoni* which is transmitted by soft ticks. The diseases are found in Asia, Africa, the Middle East and South America.

The symptoms of fever, myalgia and headache begin after an incubation period of up to 10 days. There may also be organic confusion, arthralgia, cough and dyspnoea, jaundice, petechial rash and conjunctivitis. The initial episode lasts for a few days but a week or so later there is a relapse caused by a fresh generation of *Borrelia* bearing different surface antigens. Generally only a single relapse occurs with louse-borne relapsing fever but there are more relapses in the tick-borne form. Diagnosis involves identifying *Borrelia* in the blood. Treatment with tetracycline or erythromycin is optimal, but Jarisch–Herxheimer reactions are not uncommon. Control involves louse eradication.

# *I*NFECTION IN THE IMMUNOCOMPROMISED HOST

Immunocompromised patients are those with some abnormality of defence mechanisms that predisposes them to increased frequency and severity of infections. All deficits do not predispose the patient to the same infections. The defects in host defences are, for convenience, often divided into specific impairment of one of four major groups: humoral immunity, cellular immunity, the complement system and phagocytosis. Each of these different forms of immunodeficiency is associated with a particular, well-recognized pattern of infective problems (Table 23.22). Many factors may interfere with the normal defence functions of the body but it is unusual for there to be a generalized susceptibility to infection, although sometimes, particularly as a result of powerful cytotoxic and immunosuppressive therapy, patients have disorders or deficits in several of their defence mechanisms.

Although some of the infections in immunocompromised hosts are due to organisms that are only capable of causing disease when resistance is lowered, most are caused by the same organisms that infect normal hosts. It is usually only the frequency or severity of infection that is altered by the defect in immunity.

# Humoral immunity

An effective antibody-mediated immune response is particularly crucial in the defence against encapsulated bacteria (especially *Strep. pneumoniae* and *H. influenzae*) and Gram-negative bacteria. Patients with hypogammaglobulinaemia typically develop chronic or recurrent infections of the middle ear, sinuses and lungs,

**Table 23.22** The principal infections in immunocompromised hosts.

| Immune dysfunction | Condition | Resultant infections |
| --- | --- | --- |
| Humoral immunity | Hypogammaglobulinaemia<br>Myelomatosis<br>Chronic lymphatic leukaemia | *Streptococcus pneumoniae*<br>*Haemophilus influenzae*<br>*Staphylococcus aureus*<br>Enteroviruses |
| Cellular immunity | Lymphomas<br>Cytotoxic drugs<br>Immunosuppressive drugs<br>AIDS | *Listeria*<br>*Salmonella*<br>*Legionella*<br>*Cryptococcus*<br>*Pneumocystis*<br>*Toxoplasma*<br>Herpes viruses<br>*Mycobacteria*<br>Opportunistic pathogens |
| Phagocytosis | Acute leukaemia<br>Chemotactic or neutrophil function<br>  defects | *Staphylococcus aureus*<br>Gram-negative bacilli<br>*Pseudomonas aeruginosa*<br>*Candida* |
| Complement system | Congenital deficiencies | *Staph. aureus*<br>*Neisseria*<br>*H. influenzae*<br>*Strep. pneumoniae* |

with or without bacteraemia. They can be helped by regular replacement therapy with intravenous immunoglobulin preparations. Immunoglobulin deficiencies are also present in patients with multiple myeloma and some forms of chronic lymphatic leukaemia. Humoral immune deficiencies are not generally associated with an increased frequency or severity of viral, fungal or protozoal infections, although selective deficiency of IgA is associated with giardiasis.

# Phagocytes

A decrease in the phagocytic function of the neutrophils, particularly when it is due to a profound reduction in circulating numbers, is usually secondary to drug therapy or malignancy. As the total neutrophil count falls below $0.5 \times 10^9/l$, the patients' risk of acquiring infection from their own endogenous flora of staphylococci, Gram-negative bacteria and

yeasts increases markedly. The infections tend to be prolonged, poorly responsive to therapy and recurrent. The spectrum of diseases is wide and includes pneumonia, skin infections (particularly perirectally), pharyngitis and bacteraemia. Similar infections occur in patients with congenital defects in chemotaxis or neutrophil function.

A defect in opsonization and phagocytosis accompanies hypogammaglobulinaemia and complement deficiency and is also seen after splenectomy or in functional hyposplenism (e.g. sickle cell disease, coeliac disease). These patients have frequent and often fulminant infections with encapsulated bacteria, particularly pneumococci and *H. influenzae*.

# Cell-mediated immunity

The pathological deficiencies of cellular immunity may be congenital or acquired. All the congenital ones are extremely rare but the acquired deficiencies are more commonly seen. They may result from malignancies such as Hodgkin's disease and certain other lymphomas, cytotoxic agents, or therapy with cyclosporin A, corticosteroids or radiation. The condition that has the most profound and persistent effects upon cellular immunity is infection with a human immunodeficiency virus (HIV), which ultimately results in the acquired immune deficiency syndrome (AIDS).

The organisms which cause infection in such patients are particularly intracellular pathogens such as viruses, protozoa and certain bacteria. They include those such as *Pneumocystis* and *Nocardia* which do not usually cause disease in normal individuals and are therefore known as opportunistic pathogens.

# Complement system

Patients with defects in one or more of the complement components have similar infections to those with hypogammaglobulinaemia (see above). They also suffer repeated or chronic bacteraemias with meningococci or gonococci.

## TREATMENT

The treatment of infection in the compromised host depends primarily upon an early diagnosis. This requires a recognition of the immune defect, aggressive investigation and often empirical therapy before the result of the investigations are available. This is especially so for patients with neutropenia when mortality is high if bacteraemia occurs. The therapy chosen should, in general, be with bactericidal agents.

# Disorders of the Skin

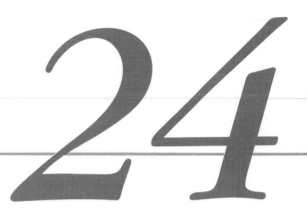

# INTRODUCTION

Skin disease accounts for a significant proportion of all diseases and in some parts of the world it is the commonest cause of consultation at primary health care level. Most dermatoses carry a low morbidity, but some can cause serious disability or death if untreated. Evidence from the UK suggests that at any time about 22 per cent of the population have at least one treatable skin condition, even though only a small proportion of these will seek treatment. In tropical areas an even higher proportion of the population may have skin disease. There are other important differences in comparing skin disease in the industrialized versus the tropical world. Whereas in the latter the majority of skin disease is infective and usually treatable if the resources are available, in industrialized countries non-infective inflammatory skin diseases such as psoriasis and eczema are more common and infectious conditions less frequent.

Skin disease is important not only because of the high prevalence rate in the general population but also because the skin often shows characteristic changes associated with internal disease. These range from those conditions which only occur in the presence of an internal disorder to those where the underlying condition affects the clinical expression of the skin condition. An example of this is the acquired immune deficiency syndrome (AIDS) in which failure of T-lymphocyte-mediated immune responses leads to a wide range of unusual or severe clinical forms of the commoner skin diseases such as candidosis, herpetic ulcers and psoriasis.

Over the past 20–30 years there have been a number of significant changes in the management of skin disease. The first of these was the introduction of topical or systemic corticosteroids for treating a range of inflammatory disorders which were previously difficult to control. Excessive use of steroids has produced certain problems, principally tolerance and local side effects. However, on balance, they remain invaluable for the treatment of skin disease. Other important changes have been the introduction of new antifungal and antiviral agents and the development of non-steroidal treatments for psoriasis. The use of hospital beds in dermatology has declined as it has been possible to discharge more patients or alternatively make use of outpatient therapies such as ultraviolet light or outpatient day treatment centres. Dermatological practice has also been the centre of a major media-backed public health campaign over cutaneous malignancy and sun exposure. The prevention of skin diseases such as this is an exciting challenge.

# Structure of the skin

The skin is the largest of the organs of the body in terms of its surface area and it should therefore be of little surprise that it may act as a mirror for events taking place in other parts of the body in health or disease. Changes in the skin may also range from physiological changes such as the waxy coating over the skin seen in newly born infants and flushing attacks in the menopause to the appearances of ageing. The skin is composed of a complex proliferating layer of epithelial cells – the epidermis, which mature from a basal zone to form, at the external surface, a zone of flattened anucleate cells, the stratum corneum supported by another layer, the dermis, containing blood vessels, nerves and lymphatics. In the process of epidermal maturation internal organelles are lost but a fibrous protein, keratin is deposited. The stratum corneum cells are dead and are eventually shed into the external environment. Certain specialized structures such as hair and nails are derived from epidermal/dermal elements. In addition, specialized glands eccrine or sweat and apocrine or sebaceous are also formed within the skin.

In recent years it has been recognized that the skin houses a unique and complex immune system. The antigen-presenting cells are called Langerhans cells and these are based in the epidermis. Immature keratinocytes can act as immunologically active cells and will express class II antigens and release cytokines. The skin is also pigmented by a network of melanocytes which provides protection against the harmful effects of ultraviolet light. Changes in the skin will involve all these structures as well as the collagen matrix which makes up the dermis.

# Ageing

In the same way as beauty is, in part, a reflection of the integrity of the skin, many of the most noticeable changes of age involve deterioration of skin structures. Ageing in the skin is dependent both on the inexorable process of wear and tear as well as other factors, notably sun damage. The term photoageing is often now used to describe this process, which may be accelerated in those who have had a high degree of sun exposure. Some of these changes are shown in Table 24.1.

Normally, light-induced damage, for instance to DNA, is repaired rapidly; but with increasing age the capacity for and efficiency of this repair process slows and abnormal areas of epidermal growth, senile or solar keratoses, may appear. In the rare congenital disease – xeroderma pigmentosum – which is characterized by severe freckling and the early development of skin cancers, there is a congenital defect affecting the repair of ultraviolet light-damaged DNA.

**Table 24.1** Cutaneous changes of photoageing.

| | |
|---|---|
| Wrinkling | Due to degeneration of elastin fibres in the dermis |
| Easy bruising | Weakening of elastic lamina in small arterioles |
| Dry scaly skin | Disorderly replication of epidermis may lead to a predisposition to skin cancer |

# $S$IGNS AND SYMPTOMS

The study of skin disease, dermatology, is dependent on the visual recognition of different patterns and their association with different disease states. Their morphology, distribution, and duration, amongst other factors, are all important in forming a diagnosis. Wrong diagnoses can be made in dermatology, as elsewhere, if the patient is not examined carefully and completely. While the patient may be concerned with one lesion, an assessment of the rest of the skin, the hair, nails and mucosa is equally important. The range of clinical expression of common skin disorders is sometimes confusing but it is generally possible to recognize the patterns of the principal disorders without too much difficulty. For this reason many dermatological conditions are dealt with by general practitioners (GPs) without hospital referral. Skin disease accounts for about 15 per cent of the work load in most European general practices. Less than 1 per cent of patients with skin disease presenting to GPs will be referred to hospitals. While this figure is small it still accounts for a large, mainly outpatient, work load in skin clinics.

# Symptoms

There are few symptoms which are seen in skin – itch and pain being two of the chief ones.

## ITCH

Itch or pruritus is the most important of dermatological symptoms. It is, however, highly subjective and there are few satisfactory ways in which this symptom can be quantified either for treatment or management. Its severity is often helpful in characterizing the disease. In scabies the itching is very severe whereas in pityriasis rosea it is either mild or absent. Pruritus gives rise to one of the most important diagnostic signs in dermatology – the presence of scratch marks or excoriations. These in turn may lead to a number of complications. Scratching is often followed by secondary infection and, for instance, in many tropical countries the commonest cause of infection with nephritogenic streptococci is scabies, simply through the introduction of the appropriate strains with scratching. Repeated scratching may also perpetuate skin lesions through a vicious cycle of scratching leading to lichenification and increased 'itchiness'.

## PAIN

Pain on the other hand is not a common dermatological symptom. It may follow certain specific conditions such as herpes zoster (shingles) or occur secondary to cracking of the skin surface, particularly on the hands and feet where chronic thickening of the skin due to either eczema or psoriasis may lead to the development of thickened but brittle plaques. Other painful lesions include eroded surfaces where the epidermis is removed, for instance, through blister formation.

## *Signs*

The morphology of skin disease is usually described by various classic terms:

- **Macule**: a localized area of discolouration of the skin without change in texture or thickening (usually up 2–3 cm).
- **Papule**: a small solid lesion up to 1 cm in diameter which is raised and palpable.
- **Vesicle**: a small fluid-filled lesion, the same size as a papule.
- **Pustule**: a pus-filled vesicle.
- **Nodule**: a circumscribed, raised and palpable thickening involving the dermis and subcutis.
- **Bulla**: a large fluid-filled lesion larger than a vesicle.
- **Plaque**: a raised, flat-topped and large lesion usually over 2–3 cm in diameter.
- **Erythema**: redness of the skin, one of the chief signs of inflammation.

- **Weal**: raised soft area of transient dermal oedema.
- **Crust**: dried serum, pus or blood on the surface of a lesion.
- **Hyperkeratosis**: thickening of the horny layer of the skin usually presenting with scaling.
- **Telangiectasia**: permanently dilated blood vessels often arranged around a central 'feeder' vessel (spider naevus) which disappear on blanching with gentle pressure under a glass slide. A small number may occur in normal subjects (Fig. 24.1).
- **Purpura**: haemorrhage about 2–5 mm in diameter into the skin from a superficial dermal blood vessel.
- **Ecchymosis**: large areas of haemorrhage into the skin.
- **Ulcer**: an area of loss of continuity of the epithelium.

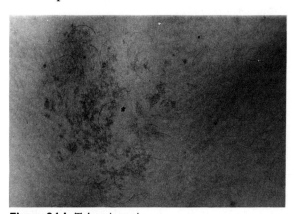

**Figure 24.1** Telangiectasia.

Like most organs the skin has a limited repertoire of pathological changes which it can produce in response to injury. One of the commonest is a process called eczema in which oedema fluid accumulates within the epidermis and inflammatory cells within the dermis. In acute forms of eczema true vesicles may develop but in chronic and slowly evolving lesions the skin appears red and thickened. Pigmentary changes are also common in skin disease with increases of pigmentation following many disorders which damage the epidermis. Vascular damage will cause bruising, ulceration or purpura, clotting disorders may also produce bruising or purpura. The infiltration of lymphocytes into the dermis may occur as a result of inflammation, for instance, in discoid lupus erythematosus, but the same can also occur as a result of a malignant process such as a lymphoma. Similar appearing lesions are therefore sometimes caused by strikingly different aetiological processes. With a reasonable knowledge of the range of appearances and access to simple methods of investigation such as biopsy it is usually possible to make a diagnosis.

# INVESTIGATIONS

Investigations used in the diagnosis of other medical conditions are also used in dermatology, for example, X-rays and blood tests. Conditions as diverse as tuberculosis and rheumatoid arthritis may present with characteristic skin lesions and these will require investigation. Other tests used in dermatology are more confined to the specialty.

## Microbiology

Skin swabs are helpful in identifying the presence and sensitivities of surface bacteria. The skin is normally colonized with *Staphylococcus epidermidis* and other bacteria such as coryneforms. The anaerobe, *Propionibacterium acnes*, is found in sebaceous follicles and is a contributory cause in the development of acne. *Staphylococcus aureus* or beta haemolytic streptococci are potential skin pathogens; both may cause infections of the skin and *Staph. aureus* is carried by many patients with extensive eczema. Skin patients are therefore an important source of cross infection by *Staph. aureus* within wards. Swabs for virological cultures are helpful for the diagnosis of herpetic infections, although electron microscopy or direct immunofluorescence using monoclonal antibody to herpes viruses of material taken from lesions may be quicker, where these techniques are available.

## Mycology

A technique peculiar to dermatology is the examination of skin scrapings or nail clippings for fungi (direct microscopy). Scrapings are taken from the edge of suspect lesions with a scalpel onto a glass slide and a drop of 5–15 per cent potassium hydroxide applied to the skin debris to clear the epidermal cells. Fungal elements are seen as round or oval yeasts or longer hyphae under the microscope. Nail clippings will take longer to soften with this technique. Material should also be cultured on mycological media. Most superficial fungal pathogens take from 2 to 14 days to grow to a stage at which they can be identified. Some cases of tinea capitis, those caused by Microsporum species for instance, will fluoresce green under filtered ultraviolet (Wood's) light. This is a useful way of screening patients for infection.

## Scabies

If scabies is suspected typical burrows can be opened with a sterile needle and by gently scraping the lesion with the tip of the needle a scabies mite can be extracted.

## Skin biopsy

Histological examination is of great importance in dermatology. Many skin conditions have diagnostic histopathological appearances and skin biopsy is a simple procedure. A knowledge of skin histopathology is a key part of the training of a dermatologist. The use of pathological techniques can be extended to include immunopathological (antibody) labelling of frozen skin sections in which the deposition of immuno-globulins or complement or the identification of the immunophenotype of infiltrating cells may help in the diagnosis.

# Patch testing

Patch testing is used in contact dermatitis in order to determine the nature of the allergen. Here the patient is challenged with a battery of common allergens in solution or ointment placed under individual patches covered with an occlusive dressing on the back. In addition to a standard range of allergens any additional suspected reactants can also be applied. Tests are read at 48 and 96 hours and the presence of erythema and vesicles under the patch test, indicating sensitivity, is noted. The common contact allergens in industrialized countries include nickel, chrome, rubber constituents and certain drugs such as neomycin.

# Phototesting

Rarely skin from some individuals reacts specifically to certain wavelengths of visible light — photodermatoses. This type of sensitivity can be tested using a special apparatus called a monochromator which can provide a source of specific wavelengths. Few centres in the UK provide such a phototesting service.

# Skin diseases

There is no simple division of skin diseases apart from their separation into endogenous and exogenous disorders depending on whether or not there is an external cause such as an infection.

Many of the common diseases such as psoriasis and eczema are largely endogenous even though exogenous forms of eczema, for instance, due to allergy, are also seen.

# Eczema

The words eczema and dermatitis have been a source of confusion for many years. While they often refer to the same condition and are therefore used synonymously, dermatitis simply refers to any inflammation of the skin and as such is the more general term. It is better therefore to refer to eczema when describing a group of itchy skin diseases which affect the outer epidermis and present with erythema, scaling and on occasions the formation of vesicles. There are different forms of eczema which share a common histopathology with involvement of the epidermis and dermis and in which vesicles may form: atopic eczema, discoid or nummular eczema, contact dermatitis, hand and foot eczema and stasis eczema. Seborrhoeic dermatitis will be considered elsewhere (page 799).

# Atopic eczema

Atopic eczema is a common condition occurring in about 4–7 per cent of all children. The aetiology is still unclear although most patients have a personal or family history of other atopic disorders such as hay fever and asthma. Raised IgE levels are found in some, but not all, affected children. While these other atopic diseases are clearly associated with allergy (immediate type hypersensitivity) to specific allergens such as grass pollen or house dust mite it is seldom possible to establish what allergy causes the appearance of the rash in patients with atopic eczema. Occasionally dietary restriction of certain foods such as eggs and milk or reduction of house dust containing mite debris from a patient's environment may produce some clinical improvement suggesting that allergic responses may contribute to the pathogenesis of this condition. Rarely atopic eczema accompanies congenital immunodeficiency diseases.

## CLINICAL FEATURES

Atopic eczema usually first appears in early childhood with the classical clinical features being seen at about the age of 2 years. It starts with itching and erythema accompanied by scaling, most frequently in the flexural sites such as the elbows, behind the knees and around the neck (Fig. 24.2). The infraorbital folds, scalp, wrists and ankles may also be affected and in extensive cases most of the body is involved.

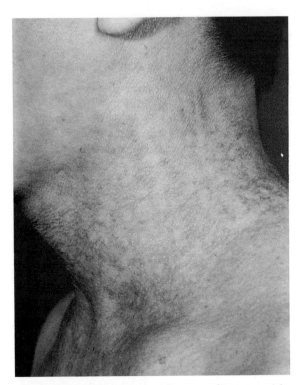

**Figure 24.2** Atopic eczema: a long standing case with lichenification around the neck.

Infantile eczema, which occurs in the first 6–24 months, is regarded as a precursor of atopic dermatitis and many cases evolve into this other variety. Children with infantile eczema often have involvement of the cheeks, and extensor surfaces such as the forearms and lower legs.

## TREATMENT

Atopic eczema is treated with weak corticosteroids such as 1 per cent hydrocortisone and emollients. Antihistamines for itching and antibiotics to control secondary infection are also helpful although this disease is subject to periodic relapse until spontaneous resolution in the teens. In about 15–20 per cent of cases skin lesions persist into late teenage and early adult life and often when this happens the pattern of involvement changes to focus on one or more sites such as the hands.

# Discoid eczema

Discoid eczema or nummular eczema is generally seen in middle-aged or elderly patients. The lesions are disc shaped and appear as large itchy plaques (4 cm or more in diameter) on the arms, legs and trunk. Itching is often intense. There is no evidence of allergy and, apart from dry skin, patients have no other skin abnormalities. The stronger topically applied corticosteroids are usually necessary, together with emollient creams.

# Stasis eczema

Many patients with varicose veins develop dry areas around the medial malleolus which can progress to involve the lower leg. This is also a potential site for the development of venous ulcers. The latter are also often surrounded by eczematous areas. It is important to ensure that these patients do not have superimposed allergic contact dermatitis, usually to one of their medications, as these will often contribute to the pathological process.

# Hand and foot eczema

Patients may present only with eczema affecting either the hands or feet or both. This may form part of the clinical spectrum of atopic dermatitis or allergic contact dermatitis or alternatively may present on its own without any obvious predisposing abnormality. If this is the case it is important to recognize that the condition may recur as an acute and painful eruption or develop into an intractable disease. Acute hand or foot eczema (pompholyx) usually presents with multiple itchy or painful vesicles along the borders of the digits and across the palm or sole. Recurrent attacks are common. In chronic hand and foot eczema the rash is plaque-like often spreading across the palms and soles. The area becomes criss-crossed with deep fissures and is often very painful. It is important to exclude contact dermatitis in these cases, if necessary by patch testing. In the acute phase potassium permanganate soaks may control the condition which is otherwise steroid responsive.

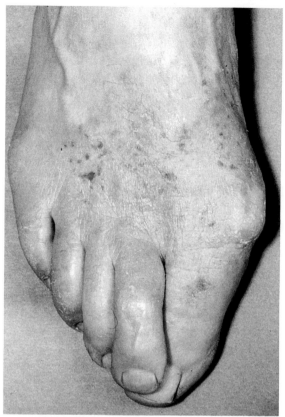

**Figure 24.3** Contact dermatitis to shoe dye.

# Contact dermatitis

There are two main types of contact dermatitis — irritant and allergic. In the former the damage is caused by a single or repeated exposure to substances which can damage the epidermis and establish an eczematous process. In allergic contact dermatitis chemical antigens mediate the damage but via an immunological mechanism involving the activation of specific T-lymphocyte-mediated immunity to the sensitizing substance. In this form of eczema prior exposure to the agent or a closely related substance is essential.

Common causes of irritant eczema include detergents, solvents and acids used at work or in the home. The rash occurs at the site of application and therefore the hands are often most commonly affected.

Allergic contact dermatitis is common (Fig. 24.3), causes include the following.

1. **Chemicals:** most topically applied substances may contain sensitizers. The most common in Europe is metal containing nickel. Chromates, for instance, in cement, are also common causes of allergy. Topical medications which contain neomycin, preservatives or antiseptics such as vioform may also cause allergy. Hair dyes and cosmetics are other sources of allergy. Certain plasticizers or industrial hardeners such as formaldehyde may cause eczema. In an industrial setting dermatitis is an important cause of disability and it may be important to visit areas to see how materials are being used and how they may affect the development of disease.
2. **Plants:** certain plants such as primulas are common sources of chemicals which induce skin allergy. To produce eczema, plant allergens may also require a change in composition under the influence of sunlight. This is photocontact dermatitis.

## CLINICAL FEATURES

The diagnosis of allergic contact dermatitis is very dependent on a good clinical history, in particular details of exposure to chemicals or other allergens and careful notes of the distribution of the rash. Contact dermatitis usually develops at sites of contact and these may well give an important clue as to the likely source of the disease. Occasionally where the reaction is severe other areas are affected. The diagnosis is confirmed by patch testing. The whole testing procedure takes three visits over 5 days.

## TREATMENT

Affected areas should be treated usually with a weak or medium strength corticosteroid such as 1 per cent hydrocortisone, betamethasone valerate or triamcinolone acetonide. Secondary infection is controlled with an oral antibiotic or antiseptic. A key part of the management is prevention. Once the allergen is identified it may be possible to eliminate it from the environment of the patient or give the individual advice on avoidance in future. This may be difficult in the case of occupational contact dermatitis where changing the job may be the only way of managing the condition.

# *P*SORIASIS

Psoriasis is a chronic scaly erythematous eruption whose clinical appearances range from the development of multiple plaques to localized pustules. While its aetiology is unknown the disease appears to follow immunological activation of epidermal cells to attract clusters of leukocytes into the epidermal layers. An immune mechanism is also supported by the responses of the rash to the immunomodulatory drug cyclosporin A and the occurrence of particularly severe forms of psoriasis in AIDS patients. There is evidence of an association between certain HLA types such as B13 and B17 with particular forms of psoriasis. It is likely that the disease is inherited as an autosomal dominant with variable transmission. Twin studies and clustering of cases in families support this view and it is important in taking a history to ask about other members of the family.

## CLINICAL FEATURES

The commonest form of psoriasis is the plaque type where large red scaly plaques develop over sites on the trunk and limbs. These are most commonly found on the knees and elbows but any site including the scalp can be involved, although facial psoriasis is less common. Each plaque is covered by silvery scales and if these are removed the lesion may bleed. Psoriasis is not usually itchy. Other areas affected include the nails where small fine pits can cover the surface of the nail plate which is separated at its distal margin from the nail bed (onycholysis) (Fig. 24.4).

Other forms of psoriasis include a guttate variety which may appear acutely to cover the body with smaller scales often after a streptococcal pharyngitis, arthropathic psoriasis where different joints may become affected and pustular psoriasis where small pustules are present on the underlying red plaques. The arthropathic form of psoriasis may resemble rheumatoid arthritis. It is commonest in middle-aged or elderly patients and presents with a polyarthritis which is destructive. Large articular joints as well as the sacroiliac or finger joints can be affected and in some cases there is severe deformity. Psoriatic arthritis is seronegative and in most cases there is at least one lesion of psoriasis on the skin or nails.

Generalized pustular psoriasis is one of the few major dermatological emergencies. Admission and rapid therapy are indicted.

## TREATMENT

Treatment for psoriasis is often difficult as it is not possible to cure the disease; rather the

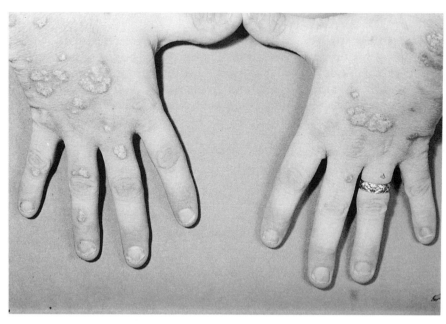

**Figure 24.4** Psoriasis of hands.

development of skin lesions is controlled. The application of tar-based ointments or those containing dithranol is useful. Topical corticosteroids are less often given and there is a danger of precipitating the acute forms of the disease by using systemic steroids. Ultraviolet light, particularly using UVA (page 807) combined with a sun sensitizer called a psoralen (PUVA) is also helpful. Newer treatments include calcipotriol, a vitamin D analogue. For severe cases methotrexate or cyclosporin may be used. Management of psoriasis involves giving advice on the control of the disease and exacerbations in the family.

# ACNE

Acne or acne vulgaris to use its full title is a disease primarily seen in adolescents although it may also persist later into adult life. It is caused by a process of obstruction of sebaceous glands which are mainly found on the face, back and chest (Fig. 24.5). Lipolytic bacteria within the glands digest lipid material releasing irritant fatty acids and other metabolites. The swollen gland may then rupture to form an inflammatory pustule.

## CLINICAL FEATURES

The main clinical features of acne are blackheads or comedones (obstructed sebaceous gland openings), pustules and papules (ruptured or inflamed sebaceous glands). The development of acne also appears to be, in part, androgen dependent, and changes in the acne during the menstrual cycle or exacerbations as well as

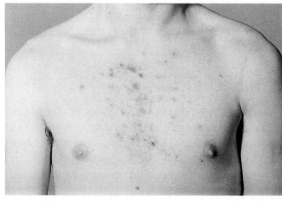

**Figure 24.5** Acne vulgaris on the chest.

improvements related to treatment with the contraceptive pill probably reflect this.

## TREATMENT

Acne is not curable but treatment is designed, often very successfully, to suppress the formation of lesions either through relief of obstructed glands with benzyl peroxide or retinoic acid,

control of bacteria with antibiotics such as tetracyclines or erythromycin, or even shrinkage of sebaceous gland secretions using 13-*cis*-retinoic acid.

Acne rosacea is not related to acne vulgaris but is a cause of a papular/pustular rash on the face of adults associated with an increased tendency to flushing in response to vasodilatory stimuli such as heat and alcohol.

# PITYRIASIS ROSEA

This condition is usually seen in young adults or teenagers. Easily recognized, it starts with a single scaly, not very itchy, area called a herald patch usually on the trunk. A week or so later more scaly patches appear over the trunk or proximal parts of the limbs. The rash follows the lines of the body on the trunk where it appears to be laid out like a conifer. Patches are usually oval

in shape. Some patients report tiredness and sometimes two or more people in a household are affected suggesting a viral aetiology. The rash generally resolves in 4–8 weeks without sequelae. Relapses are rare. Treatment is therefore seldom necessary unless lesions itch in which case a dilute weak topical corticosteroid will relieve the symptoms.

# BULLOUS DISEASES

Certain skin diseases present with blisters. Some of these are congenital or inherited disorders of keratin formation and epidermal anchoring (epidermolysis bullosa) whereas others follow immunological damage within or beneath the epidermis. Three of the latter are pemphigus, pemphigoid and dermatitis herpetiformis.

**Pemphigus vulgaris** is a blistering disease which usually appears in middle to old age. The appearance of the rash is associated with the deposition of antibodies reactive with intracellular proteins of the epidermis. Lesions develop in the mouth and over the body in crops. Severe involvement may be fatal unless the disease is treated. Treatment is with systemic corticosteroids.

By contrast, **pemphigoid**, generally seen only in the elderly, is usually very itchy and mouth lesions are uncommon. The blisters are large and flaccid (Fig. 24.6). Treatment with systemic corticosteroids is important. There has been some controversy over the connection be-

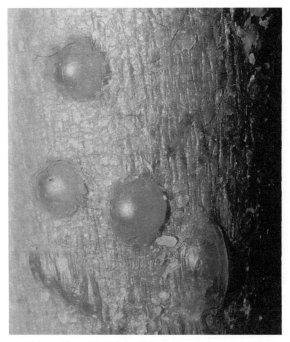

**Figure 24.6** Bullous pemphigoid.

tween cancer and pemphigoid. While there are patients in whom this condition will appear coincidentally with the finding of a cancer, it is also argued that the disease occurs in an age group in which cancer is commonest. In pemphigoid, antibodies are deposited in the basement membrane zone of the epidermis.

**Dermatitis herpetiformis** presents with multiple lesions over the scalp, elbows, base of spine, knees and shoulders. Itching is often intense. The blisters frequently have a surrounding erythematous halo and may seem urticarial. A proportion of patients have diarrhoea and appear to have a gastrointestinal condition identical to coeliac disease. The pathological appearances of coeliac disease may be found on jejunal biopsy. Part of the treatment of dermatitis herpetiformis is a gluten-free diet, although the drug dapsone is also given. In skin biopsies immunoglobulin A is deposited at the basement zone of the epidermis.

There are other ways in which patients may present with blistering. These include congenital disorders such as epidermolysis bullosa, but severe inflammation whether caused by eczema, physical injury (burns), allergy (insect bites) or infection (bacterial: staphylococcal impetigo; viruses: orf) may also cause skin blisters.

Key steps and questions in making the diagnosis are:

- The examination of the mouth for oral lesions
- The age of the patient
- The presence of a history of diarrhoea
- Skin biopsy together with immunopathology will provide the definitive answer

# LICHEN PLANUS

Lichen planus is a common condition which presents with streaks and ulcers in the mouth and a micropapular rash. The latter is very itchy and appears on the wrists and other areas on the arms and legs (Fig. 24.7). The appearance of the rash of lichen planus with pink to violet coloured papules which often develop in a scratch or scar (**Koebner's phenomenon**) is typical. The oral lesions are often silent and the mesh of white streaks on the buccal mucosa needs to be looked for. Generally this clears up within 6 to 18 months although occasionally it may persist for years.

A similar rash may be caused by ingestion or exposure to some drugs or chemicals such as diuretics (thiazides), colour developers, gold or mepacrine. It is of interest that the appearances and histopathology of the rash of acute graft versus host disease (GVHD, page 99) may be very similar to lichen planus suggesting that the latter may follow an antigenic change in epidermal cells triggered, for instance, by a drug or viral infection, leaving them liable to immunologically mediated damage.

Generally treatment is given to relieve symptoms including itch. The rash may respond to medium to high strength topical corticosteroids.

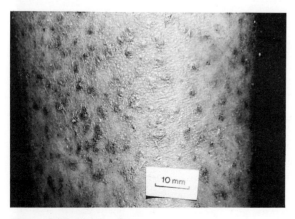

**Figure 24.7** Lichen planus.

# *I*NFECTIVE SKIN DISEASES

In most temperate climates infections account for a significant proportion of skin diseases although many are now curable and relatively easy to treat. By contrast, in the tropics infections completely dominate the picture of skin disease. The main infections are those caused by bacteria, fungi and viruses. Ectoparasites such as lice or mites (scabies) are also common.

# *Bacterial infections*

The main pathogens amongst the bacteria in skin are *Staphylococcus aureus* and beta haemolytic streptococci. They account for most infections although less commonly Gram negative bacteria cause infection in specific sites such as in the toe webs or beneath the nails.

## PYODERMA

Pyoderma is the name given to superficial bacterial infections of the skin such as **impetigo**. In this infection the main site of skin invasion is the epidermis which becomes eroded and covered by golden crusts or is the focus for the development of a bulla or blister. The two main clinical types of impetigo are therefore crusted or bullous. The principal sites for infections are the face and exposed sites as well as the trunk. Impetigo is commonest in children. Often there is some predisposing feature such as scabies or head lice infestations.

While bullous impetigo is more often caused by *Staph. aureus* and the crusted form by Streptococci in practice a clinical distinction is hard to make. Impetigo in industrialized countries is generally caused by *Staph. aureus*. In the tropics streptococcal skin infection is a significant cause of glomerulonephritis (page 455). Spread of impetigo within families is common and this is a contagious disease, although easily controlled by antibiotic therapy.

## BOILS

Boils are superficial abscesses caused by *Staph. aureus* which have invaded a hair follicle. The resulting infection is a localized tender swelling or furuncle which eventually ruptures to discharge pus. Recurrent attacks are common and infections within families are also seen. While recurrent boils may occur as a sign of an immunodeficiency state where there is defective neutrophil function such as in chronic granulomatous disease (page 94), in practice few patients with this common problem have evidence of underlying disease. In the early stages it is possible to prevent the emergence of a boil by antibiotic therapy using flucloxacillin or erythromycin; however, once formed the best treatment is to incise the lesion.

## OTHER BACTERIAL INFECTIONS

Cellulitis affecting either the legs or face (erysipelas) is not common now, although secondary complications of the latter such as cavernous sinus thrombosis may still be feared. Usually cellulitis is caused by Streptococci. A severe form of streptococcal infection results in necrotizing fasciitis. This produces gangrene and requires surgical resection as well as antibiotics.

*Staphylococcus aureus* is also a cause of other conditions such as acute infection of the nail fold, acute paronychium, and a generalized erythroderma usually seen in neonates – the scalded skin syndrome (SSS). In SSS the infection, which is originally located on the skin surface, results in the production of a specific epidermolytic toxin which causes splitting within the epidermis followed by extensive exfoliation. Toxin producing strains of *Staph. aureus* can be isolated. A generalized macular rash is a feature of the early phases of the toxic shock syndrome, also caused by Staphylococci.

# Fungal infections

The superficial mycoses are common fungal infections of the skin or mucous membranes which include athlete's foot or thrush. These are seen in both temperate and tropical climates although the prevalence of disease is higher in a hotter environment.

## DERMATOPHYTOSIS

The dermatophyte or ringworm fungi belong to three genera called *Trichophyton, Microsporum* and *Epidermophyton*. These fungi can invade the outer stratum corneum but do not penetrate further. They also attack hair and nails. Some of these fungi are acquired by transmission from other humans whereas others, chiefly those affecting children, are passed from animals or soil to humans. These infections are named tinea generally followed by the appropriate part of the body (in Latin); hence tinea corporis (body), tinea cruris (groin) and tinea pedis (feet).

## Clinical features

Tinea pedis is a common infection affecting the web spaces of the feet. It may be acute and itchy or chronic and in the latter phase may cause generalized dry scaling over the sole of the foot. Invasion of the toe nail may follow (Fig. 24.8). Web space infections can be caused by other organisms including *Candida*, coryneform bacteria (erythrasma) and Gram-negative bacteria.

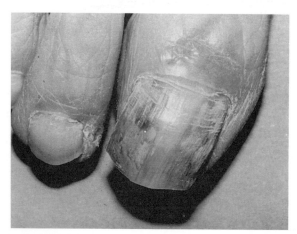

**Figure 24.8** Onychomycosis due to a dermatophyte fungus *Trichophyton rubrum*.

Tinea pedis is a sporadic disease but is particularly important in certain industrial settings. For instance, in some coal mines over 30 per cent of face workers have chronic foot infections.

Tinea cruris and tinea corporis are less common. Tinea corporis is often diagnosed in mistake for other skin diseases such as eczema which produce annular scaly lesions. Tinea capitis or scalp ringworm was once common in schools but is now generally a sporadic infection except in parts of Africa and the cities of Central and Eastern USA. There is scaling, local itching and loss of hair. As it can be transmitted from child to child, inspections for tinea capitis are still carried out in schools and, if found, both case and contacts are treated.

## Treatment

The main treatments for dermatophytosis are antifungal creams or ointments such as azole creams (miconazole, clotrimazole, econazole). In extensive infections or where there is hair or nail invasion oral antifungals are used (griseofulvin, itraconazole, terbinafine).

## CANDIDA INFECTIONS

*Candida albicans* is a yeast fungus which affects the outer layers of the skin and mucous membranes. In normal hosts it is carried as a commensal in the mouth, gastrointestinal tract and vagina; but where there is a reduction in local resistance it can invade to cause disease. Candidosis is an infection of the mouth, vagina or skin. It may also be a systemic infection in severely ill or immunocompromised patients, although this seldom originates from a superficial infection.

Thrush or oral candidosis is a common infection of the oral and buccal mucosa which presents with soft white patches on a background of erythema. A similar appearance is seen with vaginal candidosis. Other sites affected include the groins, beneath the breasts and around the nail folds.

Patients presenting with thrush generally have some other abnormality with the exception of women with vaginal infections. Predisposing abnormalities include local epithelial damage (ulcers, leucoplakia), antibiotic therapy, immunodeficiency affecting neutrophil or T-lymphocyte functions and certain endocrine diseases such as diabetes. Persistent oral candidosis may be one of the earliest signs of the development of AIDS.

## DISEASES DUE TO *PITYROSPORUM* YEASTS

*Pityrosporum* yeasts are skin surface commensal organisms found particularly on lipid-rich areas of the trunk, face and scalp. They have been associated with a number of diseases of which the commonest are pityriasis versicolor and seborrhoeic dermatitis.

### Pityriasis versicolor

Pityriasis versicolor is a common infection producing hypo- or hyperpigmented scaly macules on the trunk and proximal limbs. Lesions are generally asymptomatic and the main complaint is the disorder of pigmentation. The rash may resemble vitiligo but differs in that it is scaly, a sign that can be elicited by gently scraping the surface of lesions with a glass slide.

Pityriasis versicolor is a disease of healthy individuals particularly if they have had recent sun exposure, for instance after a holiday. It is also seen in patients who have Cushing's syndrome. It is treated with a topically applied azole antifungal cream or lotion.

### Seborrhoeic dermatitis

Seborrhoeic dermatitis is a common scaly condition in which the principal sites of lesions are the face, scalp (dandruff), chest and back. Patients are usually in their early 20s or 30s. The role of *Pityrosporum* yeasts in this condition has long been the subject of debate. However, this rash responds well to treatment with antifungal agents and this coincides with disappearance of these organisms. It is best regarded as an inflammatory dermatosis in which the chief trigger factor is an abnormal response to *Pityrosporum* yeasts on the skin surface.

### Clinical features

The main clinical signs are scaling and itching of the scalp or dandruff. This may also involve certain areas of the face particularly the nasal folds, eye brows, behind the ears and the scalp margin. Other sites affected include the central presternal area and the back. Lesions are usually erythematous and are covered with greasy-looking scales. On the back multiple follicular papules and pustules may appear.

Seborrhoeic dermatitis can develop in most individuals and appears to vary in clinical expression. It is also commonly seen in certain patients with neurological diseases particularly parkinsonism and may be exacerbated by stress. Severe seborrhoeic dermatitis of rapid onset may develop in patients with AIDS and is an important and early clinical sign of the disease, often appearing in the early stages of established AIDS.

### Treatment

Seborrhoeic dermatitis responds to treatment with topical antifungal agents such as clotrimazole or miconazole or to weak topical corticosteroids. This is a recurrent condition and periodic relapse is to be expected.

# Viral infections

Viral infections of the skin are also common. They include infections due to the herpes viruses, herpes simplex and herpes zoster (pages 728 and 729) as well as human papilloma viruses or warts. Molluscum contagiosum is also caused by a virus which has not yet been isolated.

## HERPES SIMPLEX IN THE SKIN

Herpes simplex virus (HSV) is a DNA virus whose chief clinical features have been described on page 728. On the skin it may present as a primary infection (rare) or more commonly with recurrent disease. Because it can establish a latent stage in a dorsal nerve root ganglion, facial lesions originating from a trigeminal focus or genital lesions from a sacral focus are the two commonest sites for infection. Non-genital and genital infections are caused by distinct subtypes of the virus (HSV-1 and -2, respectively).

### Clinical features

Cold sores are common recurrent infections with herpes simplex virus. They appear after a prodromal period in which the site becomes hyper-aesthetic or tingles. The lesions are papules or vesicles often on the lip which crop over 3–4 days before developing crusts. They may be triggered by a number of stimuli such as febrile illness, sunlight or menstrual cycle. Severe herpes simplex infections can develop on children with atopic eczema – eczema herpeticum. Prolonged ulcerative herpes simplex infections may also develop in patients with immuno-deficiency states including AIDS in which perianal ulceration due to HSV is well recognized.

### Treatment

Cold sores respond to acyclovir but this does not have any significant effect on the development of recurrences.

## HERPES ZOSTER

Herpes zoster or shingles is caused by the varicella-zoster virus (VZV), the cause of varicella or chickenpox. Like HSV it results from reactivation of a focus of latent infection in a nerve root ganglion. Usually patients only have one episode of reactivation.

### Clinical features

The rash of herpes zoster is usually preceded by an episode of severe pain in a localized zone on the skin surface. This is followed in 2 to 5 days by the emergence of a vesicular rash in one dermatome, commonly the trunk or face. If it occurs in the ophthalmic division of the trigeminal nerve it may cause severe infection and pain affecting the eye (ophthalmic zoster). It may also cause Bell's palsy if the geniculate ganglion is involved. A major problem is the occurrence of severe pain – postherpetic neuralgia – after the infection has resolved.

### Treatment

In the acute phase the rash can be treated with high-dose acyclovir or topical idoxuridine, although in most mild cases treatment is not given. Herpes zoster is also seen in immuno-compromised patients including transplant and leukaemic patients and those with AIDS. Here spread beyond the normal dermatomal distribution is seen and this occurrence should alert the physician to the possibility that the patient is in some way immunocompromised.

## HUMAN PAPILLOMA VIRUS INFECTIONS

Human papilloma viruses (HPV) are DNA viruses which cannot replicate in normal synthetic medium. They can therefore not be grown under conventional laboratory conditions. They cause common infections which usually present on the skin surface as warts.

Warts are usually classified by appearance on the skin and site of infection. Some of the features of common HPV wart infections are shown in Table 24.2.

**Table 24.2** Warts and human papilloma viruses (HPV).

| Wart type | Site | HPV type |
|---|---|---|
| Common (verruca vulgaris) | Hands, limbs | 1,2,3,4 |
| Plantar | Soles | 1,2,4 |
| Plane | Face, trunk | 3,5,8 |
| Genital | External genitalia | 6 |

### Clinical features

Typical warts are papules which have a pebbled surface often dotted with tiny areas of haemorrhage. On the soles they are often painful and in this site show in-growth.

Human papilloma viruses are known to contribute to carcinogenesis, for example, HPV-16 and -18 and cervical cancer. There is some evidence that they can also contribute to the development of skin cancer in patients with a rare inherited predisposition to severe and atypical wart infections combined with immuno-deficiency known as epidermodysplasia verruciformis. It is believed that they may also play a part in the appearance of skin cancers in solid organ transplant patients.

### Treatment

Warts are generally treated by cryotherapy using liquid nitrogen or with strong keratolytics or acids such as salicylic acid or glutaraldehyde. Recurrences however are very common.

## MOLLUSCUM CONTAGIOSUM

Molluscum contagiosum is also an infection with an uncultivable pox virus. It causes a common infection seen in children or young adults in which small pearly papules with soft centres develop in clusters on the skin. Severe molluscum contagiosum infections may develop in AIDS patients. While the clinical features are typical, other infections can mimic molluscum contagiosum in immunocompromised patients, particularly deep fungal infections such as cryptococcosis. If the lesions are widely scattered and there is doubt about the diagnosis they should be biopsied.

# Parasitic infections

## SCABIES

Scabies is the commonest of the ectoparasite infections of the skin. It is caused by a human mite, *Sarcoptes scabei*, which can be transmitted by close contact from person to person. It causes disease in all age groups. The occurrence of scabies in communities varies in a cyclical pattern over a number of years so that every 10–20 years there is a peak incidence of this infection.

### Clinical features

The main symptom of scabies is itching which is usually worse at night. An important diagnostic pointer is that other members of the household are also itchy. The rash consists of multiple papules around the wrists, fingers, elbows, shoulders, buttocks, scrotum and ankles. In adults, but not infants, the infection does not affect the scalp. A diagnostic feature is the burrow which is formed by the adult mite excavating into the stratum corneum to cause a small shallow tunnel visible on the skin surface as a pale wavy line culminating in a small papule where the mite lives. In immunocompromised patients and in those with Down's syndrome a peculiar form of scabies known as Norwegian or crusted scabies may develop. Here itch may be minimal and the main signs of infection are scaly crusts over the hands, face and limbs. This form of scabies is highly contagious and can lead to transmission of the infection to staff and other patients.

### Treatment

Treatment of the entire family or household is necessary. The main treatments are lotions which are applied once or twice only to the entire skin surface. Gamma benzene hydrochloride, benzyl benzoate, malathion and permethrin are all used for this purpose.

## PEDICULOSIS (HUMAN LOUSE INFECTIONS)

Whereas infestations with the human body louse are now less common, head lice are endemic in many schools. The disease caused by lice is known as pediculosis. Pediculosis corporis affects the body and the adult lice live in clothing. These can spread other infections such as typhus although this usually only happens where there is overcrowding and breakdown of hygiene. Body louse infestations are mainly seen in the poor and disadvantaged or in times of war or captivity.

Head lice are very common and can occur in children or adults of any social class. They develop irrespective of standards of personal hygiene. Transmission is by direct contact from infected scalps. Lice become attached to hairs and feed from the scalp surface. Eggs are laid attached to the hair shaft and can be seen as pale structures adhering to hairs, nits. These are often grouped on the sides of the scalp particularly around the ears.

Treatment of head lice should include the whole household and involves the application of lotions such as malathion, permethin, gamma benzene hexachloride or carbaryl to the scalp. Single applications are generally sufficient with a repeat treatment after 2 weeks. In many schools children are regularly inspected for head lice.

## OTHER PARASITIC INFECTIONS

On a worldwide basis one of the commonest causes of infectious skin lesions is the parasitic infestation due to the filarial worm *Onchocerca volvulus* – onchocerciasis. This is occasionally seen as an imported disease presenting with itching. The skin inflammation proceeds from a reaction to larval worms or microfilaria released from encysted adults in subcutaneous tissue.

One of the features of the itching is that it is often localized to one segment or limb.

Other tropical diseases caused by parasites which are seen in Europe include **leishmaniasis** which may present in patients who have taken holidays in endemic areas (page 773). Knowledge of the geographic distribution of these diseases is useful as a pointer to unusual causes of skin infection.

# THE ITCHY PATIENT

One of the commonest clinical problems is the investigation of the itching patient. It is important firstly to separate those who present with irritation accompanied by a rash which occurs in eczema, scabies, lichen planus and dermatitis herpetiformis from those without a rash which is generally due to internal disease. One possible diagnostic catch is the disease urticaria where the rash is transient and may well not be present when the patient is examined.

# Urticaria

Urticaria is an itchy dermatosis accompanied by wealing on the skin. While it may be caused by exposure to certain drugs such as aspirin or to physical stimuli including sun, cold and mechanical pressure the majority of cases have no underlying cause. Urticaria is seen most frequently but not exclusively in atopic subjects.

## CLINICAL FEATURES

The rash of urticaria consists of crops of weals, soft transient swellings in the dermis which are very itchy (Fig. 24.9). They resemble the lesions caused by nettle stings, hence their common name – nettle rash. Patients may also refer to them as hives. The rash and itching is worse at night and even if lesions are not present when the patient is seen the rash usually lasts no longer than 6–8 hours. Some patients with urticaria will demonstrate dermographism (skin writing): when the skin is firmly stroked with a blunt point a weal is produced.

If an underlying cause can be identified this can be eliminated. Otherwise the best treatment

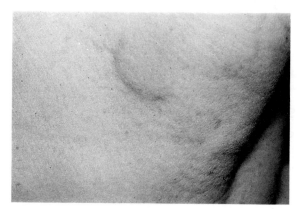

**Figure 24.9** Urticaria.

is suppression of the rash using antihistamines. One severe form of urticaria is angioedema when the swelling may involve the eyes, lips and even larynx. Laryngeal stridor may occur and its relief with adrenaline is an acute emergency. Angioedema may occur in families and this can be identified by the absence or decrease in serum levels of C1 esterase inhibitor. Patients can be taught to self-administer drugs including adrenalin to prevent potentially fatal attacks of oedema.

**Table 24.3** Causes of itching.

Renal: chronic renal failure
Endocrine: diabetes mellitus, hyperthyroidism, hypothyroidism
Hepatic: any cause of biliary obstruction
Blood diseases: iron deficiency, polycythaemia, leukaemia, Hodgkin's disease
Neurological: tertiary syphilis, brain tumours
Carcinomatosis
Pregnancy
Anxiety states
Drugs: cocaine, morphine

# Other causes of itching

If there is no evidence of skin disease there are other potential causes of skin irritation which may occur in the absence of a rash. Some of these are listed in the Table 24.3.

Appropriate investigations for these conditions will have to be instituted. Itching in pregnancy (pruritus gravidarum) occurs in some women and may be repeated after successive pregnancies. It disappears in the third trimester.

# Disorders of pigmentation

Changes in pigmentation are often profoundly distressing for many patients. Pigmentary change may be a natural sequel to any skin disease or process that damages the basal layer of the epidermis. However, others diseases such as acne may also cause pigmentary changes, particularly in black patients. Internal diseases which may cause increased pigmentation include Addison's disease and hyperthyroidism. One specific condition which presents with increased pigmentation is acanthosis nigricans. This appears as an area of pigmented, thickened, velvety skin often in the body folds or around the mouth or lips. It is asymptomatic. It is associated with internal malignancy in some cases. A similar but less extensive rash not necessarily associated with malignancy may also be seen in the overweight.

Conversely loss of pigment may be equally embarrassing for patients. The commonest of the diseases in which pigment is lost is **vitiligo**. Here small macular areas of total loss of pigment occur. The hands are often affected first and in some patients the changes are seen around the eyes. However in certain cases the loss of pigment progresses over months or years until it is almost complete. Some patients have associated autoimmune diseases, such as hypothyroidism, or anti-organ antibodies may be found. There is no effective therapy although topical corticosteroids or PUVA may be tried in some cases. Areas of extensive depigmentation have to be protected from the sun.

Other conditions may also result in loss of pigment. Pityriasis versicolor has already been mentioned (page 799). In the tropics lesions of tuberculoid leprosy may be first noticed because of pigment loss.

# Hair loss

Loss of hair is one of the commonest dermatological complaints. There are numerous causes but the first point to establish is whether the hair loss has been accompanied by skin lesions in the scalp. While there are a number of causes, lichen planus or discoid lupus erythematosus are two potential underlying diseases. In many cases, however, there is no evidence of skin disease and then loss of hair is generally either caused by abnormal hair growth or internal disease.

The common diseases affecting the hair are male pattern or androgenetic alopecia and alopecia areata. Androgenetic alopecia which is responsible for male pattern baldness may affect both men and women although females are usually affected at an older age. The tendency to produce this pattern is often seen in families, hence taking a good family history is important. The pattern of hair loss is typical as it generally presents with bitemporal recession of the hair line or thinning in this area or the vertex. Androgenetic alopecia appears to follow failure of adequate hair replacement through natural wastage due to failure of the hair germ to respond to circulating androgens.

Alopecia areata presents with circumscribed areas of hair loss which develop suddenly and may spread across the scalp. In some patients total hair loss is seen and the eyebrows, lashes and beard are also affected. A typical feature is the presence of some broken hairs with a tapering segment nearest the skin, the so-called exclamation mark hairs. Treatment is unsatisfactory although the hair returns spontaneously in many patients.

Internal causes of hair loss are rare but include iron deficiency, hypothyroidism, chronic liver disease, carcinomatosis and drug therapy (anticoagulants, cytostatic drugs, carbimazole). While oral contraceptives have been cited as causes of diffuse hair loss there is no consistent evidence to support this. Reversible hair loss may occur after the end of pregnancy.

# COLLAGEN VASCULAR DISEASES

The skin is an important focus for inflammatory diseases which destroy specific cell types. The collagen vascular diseases are important in this respect as the inflammatory reaction involves blood vessels, epithelial cells and collagen fibres. Skin signs are therefore important in the presentation of these conditions.

## Lupus erythematosus

The disease spectrum of lupus erythematosus includes a number of clinical variants whose distinction is important because this determines the likely course and prognosis of the underlying disease. Two main types of lupus erythematosus are distinguished: discoid (DLE), which is a localized variety affecting the skin and structures arising from it such as hair and nails, and systemic lupus erythematosus (SLE), which is a multisystem disease affecting internal organs as well as the skin.

### DISCOID LUPUS ERYTHEMATOSUS

This disease is mainly seen in the middle-aged or elderly patient and appears to be commoner in females than males. Variants, however, can occur at younger ages. The classical form presents with erythematous plaques on the face or hands, but other sites such as the trunk or scalp can be affected. Individual lesions are itchy and spread only slowly. In their early stages they are juicy and red but with time they become dry with superficial scaling, plugging of hair follicles is prominent. The process causes severe scarring in the skin and hair loss in hair-bearing areas. Patients with this disease often have poor circulation and a history of chilblains (perniosis) or Raynaud's disease. Around the base of the fingers prominent dilated nail-fold capillary loops may also be seen.

In addition to this more classical variety there are other clinical forms including one in which widespread involvement of other skin sites is seen (Fig. 24.10). A subacute form is often seen in younger women. Here the rash is annular and patients are often photosensitive. In this form of disease patients may have anti-nuclear antibodies, but in addition they have the anticytoplasmic antibody, anti-Ro. Children born to mothers with this type of lupus erythematosus may have neonatal heart block.

Patients often respond to strong topical corticosteroids which will prevent further scarring. Alternative drugs include chloroquine or hydroxychloroquine which may stop progression of the disease in some patients.

### SYSTEMIC LUPUS ERYTHEMATOSUS

The systemic features of this disease are described on page 571. This disease is also commoner in females than males who are seldom affected. On the skin the appearances are more variable with the rash being erythematous without the chronicity and scarring. It appears in light exposed areas and may be triggered by sun exposure. The centrofacial areas are often affected giving rise to 'butterfly' rash, although in

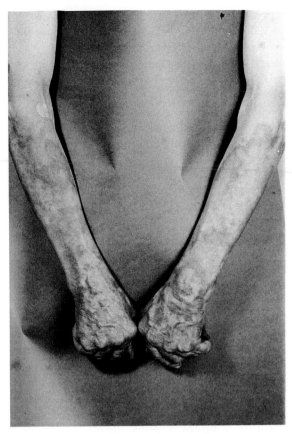

**Figure 24.10** Subacute lupus erythematosus.

the early stages only one side of the face may be involved with less scaly lesions. The arms may also be affected. Other skin features include diffuse hair loss, Raynaud's phenomenon and chilblains. Dilated nail-fold capillaries are much commoner in SLE.

Systemic lupus erythematosus may be triggered by a number of factors from sun exposure to drugs. The commonest of these are hydralazine, the contraceptive pill and griseofulvin. Patients with SLE have several abnormal blood tests such as anaemia and thrombocytopenia, and the presence of one or more anti-nuclear antibodies. In active disease anti-DNA antibodies are almost always present.

The rash of SLE does not respond well to topical therapy alone and management of the systemic disease with systemic steroids and azathioprine is necessary in order to obtain adequate control of the skin disease.

The relationship between DLE and SLE is a complex one. But the risk of DLE evolving into the systemic variety is low (less than 5 per cent). There is debate as to whether they are variants of the same process. In favour of this is the clinical and histological similarity of the skin lesions in both forms, the rare progression of the discoid to the systemic variety and similar haematological and antibody abnormalities in some patients, although these are generally found at a much lower frequency in patients with DLE. However, the low incidence of conversion of the localized to the systemic variety has also been cited as evidence in favour of these not being part of the same disease process. Generally patients with DLE are given a good prognosis and respond well to treatment of their skin lesions alone.

# Scleroderma

Scleroderma or hardening of the skin is a characteristic feature of a number of different collagen diseases; but as with lupus erythematosus there are two main clinical forms. In the first, known in dermatology as morphea, the changes are confined to the skin. The second type, systemic sclerosis, is a multisystem disorder with manifestations in the lungs, kidneys and oesophagus as well as the skin.

Morphea is a localized hardening of the skin. This may appear in plaques or bands and is called linear morphea. Generalized morphea involves large areas of the body surface and the skin is often bound down around the fingers and over the face. There is no effective therapy.

In systemic sclerosis (page 577) the skin is also hardened in places although this may be confined to certain areas such as the face and hands. Pulmonary fibrosis, progressive renal impairment and oesophageal fibrosis may all occur.

The difference between the two is based on clinical observations although occasionally a patient originally diagnosed as having severe morphea will progress to systemic sclerosis. Localized sclerotic changes on the hands are known as the CREST syndrome because the essential features are calcium deposition (calcinosis), Raynaud's phenomenon, oesophageal involvement, sclerodactyly and multiple telangiectasia.

# Dermatomyositis

Dermatomyositis is another combined system disease which may present with skin lesions. The disease affects the skin and striated muscles and may be a presenting feature of an internal malignancy. The skin changes consist of a vio-laceous rash on the face around the eyes and on the dorsum of the hands where erythema and oedema are prominent. Progressive proximal muscle weakness will herald the onset of the myositis. The disease has a characteristic histo-pathology in skin biopsies and serum creatinine kinase levels are raised. The muscle biopsy changes are also diagnostic as they show diffuse infiltration of lymphocytes and destruction of muscle tissue.

Dermatomyositis responds to systemic corticosteroid therapy with improvements in both the rash and the muscle weakness.

# ULCERATION OF THE SKIN

The development of ulcers on the skin follows destruction of the epidermis and dermis. In some cases the ulcer may extend through the sub-cutaneous tissues to deep fascia. The causes of ulceration range from infection to trauma. Infective causes of ulceration include deep sta-phylococcal or streptococcal infections called ecthyma or severe herpes simplex. In many tropical areas a major cause of disease in children and young adults is a condition called tropical ulcer which presents with acute regular ulcers on the lower limbs and feet. It is probably caused by a synergistic bacterial infection. Rarer infectious causes of ulceration of the skin include leish-maniasis, tuberculosis, syphilis and amoebiasis. Trauma from a superficial wound or a burn will also result in ulceration. It is particularly import-ant in such cases to note the presence of any sensory nerve defect in the area as trophic ulcera-tion caused by minor episodes of trauma can follow denervation. This is seen in diabetic patients and those with leprosy.

In addition to these causes of ulceration acute vascular damage, venous stasis and self-inflicted trauma may cause similar lesions.

of skin changes usually around the medial or lateral malleoli. These include deposition of haemosiderin which appears as red/brown pig-mentation, dryness of the skin and ulceration.

## CLINICAL FEATURES

The formation of venous ulcers may follow minor trauma or they may appear spon-taneously. These large indolent and irregular lesions may extend deeply to involve the per-iosteum of the tibia. They are mainly seen in elderly patients. It is important in such cases to make sure that the lesions are not arterial in origin by carefully examining for peripheral pulses and the temperature of the feet. Diabetics may also develop ulcers and patients should be screened for diabetes.

## TREATMENT

Venous ulcers are always difficult to treat. They heal with appropriate antisepsis, sterile dress-ings and compression bandages. Unfortunately, relapses are common.

# Venous (stasis) ulcers

Venous stasis following defective drainage through incompetent veins leads to a number

# Vasculitis

Inflammation of blood vessels usually secondary to the deposition of immune complexes may cause a variety of different changes depending on the size and location of the blood vessels involved. Some of these are listed in Table 24.4.

Many of these conditions are associated with internal disease and other organ systems have to be screened (renal function, clotting studies, platelet counts, antinuclear factor). The development of purpura may signify a defect in clotting and in particular in platelet numbers or function. The investigation of the patient with purpura will include platelet counts as well as a skin biopsy which will show inflammation of the blood vessels in vasculitis. Erythema nodosum may be a presenting feature of a number of diseases such as sarcoidosis, streptococcal infections, tuberculosis and coccidioidomycosis.

# Pyoderma gangrenosum

Pyoderma gangrenosum is a form of severe episodic ulceration of the skin. The initial lesions are purple, irregular, nodular thickenings which rapidly break down and ulcerate. Any site may be affected. There is no evidence of infection and the skin biopsy merely shows necrosis of the epidermis and dermis. Pyoderma gangrenosum is an important condition to recognize because it may be associated with internal disease such as ulcerative colitis, Crohn's disease, rheumatoid arthritis, diabetes, myeloma or leukaemia. It responds well to systemic corticosteroids.

**Table 24.4** Skin changes in vasculitis.

| Vessel type | Skin changes | Diseases |
| --- | --- | --- |
| Small arterioles | Purpura, bruising | Idiopathic vasculitis, Henoch–Schönlein purpura |
| Larger arterioles/arteries | Nodules, ulcers | Polyarteritis nodosa |
| Larger arteries in subcutaneous fat | Large nodules | Erythema nodosum |

# $S$KIN DAMAGE

# Photosensitivity

The visible spectrum forms only a small part of the complete electromagnetic spectrum. In particular some of the short wavelength ultraviolet (UV) waves are potentially harmful to humans. The UV spectrum consists of three main bands: UVA (320–400 nm), UVB (290–320 nm) and UVC (<290 nm). Ultraviolet and visible light can induce photochemical changes and significant amounts of UVB can penetrate through the epidermis into the dermis. By producing pyrimidine dimers in DNA chains absorbed UV light can cause significant damage to fundamental processes. The normal responses to sun exposure in the human skin are erythema (largely UVB induced), pigmentation (due to UVA and UVB) and an increase in skin thickness. The chronic changes are photoageing (page 787) and skin cancer (page 808).

The commonest form of skin damage due to sunlight is sun burn. However, in addition to this there are some specific disorders which are specifically related to light exposure. These can be classified as follows:

1. Metabolic, for example, porphyrias, pellagra
2. Drug or chemical induced (Fig. 24.11), for example, topical (tars, plant oils) or systemic (sulphonamides, phenothiazines, demethylchlortetracycline). Drugs or chemicals may also cause allergic contact dermatitis after transformation to a sensitizing chemical structure through light exposure.

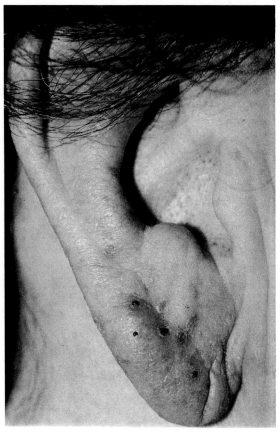

**Figure 24.11** Photodermatitis on the ear lobe due to thiazide diuretic.

3. Idiopathic, for example, polymorphic light eruption, solar urticaria.

In addition, some diseases are characteristically aggravated by sunlight, for example, discoid lupus erythematosus.

Some of these conditions have already been described. Generally the main presenting sign in most of these diseases is erythema. In the case of polymorphic light eruption the rash consists of macules, papules or plaques of erythema with some vesiculation. In the commonest form of porphyria (page 498), porphyria cutanea tarda, the main features are small blisters on the hands and face, scarring in these areas, milia and increased facial hair growth. With the rare erythropoietic porphyrias the earliest feature may be the development of severe sun burn or tingling on sun exposure.

The key to the diagnosis of photosensitivity rashes is that they are limited to light-exposed areas such as the face, neck and hands. Within these areas there are also additional clues such as sparing of the upper lids or an area under the chin which are normally shaded. Specific investigations for photosensitivity would include full blood count, erythrocyte sedimentation rate, antinuclear factors, skin biopsy and tests for porphyrins in serum or urine. In occasional cases testing for sensitivity to specific light wavelengths may be necessary.

## *Physical stimuli*

Skin disease may also be caused or aggravated by physical stimuli such as cold (Raynaud's disease, cold urticaria, perniosis or chilblains, vasculitis) or pressure (dermographism). Of these cold injury is the most frequently seen. Again clues to the presence of cold-induced disease is that the rash is usually, but not always, located on the extremities such as the fingers, toes or the tip of the nose. Other signs or symptoms include a history of Raynaud's disease, bluish discolouration of the skin and livedo reticularis.

## $S$KIN CANCERS

The skin is an important site for cancers which are becoming increasingly common. The development of many skin cancers from basal cell epitheliomas to melanomas is partially dependent on sun exposure. Genetic predisposition, papilloma virus infection and immunosuppression also play a part in the process of carcinogenesis in some cancers. The increasing popularity of acquiring a sun tan combined with the progressive erosion of the protective ozone layer which filters out potentially harmful wavelengths of light are probably responsible for much of the increase. Generally the most harmful of the sun's rays are those on the UVB end of the light spectrum. Risk factors which are important in determining the reaction to sun are a tendency to sun burn and the skin colour. Fair-skinned individuals who burn easily in the sun are the most susceptible.

# Basal cell carcinomas

Basal cell carcinomas or **rodent ulcers** are small slowly growing skin tumours with a very low capacity for metastasis. They usually arise on the face or other light-exposed areas. The initial lesion has a smooth pearly edge with a rounded appearance and central depression. With time the centre becomes ulcerated, the best method of management is excision, although for large lesions radiotherapy is indicated. The prognosis is generally very good, metastasis being extremely rare.

# Squamous carcinomas

Squamous carcinomas are malignant tumours derived from maturing epithelial cells. In the skin they usually arise on light-exposed areas. Immunocompromised patients, particularly those receiving long-term immunosuppression such as renal transplant patients, are particularly prone to develop these tumours. Once again excision is the best approach. Metastatic lesions can occur in late stage lesions.

# Melanomas

The incidence of malignant melanomas is increasing. The highest incidence in the world is in Queensland where they occur at a rate of 40/100 000; in the UK the incidence is up to about 5/100 000. These cancers are derived from melanocytes occurring in the skin or elsewhere (e.g. the retina).

The main features of melanoma depend on their gross and microscopic morphology. Lentigo maligna melanoma (*in situ* melanoma) or Hutchinson's freckle is a slowly evolving flat lesion resembling a large freckle most commonly found on the face in the elderly and it carries the best prognosis. Superficial spreading melanomas are small irregular pigmented macules which slowly enlarge. Here invasion in the early stages is usually confined to the upper layers of the dermis. Nodular melanomas carry the worst prognosis and are most likely to metastasize early.

The prognosis of melanomas is largely based on their clinical classification described above and the depth of penetration of malignant cells into the dermis (Breslow thickness).

The most difficult aspect of the diagnosis of melanoma is to separate benign lesions of pigmented naevi from melanomas. The following features of a pigmented skin lesion should arouse suspicions about melanoma: change in size, shape or pigmentation, bleeding, itching or tingling over the lesion. The changes of melanoma can be seen on skin biopsy material, and excision with careful histology will reveal the diagnosis clearly.

# Naevi

Naevi are displaced accumulations of cells which are derived from skin elements in the dermis or epidermis. They include abnormal clusters of epidermal cells (epidermal naevi), hair bud cells (hairy naevi) or melanocytic cells (pigmented naevi), amongst others. Pigmented naevi or moles are the commonest of these forms and they are generally benign. Some congenital naevi do have an increased frequency of malignant change and there is also a risk of the development of malignant melanoma in others. The criteria for recognizing sinister changes in moles are as for melanoma described above. This is one of the commonest reasons for referral to a skin department.

# Other malignant diseases affecting the skin

The two other malignant conditions which may present in the skin clinic are **cutaneous T-cell lymphoma** (Fig. 24.12) and **Kaposi's sarcoma**. There are a variety of different forms of cutaneous T-cell lymphomas which vary in clinical appearance. A key point is that they often remain unchanged for years before becoming more invasive. Kaposi's sarcoma is a tumour derived from blood vessel precursors. While classically it presents with large bluish/purple nodules on the skin, often the feet or legs, it may appear in a more subtle form with diffuse bluish patches resembling large bruises which may be difficult to see. This pattern is the presentation of Kaposi's sarcoma most often seen in AIDS patients.

# Solar keratoses

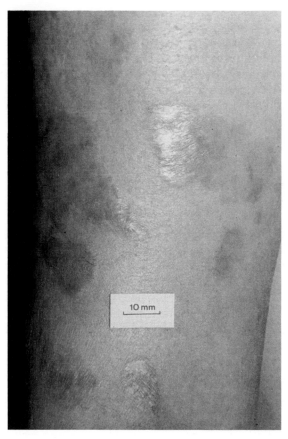

**Figure 24.12** Cutaneous T-cell lymphoma – mycosis fungoides.

One of the earliest signs of sun-induced skin damage or of the same changes seen in old age is a solar or senile keratosis, a small warty lesion on light-exposed areas such as the face, hands and the ear lobes. The bald scalp is another site. The lesions are small crusty papules which may also itch. There are often multiple lesions and other signs of photoageing such as wrinkles and telangiectasia are seen. There is a small risk of the development of squamous cell carcinomas in such lesions and individuals with multiple solar keratoses may also develop *de novo* squamous carcinomas or other light-related malignancies such as melanomas.

# CUTANEOUS SIGNS OF INTERNAL DISEASE

While most of these are discussed throughout this volume under the appropriate disease itself, it is important to remember that some internal diseases may present with skin manifestations which are either specific or give a clue to the diagnosis. Although the list in Table 24.5 is not exclusive it contains some of the commoner cutaneous signs of internal disease.

**Table 24.5** Cutaneous signs of internal disease.

| | | | |
|---|---|---|---|
| **Endocrine disease** | | **Liver disease** | Itching, urticaria, telangiectasia, palmar erythema, hyperpigmentation, nail clubbing in cirrhosis |
| Diabetes mellitus | Necrobiosis lipoidica, skin ulcers, trophic change secondary to neuropathy, superficial candidosis | | |
| Hyperparathyroidism | Calcium deposition | | |
| Acromegaly | Thickened skin, may show secondary changes due to hypogonadism | **Renal disease** | Brown pigmentation, itch, dry skin, in addition specific defects such as calcinosis may appear |
| Cushing's syndrome | Facies, striae, bruising | | |
| Addison's disease | Hyperpigmentation | | |
| Hyperthyroidism | Flushing, hyperpigmentation, pretibial myxoedema | | |
| Hypothyroidism | Pale, dry skin, oedema of face/hands, sparse hair | **Primary immunodeficiency** | Eczema, recurrent staphylococcal infections, viral warts, herpes simplex, herpes zoster, oral candidosis, other abnormalities such as purpura and urticaria can occur |
| **Markers of internal malignancy** | Acanthosis nigricans, dermatomyositis, itching, acquired ichthyosis, migratory thrombophlebitis (pancreatic cancer), sudden unilateral lymphoedema | | |

The examination of the skin is therefore an important part of the process of making a diagnosis. Clues to internal disease as well as a variety of common and treatable disorders can be found without lengthy investigation.

# Poisoning and Adverse Reactions to Drugs and Physical Agents

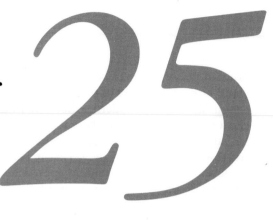

# *Poisoning*

## *I*NTRODUCTION

Human poisoning may be acute or chronic and could be caused by any of the enormous range of chemicals used by modern society. It might be expected, therefore, that there would be a similar range of toxic effects and a wide variety of treatments. In practice, however, it is possible to develop a basic, systematic approach to the assessment and initial management of all cases. Once this has been done it is possible to seek further information and advice on the specific problem using reference sources, including Poisons Information Services.

## *Classification*

Most poisoning is *acute* and may be classified as:

1. **Intentional**: these cases occur from the early teens onwards and represent the predominant group in adults. Most cases are self-poisoning and only a minority of these are truly suicidal.
2. **Accidental**: these cases occur mainly in children aged 5 years or less although adults are also liable to accidents at work or in leisure pursuits. Poisoning may occur because of errors in the prescription or administration of drugs and may be caused by doctors, relatives or patients.

## *P*RELIMINARY ASSESSMENT AND MANAGEMENT

The *history* can be impossible or difficult to obtain because the patient is unconscious or unwilling. All possible sources of evidence should be considered including reports from relatives, friends, the emergency services and the general practitioner, especially about prescribed drugs. All available information about the suspect poison or poisons should be collected, including samples of any chemical, plant or animal. With deliberate poisoning mixed exposure is frequent.

The examination must first take note of the vital signs, and immediate first aid should be given as necessary. A prediction of course and outcome can then be based upon the likely dose or doses of the poisons, the route or routes of exposure, and the time since exposure. It is important to remember that poisoning can occur from inhalation, skin absorption or injection as well as from ingestion. Exposure by more than one route may occur, especially in occupational incidents. Delayed effects may occur from sustained release formulations and when toxic effects are due not to the substance ingested but to a metabolite.

Low risks can be ascribed in some cases, particularly in children, and experience has even made it possible to draw up a list of substances which can be considered as non-poisonous (Table 25.1). Such cases need not be admitted to hospital provided there is satisfactory supervision available and that in adults there is no risk of further suicide attempts.

Moderate risks can often be managed satis-

**Table 25.1** Non-poisons. Examples of products which are unlikely to cause other than minor toxic effects in overdose. This list is based on the experience of the National Poisons Information Service over 30 years. However, if a patient appears to be suffering from unexpected symptoms after such an exposure the reader is advised to contact a Poisons Information Centre.

| **Drugs** | **Bland skin creams** |
|---|---|
| Oral contraceptives | Zinc oxide, titanium oxide |
| Vitamins (without iron) | Calamine lotion |
| Antacids | Petroleum jelly, Vaseline |
| Homeopathic preparations | Lanolin, silicon |

**Household products**

| *Soaps and detergents* | *Cosmetics* |
|---|---|
| Bubble bath | Bath oil |
| Carpet cleaner | Bath foam |
| Dishwashing liquid (hand) | Cleansing cream |
| Dishwashing rinse aid | Cream for hands, body and hair |
| Fabric soakers | Hair conditioner |
| Fabric washing powder and flakes | Lipstick |
| Fabric rinse conditioners | Make up for face and eyes |
| Shaving foam and soaps | Oils for skin and hair |
| Scouring powders and scourers | Suntan preparations |
| General purpose cleaning liquid and powders | Toothpaste without fluoride |
| | Talc (can cause acute bronchitis if inhaled) |
| | |
| *Paints and hobbies* | *Miscellaneous* |
| Chalk | Candles (beeswax or paraffin) |
| Crayon | Lubricants, mineral oil |
| Felt-tip pens | Modelling clay, Plasticine, Buddies, Blu-tac, putty |
| Indelible markers | Newspaper |
| Children's water colour paints | Silica gel |
| Colour blocks, powder colours | Sweetening agents such as saccharin |
| Emulsion paint | Starch |
| | Thermometer contents (mercury, alcohol, glass) |
| | Water-based pastes, gums and adhesives |

factorily in an emergency department or observation ward before discharge with appropriate follow-up.

High risk cases need to be admitted and the most serious cases will require intensive care.

## CLINICAL FEATURES

Whatever the risk associated with a particular chemical, management is based first and foremost on the clinical findings.

### Central nervous system effects

The level of consciousness must be assessed and monitored according to a standardized simple rating scale (Table 25.2). Some poisons are proconvulsants (Table 25.3).

### Cardiovascular effects

Circulatory failure may occur due to depression of myocardial function, cardiac arrhythmias, vasodilation and dehydration occurring singly or in combination. Pulse, blood pressure,

**Table 25.2** Clinical grading scale for level of consciousness in the case of acute poisoning.

**Grade**

1. Drowsy, responds to commands
2. Responsive to mild painful stimulation
3. Minimal response to maximal painful stimulation
4. No response to maximum painful stimulation

**Table 25.3** Drugs and chemicals which may provoke convulsion.

Alphachloralose
Amphetamines
Carbon monoxide
Cyanide
Ethylene glycol
Hypoglycaemic agents
Isoniazid
Lead
Lithium
Mefenamic acid
Monoamine oxidase inhibitors
Opioids
Organochlorine insecticides
Organophosphate insecticides
Phenothiazines
Salicylates
Strychnine
Theophylline
Tricyclic antidepressants
Withdrawal states

peripheral perfusion, and if necessary the electrocardiogram (ECG), should all be monitored.

## Respiratory effects

Respiratory effects may be due to depressed respiration, direct chemical damage to the lungs, left ventricular failure or aspiration.

## TREATMENT

### Immediate treatment

Starts with basic first aid including prevention of further exposure and removal of contaminated clothing. In the unconscious patient the airway must be kept clear and aspiration of vomit should be avoided by nursing in the semiprone (coma) position. If cardiorespiratory arrest occurs resuscitation should be started, remembering that poisoning often occurs in otherwise fit adults and children and that prolonged resuscitation can sometimes be justified (even for several hours).

### Supportive management

Further supportive management includes intravenous plasma or saline to correct hypovolaemia and the use of a cuffed endotracheal tube to protect the airway and permit mechanical ventilation if necessary.

### Drug treatment

Any drug treatment should be used with caution, remembering that the drugs may produce further toxic effects. However, intravenous diazepam may be needed as an anticonvulsant and dopamine or dobutamine may be justified to raise the blood pressure. Anti-arrhythmic drugs are best reserved until it is clear that resuscitative measures alone are not sufficient (page 216).

### Specific treatments

Such treatments include the use of measures to prevent absorption or enhance removal of the poison and the use of antidotes.

#### Prevention of absorption

Prevention of absorption of ingested poisons may be attempted by the use of measures to empty the stomach or by administration of activated charcoal to adsorb the poison. Emesis (induced vomiting) or gastric lavage (stomach washout) have been widely used and can remove some of the stomach contents. There is less evidence however that they remove significant amounts of the poisons and they can have unwanted effects of their own, for example, aspiration into the lungs or prolonged vomiting. Occasionally such treatments appear to remove significant amounts of tablets or capsules but such effects decline with time after absorption and in most cases the procedure cannot be justified more than 4 hours after ingestion. A reasonable practice is, therefore, to restrict their use to those cases where there is a high risk of toxic effects and where presentation is early, for example, in case of paracetamol overdose. Gastric lavage is generally preferred in adults and can even be used in a comatose patient provided the airway is protected by an endotracheal tube. Lavage is not well tolerated in children for whom syrup of ipecacuanha (ipecac) is the recommended emetic providing that there is no impairment of consciousness. Ipecac may also be used in conscious adults but if given the choice, patients usually prefer the stomach tube!

Activated charcoal is a fine powder which meets specified requirements for purity and adsorbance. It may be taken as a drink mixed with water or fruit juices, or given down the gastric lavage tube before it is removed. Most adults tolerate its gritty feel and lack of taste but children are much more likely to vomit back the charcoal so the addition of flavouring is advisable.

Activated charcoal can be shown *in vitro* to adsorb most poisons (Table 25.4) and volunteer studies have demonstrated a clear effect *in vivo*. Data from actual poisoned patients are less convincing but activated charcoal is now generally accepted to be safe and capable of reducing the severity of poisoning.

### Enhanced elimination of absorbed poisons

Once the poison has been absorbed it may be possible to increase the rate of its elimination by promoting excretion in the urine or the faeces or by using an extracorporeal technique, for example, haemodialysis or haemoperfusion, to remove the poison directly from the blood. In practice, logical though these approaches may seem, their efficacy in clinical use is limited and

**Table 25.4** Poisons *not* effectively adsorbed by activated charcoal.

| |
|---|
| Strong acids and alkalis |
| Copper |
| Cyanide |
| Ethanol |
| Ethylene glycol |
| Iron |
| Lithium |
| Mercury |
| Methanol |
| Organic solvents, e.g. toluene |

Note that oral activated charcoal may adsorb oral antidotes, e.g. methionine, syrup of ipecacuanha, and interfere with their actions

with the exception of the use of repeated doses of activated charcoal they should generally only be embarked upon after careful consideration, including consultation with the Poisons Information Service and/or a clinical toxicologist.

### Forced diuresis

If the poison or its active metabolites is excreted in the urine, it is possible to increase the rate of excretion by increasing the urine output, a procedure known as forced diuresis. Renal excretion can be further enhanced by altering the pH of the urine to render the excreted poison in its ionized form in order to prevent its reabsorption by the renal tubules. Thus for acidic drugs, for example, salicylate or phenobarbitone, raising the urine pH by including sodium bicarbonate in the intravenous fluid regime will increase the concentration of the ionized drug in the urine and promote excretion. Similarly, basic drugs such as amphetamine and pethidine are excreted more rapidly in acid urine. However, this procedure is not without risks since it involves giving large volumes of fluid to patients whose cardiovascular and renal status may be impaired and there is a risk of serious electrolyte imbalance and fluid overload with left ventricular failure. In addition, it has to be remembered that most drugs are inactivated by hepatic metabolism rather than excreted as unchanged drug or active metabolites so that the potential for the technique is limited. In practice the only regular indication for forced alkaline diuresis is salicylate poisoning. Phenobarbitone poisoning is also an indication for alkaline diuresis but such cases are now rare, in line with the much reduced use of that drug. Likewise, amphetamine poisoning can be adequately treated by supportive measures and forced acid diuresis has never been widely practised.

### Dialysis and haemoperfusion

The excretion of some poisons can be increased by peritoneal dialysis or haemodialysis but the range of molecules for which this is applicable is limited to those which can cross the dialysis membranes. In practice peritoneal dialysis is relatively inefficient and haemodialysis in the treatment of poisoning is usually indicated only for the support of renal function. The most obvious exception is severe, life-threating salicylate poisoning, particularly when impaired renal function makes forced alkaline diuresis impractical.

Haemoperfusion involves the passage of blood through a device containing an absorbent material such as activated charcoal or an ion exchange resin. This technique can remove significant quantities of a much wider range of poisons than that covered by dialysis and in the late 1970s/ early 1980s it had an important role in the treatment of some of the most serious cases of poisoning due to barbiturates and other hypnotics, all of which have now been removed from clinical practice. In consequence the technique is now seldom used.

### Repeated dose activated charcoal

It is now apparent that in addition to adsorbing poisons before they are absorbed from the gastrointestinal tract, activated charcoal can also remove absorbed poison by promoting back-diffusion from blood vessels through the gut wall. This has been well demonstrated in experimental situations, and clinical experience has provided increasing evidence that administering activated charcoal repeatedly (say 25 to 50 g

every 4 hours for 12 to 24 hours) can markedly reduce the elimination half-life of certain poisons (Fig. 25.1).

Unlike the other procedures outlined above repeated dose activated charcoal is simple to administer, tolerated by most patients and causes few problems. It is likely to be used increasingly in the future.

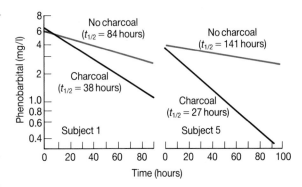

**Figure 25.1** Effect of repeated doses of activated charcoal upon the elimination half-life of intravenous phenobarbitone in two volunteer subjects. Least square regression lines are shown. Reproduced with permission from Berg *et al. N Engl J Med* 1982; **307**: 642–4.

## $B$RIEF NOTES ON SOME COMMON POISONS

This section is intended to give an introduction to some of the most common causes of poisoning in the UK. When necessary the reader is encouraged to consult more detailed references or to seek information and advice from a Poisons Information Service.

It is convenient to classify poisons by use or occurrence, for example, drugs, household chemicals, industrial chemicals, agrochemicals and natural toxins but it should be remembered the same chemical may occur in different situations, for example, ethanol may be used as a drug or as an industrial chemical.

## *Drug poisoning*

Drug poisoning is influenced by the pattern of prescribing, for example, antidepressants are

prescribed to patients who may be suicidal, and of availability, for example, analgesics which are widely available without prescription. It is also influenced by the toxicity of the drug such that some can be considered non-toxic (Table 25.1) while some can readily produce symptoms of poisoning, for example, drugs used to treat cardiac arrhythmias and cytotoxic drugs.

### ANALGESICS

The mild analgesics aspirin, paracetamol and more recently ibuprofen can be obtained over-the-counter without prescription in the UK and it is those products which feature most commonly in cases of poisoning.

### *Aspirin*

Poisoning by aspirin (or occasionally other salicylates) has decreased in frequency following the withdrawal of aspirin for use in children and in response to the increased use of paracetamol and ibuprofen. Nevertheless, serious cases are still quite frequent and as little as 25 g can be fatal in an adult whilst doses of only 2 to 4 g have proved lethal in children (most tablets are 300 mg).

In mild cases the main symptoms are nausea, vomiting, tinnitus and an increased rate of respiration. After larger doses there is mental confusion, the patient is flushed and sweating with a raised temperature and a full pulse. The overbreathing is very striking and in the early stages hyperventilation lowers the $Pa\,CO_2$ and leads to respiratory alkalosis (page 509). With increasing absorption of salicylate a metabolic acidosis develops with the fall in plasma bicarbonate. In children acidosis is common whereas in adults a raised blood pH is more usual. In addition vomiting and sweating lead to dehydration and oliguria.

Because large doses of salicylate tend not to dissolve in the stomach but to remain as a mass or even a 'lining', gastric aspiration and lavage can be useful up to 24 hours after ingestion. In mild to moderate cases rehydration and the promotion of an alkaline urine, with emphasis on a good urine output rather than an excessive forced diuresis, is usually adequate. Potassium usually needs to be added to the intravenous fluids to prevent hypokalaemia. Treatment can then be adjusted according to clinical findings and laboratory measurement of salicylate concentrations and electrolytes. In severe cases where plasma salicylate concentrations exceed 800 mg/l in an adult and 500 mg/l in a child, it may be necessary to use haemodialysis, especially if there is evidence of impaired renal function.

## Paracetamol

Paracetamol has a well-deserved reputation for safety in the correct dosage (1 g repeated 4 hourly to a maximum of 6 g in 24 hours) but a single overdose of over 15 g can produce serious liver damage whilst doses over 25 g are potentially fatal. The toxic effects come not from paracetamol itself but from a toxic metabolite. In therapeutic doses the liver metabolizes most paracetamol by conjugation to form glucuronides and sulphates. At the same time a small amount is converted to a highly reactive intermediate n-acetyl-p-benzoquinonemine (NAPQI) by the mixed-function oxidase enzyme system, cytochrome P450. The NAPQI is rapidly detoxified by glutathione to produce other non-toxic conjugates.

In overdosage the main pathways of metabolism are overwhelmed with the consequence that more NAPQI is produced and glutathione stores are depleted. The NAPQI is then free to combine covalently with hepatic cell macromolecules to cause necrosis with progressive liver failure which can lead to death. A similar mechanism can also lead to renal damage.

For the first 12 to 24 hours after ingestion there are few symptoms except perhaps for nausea, vomiting and some abdominal discomfort. In severe overdosage signs of liver involvement start with hepatic tenderness after 24 to 36 hours after which time jaundice may develop. If renal failure occurs it usually becomes apparent at around the same time as the liver damage.

Assessment of the severity of poisoning is dependent upon measurement of the plasma paracetamol concentration which from 4 hours after ingestion can be used to predict the severity of poisoning (Fig. 25.2). Subsequently an increase in the prothrombin time is the first test of liver function to show deterioration, usually after 18 hours, whilst enzyme and bilirubin changes are seldom marked until after 36 hours.

Treatment should start with emptying the stomach up to 4 hours after ingestion of the drug and administration of methionine or acetylcysteine, both of which act as glutathione precursors and thus support the normal mechanism of detoxification. Methionine is given by mouth and is simple to administer but is less effective if the patient presents late and should not be used if the patient is vomiting. Acetylcysteine is given intravenously and is highly effective during the first 8 to 10 hours after ingestion with a rapidly decreasing efficacy over the remainder of the first 24 hours. Acetylcysteine can provoke histamine release to produce a pseudo-allergic reaction with flushing, urticaria and bronchospasm. If these symptoms occur it may be necessary to change treatment to methionine or to continue under cover of a drug to block histamine type 1 receptors.

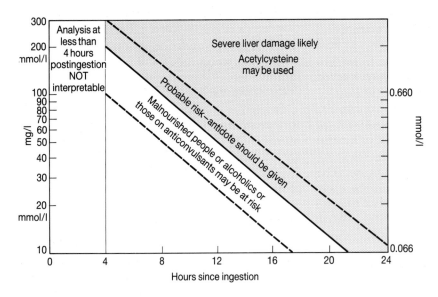

**Figure 25.2** Nomogram for use of antidotes in paracetamol poisoning.

## Ibuprofen

Ibuprofen has now been available for 24 years as an anti-inflammatory agent and 10 years as an over-the-counter general-purpose analgesic. There is now convincing evidence that it is less toxic in overdose than either aspirin or paracetamol and even extremely large doses have caused little more than mild drowsiness and gastrointestinal symptoms. The few serious overdoses that have been reported have involved mixed overdosage with other drugs or patients with serious underlying physical disease.

## Mefenamic acid

This is commonly prescribed for treatment of dysmenorrhoea and is therefore most frequently taken in overdose by young women. There is a high incidence of grand mal convulsions which may occur as late as 12 hours postingestion. These are treated with diazepam and supportive care.

## Opioids

This term covers all drugs with opiate-like actions from the original morphine and diamorphine to the newer synthetic molecules including opioid agonists/antagonists such as buprenorphine to the weaker molecules including codeine, dextropropoxyphene and diphenoxylate which is used for its constipating effect and not for analgesia.

The features of opioid overdosage are common to all of these drugs, providing that a sufficient dose is taken, and include coma which may be deep with respiratory depression and pin-point pupils. In addition the skin is cyanosed, cold and clammy. The blood pressure is low in severe poisoning and convulsions or acute pulmonary oedema may be serious complications. Death usually results from respiratory depression. Overdosage can occur not only from licensed medications but also from street drugs where the potential for overdosage is exacerbated by uncertainty as to the quality of the drug (and hence the dosage) and the sensitivity of the individual (tolerance and therefore use of increasing doses develops in regular users but a period of abstinence may result in a return to the original sensitivity).

If respiratory or cardiac arrest has occurred this takes priority and should be treated in the usual way. Naloxone is a specific opioid antagonist and competes for opioid receptors in the central nervous system (CNS). It is administered intravenously with a normal dose of 0.4 to 1.6 mg. If opioid poisoning is seriously suspected it is important to give at least 1.6 mg before abandoning the diagnosis. The administration of naloxone will not complicate the management of non-opioid poisoning and in severe overdosage there may be only slight improvements with the normal doses. In these cases much larger doses of naloxone may be given and it should be remembered that this drug has a short half-life (about 30 minutes) so that with long-acting opioids repeated doses may be necessary. There is a danger in narcotic addicts that naloxone may precipitate acute withdrawal symptoms including convulsions. This consideration should not lead to withholding naloxone but rather to its administration more cautiously. Partial opioid agonists such as buprenorphine usually respond less well to naloxone and more prolonged and intensive supportive care may be required.

## ANTIDEPRESSANTS

### Tricyclic antidepressants

This group includes amitriptyline, clomipramine and dothiepin. The clinical picture is the result of cholinergic blockade, increased adrenergic activity and direct cardiac and CNS depression. It is essentially one of excitement followed by coma.

In moderate poisoning the patient is flushed with hot dry skin, tachycardia and dilated pupils. With more severe poisoning there is confusion leading to convulsions and coma. The reflexes are usually brisk and the plantar response may be extensor. Sinus tachycardia is universal and more serious cardiac arrhythmias are possible, especially in patients with pre-existing heart disease. The ECG shows prolongation of the QRS interval and cardiac arrest may occur, even several days after the drug was taken.

There is no specific antidote and treatment is essentially supportive. Gastric lavage may be useful up to 8 hours after ingestion because the anticholinergic effects of the drugs may delay gastric emptying. Oral activated charcoal is an effective adsorbent and should be used both initially and in repeated doses. The electrolytes should be monitored along with blood gases and appropriate actions, including ventilation if necessary, should be undertaken without delay. Sinus tachycardia can usually be left untreated. Other arrhythmias may have to be treated in the normal way but with caution since all anti-arrhythmic drugs can cause further arrhythmias. Hypotension may require the use of plasma expanders and dopamine/dobutamine to increase cardiac output. Convulsions can be con-

trolled by diazepam but the suggestion that physostigmine acts as an antidote has been disproven and should be ignored.

### Newer antidepressants

The more recently introduced antidepressants including the tetracyclic molecule mianserin, 5-hydroxytryptamine antagonists such as trazodone and more surprisingly lofepramine, even though it is metabolized to the tricyclic molecule desipramine, are less cardiotoxic and less likely to cause convulsions. Treatment is supportive.

### Monoamine oxidase inhibitors

These drugs are well known at normal doses to interact with monoamines taken as drugs or as constituents of food, for example, in cheese, red wine and chocolate, to produce a sudden and severe increase in blood pressure. This is not a major feature of overdosage unless the patient deliberately provokes the interaction. In fact the patient may remain quite well for the first 12 hours or so followed by a gradual build up of muscle twitching leading to spasm. There is usually a sinus tachycardia and blood pressure may be high or low. At the same time the core temperature may increase to develop life-threatening hyperthermia. Rhabdomyolysis may develop from the muscle spasms and can cause renal failure.

Whilst supportive measures may be adequate in mild cases evidence of hyperthermia should be taken seriously and if necessary the patient should be paralysed (e.g. with pancuronium or dantrolene) and mechanically ventilated. Other measures are supportive.

## HYPNOTICS AND ANXIOLYTICS

Now that the earlier more toxic drugs have been withdrawn this group is dominated by the less toxic benzodiazepines and it can be expected that any non-benzodiazepine drugs which are introduced are likely to be even less toxic. In overdosage the picture is one of CNS depression leading to coma but without severe respiratory depression or circulatory failure. Supportive treatment is usually adequate and the duration of coma can usually be predicted from the half-life of the drug, remembering that some have active metabolites such as desmethyldiazepam from diazepam (half-life 36–200 hours compared with 20–50 hours for the parent drug).

More serious toxicity may occcur when the benzodiazepine drug is taken as part of a mixed overdose or when there is serious underlying respiratory or cardiac disease. Providing that such problems are adequately treated by supportive measures the prognosis remains good. Recently a specific benzodiazepine antagonist, flumazenil, has been licensed for the reversal of the effects of benzodiazepines used for anaesthesia. The role of flumazenil in benzodiazepine overdose is less certain and a number of problems have been described including the precipitation of convulsions from a coexisting antidepressant overdose.

## PHENOTHIAZINES

The dose–response curve of the phenothiazines is relatively flat so there is a wide margin of safety. Overdosage produces unconsciousness associated with extrapyramidal signs and with torticollis. Cardiac arrhythmias, hypotension and hypothermia may occur. The extrapyramidal symptoms, which may be delayed up to 24 hours, can be treated with benztropine and treatment is otherwise supportive.

## ETHANOL

Most subjects with acute alcoholic intoxication will sleep it off, including young children. Hypoglycaemia can be a complication in fasting patients or children, and blood glucose should be monitored. Rarely lactic acidosis (page 512) may develop in patients with liver disease or those who are taking biguanides.

The combination of ethanol and other centrally acting drugs is additive and can be very dangerous. There is no specific treatment but careful monitoring and supportive measures are indicated.

## β-ADRENOCEPTOR BLOCKERS

As would be expected these drugs cause bradycardia and a low cardiac output in overdose. The bradycardia can be reversed by intravenous atropine or, if this fails, by a pacemaker. Intravenous glucagon may reverse the cardiac effects by activating myocardial adenyl cyclase by a different mechanism than that of the β-adrenoceptor agonists. However, the symptoms can also be reversed by an infusion of isoprenaline.

## THEOPHYLLINE

Theophylline and related bronchodilator drugs may cause life-threatening toxicity in overdose. Symptoms include abdominal pain, vomiting and haematemesis and hyperventilation; cardiac arrhythmias are common and the latter may be exacerbated by hypokalaemia. In the most severe cases there may be convulsions and mortality is high. All theophylline overdose patients should be closely monitored for cardiac arrhythmias and other complications. Gastric lavage should be followed by oral activated charcoal in repeated doses and supportive treatment may include the use of β-blockers (caution if the patient is asthmatic) or verapamil.

# *S*USTAINED RELEASE FORMULATIONS

Theophylline in particular is usually prescribed as a sustained release formulation. In overdosage this has the effect of delaying the onset of symptoms and inducing a false sense of security in the attending physicians. It is vital that the use of such formulations is noted when the history is taken and that the need for an appropriate period of monitoring is stressed to both nursing and medical staff. This applies just as much to other drugs in sustained release formulations.

# HOUSEHOLD CHEMICALS

The modern household, and for that matter the garage and the garden shed, contain a wide range of chemicals for use in maintenance, hobbies or other special interests. Various licensing procedures ensure that these chemicals are selected for safety as well as for efficacy but needless to say no chemical is totally without toxic effects and all should be regarded as potentially dangerous to children or to those who misuse them by failing to follow instructions. Poisons Information Services have plenty of experience of both types of incident and should be consulted if there is any cause for concern. However, a few generalizations are possible:

*Soaps, detergents and other household cleaning products* generally cause little toxicity when ingested in small amounts by children although there is a small risk of aspiration of foam during vomiting. Even domestic bleach, sodium hypochlorite, generally produces only minor gastrointestinal symptoms because it is available only at a low concentration (not more than 5 per cent).

Commercial *cleaning agents* may be used in higher concentrations and occasionally contain more toxic chemicals than those used domestically.

Most *cosmetics* are relatively non-toxic but often contain ethanol as a solvent which may occasionally cause clinical effects.

*Products used for decorating*, including paint strippers and solvents, and those used for *motor-car maintenance* including screen wash additives and antifreeze are potentially toxic and all cases of suspected poisoning should be regarded seriously. Ethylene glycol (antifreeze) is broken down to toxic metabolites. Ethanol is a competitive inhibitor of the metabolism and can be used in treatment.

*Garden chemicals* are generally selected from the least toxic members of the groups of chemicals used in agriculture or are available only at lower concentrations. For example, most domestic insecticides use pyrethoids, a group of chemicals with extremely low toxicity for humans, rather than the cholinesterase-inhibiting organophosphates, a series of chemicals which also includes the 'nerve agents' used as chemical weapons. In fact the organophosphate insecticides that are used in homes and gardens are not only selected as being those with the lowest toxicity for humans but are also formulated in such a way as to reduce greatly the chances of accidental poisoning.

Much of the information listed above is reassuring but remember that, occasionally, more toxic chemicals from industry or agriculture may be taken home by the worker, usually without permission and often in inappropriate containers.

# CARBON MONOXIDE

Carbon monoxide can be a cause of both accidental and suicidal deaths. The introduction of natural gas removed the potential for using the domestic gas supply for suicidal purposes but car exhaust gases are readily available to most households and suicide by that mechanism is currently increasing in frequency. It is also important to remember that any heater using carboniferous fuels (including natural gas, smokeless fuel, wood and oil) can produce carbon monoxide if there is inadequate combustion. Such problems are particularly likely to occur if the flue is blocked in which case the carbon monoxide may escape back into the dwelling or even into neighbouring dwellings.

Carbon monoxide is colourless and lighter than air, it has a far greater affinity for oxygen than haemoglobin and forms carboxyhaemoglobin which is bright red in colour. It cannot carry oxygen and tissue anoxia results.

Small elevations of carboxyhaemoglobin occur from environmental exposure, for example, in a policeman on point duty, or in smokers who may tolerate a concentration of up to 8–10 per cent. Symptoms are minimal if less than 30 per cent of the haemoglobin is combined with carbon monoxide and consist of nausea, lassitude and headache. With higher concentrations the onset of symptoms is rapid and there is a transient increase in pulse rate and respiration followed by weakness, dimness of vision and finally coma, respiratory depression and death.

The patient with carbon monoxide poisoning is often pale and cyanosed. The typical cherry red colour that has classically been described as being associated with carboxyhaemoglobin is usually seen only at *post mortem*. The presence of carboxyhaemoglobin in the blood may be confirmed by its characteristic absorption spectrum and the concentration of carboxyhaemoglobin can be used as a guide to treatment.

The patient must be removed from the poisoned atmosphere as quickly as possible and artificial respiration should be started if necessary. Pure oxygen is an antidote and should generally be available in the ambulance. Severe cases are complicated by cerebral oedema which may be detected by papilloedema. This may be treated by conventional means including the use of mannitol and bed rest. Some patients show evidence of permanent cardiac or CNS damage after recovery. Some authorities believe that hyperbaric oxygen can reduce the severity of such damage but this treatment is available only at a limited number of centres and remains controversial. The Poisons Information Service will advise on the current criteria for such treatment and the location of treatment centres.

# INDUSTRIAL POISONING

The use of chemicals at work has come under increasing scrutiny and adequate information including advice on prevention, for example, use of protective clothing together with outline details of toxic effects and first aid measures should be available to both employer and employee. Furthermore, the Health and Safety Executive has legal powers to inspect premises and demand that actions are taken for safety or even to close down the process.

However, no legislation can ever work perfectly or take account of accidents or deliberate self-poisoning on the part of the worker. Examples of industrial chemicals which can cause severe acute poisoning include chlorine gas, hydrogen cyanide and other cyanides, organic solvents and strong acids such as hydrofluoric acid.

The large industrial concerns should have an occupational health department or at least should ensure that some staff have first aid training. Thus the patient should have received some treatment before arrival at hospital, even to the level of administration of antidotes as in the case of cyanide poisoning which is discussed below as an example.

## Cyanide

Hydrocyanic acid and potassium or sodium cyanide are very powerful poisons which act by

**Table 25.5** UK recommended antidotes for use in cyanide poisoning.

**First aid**

*Oxygen* 100% increases oxygen carried in blood other than as oxyhaemoglobin

*Amyl nitrite* inhalation converts haemoglobin to methaemoglobin which has a high affinity for cyanide

**Occupational health centre/hospital**

*Sodium thiosulphate* i.v. replenishes thiosulphate stores necessary for conversion of cyanide to non-toxic thiocyanate

**Plus**

*Dicobalt edetate* i.v. produces non-toxic chelates of cyanide

or

*Sodium nitrite* i.v. produces methaemoglobin

inhibiting a number of enzymes but most importantly cytochrome oxidase. They are used in a number of industrial processes and are manufactured in large amounts on a very small number of sites.

The inhalation of hydrocyanic acid (which is a gas) results in death within a few minutes unless treatment is instituted immediately. After ingestion of cyanide salts death may occur in anything from a few minutes up to several hours

depending on the salt and the dose. Generally speaking the absorption of about 1 mg cyanide is fatal.

The aim of treatment in cyanide poisoning is to give substances which combine with cyanide and prevent interference with the enzyme systems. A number of antidotes exist and currently there is a variation in the preferred treatment from country to country. Recommendations in the UK are listed in Table 25.5.

# Agrochemical poisoning

Agrochemicals are most easily classified by their intended use rather than by chemical grouping (Table 25.6). If they are used correctly, toxic effects from agrochemicals in humans should not occur. Problems arise infrequently from accidents, misuse or even deliberate exposure and the most serious of these cases will require hospital treatment. Poisons Information Services have accumulated experience of such cases and will advise.

Ingestion of the herbicide paraquat in its concentrated liquid form has, in the past, been notable as a cause of serious poisoning both from local corrosive effects and from systemic effects including impairment of renal, hepatic and respiratory function. Survivors of the acute effects may then die over the next few days from respiratory failure due to pulmonary fibrosis. There is no antidote and treatment is supportive. Fortunately accidental exposure seldom involves a fatal dose and overall the incidence of serious cases is declining.

**Table 25.6** Basic classification of pesticides.

**Insecticides**
Organophosphates
Carbamates
Organochlorines
Pyrethroids

**Rodenticides**
Anticoagulants
Alphachloralose
Calciferol

**Herbicides**
Paraquat
Diquat
Chlorphenoxy compounds

**Fungicides**
Benomyl
Captan

**Molluscicides**
Metaldehyde
Methiocarb

**Insect repellants**
Diethyltoluamide

# Environmental poisoning

Recently the media, the public and politicians have taken an increasing interest in the possibility of poisoning from environmental sources via food, water or air and there has been an

increasing recognition of the potential for poisoning from major chemical accidents. It is right that doctors in hospitals and general practice should be aware of the potential for such problems but it must be recognized that in many cases it is possible to disprove the link or the verdict will be 'open'. Our knowledge of this subject can be expected to develop during the next few years but in the meantime the following points are worth noting.

For any incident of suspected environmental poisoning:

1. A detailed history is essential.
2. Legislation and regulatory mechanisms exist to prevent and monitor risks to the population from environmental exposure be it from food, water or air. Proven incidents may need reporting.

3. Sample collection is important for the proper toxicological evaluation of the incident and carefully labelled samples should be collected as soon as possible and placed in appropriate storage.
4. If it is certain that there is no toxic risk, patients should be given a careful explanation and reassurance. Failure to do this could lead to prolonged complaints which with time become more difficult to treat.
5. If there is a real possibility that toxic effects have occurred consider referring the patient to a specialist in medical toxicology.

# Adverse reactions to drugs

# *I*NTRODUCTION

Modern drugs are the result of intensive and expensive research programmes which take a number of years to complete. Before a product licence can be granted by the regulatory agencies (e.g. the Medicines Control Agency in the UK and the Food and Drugs Administration in the USA) they have to review and accept comprehensive reports on the drug including pharmaceutical, preclinical and clinical data (Table 25.7). The requirements of the licensing authorities are based on many years accumulated experience and are designed to ensure that everything that could reasonably be expected has been done to ensure that the new drug will be used in the correct way and that any adverse effects will be minimized.

Nevertheless, adverse drug reactions are an everyday experience in medicine and probably affect about 10 per cent of hospital inpatients and 10–15 per cent of consultations in outpatients or in general practice. Many of these reactions are minor and short-lived with about 80 per cent lasting less than 1 week. Conversely, however, some adverse drug reactions can have

**Table 25.7** Testing for drug safety. Before licensing all drugs must undergo rigorous testing which may be considered under three headings.

**1. Pharmaceutical**
Quality control and purity of drug substance
Biovailability and stability of dosage form.*

**2. Preclinical**
Pharmacology: Pharmacokinetics and
　pharmacodynamics
Toxicology: Single dose and repeat dose
　　　　　　Mutagenicity and reproductive toxicology
　　　　　　Carcinogenicity

**3. Clinical**
Healthy volunteers and patients
Pharmacokinetics and pharmacodynamics
Efficacy and safety
Safety in pregnancy
Efficacy and safety in special groups, e.g. the elderly
Effects (or likely effects) in overdose
Safety in long-term use

*Biovailability is defined as the extent to which, and the rate at which, the drug product is taken up by the body in the form which is physiologically active.

serious consequences and can result in failure of treatment and/or harm to the patient.

To use drugs safely does not require an encyclopaedic knowledge of adverse reactions but rather an understanding of their underlying mechanisms, an awareness that they may be the cause of all or part of the patients' complaints and a knowledge of information sources which may be used to assess a particular problem (Table 25.8). The ultimate aim is prevention and all doctors are encouraged to play a part in the monitoring of adverse drug reactions since the results of such monitoring can be used to influence safety through the actions of the regulatory agencies or through continuing medical education.

**Table 25.8** References on adverse drug reactions.

### Regularly updated resources available to all doctors
British National Formulary (BNF)
Manufacturers' Data Sheets
Data Sheet Compendium (ABPI)
Drug and Therapeutics Bulletin (Consumers' Association)

### Reference library books
Davies, Textbook of Adverse Drug Reactions
Martindale, The Exta Pharmacopea
Meyler, Side Effects of Drugs
Goodman and Gilman, Principles and Practice of Therapeutics

### Information Services
Pharmacy Drug Information Services: see BNF for telephone numbers for regional centres
Manufacturers Information Services: see address list in BNF or Data Sheet Compendium
CSM Adverse Drug Reaction Section: freephone CSM (Committee on Safety of Medicines)
Poisons Information Services: see BNF

# CLASSIFICATION OF ADVERSE DRUG REACTIONS

It is useful to think of drug reactions under two main headings.

1. Type A reactions which can be predicted from the known pharmacological action of the drug.
2. Type B reactions which are unpredictable and include allergies, idiosyncratic reactions and those due to some genetically determined abnormal response to the drug.

## Type A reactions

In this type of reaction the pharmacological effects of the drug are excessive. This can be due to overdose or to undue sensitivity of the patient to the drug's action – an example being the undue respiratory depression produced by morphine in a patient with long-standing respiratory disease. Pharmacokinetic factors may be important, usually because the patient is unable to eliminate the drug as a result of disease, a good example being the patient with renal failure who fails to excrete digoxin with subsequent toxicity.

Sometimes adverse effects are inherent in the action of the drug even when given in normal doses and without undue sensitivity on the part of the patient. Most people taking tricyclic antidepressants will complain of dry mouth and other anticholinergic effects, and many of the patients taking the vasodilator nifedipine will develop some ankle swelling. Generally this type of side effect can be predicted and often avoided if the possibility is considered before prescribing. For example, when an antidepressant has sedative effects these can be used to advantage if the drug is taken at night shortly before going to bed.

# Type B reactions

This is a more heterogeneous group where the reaction is unrelated to the drug's pharmacological action and is usually unpredictable. They can be considered as drug allergies, genetically determined reactions and idiosyncratic reactions.

## DRUG ALLERGIES

Some reactions to drugs are known to be mediated by immune mechanisms. This means that the patient has been previously exposed to the drug or to some closely related substance. Most drugs are of a low molecular weight and are therefore not antigenic. They can, however, combine covalently with a large molecular substance, usually a protein, and the combination which is known as a hapten acts as an antigen.

Four types of allergic reaction are now recognized and it is possible for a single drug to cause more than one type of allergy.

## Type I (immediate anaphylactic) reactions

This is mediated by the IgE fraction of the immunoglobulins which induce antibody/antigen reactions on the surface of the mast cells and release pharmacologically active substances including histamine, bradykinin and 5-hydroxytryptamine (page 97). The effects may be seen in the skin (acute urticaria), the respiratory tract (bronchospasm), the gastrointestinal tract (abdominal pain and vomiting) or as a generalized anaphylactic reaction. These types of reactions are seen typically with penicillin or streptomycin and the most severe reactions are likely with antisera raised in animals. Anaphylaxis is not a problem with immunoglobulins from human sources.

The reaction occurs within a few minutes of administration of the drug. The main features are chest pain, dyspnoea, cyanosis and a rapid fall in blood pressure with collapse. The attack may be fatal and therefore it is important to work towards prevention and to be prepared for emergency treatment. Therefore, the patient should be carefully questioned about known sensitivity to the drug about to be given or to other drugs. Particular attention should be paid to any past exposure to an antiserum raised in animals. It is also helpful to know whether he or she suffers from atopy (hay fever, asthma, infantile eczema or urticaria) since type I reaction is more frequent in atopic subjects.

When there is a positive history of a reaction to serum, test doses of the serum-based product should be used before the full dose is given and the immediate treatment for anaphylaxis (intramuscular 0.5 ml of 1:1000 adrenaline and 10 mg of intravenous chlorpheniramine) should be ready. If a reaction occurs intravenous hydrocortisone may also be used along with supportive measures as necessary.

## Type II reactions

These are mediated by antibodies of classes IgG and IgM which combine with antigens on the surface of cells and fix complement. Drug-induced haemolytic anaemia and transfusion reactions are of this type.

## Type III reactions

Reactions such as serum sickness and drug-induced systemic lupus erythematosus are less acute and are due to damage caused by circulating immune complexes [antigen/antibody (IgE, IgM)/complement] which lodge in blood vessels causing local inflammation and systemic effects.

Serum sickness usually develops 7 to 10 days after the patient has received serum and is manifested by an urticarial rash, pain and swelling in the joints and usually a fever. There may be transient lymphadenopathy and albuminuria and occasionally there may be a shock-like state with hypotension. The reaction usually resolves within a few days but treatment with topical calamine lotion and a short course of oral chlorpheniramine plus prednisolone will usually relieve symptoms.

## Type IV (delayed hypersensitivity) reactions

The typical example of this type of reaction is a contact dermatitis. When the drug is applied to the skin it forms an antigenic conjugate with the dermal proteins which stimulates the formation of sensitized T-lymphocytes. If the drug is applied again a rash develops. The rash clears when the application of the drug is stopped but a topical corticosteroid cream can be used to relieve symptoms and promote healing.

# GENETICALLY DETERMINED DRUG REACTIONS

Hereditary differences in response to drugs may be due to *polygenic* influences resulting in a continuous variation, for example, in metabolism/elimination as seen with aspirin, phenytoin and warfarin.

Other effects are due to *polymorphism* where the variation is not continuous but results in distinct groups of subjects with respect to their response to particular drugs. Mostly such variation is due to a relative enzyme deficiency which reduces the rate of metabolism and delays the elimination of the drug with prolongation of its effects. Examples include:

1. A relatively deficiency of an N-acetyl-transferase which occurs in about 60 per cent of caucasians in the UK. These 'slow acetylaters' are more likely to suffer adverse reactions to drugs which are metabolized by acetylation, for example, peripheral neuritis with isoniazid (page 691) and the systemic lupus erythematosus-like syndrome from hydralazine, isoniazid and procainamide (page 572). The effects can be avoided or reduced by using lower doses or using specific treatment such as pyridoxine to prevent the peripheral neuritis from isoniazid.

2. A relative deficiency in hydroxylating enzymes which affects 10 per cent of the UK population. This was first noted with debrisoquine which is now seldom used as an antihypertensive but is employed in a test of hydroxylating capacity. Poor hydroxylation can increase the toxicity of some commonly used drugs including metoprolol, propranolol and nortriptyline.

3. Deficiencies of cholinesterase enzymes affect only a small number of people but can have serious effects when suxamethonium or similar muscle relaxants are used in surgery. In such cases the drug is not metabolized, effects are prolonged and postoperative recovery from the paralysing effect is delayed.

Polymorphism can also alter the response to a drug as seen in glucose-6-phosphate dehydrogenase deficiency which is found in some African and Mediterranean races as well as in 10 per cent of black Americans. In such patients some drugs, for example, anticonvulsants or oral hypoglycaemic agents, can precipitate acute porphyria (page 498), whilst other drugs can induce haemolysis (page 615).

# IDIOSYNCRATIC ADVERSE DRUG REACTIONS

For many drugs it is not possible to demonstrate either an allergic or a genetic mechanism for what is otherwise a dose-unrelated effect. Such reactions may have mixed causes and are best regarded as idiosyncratic and classified by the system involved, for example, the haematopoetic system, the liver or the kidney.

## Haematopoetic system

Drug effects on the bone marrow and on the blood cells are amongst the most dangerous and probably involve both allergic and direct toxic effects. The danger lies in susceptibility to infection due to neutropenia and bleeding due to thrombocytopenia, either can be fatal. The range of possible effects merits careful consideration but the large number of drugs implicated in such reactions cannot be memorized and access to reference sources is essential for the assessment of most cases.

### Agranulocytosis

This may occur with a number of drugs of which the commonest are the cytotoxic drugs which produce agranulocytosis as part of their pharmacological action. In addition sulphonamides, carbimazole, isoniazid, phenylbutazone, chloramphenicol and gold occasionally cause agranulocytosis. With most drugs the agranulocytosis is reversible, provided the drug is not continued for too long, but with chloramphenicol recovery may not occur.

There may be no symptoms and the depression in the granulocytes may be found by routine blood count. Such patients are susceptible to infection and may present with general malaise, fever, and some infective process, often a severe throat infection.

Patients should always be asked if they are susceptible to the drug before it is given. Certain drugs such as phenylbutazone and chloramphenicol should be avoided if at all possible and the former is in fact licensed only for limited use. It is doubtful if routine blood counts are of much help since the fall may be sudden. Patients must, however, be told to report to the doctor if they become ill and in particular if they develop a sore throat. A blood count must then be performed.

When there is a reaction the drug must be stopped immediately. If the white cell count does not improve within a few days, prednisolone, 30 mg daily, should be given. Infections should be treated as they arise with the appropriate antibiotics. The majority of patients will recover on this treatment.

### Thrombocytopenia

This has been described with chloramphenicol, thiazides, gold, sulphonamides and quinine. It may occur with excessive doses of cytotoxic drugs. Clinical features include purpura and bleeding from various sites. The drug should be stopped immediately. Prednisolone, 30 mg daily, sometimes helps. Platelet transfusions can be used to raise the platelet count for a few days and may allow the bone marrow to recover.

### Aplastic anaemia

This is only infrequently associated with drugs but examples include reactions to chloramphenicol, gold and sulphonamides. Such reactions are usually delayed and occur only after days or weeks of treatment.

The drug should be stopped. Repeated blood transfusions may be required. Prednisolone is not usually very helpful but it is worth a trial in patients who are not improving. Provided the drug is stopped quickly recovery usually occurs but the exception is chloramphenicol which on rare occasions, and usually after repeated doses, causes bone marrow failure.

### Haemolytic anaemia

Drugs can occasionally cause haemolysis. A number of mechanisms may be responsible (page 615). Quinine has long been known to precipitate acute haemolysis occurring in association with malaria and called blackwater fever (page 768). Haemolytic anaemia may also occur in patients with a deficiency of glucose-6-phosphate dehydrogenase, an enzyme which is responsible for the integrity of the red cells. Deficiency can result in acute haemolysis when such subjects take primaquine, sulphonamides or nitrofurantoin.

### Methaemoglobinaemia and sulphaemoglobinaemia

These changes in the haemoglobin may occur with certain drugs including phenacetin, lignocaine, sulphonamides, dapsone and rarely phenytoin. The patient appears cyanosed but is not distressed or dyspnoeic. The diagnosis is confirmed by finding the absorption spectra of methaemoglobin or sulphaemoglobin in the blood. Usually the only treatment required is to stop the offending drug. Methaemoglobinaemia can however be temporarily reversed by giving methylene blue intravenously.

### Megaloblastic anaemia

Certain drugs including pyrimethamine and the anticonvulsants primidone and phenytoin may produce a megaloblastic anaemia which can be reversed by folic acid, 10 mg daily.

## OTHER ORGAN-SPECIFIC DRUG-INDUCED DAMAGE

Any organ in the body can be subjected to idiosyncratic drug-induced damage. Such reactions occur more frequently in those organs associated with drug metabolism and excretion and thus involve most frequently the liver and kidney. These are discussed in more detail in chapters 15 and 17.

## DRUG REACTIONS AND CONNECTIVE TISSUE DISORDERS

Although some authors include a wide variety of syndromes under the term collagen diseases, this term should be confined to inflammatory disorders of connective tissues such as rheumatic fever, rheumatoid arthritis, systemic lupus erythematous (SLE), vasculitis, dermatomyositis, and giant-cell arteritis. There has been considerable discussion about whether drug reactions can cause these conditions. There is no doubt that a clinical picture similar to that of SLE can be produced by both hydralazine and procainamide, but it differs from the true disease in that recovery occurs when the drug is stopped. It is of interest that the development of drug-induced SLE is also related to the sex of the subject, acetylation status and tissue type. In addition, transient arteritis can occur in association with hypersensitivity reactions to a number of drugs, including penicillin and sulphonamides. Whether such reactions play any part in the pathogenesis of vasculitis is more doubtful, and it is unlikely that drug reactions are causal to any of the other collagen diseases.

Other types of connective tissue disease can be drug-induced. Fibrosis in the peritoneum or mediastinum is a rare complication of certain drugs of which the best documented are the rarely used methysergide and the β-blocker, practolol, now withdrawn as an oral preparation for this reason.

## OTHER DRUG REACTIONS

Fever is quite common and should always be remembered in patients with pyrexia of unknown origin (PUO).

Lymphadenopathy can be caused by drugs, particularly phenytoin, and the histological picture resembles a lymphoma.

Rashes are often caused by drugs and are considered on page 786.

Non-productive cough is now recognized as a frequent adverse effect from angiotensin-converting enzyme (ACE) inhibitors.

# DRUG INTERACTIONS

When more than one drug is prescribed then each drug may affect the pharmacokinetics or the pharmacological affect of another drug in many different ways. The increasing use of drugs has made these interactions an important problem. For example, there is about a 20 per cent chance of an interaction if five drugs are prescribed together. However, many interactions are of little clinical importance, either because the variations in drug handling or action are small or because the concentration of the drug is not critical. The difficulty is to know which interactions are potentially dangerous in a particular patient. In general, serious adverse effects are more liable to occur if the therapeutic ratio of the drug is small.

Interactions may occur at several stages during the passage of a drug through the body.

## THE GASTROINTESTINAL TRACT

Drugs may combine or their physical state may be altered so that absorption is modified. For example, iron combines with tetracycline, decreasing its absorption and leading to lower blood levels of the antibiotic.

## COMPETITION FOR TRANSPORT SITES ON THE PLASMA PROTEINS

Many drugs are transported to their sites of action partially or almost totally bound to plasma proteins. When bound in this way they cannot produce their pharmacological effects and are not available to be metabolized or excreted. The activity of the drug depends on the unbound fraction.

When two drugs compete for a limited number of protein-binding sites, there is a decrease in the bound fraction of each and an increase in the amount of free drug, with a corresponding enhancement of the pharmacological effect. Examples of this type of interaction are the displacement of bilirubin by sulphonamides in the newborn causing kernicterus, the displacement of tolbutamide by salicylates leading to hypoglycaemia, and the displacement of warfarin by salicylates causing haemorrhage.

## MODIFICATION AT SITES OF ACTION

The pharmacological action of a drug can be modified in several ways by the concurrent administration of another drug. For example:

1. Hypokalaemia produced by diuretics enhances the toxic effects of digitalis on the heart.
2. Tricyclic antidepressants reverse the effect of adrenergic-blocking hypotensive agents, possibly by increasing the amount of noradrenaline at the adrenergic nerve endings. They also enhance the effect of sympathomimetic amines which could be

used for a separate treatment, for example, adrenaline added to a local anaesthetic.

3. The action of central nervous depressants such as benzodiazepines and alcohol is additive.

4. Monoamine oxidase (MAO) inhibitors interact in two ways. First, certain drugs, particularly sympathomimetic drugs such as phenylpropanolamine or tyramine, release the excess noradrenaline which accumulates in nerve endings of the subject taking MAO inhibitors, resulting in a hypertensive crisis. Tyramine is found in certain foods which should be avoided in patients on MAO inhibitors. Second, the effect of some central depressants, particularly pethidine, is enhanced.

## ENZYME INDUCTION

Many drugs are metabolized by enzymes, usually in the liver. Certain drugs increase the activity of these enzymes so that drug breakdown is enhanced. For example, if a patient on an oral anticoagulant is given phenobarbitone, the barbiturate increases the enzyme activity and the anticoagulant is metabolized more rapidly. An increased dose is therefore necessary to produce a satisfactory anticoagulant effect. Conversely, if the phenobarbitone is stopped enzyme activity decreases and signs of anticoagulant overdosage may appear.

## ENZYME INHIBITION

Sulphonamides decrease the rate of breakdown of the oral hypoglycaemic tolbutamide increasing the risk of hypoglycaemia. Allopurinol decreases the rate of breakdown of the immunosuppressive drug azathioprine.

## RENAL EXCRETION

Competition for pathways in the kidney by two drugs given together may reduce the rate of excretion of both. Use is made of this phenomenon when probenecid is given with penicillin to reduce its excretion and so achieve a higher level of penicillin in the blood.

## THE ROLE OF NON-PRESCRIBED MEDICINE

When the possibility of adverse drug reactions or interactions is included in a differential diagnosis it is important to remember that not all drugs are prescribed and the patient may forget or even try to hide the use of non-prescription drugs. The range of such drugs extends from licensed over-the-counter products through homeopathic and ethnic medicines to drugs of abuse, including the so-called 'designer drugs'. With the exception of the properly licensed drugs most are not subject to adequate quality control and may contain drugs which are not declared (e.g. some 'homeopathic' medicines from the Far East which have been recommended for treatment of arthritis have been shown to contain steroids or non-steroidal anti-inflammatory agents) whilst others contain impurities or dangerous additives as in the case of street heroin cut with strychnine.

## $P$HARMACOVIGILANCE

## Information sources on adverse drug reactions

The assessment of adverse drug reactions (ADRs) may require access to information which is held in Pharmacy or Poisons Information Services, by manufacturers or by the adverse drug reaction section of the Committee on Safety of Medicines (CSM). Key references are listed in Table 25.8.

## Surveillance of adverse drug reactions (pharmacovigilance)

A number of methods have been developed for monitoring ADRs including spontaneous reporting, hospital surveillance, prescription event monitoring (from general practitioners) and various industry-sponsored postmarketing projects related to specific new drugs. They vary in their effectiveness and each has its own advantages and disadvantages, including costs. Doctors are encouraged to report suspected ADRs to such schemes and in particular to make full use of the CSM yellow card system. Copies of the yellow card can be found amongst other places at the back of the British National Formulary. A yellow card should be completed and sent to the CSM when an ADR is suspected so that the CSM can investigate further.

## Prevention and education

Pharmacovigilance implies more than observation for ADRs, it also embodies the idea that appropriate action should be taken for prevention. Thus the CSM issues regular newsletters to doctors advising them of actions taken (e.g. the withdrawal of the drug or changes in the licence) and highlights drugs where suspicions have been raised and where further reporting is encouraged in order to clarify the situation. For example, when cardiac arrhythmias may be occurring with a drug which was initially thought to be free of cardiac effects. The CSM uses the symbol of an inverted black triangle ($\blacktriangledown$) to denote those drugs which are currently the subject of special monitoring. This symbol is also used in the British National Formulary.

## Summary

In summary ADRs are common and doctors need to keep them under consideration in many differential diagnoses. However, there is no need for the individual doctor to feel overwhelmed by the frequency and range of ADRs. In practice most doctors become fully familiar with use of a small range of drugs and are well aware of their potential for causing adverse reactions. For new drugs and older drugs with which one is less familiar this chapter offers an aid to ADR assessment but remember that suspected reactions must be reported if the quality of the safety database is to be maintained and improved.

# Diseases Due to Physical Agents

In contrast to the problems caused by chemical agents which are described in the preceding two sections there is also a spectrum of diseases caused by physical changes in the body's environment, changes in temperature, pressure and movement.

# Extremes of temperature

## Cold

### LOCAL EFFECTS

In cold or temperate climates complaints of Raynaud's phenomenon or chilblains are common and are exacerbated by smoking and β-adrenoceptor-blocking drugs. These problems can be avoided or at least minimized by appropriate use of clothing and footwear, especially the so-called 'thermal systems' which ensure that a thin layer of air is trapped and heated close to the body whilst the outer layer prevents heat loss by being windproof and waterproof. Some fabrics conduct moisture away from the body keeping the skin dry and either breathing or trapping the moisture in an outer layer. Such clothing was originally designed for outdoor enthusiasts and was, and still can be, expensive. Nevertheless, cheaper alternatives are now available and can be afforded by most patients. Where funds are lacking they can be sought from social services or charitable assistance. Patients who suffer peripheral symptoms need to be encouraged to stop smoking. β-Adrenoceptor blockers, however, may be continued in the first instance and only need to be stopped if the problem is not relieved by suitable clothing.

### FROSTBITE

Frostbite occurs when the local temperature in a part of the limb falls below 0.5°C, causing tissue damage. Actual freezing of the tissues occurs at even lower temperatures and can cause extensive loss of tissue. The treatment of such injuries is symptomatic and supportive including the use of analgesics, antibiotics and physiotherapy.

### HYPOTHERMIA

Hypothermia is defined as a deep body temperature (usually rectal) of less than 35°C and results from progressive cooling of the body. In the UK it occurs most frequently during the occasional, 'unexpected' spells of cold weather when the victims are usually the elderly, the poor and the homeless who have insufficient means to afford access to adequate heating. It may also occur in milder weather as a secondary feature to other diseases such as a fractured hip, stroke, excess alcohol, drug overdose or as a complication of myxoedema.

Hypothermia may also occur in young and fit individuals who pursue outdoor activities, usually but not always when wearing appropriate clothing, and then suffer from the effects of an unexpected blizzard or a prolonged immersion in water. In many such cases there is a failure to recognize the extent to which heat is lost through the head (up to 30–40 per cent of total body heat loss, especially if the victim is bald!) and to appreciate the relevance of the wind chill factor. Even a gentle breeze of 10 knots drops the effective ambient temperature by 5° to 6°C, a finding further exacerbated by the wearing of wet clothing. In addition, when hypothermia begins, the subject's mental reactions and manual ability may deteriorate very quickly raising the potential for accidents and inappropriate actions. Factors influencing the effects of cold upon an individual include the rate of heat production at the onset of exposure, body shape, the level of fat insulation (Fig. 25.3), age and sex. Thus women and young adults are likely to survive longer than children or the elderly.

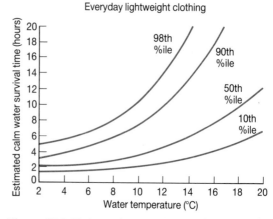

**Figure 25.3** Estimated survival time after immersion in cold water for four levels of body fat. Reproduced with permission of Dr J. R. Allen.

The clinical features of hypothermia are summarized in Fig. 25.4 which also lists the physiological changes. If the body temperature falls below 35°C the patient becomes confused, sluggish, clumsy and ultimately unconscious. Outdoor enthusiasts should be trained to recognize these effects and to take action when possible, for example, by building a shelter. However, mental confusion may undermine even the best training.

The heart is particularly vulnerable to low temperatures and there is a fall in heart rate, blood pressure and cardiac output. Cardiac arrhythmias may then supervene, typically with J waves at the end of the QRS complex (Fig. 26.9, page 854) but in fact the whole range of tachy- and brady-arrhythmias may be seen. With further falls in body temperature renal function is impaired with the failure of tubular reabsorption leading to a diuresis and further heat loss in the urine. The patient may thus be fluid depleted by the time the treatment is started. Respiratory depression also occurs but at lower temperatures there is less oxygen demand and the direct consequences may be less severe. Lactic acid production is increased however and usually leads to acidosis.

## Management of hypothermia

First it is necessary to recognize that with good protective clothing a victim may survive for many hours and that prolonged searches for individuals lost in bad weather conditions can be justified. Once the victim is discovered, first aid should include assessment of vital functions, insulation to permit passive or spontaneous rewarming, immobilization to minimize movement and careful monitoring. In particular, it is necessary to watch for postrescue collapse after immersion in water where the cardiac output has been sustained by the external pressure of the water and where loss of the hydrostatic squeeze may result in a drop of cardiac output of up to 30 per cent. Hot drinks may be offered to conscious casualties but should not be offered to the semi-conscious nor indeed poured into the mouths of the unconscious. Active rewarming may be considered in hospital, for instance by immersing the victim's trunk in water of 40 to 44°C. However, this is suitable only for otherwise fit young adults and may lead to complications with a profound drop in blood pressure. Where the victim is frail or elderly rewarming should be achieved gradually at room temperature and with careful monitoring of vital functions.

# Heat

The syndromes related to heat are more likely to occur when the subject has not been able to become acclimatized or when inappropriate exertion is undertaken. The young, the elderly,

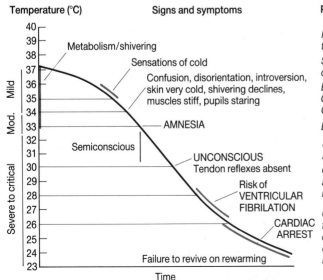

| Temperature (°C) | Signs and symptoms | Physiology |
|---|---|---|
| | Metabolism/shivering | Heat production rises then declines |
| | Sensations of cold | Skin blood vessels constricted |
| | Confusion, disorientation, introversion, skin very cold, shivering declines, muscles stiff, pupils staring | Blood to brain cool / Cold penetrates muscles / Cardiac arrhythmias |
| | AMNESIA | Blood to brain very cool |
| | Semiconscious | Spinal cord cooled / Atrial fibrillation |
| | UNCONSCIOUS / Tendon reflexes absent | Cardiac muscles cooled and cannot maintain rhythmic contractions |
| | Risk of VENTRICULAR FIBRILLATION | |
| | CARDIAC ARREST | Cardiac muscles too cold for contractions and electrical impulse conduction. Muscle hypoxic |
| | Failure to revive on rewarming | |

Mild / Mod. / Severe to critical

Time

**Figure 25.4** Symptoms, signs and physiology of exposure hypothermia. Reproduced with permission of Dr W. Guild.

the fair skinned and the bald are more vulnerable. For purposes of discussion the problems may be divided into those related to direct exposure to the sun and those due to the effects of exhaustion, although in practice many patients would suffer mixed effects.

## SUNBURN

Sunburn is due to the ultraviolet fraction of sunlight notably the UVB range 290–320 nm which produces tissue damage compared with the tanning effect of UVA at 320–400 nm. However, even UVA can cause damage in the presence of photosensitivity caused by drugs or porphyria. Burning can be prevented by avoiding exposure through judicious use of clothing, hats and even the glass in windows including car windows. Exposure may also be controlled through sun screens which are available in complete ranges from light screen to total sunblocks as well as in water-resistant formulations. Exposure can also be controlled by the recognition that the UVB content of sunlight is greatest in the middle of the day and by restricting exposure to the morning and the evening.

If sunburn has occurred there is usually redness and discomfort starting within 2 to 8 hours after exposure, varying according to the intensity of the exposure and vulnerability of the skin. Treatment consists of avoiding further exposure and the application of soothing aftersun creams or oily calamine.

## PRICKLY HEAT

Prickly heat is due to excessive sweating and inflammation of the sweat glands. It is a fine papular rash which sometimes becomes vesicular, usually with a sensation of prickling (thus the name). It may become infected. Treatment is removal to a cooler and less humid atmosphere.

## HEAT EXHAUSTION

Heat exhaustion may be related to water deficiency, salt deficiency or to anhydrosis (failure of adequate sweating), but it may also occur without definite evidence of any mechanism. Un-

treated it may progress to *heat stroke* which is a medical emergency.

1. Water deficiency heat exhaustion occurs when water is not replaced in a hot climate. Thirst and signs of dehydration occur and treatment is with oral or intravenous replacement.
2. Salt deficiency heat exhaustion is due to salt loss without adequate replacement through exercise or work in hot climates. It results in the symptoms associated with hyponatraemia and hypochloraemia, i.e. weakness, cramps, collapse and low blood pressure. Treatment should aim to replace the salt loss by mouth if possible but the intravenous route may be needed if vomiting persists. Prevention is possible if the risk is recognized and the dietary intake of salt increased or supplemented.
3. Anhidrotic heat exhaustion is characterized by an early onset of weakness and irritability when moderate exercise is attempted and follows prickly heat. Examination shows failure of sweating over all parts of the body except for face, axillae and sometimes the hands and feet. If the subject persists in exercise for longer or attempts an even higher level of exercise this may lead to collapse and heat stroke.

Treatment of the earlier stages requires removal to a cool environment and rest. Prevention is possible if those at risk are trained to recognize the symptoms.

## HEAT STROKE

Heat stroke (heat hyperpyrexia) is defined by hyperpyrexia which often exceeds 41°C, associated with headache, confusion, coma and convulsions. It occurs when heat production exceeds heat loss due to either (1) excessive production from exercise, for example, marathon running, or feverish illness, such as malaria, or (2) when there is a failure of heat loss due to failure of sweating in high ambient temperatures and dry humidity.

It may be further complicated by diversion of blood from skin to muscles during heavy exercise.

In addition to the raised temperature the victim will have hot dry skin with signs of high cardiac output. There may also be purpuric haemorrhage due to failure of the production of clotting factors which can progress to disseminated intravascular coagulation and ultimately failure of cardiac output. Emergency treatment should include cooling by removing clothing, provision of moisture via sprays and the use of fans or natural ventilation to increase evaporation. An ice pack may be used and the early objective is to reduce the rectal temperature to 39°C. Close observation is then essential with access to resuscitation facilities since the mortality can be as high as 25 per cent.

# ALTERATIONS OF ATMOSPHERIC PRESSURE

Mountaineers and divers expose themselves to extremes of atmospheric pressures and run the risk of illnesses which can be serious or even fatal unless adequate precautions are taken.

## Reduced atmospheric pressure

Reduced atmospheric pressure becomes noticeable above 2500 m and may result in acute mountain sickness or the more serious conditions of high altitude cerebral oedema and pulmonary oedema.

Acute mountain sickness is associated with rapid ascent from lower altitudes to above 2500 m and is a benign syndrome consisting of headache, nausea, anorexia, dizziness, dyspnoea and insomnia. The incidence of symptoms relates to the speed of the climb and the susceptibility of the individual so that the elderly and those with cardiac or respiratory disease are more vulnerable. In practice it affects over 50 per cent of those climbing above 4000 m. The illness is usually short lived providing that the sufferer descends immediately or rests before continuing to climb more slowly. It is probably caused by salt and water retention and can be prevented by acetazolamide (500 mg sustained release daily).

High altitude cerebral oedema may occur suddenly but more commonly represents a deterioration in a victim of acute mountain sickness and is manifest by ataxia, irritability, hallucinations, clouding of consciousness and coma.

Treatment is urgent and should include dexamethasone and supplementary oxygen as well as descent.

High altitude pulmonary oedema is characterize by a rapid onset of breathlessness, nocturnal dyspnoea, cough, chest pain, headache and even haemoptysis. Treatment should include oxygen, frusemide and rapid descent, but if descent is not possible nifedipine (20 mg sustained release 6 hourly) may be of value.

Each of these syndromes may also compromise the skill of mountaineers and make accidents more likely to occur. It is thought that they play a major part in high altitude deaths which have been calculated as over 4 per cent in British Expeditions over 7000 m. Prevention is possible if climbing above 3000 m is restricted to 300 m a day for 2 days and 150 m per day thereafter. However, it seems inevitable that some individuals will exceed this limit and there are likely to be increasing problems with the expanding popularity of package holiday treks in the Himalayas where the tour companies have to balance their travel schedules against the health and safety of their customers.

## Increased atmospheric pressure

Increases in atmospheric pressure occur underwater and may represent a hazard for divers. The barometric pressure at sea level is 100 kPa (the equivalent of 1 atm) and this increases linearly with descent underwater so that every 10 m (33 feet) adds a further 100 kPa. Divers are at risk of a number of diseases or syndromes associated with these pressure changes and it must be remembered that these conditions effect not only professional divers but also the far more numerous recreational scuba divers. It may be thought that such patients would be confined to warm, clear waters but in fact many of the UK's cold and cloudy lakes and in-shore waters are used for recreational diving so that the problem could well confront doctors practising throughout the country.

Since the direct cause of illnesses related to diving can be traced to the behaviour of gases under pressure it is useful to remember two laws: Boyle's law states that at a constant temperature, the volume of gas varies inversely with the pressure applied, and this explains the changes underlying the pressure-related disease or barotrauma. Henry's law states that the amount of a given gas that is dissolved in a liquid at a given temperature is directly proportional to the partial pressure of that gas and this explains the problems of nitrogen narcosis and decompression sickness.

Barotrauma is damage which results from failure of the gas-filled body spaces – lungs, middle ear and sinuses – to equalize their external pressure to correspond to changes in ambient pressure. Thus during descent increased ambient pressure leads to a decrease in the volume of the gases in the spaces and since the bony cavities around the spaces cannot collapse, the increased space is filled by engorgement of the mucous membranes which in turn may lead to haemorrhage.

Such injuries are more common near the surface where a small change in depth may cause a large change in relative gas volume.

Pulmonary barotrauma occurs during ascent and may cause mediastinal or subcutaneous emphysema, pneumothorax and arterial gas emboli. The most severe cases occur with a rapid, emergency ascent and may be associated with impaired cardiac and central nervous system (CNS) function. Treatment centres upon the maintenance of respiration and adequate arterial oxygenation using high concentrations of oxygen. A chest drain may be needed for a large pneumothorax and hyperbaric oxygen may be useful in treating air embolism.

Middle ear barotrauma occurs on descent and results from inability to balance pressure via the Eustachian tube due to poor technique, upper respiratory tract infection and anatomical abnormalities of the nasal skeleton. It is manifest by pain and conductive hearing loss which may be followed by rupture of the tympanic membrane with pain relief and vertigo. Treatment includes topical and systemic decongestants together with antibiotics if there is evidence of infection.

Inner ear barotrauma probably results from forceful efforts to equalize middle ear pressure and results in vertigo, sensorineural hearing loss and tinnitus. It may lead to rupture of inner ear membranes. Treatment consists of complete bed rest with the head elevated to reduce cerebrospinal fluid pressure. Deteriorating hearing and balance may indicate a need for surgery.

Paranasal sinus barotrauma is usually related to pre-existing chronic sinusitis and is manifest as pain over the sinuses and epistaxis. Treatment includes the use of topical and systemic decongestants with antibiotics if there is evidence of infection.

Nitrogen narcosis results from increased partial pressure of nitrogen in the CNS tissues and produces symptoms that resemble ethanol intoxication. If recognized and contained it is not unpleasant but if allowed to impair intellect and performance it can be a prelude to accidents. It occurs at any depth greater than 30 m and by 100 m may lead to hallucinations, coma and death. Recovery is rapid following ascent and prevention is easy if diving is limited to 30 m.

# Decompression sickness barotrauma

When air is breathed in at high pressure the tissues take up increased quantities of gas. Oxygen is used up in metabolism but nitrogen, being inert, is left behind and accumulates, especially in fatty tissues including the brain. When the diver returns to the surface the gases come out of solution in the tissues and expand as the pressure decreases. Any oxygen or carbon dioxide rapidly diffuses away but nitrogen does not clear so quickly and the bubbles cause symptoms by blocking blood vessels and lymphatics or by inducing direct tissue damage. The symptoms of decompression sickness are divided into two types:

**Type 1** is characterized by pain in the joints and muscles (the bends) and most frequently involves the elbows and shoulders. Symptoms begin within 1 hour after surfacing and may increase over 1 to 2 days. The pain varies from mild to severe and may be associated with itching, rashes and lymphadenopathy.

**Type 2** is more serious and begins with malaise which proceeds to CNS symptoms including parasthaesiae, weakness, headache,

visual disturbance, mental disturbance, altered consciousness, convulsions and death. These symptoms can be related to cerebral lesions which can be seen in computed tomographic and nuclear magnetic resonance scans.

Treatment should start with immediate first aid using inhaled high concentrations of oxygen plus rehydration. The patient should be transferred as soon as possible for administration of hyperbaric oxygen in a pressure chamber. Even quite late treatment seems effective in relieving symptoms and preventing long-term CNS damage. Prevention of symptoms is possible if divers surfacing from deep dives do so in stages according to protocols established by the navy and taught in diving schools.

# Motion sickness

Motion sickness may occur as a result of sea, land or air travel. Although the exact mechanism is not known it would seem that repetitive stimulation of the vestibular apparatus plays a large part; it is not possible to produce sickness in animals who have had their vestibular apparatus removed, nor are deaf and mute people seasick. Susceptibility to motion sickness varies, but is particularly common in migrainous subjects.

The victim of motion sickness complains of feeling unwell with nausea, headache and sometimes faintness. Finally symptoms are such as to require a rapid withdrawal from company and terminate in severe vomiting. The duration of the attack is variable and may last only a few hours, although susceptible subjects may be prostrate for several days.

People susceptible to motion sickness should avoid undue movement. When at sea they should remain near the centre of the ship and if possible lie down with the eyes closed. In an aeroplane the head should be rested back on the head rest. Some food should be taken.

Certain drugs diminish the liability to sea-

sickness. They are the hyoscine group and the antihistamines. The most satisfactory drug is not decided, but there is a little evidence that hyoscine is better for short journeys and the antihistamines for longer ones.

1. Hyoscine (0.3–0.6 mg according to weight) taken 20 min before starting out is suitable for journeys lasting up to four hours. Side effects include dry mouth and paralysis of accommodation.
2. Cyclizine (50 mg three times daily) or meclozine (50 mg daily) are suitable for longer journeys.
3. Cinnarizine (30 mg) 2 hours before travelling (and then 15 mg 8 hourly) is also suitable but can cause drowsiness.

These drugs can be used for children in reduced dosage.

Anxiety even before the journey begins may upset some people and diazepam (2–5 mg) taken before setting out is sometimes helpful.

# Disorders of the Elderly

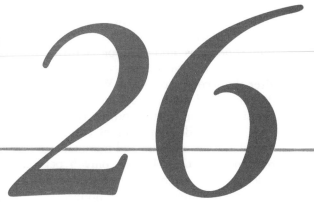

# 26

# INTRODUCTION

The term 'geriatrics' was first used by Nascher in America in 1907 to denote the branch of medicine dealing with care of the elderly. In England in 1935 Marjorie Warren wrote about the terrible conditions and lack of facilities for the elderly in the workhouse wards. During and after the second world war Warren and Howell demonstrated that many frail and ill elderly people could be treated and returned to society.

A gradual development of community services has allowed more and more elderly people to remain in their homes: only 5 per cent of elderly people are now to be found in hospitals, residential homes or nursing homes.

The physicians for the elderly assess and manage patients during acute admissions to hospital, during rehabilitation, in the outpatient department and day hospital and sometimes in their own homes. Their rôles include close liaison with general practitioners, medical specialties, orthopaedic surgeons and psycho-geriatric physicians; multidisciplinary teamwork with physiotherapists, occupational therapists, social services, community health services and many other agencies; and teaching and research. All of this is designed to ensure the highest quality of life for all patients – in their own homes if at all possible.

The wellbeing of the elderly is determined by the extent to which they have undergone the natural processes of ageing, by their social circumstances and by the type and severity of their past and present illnesses. In addition, an acute illness affecting one system may interact with long-standing impairment in another, for example, difficulty in rehabilitation after a hip fracture in a patient with Parkinson's disease.

Research is taking place into the process of ageing and the changes in control of cell growth and repair. This may lead to new approaches to the disorders of the elderly in the future.

# NORMAL AGEING

## Epidemiology and life-span

During the present century average life expectancy has increased steadily, mainly as a result of decreased infant mortality (Fig. 26.1), but maximum achievable life-span has not increased significantly. Death in middle life has also become less frequent, and thus the human survival curve has become increasingly 'rectangular' (Fig. 26.2). The proportion of people aged over 85 years or more, the majority of whom are women, has increased by 46 per cent, and the proportion aged 75–84 years has increased by 33 per cent. The number of individuals over 75 years of age is expected to continue to rise into the next century (Fig. 26.3).

It is the oldest age group who require the largest proportion of medical and social services. In 1988 40 per cent of people aged 65 years or older had chronic limitations of activity, and in 1985 43 per cent of hospital beds were occupied by those aged over 75 years. Traditionally, the definition of 'elderly' included all those over the male retirement age of 65 years, but many Departments of Medicine for the Elderly are now concentrating on those aged 75 years or more.

## Theories of natural ageing

A number of theories have been proposed to account for individual variability in natural lifespan. There is evidence for genetic deter-

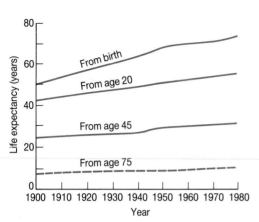

**Figure 26.1** Changes in life expectancy in the USA from 1900 to 1980. The figure shows the expected years of life remaining to individuals from birth, and from the ages of 20, 45 and 75 years. The greatest increase in life expectancy has occurred from birth (26 years), and the smallest increase for those who have reached the age of 75 (3 years). (Reproduced from Fries JF. Aging, natural death, and the compression of morbidity. *N Engl J Med* 1980; **303**: 130–5.)

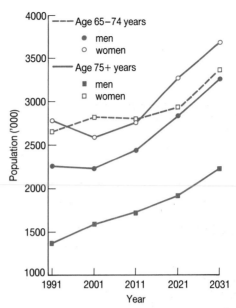

**Figure 26.3** The predicted increase in the numbers of retired and elderly people in the UK in each decade until 2031. (Office of Population Censuses and Surveys.)

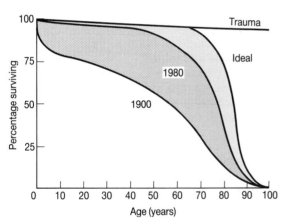

**Figure 26.2** The survival curves of the population in 1900, 1980 and in a hypothetical 'ideal' population. The curve has become increasingly 'rectangular' during the present century. The disappearance of the high infant death rate is shown and the continued mortality due to trauma, at all ages. (Reproduced from Fries JF. Aging, natural death, and the compression of morbidity. *N Engl J Med* 1980; **303**: 130–5.)

mination in that longevity runs in families and monozygotic twins die nearer to the same age than do dizygotic twins. Alternatively, accumulation of abnormalities in DNA during cell division or other 'wear and tear' abnormalities may lead to cell malfunction and degeneration or to neoplastic change. Finally, some form of biological clock has been proposed, perhaps dependent upon involution of the thymus, leading to failure of the immune system to recognize 'self' and thus to cell destruction which contributes to ageing.

# Physiology of ageing

The function of most organs of the body declines steadily after 30 years of age, even in the absence of any disease. The effects of ageing on individual organs are summarized in Table 26.1.

**Table 26.1** The physiology of normal ageing (after 30 years of age).

**Cardiovascular system**
Fibrosis of ventricles and of conducting system
Fall in cardiac output by 1% per year
Smaller increase in heart rate in response to stress
Decreased maximum heart rate
Thickening and rigidity of heart valves
Thickening and rigidity of media of arteries
Increased peripheral resistance and systolic blood
pressure

**Respiratory system**
Decreased elastic recoil, and early small airways closure
Increased ventilation/perfusion mismatch.
25% decrease in vital capacity and 50% increase in
residual volume by 70 years of age
Increased stiffness of chest wall
Wasting and weakness of respiratory muscles
Decreased alveolar wall area and gas transfer
Decreased number and function of cilia and slower
tracheobronchial clearance

**Alimentary system**
Loss of teeth and decreased production of saliva
Failure of normal oesophageal peristalsis
Atrophic gastritis and decreased gastric acid output
Increased gastric colonization with coliform bacteria
Increased gut transit time and constipation
Decreased liver size
Decreased hepatic blood flow
Delayed induction of hepatic enzymes

**Kidneys**
Reduction of glomerular filtration rate by 1% per year
after age 35
Loss of 50% of nephrons between the ages of 30 and
70 years
Decreased renal blood flow
Decreased concentration gradient in loop of Henlé
Decreased sodium resorption
Decreased ADH response
Reduced free water clearance

**Nervous system**
Slowing of learning but accurate recall
Decreased vibration sense and joint position sense
Alteration in gait with increased body flexion and short
steps
Loss of ankle jerks (may occur); loss of abdominal
reflex

**Vision and hearing**
Central cataract
Vitreous opacities
Macular degeneration
Presbyopia
Presbycusis (degeneration of the cochlea)

**Immune system**
Decreased level of primary and secondary antibody
responses
Decrease in T-lymphocyte function (normal total
number)
Possible decline in neutrophil function
Decreased T-helper cell numbers and interleukin-2
production
Involution of the thymus and secondary lymphoid
organs
Increase in natural killer cell numbers and activity

**Bones, muscle and joints\***
Osteoporosis (too little bone, of normal composition)
Decrease in muscle mass and strength
Increase in collagen, and decrease in proportion of
slow muscle fibres

**Skin**
Loss of flexibility of dermal collagen
Senile purpura due to blood vessel rupture
Greying and loss of hair

**Endocrine system**
Progressive impairment of glucose tolerance
Decreased serum T3 level but normal TSH and T4
Decreased rate of secretion of T4
Slightly reduced hypothalamo–pituitary–adrenal
response to stress
The menopause; atrophy of uterus and vagina
Nodular hyperplasia of the prostate

---

\*Osteoarthrosis is not a normal ageing process but a pathological process affecting cartilage with thinning and disruption due to 'wear and tear'.

## Medicine in the Elderly

# *Principles of the history and examination*

The symptoms produced by an illness often alter with advancing age and much may be mistakenly attributed by the patient to ageing itself, for example, the insidious onset of hypothyroidism. Similarly, the distinction between physiological ageing and pathological processes may be difficult for physicians to make unless they are accustomed to the presentation of disease in the elderly. Minor symptoms may indicate significant disease, and nonspecific symptoms such as confusion and 'loss of function' may occur in widely differing conditions. Physical signs may differ in significance compared with the same signs in a younger person. If possible the history should be obtained initially from the patient. This may take time and gentle persistence, and good rapport is essential. The environment should be quiet and private, the patient should be comfortable, and hearing aid, spectacles and dentures should be in place. Sufficient time must be allowed to cope with visual, hearing and mental impairment.

Corroboration of details should be sought from a relative or carer, particularly regarding past and present mental state and functional abilities. Marked discrepancies between the accounts may provide information about both the patient and the carer. Sometimes no history is obtainable from the patient and this fact should then be recorded, together with the reasons. Previous notes and X-rays, and information from the patient's general practitioner should be obtained.

## SOCIAL HISTORY

This should be obtained in detail along the lines given in Table 26.2. These aspects are important to a full understanding of the patient's current problem as well as being vital knowledge in relation to further care at home. While it may be inappropriate to seek all these details at the time of an acute hospital admission, they should certainly be obtained well ahead of discharge.

## DRUG HISTORY

Enquire whether the patient knows and understands the medication, and check the details by asking to see all medications or by obtaining confirmation from the carer. Beware of over-the-

**Table 26.2** Aspects of social history.

**Social situation**
Does the patient live alone, or with a carer? Are there any pets?

Are family members alive, and where are they?

**The home itself**
Is home a house or flat? Which floor? Is there a lift or stairs?

Consider cooking, toilet and sleeping facilities

**Aids and appliances**
Frame, rails

**Support at home**
Home help, meals on wheels, district nurse, voluntary organizations, neighbours

Who does the shopping?

**Activities of daily living**
Can the patient wash, bath, dress, get to and use the toilet?

Can the patient cook, feed, manage stairs and use wheelchair?

Can the patient transfer from bed to chair, get in and out of bed unaided, get to the front door, go safely outside?

**Recreation/hobbies**
Day centre
Luncheon club
Other hobbies and activities

counter medications, and treatment left over from previous conditions. Ask about previous adverse drug reactions (not just 'allergies') and use of 'alternative' medicines.

## PHYSICAL EXAMINATION

Again, adequate time must be allowed. The responses of an elderly person may be slow, and more explanation is likely to be required than in the young (and is especially important since accurate interpretation depends upon correct performance). Patients should be fully undressed (with their agreement), even though they will probably be found in the ward fully clothed. This also takes time, but useful functional observations may be made during the process. Gentleness and preservation of the patient's modesty and dignity are essential throughout. Parts not being examined should be covered and a nurse should be present at least during any potentially embarrassing phase of the examination.

Particular attention should be given to difficulties in speech, vision, hearing and higher mental function. General appearance, mood, and the state of the skin including any pressure sores, ulcers or bruises should be noted. Lying and standing blood pressure, respiratory rate, rectal examination, and observation of gait are all essential. If aids, such as hearing aids or spectacles, are used their adequacy for their purpose should be checked.

# Significance of symptoms and signs in the elderly patient

## CARDIOVASCULAR SYSTEM

In the elderly, sinus node disease is relatively common, and the intermittent tachycardia or bradycardia may present typically as 'dizzy spells' or atypically as recurrent attacks of breathlessness. Valvular heart disease may be more severe than clinically apparent, while an aortic ejection murmur is common and may represent thickening of the valve and a possible source of cerebral emboli. Peripheral oedema may result from venous stasis or insufficiency.

Myocardial infarction may present with confusion, syncope or breathlessness but without chest pain. A fourth heart sound is common, caused by decreased ventricular compliance due to ageing. Bruits over the carotid and femoral arteries and over the abdominal aorta generally indicate atheromatous narrowing.

Peripheral vascular disease produces intermittent claudication and may affect tissue viability. Vasculitis may present with non-specific features such as fever, weight loss and muscle aches. Temporal arteritis (page 575) should always be remembered as a cause of persistent headache in the elderly.

## RESPIRATORY SYSTEM

The regular productive cough of chronic bronchitis may be attributed to 'old age' by the patient. In the elderly cardiac failure and pulmonary embolism are more likely to present as intermittent wheezing than in younger patients. Basal crackles are common and do not necessarily represent significant pathology. Bronchopneumonia becomes more common with age, and may present as confusion or falls.

## ALIMENTARY SYSTEM AND NUTRITION

A patient's complaint of 'diarrhoea' or 'constipation' may represent one extreme of the range of normal variation. Progressive loss of weight is usually the result of significant pathology, for example, neoplasia, peptic ulceration or thyrotoxicosis. Rarely it may be due to simple disinclination to eat, or to difficulty in preparing food or in feeding. Dentures and diet should be checked. Malnutrition is not uncommon in the elderly and is often secondary to other disorders including dementia. There may be deficiency of vitamin C, vitamin D, folic acid or iron. Examination of the abdomen should always include a rectal examination to check for faecal impaction, prostatic hypertrophy or occult neoplasia.

In the elderly an acute abdomen may present simply as absent bowel sounds without guarding or rigidity. Gallstones are present in 30 per cent of females over the age of 70 years and may be found in the common bile duct some years after cholecystectomy. Pain may be relatively mild, and subacute or recurrent cholangitis may cause fever, malaise, weight loss and mild jaundice. Acute pancreatitis may also be milder than in the young, and the serum amylase should be determined whenever abdominal discomfort, hypotension or fever are otherwise unexplained.

Peptic ulceration or ulceration induced by non-steroidal anti-inflammatory drugs (NSAIDs) may be clinically silent until perforation or bleeding occurs. Anorexia and weight loss may be the only indication of a peptic ulcer or a gastric carcinoma, while carcinoma of the caecum and colon often present as iron-deficiency anaemia.

## GENITOURINARY SYSTEM

Frequency, nocturia and incontinence are common and may result from recurrent urinary tract infections, prostatic hypertrophy, vaginal prolapse or atrophic vaginitis. Painless chronic urine retention with a palpable bladder is frequent, but if found should lead to a careful neurological examination to exclude spinal cord compression.

## METABOLIC AND ENDOCRINE FUNCTION

The frequency of non-insulin-dependent diabetes mellitus increases with age. Patients may develop non-ketotic hyperosmolar coma rather than diabetic ketoacidosis. Thyroid dysfunction is common and frequently goes undetected until it is severe. Many of the features of hypothyroidism are mimicked by changes in normal ageing, such as thinning hair, dry skin and constipation, and hyperthyroidism may present atypically with general debility.

## NERVOUS SYSTEM

Loss of vision and hearing may be major impediments to independence. Any foreign body or wax in the ears should be removed, and the adequacy of any hearing aid and/or spectacles should be checked.

Impairment of joint position and vibration sense in the lower limbs is common, and there is increased postural sway, especially with the eyes closed. A positive Romberg's test is abnormal. Muscle wasting commonly accompanies ageing. Otherwise it is most commonly secondary to arthritis (usually osteoarthritis). Parkinson's disease may be missed if it presents as simple immobility or if the diagnostic signs are unilateral or minor.

## SKIN

Ulcers and pressure sores (Fig. 26.4) occur frequently in elderly patients, but the incidence is reduced by accurate assessment and early management of any underlying medical condition, together with committed and expert nursing care. Intrinsic causes (including paralysis, loss of sensation, sedation, coma, hypotension, malnutrition and peripheral vascular disease) com-

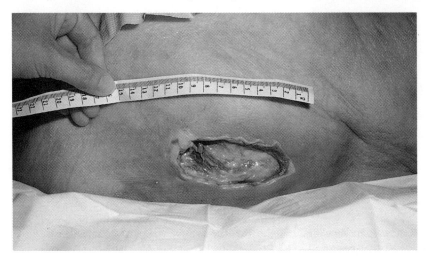

**Figure 26.4** Deep sacral pressure sore with necrotic slough down to the paraspinal muscles. Lesions of this severity may develop rapidly once the skin and subcutaneous tissues have become non-viable after several hours of unrelieved pressure.

bine with extrinsic causes (a hard bed or casualty trolley, moist skin due to urinary incontinence) to cause superficial or deep tissue necrosis, sometimes within hours. Breakdown and sloughing of the necrotic tissue follows. Treatment is by relief of pressure allowing re-establishment of blood flow, removal of dead tissue, correction of predisposing causes and maintenance of a clean, moist wound with appropriate dressings. Prevention is much easier than cure and at-risk patients should be nursed on an appropriate alternating pressure air mattress.

## JOINTS, BONE AND MUSCLE

Eighty per cent of people aged 65 or over have a major or minor joint disorder and the effect of this on the ability to carry out normal daily tasks should be noted (Fig. 26.5). Impairment of joint mobility may be worsened by the rapid

development of flexion contractures if a patient becomes immobile in bed or chair. Osteoporosis is found almost exclusively in elderly people (Fig. 26.6), and polymyalgia rheumatica (page 586) is a disorder of those over 50 years of age. The possibility of osteomalacia should be remembered.

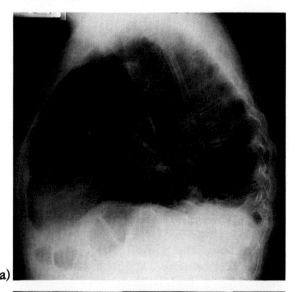

(a)

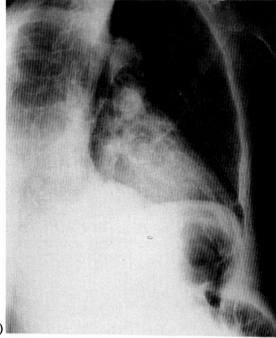

(b)

**Figure 26.5** Osteoarthrosis of the lumbar spine showing osteophyte formation in the spine.

**Figure 26.6** Osteoporosis. (a) The lateral chest radiograph shows generalized rarefaction of the vertebrae with wedge fractures, and loss of thoracic height. (b) The oblique view shows multiple rib fractures on the left, following a fall.

## INFECTIONS

Patients may present atypically with confusion, falls or 'loss of function'. A pyrexia may or may not be present in the early stages of an infection, although pyrexia usually develops eventually in the absence of treatment.

In the urinary tract structural abnormalities, catheters and calculi predispose to infection. In the chest there is an increased frequency of Gram-negative organisms as well as the more common *Pneumococcus* and *Haemophilus influenzae*. Poor tracheobronchial clearance and increased spillover from the upper gastrointestinal tract contribute to the frequency of broncho-pneumonia.

## SOME PARTICULAR DISORDERS IN ELDERLY PATIENTS

# Hypertension

## DIAGNOSIS

'Normal' blood pressure has been regarded as increasing steadily with age, and yet a number of elderly people have unusually low blood pressure, and a number of individuals who had hypertension in their fifties and sixties become normotensive in their seventies and eighties. Pragmatically, hypertension may be regarded as that blood pressure above which there is an identifiable increased risk of cerebrovascular disease, coronary artery disease or renal impairment (page 220).

Almost all hypertension in individuals up to the age of 50 years is diagnosed on the basis of an elevated diastolic pressure. With increasing age, elevations of systolic pressure become commoner, and in those aged 70–79 years over two-thirds of hypertensive patients are diagnosed on the basis of elevated systolic blood pressure alone. These individuals with isolated systolic hypertension have a significantly increased cardiovascular mortality and may also be at increased risk from cerebrovascular disease. Clinical trials are in progress to determine whether the excess mortality can be reduced by treating isolated systolic hypertension.

## MANAGEMENT

Management of hypertension without drugs is especially important in the elderly because of the high incidence of drug-related side effects. Weight reduction to within 15 per cent of ideal body weight, dietary sodium restriction to 70–100 mmol/day, regular exercise training, which may lower average blood pressure by 20 mm Hg, and stress management programmes can all be employed.

Drug therapy in the elderly has some points of difference from that of younger hypertensives (Table 26.3). β-blockers are markedly less effective in the elderly than in the young, and calcium channel blockers are more effective. This is because, in the elderly, increased peripheral resistance contributes more to hypertension than does increased cardiac output, the reverse of the situation in the young. In addition β-blockers may precipitate congestive cardiac failure.

Elderly hypertensive patients may have significant cerebral arterial disease as well as coronary artery disease. Some care is needed when treating hypertension in these patients in order to avoid precipitating cerebral or coronary ischaemia.

Persistantly raised diastolic pressure above 95 mm Hg requires drug treatment in most patients. Isolated systolic hypertension is associated with an increased risk of vascular disease and treatment should be considered with systolic pressures over 180 mm Hg.

# Stroke

The incidence of stroke and transient ischaemic attacks increases with age, 75 per cent occurring

**Table 26.3** Medical management of hypertension in the elderly.

| Drug | Advantages | Disadvantages |
|---|---|---|
| Calcium channel blockers | Lower peripheral resistance<br>Useful in peripheral vascular disease<br>No metabolic effects | Occasional reflex tachycardia |
| Angiotensin-converting enzyme inhibitors | Lower peripheral resistance<br>Increase renal blood flow<br>Diminish preload, useful in left ventricular failure | Reduce renal function in renal artery stenosis |
| Thiazide diuretics | Effective in subdiuretic dosage (e.g. bendrofluazide, 2.5 mg) | Increase lipid and glucose levels<br>Loss of $K^+$, $Mg^{2+}$<br>Reduce plasma volume and renal blood flow |
| β-Blockers | Not a first-line treatment in the elderly | Reduce cardiac output<br>Effective in only 20%<br>Worsen peripheral ischaemia |
| Methyldopa | No advantages<br>Not recommended as first-line therapy | Reduce cardiac output in elderly<br>Depression and lethargy<br>Constipation |
| Arteriolar vasodilators | Lower peripheral resistance | Increase heart rate and renin levels<br>Postural hypotension |
| α-Blockers | Lower peripheral resistance<br>Maintain cardiac output<br>No increase in plasma renin | Postural hypotension |

in those over 65 years of age (Fig. 26.7). Stroke is defined as a focal neurological deficit of presumed vascular origin, lasting more than 24 hours. In a transient ischaemic attack (TIA) the deficit resolves completely within 24 hours. Nearly all TIAs are due to cerebral embolism, over 90 per cent being from platelet aggregates or atheromatous plaques in the common or internal carotid arteries.

Eighty per cent of all strokes are ischaemic, and most of the remainder are due to intracranial haemorrhage. A number of less common conditions masquerade as a stroke (Table 26.4). Subdural haematoma is an important differential diagnosis. It can occur after minor trauma which may not be remembered. The distinction between haemorrhagic and ischaemic stroke cannot be made clinically, and if anticoagulant treatment is being considered for presumed embolic stroke a computed tomographic (CT) scan should be performed to exclude haemorrhage (Fig. 26.8). A CT scan should also be

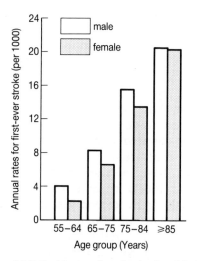

**Figure 26.7** Incidence of stroke in the elderly.

performed if the clinical features are atypical, if there is any suggestion of antecedent head injury, if conscious level is markedly impaired in the presence of only minor lateralizing signs

**Table 26.4** Differential diagnosis of a stroke.

Epileptic fit (may be caused by scar from earlier stroke)
Worsening of previous stroke due to intercurrent
  illness
Neurosyphilis
Infective endocarditis (may present as mycotic
  embolism)
Subdural haematoma
Hypoglycaemia
Cranial arteritis
Intracerebral tumour (primary or secondary)
Cerebral abscess
Meningitis

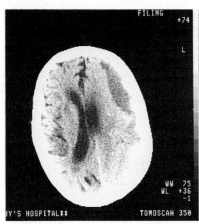

**Figure 26.8** Computed tomographic head scan showing a large left-sided subdural haematoma. The patient was a 95-year-old man who had been diagnosed as having a mild stroke 9 days earlier. He had atrial fibrillation, and had been started on soluble aspirin. During the 9 days his weakness had worsened and he had become confused.

(suggesting raised intracranial pressure), if there is a history of recurrent 'strokes' with partial recovery (which may indicate the presence of a tumour) or of vertigo, vomiting and ataxia suggest a cerebellar haematoma (possibly requiring surgical intervention).

## ACUTE STROKE MANAGEMENT

Management of a patient with stroke provides an excellent example of multidisciplinary team management. Maintenance of hydration and, in the longer term, of nutrition are required together with treatment of intercurrent medical problems. Careful nursing will prevent pressure sores and physiotherapy is aimed at avoiding contractures and preventing orthostatic pneumonia. During recovery the continued involvement of the physiotherapist is needed to ensure that sitting and standing balance, transfers and walking are developed in sequence. Functional disabilities are assessed and managed by the occupational therapist using appropriate aids and appliances. The speech therapist should advise on swallowing, speech and communication difficulties. Community services and social services are likely to become involved as the time of discharge home approaches.

## PROPHYLAXIS OF STROKE

Primary and secondary prophylaxis of stroke is directed at minimizing known risk factors (Table 26.5). For TIAs or minor strokes, secondary prophylaxis with soluble aspirin should be started immediately after the event, but in established ischaemic stroke there is a small risk of secondary haemorrhage, so that it is better to delay starting aspirin for 2 weeks. In the long-term aspirin prophylaxis reduces the risk of a further vascular event from 22 to 18 per cent over 2 years. Doses of 75–300 mg daily have been successful but the incidence of gastric side

**Table 26.5** Risk factors for transient ischaemic attack and stroke.

**Non-cardiac risk factors**
Hypertension (systolic and diastolic)
Atheromatous arterial disease
Smoking
Alcohol
Diabetes mellitus
Hyperlipidaemia
Raised haematocrit

**Cardiac risk factors**
Emboli from – Mural thrombus in left atrium (atrial
              fibrillation, rheumatic mitral valve
              disease)
              Mural thrombus following transmural
              myocardial infarction
              Mural thrombus in cardiomyopathy
              Prosthetic heart valve
              Infective endocarditis of mitral or aortic
              valve

effects is dose related and therefore the lowest effective dose should generally be used.

Patients with atrial fibrillation and mitral valve disease should receive anticoagulation treatment. In patients with atrial fibrillation without mitral stenosis anticoagulation is more effective than aspirin in long-term prophylaxis when there is any cardiac abnormality. In the absence of mitral valve disease lower levels of anticoagulation are probably sufficient.

The risk of intracranial haemorrhage in patients receiving anticoagulant drugs increases with age. This is partly through poor control of anticoagulation, resulting from altered drug metabolism and physical difficulty in attending clinics. At the same time the projected benefit obtainable declines with the years of remaining life. Thus, long-term oral anticoagulation should only be undertaken with great caution in those over 80 years of age.

The place of carotid endarterectomy in elderly patients with stroke is also controversial. A reduction in the 3-year incidence of further strokes has been shown in patients in their sixties who have already had a minor stroke and who have a 70–99 per cent ipsilateral carotid stenosis. However, there is a significant risk of stroke associated with the surgical procedure itself, and it is still unclear at what age this risk begins to outweigh the possible later benefits of surgery.

# Movement disorders

## PARKINSON'S DISEASE

Parkinson's disease (page 678) is a syndrome of akinesia (paucity of movement), rigidity, resting tremor and postural abnormalities. The onset is usually with tremor, at 4–6 cycles per second, affecting one or both hands. The other features of the disorder develop later, with loss of postural control, mask-like facies, dribbling of saliva, difficulty in speech and in swallowing. Posture becomes stooped, there is difficulty starting and stopping walking, and the gait becomes shuffling with small rapid steps.

The underlying deficiency of dopamine in the substantia nigra is treated by supplementation with levodopa. L-Dopa is usually combined with a dopa-decarboxylase inhibitor to prevent peripheral breakdown and to enhance levels of dopamine in the central nervous system. Side effects include postural hypotension, nausea, hallucinations and dyskinesias. Anticholinergic drugs are more effective against tremor than against rigidity, but have limited use in the elderly because of side effects, particularly confusion and constipation. Bromocriptine is a dopamine agonist, and selegiline is a monoamine oxidase B inhibitor which prevents dopamine breakdown.

## NON-PARKINSONIAN MOVEMENT DISORDERS AND PARKINSONIAN SYNDROMES

Several movement disorders become more common with increasing age and may severely impair a patient's functional abilities (Table 26.6).

# Hypothermia

Hypothermia (a body core temperature below 35°C) occurs most frequently during the winter months in elderly people who live alone at home and have inadequate heating. There is usually some additional predisposing abnormality (Table 26.7). The predominant clinical features include cold, pale skin; confusion, disorientation and eventually coma; hypotension, bradycardia or cardiac arrhythmia (eventually ventricular fibrillation), slow respiration, gastric dilatation and sometimes acute pancreatitis, decreased glomerular filtration rate and oliguria. The electrocardiogram (ECG) may show a bradycardia, an arrhythmia or the characteristic J waves (Fig. 26.9) (page 854).

## MANAGEMENT

Management includes identification and treatment of the primary cause, rewarming and the treatment of complications. Rewarming from mild hypothermia (32–35°C) is generally possible by nursing in an ambient temperature of

**Table 26.6** Parkinsonian syndromes and non-parkinsonian movement disorders.

| Disorder | Features | Treatment |
|---|---|---|
| **Akinetic rigid syndromes** | | |
| Drug-induced parkinsonism | Phenothiazine usage | Stop offending drug Anticholinergic agents |
| Arteriosclerotic pseudoparkinsonism | Stepwise progression Upper motor neuron signs Multiple lacunar infarcts | Little or no response to levodopa |
| Shy–Drager syndrome | Postural hypotension, failure of sweating, urinary incontinence, impotence, Parkinson-type rigidity, sleep apnoea | Symptomatic |
| Postencephalitic parkinsonism | Now very rare | Poor response to levodopa |
| **Choreiform movements (irregular twitching)** (Due to enhanced dopaminergic activity) | | |
| Senile chorea | Loss of cells in putamen or caudate nucleus | Dopamine antagonist, e.g. tetrabenazine, haloperidol |
| **Athetosis (writhing movements)** | | |
| Levodopa-induced dyskinesias | Abnormal movements of trunk and limbs | Stop levodopa |
| **Hemiballismus** | | |
| Cerebrovascular disease of contralateral subthalamic nucleus | Outward projection of ipsilateral arm and leg | Stop levodopa |
| **Tardive dyskinesia** | | |
| After many months of treatment with neuroleptic drugs (phenothiazine and haloperidol) or many months after stopping. Also induced by metoclopramide and prochlorperazine | Abnormal movements of face, tongue and mouth (orobuccofacial dyskinesia) Abolished during sleep | Withdraw causative agent (often exacerbates condition). Tetrabenazine |
| **Tremor** | | |
| Idiopathic tremor | Mainly an action tremor | — |
| 'Benign essential tremor' | 50% have positive family history Affects hands particularly Resting tremor, may mimic Parkinson's disease | — |
| Intention tremor | Cerebellar disease | — |
| Drug-induced tremor | Phenytoin Salbutamol Sodium valproate | Withdraw causative agent |

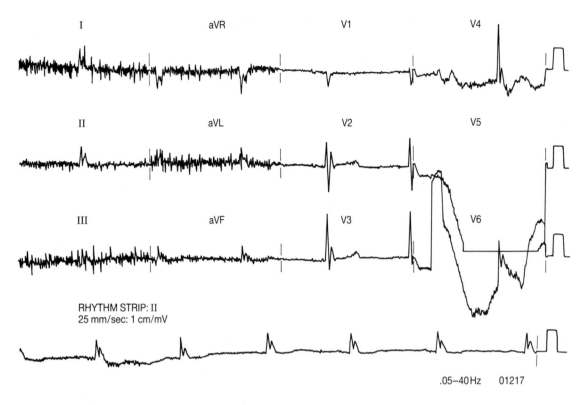

**Figure 26.9** Electrocardiogram from a patient with hypothermia (core temperature was 29°C). The characteristic J waves are seen immediately after the QRS complex. Note the absence of P waves, bradycardia and the shivering artefact affecting the baseline.

**Table 26.7** Underlying causes of hypothermia.

| | |
|---|---|
| Impaired mobility | Stroke |
| | Parkinson's disease |
| | Arthritis |
| | Fracture |
| | Myocardial Infarction |
| Unconsciousness | Epilepsy |
| | Sedation/drug overdose |
| | Diabetic coma |
| Impaired mental state | Depression |
| | Delirium |
| | Dementia |
| Impaired temperature regulation | Hypothyroidism |
| | Hypopituitarism |
| | Drugs including alcohol, neuroleptics, tricyclics |
| Infection | Sepsis |
| | Bronchopneumonia |

25–30°C, covering the patient in a space blanket and possibly with the addition of warmed blankets inside. A rise in temperature of 0.5 to 1.0°C per hour should be achieved. If the temperature is below 30°C spontaneous rewarming may be very slow. Warmed intravenous fluids, (with care taken to avoid pulmonary oedema), warmed inspired air or oxygen and warmed bladder or gastric irrigation may be used.

The mortality rate is high, and the lower the core temperature the greater the risk of death. Prophylactic antibiotics should be given and the quite frequent occurrence of vasodilatation causing hypovolaemia on rewarming should be treated with intravenous colloid infusion. Patients should be disturbed as little as possible, since cardiac arrhythmias may be precipitated by violent movement or by the injection of positive inotropic drugs.

# COMMON SYMPTOM COMPLEXES IN THE ELDERLY: THE 'GERIATRIC GIANTS'

The term 'geriatric giants' was coined by Isaacs for a number of commonly presenting symptoms, each of which may represent a wide variety of underlying disease processes. They include intellectual impairment, incontinence, instability and immobility.

# *Intellectual impairment*

This may be chronic (dementia), acute (delirium) or acute superimposed on chronic (page 872). Patients with dementia are awake and alert and are apparently in touch with their surroundings. Quite significant intellectual impairment may be masked by a few cleverly utilized social skills, vague answers to questions, and confabulation. Brief but formal testing is needed in all elderly patients using the Abbreviated Mental Test score (Table 26.8). It is important to establish the duration of any mental impairment in order to separate delirium from dementia.

**Table 26.8** Abbreviated Mental Test (AMT).

| | |
|---|---|
| 1. | Age |
| 2. | Time (to nearest hour) |
| 3. | Address for recall at end of test–this should be repeated by the patient to ensure it has been heard correctly: *42 West Street* |
| 4. | Year |
| 5. | Name of institution |
| 6. | Recognition of two persons (doctor, nurse etc) |
| 7. | Date of birth (day and month sufficient) |
| 8. | Year of First World War |
| 9. | Name of present monarch |
| 10. | Count backwards 20 to 1 |

*Scoring:* Each correct answer scores one mark

A guide to rating cognitive funtion: 0–3 severe impairment; 4–7 moderate impairment; 8–10 normal

Source: Hodkinson. *Age and Ageing* 1972; **1**: 233–8.

Dementia is most commonly due to Alzheimer's disease (senile dementia of Alzheimer's type, SDAT) or to multi-infarct dementia. Neither condition is reversible. In Alzheimer's disease deterioration is progresive, and the CT scan will show cortical atrophy although this finding is neither specific for, nor diagnostic of, SDAT (Fig. 26.10). In multi-infarct dementia deterioration is stepwise, there is an association with stroke, and with the risk factors for stroke including hypertension. The CT scan shows multiple cerebral infarcts. Some rarer causes of apparent dementia are reversible and should be sought (Table 26.9).

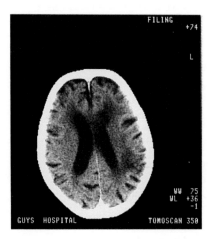

**Figure 26.10** A computed tomographic head scan of a 90-year-old lady with memory loss. The appearances of widened sulci and expanded lateral ventricles are typical of age-related cerebral atrophy.

**Table 26.9** Treatable causes of dementia.

Hypothyroidism
Depression ('pseudodementia')
Vitamin deficiencies ($B_{12}$, thiamine)
Intracranial space-occupying lesion
Normal pressure hydrocephalus
Chronic subdural haematoma
Drugs such as long-acting tranquillizers
Chronic alcohol abuse

**Table 26.10** Causes of delirium.

**Drugs**
Tranquillizers and hypnotics, e.g. benzodiazepines
Cardiovascular agents, e.g. diuretics
Anticholinergic drugs, e.g. anti-parkinsonian agents
Dopamine agonists, e.g. methyldopa
Anticonvulsants, e.g. phenytoin
Oral hypoglycaemic drugs, e.g. chlorpropamide and
    glibenclamide
Alcohol and alcohol withdrawal

**Infection**
Urinary tract
Pneumonia
Bacteraemia
Infective endocarditis
Intracranial infections

**Metabolic and endocrine dysfunction and
    malnutrition**
Diabetes mellitus
Renal or hepatic failure
Dehydration or water overload
Hypopituitarism, hypothyroidism, thyrotoxicosis

**Cardiovascular and respiratory disorders**
Congestive cardiac failure
Myocardial infarction
Hypoxia or hypercapnia

**Intracranial lesions**
Trauma
Stroke and subarachnoid haemorrhage
Tumour
Epilepsy

**Intra-abdominal causes**
Perforated peptic ulcer
Other causes of acute abdomen
Ascending cholangitis
Upper gastrointestinal haemorrhage

**Surgery and anaesthesia**

Delirium is a reversible condition and is caused by an underlying acute event that requires treatment (Table 26.10). Patients with delirium typically exhibit clouding of consciousness and are out of touch with their surroundings. A few moments thought should enable the two conditions to be separated clinically (Table 26.11).

# *Incontinence*

Urinary or faecal incontinence may be the presenting symptom of a number of underlying conditions (Table 26.12). Because incontinence is socially stressful it is often the first symptom to bring the patient or carer to medical attention. Management of incontinence is directed at the primary cause when this can be established, and expert urological or gynaecological advice may be required.

Anticholinergic drugs may help those with an unstable bladder. Re-education with a 2-hourly toileting regime may be helpful, and long-term catheterization should only be employed when other approaches have failed. Pads and other aids, for example, penile sheaths, are available.

Faecal incontinence is also managed by identifying and treating any primary cause. If the cause is untreatable (e.g. late dementia) then a regimen of codeine phosphate orally, with regular enemas, may allow continence most of the time, but at the expense of some inconvenience and discomfort to the patient.

**Table 26.11** Distinguishing delirium and dementia.

|  | **Delirium** | **Dementia** |
| --- | --- | --- |
| Clouding of consciousness | Yes | No |
| Duration of onset | Hours/days | Months |
| Course | Fluctuating | Steady, or stepwise decline |
| Poor short-term memory* | Yes | Yes |
| Hallucinations and delusions | Yes | Sometimes |
| Agitation and restlessness | Yes | Sometimes |
| Evidence of underlying primary disease | Yes | Usually not |
| Rambling incoherent speech | Yes | No |

*The Mini-Mental Test (page 654) does not in itself distinguish delirium from dementia, but a steady improvement in the score is against a diagnosis of dementia.

**Table 26.12** Causes of urinary and faecal incontinence.

### Urinary incontinence
Urinary tract infection

Bladder outflow obstruction with overflow, due to constipation, prostatic hypertrophy

Acute or chronic cerebral disease

Drugs (sedatives or diuretics)

Stress incontinence, uterine prolapse, atrophic vaginitis

Detrusor instability

Specific neurological deficit including spinal cord compression (neurogenic bladder with automatic voiding)

Normal pressure hydrocephalus

Autonomic neuropathy due to diabetes mellitus

### Faecal incontinence
Faecal impaction with overflow

Acute or chronic brain failure

Spinal cord disease

Carcinoma of the colon or rectum

Ulcerative colitis

Autonomic neuropathy

Laxative abuse

**Table 26.13** Common causes of falls.

### Neurological disease
Stroke, transient ischaemic attack, Parkinson's disease, cerebellar disease

### Cardiovascular disorders
Myocardial infarction, cardiac arrhythmias, postural hypotension

### Musculoskeletal disorders
Generalized muscle weakness, arthritis and secondary wasting, unstable knee or painful hip, proximal myopathy

### Drugs
Psychotropic drugs, diuretics, antihypertensives, levodopa, alcohol

### Premonitory falls
These occur in the preliminary phase of an acute illness, usually an infection

### Miscellaneous causes
Hypoglycaemia, electrolyte abnormalities, acute labyrinthitis, impaired vision, cervical spondylosis, physical abuse

possible. The patient's gait after the fall may suggest Parkinson's disease, hemiparesis, ataxia, or arthritis. Physical examination after a fall should include a careful check for injury: pain in one hip on walking may be indicative of a femoral fracture, and if there has been a head injury the skull should be X-rayed to exclude fracture.

# Instability (falls)

Up to 30 per cent of elderly people fall each year, and 20 per cent of falls are associated with syncope (Table 26.13). Falls may cause injury or fracture, loss of confidence and a vicious circle of increasing dependency.

It is important to establish whether the patient has had previous falls, has tripped, whether there was any warning (if not, a cardiac or cerebrovascular cause is suggested), and what the patient was doing immediately before the fall. If the fall occurred after standing up, postural hypotension is suggested and if after looking upwards, vertebrobasilar insufficiency is

# Impaired mobility

The usual complaint is that the patient has 'gone off her legs' or is 'unable to get out of bed'. A careful history of the time course of the loss of mobility may give clues to the cause (Table 26.14). Often there is long-standing impairment, and confinement to bed or a chair is precipitated by intercurrent illness, by a diminution in social support at home, or by loss of vision.

**Table 26.14** Causes of impaired mobility.

| | |
|---|---|
| **Joint disease** | **Muscle disease** |
| Osteoarthritis of the knees, hips or spine | Myopathy (e.g. osteomalacia or thryotoxicosis) |
| | Atrophy |
| | Polymyalgia rheumatica |
| **Neurological disease** | |
| Stroke | **Contractures** |
| Parkinson's disease | The patient has become 'chair-shaped' |
| Motor neurone disease (rarely) | |
| Ataxia | **Other examples of precipitating causes** |
| | Pneumonia |
| | Cardiac failure |

# INVESTIGATION OF THE ELDERLY PATIENT

Establishment of the diagnosis is the first step on the road to successful treatment, at any age. However, age may alter subsequent decisions about the most appropriate treatment. Investigations should be requested as in younger patients. The principles governing investigations in the elderly are the same as in any other age group.

# TREATMENT OF THE ELDERLY PATIENT

Treatment should be designed to achieve cure, but this may not be possible, and maximization of function with preservation of independence and quality of life should be the chief aims. In most, although not all, disorders medical therapy is with the same drugs as in the young but often in lower dosage because of impaired metabolism and excretion (Table 26.15).

If surgical treatment is indicated it is usually best to proceed sooner rather than later, provided that the patient is fit enough for an anaesthetic. Delay usually worsens the prognosis (e.g. in severe upper gastrointestinal haemor-rhage or fractured neck of femur), and if preliminary medical treatment is needed this should be carried out as rapidly as possible.

# Rehabilitation

The role of the rehabilitation team is to maximize the patient's functional abilities and to return the individual to independent life at home if at all possible.

To achieve this, rehabilitation must begin as soon as possible after disability or illness are diagnosed at home, or after a patient is admitted to hospital. Waiting for an acute illness to resolve fully before starting rehabilitation is usually counter-productive. The physiotherapist will re-establish mobility and muscle and joint function, and the occupational therapist will ensure that activities of daily living can be carried out safely. Appropriate aids to mobility and to daily activities, respectively, may be provided as necessary (Fig. 26.11).

**Table 26.15** Rules for prescribing in the elderly.

1. Use a few, well-known drugs
2. Use low starting doses
3. Simplify dosage and regimen
4. Clear labelling and accessible containers
5. Regular review of medication
6. Check for compliance
7. Communicate with family doctor
8. Careful explanation to patient and carer
9. Written instructions

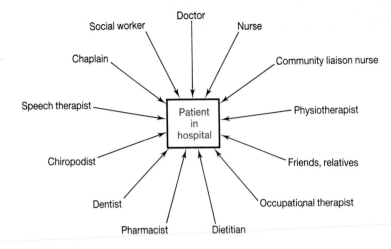

**Figure 26.11** Make-up of the teams involved with the care of elderly patients in hospital. (Modified from Davies J (ed.). Practical Clinical Medicine. Oxford: Butterworth-Heinemann, 1992: 357.

# DRUGS AND THE ELDERLY PATIENT

Elderly people comprise 12 to 18 per cent of western populations, but receive 30 to 40 per cent of prescriptions. Elderly people are more prone to develop adverse drug reactions, even allowing for their increased medication, and 80 per cent of these reactions are dose dependent and therefore theoretically avoidable if a few simple rules for prescribing are followed (Table 26.15).

## Compliance

Age itself does not limit compliance, but cognitive impairment and multiple prescribing do. Failure of compliance is associated with therapeutic failure, and often the prescription of additional medication follows. Regimens should be simple, time must be given for adequate explanation of therapy to the patient and carer, and liberal use should be made of written instructions, diary cards and containers labelled with day and time.

## Altered pharmacokinetics and pharmacodynamics

Many changes in the absorption, metabolism and excretion of drugs occur with ageing, even without any disease process (Table 26.16).

**Table 26.16** Alteration in pharmacokinetics with age.

| Nature of change | Effect on pharmacokinetics |
|---|---|
| Absorption from gut slowed but complete | Reduced peak drug levels |
| First pass hepatic metabolism decreased | Increased bioavailability of propranolol, nifedipine and nitrates |
| Altered lipid/water distribution and decreased protein binding (small effect usually) | Polar drugs less widely distributed (cimetidine)<br>Non-polar drugs more widely distributed (barbiturates and benzodiazipines)<br>Greater free fraction of protein-bound drugs (diazepam) |
| Reduced renal clearance | Increased plasma levels of atenolol, sotolol, digoxin, aminoglycosides, lithium and chlorpropramide |
| Reduced hepatic clearance dependent on liver mass and blood flow | Drug clearance by cytochrome P450 and by conjugation reduced in parallel with reduced liver mass (cimetidine and warfarin) |

Drugs which affect systems already impaired by the ageing process or disease should be used with caution. The following are examples:

1. Orthostatic circulatory response is affected by tricyclics, benzodiazepines and anti-parkinsonian drugs
2. Thermoregulation is affected by tricyclics, alcohol, neuroleptics and barbiturates
3. Postural control is affected by hypnotics and tranquillizers
4. Mental state is affected by hypnotics, tranquillizers and many other drugs

Some reduction in $\beta$-receptor activity occurs in the elderly, so that $\beta$-blockers and $\beta$-stimulants become less effective. Cholinergic receptors are maintained and anticholinergic agents remain useful.

# $S$OCIAL SUPPORT OF THE ELDERLY

## *Discharge home*

One major objective of the practice of medicine in the elderly is to maintain the individual's independence in his or her own home for as long as possible. Not all elderly people require hospital admission for diagnosis and treatment. Some may be managed in the outpatient department, and others in the day hospital, where input from the multidisciplinary team is directly available. In all cases it is vital to assess fully the patient's social background, and current and future care needs at home.

If admitted to hospital a discharge plan incorporating these considerations should be made as soon as possible in order to avoid any unnecessary delay in discharge. The plan may be modified and refined as rehabilitation proceeds, and input should be obtained from all disciplines. A predischarge home visit with the occupational therapist and sometimes the physiotherapist, may be an important part of discharge planning. Functional abilities in the patient's own environment can be assessed, together with any potential hazards and the need for, and practicability of, aids, appliances and adaptations. The visit should be timed so that rehabilitation is well advanced (Fig. 26.12).

The date of discharge should be agreed between the multidisciplinary team, the patient and any carers. Adequate time must be allowed for the instigation of support from social services, district nurse and other agencies. If a dependent person lives alone, discharge on a Friday should be avoided. The patient's general practitioner should be informed of the impend-

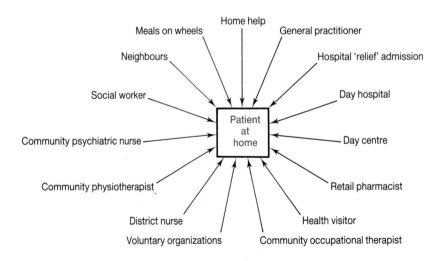

**Figure 26.12** Support available for elderly people and their relatives or carers in the community. (Modified from Davies J (ed.). Practical Clinical Medicine. Oxford: Butterworth-Heinemann, 1992: 357.

ing discharge of a disabled patient, together with the arrangements made for support at home, and details of planned follow-up. Readmission to hospital within 48 hours should be regarded as a failure of discharge planning unless another reason can be identified.

# Care in institutions

Those who are unable, or occasionally unwilling, to return to their own home will need care in an institution or 'Home'. Individuals who are mobile, with appropriate aids if necessary, who are continent and who require minimal help with washing, dressing and eating are generally suitable for residential accommodation. This is available in local authority residential homes, established under Part 3 of the 1948 National Assistance Act ('Part 3 Homes'), or in privately run or charitably funded residential homes, licensed by the local authority. Residential homes do not have resident nursing staff, and cannot manage people with severe disability.

More severely disabled individuals who need care frequently or for prolonged periods are appropriately cared for in nursing homes or sometimes in a hospital long-stay ward: such individuals may be bedbound, chairbound, incontinent or severely mentally impaired. Hospital long-stay wards rarely provide an ideal environment and privately run nursing homes are of variable standard and experience. Nursing homes are obliged to have a minimum number of qualified nurses on duty but overall staffing levels may be low. Nursing homes are registered with the health authorities, who are responsible for monitoring standards.

For those receiving supplementary benefit a grant from the Department of Social Security is available, although it does not fully cover the fees charged by many private nursing homes. The current system changed in April 1993 so that the local authority now manages the budget for all forms of institutional care outside hospitals, as well as for home care.

# Psychiatric disorders

# 27

# INTRODUCTION

Psychiatry is a medical specialty concerned with behaviour which may be distressing, difficult, problematic or eccentric. 'Behaviour' includes everything people think and say as well as what they do, covering subjective experience as well as observable action, and is the subject matter of the various branches of psychology as well as psychiatry. Psychological or psychiatric problems may arise in connection with any illness.

The field of psychiatry includes three groups of problems: (1) psychological aspects of medical practice, (2) coexisting medical illness and psychiatric disorder, and (3) psychiatric disorders. This chapter deals largely with the first two of these; the third category, the 'psychiatric disorders', includes conditions where the physical medical aspect is relatively minor, and care is usually given by specialists rather than by general physicians.

# PSYCHIATRIC ASSESSMENT

## General considerations: formulation

The general principles of psychiatric assessment should be known by every doctor because they apply to the evaluation of behaviour problems in any field of medicine.

The main task is to understand the patients and their problems, and make sense of their behaviour. This is done as elsewhere in medicine by history taking and examination, although the examination is principally by observation and through conversation in clinical interviewing. Clinical interviewing skills are therefore particularly important in the psychiatric assessment. This assessment summary, or **formulation**, has four parts:

- Description
- Diagnosis
- Problems
- Explanation

which together form the basis of management.

The **description** is a summary of the significant symptoms and signs (often called phenomena in psychiatry) noted on psychiatric examination. It comes first because description should precede explanation, and the problem behaviours should be known before attempts are made to account for them.

**Diagnosis** comes next because psychiatric diagnostic categories represent collections of symptoms and signs, that is, syndromes defined according to agreed rules of thumb set out in various official manuals. Diagnosis is important because (a) it represents a communicable summary of examination findings; (b) it indicates problems which the patient does not have; and (c) it provides some, albeit often limited, pointers to prognosis. Diagnosis in psychiatry is sometimes devalued by people who expect it to do what the problem formulation actually does.

The psychiatric assessment should arrive at statements of the patient's **problems** which suggest and lead to action. To be most useful the problem statements must make maximum sense to both patient and interviewer. The assessor will need to be able to consider problems in psychological, biological or social terms as appropriate, for no single conceptual framework (brain chemistry, psychoanalysis etc.) is applicable in all psychiatric circumstances.

**Explanation** is an attempt to account for the symptoms, signs and problems which have been identified, indicating how they have arisen and how they may be linked together. Again, this will often have psychological, biological and social aspects. It should make sense to interviewer and patient, with whom it should often be shared.

These phases of assessment may suggest a **management** plan, or additional investigations may be needed to inform the choice between alternative plans of action.

# *History taking*

The psychiatric history should provide an account of the behavioural changes, problems and symptoms which the patient has recently experienced or encountered, and of current and past relationships relevant to understanding these as well as some degree of understanding of the patient's personality.

Sometimes patients are unaware of the impact of their behaviour on others, or even of problems altogether, and symptoms may be minimized or concealed and appear to be ill-defined. Many symptoms concern sensitive areas of personal life about which conversation does not come easily – sexual difficulties for instance.

Hence, history taking can be difficult. Three principles should be borne in mind: (1) self-disclosure is facilitated by sensitive, empathic interviewing; (2) symptoms and problems can be defined clearly if sufficient attention is paid to detail; and (3) an account from another informant often clarifies a clinical mystery associated with a self-reported history.

The history includes five headings:

1. Reason for referral
2. Present problem
3. Family history
4. Personal history
5. Personality

Enquiry into the **reason for referral** ascertains who identified that a problem exists, and when, and what previous steps at seeking help have occurred. Often, asking for help with a behavioural problem occurs when someone, either the person themselves or someone closely concerned with them, is having difficulty coping

with the situation rather than that the problem itself has become worse.

The **history of the present problem** should usually be obtained next. This amplifies the presenting complaints. Special attention should be paid to details of the onset of symptoms as well as to their nature, because illnesses have onsets whereas long-standing personality problems do not and may require a different therapeutic approach. A clear onset of symptoms tends to point to a state of illness. Symptoms of psychiatric disorder are often changes in degree from normal experience rather than qualitatively novel departures from it, and a degree of anxiety, sadness etc. which may not appear excessive at interview may yet represent for that individual a change indicative of illness.

As well as enquiring about the onset, nature and development of symptoms, the interviewer should note their temporal relations to possible precipitants. Many behavioural problems arise at least in part in response to stressful life events, commonly associated with changes in interpersonal relationships, living or work arrangements. It can be very helpful to ask the patient to describe a typical day in their life.

The problem can be set in its personal and social context by enquiry into the **family and personal history**. Common-sense and the time available determine the extent to which particular items should be pursued.

The term **personality** refers to the sort of person this is. If a set of acute symptoms constitute an illness then we are interested in the person's habitual ways of behaving before the illness, the premorbid personality. In other instances, the focus may need to be on the progression of the individual's characteristics from early life to the present time without any illness discontinuity.

Personality assessment should cover habitual patterns of social and personal behaviour, including sociability and interests, emotional responsiveness, stability, ability to cope with stressful events, general levels of drive and energy, ambitions and moral standards, and overall evaluation of the self (Table 27.1).

A person's self-description is often complemented usefully by the descriptions of others who know them well.

**Table 27.1** Family and personal histories.

### The family

1. Parents and 2. siblings: ages, state of health, occupation

3. Family relationships: parental discord, separation, divorce; abusive experiences; overall evaluation of home; present state of relationships

4. Family health: psychiatric disorder in blood relatives

### Personal

1. Origins: where born and brought up

2. Education: highest level reached; overall evaluation; any problems

3. Occupation: work record; overall evaluation

4. Health: previous medical and psychiatric disorders

5. Relationships: friendships and close relationships, including psychosexual history; present domestic arrangements and current relationship pattern.

# Examination of mental state

The mental state examination is based on the patient's self-report and the observations made of the patient's behaviour. It should be set out under five headings:

1. General behaviour
2. Thought and talk
3. Emotion
4. Perception
5. Cognitive functions

## GENERAL BEHAVIOUR

The observer should attend to the patient's dress, gestures, facial expression and general activity level, which may be increased as in states of excitement or reduced as in severe depression. The appropriateness of the patient's behaviour to the interview situation should be noted – a patient may be flippant, aloof and unconcerned, or suspicious and on their guard.

The examiner may fail to develop a customary sense of contact with the patient; this important phenomenon always *raises the possibility* of a schizophrenic disorder (page 891).

## THOUGHT AND TALK

Disorders of thought have four aspects: stream, possession, form and content.

The stream or flow of thought may be accelerated, as sometimes in anxiety or agitation; or slowed (e.g. in depression); or interrupted, as in schizophrenic thought blocking. The flow of thought is usually accelerated in agitated depression and slowed in retarded depression.

Normally, people experience their thoughts as controllable, and their own. Distortions of this arise with obsessional thoughts which are intrusive, unwelcome and repetitive, or when thoughts may be felt to be withdrawn from the self, or forced into the mind from outside, by some alien force, as occurs typically in schizophrenia.

The form or structure of thought may be distorted. Sentences may be ill-formed, sometimes with newly invented words mixed with familiar ones, or sentence construction may be normal but the transmission of ideas faulty, which can produce the disconcerting effect of an earnestly spoken sequence of apparently normal sentences which yet convey no meaning and lead nowhere.

Three important problems may arise with the content of thought. First, preoccupations – things people think about a lot – may be morbid or normal. Second, overvalued ideas may occur. These are like preoccupations which go beyond the normal range or are about things which would not normally preoccupy a person.

Third, there may be delusions. A **delusion** is a demonstrably false belief, held with absolute certainty, inappropriate to the person's socio-cultural background. Primary delusions arise spontaneously and cannot be understood empathically. Secondary delusions emerge from a coexisting mental experience, most frequently an intense mood state, in terms of which they can be understood. In depression, secondary delusions may extend to beliefs about being of no worth, or having an incurable disease, or being already dead – such beliefs may be termed nihilistic. Persecutory and grandiose delusions of exalted status are referred to as paranoid. Paranoid delusions may occur in many illnesses, including organic states, depression and schizophrenia.

## EMOTION

The assessment of the emotional state of a patient is important and is frequently difficult. Mood is gauged from what the subject reports, what is observed of behaviour, and what the observer feels empathically is the other person's feeling state. Subjects' reports may be halting and uncertain, because many people find it hard to recognize their own feelings and to put words to them. Behavioural observations are always easier to interpret in people one knows than in new acquaintances, or may be hard to interpret if for instance mechanisms underpinning facial expression are impaired.

Most emotions are experienced as pleasant and positive or unpleasant and negative; as having some degree of intensity; and in relation to a particular event, person, object or experience. Naturally, clinical problems more often focus on negative feelings than on positive ones. Most problem emotions concern anxiety, sadness, guilt, anger, jealousy, apathy or mixtures of these; but emotional experience may be complex and richly described and care should be taken not to oversimplify it. Some patients are unnaturally elated, blissful or ecstatic. Nevertheless, it is sadness, misery, dejection, pessimism and an overall feeling of unhappy wretchedness which are commonplace, particularly in the various depressive disorders, and every doctor should be able to identify such states of mind.

It is important to assess the appropriateness of the patient's state of feeling to the rest of the mental condition, and if it is constant or variable. Shallow emotional responses, or lability of mood, are important and should not be missed.

Feelings can be thought of as having three components: behaviour, physiology and cognition. A person may talk about feelings and refer to any of these domains, or a mixture of them, for example, depression may mean immobility and sad expression (behaviour), constipation and early morning waking (physiology) or sadness or hopelessness (cognition). It is vital that when a feeling word like 'depression' is used in a clinical context, patient and doctor should use the word to refer to the same aspects of experience.

## PERCEPTION

Perceptual processes organize sense data from all the modalities which form the basis of interaction with the environment. Perceptions may be heightened or dulled as in some toxic and delusional states, or as under the influence of hallucinogenic drugs. **Illusions** are distortions of environmental stimuli; they can occur in states of fatigue and anxiety as well as in organic illnesses and in schizophrenia.

**Hallucinations** are false perceptions; they occur in the absence of outside stimuli. Hallucinations do not always signify mental illness – they may occur after sensory deprivation, while going to sleep (hypnogogic) and waking up (hypnopompic), and during normal grief.

Hallucinations may arise in any sense modality, but auditory and visual hallucinations are much commoner than hallucinations of taste, touch or smell. Visual hallucinations should suggest an organic mental state, although they are not uncommon in schizophrenia. Auditory hallucinations may occur in many mental illnesses, but complex voices, including third-person conversations about the subject, or commentaries on their actions, are uncommon except in schizophrenia.

## COGNITIVE FUNCTIONS

Cognition is the means whereby information is stored and retrieved. It involves several functions and processes (Table 27.2). Cognitive function is always impaired in organic mental states. If the level of consciousness is altered or

**Table 27.2** Cognitive functions.

1. Conscious level
2. Orientation
3. Memory
4. Concentration
5. General information
6. Intelligence
7. Insight

fluctuates, and whenever there is disorientation and/or impaired recent memory (even with unimpaired consciousness), then there is some cerebral malfunction.

Orientation includes orientation for time (time, day, month, year), for place (where (s)he is), and person (name, personal details). Disorientation may fluctuate and may be marked at one assessment and absent a few hours later. Hence, repeated observations are of value. In hospital cases, nurses' observations are invaluable.

Memory functions include the learning of new material and the retrieval of newly learned and familiar material. The most important clinical distinction is between recent and distant memory, because organic brain dysfunction invariably interferes with recent memory and the learning of new material first, so that organically impaired patients usually remember things from childhood better than the events of yesterday or today. Simple and useful tests are to give the patient a name and address, making sure that they have repeated it, and test its recall after 5 minutes; and asking them to describe what they did yesterday.

Impairment of concentration is common in organic and 'functional' mental disorders and hence non-specific. Very good concentration usually means the absence of serious mental illness however. So long as arithmetic ability is unimpaired, it can be tested by asking the patient to subtract 7 from 100 and to go on subtracting.

General information is usually assessed as the history is taken, but can also be tested by asking the names of six countries, the names of public figures, some recent important events in the news etc. The patient's educational and cultural background need to be taken into account.

Intelligence is usually assessed during interview, although formal tests may be very informative. Important simple pointers are (a) is the patient literate? and (b) what was their best level of educational attainment?

Insight is a complex notion. It refers to the ideas (and feelings) which the patient has about what is the nature of their problem, for instance, whether they think they are ill in any way. Often a difference between the patient's and the doctor's view of the problem is more important than the details of either opinion, because such disagreements make compliance with treatment more difficult to sustain.

Cognitive assessment is mandatory (with physical examination and appropriate medical investigations) whenever there is any suspicion of organic mental disorder, although it is not required in all other cases (Table 27.3).

**Table 27.3** Psychiatric indications for medical tests.

1. Disorientation ± loss of recent memory or clouded consciousness
2. Lability of mood or other aspects of mental state
3. Paranoid ideas without prehistory
4. Variable delusions of any sort
5. Visual hallucinations
6. Failure of depression to respond to drugs as expected
7. Hysteria or hypochondriasis arising *de novo* over the age of 40

# CLASSIFICATION

Past disagreements about pyschiatric diagnosis and classification have been resolved by the general use of standard systems. In the UK, the ninth and tenth editions of the International Classification of Diseases are most widely used, although a useful alternative is the American Diagnostic and Statistical Manual, 3rd edition revised (DSM-3R). These systems are based on the principle that psychiatric disorders should be operationally defined as syndromes (collections of clinical phenomena).

Classification is often on the basis of syndromes, collections of symptoms which are not in themselves unique to each condition. The delineation of disease entities, where clinical features, pathological and aetiological processes, and prognosis, are all linked together, is not yet possible in psychiatry except in the 'organic' disorders.

Another principle of classification is to define the dimensions in which the study population varies. In this method, people are described in terms of continuous variables (like height or weight) rather than discontinuities (categories) which imply qualitative differences from normal. For instance, unhappiness, grief and sadness, and the various depressive illnesses form a continuum of increasing severity. Dimensions have much to commend them, and make intuitive sense, but categories are easier to use in practice, provided one remembers that they may oversimplify things.

Table 27.4 lists broad categories of psychiatric disorder; the psychiatric assessment should

**Table 27.4** Classes of disorder.

1. Organic disorders
2. Personality disorders
3. Neuroses
4. Disorders allied to neuroses
5. Affective disorders
6. Behaviour disorders
7. The schizophrenias

allow the patient to be placed in one or more of these with confidence. (Classification within these major classes is often not necessary for the non-specialist.) Particular emphasis is given in this chapter to neuroses and disorders allied to them, and the personality and affective disorders.

# AETIOLOGICAL PRINCIPLES

Some general aetiological principles apply to all psychiatric disorders (Table 27.5). Causation of psychiatric disorder is always multifactorial, and biological, psychological and social factors should always be considered.

Different causal influences have different time relations to the onset of psychiatric disorders;

Table 27.6 lists predisposing, precipitating and maintaining aetiological factors. Predisposing factors make the occurrence of a disorder more likely in the presence of other factors required to precipitate or 'bring on' the illness. Once started, a disorder may be 'kept going' by other factors.

The term 'system' in Table 27.5 refers to the

**Table 27.5** Aetiological principles.

1. Multifactorial nature
   Biological
   Psychological
   Social

2. Time course of influence
   Predisposing
   Precipitating
   Maintaining

3. Type of influencing system
   Individual
   Couple
   Family
   Society

4. Relevance of life events and difficulties

5. Relevance of system life-cycle (see text)

**Table 27.6** Aetiological factors.

**Predisposition (risk factors)**
1. Epidemiological influences
2. Genetic constitution
3. Early childhood experience
4. Personality
5. Current psychosocial environment
6. Current biological status

**Precipitation**
1. Acute life events
2. Biological factors

**Maintenance**
1. Social difficulties
2. Personality and psychological influences
3. Biological factors
4. Treatment factors

importance of family, marital and other social relationships as well as individual characteristics in causing ill-health. A 'system' is something that functions as more than the sum of its parts. Couples and families as such, in addition to the individuals in them, have 'lives of their own'.

Principles 4 and 5 in Table 27.5 are important but easily forgotten. Life events *do* often precipitate illness, but illnesses can arise without stressful events, and events which might plausibly have done so, do not always provoke problems.

Individuals, marriages and families, progress through life-cycles, with stages for instance from infancy through childhood and adolescence to adulthood, middle age, old age and death. The life-cycle stage the person is at, or the stage the marriage or family is at, not infrequently precipitates or maintains illness.

# Clinical problems

## PSYCHIATRIC ASPECTS OF MEDICAL PRACTICE

Table 27.7 lists classes of psychiatric problems of importance in the practice of general medicine. The 'organic states' are caused by acute or chronic dysfunction at the cellular level, and are 'psychiatric' as well as medical because they have major effects on emotion, intellect, personality and social relationships.

Affective disorders span the medical and specialist pyschiatric field. Depressive illnesses are extremely common in the community, in primary care, psychiatric clinics and general medical settings, where depression is a most important cause of somatic symptoms unexplained by somatic pathology. Anxiety states are also common, and occur in many specialist medical departments depending on which manifestations of anxiety dominate the clinical picture.

Table 27.7 lists 'somatoform' disorders, a concept which draws together conditions which all involve the presentation of bodily complaints unexplained by somatic pathology. These problems are generally treatable but if not well dealt with may lead to wasted time and resources through repeated clinic attendance and fruitless medical investigation. Appetite problems, also mentioned in the table, are also common and associated with enough morbidity to be of considerable public health significance. In some general hospitals, up to about one-third of acute

**Table 27.7** Psychiatric aspects of clinical problems in medical practice.

1. Organic states
   Acute organic reactions
   Chronic states

2. Affective disorders
   Depression
   Anxiety
   Hypomania

3. Somatoform disorders
   Hysteria
   Hypochondriasis
   Somatization
   Pain

4. Appetite problems
   Eating disorders
   Alcohol problems
   Drug misuse
   Sex problems

5. Suicide and attempted suicide

6. Psychiatric emergencies

7. Post-traumatic stress disorder

mental admissions may be alcohol related in some way.

Self-destructive behaviour, whether or not

leading to completed suicide, has always involved both medical and psychiatric care systems. Self-poisoning is particularly common in many supposedly developed societies, including the UK, and in some places it is the second or third commonest cause of acute medical admission. Acute behavioural emergencies, which may occur in general medical wards or in accident departments, are also at the medical/psychiatric interface.

The results of disasters both man-made and natural (e.g. terrorism, wars in the Middle East and former Yugoslavia, and extensive earthquakes) have increased awareness of troublesome sequelae which may occur. Post-traumatic stress disorders may follow bereavement, or physical or sexual assault, as well as torture, civil accidents, terrorist acts or war experiences.

Every doctor should know how to use psychotropic medication, and understand basic counselling. All more complicated psychological treatment methods build upon the principle of concerned attentive respect which should guide doctors in their interactions with patients.

# $O$RGANIC STATES

## *General aspects*

Organic psychiatric states are caused by dysfunction at the cellular level, and hence by any process which may affect the brain. The clinical manifestations are more the result of (a) the location, (b) the extent of cerebral damage, and (c) the acuteness of the affliction, than (d) the specific pathology involved, although this does play some part. Classification begins by distinguishing acute and chronic states (Table 27.8).

The symptoms of organic states may include a range of impairments of cognitive abilities, emotional and personality functioning, perception and thought content, and also focal signs and symptoms. Nevertheless, the fundamental

**Table 27.8** Organic psychiatric disorders.

**Acute and subacute conditions**
Delirium (acute)
Confusional state (subacute)

**Chronic conditions**
Dementia
Amnesic syndrome
Personality change
Other focal syndromes

rule is that, if the patient is disorientated and has impaired short-term memory, then cerebral dysfunction is present, even without altered consciousness or other symptoms.

## *Clinical features of acute organic states*

In the most acute organic disorder, called **delirium**, consciousness is clouded, and concentration and attention are fleeting and narrow. Onset is usually acute. The patient is disoriented and the environment appears strange and frightening and may be misinterpreted, and fragmentary delusions may develop. The dominant emotion is usually fear, and frightened uncertainty leads to excited overactivity. Symptoms are often worse at night, because perceptual clues may be ambiguous.

In a subacute organic state, consciousness is usually clear, and onset may be slow and the course prolonged. The patient is disorientated and may be perplexed and incoherent, labile or unsettled in mood and unable efficiently to complete sequences of goal directed action. Subacute delirium is very common in medical and surgical wards, and is often missed for days or weeks until the patients slips into frank delirium. Sometimes, a 'difficult' or 'uncooperative' patient is found on careful examination to be vague and muddled, or anxious and querulous, on account of perplexity and misinterpretation of the environment.

# Clinical features of chronic organic states

## DEMENTIA

This clinical syndrome is defined as an acquired global impairment of intellect, memory and personality (Table 27.9). Consciousness is typically clear.

Failure to retain and remember newly registered information, with past information both retained and retrievable until the disease is well advanced, is a constant feature of dementing illnesses, whatever their pathological basis. At first the patient cannot remember to keep appointments, but can get by with a notebook. Later, the patient may become lost while away from home, or so forgetful that everyone else is concerned, even though the person may be unaware themselves of the problem. Concentration fails, and thought becomes vague and muddled. Talk may be repetitive and sparse, and importu-

**Table 27.9** Common clinical features of dementia.

**Cognition**
Disorientation
Poor recent and increasingly also distant memory
Vague, repetitive, importunate, talk

**Emotion**
Lability
Shallowness
Irritability, uncontrolled outbursts
Depression

**Personality and behaviour**
Disinhibition
Loss of self-care
Social failure
Aimless wandering

nate repetitive questioning, especially of basic items such as 'what is for dinner?', is not only common but a very difficult phenomenon for carers to tolerate for long periods of time. As dementia progresses, disorientation increases to include inability to recognize close relatives, or to know one's own personal details such as name and date of birth.

Affective symptoms may develop early in dementia, when the patient is aware of failing powers. Anxiety and sadness, indeed increased arousal of any kind, tends to make cognitive function temporarily even worse. Later, emotional symptoms are caused by lack of higher cerebral control, making mood labile and inappropriately expressed, even to the point of 'emotional incontinence' where feelings are expressed noisily and without any social control, and outbursts of tears, rage or laughter may be sparked off by trivia.

Personality change is probably related to frontal lobe damage. Initially, pre-existing personality traits appear to be exaggerated, but later behaviour becomes coarsened, and increasingly unresponsive to social situations and niceties. Social behaviour becomes uninhibited and inappropriate; tactlessness and rudeness go beyond eccentricity and cause embarrassment. The patient may appear driven to walk about and wander, often more or less aimlessly, and diurnal rhythms may break down. Control of bowel and bladder, and the ability to feed oneself, may cease. The onset of nocturnal wandering, particularly with incontinence, is exceedingly stressful for carers. The end-point may be babbling helpless incoherence, with little remaining of recognizable personality.

## AMNESIC SYNDROME

This focal cerebral disorder arises from the parts of the brain subserving memory (posterior hypothalamus and nearby mid-line structures). Severe loss of memory for recent events is the main feature. A total failure to retain and recall immediate impressions is associated with disorientation for time and place and, very strikingly, a tendency to invent answers to make up for memory gaps (confabulation). Manifestations of dementia which arise from generalized brain damage may be largely absent. In the classic Korsakov's syndrome, the amnesic syndrome and peripheral neuropathy occur in chronic alcoholism with thiamine deficiency. The onset may follow an acute neurological illness with ocular palsies and other deficits, the encephalopathy described by Wernicke. A Korsakov-like picture can be caused by injury, ischaemic disease and various toxins.

## PERSONALITY CHANGE AND OTHER FOCAL SYNDROMES

Frontal lobe damage, for instance, after head injury or subarachnoid haemorrhage, may lead to personality changes similar to those found in dementia but unaccompanied by signs of damage to other parts of the brain. The effects of focal damage to occipital, parietal and temporal lobes are discussed in the chapter on neurology.

It should be noted that some symptoms in organic states express the acuteness of the cerebral malfunction, while others express the extent or the site of it. Organic syndromes indicate that the brain is malfunctioning, but not why this is so.

# *Diagnosis*

This has two steps: first, the identification of an organic psychiatric state; and second, the investigation of its cause(s).

The detection of an abnormal organic mental state should not usually be difficult, provided that the examiner remembers to enquire about orientation and memory, and assess the level of consciousness. Depression may resemble dementia, especially in old people where slowness, apathy and forgetfulness are common in both conditions. Since depression is treatable, a diagnosis of dementia should always have excluded depression. Paranoid and schizophrenic illnesses, and personality disorders, sometimes give rise to diagnostic difficulty and should always be included in the differential diagnosis.

# *Investigations*

Physical examination and appropriate medical investigations will point to the causes of organic psychiatric syndromes. Modern scanning techniques have greatly reduced the need for invasive cerebral investigations such as electroencephalography and lumbar puncture (page 652).

Psychological testing is invaluable in establishing the extent and variety of functional impairment and, when repeated in chronically ill patients, can usefully point to the rate of deterioration.

# *Particular organic syndromes*

As a rough guide, every serious medical disease process should be thought of as liable to cause both acute and subacute or chronic organic psychiatric states, and also disturbances, usually chronic, peculiar to itself. As noted, the clinical features of acute and chronic organic mental syndromes point to *some* medical condition, but not to any particular one. However, signs and symptoms which commonly coexist with abnormal mental states may suggest one medical cause rather than another (Table 27.10). The following clinical points are arranged alphabetically. (Note that this section deals only with organic psychiatric *illnesses* associated with medical disorders; other psychological effects of medical conditions are noted later.)

## CEREBROVASCULAR DISEASES

Subarachnoid haemorrhage may be followed by depression, intellectual deterioration or personality change, particularly if the frontal lobes have been damaged, for instance, by bleeding from an anterior communicating aneurysm.

After cerebral infarction, some degree of emotional, volitional or intellectual impairment, or personality change, is common, and tends to increase with the extent of cerebral damage.

**Table 27.10** Particular organic states.

1. Intoxications
   Drugs
   Barbiturate
   Benzodiazepines
   Steroids
   Alcohol
   Lead
   Mercury
   Manganese

2. Infections
   Acute infections
   Chronic: neurosyphilis, HIV infection

3. Metabolic and endocrine disorders
   Renal failure, hepatic failure
   Thyroid disorders
   Adrenal, pituitary disorders
   Diabetes mellitus
   Electrolyte imbalances
   Porphyria

4. Deficiency diseases
   Pellagra
   Anaemias
   Folate deficiency

5. Cardiac failure

6. Respiratory failure

7. Hepatic and gastroenterological diseases

8. Neurological diseases
   Cerebral tumour
   Multiple sclerosis
   Epilepsy
   Parkinson's disease
   Cerebrovascular disease

9. Presenile and senile dementias

10. Degenerative and traumatic disorders
    Head injury

Depression is common, and also easy to miss when the mechanisms of emotional expression are damaged as is frequently the case.

## DEFICIENCY DISEASES

The weakness, malaise and fatigue of severe anaemia may be mistaken for a depressive or other psychiatric disorder. Folate deficiency should always be remembered in patients on anticonvulsant drugs.

Pellagra (nicotinic acid deficiency) is rare in the UK although occasionally it is seen in alcoholics. The triad of 'diarrhoea, dermatitis and dementia' is classical, although psychiatric symptoms may mask everything.

In pernicious anaemia, anaemia and neurological deficits usually present first, but an organic mental state occasionally dominates the picture.

## DRUG-INDUCED STATES

Alcohol and recreational drugs such as cocaine and amphetamine and their derivatives may cause acute psychotic states with excitement, mood changes, disinhibition, hallucinations and trance-like states.

Barbiturate dependence is associated with withdrawal symptoms, including fits, and also ataxia, nystagmus and dysarthria. Chronic hypnotic use may lead to a paranoid hallucinosis.

Beta-blocking drugs may produce hallucinations and unpleasant mood changes.

Corticosteroids can cause delirium, elation or even manic-like excitement, lability of mood, and paranoid symptoms ('steroid psychosis'). Vague if real symptoms such as weakness or tiredness are often clarified by changing or stopping a drug.

## ELECTROLYTES

Periods of disorientation and altered awareness, often associated with 'feeling generally unwell' and attributable to short-term changes in electrolyte balance, and often also to the effects of drugs and of cerebral anoxia, are common in many acute and chronic afflictions, including congestive cardiac failure and postoperative states.

## ENDOCRINE DISORDERS

These are frequently associated with psychiatric symptoms. Hypothyroidism is often accompanied by depression, which may fail to respond to antidepressant drugs if the medical diagnosis is missed, and may also cause a paranoid psychosis (myxoedema madness). Hyperthyroid patients often have high levels of anxiety, and less often a paranoid or affective illness. In Cushing's syndrome, as with exogenously administered steroids, affective syndromes (including anxiety, depression and elation) and also delirium or a paranoid psychosis may occur.

## EPILEPSY

A confusional state is usual immediately after a grand mal fit, when of course the diagnosis is usually obvious. Psychiatric and behavioural phenomena are, however, particularly associated with focal epilepsy. Temporal lobe fits often start in early life following birth injury and may adversely affect psychosocial development, leading to personality disorder. Episodic aggression, ecstasy or excitement may indicate temporal lobe epileptic activity, and postictal fugue states (wanderings) and memory lapses may occur. A psychosis closely resembling paranoid schizophrenia occurs in some chronic temporal lobe epileptics.

## HEAD INJURY

After open or closed head injury (not severe enough to cause coma) the immediate sequel is often delirium, and depending on the extent of the brain damage the effects may be permanent. Progressive encephalopathy occurs in boxers who have been knocked out repeatedly, and may become known as 'punch drunk' because of the similarity of their slurred speech and staggering gait to the phenomena of alcohol intoxication.

Subdural haematoma should not be overlooked as a cause of a confusional state, or of an apparent dementia, especially in elderly patients, alcoholics and anyone with a history of repeated head injury.

## HEPATIC FAILURE

This causes subacute delirium and coma as part of the syndrome of portal systemic encephalopathy. A flapping tremor and incoordination are well-known signs, and parietal lobe function is often defective. The subacute delirious state may mimic irritable depression.

## INFECTIONS

Acute infections produce delirium in high fevers, but these disappear when the infection is controlled. Chronic infections which affect cerebral function may produce very varied psychiatric pictures dominated by emotional symptoms (depression, mania or mood lability), paranoid or other psychotic states, or dementia. Neurosyphilis is a classic example. Human immunodeficiency virus (HIV) infection affects brain function, and acquired immune deficiency syndrome (AIDS) may also be accompanied by a range of psychiatric syndromes. It seems likely that when clinical AIDS can be diagnosed, some degree of neuropsychological impairment can invariably be found, if carefully sought for.

## INTOXICATIONS

These are rare causes of organic psychiatric states, but should not be forgotten. Lead can produce encephalopathy or dementia; manganese and carbon monoxide extrapyramidal signs and dementia; and mercury tremor and dementia.

## PORPHYRIA

Acute intermittent porphyria (page 498) is a rare inherited metabolic disorder, the symptoms of which include peripheral neuropathy, abdominal pains, skin changes, and also psychiatric states akin to neurosis, depression or hypomania, although delirium is most frequent. Attacks may be precipitated by drugs such as barbiturates, alcohol, sulphonamides or chloroquine.

## RENAL FAILURE

This causes subacute delirium and coma.

## TUMOURS

There is nothing specific about organic psychiatric states caused by cerebral tumours. If there are focal signs, or signs of raised intracranial pressure, then the diagnosis is more easily made, but about 30 per cent of brain tumours start in 'silent' areas and psychiatric symptoms are present in about 60 per cent. Patients presenting – especially in middle age or later – with unexpected cognitive or personality deterioration should always be investigated for subacute cerebral pathology, particularly tumour or subdural haematoma.

# Presenile dementia

As already noted, dementia is a syndrome. Dementias are classified in terms of the age at which they occur; presenile dementias occur before, and the dementias of later life after, the age of 65 years.

Presenile dementia can be caused by the wide range of disorders mentioned in the preceding section if their effects are severe and prolonged enough. In addition, there are several types of primary cerebral degeneration, all rare, which give rise to specific forms of presenile dementia. Pick's and Alzheimer's diseases are clinically somewhat similar, although with different pathologies: in **Pick's disease**, frontal lobe signs predominate with cortical atrophy; the neuronal loss in **Alzheimer's disease** affects the whole brain with amyloid plaques and neurofibrillary tangles. Huntington's disease is a rare autosomal dominant disorder which most usually presents in the 40s or 50s with involuntary movements and perhaps also depression and memory impairment. Suicide is a feature, and sometimes the first and last sign of illness. In due time, dementia inevitably supervenes, and survival rarely exceeds 10–15 years beyond diagnosis. Jakob–Creutzfeldt disease is rare but of interest because of its similarities to bovine spongiform encephalopathy, known to be due to a slow virus. Dementia is associated with myoclonus, epilepsy, extrapyramidal signs and a rapidly downhill course. Normal pressure hydrocephalus is a rare cause of presenile dementia, but important because surgical treatment may be curative.

# Dementing illness in old age

This is a major and increasing public health problem wherever increasing numbers of people are surviving into their 70s and beyond. There are two common forms of dementia in old age.

Multi-infarct dementia (formerly 'arteriosclerotic') tends to start in the 60s rather than later. The onset may be insidious, or marked by an apparently recovered focal 'stroke' or an episode of delirium. The course is typically progressively generally downhill, although with episodic worsenings ('little strokes') with partial recovery. Survival once the disease is clearly established is rarely beyond 2 years. 'Organic' mental state signs (disorientation etc.) which become progressively more marked may be accompanied from time to time by other symptoms such as marked anxiety, hypochondriacal complaining, or querulous, paranoid behaviour.

What used to be known simply as 'senile dementia' is now referred to as **senile dementia of Alzheimer type** (SDAT) because of the neuropathological similarities with (presenile) Alzheimer's disease. Senile dementia of Alzheimer type is increasingly common over age 75 – upwards of one-quarter of the over 85s may suffer from it. Women tend to live longer than men, so there are more women than men with this disease. Pathologically, there is progressive reduction in numbers of cortical cells and consequent cerebral atrophy, reduced brain mass, and increased ventricular size. Microscopic examination shows 'neurofibrillary tangles' of the twisted fibrils of degenerated nerve cells, and 'senile plaques' containing amyloid. The cholinergic transmitter system in the cortex fails, with reduced synthesis of choline acetyl transferase. There is evidence of a genetic contribution to this disease, and attention has recently focussed on chromosome 21 because an excess of early Alzheimer's disease has been found to occur in individuals with Down's syndrome in which trisomy of chromosome 21 occurs.

Clinically, the onset is usually insidious and the course progressive over 3–5 years or even longer, usually depending on the person's physical health. The care of demented people often makes enormous demands on carers, most of whom are relatives who may sacrifice much to keep the person at home as long as possible. Continual questioning, unpredictable wandering, incontinence, nocturnal restlessness and aggressive attacks are some of the behaviours which may be particularly hard for relatives to cope with.

## PERSONALITY AND PERSONALITY DISORDERS

Personality is like a coin with the two sides being the person's view of themselves, and others' views of them. It is what people refer to when they ask, 'what sort of a person is this?' It is helpful to think of personality under three headings

1. Attribute
2. Problem
3. Disorder

Personality attributes are just that, and are often relevant to an understanding of a patient's current difficulties. Personality attributes become personality problems when they are regarded as in some way unsatisfactory by the person themselves or by others with whom they interact. Personality disorders represent more extreme variations from normal, and represent clusters of attributes which form syndromes of clinical importance (Table 27.11). People with severe personality disorders often find it difficult to fit into society.

### SCHIZOID PERSONALITY

Schizoid people are inward looking and tend to be shy, self-absorbed and withdrawn, perhaps with eccentric interests. They may be aloof and yet have a vivid fantasy life or a dreamy intellectualism making them very ineffective at complex tasks when emotion interferes with performance. If depressed, the schizoid person may have atypical symptoms.

### OBSESSIONAL PERSONALITY

Obsessional people are troubled by guilt and self-doubt and are perfectionist and over-conscientious, sometimes to a handicapping

**Table 27.11** Varieties of personality disorder.

1. Schizoid
2. Obsessional
3. Paranoid
4. Hysterical
5. Antisocial
6. Asthenic
7. Others

Note: These are categories from the International Classification of Diseases (ICD) system. Different terms appear, including 'Borderline personality disorder', in the American Diagnostic and Statistical Manual (DSM) system, currently in its third edition, revised (DSM-3R).

degree. The obsessional person tends to make a good subordinate but a bad leader, a combination which runs the risk of promotion beyond one's competence and hence breakdown. There is a sense of being driven to attain perfection with its inevitable sense of failure despite the approval of others. Obsessional people are prone to depression and hypochondriasis, and tend to be overcontrolling and worried parents who engender insecurities and anxiousness in their children.

### PARANOID PERSONALITY

The paranoid person is suspicious, touchy and oversensitive, and overreacts to criticism either real or fancied. A basic sense of injustice may be channelled into a 'cause' but this can be carried to extremes which embarrass friends. The paranoid tendency to overvalue ideas and resent criticism can build up into bitterness and even violence.

### HYSTERICAL PERSONALITY

Applied to personality, the term 'hysterical' means 'histrionic' not 'prone to conversion hysteria' (see later). The histrionic person is egocentric, emotionally shallow and labile and prone to outbursts or displays of emotional activity. Sudden bouts of gloom may pass to be replaced by an unexpected infatuation or enthusiasm which fails to last. Behaviour tends to be dramatic and importunate, and relationships to be unstable.

## ANTISOCIAL (PSYCHOPATHIC) PERSONALITY

Nowadays the terms 'antisocial personality' and 'psychopath' are synonymous. The person with an antisocial personality presents society with many problems (Table 27.12). In many ways, the behaviour is reminiscent of a child who flies into a rage when its immediate wish is not granted. A major task for health and social services is to minimize the damage which psychopathic individuals can do, especially in the realm of domestic relationships.

## ASTHENIC PERSONALITY

This category has been losing fashion but the idea of 'lack of vigour in facing life's challenges' is a very helpful one in understanding people who seem to be surrounded by an unending sequence of social and personal disorders.

## OTHERS

In the American DSM system, personality disorders are called 'Axis 2' problems, illnesses (i.e. states) being rated on Axis 1. Several categories unfamiliar in the UK are used in DSM, but borderline personality is being more widely used. This term draws attention to the tendency of some people to have problems through having an inconstant sense of 'self' and hence a tendency to move from time to time into different states of mind and behaviour which may include alcohol or drug abuse, and relationship difficulties, so that there is some overlap with antisocial personality.

Table 27.13 summarizes the clinical importance of personality and its disorders.

**Table 27.12** Antisocial (psychopathic) personality: clinical importance.

| Problem | Notes |
| --- | --- |
| 1. Aggression | Violence to wife/partner/child; damage to property. Hence criminal contacts |
| 2. Acquisitiveness | Stealing property and money |
| 3. Alcohol + drug abuse | Medical and psychosocial effects |
| 4. Psychiatric illness | Depression, paranoid disorders, anxiety |
| 5. Relationships | Marital breakdown, child abuse, infidelity |
| 6. Social | Unemployment, money problems |
| 7. Medical | Injuries, intoxicant consequences |

**Table 27.13** Clinical importance of personality.

1. Personality disorders cause much suffering
2. They make psychiatric diagnosis more difficult
3. They predispose to psychiatric illness and behaviour difficulties
4. Personality attributes affect the content of every psychiatric illness; coping with the illness; compliance with treatment
5. Illness may be precipitated by personality problems

# AFFECTIVE DISORDER AND NEUROSIS

Affective disorders all have a primary disturbance of mood, with symptoms in the areas of cognition, behaviour and physiological function. The mood is elevated in mania, and lowered in the depressive disorders.

All emotions, not just elevated and lowered

moods, have cognitive, behavioural and physiological components. Different emotions may coexist or lead to one another, yet tend to have specific cognitive and behavioural features. However, physiological patterns are similar in different emotions because of their common substrate of autonomic and central arousal, and hence some symptoms are common to all emotional states.

Depression, hypomania, the anxiety disorders and obsessive-compulsive disorders are considered in this section. Hysteria, often dealt with under 'neurosis', is considered under 'somatoform' disorders.

# Depression

In clinical practice, depression is common, important, potentially serious and often confusing. The core feature of depressive illness is persistent lowered mood, but this is not only associated with depressive illness (Table 27.14), and clinicians deal with it whether or not it amounts to illness. People sometimes seek help in coping with normal sadness, usually if they lack the domestic or family support of confiding relationships which ordinarily enable people to manage their distress. Clinicians should be willing and able to respond to distress, usually by some means of counselling, without misidentifying it as amounting to depressive illness.

The commonest circumstance in which lowered mood amounts to illness is when it is more prolonged or more intense than it should be in response to something 'depressing'; but it can be hard to be sure about this in practice because so often the 'something depressing' is a long-standing set of depressing difficulties rather than an acute trauma. Sometimes, the mood in depression is unlike that of normal sadness, but (except when depressive illnesses are at their most severe) this is not common and it more often makes sense to think of sadness and depressive illness as on a continuum of severity.

The events which tend to provoke sadness and depression are those which represent significant loss to the person. Hence the effect of bereavement depends on the closeness and kind of relationship the survivor had with the dead person, and for some the death of a pet or failing an examination may be as catastrophic as any loss through death. Sometimes people wrongly attribute their feelings to one event rather than another, an easily understood tendency because several stressful events may impinge on a person at the same time, and also because of the natural tendency to try and convince oneself that the event has not happened (the mechanism of 'denial').

If a lowered mood state amounts to a depressive illness, then a diagnosis of the type of

**Table 27.14** States of lowered mood.

|  | Depressive illness | Normal sadness | Normal grief |
|---|---|---|---|
| 1. Mood intensity | Usually > normal | Normal | May be > normal |
| 2. Mood duration | > Normal | Normal | If prolonged = abnormal |
| 3. Quality | Usually normal | Normal (variable) | Relatively constant |
| 4. Onset | Definite ? gradual | After sad event | After bereavement |
| 5. Relationship to events | (a) Absent<br>(b) As with sadness<br>(c) Other event<br>(d) Unusual timecourse<br>(e) Attribution problem | Constant; notable time relationship | Constant; notable time relationship |

depression is required (Table 27.15). The depressed phase of a bipolar disorder, and an episode of unipolar depression, can be distinguished only in terms of the presence or absence of a history of mania, for their clinical features are identical. The student may encounter the terms 'psychotic' and 'endogeneous' depression; episodes to which these terms are applied are those which here are called unipolar or depressed bipolar. 'Psychotic' refers to symptoms such as delusions and hallucinations, and 'endogeneous' to disturbances of sleep, nutrition etc. which are all largely consequences of severity of depressive illness. Sometimes, 'endogenous' has in addition been used misleadingly to draw attention to the mistaken but supposed non-precipitation of this form of depression by life events. The student should assume that all forms of depression may be 'reactive' in the sense of being precipitated by loss-mediating life events.

Many patients with a depressive state and no history of hypomania are difficult to allocate to 'unipolar' rather than 'neurotic' depression. The author's practice is to reserve the 'unipolar' category for patients with a definite family history of depression (but not mania) and marked 'biological' and/or 'psychotic' features, with 'depressive neurosis' for others. Within 'depressive neurosis', it is sometimes helpful to distinguish subsyndromes in terms of (a) anxious depression, (b) hostile depression, and (c) depression with personality disorder.

## AETIOLOGY

About 15 per cent of women have significant clinical depression (often unrecognized by doctors and untreated) in some community studies. This is usually associated with some if not all of the predisposing factors listed in Table 27.16.

**Table 27.15** Varieties of depressive illness.

| Diagnostic category | Distinguishing features |
|---|---|
| 1. Depressive phase of manic-depressive illness | For a bipolar diagnosis, a hypomanic episode must have occurred. Bipolar family history is suggestive |
| 2. Unipolar depression | Definite onset; state out of proportion to any precipitant<br>Unipolar family history is suggestive |
| 3. Depressive neurosis | Onset may be gradual, linked with chronic social ± personality difficulties |
| 4. Secondary depression | Severe ± prolonged enough to be an illness, but another illness present |
| (a) Other psychiatric disorder present | Schizophrenia, alcoholism, drug misuse, anorexia nervosa, post-traumatic stress disorder, adjustment reactions, anxiety and obsessive illness |
| (b) Physical disorder present | Many, but note especially cancers, strokes, dementias, Parkinsonism, endocrine disorders etc. |

**Table 27.16** Aetiology of depression.

**A. Predisposition**
1. Genetic vulnerability (bipolar and unipolar disorders)
2. Gender: women > men
3. Race: Jews > others
4. Class: working > middle class
5. Early experience: loss of parent in childhood
          abuse
          deprivation
6. Personality: habitual low self-esteem
         marked obsessionality
         cyclothymic traits
7. Life transitions: childbirth, retirement
8. Psychosocial stresses: chronic relationship problems
          long-standing deprivation

**B. Precipitants**
1. Acute loss events
2. Acute physical illnesses
3. Certain drugs

**C. Protective factors**
1. At least one rewarding close relationship
2. Satisfactory family structure
3. Biological status

The commonest pattern is when the woman has been sensitized to loss in childhood by deprivation or abuse which may be physical, sexual or mental. Early parental loss is particularly hard to cope with, leading to chronic low self-esteem and perhaps also other personality problems. This makes the person vulnerable to respond to later acute loss events with lowered mood beyond the normal, i.e. depressive illness. The fact that a good current confiding relationship protects against this sort of depression points to the importance of marital therapy in helping to prevent depression in vulnerable women.

The importance of biological factors should be remembered. Illnesses such as jaundice and other virus infections are very debilitating and associated with depression often enough for this to be on occasion a true causal connection. 'Depressogenic' drugs include methyl dopa, phenobarbitone and reserpine, now infrequently or never used but of considerable theoretical interest because they point to the importance of central nervous system (CNS) transmitters (catecholamines and indoleamines) in mediating mood experiences and in the ways people respond to stress.

## CLINICAL FEATURES

Words do not easily do justice to the wide range of feelings that can contribute to the core experience of lowered mood in depression. Despair, pessimism, guilt, apathy, tearfulness, gloom, endless self-scrutiny, multiple somatic symptoms, or morbid intrusive thoughts may all at times be dominant (Table 27.17). Negative evaluation of self, the world, the past, the future and other people are usually conspicuous features. It is important to remember that changes in energy level, sense of volitional purpose, or the ability to enjoy things, may be more prominent than any actual sadness. A clear dated onset of a state that is abnormal for that individual is the most important feature of all.

Psychomotor retardation and agitation represent opposite poles of a single activation—inhibition dimension. Retardation is shown by delayed answers to questions which are to the point although usually brief when they do come. Retardation and agitation, and the painful experience of mood change which is the core depressive experience, may all colour and also be obscured by behavioural problems such as alcohol or drug excesses, diminished sexual, work or

**Table 27.17** Clinical features of depression.

| | | |
|---|---|---|
| 1. Mood: | Lowered | |
| | May show diurnal variation | |
| | May lose responsiveness to outside events | |
| | Anhedonia or anergia may be more obvious than sadness | |
| | Malaise | |
| | Irritability, anxiety, tension | |
| | Feelings of apathy, inertia, loss of volition | |
| 2. Behaviour: | Increased in amount, and faster, in agitation | |
| | Reduced in amount, and slowed, in retardation | |
| | Depressive posture and gait | |
| | Altered and deteriorated work performance | |
| | Changed sexual behaviour (quantity ± quality) | |
| | Altered relationship behaviour | |
| | Misuse of alcohol and/or drugs | |
| | Reduced self-care | |
| 3. Thought process: | Speeded in agitation; slowed in retardation | |
| | Poverty of thought (can be without retardation) | |
| | Poor concentration | |
| | Memory impairment | |
| 4. Thought content: | Hopelessness, helplessness, worthlessness | |
| | Delusions – hypochondriacal, nihilistic, paranoid | |
| | Self-destructive thoughts, suicidal plans | |
| | Somatic preoccupations – bowels, pains, headaches | |
| 5. Perception: | 'Depressive' view of the world | |
| | Mood congruent hallucinations | |
| | Slowed subjective sense of time passing | |
| 6. Physical symptoms: | Weight loss (sometimes increase) | |
| | Appetite reduction (sometimes increase) | |
| | Disturbed sleep | |
| | Diurnal variation of mood | |
| 7. Insight: | Impaired (depressive view of things) | |

relationship performance, or reduced self-care.

Problems of thought process and content are some of the most important manifestations of depression. The 'cognitive triad' of hopelessness, helplessness and worthlessness predisposes to depression when it exists as a personality factor but also is a feature of acute depressive states. Somatic preoccupations are extremely common, and may dominate the clinical picture, especially in cases presenting in general medical settings. Preoccupations may have the quality of obsessional ruminations and are experienced as fitting in with the general mood state. If the patient has physical symptoms of the kind common in depression, but the mood is not experienced as lowered, then the diagnosis should not be depression, but some sort of somatoform disorder.

The so-called biological symptoms of depression, by which is usually meant early morning waking, diurnal variation of mood (typically worse in the morning), reduced appetite and weight, and disturbed sleep and sexual function, are not necessary for the diagnosis, and often reflect either severity (worse in more severe cases) or age (more common in older patients).

Insight is always important when depression is in question. Frequently the patient appears reasonable and able to make sensible decisions, yet is transpires that their view of everything has a pervasive negative bias which renders their judgement unreliable. Of course, when suicidal sentiments are dominant, special care is required to assess risk of self-harm.

## DIAGNOSIS

The steps here are first, to see if a state of illness/distress exists; second, to see if the state amounts to a depressive illness; and third, to identify the variety of depressive disorder being dealt with. After that, the formulation should summarize the factors relevant to the genesis and maintenance of the illness. The most important pointers are first, the presence of a dateable onset of a change in personal functioning (which distinguishes between a 'state' and a personality phenomenon, though chronic illnesses cause difficulties here); second, distinguishing the state as outside the limits of normal sadness; and third, a history of hypomania, a positive family history, or the coexistence of another physical or mental disorder.

## HYPOMANIA

The term 'mania' is rarely used today because patients are usually treated before they reach the extreme states to which 'mania' applies. Hypomania simply means somewhat less than mania; it can still be an extremely disturbed state, until treated.

The basis of hypomania is elevation of mood leading to increased activity and energy, elation and disinhibition. In the milder states, the patient undertakes and achieves more than usual, and is more self-confident and decisive. The patient becomes wakeful and perhaps begins new projects at night. There may be little apparent need for food. As mood elevation increases, judgement becomes impaired and activity becomes more disinhibited and tends towards grandiosity. By this stage it becomes important to protect the patient from the personally damaging consequences of the fiscal, sexual or other imprudence to which the morbid state leads. In the extreme case, there may be grandiose delusions, uncontrollable activity and excitement, continuous noise and movement, and ultimately a risk of physical exhaustion.

Hypomania is of clinical importance as a major part of the clinical picture of bipolar illness. This, with schizophrenia, is the heartland of specialist psychiatry and not dealt with in further detail here. The general hospital clinician needs to be aware that bipolar patients may present with episodes of hypomania in various ways, and that states of excitement resembling hypomania states may occur (Table 27.18).

**Table 27.18** Clinical implications of hypomanic states.

1. Bipolar illness – presentations in general hospital
   Accident department emergencies
   Alcohol-related problems
   Concurrent medical/surgical illness

2. Other causes of elated excitement
   Intoxications – illicit drugs
   Side effects of prescribed drugs, e.g. steroids
   Encephalopathies, e.g. hepatic and renal failure
   Infections, e.g. AIDS, neurosyphilis

# Anxiety disorders

Anxiety is the experience of the possibility, but not the certainty, of something happening. In itself it is normal and adaptive, tending to occur when the person needs to consider what might be done in a situation and serving to mobilize biological and psychological resources in readiness for appropriate action. In anxiety and panic disorders, the anxiety is abnormal in being more intense, or more prolonged, than the occasion demands, or in having no discernible relationship to external stimuli. In **phobias** anxiety is occurring in response to something which is objectively not at all dangerous. A phobia is an irrational (i.e. an unnecessary) fear; anxiety not associated with an object is sometimes called 'free-floating'. High levels of anxiety can also occur as part of other clinical syndromes, notably depressive and obsessional illnesses and somatoform disorders. Normal and abnormal anxiety are linked in a curvilinear relationship with performance in the so-called Yerkes–Dodson law: performance suffers if anxiety is too low *or* too high.

## CLINICAL FEATURES

The clinical features of anxiety are summarized in Table 27.19.

Cognitive and behavioural aspects of anxiety are relatively specific to the anxious experience; but the physiological manifestations resemble those of other causes of autonomic arousal, including every variety of emotional experience. Also, environmental demands on a person stimulate arousal, and this serves to facilitate appropriate responses, including 'fight or flight'. Whether or not arousal is experienced as any particular emotion appears to depend on the cognitive structure attached to it, and arousal which orients the person to the environment is not always experienced as emotional at all. When arousal is neither experienced as emotion nor effectively adapts the individual to the environment, it may lead to impressions of changed bodily function and (if complained about) somatic symptoms without somatic cause or characteristic emotional signs (see somatoform disorders below).

**Table 27.19** Clinical features of anxiety.

**1. Cognition–experience**
Mood: scared
Thinking: speed increased, disjointed trains of thought
Preoccupations: with the objects of fear/anxiety, or unfinished business, or future uncertainty

**2. Behaviour**
Expression: worried, furrowed brow
Motor activity: increased
Goal-directed activity: interrupted
Avoidance: of objects of fear

**3. Physiology**
Sleep: interrupted, restless
Autonomic arousal: increased (tachycardia, tachypnoea, urinary frequency, diarrhoea, pupillary dilation, tremor, headache, muscular tension, sweating, skin colour change, fainting, giddiness, tingling in extremities)

In anxiety, panic and phobic disorders, the predominant symptoms are, respectively, free-floating anxiety, panic attacks, and phobic anxiety and avoidance. Established free-floating anxiety usually evolves into depression in time, and panic attacks are rare without some degree of generalized anxiety. Also, the most severe phobic illness, agoraphobia, not infrequently includes both free-floating anxiety and panics, and also depression, as well as the characteristic pattern of anxiety in relation to situations which involve being away from the home and safety, and avoidance of these.

Agoraphobia occurs most often in young women aged 18–35. The typical patient is anxious about travelling by car, bus, train or even on foot; about shopping or being in crowds; and perhaps about being trapped in enclosed spaces as well as being exposed in open ones. Anxiety is usually reduced by being accompanied by a close relative or friend, or even a pet or talisman.

Other phobic disorders include social and specific fears. Social phobias are equally common in men and women and include anxieties about speaking, vomiting, eating or drinking, being seen, or (in men) urinating in public. Specific phobias are common in childhood up to puberty, and are more likely to persist into adulthood in women, usually unaccompanied by other psychiatric problems. Most fears are of animals such as cats, dogs, rats, mice, spiders or snakes, to which the patient responds as if exposed to objective danger. Phobias are usually responsive to psychological treatments.

# Obsessional disorder

Obsessions include ideas, phrases and actions which a person feels compelled to repeat against a feeling of inner resistance. Obsessions are unpleasant for the sufferer and may cause anxiety and depression. They are intrusive, very like the common childhood experience of 'having to' avoid cracks between paving stones. Obsessions occur in many abnormal mental states, but in obsessional disorder they dominate the clinical picture. The disorder usually begins early in life and tends to run a chronic course, sometimes with a relentless state of shame and tension perpetuated by the obsessions and rituals. However, the prognosis is less bad than was once thought and long periods of remission may occur. Depression is a common complication.

Obsessions are regularly helped by treating any concurrent depression; by admission to hospital, where the externally imposed routine allows less time for obsessional behaviour; and by behavioural psychotherapy.

# SOMATOFORM DISORDERS

These disorders are varieties of medically un-explained bodily distress. They may be very dis-abling, and are often associated with repeated, time-consuming, and unrewarding contact with doctors and hospitals.

# Conversion disorder (hysteria)

This disorder involves loss of function of some bodily part without structural damage to ac-count for it. Typically the presentation resem-bles, but is not identical to, some physical condition. Well-recognized varieties include hysterical paralysis, loss of sensation, blindness and deafness, and amnesia. The diagnosis re-quires the identification of a conflict to which the development of the physical symptom is a response. The idea of 'conversion' is that the pain and distress of the conflict is somehow changed (converted) into or expressed as the physical symptom; the (primary) gain is relief of distress, but at the cost of the disability from the symp-tom. An established symptom may evoke con-cerned attention from relatives, friends, and medical and nursing personnel, or allow the patient 'sick leave' from work, which may represent 'secondary gains' for the patient.

The term 'hysteria' is used in distinct ways which should be distinguished from each other (Table 27.20).

**Table 27.20** Meanings of 'hysteria'.

1. Conversion hysteria

2. Somatization ('Briquet's syndrome')
   Multiple somatic symptoms vaguely called 'hysterical'

3. Anxiety hysteria
   Freud applied this term to patients who would nowadays be assigned a specific syndrome diagnosis

4. Mass hysteria
   Distressing and unusual crowd beliefs and/or behaviour

5. Hysterical personality traits and disorder

6. Lay uses of 'hysteria' (typically vague)

# Hypochondriasis

What makes an experience hypochondriacal is overconcern, often associated with worry and anxiety, about some aspect of health or personal functioning. The word 'fascination' conveys the essential point. Hypochondriasis is not simply a matter of imagining you have a disease when you do not; it is quite possible to have a hypochondriacal attitude to a definitely existing disease. Nor is hypochondriasis confined to concerns about bodily disease; concern about psychological function ('psychiatric hypochondriasis') is nowadays not at all uncommon.

Nevertheless in terms of management it is important to distinguish between states in which hypochondriacal experiences may occur (Table 27.21). Patients with psychotic hypochondriacal states unaccompanied by other signs of serious pyschiatric disorder usually attend physicians and are often reluctant to be assigned a psychiatric diagnosis. Examples are delusions that the hair is falling out, or about the emission of a smell, or of parasites under the skin.

Many non-psychotic hypochondriacal experiences have phobic or obsessional characteristics as well as the essential fascination which makes them hypochondriacal, and anxiety is usually linked with them in some way. A common variety is a phobia of cancer which is associated with recurrent thoughts about the possibility of serious illness and death.

**Table 27.21** Hypochondriacal states.

**Hypochondriacal worrying ± obsessions ± phobias**
1. With physical disease
2. Without physical disease

**Hypochondriacal delusions**
1. In depressive illness
2. In schizophrenia
3. In organic psychoses
4. With no other signs of depression, schizophrenia or organic psychosis

# Somatization disorder

This category includes patients who may have very varied somatic symptoms over long periods of time, and engage in exceedingly extensive help-seeking behaviour. Typically, the experience of a troublesome sensation in some part of the body leads to consultation and then referral for the relevant specialist investigation. When 'nothing abnormal is found', a symptom in another body part may develop, leading to further consultation and referral. The whole process is exceedingly wasteful of patient and professional time.

Not uncommonly, one or more investigations disclose some degree of abnormality, perhaps warranting specialist attention even if insufficient to explain all symptoms and the associated disability. These cases tend to become particularly entrenched hospital attenders.

While as indicated, many somatizing patients attend multiple hospital departments, some develop a somatizing state which is more department and system specific. In fact all medical specialties have their own variety of this — and new specialties soon develop theirs. Some examples are in Table 27.22.

Somatizing disorders are treatable, but require time and that the patient's concerns and

**Table 27.22** Varieties of somatization disorder.

1. Cardiac: 'effort syndrome', 'chest pain with normal coronary arteries'
2. Respiratory: hyperventilation
3. Gastroenterological: 'irritable bowel'
4. Neurological: 'hysteroepilepsy'
5. Rheumatological: 'back pain', 'fibrositis'
6. Other medical: 'myalgic encephalomyelitis', complaints of allergies to foods, computers, various environmental features or of being poisoned by such
7. Surgical: 'Munchausen's syndrome'
8. Dental: successive removal of normal teeth
9. Pain syndromes

symptoms are taken seriously and adequately discussed. Treatment is usually more acceptable to the patient when psychiatrist or psychologist collaborate closely with physician; patients can with advantage be seen on medical rather than psychiatric territory.

# Pain

Pain often originates in a body part which is injured or threatened, and serves to draw this to the attention of the sufferer, who is stimulated to behave accordingly, usually to reduce damage or danger. Often, this action sequence involves other people associated with the sufferer, including health care personnel. This is inevitable whenever pain of any cause continues for more than a few hours.

These social dimensions of pain mean that social rewards or disincentives follow pain behaviour and hence tend to increase or decrease it (act as positive or negative reinforcers). *This is so whatever the origin of the pain.* Not infrequently, pain complaints and behaviour are more than justified by the physical pathology which is present. On these occasions, full psychosocial assessment and psychological treatment measures may be invaluable. Commonly, depression of mood (which invariably makes pain feel worse) is found to be present; or problems may have arisen from the association of significant personal rewards with the whole complex of pain behaviour (e.g. it may be gratifying to find people more solicitous and expecting less of one than before the pain began).

# Appetite and Behaviour Disorders

An important group of problems is associated with the ways in which people deal with appetite. Complex psychological and social arrangements can be built upon fundamental biological drives. Eating and weight regulation, the satisfaction of thirst and the self-administration of chemicals with mental effects, and the expression of sexuality share a sense of drive with the capacity to generate problems via actions later or concurrently regretted. The theme of 'how do I control myself' is common to all these areas.

# Eating disorders

Three main disorders are of clinical importance: anorexia nervosa, bulimia and obesity.

## ANOREXIA NERVOSA

Anorexia nervosa was described by Sir William Gull in the late nineteenth century. It is a syndrome characterized by food refusal which leads to weight loss and (in girls) amenorrhoea. (In some cases the amenorrhoea precedes any substantial weight loss, so clearly more than one mechanism may operate.) Usually the anorectic has a normal appetite; the problem is of refusal to eat and the development of various abnormal food-related behaviours. The patient may hide food or throw it away, or make themselves vomit or ingest large quantities of purgatives. Intense physical activity is remarkable, and characteristic; in an advanced case continued overactivity contrasts with the emaciated bodily appearance.

The weight loss in anorexia nervosa may be severe and lead to marked electrolyte disturbances with dehydration and dangerously low potassium levels. There may be significant depression of mood or distressing obsessional ruminations.

The food refusal is based upon a morbid fear of being fat. The anorectic sees herself (her self-image) as fatter than she really is. The fear is partly determined by social pressures, including advertizing which exhorts the virtues of slimness, and partly by developmental and family pressures, for instance, related to the transition from childhood to adulthood in adolescence.

Anorexia is commoner in girls than boys (10:1) and usually begins before the age of 20, although cases starting much later have been reported. It is a serious condition, with a mortality of about 4 per cent. Some patients continue in a chronic anorexic state for years, while others recover to normal weight and mature both physically and psychologically. Treatment is primarily psychosocial; drugs play only a minor part.

Anorexia often presents to physicians rather than psychiatrists, perhaps with amenorrhoea or gastroenterological complaints such as diarrhoea or vomiting with the self-induced nature of the phenomenon concealed. A detailed behavioural analysis of the patient's food-related behaviour is the best pointer to the diagnosis.

## BULIMIA

Bulimia overlaps with anorexia to the extent that self-induced vomiting is a feature. However, normal weight is often maintained, and episodic bingeing and chaotic dietary habits generally are conspicuous. The patient is usually exceedingly ashamed of their behaviour, and preoccupied with what they regard as their inability to control themselves. Once again, treatment is psychological in nature.

## OBESITY

Obesity is a major health problem in all affluent countries, the problem increasing greatly as the weight increases beyond norms based principally on age and gender. As weight increases, its psychological implications also tend to increase; weight and eating become associated with mood and emotional interchange in the family and weight reduction may be difficult because of adverse emotional consequences which have negative feedback effects. Severe obesity always warrants a thorough psychosocial assessment.

# Alcohol

Alcohol has pleasurable effects and its use is condoned by many societies despite its dangers.

Acutely, alcohol taken in large enough amounts can produce coma and death. Very small doses can be shown to impair cognitive efficiency (for instance, motor driving skills), and the social disinhibition which can be one of alcohol's attractions is accompanied by impaired awareness of the impact of one's behaviour. As many as one-third of acute medical and surgical admissions to general hospitals are related to the physical, psychological or social effects of alcohol. Chronic alcoholism is a state in which a person is unable to control the amount they drink and so develops physical, psychological and social handicaps in consequence. The harmful effects of chronic alcohol misuse are listed in Table 27.23.

Severe alcoholism is not really hard to diagnose, but doctors still sometimes have a blind spot for someone whose drinking is getting out of control, especially someone reasonably high in the social scale, such as another doctor. Warning signs for drink becoming a problem are listed in Table 27.24.

# Drug misuse

'Non-medical use' distinguishes the use of drugs for pleasure or to relieve distress from the therapeutic administration of drugs. Care must be taken to ensure that people do not become dependent on drugs prescribed for them by doctors. **Dependence** is a state in which a person has to go on taking a drug (the same applies to alcohol) because of the pleasurable effects when they take it and/or the unpleasant effects if they stop taking it. Most drugs which can make people feel better are potential drugs of dependence.

Drug dependence has physical and psychological aspects. The relative importance of these vary from one dependence-producing substance to another. Thus in the case of opiate dependence, physical dependence is usually severe but presents no risk to life; in alcohol and barbiturate dependence, chronic dependence produces a state in which acute withdrawal may lead to fits which may be fatal.

Which substances are misused, and how they

**Table 27.23** Harmful effects of chronic abuse of alcohol.

## Medical
1. Increased mortality from increased incidence of many diseases, especially ischaemic heart disease, hypertension and cerebrovascular disease
2. Cardiac
   Heart muscle disease
3. Gastrointestinal
   Peptic ulcer
   Pancreatitis
   Cirrhosis
4. Thoracic
   Liability to tuberculosis
5. Neurological
   Cerebellar failure
   Peripheral neuropathy
   Amnesic syndrome
   Subdural haemorrhage
   Wernicke's encephalopathy
   Dementia
6. Withdrawal phenomena
   Tremor
   Memory lapses
   Delirium tremens
   Epileptic fits
   Auditory hallucinations

## Psychiatric
1. Depressive illnesses and anxiety states
2. Suicide
3. Morbid jealousy
4. Sexual dysfunction

## Social
1. Road accidents
2. Marital distress, violence, breakdown
3. Child violence
4. Absenteeism, loss of job
5. Financial difficulty
6. Criminal offences
   Acquisitive
   Traffic
   Violence

**Table 27.24** Pointers to alcoholism and screening test.

1. Increased intake (> safe weekly limits of 21 'units' for men and 10 for women)
2. Drinking daily
3. Drinking in the mornings
4. Lying about drinking behaviour
5. Becoming preoccupied with drink matters, the availability of drink, arranging to have the next drink
6. Regularly craving drink
7. Any withdrawal symptoms
8. Any drink-related criminal offence
9. Any intoxication in a public place, or in the workplace
10. Binges becoming more frequent, with associated drunkenness
11. Any serious marital or intrafamily dispute or violence

### Screening test (CAGE test)
A drinking problem should be seriously investigated if a person answers 'yes' to two or more of the following:

**C** Have you ever felt you should cut down your drinking?

**A** Have you ever been annoyed by criticism of your drinking?

**G** Have you ever felt guilty about your drinking?

**E** Do you drink in the morning?

cocaine and its derivatives, and latterly also of amphetamine-like substances, has greatly increased. Multiple drug misuse, often with alcohol, is common. Currently, there is much public health concern about the transmission of important viruses, notably hepatitis B and HIV, among intravenous drug users who share needles.

The serious problem of benzodiazepine dependence is iatrogenic, emerging from the ill-advised use of these drugs in response to complaints suggesting anxiety.

Assessment of individuals with alcohol and drug problems requires adequate physical, psychological and social evaluation. This is often

are misused, are subject to fashion and availability, and vary greatly from place to place, not just from one country to another but from one street to another in the same town. This is because drug dependence often spreads by personal contact, much like an epidemic. Opiate and alcohol dependence are well established in many countries; since the 1980s the use of

difficult, for the patient may be secretive, not easily trusting of others, defensive, and at best ambivalent about giving up the habit. It may be very helpful to involve relatives in the assessment.

Personality is important in the case of drug and alcohol dependence. These habits often develop in part as attempts to cope with life problems or stressful events. If the personality has few weaknesses or vulnerabilities, then relatively more environmental stress will be needed to push the person into dependence. Whether or not a person becomes physically dependent when exposed to drug use depends upon their state of physical health as well as upon pyschosocial factors. Thus some very fit men exposed to heroin (or alcohol) abuse during military service have been able to control their habit on return to the different culture of civilian life.

Ways in which opiate misuse may impact on general hospital practice are listed in Table 27.25.

Treatments are often a combination of specialist and self-help measures, which are particularly valuable in this field.

**Table 27.25** Opiate dependence problems in general hospital practice.

1. Concurrent medical illness related to drug habit
   Hepatitis
   HIV infection and genitourinary diseases
   Septicaemias

2. Direct medical effects of drugs
   Coma and death from overdose
   Convulsions etc. from other substances taken concurrently
   Withdrawal symptoms

3. Drug-related behaviour
   Attempts to obtain supplies by mimicking illness

4. Effects on other people
   Drug-dependent infants
   Domestic strife, abuse, violence
   Acquisitive or violent crime

# Sexuality and its disorders

These are summarized in Table 27.26. Sexual dysfunctions are problems which make coitus

**Table 27.26** Sexual disorders.

1. Sexual dysfunctions
   Male: impotence, premature or retarded ejaculation
   Female: orgasmic and arousal dysfunctions, vaginismus

2. Drive problems: increased or decreased drive

3. Sexual preference problems

4. Gender identity problems

difficult or impossible, or unsatisfactory. Common problems are impotence and premature ejaculation in the male, and orgasmic difficulties in women. Causes invariably include psychological and relationship components; anxiety usually (though not always) impairs sexual performance, and few couples continue active sexual lives when their general relationship is bad. However, erection problems in particular are often caused at least in part by physical factors leading to structural or functional interference with local nervous or vascular pathways. Important causes include diabetic autonomic neuropathy, antihypertensive and antidepressant drug therapy, atheromatous vascular disease and alcohol (which has both physical and psychosocial effects on sexuality). Hypogonadism is a rare but important hormonal cause. It is important to recognize the presence of sexual dysfunctions because they are treatable.

Loss of sexual desire is a common complaint, most usually associated with some dysfunction but occasionally a pointer to a hormonal disorder. Complaints of excess sexual activity are uncommon but may be a symptom of hypomania or point to relationship or personality difficulties. The term sexual *preferences* refers to the sorts of people, or substitutes for people, which arouse erotic responses in a person. Sexual preferences may be problematic (a) if they have legal consequences, for instance when sexual attraction is for children or involves violence; or if they involve behaviour unacceptable (b) to the individual or (c) to the partner or family. People's views in these matters vary greatly and fetishistic, masturbatory or cross-dressing behaviour (for instance) may or may not be a problem, depending on its acceptability to the individuals concerned. Similarly, a homosexual preference is not a problem *per se*, and does not itself represent any psychological disorder, although it may of course involve difficulties in individual cases.

Gender problems involve a person's sense of themselves as male or female, and may accompany the various endocrine illnesses which affect genital development, such as Turner's and Klinefelter's syndromes, or testicular feminization. The rare disorder of transsexualism, where individuals experience themselves as of the gender discordant with their anatomical sex, is not usually associated with any physical abnormality.

# $S$UICIDE AND ATTEMPTED SUICIDE

The correlates of completed suicide include being male, age over 50, social isolation (living alone, being widowed, divorced or separated), recent significant loss (bereavement, retirement), presence of serious (especially painful) physical illness, history of depressive illness and perhaps also recent treatment for depression, and presence of alcoholism or (less commonly) schizophrenia or Huntington's disease.

There is partial overlap between the 'suicide' and 'attempted suicide' populations, for many patients who commit suicide have a history of unsuccessful attempts, and some attempters will later complete suicide. Nevertheless, the statistical associations of attempted suicide (self-poisoning in most instances) differ from those of suicide. Suicide attempts correlate with being female, aged under 30, current interpersonal difficulties (e.g. arguments with boyfriend or parents, or unwanted pregnancy), social unsettlement (no steady job or stable living arrangements), and personality disorder rather than psychiatric illness. Only a minority of suicide attempters have schizophrenia, depressive illness or alcoholism. Most suicide attempts are best understood as maladaptive responses to stressful life events.

Self-poisoning is the commonest medical emergency in those under the age of 30. Each patient requires a psychosocial assessment which is best done as a collaborative effort between psychiatric and medical teams. Intensive psychiatric treatment after self-poisoning is likely to be needed for patients who articulate suicidal intentions; are depressed, alcoholic, or pyschotic; have major problems of social adjustment (e.g. with respect to relationships, living arrangements or finances); or have unresolved life crises (e.g. an unwanted pregnancy or a pending court appearance).

Some self-poisoning patients need only sensible counselling and advice; admission to hospital is not necessary in every case.

# $E$MERGENCIES

Common emergencies are listed in Table 27.27. In general hospitals, psychiatric emergencies often present in the accident department, and casualty staff must be familiar with the principles of psychiatric assessment. Often, tranquillizing medication will play a part in management, but a calm, confident demeanour can defuse many anxiety-laden situations. The first step is always to attempt to talk to the patient to try and understand what they are experiencing.

**Table 27.27** Common psychiatric emergencies.

| | |
|---|---|
| 1. Attempted suicide | 4. Other acute 'psychopathological' states<br>Amnesia, fugue states<br>Paranoid states<br>Cognitive decompensation<br>Self-imposed starvation |
| 2. Acute excitement (increased motor and verbal<br>activity)<br>Organic, manic or schizophrenic psychoses<br>Intoxication with alcohol or drugs | |
| 3. Acute emotional states<br>Panic, hyperventilation, rage/temper | 5. Psychosocial crises<br>Flight from domestic violence<br>Homelessness |

# POST-TRAUMATIC STRESS DISORDERS

Everyone is exposed daily to environmental events. Some are pleasant, some unpleasant; some are easy to cope with, some difficult. *Stressful* events are those which make demands on a person who has to exert effort to respond appropriately to them. In certain circumstances, a person may deal in some less than ideal fashion with a stressful event. Then, the event may have more or less long-lasting effects on psychological and physical health. The circumstances which are likely to make an event hard to cope with are (a) when the event is *exceedingly* stressful (for instance, being tortured or held as a hostage, being involved in a natural disaster, or being beaten or mugged; and (b) when the individual is especially vulnerable (for instance, when a child is physically or sexually abused by an adult).

Post-traumatic stress disorder (PTSD) may arise when a person has not 'got over' a stressful event, or when something happens to activate troubled memories or feelings connected with a past event. For instance, in recent years many people have had long-buried memories of abusive childhood experiences activated by watching television programmes concerned with child sexual abuse.

Post-traumatic stress disorder may present with anxiety, irritability, insomnia, guilty feelings, depressed mood, troubled memories of the traumatic event and a sense of paralysis of action. The emotional arousal may generate somatic symptoms in any body system, so that PTSD patients may find their way to any medical department. A careful psychosocial history will suggest the diagnosis.

# SCHIZOPHRENIA AND PARANOID STATES

## *Schizophrenia*

The schizophrenic illnesses are the meat of the specialist subject of psychiatry, but of peripheral interest in the context of general medicine, and therefore only a summary is given here.

In schizophrenic illnesses, there occur, in clear consciousness, disturbances of thought, perception, mood, behaviour and personality which may together give rise to deeply distressing experiences and multiple psychosocial disabilities.

The incidence of schizophrenia in the general population is 0.85 per cent, a figure which is fairly constant worldwide, and the illness is equally common in males and females. Most cases begin in late adolescence, with illnesses starting after the age of 35 usually having predominantly paranoid symptoms. Genetic factors undoubtedly play a part in many cases, although non-familial cases occur and in these it is likely that perinatal birth trauma may be causative. Cerebral abnormalities can be demonstrated in many cases of schizophrenia, for instance, in the relative activity levels of different brain areas, and a schizophrenia-like psychosis can occur in temporal lobe epileptics or in amphetamine addicts, so that brain malfunction undoubtedly contributes to the picture in established schizophrenia. Psychologically, there are major problems with information processing, and many symptoms can be thought of as arising from an inability to distinguish between what should relate to 'me' and what to 'persons outside me'.

Symptoms of schizophrenia include the delusions and hallucinations that give rise to general notions of 'madness', and there may be interruptions in thought process such that the individual thinks people are putting thoughts into his mind, removing his thoughts, or distributing thoughts to others. Other less obvious symptoms may however be exceedingly disabling. There may be a difficulty with intending acts so that sequences of goal-directed action fail to occur and the patient drifts aimlessly through life, achieving nothing. The normal apparatus of emotional expression may fail, so that the person becomes unable to share in the normally rewarding exchanges of close relationships. On occasion, unusual motor movements, odd mannerisms or self-care habits, or socially undesirable behaviour may make it hard for a schizophrenic patient to fit easily in to the community.

Schizophrenic illnesses which start in late teenage are most likely to include a full range of symptoms and to lead to chronic disablement and deterioration. Paranoid patients who may become ill from middle life may remain relatively undamaged in many areas of life and continue ordinary social lives for many years.

The diagnosis of schizophrenia need not be difficult. If a person appears to be 'mad', then systematic search should be made in mental state examination for specific symptoms, checking particularly that the person is not suffering from a depressive illness. If the mental state is indeed 'schizophrenic', then investigations are required to establish whether or not organic factors are relevant.

# Paranoid states

Experiences are paranoid when they involve a misinterpretation of the subject's relationship to the world; most commonly this takes the form of a mistaken sense of being persecuted, for instance, by neighbours, family members, or workmates. The circumstances in which paranoid symptoms may occur are listed in Table 27.28. For the general hospital clinician, the most important point is that paranoid symptoms may draw attention to a medical illness. Causes of acute paranoid symptoms important in general hospital practice include hypothyroidism, hypovitaminosis $B_{12}$, HIV infection, alcoholism, intoxication with illicit drugs such as cocaine and amphetamine, adverse reactions to prescribed drugs such as steroids and disorientation due to brain malfunction from any cause. A good description of a subacute organically caused paranoid state is to be found in E. Waugh's *The Ordeal of Gilbert Pinfold*.

Of the other illnesses listed in Table 27.28, systems of delusional ideas are common to the

**Table 27.28** States in which paranoid symptoms occur.

1. Paranoid schizophrenia
   (thought disorder + hallucinations + delusions)

2. Paraphrenia
   (hallucinations + delusions)

3. Paranoia
   (delusions only)

4. Induced (shared) paranoid disorder
   (so-called *folie a deux*)

5. Morbid jealousy

6. Affective disorder
   (hypomania or depression: mood congruent symptoms)

7. Paranoid personality disorder

8. Organic states

first three. In paraphrenia and paranoid schizophrenia there are hallucinations (usually auditory) as well, and in schizophrenia additional problems of disordered thinking. Occasionally, systematic delusions believed by one person may come to be shared by another, usually a family member who is generally submissive to the originally symptomatic individual. Morbid jealousy is a state of delusions of infidelity and associated with serious domestic difficulties.

# PRINCIPLES OF TREATMENT

The treatment of psychological problems and disorders should be thought of under four headings (Table 27.29). All these kinds of intervention should be considered in every case, even when one treatment turns out to be sufficient, because their effects often complement each other. There is no contradiction in advising a form of counselling *and* medication *and* altered social arrangements.

Doctors have psychological effects on patients in every clinical setting. So do other health workers, including nurses, occupational therapists, physiotherapists etc. The psychological effects which may accompany surgical, nursing, pharmacological and other medical procedures are neither negligible nor unimportant. They affect patients' compliance with, and responsiveness to, physical treatments, and their compliance with technical procedures. For instance, relief of preoperative anxiety tends to reduce postoperative pain intensity and analgesic intake, to increase the benefit from postoperative physiotherapy and to reduce the length of hospital stay.

Many patients benefit from the focussed attention of a concerned person, a caring attitude which tends to reduce distress independently of the person's professional knowledge or affiliation. All doctors need to be able to provide this **level 1** intervention. Somewhat more complex, but also required of every doctor, are **level 2** treatments which include various ways of advising people how to solve their problems, for example, by revising their ideas about the problem, acting to mitigate its environmental causes, or systematically reviewing alternative courses of action.

Many doctors also become competent to provide one or more varieties of **level 3** psychological treatments, which require some more formal training in techniques allowing interventions to be directed at problems not amenable to simpler procedures. Such measures can be categorized by aim, modality, length or theoretical basis (Table 27.30). In most health service settings, brief

**Table 27.29** Varieties of treatments used in psychiatry.

1. Psychological treatments
   (a) Psychological effects
   (b) *Level 1*: non-specific attention
   (c) *Level 2*: simple problem-solving
   (d) *Level 3*: specific treatments

2. Biological treatments
   (a) Drug treatments
       Neuroleptics, antidepressants, lithium, sedatives
   (b) Electroconvulsive therapy (ECT)

3. Social and rehabilitation treatments

4. Service organization

**Table 27.30** Specific psychological treatments.

**By aim**
Relief
Behaviour change

**By modality**
Individual
'Natural group' (family, couple)
Group

**By length**
Brief
Prolonged

**By theoretical basis**
Cognitive-behavioural
Psychodynamic
Other

methods are chosen because they are more economical of resources and are often preferred by patients. They are often incidentally more effective! The insights of cognitive and behavioural psychology have greatly enhanced the effectiveness of psychological treatments, especially as applied to depressive and anxiety disorders and other neurotic problems. They are particularly helpful when interpersonal difficulties are involved, or the patient is troubled by the current implications of difficult early life experiences.

Four groups of drugs are important in the field of psychiatry. In general the *neuroleptics* slow psychomotor overactivity, damp down feeling and block hallucinosis, at least in part through their effects on CNS arousal via the reticular activating system. Of the phenothiazines, chlorpromazine, 75–400 mg daily, is the most widely used. Thioridazine, 30–600 mg daily, has some antidepressent effect, and trifluoperazine, 3–40 mg daily, has some alerting effect. The butyrophenones are the other major group of neuroleptics, haloperidol, 5–50 mg daily, being the most widely used. All these neuroleptics are liable to cause troublesome extrapyramidal side effects. Nevertheless, they are the drugs of choice when medication is required for the symptomatic control of excitement, excess elation or euphoria or other manifestations of overarousal.

The availability of *antidepressants* has greatly reduced the need for electroconvulsive therapy (ECT). There are three main groups of antidepressants: the early monoamine oxidase inhibitors (relatively little used today), the tricyclics and the more recent 5-hydroxytryptamine (5HT) inhibitors.

Common practice is to start antidepressant treatment with a tricyclic drug although recently many prescribers start with one of the new 5HT inhibitors. The student should know of two or three of these drugs, despite the fact that more than 30 compounds are available for prescription. Of the tricyclics, amitriptyline and imipramine are well tried with imipramine

being less sedating. Both are given in doses up to 150–200 mg daily. Atropine-like side effects (dry mouth, constipation, delayed micturition, poor erection) are common with all tricyclics and their cardiac effects make them dangerous in overdose. The newer 5HT inhibitor drugs such as fluoxetine, 20–40 mg daily, have fewer side effects.

*Lithium* is an invaluable mood-stabilizing drug and an important part of the treatment of manic-depressive disorders. It may cause hypothyroidism (page 526) and renal damage (page 470) and specialist supervision is essential, with regular blood level monitoring.

*Sedatives* have in the past been much used to treat anxiety, but have caused major problems through inducing dependence on the anxiolytic drug. A good rule is to give drugs to relieve anxiety, for instance, diazepam, for the briefest possible periods of time, if at all.

Social measures often form a crucial part of the treatment plan for a patient. Thought should always be given to the effect of the patient's living and working environment on their symptoms and illness. The amelioration of such difficulties often requires liaison with other agencies, such as local social services or housing departments.

Rehabilitation means maximizing the patient's assets and minimizing the effects of disabilities on personal and social life. A rehabilitation programme requires proper assessment of these disabilities, which may be *primary* (directly due to the illness itself), or *secondary* (effects such as social stigma, family rejection or discrimination by employers).

Nowadays a comprehensive management plan must take detailed cognisance of the way services are arranged, in hospital and in the community. Doctors inevitably interact with management in these matters, whether they like it or not, and need to inform themselves about local details which vary considerably from place to place.

# Appendix
# Normal Values

This section gives the results of tests in relatively common use. The values given can generally only be taken as the approximate normal range. There will be differences between techniques and machines used in the analysis. In many cases laboratories will build up their own range of normal values which should be used in preference to those given here.

## HAEMATOLOGY

Total blood volume                                   65–85 ml/kg (male)
60–80 ml/kg (female)

### Red cells

| | |
|---|---|
| Red cell mass | 25–35 ml/kg (male) |
| | 20–30 ml/kg (female) |
| Haemoglobin | 13.0–17.0 g/dl (male) |
| | 11.5–15.5 g/dl (female) |
| Red cell count | $4.5–6.5 \times 10^9/l$ (male) |
| | $3.9–5.8 \times 10^9/l$ (female) |
| Mean corpuscular haemoglobin (MCH) | 27–32 pg |
| Mean corpuscular haemoglobin concentration (MCHC) | 32–36 g/dl |
| Mean corpuscular volume | 80–96 fl |
| Packed cell volume | 0.40–0.54 l/l (male) |
| | 0.37–0.47 l/l (female) |
| Reticulocyte count | 0.2–2.5% of red cells |

### White cells

| | |
|---|---|
| Total white cell count | $4.0–11.0 \times 10^9/l$ |
| Neutrophils | $2.5–7.5 \times 10^9/l$ |
| Lymphocytes | $1.5–3.5 \times 10^9/l$ |
| Monocytes | $0.2–0.8 \times 10^9/l$ |
| Eosinophils | $0.04–0.44 \times 10^9/l$ |
| Basophils | $0–0.10 \times 10^9/l$ |

### Coagulation

| | |
|---|---|
| Prothrombin time | 10–14 s |
| Partial thromboplastin time | 30–40 s |
| Bleeding time (Ivy) | 3–8 minutes |

## OTHER HAEMATOLOGICAL VALUES

| | |
|---|---|
| Platelet count | $150–400 \times 10^9/l$ |
| Serum folate | 5–63 nmol/l |
| Red cell folate | >160 µg/l |
| Serum $B_{12}$ | 200–800 pmol/l |
| Fibrinogen | 2–4 g/l |

# *Biochemistry*

| | |
|---|---|
| Acid phosphatase | 1–5 U/l |
| Alanine aminotransferase | <45 IU/l |
| Albumin | 34–50 g/l |
| Alkaline phosphatase | 30–115 IU/l |
| Alpha-fetoprotein | <10 kU/l |
| Ammonium | 37–84 µmol/l |
| Amylase | 0–180 U/l |
| Aspartate aminotransferase | <41 IU/l |
| Bicarbonate | 25–35 mmol/l |
| Bilirubin (total) | 3–20 µmol/l |
| Bilirubin (direct) | 0–3 µmol/l |
| Calcium (Calcium should be corrected for abnormal levels of albumin) | 2.1–2.6 mmol/l |
| Carcinoembryonic antigen (CEA) | <10 µg/l |
| Chloride | 98–108 mmol/l |
| Cholesterol | <6 mmol/l |
| Cortisol (09.00h) | 280–700 nmol/l |
| Cortisol (24.00 h and asleep) | 140–280 nmol/l |
| Creatinine | 45–120 µmol/l |
| Creatinine clearance | 105–132 ml/minute per 1.73 m² surface area |
| Creatinine phosphokinase (CPK) | 24–195 U/l |
| Gamma glutamyl transpeptidase | (male)<60 IU/l (female)<40 IU/l |
| Globulin | 25–35 g/l |
| Glucose (fasting) | 4.0–5.8 mmol/l |
| Glycosylated haemoglobin (HbA1c) | 3.8–6.4% |
| Hydroxybutyric dehydrogenase (HbD) | 40–125 U/l |
| Iron | 12–30 µmol/l |
| Iron binding capacity | 42–80 µmol/l |
| Lactate | 0.3–0.8 mmol/l |
| Lactic dehydrogenase (LDH) | 240–525 U/l |
| Magnesium | 0.7–1.1 mmol/l |
| Osmolality | 280–296 mOsm/kg |
| Phosphate | 0.8–1.5 mmol/l |
| Potassium | 3.4–5.0 mmol/l |
| Protein (total) | 60–80 g/l |
| Sodium | 135–150 mmol/l |
| Thyroid function | |
| Thyroxine ($T_4$) | 60–160 nmol/l |
| Triiodothyronine ($T_3$) | 1.2–3.1 nmol/l |
| Free thyroxine (free $T_4$) | 9–23 pmol/l |
| Free triiodothyronine (free $T_3$) | 3–9 pmol/l |
| Thyroid stimulating hormone (TSH) | 0.3–3.0 mU/l |
| Triglycerides | 0.8–2.0 mmol/l |
| Urate | (male) 250–520 µmol/l (female) 165–400 µmol/l |
| Urea | 2.5–7.5 mmol/l |

## URINE

*Values per 24 hours*

| | |
|---|---|
| Volume | 600–2500 ml |
| Protein | <150 mg |
| Potassium | 80–160 mmol |
| Sodium | 10–200 mmol |
| Calcium | 2.5–7.5 mmol |
| Phosphate | 16–48 mmol |
| Creatinine | 9–17 mmol |

## ARTERIAL BLOOD GASES

| | |
|---|---|
| $PCO_2$ | 4.8–6.1 kPa (36–46 mmHg) |
| $PO_2$ | 10–13.3 kPa (75–100 mmHg) |
| pH | 7.35–7.45 |
| $[H^+]$ | 35–45 nmol/l |

## CEREBROSPINAL FLUID

| | |
|---|---|
| Pressure | 70–160 mm of csf |
| Lymphocytes | 0–5 mm³ |
| Polymorphs | 0 |
| Red cells | 0 |
| Protein | 20–45 g/l |
| IgG | <15% total protein |
| Glucose | >50% blood glucose |
| Chloride | 122–128 mmol/l |

# Index